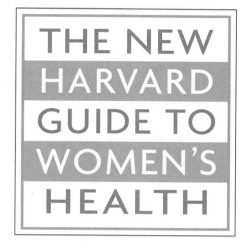

THE NEW HARVARD GUIDE TO WOMEN'S HEALTH

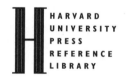
HARVARD
UNIVERSITY
PRESS
REFERENCE
LIBRARY

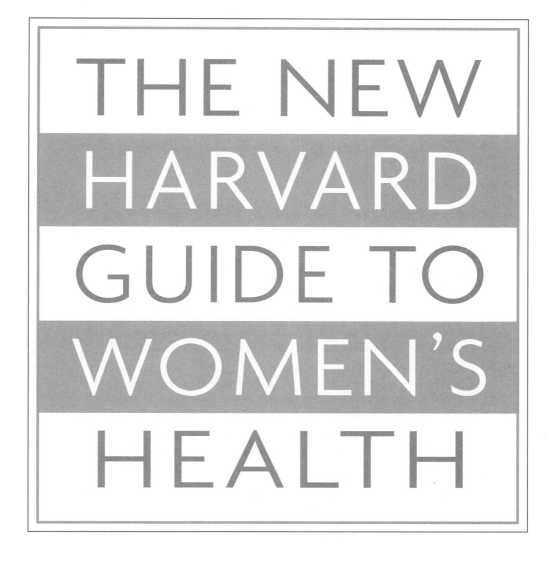

THE NEW HARVARD GUIDE TO WOMEN'S HEALTH

Karen J. Carlson, M.D.

HARVARD MEDICAL SCHOOL

Stephanie A. Eisenstat, M.D.

HARVARD MEDICAL SCHOOL

——— Terra Ziporyn, Ph.D. ———

HARVARD UNIVERSITY PRESS

CAMBRIDGE, MASSACHUSETTS, AND LONDON, ENGLAND   2004

This book is meant to educate, but it should not be used as a substitute for personal medical advice. The reader should consult her clinician for specific information concerning her individual medical condition. The authors have done
their best to ensure that the information presented here is accurate up to the
time of publication. However, as research and development are ongoing, it is
possible that new findings may supersede some of the data presented here.

Many of the designations used by manufacturers and sellers to distinguish their
products are claimed as trademarks. Where those designations appear in this
book and Harvard University Press was aware of a trademark claim, then the
designations have been printed in initial capital letters (for example, Tylenol).

The New Harvard Guide to Women's Health is available at quantity discounts
with bulk purchases for educational, business, or sales promotional use. For
information please contact:
SPECIAL SALES DEPARTMENT, Harvard University Press
79 Garden Street, Cambridge, Massachusetts 02138-1499
Tel. 1-617-495-2606, Fax 1-617-496-2550

Library of Congress Cataloging-in-Publication Data

Carlson, Karen J.
The new Harvard guide to women's health /
Karen J. Carlson, Stephanie A. Eisenstat, Terra Ziporyn.
p.   cm. — (Harvard University Press reference library)
Includes index.
ISBN 0-674-01282-8 (cloth : alk. paper). — ISBN 0-674-01343-3 (pbk. : alk. paper)
1. Women—Health and hygiene. 2. Women—Diseases. 3. Medicine, Popular.
I. Eisenstat, Stephanie A. II. Ziporyn, Terra Diane, 1958– . III. Title. IV. Series.
RA778.C2164   2004
616'.0082—dc22   2003063680

To our families:
Richard, Nicholas, and Christopher Mollica
Russell, Benjamin, Samuel, and Joshua Eisenstat
James, Pallas, Sage, and Solon Snider

Preface

For most women, being well informed is an essential element of good health. Research has shown clearly that when a woman goes to her doctor with a health problem, the two most important factors in achieving a good outcome are the amount of information communicated between the patient and her doctor and the active participation by the patient in making decisions about her care. Unfortunately, in today's managed care environment, physicians often have more information to share than they have time to share it. We wrote this book to help bridge that gap: to give women the knowledge they need to communicate effectively with their doctor, and to become partners in taking good care of their health.

Since the publication of the first edition of this book in 1996, we've seen both advances and reversals in women's health care. On the positive side, we've seen improved approaches to detect, prevent, and/or treat osteoporosis, diabetes, Alzheimer's disease, and breast, ovarian, and cervical cancers. We've seen a variety of new contraceptive options and an increased awareness of colon cancer and steps required to prevent it. We've integrated more "alternative treatments" into mainstream medicine while, at the same time, gathered better evidence about what works, what doesn't work, and what may be unsafe. We have increasing evidence about the effects of drugs on women in particular, and, as a result, we're finally seeing medication for certain conditions approved for use solely in women.

We've also had some surprises and frustrations. Evidence from the Women's Health Initiative has turned upside down many of our assumptions about the value of estrogen replacement therapy (ERT) for the prevention of disease, resulting in widespread confusion and disillusionment. Women are stopping their ERT abruptly only to find their symptoms recurring and their faith in the medical establishment shaken once again. Meanwhile, the same chronic diseases responsible for the most deaths in women – heart disease and cancer – remain the primary causes of mortality. Ever-increasing time demands and economic pressures continue to put women under as much, if not more, stress than a decade ago. Violence against women in general and domestic violence in particular remain major concerns. Many women of color continue to suffer disproportionately from premature death, disease, and disabilities with a greater prevalence of chronic disease and higher infant mortality rate compared to white women. Many women still do not go for routine preventive tests such as mammography, and many still do not get sufficient exercise. We're seeing an increased number of obese Americans (both men and women), particularly among Hispanics, African-Americans, and adolescents, and, partly as a result, diabetes has become a growing problem among women.

Progress itself has also brought new challenges along with it. Sexual dysfunction in women emerged, in part as a result of the attention following the successful launch of Viagra, but scientific understanding of the complexity of this problem or how to treat it is still in its infancy. Many new diagnostic tests are available but we still have made only small advances in addressing the behavioral problems (overeating, inactivity, smoking) that underlie these diseases. And too many of our new technologies represent only a marginal improvement over existing methods, at astoundingly high cost (e.g., getting an MRI whenever something hurts). Unless we quickly resolve the crisis of how we pay for health care as a nation, all other advances in health care for women will be moot.

The New Harvard Guide to Women's Health incorporates these recent advances, reversals, surprise, and challenges. At the same time, as in the first edition, it still aims to answer the kinds of questions physicians hear every day from their female patients—questions such as "Is this normal?," "Do I need to worry about this?," "What can be done about this?," and "What's going to happen to me now?" With each of the health concerns listed in this A-Z Guide (encompassing over 300 entries), we try to explain who is likely to develop the problem, what the typical symptoms are, and how the condition is evaluated and treated. We also outline any preventive steps a woman can take to improve her chances of avoiding the problem or its recurrence.

Some kinds of questions on the minds of women patients often do not get addressed in a busy office visit—questions about anxiety, depression, occupational hazards, postpartum issues, and stress. Other questions are never clearly articulated, often out of a sense of privacy, embarrassment, or perhaps even denial—questions about domestic violence, sexual orientation, sexual response, and substance abuse, for example. In this book we attempt to answer some of the unspoken questions about these issues and other psychological and social factors that so often have a profound effect on a woman's physical well-being. The reader will find informative entries on antianxiety and antidepressant drugs, panic and phobias, posttraumatic stress and psychosomatic disorders, sexual abuse and incest, and other vital topics in the area of women's emotional and mental health.

Sometimes what worries a woman most is a single symptom: a sudden pain in her abdomen, back, chest, or head; fatigue, hair loss, incontinence, or insomnia; the appearance of an unusual mole or varicose veins. Many entries in *The New Harvard Guide to Women's Health* look at specific symptoms such as these and explain the range of disorders that could account for them.

A major focus of this guide is, naturally, on diseases that may affect a woman's reproductive system. Topics range from breast lumps, cervical cancer, endometriosis, and ovarian cysts to pelvic inflammatory disease, uterine fibroids, and yeast infections. The symptoms, treatment, and prevention of sexually transmitted diseases are described in detail, and the pros and cons of birth control options are assessed, including natural birth control methods and the many different forms of hormonal contraception available today.

But disorders of the reproductive system are not the whole story when it comes to women's health. In the last decade, researchers and physicians alike have recognized that many diseases common to both sexes manifest themselves differently in women. For example, heart diseases—angina, aortic stenosis, congestive heart failure, coronary artery disease, even high blood pressure—sometimes follow a different course in women than in men, for reasons that are biological, social, or, often, both. For every common condition described, we try to call attention to the ways in which the incidence, symptoms, evaluation, and treatment may be different in women.

We pay special attention to the impact of common diseases on the outcome of pregnancy, and to the effect of pregnancy itself on the course of a disease. Autoimmune disorders such as lupus and multiple sclerosis, as well as diabetes, epilepsy, kidney disorders, and thyroid disease, are among the dozens of conditions with special implications for women who are pregnant or are thinking about becoming pregnant. Among the other reproductive issues discussed are abortion, breastfeeding, genetic counseling, infertility, midwifery, morning sickness, postpartum psychiatric disorders, and pregnancy after age 35.

The health needs of women change dramatically over the lifespan. Entries on such topics as body image, depression, exercise, and nutrition are organized around the changing circumstances of women as they age and their impact on health. We also try to examine some of the special health issues that may concern younger and elderly women as well as the family members who may care for them. Anorexia nervosa and Alzheimer's disease are just two of many examples.

In entries on standard clinical practices such as blood tests, immunizations, Pap tests, physical examination, and other screening procedures, we point out the importance of taking into account a woman's age and reproductive status. In addition, many techniques used in the diagnosis and treatment of disease are described, and their risks and complications are assessed. These include biopsies, colposcopy, cryosurgery, hysterectomy, hysteroscopy, laparoscopy, laser surgery, lumpectomy, mammography, MRI, and others.

And finally, the health of modern women has been inextricably linked with appearance. In discussion of such topics as breast implants, cosmetics, dieting, foot care, hair dyes, liposuction, nail care, orthodontia, sclerotherapy, and skin care, we try to take an honest look at potential benefits and risks so that women can make informed decisions about the products they buy and the procedures they choose to undergo.

The main topics covered in *The New Harvard Guide to Women's Health* are listed alphabetically in the table of contents at the beginning of the book. The Index at the back directs the reader to discussions of hundreds of additional topics that are not main entries (such as biofeedback, bunions, migraines, pleurisy, and so on), or to topics that appear under another name (such as high blood pressure instead of hypertension). At the end of each entry, "Related entries" lists other topics that expand on some aspect of the discussion. The section entitled "For More Information," which begins on page 631, lists organizations and online resources that offer additional information on topics of special interest.

This guide draws on the expertise generously shared by physicians at Harvard Medical School, Massachusetts General Hospital, Brigham and Women's Hospital, and elsewhere. Their specific contributions are described in the Acknowledgments. To the many colleagues, friends, and especially patients who have inspired this project, we would like to express our hope that *The New Harvard Guide to Women's Health* will be useful in promoting the good health and well-being of women everywhere.

Karen J. Carlson, MD
Stephanie A. Eisenstat, MD
Terra Ziporyn, PhD

Contents

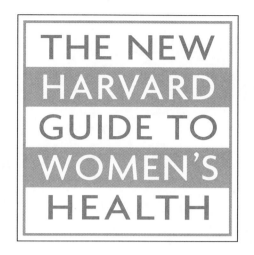

THE NEW
HARVARD
GUIDE TO
WOMEN'S
HEALTH

Abdominal Pain

The abdomen is not a single organ but rather a section of the body that contains a number of different organs and other tissues. Pain in this area can signal hundreds of conditions, ranging from mild intestinal gas to severe inflammations, infections, and cancers. Usually a temporary abdominal twinge or cramp is no reason for concern, but any incapacitating or unremitting pain could indicate a surgical emergency that requires immediate medical attention. *Anyone who suddenly develops severe abdominal pain that lasts more than an hour should consult a clinician (by telephone or otherwise) as soon as possible.*

Doctors divide the abdomen into four quarters or quadrants by drawing an imaginary line down through the navel from the bottom of the chest to the top of the pubic area, and then crossing this line with a horizontal line that runs through the navel (see illustration). Pain can then be said to occur in the right upper quadrant, for example, or in the left lower quadrant. It is also possible for pain to occur right in the middle of the abdomen, either above or below the navel.

Treatment varies with the nature of the condition underlying the pain. The patient can speed up the process of selecting the right treatment by supplying information about the timing, severity, and location of the pain—which helps the clinician narrow down its cause.

Pain in the lower abdomen

Abdominal pain in the lower two quadrants of the abdomen is not clearly distinguishable from pelvic pain and can result from a large number of disorders of the reproductive organs: pelvic inflammatory disease, endometriosis, adenomyosis, ovarian cysts, ovarian cancer, fallopian tube cancer, endometrial polyps, endometrial cancer, menstrual cramps, premenstrual syndrome, miscarriage, urinary tract infections, and uterine fibroids, to name a few (see entries under these disorders, and see also pelvic pain).

Here is a brief description of some common conditions, in addition to those just listed and described elsewhere, which may account for lower abdominal pain in women.

Bowel disorders. Many women with lower abdominal pain, crampiness, and gas have some kind of bowel disorder, which may include constipation, irritable bowel syndrome, diverticular disease, and colon and rectal cancer (see entries), as well as ulcerative colitis, Crohn's disease, celiac disease, polyps, and arteriosclerosis of the bowel (see bowel disorders). Often bowel disorders are marked by a noticeable change in the frequency of stool or a change in consistency or ease in elimination.

Appendicitis. Severe or persistent abdominal pain may sometimes indicate appendicitis. A good rule of thumb is to assume it does until proven otherwise. This is particularly true if the pain occurs in the lower right or moves from

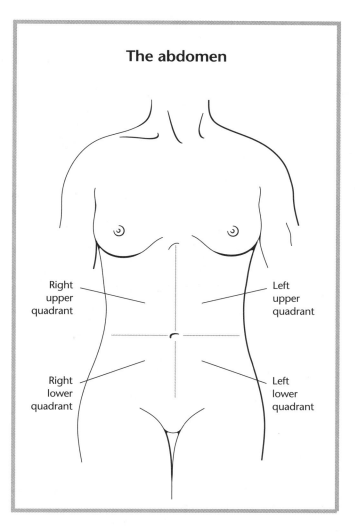

The abdomen

Right upper quadrant

Left upper quadrant

Right lower quadrant

Left lower quadrant

around the navel to the lower right side. The appendix is a small sac attached to the first part of the large intestine (the cecum; see illustration). It has no known function, but it frequently becomes infected or inflamed and must be removed surgically as soon as possible. Otherwise it may rupture and cause life-threatening infection of the abdominal lining (peritonitis).

Often the first sign of appendicitis is a dull pain or tenderness around the navel or on the lower right side of the abdomen. If any abdominal pain is specific to these areas, a clinician should be consulted. Even a dull pain in this area, particularly if it persists for more than 12 hours, may signal appendicitis. Other symptoms may include nausea, lack of appetite, fever, vomiting, and constipation. Appendicitis is particularly common in teenagers and young adults, but it can occur in anyone. If it is diagnosed and treated promptly, it is rarely fatal.

Lactose intolerance. People who develop lower abdominal pain, cramps, diarrhea, and gassiness after they consume milk or other dairy products may have a deficiency of lactase. This enzyme normally metabolizes lactose, a sugar found in

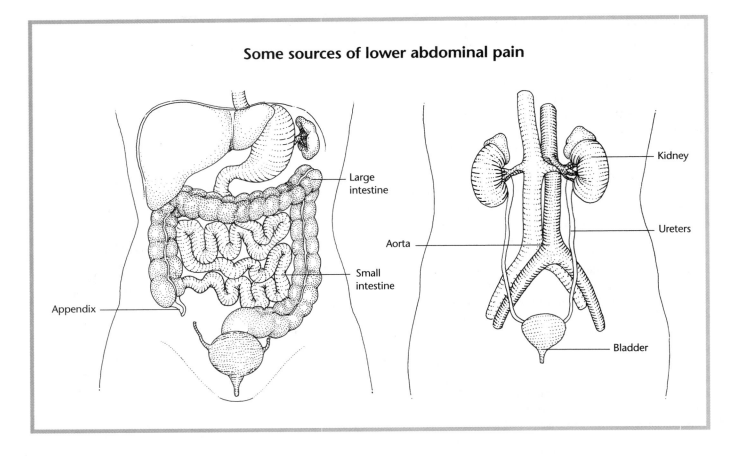

Some sources of lower abdominal pain

Large intestine

Appendix

Small intestine

Kidney

Aorta

Ureters

Bladder

milk and other dairy products, as well as prepared foods that contain these substances. Lactose intolerance is most easily diagnosed by observing the effects on symptoms of a lactose-free diet. Usually it is possible to control the symptoms by making a few simple dietary changes (see irritable bowel syndrome). Many people with lactose intolerance find that they can tolerate eating yogurt, as well as milk products that are pretreated with lactase (Lactaid and Dairyease).

Ectopic pregnancy. Another life-threatening source of lower abdominal pain that needs to be considered by any woman with even a remote chance of being pregnant is an ectopic (tubal) pregnancy (see entry). Symptoms of this condition include sharp or constant one-sided pain in the lower abdomen, shoulder pain, or irregular vaginal bleeding or staining after a light or late menstrual period.

Aortic aneurysm. As women grow older, they also have to consider the possibility that sudden, severe abdominal pain may signal a ruptured aortic aneurysm. In this condition—which also requires immediate medical attention—the walls of the abdominal branch of the aorta (the major artery in the body; see illustration) balloon out and eventually leak or burst. This is thought to occur after the aorta has been subjected to many years of arteriosclerosis (hardening), a process probably exacerbated by untreated high blood pressure. Although it is quite common to have an aneurysm in the aorta

without any symptoms—or with only a sort of pulsating sensation in the abdomen—a ruptured aorta is catastrophic and can quickly result in severe pain, shock, unconsciousness, or even death.

In some people, however, a slow leak may occur rather than an abrupt rupture, in which case the more serious consequences may be presaged by a few days of mild abdominal aching. This condition needs to be promptly evaluated so that it can be repaired surgically before major damage occurs.

Kidney disorders. Lying on either side of the spine at the back of the abdominal cavity (see illustration), the kidneys can sometimes develop problems that produce pain in the abdomen. This is usually accompanied by pain in the back or flank and often fever, chills, and pain or bleeding during urination. Among the kidney disorders (see entry) that can cause abdominal pain are infections, chronic kidney failure, and kidney stones (the last are most likely to produce waves of pain).

Right upper quadrant pain

Gallstones and other gallbladder disorders. The gallbladder is a small organ that sits behind the liver and stores bile which the liver has produced. An infected or diseased gallbladder—particularly common in middle-aged or pregnant women—very frequently causes right upper abdominal pain. Sometimes the pain, which can involve the shoulder or back as well, is caused by crystalline structures that form inside the gallbladder called gallstones (see entry). Gallbladder attacks are most common at night and after eating and, if complications have begun to develop, may include other symptoms such as high fever, chills, and jaundice (yellowing of the skin).

Liver disease. Exposure to infectious microorganisms, alcohol, toxic chemicals, and certain medications can all lead to liver inflammation, a condition called hepatitis (see entry). Whatever the specific cause, an inflamed liver sometimes results in the gradual development of an ache deep inside the upper abdomen (see illustration). This is often accompanied by various flulike symptoms, including low-grade fever, nausea, vomiting, diarrhea, lack of appetite, muscle aches, and headache.

Pancreatic disorders. The pancreas is a glandular organ extending across the upper portion of the abdomen, behind the stomach (see illustration). In addition to manufacturing the hormone insulin, it also supplies enzymes that help accelerate digestion. Sometimes as a complication of gallbladder disease—or alcohol consumption, or exposure to certain drugs—the pancreas becomes inflamed, producing an extremely painful condition known as pancreatitis.

In its acute (sudden and severe) form, pancreatitis results in intense, constant, and deep-seated abdominal pain, which sometimes radiates to the back and chest and can persist unabated for hours or even days. Unlike the pain of a gallbladder attack, pain from pancreatitis usually worsens when the person is lying down and sometimes diminishes when she is sitting, standing, or leaning forward. The abdomen is tender, and there may be a low-grade fever, sweating, nausea, vomiting, rapid pulse and breathing, and skin clamminess as well. Because severe pancreatitis can be life-threatening—particularly if a cyst or abscess develops or if pancreatic fluid leaks into the abdomen—anyone with these symptoms should quickly contact a clinician.

Sometimes a chronic form of pancreatitis develops in people with a history of alcohol abuse, people who have been using certain drugs for long periods of time—including valproic acid (an anticonvulsant), azathioprine (an immunosuppressive agent), furosemide (a diuretic), and sulfasalazine (used to treat inflammatory bowel disease)—and in other people for unknown reasons. This condition involves frequent or intermittent attacks of intense abdominal pain over a number of years. Accompanying symptoms may include fever, nausea, vomiting, clammy skin, abdominal bloating, and weight loss. Eventually people with this condition may start excreting fat-containing feces—as marked by unusually bulky, foul-smelling, and buoyant stools. Chronic pancreatitis develops when the pancreas gradually loses its ability to secrete digestive enzymes. This in turn leads to malabsorption problems—which explain the weight loss and fat-containing stools, since nutrients not absorbed by the intestine are excreted in the stool. Damage to the part of the pancreas that secretes insulin can also lead to the development of diabetes.

A variety of dietary, drug, and surgical treatments can be used for pancreatitis, depending on the underlying cause and the extent of damage. In all cases, however, part of the treatment involves elimination of alcohol.

In rare cases advanced cancer of the pancreas may also un-

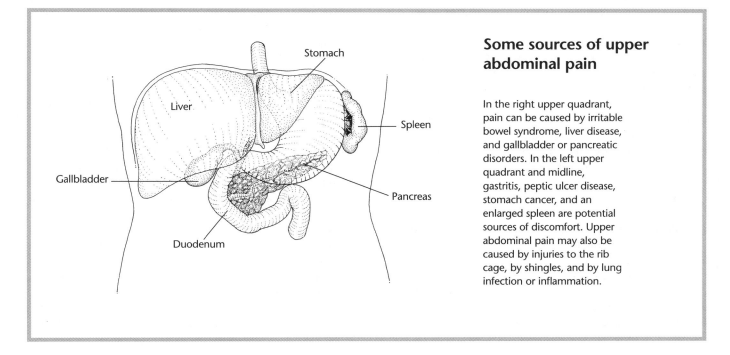

Some sources of upper abdominal pain

In the right upper quadrant, pain can be caused by irritable bowel syndrome, liver disease, and gallbladder or pancreatic disorders. In the left upper quadrant and midline, gastritis, peptic ulcer disease, stomach cancer, and an enlarged spleen are potential sources of discomfort. Upper abdominal pain may also be caused by injuries to the rib cage, by shingles, and by lung infection or inflammation.

Stomach

Liver

Spleen

Gallbladder

Pancreas

Duodenum

derlie upper abdominal pain. Although more common in men than in women, pancreatic cancer remains a leading cause of death in this country, and often goes undiagnosed until it is well advanced. Frequently the first symptoms in a person with advanced pancreatic cancer are unexplained weight loss and yellowing of the skin without abdominal pain (painless jaundice).

Irritable bowel syndrome. Sometimes this disorder of bowel function can produce pain in the upper portion of the abdomen. Just where the pain occurs depends on which part of the gut is affected (see irritable bowel syndrome).

Pneumonia and pleurisy. If upper abdominal pain was preceded by a respiratory infection, it may be due to inflamed or infected lungs—which occasionally can irritate the diaphragm (a muscle that separates the lungs from the abdomen) and the upper portion of the intestines. The sharp pain caused by pneumonia and pleurisy tends to be particularly noticeable after taking a deep breath (see breathing disorders).

Rib cage pain. If a rib in the abdominal region is fractured, a simple cough, sneeze, or movement can result in considerable pain in the upper abdomen. The result may be sharp pain that increases with every inhalation of air or when the affected area is pushed (see chest pain).

Shingles. This condition, which is most likely in older people or those experiencing ill health or severe stress, first produces a sensitivity or tingling in the affected nerves and then sometimes progresses to excruciating pain. The exact location of the pain depends on which nerves are affected. For this reason, shingles in the abdominal region can easily be confused with many other conditions—until several days later, when characteristic blisters erupt along the nerve path and make the condition unmistakable. Both the pain and rash of shingles (see entry) usually disappear after a few weeks, but some people continue to have pain in the affected area for many more months.

Pain in the left upper quadrant and midline

With the exception of liver or gallbladder problems, the conditions that may account for right upper quadrant pain are also possible explanations for pain in the upper left and upper midline sections of the abdomen. Below are listed several other conditions that may account for pain in these areas.

Functional dyspepsia. Persistent or recurring pain in the upper abdominal region without an identifiable cause affects about 25 percent of the population in Western countries. This condition is called functional dyspepsia. Symptoms may also include indigestion, bloating, and a sense that the stomach is full while eating.

Although by definition the exact cause of functional dyspepsia is unclear, in some cases the symptoms may be related to food intolerances, various abnormalities of gastrointestinal motor function, a low threshold for pain, and, possibly, infection with the bacterium *Helicobacter pylori* and/or various mood disturbances such as anxiety or depression. Whatever the cause, the condition is generally diagnosed by ruling out more serious causes of abdominal pain. Just how this is accomplished, however, is somewhat controversial. While some experts contend that any patient with symptoms of functional dyspepsia should be given various invasive tests to rule out more serious conditions such as peptic ulcer disease or stomach cancer, others believe that these tests should be used only after more conservative measures (such as altering the diet or taking antacids) fail to solve the problem. The course of action depends partly on the patient's age and risk factors, as well as the severity of symptoms.

Functional dyspepsia is often treated with dietary and life-style changes, including limiting fatty foods, eating small, frequent meals, and avoiding specific foods (such as coffee or alcohol) that aggravate symptoms. Avoiding smoking and certain medications (such as aspirin and nonsteroidal anti-inflammatory drugs) that may irritate the stomach lining can also help. Over-the-counter antacids can provide relief as well. If these steps fail, a clinician may prescribe stronger medications including H2 blockers that inhibit stomach acid, medications that improve stomach emptying, and low doses of antidepressants (even in patients without symptoms of depression). Researchers are also trying to determine if visceral analgesics—medications that relieve sensitivity to pain—may be helpful as well.

Gastritis. A stomachache, sometimes together with nausea or vomiting and occasionally diarrhea, can be a sign of gastritis (often called "burning" or "sour" stomach). This usually mild and temporary condition occurs when the lining of the stomach is irritated (see peptic ulcer disease). It is the rare person who goes through life without at least some experience of gastritis. Most often the cause is simply excessive eating or drinking. Taking daily doses of aspirin—as is sometimes recommended as a way to help prevent heart disease—can also irritate the stomach, as can excessive alcohol consumption or cigarette smoking.

Asymptomatic gastritis also occasionally develops in people with pernicious anemia (vitamin B_{12} deficiency) when the lining of the stomach starts to waste away. If symptoms of gastritis are ever accompanied by black stools (a sign of blood in the stool), a woman should consult her clinician, as there may be an area of the stomach that is bleeding.

Over-the-counter antacids can often help relieve the discomfort of gastritis. If they are ineffective, a physician can prescribe drugs that reduce the secretion of stomach acids (such as cimetidine, ranitidine, or omeprazole) or antiulcer drugs (such as sucralfate) which help protect the stomach lining. Cimetidine, ranitidine, and omeprazole are available without a prescription. Cutting down on cigarettes, caffeine, and alcohol may also help, as can regular injections of vitamin B$_{12}$ in people with pernicious anemia.

Heartburn. Heartburn (see entry), or gastroesophageal reflux disease (GERD), occurs when acid contents of the stomach wash back up (reflux) into the esophagus (food tube). It is particularly common during pregnancy, as well as in women who are obese or who have a hiatus hernia, a disorder in which part of the stomach protrudes into the chest area. Taking calcium-channel blockers or other smooth muscle relaxants can also precipitate heartburn. The abdominal pain associated with heartburn usually begins as a gnawing or burning sensation in the chest that may radiate to the arms or jaw. Sometimes sour-tasting materials back up as far as the throat or even the mouth. Over time the irritating acid may lead to esophagitis, or inflammation of the esophagus, a condition that can make swallowing difficult and result in bleeding. Occasionally there may be hoarseness, coughing, or wheezing as well. Symptoms of heartburn generally occur soon after eating and when a person is lying down.

Peptic ulcer disease (PUD). Erosions (ulcers) in the lining of the gastrointestinal tract are sometimes the source of pain much like that of gastritis—except that it lasts a lot longer. They are particularly likely to develop in women who take nonsteroidal antiinflammatory drugs on a regular basis, use alcohol excessively, smoke cigarettes, or are infected with the *Helicobacter pylori* bacterium. Symptoms commonly include pain in the stomach area which improves with eating (see peptic ulcer disease).

Stomach cancer. In rare instances a stomachache may stem from a malignant growth in the stomach. The associated pain is not relieved by either dietary changes or antacids. Depending on the exact site of the tumor, there may be a number of other symptoms, including difficulty swallowing, black stools, anemia, a feeling of fullness or slight pain, vomiting after eating, vomiting blood, and weight loss. Many people with stomach cancer have no symptoms until the disease has spread. Others have symptoms indistinguishable from those of peptic ulcer disease.

For this reason, a clinician will often consider the possibility of a stomach tumor in someone who has recently developed persistent indigestion, unexplained weight loss, and nausea, particularly if that person is over the age of 50. Tumors of the stomach rarely occur in people under 40 and are about twice as common in men as in women. In this country they are also most common among African Americans and among the poor. These tumors can often be removed surgically, though complete cure is most likely if this is done before the cancer has spread beyond the stomach.

Enlarged or ruptured spleen. The spleen is an organ lying close to the surface of the abdomen which helps recycle red blood cells. In a number of different conditions (including inflammatory diseases such as infectious mononucleosis, hepatitis, and lupus; see entries), the spleen can enlarge, stretching the capsule that covers it to the point of causing pain. In addition to pain in the left upper quadrant of the abdomen, an enlarged spleen sometimes results in a feeling of fullness after eating and in otherwise unexplained bruising.

An enlarged spleen is also prone to rupture. Since the spleen is so close to the surface of the body, anyone who knows she has an enlarged spleen must take particular care to avoid contact sports or other activities that might injure the organ. A ruptured spleen can be life-threatening and requires immediate medical attention. It is usually marked by sudden, brief, and sharp pain in the upper left abdomen and a blue discoloration around the navel.

How is abdominal pain evaluated?

Abdominal pain can signal anything from a life-threatening emergency to simple indigestion. A good description of the pain will help the clinician focus on the most likely causes. A woman should note the location and character of the pain (for example, dull, sharp, or burning), its duration and timing (after meals or in connection with specific foods, near the end of the menstrual cycle, before breakfast), and any accompanying symptoms (diarrhea, vaginal bleeding, chills and fever). In addition to focusing on the pain itself, the physician may ask questions about medications being taken, any recent chemical exposures or occupational hazards, use of alcohol and other substances, and any stressful changes in life circumstances. After a physical examination, often including a pelvic exam, blood tests and urine tests may be performed, particularly if the pain is acute or severe.

Sometimes the evaluation of abdominal pain requires a period of observation to determine whether symptoms respond as expected to a trial of treatment. For example, a woman with suspected irritable bowel syndrome may be able to avoid the discomfort and inconvenience of further testing if her symptoms respond well to dietary changes.

A variety of imaging tests may be done once the initial evaluation narrows down the possibilities. Ultrasound examination of the right upper quadrant is usually the best test if gallstones are suspected. Ultrasound (see entry) can also be used to detect kidney stones or certain pelvic disorders. Plain x-rays of the abdomen are not helpful in most cases of abdominal pain, but x-rays combined with a barium enema can often pick up abnormalities of the lower intestine (see bowel disorders), and, similarly, an upper GI series can detect many problems of the esophagus and stomach (see heartburn, peptic ulcer disease). More complicated tests, including endoscopy or colonoscopy, which involve visual inspection of the stomach or colon using a narrow lighted tube, and CT scans (see entry), are sometimes necessary for a firm diagnosis.

Related entries

Bowel disorders, chest pain, colon and rectal cancer, constipation, diverticular disease, ectopic pregnancy, gallstones, hepatitis, irritable bowel syndrome, kidney disorders, pelvic pain, peptic ulcer disease, shingles

Abortion

Abortion is the termination of a pregnancy before the embryo or fetus can live independently. Among physicians a miscarriage—the involuntary, spontaneous loss of a pregnancy for some physical reason—is also called an abortion, but in nonmedical circles the term is generally used to describe a voluntary procedure that ends a pregnancy before the fetus is viable.

Each year since 1980 approximately 1 million abortions have been performed in this country, with 1 in 4 of all pregnancies in the United States terminated. These numbers do not include the uncounted "menstrual extractions"—procedures performed very early in pregnancy to remove products of conception. By the time they have reached 45 years of age, almost half of all women in the United States have had at least one abortion.

Obtaining accurate estimates is difficult, in part because of incomplete reporting. About a fifth of all abortions in the United States are performed in clinicians' offices. Others are performed in unlicensed facilities, and these may not be as rigorously reported as those performed in family planning and abortion clinics or hospitals. Determining the frequency of illegal abortion with any accuracy is even more difficult, if not impossible. (An illegal abortion is one performed by an unlicensed person.)

Why are abortions performed?
Women choose abortion for a number of different social, economic, medical, and moral reasons. Despite the raging religious and political controversy surrounding it, abortion continues to be legal in this country and, for many women, represents a valuable option in dealing with an unintended or unwanted pregnancy.

Among the many factors that may influence a woman's decision to terminate a pregnancy are her age, financial status, educational or career plans, relationship to the father, number of other children, emotional stability, sources of family and professional support, health, religious and political values, and, in the case of adolescents, relationship with parents. Some women have an abortion as a result of inadequate access to (or inaccurate information about) contraception or because of contraceptive failure. Women who become pregnant through rape or incest frequently opt for abortion, while other women terminate a pregnancy to save their own life. Many women ultimately choose abortion after weighing the impact of structural or chromosomal defects that are revealed during amniocentesis, ultrasound, or other prenatal screening tests during a wanted pregnancy. The number

of abortions performed for this reason will undoubtedly increase as such screening tests become more routine and as the number of detectable anomalies continues to grow.

Most women in this country do not use abortion as a substitute for contraception. For many women, determining whether or not to have an abortion is an agonizing emotional decision made only after considering the welfare of both the mother and the potential child, as well as that of everyone else who would be affected (particularly the father and any other children).

How are first trimester abortions performed?
Several different types of abortion procedures can be performed during the first trimester of pregnancy—that is, between 5 and 13 weeks after the beginning of the last menstrual period. Usually these involve a form of surgery in which the cervix is dilated (or widened) and the contents of the uterus are removed.

The exact procedure varies somewhat depending on how far the pregnancy has progressed. This progression is measured in "gestational age," a figure derived from the number of weeks that have passed since the pregnant woman's last menstrual period (which is approximately 2 weeks earlier than the actual time of fertilization). A woman who is 1 week late getting her period, for example, would generally be considered about 5 weeks pregnant in terms of gestational age.

Menstrual extraction. Between 5 and 7 weeks of gestation, the contents of the uterus can often be suctioned out without dilating the cervix. This procedure—sometimes called menstrual extraction, menstrual regulation, minisuction, or miniabortion—is usually performed in a doctor's office by either the physician or an assistant. A flexible plastic tube (called a cannula) 3 to 4 mm in diameter is inserted through the cervix and into the uterus. Then the contents of the uterus are suctioned out by the vacuum power of either a bulb syringe or a small pump. Sometimes this procedure is called a preemptive abortion or endometrial aspiration if it is done before the pregnancy has been confirmed and if the uterine contents are sucked out with a nonmechanical syringe. The entire procedure takes only a few minutes and often requires no anesthesia.

Menstrual extractions are generally considered safer procedures than later abortions, but they have a greater risk of failing, thus allowing the pregnancy to continue (a result called an incomplete abortion). This failure occurs because there is so little fetal tissue so early in a pregnancy that it is relatively easy to miss it. Therefore, even though it may seem appealing to terminate a pregnancy as soon as possible, it may be wise to wait another week or two. Women who do choose menstrual extraction should be sure to have a follow-up examination and blood test 2 or 3 weeks after the procedure to make sure that they are no longer pregnant.

Dilatation and evacuation. After week 6 or 7 of a pregnancy, the cervix usually has to be dilated somewhat before suction evacuation can be performed. A procedure that involves dilation of the cervix, followed by suction evacuation of the contents of the uterus, is called a dilatation and evacuation, or D&E. Depending on the specific procedure used to evacuate the uterus, a D&E performed during the first trimester may also sometimes be referred to as a vacuum aspiration (see entry), a vacuum curettage, a suction curettage, or a suction D&C.

A D&E is almost always a one-day outpatient procedure. Because opening the cervix can be painful, sedation (such as short-acting tranquilizers) may be given to help reduce anxiety.

Sometimes laminaria—long rods of kelp which absorb moisture—are inserted into the cervix 2 to 24 hours before a first trimester abortion to help dilate the cervix slowly. As the cervix dilates, there may be some crampy pain. Having a specially trained nurse, counselor, family member, or friend present during the procedure may provide emotional support, and deep breathing, verbal distraction, and other relaxation techniques can help offset anxiety.

Once the sedative has taken effect, the woman will be helped to lie back on a table with her legs elevated and her heels in stirrups. After the surgeon examines the uterus to confirm the stage of the pregnancy (which determines the size of the cannula required) and removes any laminaria that may have been used, he or she inserts a metal speculum and washes the cervix with an antibacterial liquid. In very early abortions (up to about 12 weeks) and during some later abortions (12 to 24 weeks) local anesthesia may also be given— usually a paracervical block, an injection of medicine which numbs the area around the cervix but does not mask uterine cramping. (Although general anesthesia is used under some circumstances, its tendency to relax the uterine muscle may increase the chance that the uterus may be perforated during the evacuation procedure.) This injection is usually only a little painful, since the cervix has few nerve endings. The surgeon then holds the cervix steady with a metal clamp called a tenaculum and progressively inserts a series of tapered metal rods of increasing diameter through and just beyond the opening to the cervix. Within a few minutes the cervix is usually sufficiently dilated, and a cannula (generally a plastic or metal instrument) is inserted into the uterus.

Once the cannula is in place, the outer end is attached to an electric or hydrostatic pump. This produces enough vacuum pressure to aspirate fetal tissue out of the uterus so that it can be collected in a bottle. Sometimes a tool called a curette may also be used to scrape the inside of the uterus or to check to make sure that all fetal tissue has been removed, although some surgeons argue that this is often unnecessary.

The level of discomfort experienced during the suction can vary considerably, depending on personal feelings about the abortion, the length of the pregnancy, and an individual's pain threshold. As the uterus contracts and empties, some women experience only mild pain, if any, while others feel intense menstrual-like cramps. Squeezing the hand of a nurse or companion, breathing deeply, concentrating on a distant object, or trying other relaxation techniques may minimize the discomfort. If tranquilizers are given before the procedure, they will blunt the intensity of the pain, reduce anxiety, and may cause mild amnesia about the abortion itself, but usually some cramping occurs.

The entire procedure takes between 5 and 15 minutes (the greater the gestational age, the longer the procedure generally takes). After resting for about an hour and receiving specific instructions for aftercare, the woman is usually able to go home.

Women with stable diabetes, well-controlled seizure disorders, or mild to moderate hypertension, as well as women infected with HIV (see acquired immune deficiency syndrome), can usually undergo abortion on an outpatient basis if special precautions are taken. Hospitalization, as well as special monitoring and medications, may be necessary for women who have heart disease, previous bacterial endocarditis (inflammation of the membrane that lines the interior of the heart), asthma, lupus, uterine fibroids, blood clotting disorders, certain mental disorders, and poorly controlled epilepsy.

Medical (nonsurgical) abortions. The drug mifepristone, marketed as RU-486, is the only drug currently approved by the U.S. Food and Drug Administration (FDA) to terminate a normal pregnancy, although drugs approved for other conditions are also being used for this purpose (see entry on nonsurgical abortion). Mifepristone works by blocking the effects of progesterone, a hormone necessary for the fertilized egg to implant and develop in the uterus. After a decade of struggles and setbacks in both the political and business arenas, mifepristone was finally approved for commercial use in the United States. With mifepristone, abortion can be safely accomplished before the 6th or 8th week of pregnancy. To be effective, the drug must be taken before the 9th week after the start of the last menstrual period.

Mifepristone is used in conjunction with the antiulcer drug misoprostol, taken by mouth two days after the mifepristone to induce uterine cramping and bleeding and promote the expulsion of the fetus and pregnancy-related tissue. The expelled tissue is usually collected by the woman herself, often at home. Approximately 96 percent of these procedures are effective, although a small percentage of women may need to have surgery to evacuate the uterus. About 1 percent of women may lose enough blood to require a blood transfusion. At present, this form of abortion is most suitable for women who live in areas where surgical abortion is unavailable or for those who prefer the privacy over a medical visit or who dislike the idea of surgery.

Another method of nonsurgical abortion, which was being performed in the United States before the approval of mifepristone, involves a combination of two prescription drugs. The first of these drugs, methotrexate, has been used for years to terminate ectopic pregnancies (as well as to treat cancer, arthritis, and psoriasis). The second drug, misoprostol, is an antiulcer medication that is also used with RU-486. The combination of these drugs is successful 90 to 95 percent of the time. Although two-thirds of women using this method abort the very first day, the rest may experience cramping and bleeding for an average of 28 more days until the abortion is complete. For the 5 to 10 percent of women for whom the combination fails to work, surgical abortion is necessary.

Occasionally another medical abortion practice known as "multifetal pregnancy reduction" is used during the first trimester to reduce the number of fetuses in a multiple pregnancy. This procedure is usually done so that the remaining fetus or fetuses will have a decreased risk of prematurity and an increased chance of survival; it is also sometimes used during the second trimester to abort a twin with multiple anomalies. Usually the reduction is accomplished by injecting potassium chloride through the pregnant woman's abdominal wall and into her uterus (with the aid of ultrasound) so that the affected fetus is terminated. Usually nothing is passed through the vagina, however. The terminated fetus is frequently resorbed, although fetal remnants can often be found at the time of delivery.

As treatments for infertility such as in vitro fertilization have increased the odds of multiple pregnancies, multiple pregnancy reduction has become more common. Complications can include bleeding, infection, leakage of amniotic fluid, the need to repeat the procedure (which can be emotionally very trying for the woman), and in rare cases losing the whole pregnancy. In extremely rare cases, a D&E or even hysterectomy (surgical removal of the uterus) may be necessary.

How are second trimester abortions performed?

More than 95 percent of abortions are performed in the first trimester (the first 13 weeks of pregnancy), a time when they are relatively safe and easy. But there are a number of reasons why second trimester abortions (during weeks 14 to 24) may be unavoidable. Some women may not realize they are pregnant until several months have passed. This is particularly true for teenage girls and for women with irregular periods, as well as for women using forms of birth control that are considered highly effective such as the pill or the IUD. It is not uncommon for adolescents to put off telling parents about a pregnancy, to deny the possibility of pregnancy for as long as possible, or to know that they are pregnant but irrationally wish the whole problem would disappear on its own. Other women simply have trouble finding access to abortion facilities or do not have the funds to pay for an abortion in the early months. Delay for whatever reason creates additional burdens, since second trimester abortions are considerably more costly and risky.

With the growing prevalence of prenatal screening—and a trend toward bearing children relatively late in life—a number of women are undergoing second trimester abortions after the results of an amniocentesis or ultrasound indicate fetal abnormalities. These results are often unavailable until the 18th week of pregnancy or later, necessitating a second

trimester abortion should the woman decide to terminate the pregnancy. Finally, some women do not discover until the second trimester that continuing the pregnancy would threaten their own health or even their life.

For a woman in any of these circumstances, the decision to terminate a pregnancy can be particularly difficult, with many women feeling that they are having to choose between a bad option and a worse one. Often already able to feel the kicks and movements of a wanted and loved fetus as she awaits the procedure, a woman in this position must sometimes endure insensitive comments about the lateness of her abortion. In some public facilities she may have to undergo the abortion procedure in the same room with women experiencing full-term childbirth.

D&E versus labor induction. There are two basic options for a woman having a second trimester abortion: a late D&E or an induction procedure. The latter essentially involves having uterine contractions induced with drugs and then going through labor until the fetus is expelled from the vagina. In contrast, a late D&E is generally quicker, safer, and, for many women, less traumatic—provided that it is performed by a skilled clinician.

For some women a D&E after about 16 weeks' gestation is not an option. First, many doctors and facilities cannot or will not do D&Es beyond a certain gestational date— often about 16 or 18 weeks—either because they do not have proper training or because they feel uncomfortable about removing the dismembered body parts of a more fully developed fetus. Some doctors also contend that beyond about 16 weeks' gestation induction of labor may be a safer procedure, and do not even offer women the option of having a late D&E. Other doctors, however, maintain that a D&E performed by a skilled and experienced clinician (and this is essential) as late as 23 weeks' gestation may be safer than an induction procedure performed at the same point. Far too often a woman simply does not know that she has this option—or does not have enough money to travel to a distant facility where late D&Es are performed safely.

For psychological and emotional reasons, some women prefer to have an induction procedure even when a D&E is an option. For example, a woman whose fetus has been diagnosed as having a genetic defect may regard the aborted fetus as a "baby" for whom it was best not to live. The pain and time involved in the labor will become part of her memory of that "child" and thus are endurable and perhaps even comforting. She may not be able to bear the thought of having the fetus dismembered during the D&E procedure. Also, for abnormal fetuses, induction procedures allow for a more accurate diagnosis of the problem, since the fetus is delivered intact.

Other women, however, find it easier to handle the loss by regarding the defective fetus as only a potential life and to view the entire episode as fundamentally different from the birth of her children or her future children. For these women a safely performed D&E procedure can be infinitely preferable to an induction, since it differentiates the abortion from the childbirth experience.

Late D&E. A D&E done after the 13th week of pregnancy is essentially similar to one done earlier, except that it takes longer to perform. It also requires more experience and skill on the part of the clinician because there is more fetal tissue to remove, the larger and softer uterus is easier to injure, and larger instruments are required. Doctors who feel that they cannot safely perform a D&E after 16 or 18 weeks may be able to refer a woman to another surgeon who can, although this is not always possible and frequently involves considerable travel and expense.

The surgery itself can usually be done in a clinic or hospital on an outpatient basis. It is often necessary to go to the hospital the day before the procedure, however, to fill out forms and have preoperative testing (such as blood tests) and discussions of anesthesia. Also, because the cervix has to be dilated to a greater extent than in a first trimester procedure, most women will need to have laminaria inserted a day before the procedure.

Some doctors may prefer to soften the cervix using synthetic dilators such as Lamisil (made of a dried polyvinyl alcohol sponge stick) or Dilapan (a polymer similar to a soft contact lens). As these agents absorb moisture and expand, the cervix softens and dilates gradually, thus reducing the chances of cervical tears, uterine perforation, and excessive bleeding.

Before inserting the laminaria—which look like small sticks of wood about 2 inches long and an eighth of an inch or so in diameter—the doctor holds the vagina open with a speculum and washes the surface with Betadine or some other antiseptic (this stains, so a sanitary pad must be worn afterward). The sticks are inserted one by one and held in place with small sponges. The woman may feel a brief stabbing sensation followed by mild to moderate cramping. The more sticks inserted, the better the dilation and the easier the procedure; with a D&E after 18 weeks, as many as 6 or 7 may be ideal.

In practice, however, the number used is often limited by the woman's pain, which tends to worsen with each additional insertion. Although dilation is usually complete within about 6 hours, the same kind of cramping often continues off and on until the abortion takes place, which can be up to 24 hours later. For many women, acetaminophen (Tylenol) can help take the edge off the pain. Painkillers such as aspirin or ibuprofen should be avoided since they can interfere with blood clotting during the abortion, but other pain medications are available if the discomfort is not adequately controlled with acetaminophen.

Because late D&Es are lengthier and more painful than earlier ones, anesthesia is often useful. One option is a paracervical block injected into the cervix, which numbs the cervix and area around it but cannot mask uterine cramps.

The cramps can be made more bearable with intravenous sedation, which will make the woman groggy and less anxious about the pain. Other women opt for general anesthesia, administered intravenously, because they want to be asleep throughout the entire operation. Some surgeons dislike doing D&Es with general anesthesia, however, because it relaxes the uterus and makes it more susceptible to perforation by a sharp instrument, thus considerably increasing the risks of the procedure. For this reason—and for women who prefer to remain conscious—having a regional anesthetic (possibly combined with intravenous sedation) can be a good alternative for a patient particularly concerned about pain and anxiety. Injected between two of the vertebrae in the spinal column, spinal or epidural anesthesia numbs the body from the waist down so that nothing more is felt than occasional light tugs during the scraping and suction. Even these tugs can be masked with light sedation.

As soon as the anesthesia has taken effect, the surgeon removes the laminaria or other cervical softening agent and, if necessary, dilates the cervix further with metal or plastic rods. Next a curette, vacuum suction, or forceps are used to remove the fetal tissue and placenta. The operation usually takes between 10 and 45 minutes.

Afterward the woman is monitored for a few hours until the anesthesia wears off and vaginal bleeding has slowed to a moderate level. Sometimes oxytocin may be given during the recovery period to help the uterus contract and to slow the bleeding.

Labor induction. Abortion through induction of labor is another option—and sometimes the only option—for women who want to terminate a pregnancy after 16 weeks' gestation. Overnight hospitalization may be necessary (depending on the length of the labor), though in many facilities women can go home on the day of the procedure. This makes scheduling easier and can help reduce the considerable cost of the operation. As with a late D&E, however, often a visit to the hospital or doctor's office is necessary the day before the procedure for tests and for the insertion of laminaria rods or other cervical softening agents to help speed up labor. The agent Lamisil in particular not only makes the cervix more amenable to gradual dilation with conventional dilating instruments but also may enhance the effectiveness of some of the agents (prostaglandins) used to induce labor.

On the day of the induction, one or more of a variety of drugs—often prostaglandin, saline (a salt solution), or, less often, urea—is injected into the amniotic sac to start uterine contractions. Saline causes fetal death as well as uterine contractions, though the contractions tend to be milder than those associated with other induction agents. If the salt enters a blood vessel, however, there is a slight risk to the woman of fluid retention, shock, or even death. Moreover, saline is relatively slow to work: when saline is used alone, contractions may not begin for up to 24 hours. Urea takes even longer to work—an obvious disadvantage. Prostaglandin, while much quicker and less risky overall, may produce intense nausea, vomiting, and diarrhea and, less often, bronchial spasms. It also frequently needs to be readministered when contractions do not begin the first time around. Thus, many doctors like to follow an instillation (injection by drops) of prostaglandin with another instillation of saline.

With a needle similar to that used for amniocentesis, the drug is instilled into the amniotic fluid. There may be a small cramp when the needle first enters the uterus and then a feeling of pressure. If prostaglandin is used, contractions generally begin within a few hours. If labor does not begin, the injection may have to be repeated; if progress is slow, other agents such as prostaglandins (administered via vaginal suppositories) or oxytocin (administered via an IV) may be used to induce contractions.

Contractions that occur during induced abortion are often milder than those of full-term labor, but many women find them more difficult to endure. This is probably because pain is, to some degree, contextual. The pain of childbirth is somewhat assuaged by the knowledge that the process is natural and that a healthy, wanted baby will result. The pain of an induced abortion, by contrast, is colored for many women by fear, ambivalence about the procedure, and, in some cases, grief over the loss of a previously desired child or guilt about choosing to abort. Thus, while some women are able to use deep breathing and other nondrug relaxation techniques to make it through the procedure, most rely on anesthesia. Anesthesia of the same sort used during childbirth (paracervical blocks, sedation, epidurals, or spinals; see anesthesia) is usually available to most women having induction abortions. Other drugs can be used to relieve the nausea, vomiting, and diarrhea that often accompany a prostaglandin instillation.

It takes an average of 8 hours of labor before the woman is ready to deliver, though in some women it may take as long as 72 hours before the cervix is fully dilated—in which case overnight hospitalization is unavoidable. In certain facilities (though this is rare today) the woman is left to deliver the fetus on her own—which can be tremendously frightening and upsetting—or with the aid of a nurse. Preferably a clinician will be present to help deliver the fetus as quickly as possible and to check the uterus after delivery to make sure the placenta and other products of delivery have been expelled completely (which they often are not, especially in abortions that involve prostaglandin alone). A D&E may be necessary to remove any remaining tissue. Most women are able to go home a few hours after the procedure.

What happens after an abortion?

Physical changes and aftercare. After the abortion is over, some women receive additional medication (either via injection or through the intravenous line) to help the uterus contract and to help control bleeding. Women at high risk of infection may be prescribed antibiotics, and women who are Rh negative should receive anti-D immune globulin such as Rhogam to prevent sensitization and possible Rh disease (see entry) in subsequent pregnancies. Immune globulin is ideally administered after menstrual extraction or drug-induced abortion as well, even though the chances of sensitization after these procedures are lower.

Normal activities can usually be resumed almost immediately after an abortion, although women often feel tired or crampy for a few days. Strenuous activity and heavy lifting are best avoided until after the 2- or 3-week checkup. Many women have vaginal bleeding for up to 3 weeks, which at the beginning may be somewhat heavier than that of a menstrual period. This bleeding should gradually diminish, although it is perfectly normal for it to stop after a few days and then start again. For about 2 weeks—or until the bleeding has stopped completely—women should avoid sexual intercourse, swimming, bathing, douching, or inserting anything into the vagina (such as tampons), since any of these may increase the odds of uterine infection.

Mild menstrual-like cramping can be relieved with acetaminophen (Tylenol), hot water bottles, or heating pads. Aspirin, ibuprofen (Advil, Motrin), and other nonsteroidal antiinflammatory drugs should be avoided, since they can increase bleeding.

Some women find that their breasts become somewhat tender or even produce a small secretion after a first trimester abortion. After a late second trimester abortion, milk may even come in and engorge the breasts, leaving them hard and swollen. Besides being quite painful, this can be deeply upsetting for many women. Breast tenderness is usually most severe on the third day after surgery and subsides on its own. In the meantime, wearing a supportive bra, taking frequent hot showers, or applying ice packs to the breasts can provide some relief.

At the postabortion checkup the clinician will make sure the uterus has returned to normal size, check for complications, provide emotional support, and answer questions about contraception and future family planning. Most women can expect their normal menstrual period to occur 4 to 8 weeks after the abortion. Because conception can occur almost immediately, however, contraception must be used as soon as sexual intercourse is resumed (see birth control).

Women who used a diaphragm or cervical cap before the abortion should have it refitted. Those who want to have an IUD inserted may be advised to wait several months and to use another form of contraception in the meantime, although some clinicians believe it is safe to insert an IUD immediately after an abortion. A woman using contraceptive pills can begin taking them the week after the abortion and should expect her period to begin sometime during the last week of pills. A backup form of contraception should be used for the first month, since the pills may not be fully effective until the second pack is started.

Some women, particularly those who have completed their families, ask to be sterilized immediately after an abortion, but most clinicians advise waiting until a less stressful time to make this often irrevocable decision (see tubal ligation).

Feelings after an abortion. Emotions can vary considerably in the first 2 or 3 weeks after an abortion. Many women feel tremendous relief once the procedure is over and done with. Often, however, these same women may also feel weepy or moody and experience grief after their loss. This grief can be profound, particularly after the termination of a planned pregnancy. There is no evidence that rapidly changing hormone levels after an abortion (particularly a first trimester abortion) produce true postpartum depression, but any woman who experiences prolonged or severe emotional distress should seek professional counseling. Talking to close friends—particularly other women who have had abortions—is often consoling as well. Some women find that disturbing feelings about a past abortion can resurface on occasion for many years to come, but these feelings are usually fleeting as time passes and are almost never incapacitating. Adverse psychological reactions are most common in adolescents who have had abortions.

Many women feel uncomfortable or even fearful about sexual intimacy for some time after an abortion. Concerns about unwanted pregnancy, mistrust of her own body, or, in some cases, new consciousness of the potential tragedy inherent in sexual intimacy all may interfere with a woman's normal sexual response. These feelings can manifest themselves for months or even longer, both with the man who fathered the aborted fetus as well as with future sexual partners (see sexual dysfunction).

Other conflicts within a relationship are common after abortion, and these can compound the sexual problems. Feelings of sadness, resentment, betrayal, or anger often arise, for example, when the man did not have the same feelings about choosing to have the abortion as did the woman. Women also may feel distanced from partners who do not seem to share—or know how to acknowledge—their strong, mixed, or negative feelings, or who, for whatever reason, were not present during the abortion.

Feelings after an abortion are often somewhat different in women who terminate a pregnancy for medical reasons or because of a fetal defect—especially for those who choose an induction abortion, which essentially involves "giving birth" to the aborted fetus. Not only are their emotions generally more intense and long-lasting, but also it is more common for women in these situations to feel a sense of loss akin to that of a woman who has had a miscarriage or stillbirth—after all, the baby had been planned and wanted—while at the same time being deprived of equivalent sources of support (although women who terminate a pregnancy for *any* reason may experience these feelings as well). Because so many people still frown on abortion, initial murmurs of sympathy for "the loss" may quickly turn to criticism for the decision. Some women who aborted a fetus with an anomaly may not even have told anyone that they were pregnant and may find themselves going through the decision-making and abortion process alone—without ever receiving any affirmation or acknowledgment of their pregnancy, their fetus (or, to some women, their baby), or their physical ordeal and grief. It is not unusual in women who have had an abortion for any reason, and at any time during a pregnancy, for an intense desire for the entire world to know about the tragedy to be mingled with the compulsion to keep it private. For many months afterward just seeing a pregnant stranger can trigger tears in a woman who has experienced this loss.

Talking to a close friend or joining a perinatal loss support group can be invaluable for some, though many women may feel uncomfortable—or unwelcome—in a group of women who lost pregnancies involuntarily. An alternative for women who live in large urban areas or near major medical centers is a group that consists solely of women who terminated pregnancies because of problems revealed by prenatal testing. A clinician or genetic counselor may be able to help locate some of these groups. There may also be support groups consisting of women who chose abortion for nonmedical reasons but who nevertheless feel a need to talk with others who have gone through a similar experience.

Some women who abort a fetus for medical reasons—particularly those who choose to regard the aborted fetus as a child who died—have also found it helpful to name the baby and hold a full-fledged funeral and burial. Acknowledging their loss to both themselves and the world is part of their way of overcoming grief. Others find this approach morbid and prefer to deal with their grief by trying to become pregnant again right away. Although it is perfectly safe for most women to attempt another pregnancy as soon as a normal menstrual period has occurred, many doctors advise waiting for a few months. The body may be physically ready, but more time may be needed for emotional healing. Also, dating of future pregnancies may be more accurate after 2 to 3 normal menstrual cycles.

What are the risks and complications?

Legal induced abortion is a safe surgical procedure in healthy women, especially when it is performed during the first trimester of pregnancy by a trained practitioner. But that may change if the opposition to safe and legal abortions continues to grow. There is already a shortage of health care providers trained and willing to perform certain procedures (particularly second trimester surgical abortions). Also, the highly publicized death threats and actual violence directed toward personnel at abortion clinics make it unappealing for younger clinicians to enter this realm of health care. Lack of universal public funding for induced abortions is already limiting access to abortion for many women, and recent Supreme Court legislation has made it easy for states to restrict access, particularly among poor women who use public hospitals or receive public aid. Laws, regulations, or constitutional amendments in 30 states endorse public financial coverage for induced abortion only if the mother's life is endangered by the pregnancy. In most states adolescents must meet parental consent or notification requirements before they are allowed to terminate a pregnancy. And in as many as 84 percent of all counties in the United States, there is no known abortion provider whatsoever.

There is no evidence that constraining access to abortion actually reduces the number of procedures performed—it only makes them more dangerous. Conversely, legalizing abortion does not seem to increase the total number of abortions performed but only makes them safer. When restrictive abortion laws in New York State, England, and Wales were repealed in the 1970s, for example, the total number of abortions did not change much. Instead, the abortions that had previously been done illegally were now simply performed legally. Furthermore, since the legalization of abortion, the number of deaths attributable to pregnancy termination has declined by a factor of 20.

Although legal abortion in the United States is generally quite safe, occasionally complications do arise. One of the most common causes in first trimester procedures (occurring in perhaps 1 or 2 out of 1,000 attempted abortions, especially those done under 6 weeks' gestation) is retained tissue—also known as an incomplete abortion. Ectopic pregnancy or the removal of only one twin may account for the continuation of pregnancy after an abortion as well. Retained tissue often complicates second trimester abortions, too, which is why many clinicians routinely check the uterus before completing the procedure. If fetal tissue is retained, the woman could still be pregnant—something she may not discover until she returns for her postabortion checkup 2 or 3 weeks later. At this time drugs can be given to stimulate expulsion of the tissue, or a second procedure can usually still be performed. The possibility of an incomplete abortion makes this follow-up exam essential even if a woman feels fine and would prefer to put the whole experience behind her. Among possible symptoms of retained tissue are heavy or prolonged vaginal bleeding, the passage of large blood clots, intense cramping, or signs of pregnancy that last longer than a week.

Another relatively common complication of surgical abortion—particularly in the second trimester—is heavy bleeding (hemorrhage) during the abortion or a few days afterward. Sometimes a transfusion may be necessary to replace lost blood, or a dilatation and curettage (D&C), in which the cervix is dilated and the uterus scraped, may be required to stop the bleeding. As in any surgical procedure there may be adverse reactions to medications used for anesthesia, including—in rare cases—seizures and allergic responses.

Occasionally surgical abortion is followed by uterine infection—signaled by pain and fever. Immediate treatment with antibiotics (and sometimes a D&C) usually stops the infection, but delaying treatment can lead to a very serious and possibly life-threatening infection which may cause chronic pain and even future infertility.

Perforation of the uterus with a surgical instrument occurs in 1 or 2 out of 1,000 abortions. The uterus often heals on its own, but sometimes surgery is necessary. Very rarely, the intestines may be injured. Occasionally the cervix may tear during a D&E, sometimes severely enough to require stitches. The odds of both uterine perforation and cervical tears are higher the later in pregnancy the abortion is performed, and the odds of a perforation are increased by use of general anesthesia.

There is no evidence that first trimester abortion in and of itself impairs a woman's future fertility, threatens future pregnancies, or raises the risk of ectopic pregnancy. As for the impact of second trimester abortions on future fertility, no definitive conclusions can be drawn until bigger and better studies are done based on the procedures of well-trained clinicians. To date there is also no scientific evidence to suggest that having an abortion in and of itself increases a woman's chances of developing breast cancer later in life.

Finally, as in any surgical procedure, abortion carries a very small risk of death. In the United States this is an extremely rare event—something on the order of 2 or 3 out of every 100,000 legal abortions. This risk is considerably lower than the risk of death associated with carrying a pregnancy to term (about 15 per 100,000 deliveries). The mortality rate is higher if the abortion is performed late in the pregnancy and eventually becomes about the same as if the pregnancy were continued to term.

A clinician should be called immediately if any of the following signs of infection or other complications occur after an abortion:

- a fever of over 100°F
- excessive vaginal bleeding (soaking a pad every 1 to 2 hours or passing large clots)
- an increase in bleeding over two consecutive days
- severe, persistent abdominal pain or swollen abdomen
- a foul-smelling vaginal discharge
- vomiting or fainting
- signs of pregnancy that last more than a week

Before calling the clinician, a woman should know her temperature, the number of pads used in the last hour, and the time of her last bowel movement.

Related entries

Alpha-fetoprotein screening, amniocentesis, anesthesia, birth control, childbirth, chorionic villi sampling, dilatation and curettage, genetic counseling, hysterectomy, infertility, miscarriage, nonsurgical abortion, postpartum psychiatric disorders, preconception counseling, pregnancy, pregnancy over age 35, Rh disease, sexual dysfunction, sexual response, tubal ligation, ultrasound, vacuum aspiration

Acne

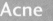

Acne is a collection of blackheads, whiteheads, pimples, pustules, or sometimes cysts on the face, chest, or back. Normally an oily substance called sebum is excreted into tiny hair follicles by sebaceous (oil) glands and rises through an open pore to lubricate the hair and skin (see illustration). If

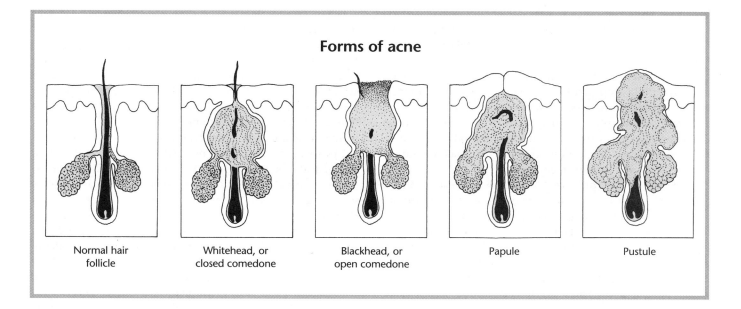

Forms of acne

| Normal hair follicle | Whitehead, or closed comedone | Blackhead, or open comedone | Papule | Pustule |

the pore becomes blocked, the sebum and dead cells can become impacted into a plug, forming what is known as a comedone.

Closed comedones (also known as whiteheads) appear when the pore is completely closed to the air. Open comedones (blackheads) are exposed to the air, which darkens their color. If bacteria invade the comedones, the surrounding skin may become inflamed and red, and tender pimples (papules) may erupt. Sometimes the pimples become pustules, and in severe cases pus may collect deep in the skin and form painful sacs of fluid called cysts.

Who is likely to develop acne?

Approximately 17 million people have some form of acne (also called acne vulgaris). Most of these people are women, although males are more likely to develop the more severe cystic forms of the condition. Acne is most common in adolescents, usually beginning around the time of puberty. This is probably because hormonal changes stimulate the sebaceous glands to increase sebum production. It generally disappears spontaneously by about age 20. Acne sometimes leaves permanent scars, but the red and brown discoloration tends to fade over time. More damaging can be the effects of severe acne on a teenager's self-esteem and social life.

Acne can also appear for the first time in adult women, sometimes because of a genetic predisposition or hormonal fluctuations. It can result, too, from reactions to certain cosmetics and hair treatments, as well as to drugs such as oral contraceptives, corticosteroids (hormone-like drugs used to treat inflammation), androgenic steroids (such as danazol, used to treat endometriosis), phenytoin (Dilantin, used to treat epilepsy), and lithium (used to treat manic depression and some other mental disorders). Other women develop acne in the week before their menstrual period begins or at the time of menopause. Generally, women notice that acne improves during pregnancy. Up to half of adult women with

acne show evidence of excess androgenic hormones that in high concentrations produce masculine traits such as beard growth, thinning of scalp hair, and deepening of the voice. These women often have other signs of high androgen levels, such as excess hair growth and irregular menstrual periods (see hyperandrogenism).

Severe acne seems to be hereditary, although why certain individuals develop worse cases than others remains unknown. Women of Asian background have a higher frequency of acne than women in other ethnic groups.

How is the condition evaluated?

A clinician evaluating acne will want to know at what age it began, which treatments have been tried, and whether any drugs such as oral contraceptives are being used. If a woman has irregular menstrual periods or excess hair growth, the clinician will probably want to do some blood tests to check for hormonal imbalances.

How is acne treated?

Treatment for acne aims at unplugging the blocked pores, as well as reducing inflammation of the surrounding skin. Some of the home practices commonly used to treat acne—such as harsh scrubbing, "skin machines," and antibacterial soaps—can actually aggravate the condition. Squeezing or picking at pimples can also further irritate the eruptions and lead to scarring. Exposure to the sun and artificial tanning devices seems to improve acne temporarily in some women, but in others it can lead to an outbreak. In any case, a temporary gain in clear skin does not justify the risks of skin cancer (not to mention an increase in wrinkles) that can result from excessive exposure to ultraviolet light.

The best skin care for the woman with acne starts with washing the face with a mild soap. Any soap or other treatment that dries the skin is valuable because it may cause some skin to shed, carrying away with it the sebum and dead cells that are clogging the pores. Washing the hair several times a week may also help control acne around the hairline. Oil-based cosmetics should be avoided because they obstruct pores.

Making changes in medications can also help, though women should stop taking a prescribed drug only under a doctor's supervision. Women whose acne seems to worsen with oral contraceptive use may want to try a low-androgen oral contraceptive or switch to another method of birth control. Usually after medications are changed it takes a month or two before any improvement occurs.

A woman who has only blackheads or whiteheads can try a lotion, gel, or cream containing benzoyl peroxide to dry up the skin, promote peeling, and unclog pores; Oxy-5, Oxy-10, and other brands are available over the counter. Because benzoyl peroxides can make skin more sensitive, women should use it only once a day until the skin adjusts, and they should avoid unnecessary exposure to other drying agents and to wind, sun, or cold. Outdoors in any season a sunscreen should be used on the face.

A physician should be consulted if there has been no improvement after 2 or 3 months of benzoyl peroxide treatment, or if there are cysts or scarring. The next step may be to try a stronger drying agent such as one containing a form of vitamin A (tretinoin, sold as Retin-A or Avita). Available through prescription, this acid, like benzoyl peroxide, can irritate the skin and should therefore be applied at first in low doses at bedtime. The dosage can be increased gradually over the next few months. Any woman using tretinoin should avoid extensive exposure to sunlight and use a sunscreen with an SPF of 15 or greater daily, because there is some evidence that this may increase the sensitivity of skin to sunlight. Use of tretinoin can lighten the color of sun spots and other irregularities in the pigment of the face, as well as minimize fine wrinkles.

If Retin-A causes skin irritation, other retinoid medications are now available in topical form as well. These include isotretinoin (Tazorac) and adapalene (Differin). Adapalene in particular generally irritates the skin less than tretinoin, although it can also increase sun sensitivity and should therefore be applied at bedtime, and used together with a sunscreen applied each morning. Just which medication should be used depends on skin type and personal preference. Women with oily skin may prefer gels, for example, because these tend to dry the skin. Women with drier skin, in contrast, may prefer creams or lotions.

Pimples or pustules generally require additional treatment involving either topical or oral antibiotics. As a first step, a clinician will usually advise washing the entire face with mild soap both morning and night and then applying one of several topical antibiotics such as clindamycin, erythromycin, or metronidazole (Flagyl or Protostat). For treating pustules or cysts, it may be necessary to take an antibiotic by mouth, to be used in conjunction with either benzoyl peroxide or Retin-A. Commonly prescribed oral antibiotics include erythromycin and tetracycline.

When considering oral antibiotics, women should take into account potential side effects, which, in the case of most antibiotics, and especially tetracycline, can include vaginitis. In addition, tetracycline and other antibiotics may interfere with the efficacy of birth control pills; an alternative form of contraception should be used while taking these drugs. After the second month of pregnancy, tetracycline can damage the bones and teeth of a fetus and so should not be taken by women who are pregnant or trying to become pregnant.

Cysts can now be cured or vastly improved with a new drug called 13-cis-retinoic acid (Accutane), which is available by prescription. This drug is very expensive and can cause severe birth defects if taken when a woman is pregnant. It should therefore be prescribed only for women who are using effective birth control measures, who have had a negative pregnancy test before starting the drug, and who have no immediate plans to try to become pregnant. Another drawback to Accutane is that it almost always produces lip peeling and cracking, dry skin, and inflammation of the eyelids; it may also lead to headaches, hair thinning, and joint pains. There is some evidence that it may increase levels of triglycerides in the blood; the long-term medical implications of this are unclear.

Other methods a dermatologist may try include superficial chemical peels or minor outpatient surgery in which cysts are drained and removed. Occasionally injecting corticosteroids directly into an acne cyst helps reduce the inflammation in a matter of days. Women with severe scarring might also consider dermabrasion (see entry), a form of cosmetic surgery in which scars are rubbed off with a rotating wire brush.

How can acne be prevented?

If a woman has a predisposition to acne, it cannot really be prevented, although it can be controlled somewhat by cleansing the face with mild soap, washing hair frequently, avoiding cosmetics than can clog pores, and not picking at pimples. There is no evidence that eating chocolate or greasy foods—or any food, for that matter, to which one is not otherwise allergic—causes or aggravates acne.

Some women prone to acne find that it becomes worse just before their period, or around the time of ovulation, or at other times when they are under extraordinary stress. Although hormones are known to cause fluctuations in the severity of acne, there is no conclusive evidence that stress per se makes acne worse or that reducing stress can prevent it. For some women, feeling stressed is part of premenstrual syndrome (see entry), and therefore it is difficult to know whether both the stress and the acne are the result of hormonal changes, or whether stress makes a separate contribution to outbreaks. These things have not been carefully studied, and indeed it would be difficult to do so.

Related entries

Antibiotics, cosmetic safety, dermabrasion and chemical peels, hyperandrogenism, menarche, menopause, menstrual cycle, premenstrual syndrome, skin care and cosmetics, skin disorders, stress, wrinkles

Acquired Immune Deficiency Syndrome (AIDS)

AIDS, or acquired immune deficiency syndrome, is caused by a virus called HIV—human immunodeficiency virus. This virus weakens the body's natural ability to fight various lethal infections and cancers. People with AIDS are prone to so-called opportunistic infections caused by certain (sometimes unusual) bacteria, viruses, parasites, and fungi which normally would not be a threat to healthy people. AIDS also affects the central nervous system and can cause gradual mental deterioration and progressive paralysis.

To date no person who has developed the symptoms of full-blown AIDS has recovered normal immune system function. Medications are available, however, to slow the progression of AIDS.

Today women constitute approximately 47 percent of the 33 million adults worldwide living with HIV/AIDS. In the United States they also continue to be the fastest-growing new group of persons with AIDS, with the proportion of women with AIDS rising from 7 percent of all AIDS patients in 1995 to 22 percent in 1997. Today women constitute about 20 percent of all AIDS cases in this country, and the Centers for Disease Control and Prevention (CDC) estimates that 30 percent of the 40,000 new HIV infections each year occur in women.

Despite advances in HIV treatment, AIDS remains among the leading causes of death for American women aged 25 to 44. Minority women are disproportionately represented in these statistics: although African American and Hispanic women make up less than 25 percent of all women in this country, they account for a full 77 percent of all AIDS cases reported in the United States.

In 1996 the overall death rate from AIDS fell for the first time in the history of this disease, but in women the death rate rose by 3 percent. This may be due in part to the fact that women tend to be diagnosed later in the course of the disease—which, in turn, may be because many HIV-infected women live in poverty and do not have access to health care. It may also be related to the fact that early in the course of the epidemic, risks to heterosexuals and women in particular were often discounted. Entering a treatment program can also be difficult for women who have trouble finding or affording good child care. Relatively late diagnosis for women may also be related to the fact that many women let the health care of their children or families take precedence over their own. In some cases, too, clinicians may not recognize the early signs and symptoms of AIDS in women. In fact, re-searchers at Johns Hopkins University recently found that HIV-infected women carry lower levels of the virus (lower "viral loads") in their blood than men during early phases of the infection but have the same risk as men of developing AIDS. Because many clinicians do not start drug therapy until viral loads reach certain levels, more men than women may be offered treatment, or may be offered it sooner. In addition, even when women receive appropriate and timely treatment, they may be less responsive than men to the standard AIDS medications.

Who is likely to develop AIDS?

Recent studies indicate that the majority of women infected with HIV are in their childbearing years, married, and monogamous. Many are poor and unemployed, and approximately half have at least one child under the age of 15 years. HIV is transmitted through the body fluids—usually blood or semen—of infected persons. Almost all known cases have resulted from intimate sexual contact, injections with contaminated hypodermic needles, transfusions of contaminated blood or blood products, or passage from mother to child. For women the most common source of HIV infection is either intravenous drug use or intimate exposure to infected partners. Intravenous drug use, by itself and through contact with drug-using partners, appears to account for approximately 57 percent of HIV infection in women.

A full 38 percent of HIV infections can now be traced to heterosexual transmission, and are often related to lack of condom use, anal intercourse, numbers of sexual contacts, advanced disease state of the partner, and genital sores in the already infected partner. Although the virus can be transmitted from man to woman, from woman to man, or between partners of the same sex, a woman is more likely to acquire the virus from a male partner than a man is from a female partner. Nearly half of all women who acquire HIV through heterosexual activity do not even know that they were exposed to the virus until infection is detected clinically. Transmission of the virus between lesbian partners is very infrequent.

Anal intercourse is particularly risky behavior because anal tissues often tear during intercourse, allowing the virus to enter the bloodstream. Women who at the time of sexual contact have open sores on their genitals—from vaginitis or herpes, for example—are also at high risk. Having many sexual partners, having frequent contacts with a single infected partner, and failing to use condoms all increase a woman's chance of becoming infected. Using spermicidal creams, foams, and jellies appears to reduce the risks of infection somewhat—because the spermicide found in these products (nonoxynol-9) destroys the AIDS virus—but still does not reduce the risk to zero. Having sexual intercourse during the menstrual period also raises the risk of transmission from the man to the woman, as does having intercourse with an uncircumcised male or with a partner who has a high level of HIV in the bloodstream. In any case, a woman in a sexual relationship with an HIV-infected man has a 20 percent chance of acquiring the virus after unprotected sex for a sustained period of time.

HIV can be transmitted from mother to child through the placenta while the baby is still in the uterus and through breast milk as well. The chances of a baby's being infected in utero are between 25 and 30 percent. This rate can be decreased by up to 50 percent with the use of certain antiretroviral medications. Symptoms of AIDS in the mother do not seem to worsen during pregnancy.

AIDS is particularly common in women of color, and in African American women in particular. As many as 77 percent of all HIV-infected women, but only 49 percent of HIV-infected men, are African American or Hispanic. Most of these differences are due to high rates of infection in African American women, who account for 56 percent of AIDS cases in females, in contrast to African American men, who account for only 32 percent of AIDS cases in males.

What are the symptoms?

Although all people with AIDS are susceptible to various lethal infections and cancers, women have a very different pattern of symptoms from men. Women appear to develop symptoms of AIDS at lower relative blood levels of HIV ("viral loads"), and also become sicker more quickly than males with equivalent viral loads. As a result, HIV-infected women meet the criteria for AIDS earlier in their illness than do men and develop various complications earlier in the course of their illness. In addition to these physiological differences, psychological and socioeconomic factors, including poverty and child care responsibilities, often keep women from seeking early diagnosis and treatment, contributing to a more rapid progression of symptoms.

In the early stages of infection either sex may sometimes experience a brief illness consisting of aches and pains, fever, and swollen glands. Other signs of infection in either men or women can include swelling of the lymph nodes (most often in the neck, armpits, and groin; see illustration), severe diarrhea, breathing difficulties, joint swelling, night sweats, weakness, fatigue, lack of coordination, muscle pain, rapid weight loss (wasting syndrome), unexplained fever, and persistent dry cough. In addition, women may have abnormal Pap tests (indicating the presence of abnormal and possibly cancerous cells in the cervix) or recurrent yeast infections. Although yeast infections occur frequently in women who are not infected with HIV, any woman who has recently started having frequent or difficult-to-cure yeast infections—and who is not using antibiotics (which can predispose any woman to yeast infections)—should discuss the need for HIV testing with her physician.

As AIDS progresses, an infected woman may develop severe genital herpes (herpes simplex II) infections. Again, although herpes is prevalent in the general population, HIV-infected women often have cases that are particularly difficult to treat. HIV-infected women also have about double the number of menstrual irregularities as noninfected women and may develop hard-to-treat forms of cervical cancer, perhaps because these cancers are detected at a later stage or perhaps because they are unusually aggressive forms of the disease. Some studies suggest that HIV-infected women may also be susceptible to cancer of the lower anal-genital tract.

In the middle stages of AIDS, both men and women may develop tuberculosis, various bacterial infections in the blood, yeast infections of the mouth, and a condition called hairy leukoplakia, in which the mucous membranes of the cheeks, gums, or tongue become coated with thickened white patches.

People in the late stages of AIDS are susceptible to diseases that are not usually found among people who do not have compromised immune systems ("opportunistic infections"). Men with AIDS are prone to Kaposi's sarcoma (a form of cancer) and *Pneumocystis carinii* pneumonia (PCP), which are relatively rare among people who do not have AIDS. Women with AIDS, in contrast, tend to develop recurrent pneumonia caused by forms of bacteria that also cause pneumonia in the general population. Whether women with AIDS are more likely than men to develop yeast infections of the esophagus (esophageal candidiasis) and herpes simplex infections remains unknown. In the final stage of AIDS, both men and women tend to develop a herpes infection that can cause blindness, pneumonia, colitis (inflammation of the colon), and esophagitis (inflammation of the esophagus), as well as various brain or lung infections caused by several different microorganisms, including a form of tuberculosis bacterium that is normally found in chickens and pigs. The latter virus damages the nervous system in 40 to 60 percent of patients. The most common symptom is progressive dementia; some patients also develop pain, weakness, and numbness in the arms and legs.

How is the condition evaluated?

Women with any of the following conditions should be referred for HIV counseling and testing: ▸ persistent, recurrent, or severe vaginal yeast infections; ▸ recurrent, severe genital herpes; ▸ syphilis; ▸ chanchroid; ▸ difficult to treat genital warts; ▸ abnormal Pap test results (moderate to severe cervical dysplasia or cervical cancer); ▸ persistent, recurrent pelvic inflammatory disease; ▸ or pregnancy.

The presence of HIV can first be detected in blood about 1 to 3 months after infection, although it is possible for results to be negative for up to a year. Actual symptoms of full-fledged AIDS may not occur for years or even a decade or more. Individual variations in immune system function are part of the explanation for differences in the course of the disease. On average, the time between initial infection and the development of life-threatening complications is 8 to 10 years. In very rare cases children who were HIV-infected have, over time, become HIV-negative; this has not been known to happen in adults.

A new test can also be used to detect if infections are new or long-standing, potentially helping researchers to determine if infection rates are rising, decreasing, or staying the same. Whether or not this test will also help patients by catching early infections remains to be seen. But it may prove useful in helping newly infected patients determine if they contracted the virus from a sexual partner or vice versa.

A person is said to have AIDS when she has developed one or more life-threatening opportunistic infections, invasive cervical cancer, severe ulcerative genital lesions from herpes simplex, or a CD4 count less than 200. CD4 cells are a type of white blood cell central to the body's immune system, and over time, levels of these cells tend to drop in people with AIDS. A CD4 count of less than 200 markedly increases the risk of developing life-threatening opportunistic infections.

How is AIDS treated?

There is still no treatment that can eradicate HIV or fully eliminate the symptoms of AIDS. Newer drug combinations used over the past several years, however, do appear to slow the progression of AIDS, control infections, and, in some cases, bring HIV down to undetectable levels—at least temporarily. Nevertheless, because even the best treatments can be complicated, costly, and physically taxing—and because the HIV seems to develop resistance to them over time—no existing treatment can be considered a surefire or permanent way to eradicate HIV or eliminate the symptoms of AIDS.

Treatment for AIDS continues to evolve as the HIV/AIDS Treatment Information Service incorporates new information into its guidelines. Current federal guidelines state that treatment for AIDS should aim at suppressing symptoms for as long as possible while minimizing side effects. These guidelines recognize that diagnosing and treating HIV infections during the first stage of the disease can often help slow the course of the disease. The problem remains, however, that many HIV-infected women tend to seek and receive medical care for their illness later than their male counterparts, although increasing recognition that women may develop symptoms of AIDS at lower HIV levels than do men is helping to change this situation. Newer guidelines suggest that clinicians consider initiating treatment for HIV-infected women at an earlier stage of infection (lower levels of HIV and/or higher CD4 counts) than they might for male patients. Currently approved treatment guidelines can be obtained by calling the HIV/AIDS Treatment Information Service (800-HIV-0440) or checking the Web site (www.hivatis.org).

Before beginning any kind of treatment, a practitioner will want to see how far the disease has progressed. An initial physical examination should include a pelvic examination and Pap test, as well as a blood test that measures current levels of CD4 cells. The CD4 count should be measured every 3 to 6 months. In the initial exam various laboratory tests will be conducted to determine any prior or latent infections. A skin test will be done to test for tuberculosis exposure. Appropriate medications will be prescribed to treat existing infections and sometimes to prevent the recurrence of latent infections (such as certain sexually transmitted diseases or toxoplasmosis; see entries). Immunizations for conditions such as tetanus, diphtheria, mumps, measles, rubella, hepati-

tis B, hemophilus pneumonia, streptococcal pneumonia, influenza, and pneumococcal pneumonia should also be updated over the course of treatment. Routine Pap tests every 6 to 12 months are especially important for HIV-infected women. Because more than 90 percent of HIV-infected women have histories of sexual and physical abuse, the clinician may also try to determine if the woman is involved in any ongoing domestic violence. If the woman is a candidate for highly active antiretroviral therapy (HAART; see below), other tests may be done to determine lipid and glucose levels, both of which can be adversely affected by some antiretroviral medications.

The most successful drugs so far in the treatment of AIDS are the three classes of antiretroviral drugs: nucleoside reverse transcriptase inhibitors (NRTIs), non-nucleoside reverse transcriptase inhibitors (NNRTIs), and protease inhibitors (Pis). NRTIs, the first class of antiretroviral drugs available, work by inhibiting an enzyme, reverse transcriptase, that is needed for the HIV to replicate. These drugs include abacavir (ABC), lamivudine (3TC), stavudine (d4T), zalcitabine (ddC), and zidovudine (ZDV, AZT). NNRTIs—which include delavirdine (DLV), efavirenz (EFV), and nevirapine (NVP)—work by binding to reverse transcriptase and, ultimately, keeping it from promoting the replication of HIV. The third class of antiretroviral drugs, the protease inhibitors, work by interfering with HIV protease, an enzyme required to promote a later stage of the HIV replication process. Protease inhibitors include amprenavir (APV), indinavir (IDV), nelfinavir (NFV), ritonavir (Norvir), and saquinavir (SQV).

While each of these drugs can be effective over the short term, the rapid changes, or mutations, in the HIV usually render them ineffective after a while; when used in combination, however, these three classes of drugs can often delay the onset of opportunistic infections and prolong survival in people with suppressed CD4+ T cell counts (less than 500 cu/mm). Currently, most clinicians use combination therapy to treat all patients with symptoms of AIDS or who have progressive disease, including pregnant women. While the safety of many of these drugs during pregnancy remains to be determined, overall consensus right now is that controlling HIV replication in a pregnant woman far outweighs any risks.

The exact combination of drugs and treatment regimen needs to be determined on an individual basis, and the effects must be closely monitored by a highly skilled clinician with experience in treating AIDS, possibly in consultation with an expert in HIV drug therapy. People on HAART should have their blood levels of HIV (viral load) measured every few months to monitor the success of therapy. Because all of the drugs currently used to treat HIV/AIDS can have serious adverse effects, close supervision and frequent consultation with a skilled clinician is important to determine if changes in drug regimen may be necessary.

New treatments, including HIV vaccines, continue to be tested and developed to treat HIV/AIDS itself as well as AIDS-related infections. While these new treatments are not yet approved, women interested in participating in clinical trials should contact the HIV/AIDS Treatment Information Service at 800-TRIALS-A (800-874-2572).

How can AIDS be prevented?

At present there is no vaccine available to prevent the spread of AIDS. Transmission of the AIDS virus can be slowed or prevented by avoiding risk factors such as sex without using a condom (see chart) and, among substance abusers, shared needles. Making an effort to practice other aspects of safer sex—including limiting the number of sexual partners and discussing sexual history with all partners—can also reduce the chance of acquiring and spreading the virus.

Women who think they may be positive for HIV should consult a physician, and those who are thinking about becoming pregnant should receive preconception counseling. People who know they are infected, or suspect it, should inform their sexual partner(s) and health care providers so that proper precautions can be taken, and they should not donate blood or blood products. Blood banks now routinely screen for antibodies to keep the blood supply safe and also help identify people at risk for spreading the virus.

Related entries

Condoms, herpes, preconception counseling, safer sex, sexually transmitted diseases, substance abuse

Adenomyosis

In adenomyosis the endometrium, or lining of the uterus, grows into the muscular wall of the uterus. Unlike fibroids—which have similar symptoms—adenomyosis involves normal tissue that just happens to be growing in the wrong place.

Who is likely to develop adenomyosis?

Adenomyosis most often develops late in the reproductive years, usually between the ages of 35 and 50. Women who have had uterine surgery (such as a dilatation and curettage or cesarean section) also have a higher than average risk of developing this condition.

What are the symptoms?

Most women with adenomyosis have no symptoms, though some may experience pelvic pain, especially painful menstrual cramps, as well as heavy, prolonged menstrual periods. Menstrual cramps associated with adenomyosis often begin a few days before menstruation and worsen as the period continues.

How is the condition evaluated?

If symptoms suggest adenomyosis, a doctor will first perform a pelvic examination to examine the uterus. In this condition the uterus is sometimes enlarged and soft, although usually no larger than the size it would be at 12 weeks of pregnancy. To rule out a possible pregnancy and uterine fibroids if the uterus is enlarged, the woman's blood or urine may be tested for human chorionic gonadotropin (hCG), a hormone produced by the placenta during pregnancy, and she will have an ultrasound examination. Sometimes it is not possible to diagnose adenomyosis definitively unless a hysterectomy is performed.

How is adenomyosis treated?

Mild cases of adenomyosis may require no treatment and often disappear spontaneously after menopause. Severe menstrual cramps can be relieved with drugs called antiprostaglandins. If cramps or prolonged periods become intolerable, however, a woman may want to consider a hysterectomy. More conservative surgery to remove only the abnormal tissue is occasionally done, although its long-term effectiveness is unclear. Synthetic hormones called GnRH (gonadotropin-releasing hormone) agonists may provide a nonsurgical alternative for treating adenomyosis, as may progestin-releasing intrauterine devices (such as Mirena). At present, however, these usually provide only temporary relief.

Related entries

Hysterectomy, menorrhagia, menstrual cramps, uterine fibroids

Adhesions

Adhesions are fibrous bands of scar tissue that extend between internal organs. In women, adhesions are particularly common between pelvic structures and may cause pelvic pain and infertility.

Who is likely to develop adhesions?

Adhesions are more likely to occur in women who have had a previous pelvic infection, such as pelvic inflammatory disease (PID), appendicitis, or any kind of abdominal or pelvic surgery. Adhesions tend to be more extensive and painful if they follow a ruptured abscess (which sometimes occurs in PID) or ruptured appendix. Women with endometriosis may also develop adhesions, and, again, if this has involved a ruptured endometrioma (a noncancerous mass composed of tissue from the lining of the uterus), the adhesions can be particularly severe.

What are the symptoms?

Adhesions sometimes cause pelvic pain, which can be either dull or sharp. Whereas some women find that the pain occurs constantly or unpredictably, others notice the pain more during activities that put tension on the adhesions, such as inter-

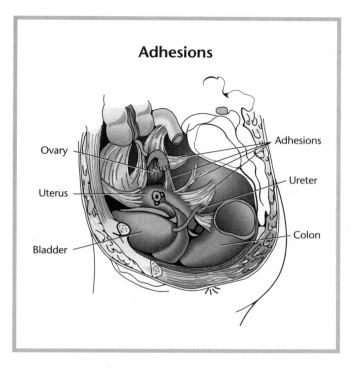

Adhesions

Ovary

Adhesions

Uterus

Ureter

Bladder

Colon

course, exercise, defecation, ovulation, or filling or emptying the bladder.

How is the condition evaluated?

Pelvic adhesions must be distinguished from other causes of chronic pelvic pain such as gastrointestinal diseases, menstrual cramps, endometriosis, and uterine fibroids. Usually a doctor will first check for these other conditions by doing laboratory tests for pregnancy and abnormal blood counts as well as an ultrasound exam. If these tests are normal, and if there are no indications of a gastrointestinal disease, then a laparoscopy (see entry) may be performed to check for either adhesions or endometriosis. Sometimes adhesions detected through this procedure can be treated at the same time.

How are adhesions treated?

Adhesions are usually surgically removed via a laparotomy or laparoscopy (see entries), depending on the experience and preference of the surgeon. In general, laparoscopy is preferable because new adhesions may develop after a laparotomy. Although most surgeons advocate excising adhesions that cause pain, they caution that the adhesions often recur, and that the surgery itself can sometimes produce new adhesions. Laser surgery may make recurrence less likely but is still not routinely available.

How can adhesions be prevented?

Pelvic adhesions caused by conditions such as endometriosis and appendicitis cannot be prevented, although prompt treatment of these conditions may reduce the chances of developing more extensive scar tissue. Other adhesions can be prevented only by avoiding the conditions that cause

them: unnecessary pelvic surgery, pelvic inflammatory disease, and the sexually transmitted diseases (STDs) that often produce PID.

Related entries

Endometriosis, laparoscopy, laparotomy, laser surgery, pelvic inflammatory disease, pelvic pain, sexually transmitted diseases

Airbags

Almost every woman these days drives or rides in vehicles with airbags on the driver's side, passenger side, or both. While these airbags have indisputably saved thousands of lives, they do pose a threat to some people. It is now known that airbags were initially tested with male-size dummies; an airbag that is built to protect a 6-foot, 200-pound man may not be as effective—or even safe—for a 5-foot-3, 110-pound woman.

Airbags work because they are deployed quickly and forcefully. They must completely inflate in the blink of an eye, before the driver's head could hit the steering wheel. The force required for such fast inflation can be dangerous if a person is too close to the steering wheel or passenger side dashboard. This is particularly true for older "first-generation" airbags found in vehicles manufactured before 1998. Many manufacturers are now installing depowered airbags, which do not inflate with as much force as traditional airbags. Future airbags may be able to eliminate the risks produced by current airbag designs by basing deployment on crash severity, occupant size and position, or seat belt use. Anyone concerned about airbag safety should consider discussing these possibilities before purchasing a new vehicle.

Safe use of airbags

In any car equipped with airbags, the U.S. Department of Transportation National Highway Traffic Safety Administration (NHTSA) recommends sitting 10-inches from the airbag—and never within 2–3 inches, where the force is the greatest. They also recommend wearing seatbelts at all times. Airbags are designed to work in conjunction with seatbelts, and the majority of airbag-related injuries and deaths have occurred in people not wearing them. Children under the age of twelve are at high risk of airbag injury and should sit in the back seat. Infants in rear-facing infant seats should never sit in front of an airbag.

Adults who happen to be relatively short or who have certain disabilities, however, have the same risk as children under 12 but cannot solve this problem by relegating themselves to the backseat. Under certain conditions, these people can obtain an on/off switch that temporarily disables the airbags but still allow other drivers and/or passengers to reac-

sometimes offer advice on who to contact. The NHTSA website also provides a list of companies willing to install on/off switches on at least some vehicles.

Safe use of airbags

The U.S. Department of Transportation National Highway Traffic Safety Administration recommends sitting 10 inches from the airbag, measured from your breastbone to the center of the steering wheel. If you now sit less than 10 inches away, you can change your driving position in several ways:

- Move your seat to the rear as far as possible while still reaching the pedals comfortably
- Slightly recline the back of the seat
- Raise the seat manually or by using a firm, non-slippery cushion
- Tilt the steering wheel downward

Most people killed by airbags would not have been seriously injured if they had worn a seat belt and sat far enough away from the steering wheel.

---

tivate them. Before making this investment, however, the NHTSA strongly encourages people to try adjusting their seating positions (see chart). However, even with these adjustments, certain drivers are at risk of airbag injuries, including:

- Drivers who must transport infants in rear-facing infant seats (in pick-up trucks that do not have a back seat, for example)

- Drivers who must transport a child under 12 in the front seat

- Drivers or passengers with unusual medical conditions, such as scoliosis or severe arthritis (a physician must be able to explain that their risk of having an airbag is greater than what may happen if they turn it off)

- Drivers who cannot sit back ten inches after adjusting seat and steering wheel

All other drivers, including pregnant women who can adjust their seat properly, are not eligible for an on/off switch.

Obtaining on/off switches

To obtain an on/off switch, people must apply to the NHTSA by filling out a form explaining why they are in an at-risk group for a specific vehicle. The application can be found at the department of motor vehicles, on the NHTSA web site (www.nhtsa.gov), or at certain automobile dealer and repair shops. If the NHTSA accepts the application, they send the applicant a letter authorizing an automobile dealer or repair shop to install an on/off switch in the specified vehicle. Even with this letter, it is often difficult to find anyone willing to install the switch. Car dealerships, local driving schools, and even the driver's ed department at a local high school can

Alcohol

In the last decade or so considerable controversy has arisen about whether women who drink moderate amounts of alcohol might actually be healthier than either nondrinkers or heavy drinkers. Until recently the evidence in favor of alcohol came largely from studies on men, and it indicated that drinking 2 alcoholic beverages a day significantly reduces deaths from clogged heart arteries—probably because alcohol increases levels of high-density (HDL) cholesterol (see entry) and reduces the formation of plaque in blood vessels. (These findings, in turn, fed speculations about the "French paradox": perhaps it was the red wine along with meals that explained why the French, with their cream-laden cuisine, were not unusually prone to heart disease.)

Most clinicians hesitated to extend any of these findings to women, however, partly because women are known to metabolize alcohol somewhat differently than men (accumulating more alcohol in their blood more readily) and partly because women who drink may be particularly susceptible to alcoholic liver disease and breast cancer. Adding to the confusion was a large-scale study from Scotland published in 1999 indicating that alcohol consumption had no apparent effect on risk of mortality from heart disease, although heavy drinking was closely linked to an increase risk of stroke.

At the same time, evidence continues to suggest that light to moderate drinking may indeed decrease deaths from all causes in women over the age of 50. A major 12-year study of 86,000 nurses aged 34 to 59 (part of the ongoing Harvard Nurses' Health Study) showed that women over 50 who had between 1 and 20 drinks per week had a lower risk of death, particularly from cardiovascular disease, than nondrinkers. Heavier drinking (more than 20 drinks per week) was associated with an increased risk of death from other causes, particularly cirrhosis and breast cancer. (One drink = 12 ounces of beer = 5 ounces of wine = 1.5 ounces of 80-proof liquor. All of these are equivalent to 0.5 ounces or 12 grams of ethanol.)

The benefits were greatest for women who were at risk for heart disease—for example, women who were obese, smoked cigarettes, or had high cholesterol levels, high blood pressure, diabetes, or a family history of heart disease. Women 34 to 39 years of age who drank had a slightly higher risk of death from all causes regardless of how much they drank, but the number of deaths in this group was small.

This large and convincing study did not suggest that a nondrinker who suddenly adds a few drinks to her diet will necessarily lower her risk of cardiovascular disease. The benefits appeared only in women over 50 who were already drinkers when the study began. As in all studies of this type, it is possible that the lower death rates were attributable not to alcohol per se but to some other (unknown) factor common among women who drink moderately over the course of their adult lives. The only way to know for sure that alcohol itself confers health benefits would be to conduct a prospective study in which a group of nondrinkers started to drink moderately and were compared over time to an otherwise similar group who continued to abstain. Such a study seems unlikely.

If one adds to this research limitation the fact that women under 50 and risk-free women in the study showed no benefit from moderate drinking, and the fact that heavy drinking substantially increases a woman's risk of death, it does not make sense for nondrinkers to start drinking alcohol for the sake of their health. But for those women who already drink in moderation, most experts believe that they can continue in good conscience without worrying about serious health complications.

Yet every woman who drinks, even in moderation, should be aware of the downside: the potential for alcohol abuse and dependence.

The downside of drinking

The percentage of women addicted to alcohol has grown by leaps and bounds since the late 1960s. Today an estimated 4.6 million American women are alcoholics—that is, dependent on alcohol—and 1 out of every 3 alcoholics in this country is female. The increase in drinking among younger women is growing at a particularly high rate. As women make strides toward professional and educational equity, some of them seem to develop a pattern of "drinking like men," thus increasing their susceptibility to alcohol-related problems.

Yet the tenacious belief that respectable women are not heavy drinkers has made women less likely to admit they have a problem with alcohol; and many of them are less likely than men to drink heavily in public, where other people may discover it. Drinking clandestinely and alone, many women alcoholics are socially isolated, demoralized by the prolonged illness of alcoholism, and less likely than men to seek treatment for it.

Women who do admit they have a drinking problem may risk losing custody of their children. In recent years, some states have prosecuted women as criminals for exposing their children in utero to alcohol and other drugs. Women aware of these risks have even greater incentives to hide or deny their alcoholism.

Women who seek therapy get much less psychological and social support from spouses and other family members than do men. Women alcoholics not only are more likely than men to have an alcoholic spouse, but also are more likely to have other alcoholic family members for whom they are the caretakers. These women often develop depression, psychosomatic disorders, or eating disorders in addition to their drinking problem. Whereas only 1 in 10 married men who seek treatment for alcoholism ends up divorced, 9 out of 10 married women alcoholics are divorced after or during treatment.

Women are still less likely than men to be diagnosed by their physician as having a problem with alcohol, and therefore less likely to be treated for it. The notion that only certain types of women drink to excess has led physicians to overlook the drinking problems of many professional and well-educated women. Misdiagnosing alcoholism as depression or anxiety, they may end up prescribing mood altering and potentially addictive drugs that do not address the problem and can in fact make it worse. These drugs include other central nervous system depressants—such as barbiturates or tranquilizers—which, when mixed with alcohol, can lead to serious side effects.

Who is likely to develop alcoholism?

In general, white women are more likely to use alcohol than are African American women, and both of these groups are more likely to drink than are Hispanic women. College graduates are more likely to drink than high school graduates.

People start drinking alcoholic beverages for many reasons, usually because drinking is part of social life in their circle. Some women may start drinking because they find that it helps them cope better with young children, job stress, separation, divorce, or bereavement. Others may begin using alcohol to relieve aches and pains or insomnia. Teenage girls with low self-esteem or impaired ability to cope with stress may drink to relieve shyness, to increase their enjoyment of dates, or simply to "get high." For reasons still not fully understood—but which probably have to do with biological differences—only some of these people will end up as alcohol abusers or alcohol-dependent.

Single, divorced, or separated women are more likely to drink heavily and have alcohol-related problems than are married women or widows (although cause and effect are not easy to disentangle). Alcohol abuse and dependence in women is often associated with depression, and more often than not the depression preceded the alcohol problems. Perhaps related to the depression is the fact that women with alcoholism attempt suicide more often than other women. Alcohol abuse seems to be particularly common among young women, although older women with a drinking problem may simply be harder to identify. Women with a history of childhood sexual abuse are more likely than others to become alcoholics later in life.

Other risk factors for alcoholism include having a personality disorder (see entry), having biological relatives who are alcoholics, and working in an environment that encourages heavy drinking.

What are the symptoms?

Alcohol abuse and dependence means the repetitive and chronic use of alcohol to the point where it significantly interferes with an individual's health or the ability to function normally. People who are dependent develop a tolerance to alcohol and require increasing amounts of it to achieve the same effects. They also suffer from withdrawal symptoms when they reduce or stop their alcohol intake. These can include the classic hangover—headache, nausea, vomiting, anxiety, or malaise. In cases of heavy drinking, the end result may be DTs (delirium tremens)—tremors, panic attacks, confusion, delirium, hallucinations, and seizures.

In addition to increased tolerance and symptoms of withdrawal, other signs of alcohol dependence include a preoccupation with drinking, excessive or frequent drinking, solitary drinking, and temporary memory lapses (blackouts). Using alcohol as a medicine or to promote sleep, making excuses for drinking, or denying that drinking is a problem despite evidence to the contrary are other signs (see chart).

Some background may be helpful. Alcohol (ethyl alcohol or ethanol) is a naturally occurring colorless liquid produced by the fermentation of sugars. A central nervous system depressant, it acts as a sedative or tranquilizer that relaxes people and releases their inhibitions. Although people may feel more confident and talkative after a drink or two, the alcohol is actually slowing down their motor coordination and reaction time, as well as impairing judgment, memory, reasoning, and self-control. These effects are more obvious when large quantities of alcohol are consumed. Too much alcohol can lead to drowsiness, stupor, and life-threatening coma.

Studies find that women have higher blood alcohol levels than men after drinking the same amount, even after adjusting for body weight. Because women generally have a higher ratio than men of body fat to water, there is proportionately less water available in the female body in which alcohol can be dispersed. Women also have relatively low levels of an enzyme called gastric alcohol dehydrogenase, which is responsible for breaking down alcohol in the stomach. Alcohol seems to be more rapidly absorbed into the bloodstream at certain points in the menstrual cycle, particularly just before the menstrual period.

Because of alcohol's effects on the nervous system, women under the influence of alcohol may engage in risky behaviors or make mistakes they would normally avoid. For example, they may forget to use birth control or neglect to insist on condom use by a new sexual partner. Women who drink heavily are more likely to become victims of alcohol-related violence, including domestic abuse and rape. In addition, 30 to 70 percent of women alcoholics are dependent on other drugs, including sedatives and minor tranquilizers.

Alcohol-related health problems appear much sooner and more severely in women than in men. Women develop cirrhosis of the liver (a progressive disease that causes permanent liver damage; see illustration) over a shorter period of time and they die from it at a younger age than do men—despite the fact that they tend to drink less overall and tend to develop a drinking problem at a later age than men do. Both Native American and African American women have particularly high rates of cirrhosis.

In addition to cirrhosis, the Harvard Nurses' Study confirmed the association between heavy drinking and a woman's risk of dying from cancer, particularly breast cancer. Cancers of the mouth, throat, larynx, esophagus, stomach,

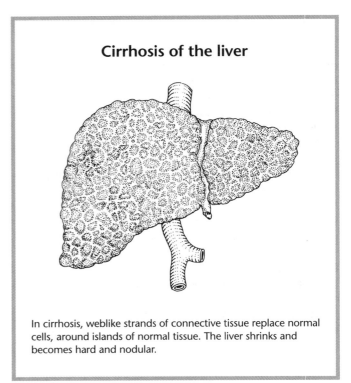

Cirrhosis of the liver

In cirrhosis, weblike strands of connective tissue replace normal cells, around islands of normal tissue. The liver shrinks and becomes hard and nodular.

and pancreas are also more common among heavy drinkers. Other health problems that have been linked to alcoholism are fatty liver, obesity, anemia, malnutrition, and peptic ulcers.

Alcohol consumption can worsen osteoporosis, a disorder leading to progressive loss of bone density and accompanying fractures. One study found that women over 65 who drank 2 to 6 drinks per week had an increased risk of hip fracture, both because they were more likely to fall and because of the effects of alcohol on bone strength.

Women who are heavy drinkers seem to have high rates of amenorrhea, abnormal vaginal bleeding, painful menstrual cramps, premenstrual syndrome, infertility, and—although drinkers may feel more aroused after a glass of wine—sexual dysfunction (including vaginal pain, lack of sex drive, and inability to have an orgasm). Whether these problems are due to drinking alcohol or are a reason for drinking in the first place remains unclear.

Recently the effects of alcohol on a growing fetus have received a lot of publicity. The most severe complication that can occur from drinking more than 4 drinks per day during pregnancy is called fetal alcohol syndrome (FAS). In this condition the affected infant develops irreversible mental retardation, which leads to learning disabilities, coordination and balance problems, and hyperactivity. Babies born with this syndrome have an unusually small head (microcephaly) and a depressed nose bridge, an elongated and flattened upper lip, abnormally small eyes, and displaced, deformed ears. Defects of the joints, limbs, or organs, including congenital heart defects or malformed hips, often occur in FAS.

Moderate drinking (under 2 drinks per day) in pregnant women has been linked to prematurity, low birth weight, and more subtle neurological problems. Even occasional social drinking may increase the risk of miscarriage, particularly during the first trimester of pregnancy. Experiments in pregnant animals suggest that binge drinking is more dangerous than consuming small amounts of alcohol over a long period of time.

In light of these serious risks, obstetricians recommend total abstinence during pregnancy, since no one knows the level of alcohol that can be consumed safely, and even this may vary from woman to woman.

How is alcoholism treated?

Only about a fourth to a fifth of all patients in treatment for drinking problems are female, even though about a third of all alcoholics are women. Many women with alcoholism are clearly not getting the treatment they need.

Once a woman has been diagnosed as having a problem with alcohol—and, most crucially, has admitted to herself that she is alcohol-dependent—treatment can begin. Women who have support at home and are not at risk of losing child custody or a job may first ask their clinician to refer them to a 12-step program such as Alcoholics Anonymous, Al-Anon (for the spouses of alcoholics), Women for Sobriety, Rational Recovery, and Secular Organizations for Sobriety. All-women, all-lesbian, and all-nonsmoker self-help groups of the 12-step variety are available.

Whether or not a woman chooses to enter a 12-step program, her clinician should also work with her to achieve detoxification (a process through which the woman is weaned from alcohol), provide any necessary medical care to aid the withdrawal process, and help her find better ways to deal with stress, anxiety, anger, and other emotions. Often family therapy is useful in educating other family members about the disease and helping them handle their negative feelings about the patient and participate in the recovery process. Psychiatric illnesses such as major depression which often accompany alcoholism need to be treated separately, usually with a combination of psychotherapy and antidepressants.

If a woman has more severe medical problems, an abusive home situation, legal issues, or a partner or other immediate family member who is a substance abuser, the clinician may refer her to an alcohol treatment clinic, detoxification center, hospital, or residential care facility, where appropriate specialists are available. Often the staff will include recovering alcoholics who serve as role models in addition to offering professional care. These facilities can provide treatment on an outpatient or inpatient basis as appropriate.

Part of the recovery program at alcohol treatment clinics involves education about balanced diet and the nature of alcoholism, and group therapy or self-help groups. Individual counseling or other psychotherapy may be provided as well. Medical supervision is necessary if drugs such as benzodiazepines (Librium, Valium) are given to help prevent DTs.

Sometimes a drug called disulfiram (Antabuse), which disrupts the metabolism of alcohol in the liver, may be useful in preventing alcohol consumption. After a person takes tablets of this drug, consuming alcohol (even the small amount contained in some foods, mouthwashes, and cough syrups) results in extremely unpleasant physical reactions, including flushing, nausea, severe vomiting, throbbing headaches, sweating, chest pain, rapid heartbeat, difficulty breathing, blurred vision, and dizziness. The purpose of the drug is to serve as a powerful physical deterrent to alcohol consumption, but it works over the long run only if the patient takes it willingly and consistently.

Almost all treatment programs view alcoholism as a chronic, progressive disease and insist on complete abstinence from alcohol and other addictive substances. Some aftercare programs are available to help recovering alcoholics remain sober and to help them if relapse occurs. Many experts recommend using a self-help group such as Alcoholics Anonymous as a support system.

Not everyone views alcoholism as treatable only with abstinence, however. A return to "social" (or "controlled" or "asymptomatic") drinking is the goal of some programs, and a handful of studies have demonstrated that a tiny minority of alcohol abusers can learn to control their drinking behavior for long periods of time. A large-scale study that sheds light on the question of abstinence versus controlled drinking—the ongoing Harvard Study in Adult Development, which has been following a sample of (male) Harvard graduates for many decades—has found that the success rate of those who have attempted to drink asymptomatically has been far from impressive over the long term. The Harvard investigators have concluded that, while it is possible for a few alcohol-dependent people to return to social drinking for a period of time, controlled drinking is, in most cases, a transient stage between abstinence and abuse. A more practical treatment goal for the vast majority of problem drinkers is to avoid alcohol entirely.

Related entries

Antianxiety drugs, antidepressants, anxiety disorders, breast cancer, coronary artery disease, depression, domestic abuse, heart disease, hepatitis, personality disorders, postpartum psychiatric disorders, psychosomatic disorders, psychotherapy, stress, substance abuse

Alpha-Fetoprotein Screening

This prenatal test measures the amounts of a substance called alpha fetoprotein in a pregnant woman's blood. Alpha fetoprotein (AFP) is produced by the fetus's liver and is present in both the amniotic fluid and the mother's blood. All that is required is a simple blood test. An alpha-fetoprotein test can also be performed directly on the amniotic fluid (see amniocentesis).

Why is the procedure performed?

Abnormally high levels of AFP often indicate the presence of defects in the neural tube, a structure that forms along the embryo's back between the 5th and 6th weeks of pregnancy and normally closes completely to form the brain and spine. When the tube fails to close, the result is either anencephaly or spina bifida. Anencephaly is a condition in which the upper part of the brain and head are absent or underdeveloped; infants with anencephaly are stillborn or die soon after birth. Spina bifida occurs when the spinal cord and nerves are pushed out through an opening in the spine. The outlook for babies with spina bifida varies depending on the location of the opening. Some forms result in death during childhood or in major handicaps; others result in weakness, paralysis from the waist down, problems with bowel and bladder control, and repeated infections. Many children with spina bifida require frequent operations to close the spinal opening. Children with an opening lower in the spine, however, often have normal intelligence and fewer medical complications.

The AFP test is now offered routinely to women between 15 and 18 weeks of pregnancy. It can help screen for certain chromosomal abnormalities such as Down syndrome as well. A small amount of blood is taken from the mother's arm and sent to a laboratory, where the levels of AFP are measured.

How accurate, reliable, and safe is AFP screening?

The results of this test, which take about 2 to 4 days, are not ironclad; accuracy is much higher when the AFP is withdrawn directly from the amniotic fluid, as generally occurs during amniocentesis. Whereas some 3 percent of women screened will have an elevated AFP on the first test, about half of these abnormal levels will turn out to be due to the presence of twins, fetal death, or incorrect estimates of gestational age. Even among the remainder only about 1 in 15 will turn out to be carrying a fetus with a neural tube defect. In other words, the test has a high rate of false positives.

It also has a high rate of false negatives; that is, the AFP test fails to detect all neural tube defects. Although it detects about 90 percent of all cases of anencephaly, it finds only about 80 percent of cases of spina bifida. And only 20 percent of fetuses with Down syndrome produce abnormally low levels of AFP, so a normal AFP test is no guarantee of a fetus without Down syndrome.

When it is combined with ultrasound, the AFP test is a more reliable predictor of neural tube defects. Generally a positive first test will be followed by a second test to see if the results are repeated. If the second test is elevated, an ultrasound examination will be done to check for twins, duration of pregnancy, and defects of the fetus's skull, spine, or abdominal wall. If ultrasound fails to reveal the cause of the abnormal AFP test, amniocentesis is the next step, although some physicians believe that ultrasound is as sensitive as amniocentesis in finding clinically significant neural tube defects.

The reliability of the AFP test for the detection of chromosomal abnormalities has been improved with a procedure known as the triple marker test. In this test, which must be done as soon as possible after the 15th week of pregnancy and no later than the 20th week, other pregnancy hormones in the mother's blood—human chorionic gonadotropin (hCG) and unconjugated estriol (UE3)—are measured in addition to AFP. Like AFP, these substances are made by the fetus or the placenta and pass into the mother's blood. In Down syndrome hCG levels are higher than expected and estriol levels are lower.

Like the AFP test alone, the triple marker test cannot definitely identify a birth defect, but it can indicate that the fetus is at increased risk to have one. Additional tests such as ultrasound or amniocentesis are therefore usually necessary after a positive triple marker test. For example, the results of the triple marker test can be combined with the mother's age to determine if her risk of carrying a child with Down syndrome is higher than would otherwise be expected for a woman her age. If her combined risk is greater than 1 in 250, she might want to consider an ultrasound to see if estimates of gestational age are correct—which, as it turns out, they often are not. In women under 35 a positive triple marker test can detect between 39 and 58 percent of Down syndrome fetuses and 85 to 90 percent of cases of open spina bifida. These women will be advised to have genetic counseling as well as amniocentesis for a more accurate prediction.

Because the AFP is a blood test, the risks to the mother or fetus from the test itself are practically nil.

Related entries

Abortion, amniocentesis, chorionic villi sampling, genetic counseling, miscarriage, preconception counseling, pregnancy, pregnancy over age 35, ultrasound

Alternative Therapies

In recent years millions of Americans have turned to chiropractic, acupuncture, homeopathy, biofeedback, visualization, and crystal healing as alternatives to conventional medicine, or have "mixed and matched" conventional therapy with other, seemingly incompatible healing options. In 1997 as many as 42 percent of all Americans used these "alternative or complementary" approaches to healing, spending an estimated $21.2 billion dollars on alternative medical professional services and paying more than half of this amount out of pocket. They made an estimated 629 million visits to providers of nonconventional therapies in that year, up from 427 million in 1990 and far exceeding the number of visits to primary care physicians within the medical "establishment." In addition, in 1997 an estimated 15 million American adults took prescription drugs together with herbal remedies and/or high-dose vitamins, but more than half of them failed to mention this fact to their physician.

Alternative therapy is reshaping medicine for patients and conventional caregivers alike. In fact, many mainstream practitioners now speak of alternative therapies as part of what they call "complementary medicine"—that is, approaches to health that are used not as alternatives but as supplements to more conventional care. Others use both conventional and alternative approaches as appropriate in what they call "integrative medicine." Nearly two-thirds of U.S. medical schools now offer courses on complementary or alternative medical practices and have begun to reexamine techniques once dismissed as quackery. It is not unusual to find traditional cancer therapy being supplemented by relaxation exercises and support groups, or to see studies in leading medical journals on the impact of yoga or biofeedback on coronary artery disease, or to encounter best-sellers written by prominent physicians about the influence of laughter or hope on the immune system.

Many physicians question the more extravagant claims of certain alternative therapies. They warn that these practices, if not downright dangerous, may keep people from seeking effective treatment. Many clinicians are increasingly concerned about undesirable interactions that can come from patients mixing alternative and conventional medications without supervision. But it is becoming harder to deny that at least *some* alternative techniques work for *some* patients— even in cases where medical science cannot explain exactly how.

Furthermore, the growing acceptance of alternative therapies has led some critics of mainstream medicine to perceive it as the harbinger of a medical revolution. They predict that Western medicine someday will evolve from its narrow biochemical model to a "biopsychosocial" one that incorporates holistic thinking: a perception—sometimes regarded as a traditionally feminine one—that the body is an integrated unity and that emotional, spiritual, social, and environmental factors are as crucial in determining illness as physical trauma or biochemical events. While acknowledging that viruses play a role in inducing colds, alternative healers may also consider stress in the workplace, mental depression, and inadequate diet equally important. Before the twentieth century such thinking was common in conventional medicine. The fact that many traditional doctors have begun to reincorporate these ideas into their studies and practices reflects the success of alternative therapy advocates, as well as the frustration that many patients feel with conventional medical care.

The appeal of alternative therapies

Conventional biomedicine has been particularly powerful in treating critical injuries and infectious diseases—broken arms or diphtheria, for example—and its stunning successes account for the relative decline in alternative therapies earlier in the twentieth century (together with active efforts by proponents of conventional medicine to marginalize and even outlaw some alternative practices and practitioners). But in recent decades, as many of our society's pressing medical problems have shifted from infectious diseases to chronic conditions such as cancer, coronary artery disease, multiple sclerosis, back pain, and diabetes, biomedicine has been somewhat less effective in dealing with them. Critics, including many baby boomers who grew up questioning authority, add that biomedicine has also been deficient in treating everyday ailments and in maintaining health. The holistic approach, with its emphasis on individual circumstances, provides an alternative for those patients who are frustrated by these limitations and by physicians who, they feel, regard them not as whole human beings but as body parts.

Other people are attracted to alternative therapies because they deemphasize drugs, surgery, and technology. "Natural" approaches to good health such as herbal preparations, lifestyle changes, healthful diets, massage, and psychotherapy appeal to patients who want to participate more in their own health care. And in this age of exploding medical costs, few can afford to ignore the potential savings that may come from emphasizing wellness over disease and prevention over treatment—an emphasis common among alternative practitioners.

What makes a therapy "alternative"?

The most obvious distinctions between alternative and conventional care are different educational standards required of practitioners; an emphasis on holistic or biopsychosocial explanations for illness, in contrast to the biomedical model that underlies conventional medicine; and, in some cases, different standards of scientific proof (although, to be fair, a number of conventional medical practices have never been held up to these standards either).

Whereas a few successful cases may "prove" the efficacy of a therapy to an alternative healer, medical scientists disregard such anecdotal evidence. They argue that a certain number of patients are bound to get well with or without treatment. Studying just a few cases leaves open the possibility that the "cure" was the result of blind chance or the placebo effect—a phenomenon in which the patient's belief that she is being treated effectively is enough to make the treatment actually work.

The gold standard in conventional medicine, though by no means yet attained in most cases, is the clinical trial—a randomized study of comparable groups of patients, some of whom receive the treatment being studied and some of whom receive an inactive placebo. In "double-blind" clinical trials, neither the patients nor the health care providers administering either therapy or placebo know which patients are receiving what until the results are revealed at the end of the study. Only this kind of controlled trial can rule out the effects of chance, from the point of view of conventional research.

From the holistic perspective, by contrast, traditional diseases are merely the symptoms of underlying spiritual or natural imbalances, which can vary from individual to individual. This explains why some alternative healers advocate remedies that have been disproved by large-scale clinical trials: if each patient's experience of illness is a product of individual diet, lifestyle, history, mental state, and so on, then a treatment that works for one sick person does not necessarily work for another, and certainly might not work for a whole group of people in a randomized trial.

Alternative practitioners argue that they treat the underlying *cause* of disease, while conventional medicine treats only its *symptoms*. Conventional medicine counters by claiming just the opposite, since biomedicine regards the true causes of disease, whether physical or emotional, to be the bacteria, tumors, biochemical imbalances, physical trauma, and the like that they study in their clinical trials.

Forms of alternative therapy

Alternative therapies can be divided into three basic categories: botanical healing, hands-on therapies, and mind–body techniques. Some schools of practice, such as naturopathy, macrobiotics, and Ayurvedic medicine (a 4,000-year-old Indian healing tradition) rely on more than one form and sometimes advocate changes in diet or exercise patterns as well. Some alternative practices are derived from mainstream medicine as practiced in other parts of the world, while others stem from contemporary "New Age" thinking.

Botanical healing. Herbal medicine uses pills, teas, or extracts from flowers, leaves, or other whole parts of plants such as peppermint, chamomile, garlic, or aloe vera to treat a wide range of ailments. In aromatherapy, essential oils from flowers and plants are massaged into the skin or inhaled. Recent evidence that certain Chinese and Indian herbs contain the same chemicals active in Western pharmaceuticals increases the likelihood that some of these medications actually work beyond their placebo effect.

But buyers should beware: even potentially effective herbs can lose potency if exposed to air, light, or moisture—as many of them are when sold in bulk or powdered into capsules. And just because a substance is "natural" does not mean it is safe: arsenic is natural, too, after all. Taken over long periods of time or in large doses, many of the plants used in herbal remedies can cause extensive damage. Comfrey, for example, which is sold as a digestive aid, may seriously damage the liver. Large doses of licorice, used to suppress coughs, can raise blood pressure and alter heartbeat. And herbal medicines may carry residues from pesticides or molds. Because they are regarded as "foods," herbal preparations are exempt from the Food and Drug Administration's stringent regulations requiring all drugs to be proven both safe and effective.

Equally distressing is the common misperception that herbal remedies and "dietary supplements" are not "drugs"; patients often fail to mention to their clinicians that they are taking these substances, and doctors often fail to ask, and as a result, patients end up taking them together with conventional medications. The danger is that the different drugs can undermine one another's effects or work together to produce dangerous, even life-threatening results. The most reasonable

attitude is to regard botanicals as equivalent to more conventional drugs: while many have the power to relieve and heal, all also have the potential to do damage as well and must be used with care.

Another botanical alternative is homeopathy, a school of thought that has been around since the late eighteenth century and is based on the premise that disease can be treated with highly diluted doses of the same substances that cause it. Extremely popular in the nineteenth century, homeopathy dwindled almost to extinction until the early 1980s. Now, according to the National Center for Homeopathy, there are over 2,500 homeopathic physicians as well as 3,000 to 5,000 licensed health professionals who practice homeopathy. Prepackaged homeopathic remedies for aches, pains, allergies, and colds are routinely sold over the counter.

Although some European studies have demonstrated a therapeutic effect of homeopathic herbs on influenza, headache, and allergies, the evidence is unconvincing to much of the American medical establishment. Because homeopathic preparations are often so dilute that no active chemicals remain, the FDA has tended not to require proof of safety and efficacy.

Hands-on therapies. Premier among the hands-on therapies is chiropractic medicine, which, with approximately 50,000 practitioners, is currently the third-largest health care profession in the United States. Once labeled quacks and impostors by conventional medical doctors, chiropractors not only have survived for a century but also have gained both legal and public acceptance. Although they do not have medical degrees, chiropractors are licensed to practice in all 50 states, and their services are covered by many insurers. Chiropractic's main therapy—the manipulation of the spine—is now generally acknowledged as a valid treatment for acute low back pain.

Nevertheless, most medical doctors still dispute the claims of many chiropractors that misaligned vertebrae ("subluxations") underlie a plethora of human conditions, from childhood ear infections to headaches to high blood pressure. They also deny that chiropractic manipulation should be used to treat or prevent these conditions. Without offering evidence convincing to the medical profession, many chiropractors maintain that misaligned vertebrae impair the nervous system, thereby lowering the body's defenses and contributing to disease. In any event, for some of the 30 million Americans who suffer from back pain, chiropractic manipulations may indeed provide relief.

Osteopaths, who have a medical education and hospital privileges similar to those of MDs, also perform hands-on manipulations, but these may involve parts of the body other than the spine, including the arms, legs, and skull to reposition bones, organs, and bodily fluids. Osteopathic manipulations have helped many patients with headaches, arthritis, back and neck pain, and sports injuries in particular. Part of osteopathy's success has a lot to do with the philosophy of care that underlies it, which emphasizes preventive medicine (including nutrition and exercise), aims to channel the body's self-healing abilities, and regards health as a reflection of mind, body, and environment.

Acupuncture, another hands-on therapy, is gaining acceptance in many circles. Still regarded as an alternative practice in the United States, it has been a conventional therapy in China for thousands of years. Acupuncturists contend that the body consists of a system of specific "vital energy" or "life force" (called *qi* or *chi*) pathways. Disease and pain result when the energy flow of these pathways is interrupted. Acupuncturists say they can rebalance the flow by inserting hair-thin needles into precise points along the pathways and then manipulating them.

Particularly impressive to many Western researchers is acupuncture's effectiveness as a pain reliever and surgical anesthetic. Western science has yet to explain how this works. The most convincing hypothesis so far is that the needle somehow stimulates nerve cells to produce chemicals called endorphins, the body's natural painkillers. A few animal studies have shown that inhibiting the release of these chemicals can block acupuncture's anesthetic effect. In other studies animals became partially anesthetized after being injected with body fluids from other animals that had undergone acupuncture. Whatever the explanation, recent reports in esteemed medical journals indicate that acupuncture can relieve chronic back pain, as well as the pain of osteoarthritis and rheumatoid arthritis. It is also used as a surgical anesthetic and to relieve withdrawal symptoms in recovering alcoholics, drug addicts, and cigarette smokers.

In acupressure the same energy points cited by acupuncturists are massaged with finger pressure, primarily to relieve stress. Shiatsu is the Japanese equivalent of this technique. Similarly, practitioners of therapeutic touch claim to unblock energy flow by moving their hands over a patient's "energy fields." Proponents insist that this technique not only improves overall well-being but also relieves pain and anxiety and even speeds wound healing.

Reflexology is yet another massage technique based on Eastern teachings, this time with emphasis on the feet. Reflexologists have mapped specific areas of the sole to every organ, gland, and body part. The heel corresponds to the lower body, the middle of the sole to the digestive organs, the ball of the foot to heart and lungs, and the toes to the head. By stimulating relevant points, reflexologists claim to be able to relieve pain and stress and improve circulation in corresponding areas of the body. Most conventional doctors are skeptical of this technique, suggesting that self-massage, Epsom salt baths, and foot exercises provide equivalent health benefits.

Even without an elaborate map of energy pathways, alternative healers use other massage techniques to relieve stress and discomfort. "Hellerwork," for example, involves numerous 1 ½-hour deep-massage sessions on the theory that pain and tension in body structures increase risk of injury. To ease muscle pain, stress, depression, ulcers, tension headaches, exhaustion, and various respiratory and digestive woes, the "Al-

exander technique" teaches patients how to improve posture in a dozen or so sessions. Conventional practitioners generally question the more grandiose benefits attributed to such practices, but many acknowledge that at the very least these techniques may relieve stress simply because the therapist is paying attention to the patient—which can also be said of many conventional practices when the doctors and patient have a mutually respectful relationship.

Increasing evidence suggests that less exotic massage techniques that simply involve systemic manipulation of the body's soft tissues may play a major role in human health and well-being. Not only can massage therapy relieve stress and sore muscles, but also there is increasing evidence linking it to the relief of certain physical symptoms associated with arthritis, backaches, migraines, high blood pressure, asthma, diabetes, rashes, and other skin conditions. Massage therapy can relieve labor pain, minimize water retention associated with premenstrual syndrome, relieve depression in people with eating disorders, and boost growth and development in premature babies. It may even boost immune function in patients with AIDS and cancer. Studies at Miami's Touch Institute, the world's first multidisciplinary research center devoted to studying the role of touch in human health and development, are increasingly documenting the relationship between touch and measurable changes in biochemical markers of depression, stress, and immune function in the bloodstream and saliva. Studies at the Touch Institute also suggest that massage therapy may speed recovery from addictions, depression, and attention deficiency hyperactivity disorder (ADHD).

Mind–body techniques. Alternative practices based on the interaction of mind and body have been entering the mainstream lately, partly because of recent discoveries in a new field called psychoneuroimmunology. Researchers in this field explore the way behavior and emotions influence the nervous and immune system, and their findings are starting to close the mind–body gap that so bothers critics of modern Western science. For example, research at Stanford University showed that women with advanced breast cancer receiving standard therapy live twice as long if they also participate in a support group.

Psychoneuroimmunology could potentially provide scientific evidence for a belief held by healers, both mainstream and alternative, from the earliest days of medicine: that healing the mind is an integral part of healing the body. The evidence gleaned so far has not convinced medical scientists that mental states can actually cause, cure, or prevent diseases. But this type of research does open new possibilities for easing the discomfort of disease, surgery, or chemotherapy.

Biofeedback is a particularly popular mind–body technique. Through it, patients learn how to regulate their ordinarily involuntary body functions such as heart rate, temperature, and muscle tension. Hooked up to machines that measure these functions, patients watch a display or listen to a tone that tells them how close their physiological responses are getting to a desired result. Eventually they learn to control responses without feedback from the machine. After ruling out physical problems, many conventional doctors now use biofeedback to treat pain and anxiety, migraine or tension headaches, incontinence, or chronic pain syndrome. Biofeedback is often a first-choice treatment for Raynaud's phenomenon, a condition mainly affecting women, in which exposure to cold turns fingers white and blue, cold, and painful (see entry). And many private insurers are willing to pay for biofeedback training sessions.

Another mind–body technique increasingly used by mainstream physicians is hypnosis—even though, as with biofeedback, understanding of the physical mechanism or even hard evidence of effectiveness remains limited. Once regarded as sheer chicanery, hypnotherapy is now practiced by thousands of medical doctors in conjunction with conventional medical techniques. It can be used to help patients break bad habits, overcome phobias and sexual dysfunction, and cope with pain. Therapists help patients go into a trancelike state in which they lose awareness of their body and become more responsive to suggestion. When the session ends, patients remember everything that happened.

The American Medical Association's Council on Scientific Affairs has called for more research into hypnotherapy to help elucidate its role and means of action. Some practitioners hypothesize that hypnotherapy stimulates the brain's limbic system, which has been linked to emotions and normally involuntary activities such as digestion and hormone regulation. This link may explain in part the observation that hypnotherapy has helped control the stomach acid secretions of ulcer patients, reduce the discomfort of chemotherapy, and even speed recovery from burns.

Other mind–body techniques aim at reducing stress (see entry), a poorly defined concept that has been linked repeatedly to a series of ailments. Therapists at the Harvard-affiliated Mind/Body Medical Institute in Boston teach relaxation techniques such as meditation and yoga to help relieve stress in patients with coronary artery disease, infertility, insomnia, chronic pain, AIDS, and cancer. Other medical centers around the country have established their own meditation or massage clinics or have simply begun to emphasize listening and touching as crucial aspects of treatment. And stress-reduction techniques such as meditation and yoga are now often taught to patients by conventional health care workers, most commonly nurses, psychologists, and social workers, to help them face pain more effectively, including the pain of labor and childbirth.

Even less conventional are New Age relaxation devices such as flotation tanks and isolation chambers, which separate patients from all environmental stimuli. The same can be said for bioenergetics, in which the therapist passes an invisible and unmeasurable "energy" to the patient. In crystal healing energized light is supposedly passed through quartz or other colored minerals. Some patients claim to relax with the help of a "synchroenergizer," which surrounds them with New Age music and pulsing lights. Others swear by the healing power of magnets. For all these practices, evidence of any therapeutic effect that satisfies the standards of conventional medicine is lacking, and consumers are wise to be skeptical.

Visualization (guided imagery) is a relaxation technique which involves learning to picture each muscle relaxing. Introduced in the 1970s to improve the performance of athletes and musicians, visualization is also used to promote healing. Therapists teach patients to imagine their body conquering microorganisms or righting a biochemical imbalance. Although evidence for successful cures remains largely anecdotal, many hospitals and private psychologists have ongoing visualization groups for patients battling serious illness.

Because some alternative therapies do not lend themselves to conventional standards of scientific proof, it is often difficult to distinguish a potentially effective therapy from a pure hoax. Still, common sense can be a fairly reliable guide—plus the recognition that a great deal of conventional medicine still stems more from tradition and hunch than from rigorous evidence. Anyone seeking alternative care should avoid healers who claim to cure everything, those who offer "too good to be true" cures for serious diseases such as AIDS and cancer, and those who require multiple visits at hefty rates. Furthermore, some forms of alternative therapy have already entered the mainstream of medicine, at least for a well-defined set of conditions. Awareness of these distinctions can help anyone trying to choose from the many options.

For now, extremely risky practices such as intravenous infusions by alternative practitioners, megadoses of vitamins and minerals ("orthomolecular medicine"), colon therapy ("high colonic cocktails"), fever-induction therapy ("hyperthermia"), deep tissue massage on injured tissue, as well as radical cleansing or anti-cancer diets should generally be avoided altogether. Also to be avoided are alternative practitioners who make extravagant claims for originally conventional practices such as enzyme therapy, chelation therapy, intravenous vitamin therapy, cell therapy, hydrogen peroxide therapy, oxygen therapy, and environmental medicine and its talk of "multiple chemical sensitivities." At the present time, none of these approaches has been shown to cure or prevent cancer, AIDS, heart disease, or any other of the countless chronic, hard-to-cure ailments for which they are often used.

Additional evidence for and against alternative practices may come from studies funded by the National Center for Complementary and Alternative Medicine (NCCAM) at the National Institutes of Health, long a champion of rigorous scientific medicine. Established by Congress in 1998, NCCAM is an expansion of the Office of Alternative Medicine, which was created in 1992 to support research that tested alternative therapies using the same methods and standards of reproducibility required of more conventional practices. The NCCAM has additional resources for stimulating, developing, and supporting this research as well as the ability to disseminate to the public reliable information about the safety and efficacy of various complementary and alternative practices. Many health care workers hope that the studies it fosters will reveal new ways of dealing with some currently intractable medical problems.

Related entries
Chemotherapy, psychosomatic disorders, psychotherapy, radiation therapy, stress

Alzheimer's Disease

Alzheimer's disease is a progressive, degenerative disease—or, more accurately, group of disorders—that results in impaired memory, thinking, and behavior. It afflicts approximately 4 million Americans and as many as 15 million people worldwide. According to the Office of Research on Women's Health at the National Institutes of Health, Alzheimer's disease is more prevalent among women than among men, and this prevalence increases with age.

Alzheimer's disease is the most common cause of dementia, which is not a disease itself but rather a group of symptoms that involve a loss of intellectual function severe enough to interfere with daily activities. Formerly called senility, dementia was once thought to be a normal and almost inevitable component of aging. Today many doctors and researchers believe that dementia occurs in the elderly only when they are afflicted with specific diseases or disorders. Some of these disorders—including nutritional deficiencies (such as B_{12} deficiency), drug reactions, depression, thyroid disorders, and alcoholism—are potentially reversible. The dementia caused by Alzheimer's disease cannot be reversed, however, and ultimately results in a loss of the ability to care for oneself. Other causes of dementia, some of which are reversible, include multiinfarct dementia (caused by vascular disease and multiple strokes), Parkinson's disease, Huntington's disease, Creutzfeldt-Jakob disease, and Pick's disease, as well as infections such as meningitis (inflammation of the membrane surrounding the brain and spinal cord), syphilis, and AIDS.

On average a person with Alzheimer's lives about 8 years beyond the time of the initial diagnosis, with some people living 20 years or more. However long the survival time, symptoms continue to worsen over the years, and the patient becomes increasingly susceptible to infections and other illnesses, which are often the direct cause of death.

As public awareness about Alzheimer's grows, so do public fears. Many people who misplace their keys or have trouble remembering the name of an acquaintance fear they may be showing the first signs of dementia. The missing information is usually recovered later, often when there is less pressure to remember it, and memory problems like these—which are neither progressive nor disabling—can easily be averted in

the first place by writing reminders or notes to oneself. In most cases these short-term memory lapses are nothing more than what some health care professionals call age-associated memory impairment. Such impairment may simply be a sign that one's mental reflexes are slowing down with age, in much the same way that physical reflexes gradually decline. A number of other health-related problems, including fatigue, grief, depression, stress, vision or hearing loss, excessive alcohol consumption, and overwork, can also impair memory function in people of any age.

About 10 percent of all Americans aged 65 or older do have actual Alzheimer's disease. And often it is as hard—or harder—on family members and other caregivers as it is on the patient. In addition to dealing with the grief of "losing" a loved one who is still alive, there is guilt over giving what feels like inadequate care and the fear of developing the disease oneself. Many caregivers are saddled with huge financial burdens, too, since the average yearly cost of caring for an Alzheimer's patient at home is $18,000, and can jump to around $45,000 a year if the patient is placed in a nursing home.

Finally, in the course of caring for the Alzheimer's patient, many caregivers neglect their own emotional and physical health. The average age of primary caregivers for people with Alzheimer's in this country is 71, and most of them have at least two chronic health problems of their own.

Who is likely to develop Alzheimer's disease?
The risk of acquiring Alzheimer's disease rises with age, although the disease sometimes occurs in middle age. The youngest documented case of a person with Alzheimer's disease involved someone who was 28 years old. The early-onset forms of the disease tend to run in families, whereas cases that develop after age 65 (which constitute the vast majority) seem to occur sporadically.

Although the cause of Alzheimer's disease remains unknown, researchers now believe that some forms of the disease—particularly those that strike people before age 65—may be linked to the inheritance of at least 3 specific genes. One of these is on chromosome 21, the same chromosome involved in Down syndrome. There seems to be a genetic predisposition for late-onset forms of Alzheimer's disease as well, although more and more researchers now suspect that, as with heart disease and cancer, most forms of the disease result from the interactions of several influences, both genetic and environmental.

People of all socioeconomic and ethnic groups are susceptible, but those with relatively higher educational levels may be partially protected. A study involving 595 people over the age of 60 found that those with the highest educational levels were least likely to be diagnosed with dementia. The investigators speculated that this may be due to the fact that educated people perform better on tests of intellectual ability and thus are not as easily identified as having Alzheimer's. Alternatively, it may be that higher levels of education somehow increase brain reserves and delay the onset of Alzhei-

Degeneration of neurons in Alzheimer's disease

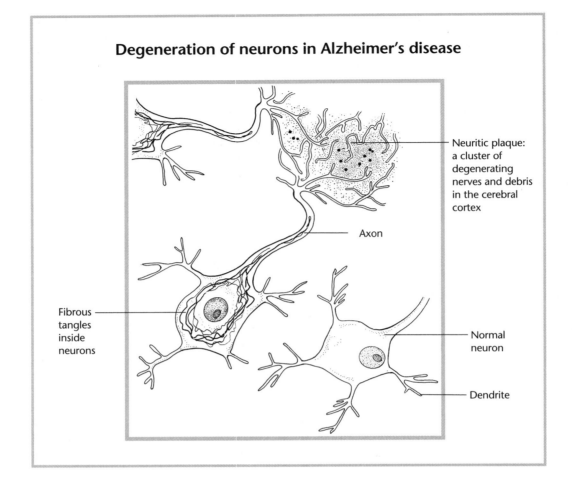

Neuritic plaque: a cluster of degenerating nerves and debris in the cerebral cortex

Axon

Fibrous tangles inside neurons

Normal neuron

Dendrite

mer's symptoms for several years. It is unlikely that higher education in and of itself can prevent someone from getting Alzheimer's disease eventually.

People with Alzheimer's disease have certain physical abnormalities that probably explain their intellectual and behavioral degeneration. In brain tissue examined at autopsy, these changes are seen in fibrous tangles inside nerve cells (neurons) and in clusters of degenerating nerves called neuritic plaques (see illustration). In living patients there is also a diminished production of certain neurotransmitters, the chemicals that send messages between nerve cells.

What are the symptoms?

Unlike various kinds of normal age-related memory impairment, the symptoms of Alzheimer's disease worsen over the years (see chart). Also, although most people with occasional forgetfulness can compensate by using reminders and notes, the memory loss associated with Alzheimer's soon makes a person unable to manage daily work and social life. Above all, the symptoms of Alzheimer's include more than forgetfulness: problems with reasoning and judgment, as well as mood and behavioral changes, always characterize the illness.

Just how quickly the disease progresses can vary considerably from one person to the next. In the early stages the patient may have trouble finding the right word, take longer to react, experience short-term memory loss, and have difficulties making mathematical calculations. She may or may not be aware that she has a problem handling these and other routine tasks. She may appear self-absorbed and insensitive and have difficulty planning and making decisions. Often there are marked changes in her ability to handle frustration and a general decrease in initiative and drive. Family members may try to cover up these problems by attributing them to stress or overwork or may not recognize that they exist.

As the disease progresses, the person will have increasing difficulty with understanding and self-expression, and will exhibit marked disorientation, behavioral changes, repetitive actions, and impaired judgment. She will frequently seem lethargic or cold emotionally, having little memory of the recent past and not recognizing familiar people while still retaining a clear memory of distant events. Often she will direct her anger and frustration at family members, who in turn may end up acting out their own feelings on her.

Even at this middle stage of the disease, many family members still deny the diagnosis or refuse help. At this stage, too,

Normal memory loss or Alzheimer's disease?

Average person	Older person	Alzheimer's patient
Is rarely forgetful	Sometimes forgets parts of an experience (may remember a shopping trip but doesn't remember stopping for an ice cream cone)	Frequently forgets entire experiences (such as shopping trips or meals)
Remembers later	Often remembers later	Rarely remembers later
Is not upset by memory lapses	Acknowledges memory lapses readily, and may ask for help in remembering forgotten information	Admits memory lapses grudgingly, only after repeated denial
Speaks fluently	May forget people's names or infrequently used words; often recalls later	Has difficulty finding words; substitutes words ("the thing" or "whatchamacallit"); loses train of thought; stutters or repeats words
Maintains skills such as reading and arithmetic	Skills usually remain intact	Loses skills gradually
Follows spoken or written directions easily; plans events and activities	Usually able to follow directions and plan activities	Becomes unable to follow directions or plan activities
Can use notes and other devices as reminders	Usually able to use reminders	Becomes unable to use reminders
Can care for self	Usually able to care for self	Becomes unable to care for self

it is particularly common for family members to begin to experience feelings of loss, guilt, and fear, and to begin to neglect their own health. It is also typical for them to isolate themselves from friends and family as they devote more time to the Alzheimer's patient, whose behavior may be a source of embarrassment which further reinforces the caregiver's isolation. This isolation often only exacerbates negative feelings and undermines the overall well-being of the caregiver.

In the final stage of the disease, the patient with Alzheimer's requires 24-hour care. She is apathetic, unaware of her state of cleanliness or dress, unable to communicate, and incontinent. She has little memory, either short-term or long-term. Eventually many patients will assume a fetal position and gradually shut down their entire mind and body. It is only at this point that many families, exhausted physically and spiritually from the ordeal, resign themselves to placing the patient in a nursing home and may experience deep feelings of guilt and grief.

How is the condition evaluated?

Currently there is no one diagnostic test available for Alzheimer's disease. Consequently, the disease is diagnosed by excluding other conditions that can cause dementia—some of which may be treatable. To do this, a physician or team of physicians usually conducts a complete physical, psychiatric, and neurologic evaluation. This examination includes a detailed medical history, a review of current medications, a mental status test, neuropsychological testing, blood work, urinalysis, and, in some cases, electroencephalography (EEG), computerized tomography (CT scan), or magnetic resonance imaging (MRI).

Health professionals believe that when this kind of detailed examination is done (and it often is not), about 90 percent of diagnoses of Alzheimer's will be confirmed. At present the only way to confirm the diagnosis is to look for tangles of nerve fibers during an autopsy.

For the time being, however, the diagnosis of Alzheimer's remains an educated guess, which leaves open the possibility that at least some of the people diagnosed with this form of dementia may instead have other, more treatable conditions. In actual practice as many as 25 to 40 percent of all Alzheimer's cases are diagnosed incorrectly. This may help explain why older women—who are especially susceptible to other, reversible causes of dementia such as depression, thyroid disorders, nutritional deficiencies, overmedication, and alcoholism—are diagnosed with Alzheimer's in disproportionate numbers. Therefore, it is important for the clinician to exclude other causes of dementia before giving the diagnosis of Alzheimer's.

Meanwhile, in many families with a history of Alzheimer's—particularly early-onset Alzheimer's, for which the genetic connection is clearer—relatives want to know their individual risks of developing this condition. They think this information might help guide future decisions, such as financial arrangements and family planning. Given our present state of knowledge, however, the medical consensus is that genetic tests for this purpose should not be done on a routine basis. This is partly because Alzheimer's appears to be caused by multiple factors, not just genetic ones, and can develop even without the presence of all three of the genes associated with the condition; for these reasons, a "clean" test may provide false reassurance. In addition, most clinicians question the value of predictive testing when the results will have little if any bearing on the course of the illness. In the case of Alzheimer's, knowing whether or not a person has genes associated with the disease cannot help predict the rate of decline or the actual age of onset, knowledge that would be essential to effective planning.

How is Alzheimer's disease treated?

In recent years several promising drug treatments have been approved by the Food and Drug Administration (FDA) to slow the progress of the dementia associated with Alzheimer's disease and possibly improve the behavioral problems associated with the disease as well. These drugs, called cholinesterase inhibitors, are tacrine (Cognex), donepezil (Aricept), rivastigmine (Exelon), and galantamine (Reminyl). While these medications cannot stop the deterioration of neurons, they can slow it and prevent or delay institutionalization of people with mild to moderate Alzheimer's.

In addition, some of the symptoms of Alzheimer's—including depression, insomnia, and behavioral disturbances—can often be managed with medications. Eating a balanced diet, getting proper health care, and engaging in regular physical exercise and social activity can make the condition more bearable.

This advice applies to caregivers as well. It is important for family members to take care of their own health, and to spend time away from the constant responsibilities—sometimes called the "36-hour day"—involved in caring for a person with Alzheimer's. This break can help protect them from depression and other health problems. Many caregivers benefit from joining a support group, often led by a professional counselor, or by taking advantage of a local respite service such as adult day care, the Visiting Nurse Association, and home care agencies. Local support groups can be found by calling the Alzheimer's Association, a national volunteer organization which not only supports research into the causes, treatment, and prevention of Alzheimer's but also provides information and assistance to both Alzheimer's patients and their families.

How can Alzheimer's disease be prevented?

Until the cause or causes of Alzheimer's are better understood, there is limited information available on how to reduce your risk of the disease. Scientists had hoped that estrogen replacement therapy might be protective, since some studies of women who had taken estrogen replacement therapy found lower rates of Alzheimer's disease compared with women who took no estrogen. However, the Women's Health Initiative, using a more reliable study design, found that postmenopausal women assigned to take hormone replacement therapy (estrogen plus progestin) had higher rates of dementia than those who did not take it. The effects of estrogen alone are still under study. At this time, hormone replacement therapy is not recommended for reducing Alzheimer's risk.

Other interventions to prevent dementia are under study, but far from proven. These include low doses of nonsteroidal antiinflammatory drugs (such as ibuprofen) and vitamin E supplements. High blood pressure has been shown to increase risk of dementia, including that caused by Alzheimer's disease. For women with hypertension, keeping blood pressure under good control makes sense. Finally, there is evidence that physical activity and exercise may protect against dementia—providing another good reason for women to make regular exercise a part of their daily routine.

Family members of an Alzheimer's patient may also be able to assess their risks of acquiring the disease later in life if they are willing to have the patient's brain autopsied after death. This not only allows the pathologist to confirm the diagnosis of Alzheimer's but also helps determine which specific disease or diseases caused the dementia. Knowing the exact cause can make a difference to family members, since some of the diseases that cause dementia, including Alzheimer's, carry a degree of genetic risk. Autopsies are sometimes performed at no charge if the brain is donated for research, but they can cost over $2,000 in some settings. Most of the cost is usually covered by insurance.

Related entries

Depression, fatigue, nutrition, stress

Amenorrhea

Amenorrhea means the absence of menstruation in a premenopausal woman. During pregnancy or breastfeeding amenorrhea is perfectly normal and is called physiologic amenorrhea. Abnormal or pathologic amenorrhea comes in two forms: primary and secondary. Primary amenorrhea is a term used if menstruation has not begun by the age of 16. Secondary amenorrhea is a term used if previously normal menstrual periods stop for more than 6 months in a woman who is not pregnant or breastfeeding and is not nearing menopause.

In most cases amenorrhea is not a cause for concern. But if it persists for more than several months it should be treated, since over time the lack of ovulation and resulting drop in estrogen levels can increase bone turnover, thus raising the risk of osteoporosis, a systemic and often debilitating skeletal disease in which the bones gradually lose their store of calcium and other minerals. As a result they become less dense and more susceptible to fracture from even slight trauma. Postmenopausal women whose estrogen levels are low are at particular risk, but young women who are not ovulating can also develop this disorder. Amenorrhea affects a woman's fertility, too, although this does not mean that women with amenorrhea cannot become pregnant or do not need to use birth control.

Who is likely to develop amenorrhea?

Primary amenorrhea is most often due to delayed puberty, a condition in which maturation is slower than average because of genetic factors or environmental factors such as poor nutrition. Sometimes, however, the first menstrual period (menarche) is delayed when a girl is undergoing excessive stress or heavy athletic training, or when she is suffering from anorexia (an eating disorder characterized by an intense fear of becoming fat; women with anorexia purposely lose weight to the point of starvation) and therefore has a low ratio of fat to lean tissue. Most adult women of average weight have a ratio of 24 percent fat to 76 percent lean tissue. If levels of fat are below 15 to 22 percent, as they often are before the growth spurt that precedes menarche, menstruation may not occur. This physiological response probably evolved as a way to reduce a woman's fertility when food was scarce and offspring were therefore unlikely to survive.

More rarely, primary amenorrhea may result from some anatomical obstruction such as an imperforate hymen, which blocks the flow of blood out of the vagina. Even more infrequently, primary amenorrhea may result from genetic disorders such as Turner syndrome, hermaphroditism, and testicular feminization syndrome (see entries); pituitary gland disorders and tumors; and thyroid or adrenal disorders.

Secondary amenorrhea, as well as infrequent periods, is common for the first few years after menarche, as well as in the years preceding menopause. This normal condition results from the imperfectly coordinated function of the hypothalamus, a part of the brain that regulates basic functions including eating, sleeping, and reproduction. Stress and acute or chronic illness can also cause amenorrhea by interfering with the normal function of the hypothalamus.

Many professional dancers, models, and actresses, as well as amateur and professional athletes such as gymnasts, figure skaters, long-distance runners, and jockeys, develop irregular periods or stop menstruating altogether as their ratio of fat to lean tissue drops. Some of these women, along with other women who have an aversion to body fat, develop anorexia nervosa and subsist on a near-starvation diet despite the high-energy demands of their profession. The lack of ovulation and resulting decline in estrogen puts these women at high risk for bone loss and severe osteoporosis, which can develop even in their 20s if amenorrhea is allowed to continue for years.

About 1 woman in 5 with amenorrhea has elevated prolactin levels. Prolactin is a hormone that stimulates the breasts to secrete milk and, indirectly, inhibits ovulation. In addition, about 5 percent of women with secondary amenorrhea exhibit hyperandrogenism, a condition in which there is an excess of hormones called androgens, which produce masculine traits. If untreated, amenorrhea and hyperandrogenism may lead to chronic stimulation of the uterine lining by estrogen hormones, which in turn has been associated with an increased risk of endometrial hyperplasia and endometrial cancer.

Another relatively common cause of amenorrhea during the childbearing years is polycystic ovary syndrome, a condition marked by multiple ovarian cysts and excessive production of androgens (male-type hormones). More rarely, secondary amenorrhea may result from cancer, radiation therapy, or scar tissue (adhesions) in the uterine lining.

Women with amenorrhea may also suffer from Cushing disease (a disorder in which a tumor of the pituitary gland causes the adrenal glands to produce an excess of the hormones called glucocorticoids), or from Cushing syndrome (a disorder resulting primarily from long-term use of corticosteroid drugs such as prednisone, which are used to treat rheumatoid arthritis, asthma, and many other inflammatory conditions).

In new mothers who are not breastfeeding, postpartum amenorrhea sometimes occurs temporarily if the hypothalamus does not inhibit the production of prolactin by the pituitary gland. In rare instances, amenorrhea may result from Sheehan syndrome, a condition in which part of the pituitary gland dies after a traumatic labor or delivery. Women who have experienced severe bleeding (hemorrhage) or shock (a life-threatening response to severe pain or injury) during or just after delivery may develop this syndrome. Because excessive postpartum bleeding is generally treated promptly, this syndrome has become quite rare.

How is the condition evaluated?

Primary amenorrhea does not usually require either evaluation or treatment until the age of 18, if there are other signs of puberty such as breast development or growth of pubic and underarm hair. It may be reassuring, however, for girls to see a clinician to rule out the few rare but serious causes of primary amenorrhea. This evaluation will include a pelvic examination to determine if there are any anatomical obstructions and a hormonal test and sometimes a CT scan or MRI (magnetic resonance imaging) to make sure there is no pituitary tumor. After age 18 these and more extensive investigations will be done to discover the causes of primary amenorrhea.

Before evaluating secondary amenorrhea, the clinician will first want to make sure that the woman is not pregnant or approaching menopause. After that he or she will usually take a detailed history, do a physical and pelvic examination, order certain hormonal tests to rule out ovarian failure, and check for underlying diseases. So that the function of the uterus and ovaries can be assessed, progesterone (Provera) may be given for 5 days to see if withdrawal bleeding occurs after it is stopped. Alternatively, blood tests may be done to measure estrogen levels and basal body temperature charting, or tests of blood progesterone levels to see if ovulation is occurring. In certain women a clinician may want to conduct additional tests for hyperandrogenism or thyroid disorders. The clinician may also order a pelvic ultrasound, a chromosome evaluation, or a CT or MRI scan as well.

All women with menstrual irregularities should have a blood test to check their prolactin level. Since prolactin is increased by eating, stress, and breast exams, any woman with an elevated level should have the test repeated at a time when she is fasting and has not just completed an examination. If levels are still elevated, an MRI scan of the head may be done to rule out a pituitary tumor.

How is amenorrhea treated?

Often amenorrhea requires no treatment whatsoever. In certain cases, addressing the underlying disease or condition (such as overexercise or an eating disorder) will often restore or initiate menstruation. Postpartum or lactation amenorrhea frequently corrects itself or can be corrected with hormone therapy.

Generally a clinician will prescribe estrogen supplements to help prevent osteoporosis in women with no underlying disorder whose amenorrhea has lasted for 6 months or more.

Birth control pills are frequently the most convenient form of estrogen replacement. Supplemental calcium is often suggested as well, even if no estrogen is prescribed. Women who want to bear children may require medications to stimulate ovulation, such as clomiphene (Clomid, Serophene) or human menopausal gonadotropins (Pergonal; see infertility).

Various herbal remedies are often recommended in popular medical literature to bring on a period, but there is little solid evidence about either the safety or the efficacy of these treatments.

How can amenorrhea be prevented?

Moderating exercise, maintaining normal body weight, and reducing stress can prevent amenorrhea that may be caused by these factors, but causes traced to other underlying disorders usually cannot be prevented.

Related entries

Anorexia nervosa and bulimia nervosa, Cushing syndrome, exercise, galactorrhea, hermaphroditism, hyperandrogenism, infertility, infrequent periods, menarche, menstrual cycle, menstrual cycle disorders, osteoporosis, stress, testicular feminization syndrome, thyroid disorders, Turner syndrome, vaginal bleeding (abnormal)

Amniocentesis

Amniocentesis is a prenatal screening procedure in which a small quantity of the amniotic fluid surrounding the fetus is removed from the uterus of a pregnant woman to allow the chromosomes of the fetus to be examined. The test is usually performed between 16 and 20 weeks of pregnancy in women considered to be at high risk for having a baby with chromosomal anomalies, although some centers are now performing it as early as 10 to 14 weeks.

Amniocentesis is most commonly used in pregnant women over the age of 35 to detect chromosomal abnormalities, particularly Down syndrome (trisomy 21). The risk of chromosomal defects is known to increase with maternal age, and generally after age 35 the risk of bearing a child with a chromosomal abnormality is greater than the risks connected with the procedure. Amniocentesis cannot determine the severity of Down syndrome or any other defect, however.

A woman under 35 might consider amniocentesis if any earlier screening procedure such as an alpha-fetoprotein test or ultrasound indicates the possibility of a genetic abnormality. Amniocentesis is also sometimes used later in pregnancy to determine the lung maturity of babies at risk because of premature labor. Although the procedure provides an opportunity for women to anticipate many potential defects, any

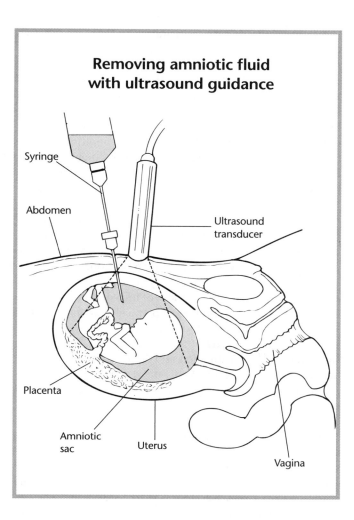

Removing amniotic fluid with ultrasound guidance

Syringe

Abdomen

Ultrasound transducer

Placenta

Amniotic sac

Uterus

Vagina

woman considering it should also bear in mind that in rare cases it can reveal abnormalities about which little is known, thus leaving her to make painful decisions about whether to carry the fetus to term.

How is amniocentesis performed?

A woman undergoing amniocentesis lies on an examination table with her abdomen uncovered. With the aid of ultrasound, the physician guides a thin needle (usually about 3 ½ inches long) through the abdomen into the uterus and amniotic sac (see illustration). About 1 ounce of amniotic fluid, which contains cells sloughed off by the fetus, is then withdrawn by a syringe attached to the needle. The actual procedure takes about 5 minutes and can be performed on an outpatient basis in either a doctor's office or a hospital. It is relatively painless.

The fluid is sent to a laboratory, where the fetal cells are cultured and analyzed for chromosomal defects through a procedure known as karyotyping. At the same time, the level of alpha fetoprotein (AFP) in the amniotic fluid is measured to determine the possibility of a neural tube defect.

It generally takes about 2 weeks for results to come in, de-

pending on what is being measured. Some new techniques not yet widely available require only 24 to 48 hours. AFP results are usually available within a few days of the test. Most women are anxious to hear from their physician as soon as possible, especially if they are considering terminating the pregnancy in the event of an abnormality.

How accurate, reliable, and safe is the test?

Amniocentesis is associated with a risk of miscarriage in 1 of 200 pregnancies as well as an even smaller risk (minimized with ultrasound guidance) that the needle may puncture the fetus. Other complications, though rare, can include cramping, vaginal bleeding, and the leaking of amniotic fluid. Thus, amniocentesis is normally offered only to women whose risk of having a genetically abnormal fetus is greater than 1 in 200. All women over the age of 35 run such a risk, as do women who know that they and their partner are carriers for genetic defects such as sickle cell anemia, Tay-Sachs disease, one of the thalassemias, or cystic fibrosis, or who have family members with a history of genetic disease (see genetic counseling). Amniocentesis is not necessary if only one member of a couple is a carrier.

Amniocentesis, even when performed as early as 10 weeks, is very reliable at detecting conditions such as Down syndrome which result from chromosomal abnormalities; but other malformations can occur during fetal development owing to nongenetic causes, and these would not be picked up by amniocentesis.

Related entries

Abortion, alpha-fetoprotein screening, chorionic villi sampling, genetic counseling, miscarriage, preconception counseling, pregnancy, pregnancy over age 35, ultrasound

Anemia

Anemia is a condition in which there is an abnormally low amount of blood, red blood cells, or hemoglobin. It can be produced by a variety of underlying causes.

Who is likely to develop anemia?

Most cases of anemia are due to iron deficiency. The body uses iron to produce hemoglobin (the iron-containing component of red blood cells which carries oxygen to body tissues), and also stores it for later use in the spleen, liver, and bone marrow. By far the most common cause of iron deficiency is bleeding, whether normal or abnormal. Women in the reproductive years often have a deficiency of iron because they lose 20 to 40 mg of iron per month in menstrual blood. Using a copper intrauterine device (IUD) can sometimes lead to particularly heavy menstrual flow and associated iron loss as well. In both men and women, bleeding from the digestive tract as a result of a stomach ulcer or colon cancer may also leach iron from the body.

Iron-deficiency anemia sometimes occurs when hemoglobin is lost through cell breakdown or when the body has trouble absorbing iron from foods. It may also occur when there is an increased demand for iron. Pregnant women are prone to anemia because iron stores are heavily drawn on to increase blood volume and to provide hemoglobin for the placenta and fetus. People with restricted diets may also be prone to iron-deficiency anemia.

Another form of anemia results from processes that interfere with the production of new red blood cells. Excess exposure to certain drugs, alcohol, metals, or chemicals can interfere with this production, as can the chronic inflammation and infection that accompany certain diseases. These diseases include cancer and rheumatoid arthritis, as well as kidney, liver, and thyroid disorders.

Certain vitamin deficiencies impair the body's ability to manufacture sufficient quantities of red blood cells. A lack of folic acid, particularly common in pregnant women, can decrease the production of red blood cells. If there is a deficiency of vitamin B_{12}, an autoimmune disorder called pernicious anemia may result. Traditionally regarded as a disorder of older people of northern European descent, pernicious anemia has probably been underrecognized in other groups, particularly young black women. In one study to detect the prevalence of pernicious anemia, about one-fifth of people with the disease turned out to be black females, a quarter of whom were under age 40. Because vitamin B_{12} is abundant in red meat and dairy products, pernicious anemia is generally due to an inadequate diet only in people who eat no meat, eggs, or dairy products. Usually it is the result of stomach surgery, a congenital abnormality, or some acquired defect that interferes with the production of a stomach secretion called intrinsic factor which is required for the intestine to absorb vitamin B_{12}.

Genetic disorders such as thalassemia and sickle cell disease cause varieties of anemia in which the body makes abnormal forms of hemoglobin (see illustration). People whose ancestors came from regions bordering the Mediterranean, Southeast Asia, the Philippines, southern China, Pakistan, and India are at particular risk for thalassemia, a condition in which the low rate of production of hemoglobin by the bone marrow can lead to severe anemia as well as fragile bones, facial deformities, growth retardation, and early death, usually from heart failure. Sickle cell anemia results from a different hemoglobin abnormality which produces crescent- or sickle-shaped red blood cells that clog blood flow in tiny capillaries and can lead to episodes of excruciating pain and chronic organ damage. Sickle cell anemia is most common in people of African descent, but people of Central American, Greek, Italian, Arab, Cuban, Puerto Rican, and Haitian backgrounds, as well as people from certain parts of India and Pakistan, also have a higher than average frequency of this gene.

Another cause of anemia includes the starvation that accompanies anorexia nervosa, a form of eating disorder.

What are the symptoms?

Mild iron-deficiency anemia may have no symptoms. Some women may notice fatigue, lightheadedness, decreased tolerance for exercise, and pallor, particularly in the nail beds, underside of eyelids, lips, and palms. As the condition becomes more advanced, women may develop a sore tongue, fissuring and dry scaling of the lips, ringing in the ears, spots before the eyes, frequent headaches, and spooned, ridged, and brittle nails. Some women have difficulty swallowing, while a few may have a condition called pica, an abnormal craving for nonfoods (most commonly ice). Ingestion of clay-rich soils or starch can be particularly dangerous since these materials can interfere with normal iron absorption.

Symptoms of folic acid deficiency and anemia owing to anorexia nervosa are similar to those of iron-deficiency anemia. In contrast, an early symptom of pernicious anemia can be a burning sensation in the tongue. Later there may be weight loss, jaundice (yellowing of the skin and eyes), lack of appetite, intermittent constipation and diarrhea, abdominal pain, and, though rarely, fever. There may also be some loss of sensation in the arms and legs and problems with muscular coordination, as well as mental changes including irritability, mild depression, or paranoia.

Symptoms of the various forms of thalassemia vary in severity depending on the particular defective genes carried by the individual. In the less severe forms, symptoms often mimic those of mild iron-deficiency anemia. In severe forms, chronic anemia may develop as early as 3 months of age, with symptoms including jaundice, an enlarged spleen, leg ulcers, thickened and distorted facial bones, gallstones, impaired growth rate, and sometimes heart and liver impairment.

Women with sickle cell anemia are predisposed to infections, jaundice, and leg ulcers. Symptoms become worse during pregnancy, increasing the risk of miscarriage, stillbirth, and premature labor.

How is the condition evaluated?

To diagnose anemia, a practitioner will draw blood and order a complete blood count (CBC), which determines, among other things, the amount of red blood cells in a given volume of blood (this percentage is called a hematocrit level) and the concentration of hemoglobin. Anemia in a woman is defined as a hematocrit level under 36 percent or a hemoglobin concentration under 12 grams per 100 milliliters (cubic centimeters) of blood. These values are slightly lower than the normal levels for men.

Once anemia itself has been diagnosed, the physician will take a history of symptoms, perform a complete physical examination, and order additional blood tests to determine the specific cause or mechanism underlying the anemia. These tests will generally include measurements of iron levels and, if pernicious anemia is suspected, B$_{12}$ levels. Immature red blood cells may be counted to see if anemia is due to decreased production of red blood cells rather than later breakdown or loss through heavy bleeding.

If a serious intestinal disorder such as colon cancer is suspected, a test to screen for blood in the stool will be ordered.

How is anemia treated?

Usually women with iron-deficiency anemia can be treated with a tablet of ferrous sulfate or ferrous gluconate taken 3 times a day an hour before meals. If this leads to bloating, constipation, or diarrhea (as it often does), the physician may change the prescription to 1 tablet a day taken with meals, or prescribe a form of iron pill that contains a stool softener. It can take up to 9 months before anemia is completely corrected and iron reserves are replenished. Another possibility is the drug Niferex, available over the counter. This drug combines iron with a low molecular weight polysaccharide to decrease the possibility of nausea and constipation. Niferex should be taken with vitamin C to increase iron absorption.

Iron supplementation should take place only under a doctor's supervision because excess iron accumulation can cause liver damage, heart disturbances, and arthritis. It can also mask symptoms of serious conditions such as colon cancer. A few women may require a single intravenous injection of iron, which can quickly replenish total body iron stores. Sometimes this can result in pain and rash at the injection site, and, in rare cases, an excessive and sometimes life-threatening allergic reaction.

Women with pernicious anemia who lack intrinsic factor will need monthly injections of vitamin B$_{12}$ for life. Severe anemia that needs immediate correction, as sometimes happens in women with sickle cell anemia or thalassemia, may require hospitalization so that packed red blood cells can be transfused. In the case of thalassemia, blood transfusions at monthly intervals are necessary for the rest of the patient's life. Hospitalization and surgery may be required if anemia is due to a loss of blood from the digestive tract, as can happen in peptic ulcer disease or colon cancer.

Anemia caused by starvation and anorexia nervosa is corrected by increasing caloric intake and gaining weight.

How can anemia be prevented?

Preventing iron-deficiency and folic acid–deficiency anemia hinges on eating foods containing adequate amounts of iron and folic acid and taking dietary supplements when indicated. The latter are particularly important for women on weight loss diets and women who are pregnant or trying to become pregnant. Because iron is commonly lost through menstruation, premenopausal women require 50 to 70 mg of iron per day, as compared with only 30 mg for men. If this level of iron is not being supplied by the daily diet, a supplement such as a mulitvitamin with iron may be necessary.

Iron is found most abundantly in red meats, liver, legumes (rice and beans), potatoes, eggs, and dried fruits. The body absorbs iron from vegetables and grain products less efficiently than from meat and fish. Drinking citrus juice at the same time as taking a supplement or eating iron-rich food can help increase absorption.

Folic acid is found mainly in green leafy vegetables and legumes. The current Recommended Daily Allowance for folic acid in women is 0.4 mg. Many women do not get this amount through diet alone, however, and may need to take a multivitamin to supply the necessary amount. Most people get enough vitamin B12 from eating beef, pork, eggs, milk and milk products, and organ meats.

To prevent anemia in pregnancy, most practitioners prescribe supplementary iron as part of routine prenatal care. Because depletion of folic acid is a cause of neural tube defects, this vitamin is routinely supplemented as well, and women who are trying to become pregnant should start taking folic acid supplements of 0.4 mg per day even before they conceive. Supplementation is also needed during breastfeeding.

Any woman who knows that she or her partner is a carrier of thalassemia or sickle cell trait should receive genetic counseling (see entry) to assess her chances of having a child with severe anemia.

Related entries

Anorexia nervosa and bulimia nervosa, dieting, fatigue, genetic counseling, iron, nutrition, preconception counseling, prenatal care

Anesthesia

Anesthesia means total loss of sensation, but the term is often used to refer to any of a number of medications used to relieve pain during medical procedures. Some of these medications are indeed anesthetics in the sense that they do obliterate all feeling—either through complete loss of consciousness or by numbing a specific part of the body. Others are pain-relieving drugs called analgesics which are used to lessen pain while leaving some degree of sensation.

The degree to which alternative practices such as hypnosis or acupuncture can be used to produce effective pain relief without drugs is still under investigation in the West. Eastern practitioners have relied on these techniques for centuries.

With the exception of topical anesthetics (which relieve a limited surface area such as the gums), anesthesia must be administered by a licensed clinician—usually an anesthesiologist (a physician specializing in pain relief), an anesthetist (a specially trained nurse who works under the supervision of a physician), or a dentist.

Most of the time a surgeon will choose a form of anesthesia most appropriate to a particular procedure and to the patient's age and individual state of health. In many gynecological and obstetrical situations, however—particularly childbirth—the woman herself often plays a major role, if not *the* major role, in weighing the risks and benefits of each option. Because many medications taken by a pregnant woman reach the baby, women can take childbirth preparation classes and learn breathing and other relaxation techniques to help them cope with the pain of childbirth without using drugs. But because such techniques sometimes turn out to be inadequate—and because, in some labor situations, they may not be possible—all pregnant women must at least consider the possibility that they will need anesthesia. Since no one can anticipate all the circumstances of an individual labor and birth, choices must necessarily be left somewhat flexible. The ultimate decision will reflect these choices, together with the options available at the particular hospital and the judgment of the physician and anesthesiologist.

Below is a brief description of the more common forms of pain relief women may encounter. These procedures can be used separately, and some of them can be used in combination.

Systemic analgesia

Systemic analgesia involves using medications to relieve anxiety and tension throughout the body, thus reducing the intensity of pain while allowing the patient to remain conscious. Often morphine-like medications are injected into a muscle or a vein during surgical procedures; they may also be given during childbirth, to "take the edge off" contractions, and during abortions.

Although the patient can still feel pain with these drugs, she is generally so relaxed that she is much less likely to mind it. Depending on the dosage, she may drift in and out of alertness, so that time seems to pass unusually fast. Of course, depending on one's perspective, the same characteristics that allow sedation to work—in particular, difficulty concentrating and drowsiness—can also be construed as potential side effects. This is especially true during childbirth if a woman wants to be aware of everything that is happening. Furthermore, because systemic analgesics can slow the reflexes and breathing of a newborn, they are used only in small doses during childbirth and discontinued as delivery approaches.

Local anesthesia

Local anesthetics numb a confined area of the body such as the gums or the eye. A local anesthetic applied to the surface of the body to relieve pain in a limited area is called a topical anesthetic. Many topical anesthetics—including mouthwashes, throat lozenges, cold sore relievers, and rectal suppositories—are available without a prescription. All other forms of local anesthesia are Novocain-type drugs and are administered by a clinician, usually by injection. Although local anesthesia is considered the safest form of pain relief, it can be used only for relatively short procedures, since its effects usually wear off after an hour or so. Occasionally, however, it may be used for more extensive procedures in pa-

tients whose age or health precludes using other forms of anesthesia.

Local anesthetics may be used during childbirth to numb the perineum (the area between the vagina and rectum) before an episiotomy (a small cut made to prevent ragged tearing). It may also be used before the clinician stitches up any tears in this area after delivery. This kind of anesthesia rarely affects the baby in any way.

Regional anesthesia

Regional anesthesia blocks pain sensation in a specific region of the body, for example, from the waist down. It is sometimes called conduction anesthesia because the anesthetic blocks the conduction of pain impulses in select nerves. It may be used together with some form of sedation (administered intravenously), along with an infusion of a sugar and salt solution to prevent dehydration. Although the patient remains conscious—as with local anesthesia—regional anesthesia can be used for more extensive procedures because it provides deeper and longer-lasting pain relief. It is also sometimes used to provide continued relief after a procedure is over.

The main forms of regional anesthesia are spinal, epidural, caudal, and major nerve blocks. The first three are used for surgeries below the navel—including operations on the reproductive organs (such as a tubal ligation, hysterectomy, or dilatation and curettage), bladder, rectum, legs, and hips—as well as during labor and delivery.

Epidural. This is a form of regional anesthesia that numbs the lower half of the body. It is called an epidural because it involves an injection into a small space just outside the spinal cord compartment called the epidural space. The degree of numbness can be adjusted depending on which drug—and how much of it—is used.

A woman having an epidural is usually asked to lie very still on her side with her back curved outward (see illustration), although the procedure can also be performed with the woman sitting. After washing the back with an antiseptic and numbing the outer skin with a local anesthetic, the anesthesiologist inserts a needle into the epidural space and places a hollow tube (catheter) through it. The needle is then withdrawn, but the catheter remains in place so that more medication can be administered later without necessitating another injection. The drug usually takes effect within 20 minutes, often sooner.

The procedure is usually only slightly uncomfortable—although, if used during labor, merely being asked to shift position during a contraction can be excruciating. Nonetheless, epidurals are among the most commonly used and safest forms of anesthesia for childbirth. They can greatly relieve the pain associated with uterine contractions, pushing, and episiotomies. And should an emergency cesarean section become necessary, a catheter is already in place to allow stronger dosages of the anesthetic to be given.

In childbirth, medication levels are kept as low as possible

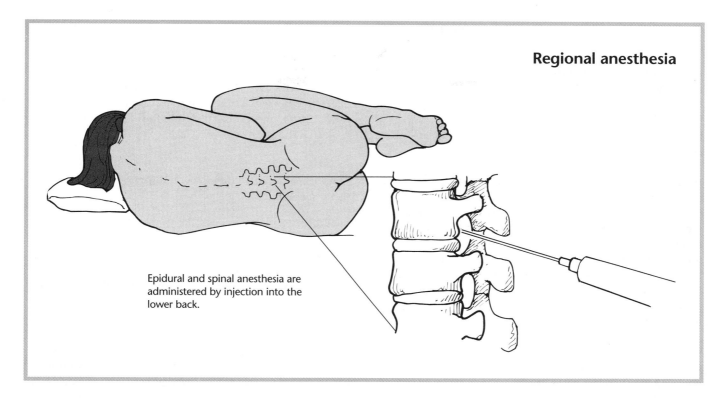

Regional anesthesia

Epidural and spinal anesthesia are administered by injection into the lower back.

to minimize side effects in both mother and baby. Often dosages are low enough that a woman can still feel the pressure—but not the pain—of a contraction. Many women can also still control their ability to bear down and push the baby through the birth canal, although the actual pushing may not be felt. Concentration and direction from a nurse or partner is required to know when to push and if the pushing is strong enough. Occasionally the clinician may need to help with either forceps or vacuum extraction.

The epidural wears off soon after delivery. Although serious complications from epidurals are rare, some women develop severe headaches afterward, lasting up to a few days if untreated. Also possible—though highly unusual—are temporary breathing difficulties (if the drug enters the spinal fluid), dizziness, or seizures (if the drug enters a vein). Epidurals can cause blood pressure to drop, which, in the case of childbirth, can slow the baby's heartbeat. To reduce the chances of this occurring, women about to receive an epidural are usually given intravenous fluids before the anesthetic is administered. The impact of epidurals on length of labor and on risk that a cesarean section will be required remains controversial.

Spinal. Like an epidural, a spinal block numbs only the lower half of the body. It is administered in much the same way as an epidural (the patient lies on her side with her back rounded), although the medication is injected directly into the spinal fluid instead of the epidural space. Within minutes the patient becomes completely unable to feel or move from the waist down, although the effect begins to wear off after an hour or two. The side effects are similar to those

of an epidural—including headache and dizziness—and are equally rare.

Whereas spinals are often used during surgeries of limited duration, epidurals are generally more desirable during labor because medications can be modified as the labor progresses. Occasionally, however, a spinal can provide quick relief during the pushing stage of labor—and even more commonly during a cesarean section—while still allowing the mother to remain conscious.

Caudal. A caudal is similar to an epidural, except that the anesthetic is injected into the epidural space around the sacral canal at the base of the back and numbs a somewhat larger area of the body. As in an epidural, a small catheter can be left in place to allow additional injection of medication should it become necessary later—either during or after the procedure. Because they require a larger dose of the anesthetic than an epidural, and therefore carry greater risks, caudals have largely been supplanted by epidurals.

Nerve blocks. Regional nerve blocks can be used almost anywhere in the body, although they are most commonly used to anesthetize the arms or, in gynecological or obstetrical situations, the perineum or the areas around the cervix (see below). Before the anesthetic drug is administered, a small needle is inserted at some distance from the area being anesthetized. This often produces a tingly feeling like a small electric shock—a sign that the needle is near the correct nerve. Once proper placement has been determined, the anesthesiologist injects the anesthetic through the needle, which keeps the nerve from sending pain signals from that region of the body to the brain.

Pudendal block. One of the safest forms of obstetrical anesthesia, a pudendal block numbs all feeling in the perineum—the area between the vagina and the anus. It is often used during childbirth just before an episiotomy is performed or before the baby pushes through the area. Serious side effects are rare.

Paracervical block. A paracervical nerve block is given by local injection to numb the area around the cervix (the entrance to the uterus). Paracervical blocks were once commonly given during childbirth to relieve pain as the cervix dilates (widens) and the uterus contracts. They are used much more rarely today because they sometimes slow the baby's heart rate—usually temporarily, but occasionally to the point of requiring an emergency cesarean section. When paracervical blocks are used, the baby's heart is always closely monitored.

General anesthesia

General anesthetics produce a complete loss of consciousness and are therefore often the anesthesia of choice for extensive and prolonged surgeries. They are administered by either inhalation or injection, often following the administration of a sedative medication. In some procedures drugs such as sodium pentothal or Diprivan may be injected to induce a quick state of light anesthesia before slower-acting drugs are administered via inhalation. In some longer operations a ventilation tube is placed through the mouth into the windpipe to facilitate breathing. Most people wake from general anesthesia feeling groggy, sometimes for many hours. For this reason, driving and other activities that require quick reflexes and good coordination should be avoided for about a day.

General anesthetics affect all parts of the body—including the brain, heart, and lungs. It is therefore standard procedure for vital signs—such as heart rate and rhythm, blood pressure, breathing, and temperature—to be monitored continually while a patient is under general anesthesia. Patients are also usually carefully screened to make sure they do not have preexisting health conditions (such as hypertension, diabetes, heart or lung disease, or allergies to the anesthetic used) which would predispose them to complications. Side effects (such as nausea, vomiting, muscle pain, or sore throat) are usually minor, temporary, and readily managed by the clinician overseeing the procedure. It is quite rare for serious complications (such as stroke, heart attack, or respiratory arrest) to result. Women who think they may be pregnant should mention this possibility to their clinician before having any procedure that might require general anesthesia.

In rare instances a patient under general anesthesia may choke when food comes up from the stomach and enters the lungs or windpipe. This is why patients are told not to eat or drink for a number of hours before they have surgery, and it is also why many clinicians advise women in labor to avoid solid food and water—on the chance that an emergency cesarean requiring general anesthesia may have to be performed. General anesthesia is no longer used during routine deliveries, but because it is the fastest anesthetic to take effect, in emergency situations requiring an immediate cesarean section to protect the health or life of the baby or mother it is often the anesthetic of choice.

Related entries

Abortion, alternative therapies, antianxiety drugs, cesarean section, childbirth

Angina Pectoris

Angina pectoris literally means pain in the chest. It generally occurs in self-limited attacks (10 or 15 minutes at most), which can be triggered by anything that increases the heart's workload and its need for blood and oxygen beyond its capacity. This includes such everyday occurrences as exercise, emotional stress, exposure to cold, or even eating a heavy meal. Pain occurs because of an imbalance between increased demand for blood and oxygen to the heart muscle and inadequate supply, a condition called myocardial ischemia.

Although angina is not always a precursor to a heart attack, even occasional attacks of angina can be a sign of serious coronary artery disease and should be called to the attention of a physician. *Any woman who experiences a heavy squeezing pain or pressure across her chest that lasts longer than 20 minutes should seek emergency care immediately. She may be having a life-threatening heart attack.*

Who is likely to develop angina?

Before the age of 75, men are more likely to have angina than women. The prevalence of angina in women increases with age, however, so that after the age of 75, angina is more common among women. Angina in women often takes a somewhat different course. Although most angina in both sexes is brought on by physical exertion, more women than men experience angina after emotional stress—or even during sleep or rest.

One explanation for this difference is that most angina in men is due to atherosclerosis—a process in which the arteries become clogged with fatty plaque. When this condition develops in the arteries of the heart, it is called coronary artery disease (CAD), and it can lead to heart attack if untreated. Angina in women under 50 may be due either to atherosclerosis or to spasms of the arteries supplying the heart (see illustration). Spasm is a sudden but temporary narrowing of the layer of smooth muscle inside coronary arteries that helps regulate blood flow. This kind of angina, characterized by pain during rest, is called variant angina, Prinzmetal's angina, or rest angina. Its prevalence in women helps explain why some younger women, whose arteries are free of coronary artery disease, still experience angina. Variant angina seems to result in serious complications or death less often than does more typical angina. In fact, 90 percent of people with this form of angina can expect to be alive 5 years after diagnosis.

No one fully understands just what triggers coronary artery spasm. Various factors are under investigation. These include overzealous platelets (blood components responsible for clotting), cigarette smoking, and stress. Whatever the ultimate cause, all spasm is preceded by an influx of the mineral calcium into the smooth muscle cells that line the arteries.

Other women with symptoms of angina may have a condition called microvascular angina. Although many people with this syndrome, most of whom are women, have characteristic abnormalities in their electrocardiogram (ECG), they often have unblocked coronary arteries and normal heart function and rarely show any signs of oxygen deprivation to the heart during exercise or stress. Some researchers suspect that microvascular angina may be due to some dysfunction of tiny arteries near the larger coronary arteries.

Although these variations in women are more common under the age of 50, most women over 50 with angina have typical angina—the same type that men have—and it is caused by atherosclerosis and coronary artery disease. Over 2.5 million American women are hospitalized each year for cardiovascular disease, and approximately 250,000 of them die each year because of coronary artery disease. It is the most frequent cause of death among women in the United States.

Since women rarely develop atherosclerosis before their late 50s or 60s, under the age of 60 men are generally more likely than women to develop this condition. The increase in atherosclerosis in women in their late 50s is likely to be related in part to decreased levels of estrogen, which decline after menopause. But women under 60 who have diabetes or high blood pressure seem to be at higher risk than men the same age, and having a close relative with atherosclerosis also increases the odds that a woman will develop this problem. In both sexes, smoking cigarettes raises the risk of atherosclerosis, as does a sedentary lifestyle.

Variant angina and microvascular angina are more likely to occur at younger ages. Microvascular angina sometimes occurs in women near or just past menopause—suggesting that it might somehow be linked to falling estrogen levels. A few women with variant angina seem to have other conditions involving arterial spasm, such as migraine headaches, Raynaud's phenomenon (a condition in which fingers or toes turn temporarily white and blue after exposure to cold or sometimes after emotional stress), and, occasionally, aspirin-induced asthma. Many are also heavy cigarette smokers, and it is possible that smoking causes arteries to go into spasm.

What are the symptoms?

Angina is itself a symptom rather than a unique disorder. It is often described as a tight, band-like, suffocating or crush-

Two causes of angina in women

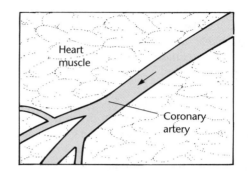

Normal flow of blood to heart muscle

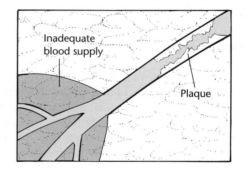

Atherosclerosis, leading to blockage of the artery, inadequate blood flow to heart muscle, and therefore chest pain

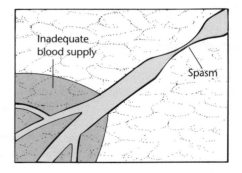

Cardiac spasm, also leading to inadequate blood flow to heart muscle and chest pain

ing sensation in the chest, which may radiate to the throat, shoulder, jaw, neck, or either arm. Typically, attacks of angina are brought on by exercise or emotional stress, generally last only a few minutes, and are relieved by rest. If pain lasts longer than about 20 minutes, a clinician should be consulted because of the possibility of long-term damage to the heart. With medications, angina can be controlled and the risk of heart attack diminished.

The pain of variant angina or microvascular angina is often indistinguishable from that of typical angina. Variant angina often occurs in frequent spurts, however, followed by long pain-free periods.

How is the condition evaluated?

Women with chest pain far too often fail to be evaluated for angina or for coronary artery disease in general. Although the likelihood of typical angina is quite low in a premenopausal woman, any woman with symptoms suggesting this problem should at the very least speak to her clinician about her personal risk factors for cardiovascular disease. If the chest pain is suggestive of angina, she should probably have an electrocardiogram done both during rest and after exercise to see if the heart muscle shows signs of damage or diminished blood flow that threatens future damage. If findings are normal, the clinician will look for causes of the pain other than heart disease.

In older women, or in women who have abnormal ECGs, further tests may be done, including echocardiography, stress testing with or without nuclear imaging, cardiac catheterization with coronary arteriography, or pharmacological stress testing (administration of various drugs that challenge the heart and other muscles; for all of these procedures, see coronary artery disease).

How is angina treated?

Until more studies focused specifically on women are done, women with otherwise uncontrollable angina should continue to use the same drugs as men. Among the most effective and best tolerated are nitrates, beta blockers, and calcium-channel blockers. Just which drug is appropriate can vary according to a woman's overall health.

Nitroglycerin. Traditionally angina has been treated simply and quickly by placing a tablet of nitroglycerin under the tongue. This drug and other nitrates, which dilate (widen) coronary arteries and increase blood flow to the heart, are also available in the form of a spray as well as ointments, slow-release patches that can be applied directly to the skin, and oral pills.

Beta blockers. This class of drugs lowers blood pressure and stabilizes heartbeat, allowing more time for the partially obstructed coronary arteries to fill with blood. These now classic medications have been shown time and again to lower the risk of heart attack in those who have angina.

Beta blockers can occasionally cause problems with blood sugar control in women with Type I (insulin-dependent) diabetes, but with close monitoring these problems can usually be managed. Since diabetic women of all ages are at the highest risk for CAD, the benefit of these drugs outweighs the risk.

Older versions of beta blockers such as propranolol and timolol sometimes cause depression or fatigue as well as slow pulse, dizziness, diarrhea, cold or tingling fingers or toes, and dry mouth, eyes, or skin. Less often, people using these older beta blockers may develop insomnia, hallucinations, anxiety, confusion, or breathing difficulties (the drugs should be used with caution by people with asthma). But newer, more "cardioselective" drugs (atenolol, metoprolol) are less likely to cause these side effects.

Calcium-channel blockers. An alternative for women with typical angina or arterial spasm is a class of drugs called calcium-channel blockers (nifedipine, verapamil, diltiazem). Calcium-channel blockers keep the arteries from going into spasm by impeding the flow of calcium through the muscle cells lining the coronary arteries. Women with microvascular angina may need no treatment at all. If chest pain is troubling, however, calcium-channel blockers often relieve it.

Aspirin. Aspirin has become a mainstay in the prevention of angina caused by coronary artery disease. It acts in part by reducing the stickiness of platelets—blood components that play an important role in the formation of blockages within arteries (see illustration in heart disease). A low dose of aspirin each day reduces the risk of future heart attacks in women with angina and CAD. Women with prolonged angina who suspect they may be having a heart attack are also now advised to chew on an aspirin to prevent further damage.

Surgery. If angina resulting from atherosclerosis does not respond to medications, procedures such as coronary angioplasty or coronary artery bypass surgery may be necessary (see coronary artery disease), although some studies have indicated that such treatments may not be as effective in women as in men.

How can angina be prevented?

Long-term treatment and prevention involves eliminating the risk factors that predispose some people to angina. For women who are overweight, this may mean losing excess pounds (which also decreases the risk of developing diabetes, another serious risk factor for CAD). For women who smoke, it means cutting out cigarettes. Controlling high blood pressure or elevated cholesterol should also be part of the plan.

Although exercise can trigger an angina attack, usually with medication and physical supervision a patient does not have to abandon it. A sedentary lifestyle may in itself increase the risk of heart disease. Although it makes sense for people with angina to stop exercising at the first sign of chest pain, there is good reason to adopt a moderate program of exercise under a clinician's supervision. Cardiac rehabilitation programs usually provide guidance in this.

Related entries

Circulatory disorders, coronary artery disease, diabetes, estrogen replacement therapy, headaches, heart disease, high blood pressure, Raynaud's phenomenon, smoking, stress

Anorexia Nervosa and Bulimia Nervosa

These two psychiatric conditions involve disturbed eating behavior that may cause irreversible damage to the heart, bones, and teeth and may be life-threatening. Women with these conditions are preoccupied with food and body weight, have poor self-esteem and a distorted body image, and often exercise excessively. Many women alternate between anorexia and bulimia throughout the course of their illness. About half of all people with anorexia develop symptoms of bulimia, and about half of all people with bulimia have histories of anorexia or eventually develop symptoms of anorexia.

What is anorexia nervosa?

People with anorexia have an intense fear of becoming fat and purposely lose weight to the point of starvation. A distorted body image leads anorectic women to perceive themselves as grossly obese despite protruding ribs, sunken cheeks, and the evidence on the scale. Although women with anorexia weigh 85 percent or less of the amount expected for their height and stop menstruating (see amenorrhea) because they lack a critical amount of body fat, they vehemently deny that they are underweight. To lose weight, an anorectic woman may severely restrict the amount of food she eats, and she may use self-induced vomiting or laxatives to purge her system of unwanted calories.

Approximately 5 to 10 percent of people with anorexia die as a result of either starvation or suicide. Most of these deaths are sudden and are probably due to cardiac arrhythmias (irregular heartbeats; see arrhythmia), although some may also be due to coma caused by low blood sugar. Chances of death are highest in anorectic women who lose more than 30 percent of their original weight and in those who rely on purges to enhance their weight loss.

What is bulimia nervosa?

Bulimia nervosa shares many features with anorexia. In bulimia, however, there is no obvious emaciation to signal an eating disorder to the world. Unlike the anorectic, the woman with bulimia is aware that she has a problem but feels compelled to conceal it. People with this condition repeatedly go on eating binges in which they eat vast quantities of food without being able to stop. A person with true bulimia has an eating binge at least twice weekly for 3 months, and

some bulimic women repeat these binges as often as several times a day. This fills the bulimic woman with shame, because in general she fears losing control over her eating behavior.

Thus, once the binge is over, she regains control over her body by ridding her system of the excess calories. Some bulimic women do this by inducing vomiting, either by sticking their fingers down their throat or by taking emetic drugs. Others use laxatives or diuretics. Still other bulimic women may follow a binge with a fast or a period of vigorous exercise. Whatever method is used, the result may be frequent fluctuations in weight but not the kind of severe weight loss seen in anorexia.

The long-term effects of bulimia are less well known than those of anorexia, partly because so many cases of bulimia are successfully hidden. What is known is that the short-term outlook is often fairly good. As many as 7 in 10 patients completing outpatient treatment programs show substantial improvement, although about a quarter relapse within the next 6 months.

Who is likely to develop anorexia or bulimia?

Over 90 percent of people affected by anorexia and bulimia are women, and most of them are white. Anorexia and bulimia are relatively rare problems among African American women and other ethnic minority groups, especially those who have newly immigrated to this country.

Approximately 0.5 to 1 percent of women between the ages of 15 and 30 have anorexia, and 1 to 3 percent of adolescent and college-age women have bulimia. In addition to these clinically recognized conditions, there is a virtual epidemic of "subclinical" eating disorders among American women, many of whom do not meet the strict criteria for anorexia or bulimia but who are nonetheless preoccupied with food and weight. Many of these women diet obsessively and use techniques associated with anorexia and bulimia—such as binging, purging, and fasting, or abusing laxatives, diet pills, and diuretics—to keep their weight under control.

That women account for over 90 percent of the cases of eating disorders is hardly surprising. The culture's emphasis on slenderness in women and their consequent obsession with weight are well known. Eating disorders are rare in cultures where food is scarce or leanness in women is not highly valued. Even in the United States there are ethnic differences in body image and desirable weight. African American women in general do not seem to be as obsessed with thinness as white women are. In a recent survey of teenage girls, 90 percent of white girls said they were dissatisfied with their bodies, and 62 percent had dieted within the past year. Among black teenagers, by contrast, 70 percent said they were satisfied with their bodies, and 64 percent said that it was better to be a little overweight than underweight.

Women have more trouble losing weight than men because they tend to have a higher percentage of body fat to begin with. A healthy woman has as much as 20 to 30 percent body fat, whereas a healthy man has only about 10 to 15 percent. Throughout most of human history this difference gave women a biological advantage during times of famine by allowing them to store the energy needed for pregnancy and breastfeeding. Today, however, it means that men burn calories faster than women and that overweight men tend to lose weight more easily than overweight women. This biological difference accounts in part for women's obsession with diets and weight loss.

There has been a great deal of speculation about just what other factors—besides a cultural emphasis on thinness and the difficulty women have losing pounds—prompt some women to develop eating disorders while other women manage to avoid them. One factor is occupational: eating disorders are common in women whose livelihood depends on thinness or appearance—for example, dancers, models, actresses, gymnasts, figure skaters, long-distance runners, and jockeys. Anorexia and bulimia are also found in young women, many of whom are discovering that their looks are connected with social acceptance and popularity. Most eating disorders begin in adolescence or young adulthood, with peak incidences occurring between 14 and 18, and a girl's genetic makeup, biology, family background, and psychology, as well as ethnicity, play a role in her vulnerability.

Some researchers have proposed that anorectic girls may lose weight in order to deny their sexuality or to avoid adulthood and independence (that is, by way of a regression to a boyish figure and lack of menstrual periods). Others have proposed that girls whose parents don't let them develop their own identities are more likely to develop anorexia as well. Still other researchers have observed that many women with eating disorders are overachievers with high expectations for themselves (and high expectations from parents) and that they have a deep-seated need to control all aspects of their lives. Some evidence even suggests that the tendency to become anorectic may be partially inherited or that some neurological or hormonal imbalance may be involved, though whether this is the cause or the result of the eating disorder is unclear.

Being obese or even slightly overweight can predispose a woman to developing an eating disorder. In almost all cases, women prone to eating disorders begin with a dissatisfaction about body shape which leads to dieting and then malnutrition. It is not uncommon for a young woman to embark on a diet to lose a few pounds only to find herself several months later hospitalized for serious emaciation. This may be due in part to certain physical and psychological consequences of starvation which perpetuate eating disorders. People who have agreed to be starved experimentally have developed many of the symptoms of an eating disorder—including a preoccupation with food, social withdrawal, loss of sex drive, and depression. Experimentally starved people also often binge temporarily when they are at last offered food.

Finally, people who have been through certain emotional and psychological experiences seem particularly likely to develop eating disorders. For example, the onset of eating disorders often coincides with a stressful event such as leaving home or losing a loved one through illness, death, or divorce. Many women with eating disorders suffer from depression or have family members who suffer from depression, although it is still not clear whether the depression is a result or a cause of the eating disorder. About 10 percent of people with anorexia have obsessive-compulsive disorder (see entry), and about half of all people with anorexia and bulimia report having a history of sexual abuse. Anxiety disorders, chemical dependency, and impulsive behaviors such as overspending, shoplifting, sexual promiscuity, substance abuse, and self-mutilation are common in people suffering from bulimia.

What are the symptoms?

Beyond their striking emaciation, many people with anorexia have no obvious symptoms. There are certain attitudes and behaviors that characterize the illness, however. Unlike people who have lost weight or are starving as a result of a medical illness, anorectic women are often proud of their weight loss and complain that they need to lose even more weight. Most anorectic women are physically restless, and some exercise. Obsessed with food, an anorectic may delight in cooking high-calorie treats for family members while abstaining from them herself.

As malnutrition progresses, certain physical symptoms begin to appear, including fatigue, difficulty sleeping, and abdominal discomfort and bloating after eating. Skin often becomes dry, pale, or yellowed, and fine downy hair (lanugo) may grow extensively over the face and arms. Anemia and a low level of white blood cells are common, as are increased blood levels of cholesterol and carotene, a building block for vitamin A.

Other changes reflect the body's response to starvation. Fat stores are depleted, and then skeletal and heart muscles begin to waste away. The metabolism of thyroid hormone changes, slowing the body's metabolism in general and generating symptoms suggestive of hypothyroidism, including intolerance to cold, slowed heartbeat, dry skin, and constipation. Blood pressure may fall, urination may be copious, and life-threatening cardiac arrhythmias may develop, sometimes resulting in sudden death.

Women with anorexia stop menstruating, often before much weight has been lost, and this amenorrhea may persist even after weight is regained, resulting in infertility. In girls who have not yet reached puberty, skeletal growth, physical development, and sexual maturation come to a halt. Unlike many other changes of anorexia, which can be reversed once body weight is restored, a young girl whose bone growth has been halted may never reach her previously anticipated height. Women with anorexia lose a significant amount of bone mass, increasing their risk of bone fracture. Even after they regain weight, bone density continues to be reduced. As a result, any woman who has had anorexia is at risk for developing osteoporosis later in life even if she manages to avoid it in her 20s, which many do not.

Anorectic women who purge may develop other symptoms depending on the mode of purging (self-induced vomiting, laxatives, emetics, or diuretics). These symptoms are also characteristic of bulimia, and result primarily from purging and not from binge eating itself. Chronic vomiting, for example, can lead to irritation, bleeding, and sometimes even tears of the stomach and esophagus, as well as heartburn and swelling of the salivary glands. It can also lead to symptoms of dehydration (such as dizziness, faintness, and thirst) and of electrolyte imbalance (such as muscle cramps and weakness, prickling sensations, copious urination, palpitations, and abnormalities in the heart's electrical activity). Repeatedly exposing teeth to stomach acids can decalcify enamel and lead to irreversible dental erosion. Women who induce vomiting with their fingers may develop characteristic teeth marks on the upper surface of their hands. Abusing ipecac to induce vomiting sometimes can lead to muscle damage and potentially fatal heart damage.

Abusing diuretics or laxatives, particularly stimulant laxatives, can also result in fluid depletion, electrolyte imbalances, and associated symptoms. Other common symptoms of laxative abuse are abdominal cramps, watery diarrhea, and rectal bleeding or prolapse (in which the rectal wall bulges into the back of the vagina because of weakened pelvic muscles). Bowel function usually returns to normal once laxative use stops, although in rare cases chronic laxative abuse can result in a "cathartic colon" that cannot produce bowel movements without stimulation.

For reasons not fully understood, many women with bulimia develop menstrual irregularities or amenorrhea even though they are not underweight.

How are anorexia and bulimia evaluated?

Anorexia is much easier to diagnose than bulimia because the evidence for it is much more obvious. Although anorectic women themselves deny that they have a problem, it is not unusual for them to be brought in for medical attention by a family member. Also, a clinician will probably suspect an eating disorder in any woman with an unexplained weight loss.

To evaluate the condition, the clinician will question the patient about her attitude toward body shape, weight loss, desired weight, and eating and exercise habits, and will often ask her to record the foods eaten over the past 24 hours. Other questions will concern previous weight loss and diets, menstrual history, symptoms of malnutrition, dehydration, and electrolyte imbalance, as well as use of laxatives, diet pills, vomiting, and emetics. A physical examination and various blood tests and other laboratory studies will be done to rule out other possible causes of weight loss and to determine the severity of malnutrition and dehydration.

The procedure is similar if a clinician suspects that the problem may be bulimia, although this eating disorder often escapes detection. A clinician may suspect it in a woman who is preoccupied with weight and food or has a history of frequent weight fluctuations. Other hints are the patient's complaints about symptoms that result from dehydration or electrolyte imbalance or certain telltale signs such as enlarged salivary glands, erosion of dental enamel, or scars on the top of the hand that has been used to induce vomiting. Some women who would be ashamed to volunteer that they have a problem will reluctantly admit that they need help if asked directly.

How are anorexia and bulimia treated?

Treating eating disorders is often a challenge because so many people with anorexia and bulimia deny that they have a problem—and often behave angrily or manipulatively toward those trying to help them. In addition, a successful treatment program not only has to help the patient regain weight and overcome the consequences of malnutrition but also must help her learn to control her abnormal eating behavior and prevent relapse by addressing underlying psychological and family problems. The best way to accomplish all of these goals is a multidisciplinary treatment approach involving a team of clinicians who together can address the medical, nutritional, and psychological aspects of eating disorders.

When it comes to anorexia, this treatment often must take place in a hospital setting—ideally in a psychiatric unit that specializes in treating eating disorders and can monitor any medical problems that develop in the course of treatment. Usually patients can be induced to gain weight with a normal diet, although sometimes they must first be force-fed through an intravenous line or a nasogastric tube. Patients hospitalized for the treatment of anorexia will also be offered psychotherapy, including family therapy (if relevant) and behavioral therapy to suggest more positive ways to achieve weight goals. Many hospitals offer supervised exercise programs as well. There is still no evidence that drugs—even antidepressants in depressed patients—are dramatically effective in treating anorexia, although fluoxetine (Prozac) may help maintain weight gain once it has occurred.

Usually patients are hospitalized until they reach a normal weight, although some anorectic women can gain weight on their own if they have close medical supervision. This is particularly true for those who have relatively few symptoms, who are highly motivated to change, and who have a strong support network at home.

Some women may recover after a single episode of anorexia, though more than half of the others repeatedly relapse or remain chronically underweight. Even after recovery many women remain preoccupied with their weight and still have unusual eating patterns and psychosocial problems. As many as 40 percent of anorectic women develop bulimia, and 15 to 25 percent develop chronic anorexia. The more weight a woman has lost, the older she is, and the longer her symptoms have lasted, the less likely she is to recover fully. Women who have coexisting bulimia are also more likely to have persistent problems.

Bulimia is usually treated on an outpatient basis with some form of psychotherapy. Although there is still limited understanding about which type of therapy works best, evidence to date supports the use of cognitive-behavioral therapy. The behavioral component helps patients monitor and change their eating behavior, and the cognitive component helps them change their attitudes toward weight and eating. In some cases bulimia can also be treated with group or family therapy, and many women with bulimia find that support groups (such as Overeaters Anonymous) can be helpful as well. Any substance abuse problem that coexists with the bulimia must be treated at the same time.

These psychological treatments are often supplemented with antidepressant medications, which seem to reduce symptoms of bulimia even in bulimic women who do not have symptoms of depression per se. Among the drugs effective in decreasing the frequency of binge eating and purging are tricyclic agents (imipramine and desipramine), trazodone (Desyrel), fluoxetine (Prozac), and monoamine oxidase inhibitors (phenelzine and isocarboxazid).

Related entries

Amenorrhea, antidepressants, anxiety disorders, body image, depression, menarche, menstrual cycle disorders, obesity, obsessive-compulsive disorder, psychotherapy, stress, substance abuse, weight tables

Antianxiety Drugs

Until the 1950s, anxiety was treated with any of a number of heavy-duty tranquilizers known as barbiturates. Although the dangers of these drugs—particularly sedation, overdose, and addiction—were well recognized, there was little alternative. Then in the mid-1950s the so-called minor tranquilizers such as Valium came on the scene. These were heralded as a safer, more effective way to combat anxiety. The benzodiazepines in particular quickly became among the most widely prescribed drugs in the United States, especially for women. Tranquilizer consumption—virtually nonexistent in 1955—reached 462,000 pounds in 1958 and 1.5 million pounds just one year later. The majority of these were prescribed for housewives—they were "mother's little helpers," as the popular 1960s song by the Rolling Stones called them.

Although benzodiazepines depress the respiratory system and relax the muscles to a lesser extent than barbiturates, they are sedatives with a strong potential for dependence. Consequently, during the decades following the drugs' introduction, addiction and overdose—especially among women—became a major problem. Current thinking about tranquilizers has consequently shifted to the side of caution, but these drugs still have an important role to play in the treatment of anxiety and panic disorders. Today, however, the preferred drugs for most forms of anxiety are the selective serotonin reuptake inhibitors, drugs also commonly used to treat depression.

Accurate diagnosis and careful prescription are the key to effective treatment, especially in complex cases in which generalized anxiety is accompanied by depression, punctuated by panic attacks, or complicated by obsessive-compulsive disorder.

Finally, whatever type of drug is used to treat anxiety, ultimately it can only relieve symptoms. To address the underlying cause of an anxiety disorder, antianxiety drugs are generally most valuable when used in conjunction with psychotherapy.

Antidepressants

In the 1980s, when Prozac (fluoxetine) and related forms of antidepressants made their appearance, they were heralded by the press, and by some practitioners and patients, as psychiatric cure-alls. The result was a decline in both the diagnosis of anxiety and the prescription of antianxiety drugs, as depression became a more common diagnosis.

Today these drugs—selective serotonin reuptake inhibitors, or SSRIs—are generally the first ones prescribed in the treatment of anxiety. In addition to fluoxetine, these drugs include citalopram (Celexa), paroxetine (Paxil), sertraline (Zoloft), and fluvoxamine (Luvox). In many cases, these drugs will first be prescribed in relatively low doses because they often cause disturbing side effects in women with anxiety—including jitteriness, nausea, insomnia, and even more anxiety. Doses will then be increased gradually to the highest tolerable level.

In many forms of anxiety, SSRIs have to be continued long after symptoms disappear to avoid relapse. This is particularly true in the case of panic disorder. As many as 50 to 75 percent of patients with this form of anxiety disorder eventually relapse after they stop taking medication, and then must be restarted on medication and treated indefinitely. Some women also seem to become habituated to the effects of SSRIs, and as a result, they need to increase the dosage or switch to different drugs.

Other forms of antidepressants, the heterocyclic (formerly called tricyclic) antidepressants (imipramine, desipramine, nortryptiline), can sometimes be helpful for anxiety disorders that are accompanied by panic attacks. A newer antidepressant called venlafaxine (Effexor) is also used to treat generalized anxiety disorder and shows considerable promise in treating both panic disorder and social anxiety disorder as well. Other promising antidepressants—though still not widely studied for the treatment of anxiety disorders—are nefazodone (Serzone) and mirtazapine (Remeron).

Benzodiazepines and other minor tranquilizers

Antianxiety medications used today include the benzodiazepines, such as clonazepam (Klonopin), diazepam (Valium), lorazepam (Ativan), and alprazolam (Xanax). The benzodiazepines are usually prescribed only in low dosages and for limited periods of time because of their potential for side effects, including dependence. A newer antianxiety drug, buspirone (BuSpar), seems to work particularly well at controlling generalized anxiety disorder and to have fewer adverse effects and little addictive potential.

Side effects from benzodiazepines are not common, but poor muscle coordination and control, drowsiness, dizziness, confusion, hallucinations, and decreased sex drive occasionally occur. Alcohol greatly increases the sedative effect of tranquilizers and should be avoided by anyone taking them. Nor should any of these drugs be used by a person operating a motor vehicle or other potentially dangerous machinery.

Some especially agitated patients and older people may become extremely nervous or excited when taking benzodiazepines, in which case the drug must be gradually discontinued. Women who are pregnant or breastfeeding should generally avoid tranquilizers as well. Finally, no matter how low the dosage, all antianxiety drugs should be discontinued gradually to avoid symptoms of withdrawal—such as nervousness, insomnia, nightmares, or seizures.

Beta blockers

Beta blockers are sometimes tried as alternative antianxiety drugs. At this point there is no evidence that they are safer or more effective than benzodiazepines, and they have the added drawback that they can aggravate depression accompanying anxiety.

The one major exception is the particular kind of anxiety attack called stage fright. Beta blockers, if taken about an hour before an anticipated attack, are often effective in preventing the trembling limbs and quavering voice that sometimes afflict performers and public speakers. A woman considering the use of beta blockers for this purpose should try them out at some time prior to the day of the "performance," in case she experiences unwanted side effects. The beta blockers most commonly prescribed to treat anxiety are propranolol (Inderal) and atenolol (Tenormin). Side effects are uncommon, but occasionally beta blockers can cause breathing difficulties in people with asthma, who should use them with caution.

Anticonvulsants

A few drugs generally used to treat seizure disorders may be useful in treating certain anxiety disorders as well. In particular, the epilepsy drug gabapentin (Neurontin) appears to be a useful, and relatively safe, alternative to benzodiazepines in treating generalized anxiety disorder. It can also be used to augment other medications such as the SSRIs. To date, however, the safety of gabapentin in pregnancy has not been established.

Related entries

Alcohol, antidepressants, anxiety disorders, depression, domestic abuse, obsessive-compulsive disorder, panic disorder, phobias, posttraumatic stress disorder, psychosomatic disorders, psychotherapy, stress, substance abuse

Antibiotics

Antibiotics are drugs used to kill or inhibit the growth of disease-causing microorganisms, usually bacteria. They are useless against diseases caused by viruses, however, such as the common cold. Many antibiotics are derived from living bacteria or molds, but a large number of synthetic antibiotics have been developed by drug companies in recent decades.

First used widely during World War II, antibiotics have saved countless lives since the 1940s and have played a major role in our triumph over various contagious childhood diseases, sexually transmitted diseases, pelvic inflammatory disease, and other life-threatening conditions. These include bacterial meningitis (inflammation of the membranes surrounding the brain and spinal cord, caused by infection) and endocarditis (inflammation of the membrane surrounding the interior of the heart, also caused by infection).

The recent resurgence of tuberculosis and other supposedly conquered diseases, however, has cast a shadow over the declarations of victory against all contagious diseases. Many people in the medical community now fear that these "untouchable" infections are due to strains of bacteria that are resistant to antibiotics, and they attribute this problem to the overprescription of antibiotics by doctors and the misuse of antibiotics by patients. In fact, since the mid-1990s, increasing evidence has confirmed the existence of strains of the *Streptococcus pneumonia* bacteria resistant to all available antibiotics—a previously unheard-of phenomenon. The World Health Organization (WHO) has concluded that almost all major infectious diseases are slowly but surely becoming resistant to existing medicines. In a recently issued report, the organization warns that once-curable diseases—ranging from sore throats and ear infections to tuberculosis, malaria, and gonorrhea—are in danger of becoming incurable, even in nations wealthy enough to afford these often expensive drugs. Medical historians add that antibiotics may not have been as powerful as they appeared to be: part of the drop in the rates of contagious diseases may have represented a temporary dip in the natural history of these diseases, something that has occurred spontaneously in the history of medicine many times before the discovery of penicillin.

None of this means that antibiotics do not play a major role in the treatment of disease. But the lesson for us is that antibiotics must be used with caution. They should be prescribed only to treat bacterial and certain fungal infections, and only in very specific cases should they be used as a preventive measure. In addition, patients should be sure to take antibiotics for the exact length of time prescribed, even if symptoms seem to have cleared up.

Women should be aware that antibiotics can produce or aggravate yeast infections because they upset the normal balance of organisms in the vagina. If this becomes a problem during the course of taking an antibiotic, a woman should consult her physician.

Penicillins

The original penicillin was first isolated by Alexander Fleming in 1929, and since then this class of drugs, which includes ampicillin, amoxicillin, and many others, has probably been the most widely used class of antibiotics, prescribed for diseases such as ear infections, pharyngitis, skin infections, and heart infections.

Some patients are allergic to penicillin, and may experience hives or other rashes, diarrhea, nausea, joint pains, fever, swelling, wheezing, or, in rare cases, severe shock. Anyone who has had an allergic reaction to penicillin or one of its relatives should alert her doctor immediately and make sure that this allergy is clearly noted in all her medical records. People who are allergic to one kind of penicillin are usually allergic to other types and occasionally to related antibiotics such as cephalosporins.

Penicillin use during pregnancy is generally considered safe, but any woman who is pregnant or considering pregnancy should discuss possible risks and benefits with her clinician. Because penicillins pass into breast milk and can cause drug sensitivity or even allergy in the infant, they, like all drugs, should generally be used with caution during breastfeeding.

Tetracycline

This class of antibiotics includes tetracycline hydrochloride and a host of other drugs whose scientific names end in "cycline." Tetracycline and various newer formulations are commonly used to treat acne, bronchitis, and certain sexually transmitted diseases (STDs), including chlamydia.

Because tetracycline increases the skin's sensitivity to ultraviolet rays, anyone taking this drug should wear a potent sunscreen outdoors, even in winter, and avoid excessive sun exposure. Also, tetracycline should generally not be taken with milk or other dairy products, which can interfere with its absorption. Supplements of iron, calcium, magnesium, and zinc can also decrease the absorption of tetracycline and so should be taken at least an hour or two before or after each dose of tetracycline.

Tetracycline should never be used by pregnant women or women contemplating pregnancy, because it may cause tooth discoloration or even permanent bone abnormalities in the fetus. Women who have myasthenia gravis or a history of kidney or liver disease should alert a clinician to these conditions before taking tetracycline.

Macrolides

Macrolides work by preventing susceptible bacteria from synthesizing protein. Among the most commonly used drugs in this class are erythromycin, azithromycin (Zithromax), and clarithromycin (Biaxin).

Erythromycin may be prescribed to women who are allergic to penicillins and who cannot take tetracycline because they are pregnant or breastfeeding. It should not be taken with acidic fruits or juices, which can diminish its effectiveness. Anyone who has liver disease or impaired liver function should avoid erythromycin altogether.

Azithromycin is often used to treat bronchitis, strep throat, ear infections, skin infections, and pneumonia, as well as many infections of the reproductive system including cervicitis, urethritis, chancroid, and pelvic inflammatory disease. Because this drug can increase sun sensitivity, women using it should avoid prolonged exposure to sunlight, and should use a sunscreen and wear protective clothing when they can't avoid the sun.

Azithromycin may interfere with certain other drugs, including seizure medications such as carbamazepine (Tegretol), phenytoin (Dilantin), and valproic acid (Depakote, Depakene); asthma medications such as theophylline; anticoagulants such as warfarin (Coumadin); and other antibiotics. For this reason, women should tell their clinician if they are taking any of these drugs before using azithromycin.

Sulfa drugs

The sulfa drugs (for example, Bactrim and Septra) work by inhibiting the growth of bacteria rather than by killing them outright. For fighting streptococcal infections, they represent another alternative for people allergic to penicillins, and they are the drug of choice for urinary tract infections.

Prolonged use of some sulfa drugs can interfere with bone marrow, liver, and kidney function. The changes in kidney function can be minimized by drinking plenty of fluids during the course of the medication. Before taking this drug, a woman should tell her doctor if she has ever developed anemia from the use of a drug and discuss any existing liver or kidney disease.

As with tetracycline, sulfa drugs may cause a rash or sunburn with exposure to ultraviolet light, but this can be minimized with a potent sunscreen. Sulfa drugs generally should not be used during the third trimester of pregnancy because of the risk of jaundice in the newborn.

Cephalosporins

These synthetic antibiotics are often called broad-spectrum antibiotics because they are effective against many different kinds of bacteria. This class of drugs is used for prophylaxis before certain surgical procedures as well as for common respiratory infections. Keflex and Ceclor are commonly prescribed brands.

Before taking cephalosporins, women with colitis, enteritis, or kidney disorders should alert their clinician to this fact. Most antibiotics, but especially the cephalosporins, can in some cases cause a severe form of diarrhea. Many people who are allergic to penicillins are also allergic to cephalosporins. Women who are pregnant or breastfeeding should discuss the risks versus the benefits with their clinician before taking cephalosporins.

Fluoroquinolones

Like the cephalosporins, this relatively new class of antibiotics—which includes the drugs ciprofloxacin (Cipro), levofloxacin (Levaquin), and norfloxacin (Oflox)—can be used to eradicate a wide range of bacteria, including many organisms that have become resistant to older drugs. Fluoroquinolones are effective for urinary tract, bladder, and kidney infections, as well as skin and bone infections, diarrhea, gastroenteritis, and pneumonia.

Fluoroquinolones should be taken on an empty stomach with plenty of water. Some people develop diarrhea, vomiting, or loss of appetite while taking certain fluoroquinolones. Combining them with alcohol or antihistamines, pain medications, narcotics, sedatives, or tranquilizers can depress alertness and reflexes, and can decrease the efficacy of the antibiotic. People with a history of epilepsy, stroke, or kidney disease should be cautious about using these antibiotics. They should not be used during pregnancy or breastfeeding because of severe effects on bone growth in the fetus or infant. Women of reproductive age should make sure they are using contraception while taking these drugs.

Related entries

Birth control, breastfeeding, epilepsy, kidney disorders, prenatal care, stroke, urinary tract infections, vaginitis, yeast infections

Antidepressants

In the past, the most commonly used drugs in treating depression had disturbing side effects that often led people to stop using them. Today, however, the options have increased greatly, allowing many people suffering from depression to find effective and satisfactory treatments.

Selective serotonin reuptake inhibitors (SSRIs)

The first line of attack against depression usually involves one of the selective serotonin reuptake inhibitors (SSRIs), a class of drugs that works by selectively raising levels in the brain of serotonin, the neurotransmitter thought to be most responsible for regulating moods. This class of drugs includes Prozac (fluoxetine), as well as the related drugs Zoloft (sertraline), Paxil (paroxetine), Celexa (citalopram), Luvox (fluvoxamine), and Effexor (venlafaxine). Because of their specificity, SSRIs have far fewer side effects than older antidepressants.

Women tend to have higher drug levels in the body and greater sensitivity to side effects of SSRIs than men. These side effects can include headaches, dizziness, and decreased sexual response—but, contrary to widespread myth, not weight gain. Often side effects can be minimized by starting with lower doses and gradually increasing the dosage over time until the lowest effective dose has been established.

Alternative antidepressants

If SSRIs fail to treat depression or cannot be used, a clinician may occasionally prescribe a heterocyclic antidepressant (HCA) such as imipramine (Tofranil), amitriptyline (Elavil), desipramine (Norpramin), or nortriptyline (Aventyl, Pamelor), as well as the newer agents maprotiline (Ludiomil) and mirtazapine (Remeron). When these fail, the monoamine oxidase inhibitors (MAOIs) phenelzine (Nardil) and isocarboxazid (Marplan) may be prescribed. These drugs often have disturbing side effects, however, including dry mouth, drowsiness, lightheadedness, and weight gain, and cannot be used by people with a variety of other medical conditions.

The new neurotransmitter uptake inhibitor venlafaxine (Effexor) can be used to treat depression, generalized anxiety disorder, or both in cases when the two conditions occur together (see entry on anxiety). Related to the SSRIs, venlafaxine inhibits the reuptake not only of serotonin but also of another neurotransmitter, norepinephrine. Shortages of both of these neurotransmitters are believed to play a role in both depression and anxiety disorders. This drug should not be taken together with any other kind of antidepressant (including herbal antidepressants) and, because it may impair judgment, thinking, and motor skills, should be taken with caution in the early stages of use. Users who suffer from depression may sometimes develop side effects that include dizziness, sleep disturbances, nausea, dry mouth, sweating, and nervousness. Users who suffer from anxiety disorders may experience other side effects as well, including anorexia and constipation.

The prescription antismoking medication buproprion (Wellbutrin, Zyban) can also be used to treat depression. Buproprion should not be used by anyone who has epilepsy or other seizure disorders or who has ever had an eating disorder. The most common side effects of this drug are skin rashes, nausea, migraine headaches, shakiness, and agitation.

Herbal remedies

Women who want to avoid side effects or who prefer treating depression "naturally" are turning increasingly to herbal remedies, most notably St. John's wort—or hypericin, the active chemical contained in this perennial plant. Now widely available over the counter, St. John's wort does appear to have some ability to relieve mild to moderate depression, at least over the short run (long-term safety and effectiveness have not yet been established).

Effectiveness aside, however, St. John's wort should never be used without the supervision of a qualified clinician who is treating the depression. In addition, herbal remedies are notorious for lack of standardization and quality control, and users run the risk of purchasing products that are adulterated or that contain inadequate levels of active ingredients (most of the studies confirming the powers of St. John's wort involved products containing 0.3 percent hypericin extract).

Choosing an antidepressant

To determine the appropriate antidepressant, a woman and her doctor must discuss her individual symptoms of depression, cost considerations, and potential side effects of treatment. Knowing, for example, that Prozac tends to promote weight loss while HCAs tend to cause weight gain may make a difference to many women. Similarly, a woman whose depression involves severe insomnia may do best with an HCA taken at bedtime because these drugs often act as sedatives. And despite the common side effects, a woman whose depression is unrelieved by other antidepressants may benefit from MAOIs taken under the supervision of a psychiatrist.

A woman with both anxiety and depression who is taking antianxiety drugs such as alprazolam (Xanax) should talk with her doctor about switching to an antidepressant. Antianxiety drugs are ineffective in treating depression, and, unlike antidepressants, they can be addictive. Much of the time, taking antidepressants alone will alleviate any associated anxiety.

Whatever antidepressant is eventually prescribed, women should schedule a physician visit within one month after starting treatment so that side effects can be monitored and dosages adjusted accordingly. After that, most women will continue to see their doctor periodically. The decision about when to stop therapy can usually be made jointly by the woman and her doctor.

After a single incident of major depression, it is often possible to stop medications gradually after 6 to 12 months, resuming treatment if symptoms recur. Some doctors feel that long-term medication may be more appropriate for patients who have a history of recurrence, a family history of manic depression, onset of symptoms before age 20, or severe, sudden, or life-threatening symptoms.

Related entries

Antianxiety drugs, anxiety disorders, depression, manic-depressive disorder, psychotherapy

Antiinflammatory Drugs

The redness, swelling, and heat that we call inflammation is part of the body's natural defensive response to infections and certain chronic diseases. Like fever and pain, inflammation is a warning sign that something has gone wrong in a part of the body and needs attention. But inflammation, when excessive, can become a problem in its own right—just as fever and pain can. Antiinflammatory drugs are designed to combat this overzealous response. For example, inflammation in the joints (arthritis) is one of the most common conditions that is treated with nonsteroidal antiinflammatory drugs (NSAIDs). The four principal types of antiinflammatory drugs are aspirin, NSAIDs, COX-2 inhibitors, and corticosteroids.

Aspirin

For most people aspirin is the kindly old lady of the pharmaceutical industry: a mild painkiller at best, a placebo at worst. But contrary to folklore, aspirin (the common name for acetylsalicylic acid) is a versatile and powerful drug. In addition to its ability to relieve inflammation, it can reduce fever, soothe pain, and prevent blood clotting. But because it can also provoke a number of undesirable side effects in some people, aspirin, though not an exotic drug, should still be used with care.

Aspirin's antiinflammatory properties have to do with its ability to inhibit the formation of prostaglandins, hormone-like substances derived from cholesterol. Prostaglandins are thought to promote inflammation and have been implicated in various types of pain, including painful menstrual cramps, some headaches, and other mild aches and pains. At larger doses (up to 10 or 15 5-grain tablets per day) aspirin is an effective and affordable drug for treating rheumatoid arthritis, although it is quickly being supplanted by better options.

The problem with high doses of aspirin, however, is that side effects become much more likely to develop. These can include ulcers, heartburn, nausea, vomiting, ringing in the ears, and kidney damage. More commonly, aspirin's ability to reduce blood clotting can promote bleeding in the gastrointestinal tract, which if prolonged can result in iron-deficiency anemia. In children and teenagers especially, aspirin should be avoided altogether because of the danger of developing Reye's syndrome, a life-threatening illness.

Many people confuse aspirin with another nonprescription painkiller, acetaminophen (Tylenol, Datril), and assume that these can be used interchangeably. Acetaminophen can effectively reduce fever and relieve pain, and it may be preferable for treating those conditions in people who cannot tolerate aspirin. But acetaminophen cannot reduce inflammation and does not inhibit the blood's ability to clot.

The many brand-name products available make it difficult for people to know just what type of analgesic they are taking. Many drug companies would have people believe that their aspirin-containing product has some special ingredient that somehow makes it more potent than regular aspirin. In fact, whether buffered or combined with other ingredients, generic or brand-name, cheap or expensive, aspirin is aspirin. There is no reason not to buy generic aspirin and take it with milk or food to prevent stomach upset.

Because aspirin can produce serious bleeding disorders in newborns, it should generally be avoided by pregnant woman (especially during the last trimester of pregnancy) and by breastfeeding women, except when prescribed for a specific disease. A pregnant woman who has taken high doses of aspirin anytime near her due date should tell her clinician because it could lead to excessive bleeding during childbirth. In some small studies aspirin has been associated with fetal malformations, but this association is controversial.

There are a number of exceptions to the rule about aspirin therapy during pregnancy. One is women who have a little-understood condition called APLA (antiphospholipid antibody) syndrome (see entry). Antiphospholipid antibodies promote blood clotting. Women with APLA syndrome have moderate to high levels of these antibodies in their blood, which may increase their risk of miscarriage and stillbirth. For this reason clinicians may advise women with APLA syndrome to take one 81-gram baby aspirin per day during pregnancy. Another situation in which low-dose aspirin therapy may be used is to prevent preeclampsia in pregnant women with a history of this condition. Aspirin can reduce the risk of preeclampsia in subsequent pregnancies from 20 percent to 2 percent.

Aspirin has many beneficial uses (see colon and rectal cancer, coronary artery disease). It should be avoided, however, by anyone who has a history of ulcers, gastritis, asthma, gout, chronic hives, or a deficiency of vitamin K or the coagulation factor prothrombin or who has a bleeding disorder.

Several other forms of salicylates, the class of drugs to which aspirin belongs, are also available by prescription. Both Salsalate (Disalcid, Amigesic) and choline and magnesium salicylates (Trilisate or generic versions) are effective and relatively inexpensive treatment for the temporary relief of pain associated with rheumatoid arthritis, osteoarthritis, and other forms of arthritis, and for some patients may provide better pain relief than aspirin. Women who are hypersensitive to salicylates should avoid these drugs, and those with peptic ulcers, porphyria, bleeding disorders, or chronic advanced kidney impairment should avoid choline and magnesium salicylates in particular. All salicylates, including aspirin, should never be used together because they can accentuate one another's effects and result in toxic levels of salicylic acid.

Nonsteroidal antiinflammatory drugs (NSAIDs)

Like aspirin, NSAIDs reduce inflammation by inhibiting the synthesis of prostaglandins. Among the NSAIDs now available are sulindac (Clinoril), ibuprofen (Motrin, Rufen, Advil, Nuprin), fenoprofen (Nalfon), naproxen (Naprosyn, Anaprox, Aleve), etodolac (Lodine), flurbiprofen (Ansaid), piroxicam (Feldene), phenylbutazone (Butazolidin), diclofenac (Voltaren), ketoprofen (Orudis), oxaproxin (Daypro), and nabumetone (Relafen).

Originally thought to have relatively few side effects, NSAIDs have been considered a promising alternative to corticosteroids in the treatment of arthritis. It now appears, however, that the doses of NSAIDs necessary to relieve arthritis pain can lead to ulcers and gastrointestinal bleeding in some people. Other side effects can include rashes, wheezing, headaches, mental status changes, liver dysfunction, tinnitus (ringing in the ears), and elevations in blood pressure. There is also some evidence that the NSAID ibuprofen can trigger asthma attacks and may possibly damage kidneys if taken together with diuretics (drugs that promote fluid loss).

Despite the potential side effects, NSAIDs overall are still often preferable to other antiinflammatory drugs. Ibuprofen, sold in both prescription and nonprescription forms, is a good alternative to aspirin and acetaminophen in alleviating pain, fever, menstrual cramps, arthritis, and other inflammatory conditions. The same can be said for naproxen sodium (Naprosyn), a longer-acting NSAID which has become available over the counter in the form of Aleve. Indomethacin (Indocin), available by prescription, seems especially good at soothing arthritis pain and muscle inflammation. Higher doses often relieve premenstrual symptoms such as cramps and migraine headaches. Pain that does not respond to one NSAID sometimes responds to another, so it may take a bit of experimenting before an effective one is found.

COX-2 inhibitors

The latest addition to antiinflammatory options are the COX-2 inhibitors, sometimes referred to as "super aspirin." (This latter term is a misnomer, however, since COX-2 inhibitors neither work exactly like aspirin—for example, they don't interfere with blood clotting—nor are they any more powerful than ordinary aspirin or any other antiinflammatory drug.) Like aspirin and NSAIDs, these drugs relieve fever, pain, and inflammation by blocking inflammation-producing prostaglandins, but, unlike aspirin and NSAIDs, they are less likely to cause stomach irritation, heartburn, bleeding, and ulcers. The first COX-2 inhibitor on the market was celecoxib (Celebrex), later joined by rofecoxib (Vioxx) and valdecoxib (Bextra).

COX stands for cycoloxygenase, a naturally occurring enzyme that helps the body make prostaglandins. This enzyme comes in two forms: COX-1, which helps produce prostaglandins that protect the stomach lining, and COX-2, which helps produce the prostaglandins involved in pain and swelling. Because COX-2 inhibitors target only the COX-2 enzymes, they seem to bypass the "good" COX-1 enzymes and leave the stomach lining intact.

Because of the relatively low risk of side effects, however, many clinicians prescribe COX-2 inhibitors to treat chronic inflammation of many sorts, including inflammation associated with arthritis, acute pain, and menstrual cramps. Some early studies also suggest that these drugs may someday be useful in preventing colon cancer and slowing the progression of Alzheimer's disease.

On the downside, COX-2 inhibitors are no more effective than classic NSAIDS, are still available by prescription only, and remain considerably more expensive than over-the-counter pain relievers. And because long-term effects remain unknown, the FDA requires COX-2 inhibitors to carry the same warning label as NSAIDs about the risk of gastrointestinal problems. As a result, they should be reserved for people who cannot tolerate NSAIDS.

Corticosteroids

The term corticosteroids (also called simply steroids) refers both to hormones produced in the outer layer (cortex) of the adrenal glands—two dissimilarly shaped glands located just above the kidneys—and to modified forms of these hormones that are used as drugs. Two of them, cortisone and hydrocortisone, serve a vast variety of functions in the body, such as regulating fat and water metabolism, helping connective tissue respond to injury, and promoting the conversion of starches into sugars. It is their ability to relieve inflammation, however, that explains much of their popularity as drugs, especially in treating conditions such as asthma, rheumatoid arthritis, lupus, kidney disorders, temporal arteritis, thyroid disorders, and tendinitis and other musculoskeletal disorders (see entries), as well as certain cancers, skin diseases, allergies, bursitis, and adrenal gland disorders. Corticosteroids are also used on a long-term basis after organ transplantations to help prevent rejection of the new organ.

Despite the name, corticosteroids should not be confused with anabolic steroids, substances that mimic the virilizing effects of testosterone and are sometimes used illegally by athletes to build up muscle mass.

Corticosteroids used as medications (which include cortisone, cortisol, hydrocortisone, prednisone, prednisolone, and beclomethasone) are available in topical, tablet, inhalable, eyedrop, nose spray, and injectable forms. The topical preparations, which can be purchased over the counter in low doses, can be used for long periods of time to relieve itching, rashes, and other minor skin irritations. Inhalable forms of corticosteroids, used daily, are very effective in treating asthma, and the nose spray forms help with other symptoms of allergies. Corticosteroid eyedrops can be used for inflammatory eye conditions. Bursitis, tendinitis, or localized arthritis can be relieved with a single injection of a corticosteroid. Additional treatments can be given over a period of months, although to avoid bone and joint damage, injections into an isolated joint or bursa are usually limited to 3 or 4.

Stronger versions of corticosteroids taken by mouth are often necessary to alleviate some of these conditions, but they can produce unpleasant and sometimes serious side effects, particularly when used continuously. These can include bone loss from osteoporosis, muscle and adrenal gland atrophy (wasting away), weight gain, skin thinning, water retention, acne, stretchmarks, cataracts, hypertension, and a characteristic rounding of the face (moon face) and upper back (buffalo hump). Mood swings and insomnia develop in many people taking steroids, and at higher doses some people experience depression and psychosis, as well as menstrual irregularities, manifestations of latent diabetes, headaches, dizziness, predisposition to ulcer, and Cushing syndrome (see entry).

A woman who becomes pregnant while taking corticosteroids should discuss the relative risks and benefits of continuing therapy with her clinician. Because drugs such as prednisone and prednisolone seem to cross the placenta poorly, they are usually considered relatively safe for use during pregnancy—especially for asthma, when the alternative is blocked airways and lack of oxygen. Using inhaled steroids for asthma or other airway disease is also considered safe during pregnancy, as are topical steroids.

Anyone taking corticosteroids on a regular basis should have the dosage carefully monitored by a clinician, since sudden termination of these drugs, even after 2 or 3 weeks of treatment, can result in life-threatening adrenal failure. In fact, for up to a year after long-term steroid treatment has ended, the adrenal glands may not respond appropriately to injury, infection, surgery, or other stress. The symptoms of adrenal insufficiency (as this condition is called) are vomiting, diarrhea, dehydration, and, in rare cases, loss of consciousness and possibly death. For this reason many clinicians advise people who are using or who have recently stopped using corticosteroids to carry with them some form of information about their medication in case emergency treatment becomes necessary. In this eventuality a clinician can administer corticosteroid drugs to compensate for the underfunctioning adrenal glands. Because of potentially compromised adrenal gland function, women using corticosteroids during pregnancy may also require supplemental steroids (stress-dose steroids) during childbirth.

Related entries

Antiphospholipid antibody syndrome, arthritis, asthma, autoimmune disorders, colon and rectal cancer, coronary artery disease, Cushing syndrome, headaches, kidney disorders, lupus, menstrual cramps, musculoskeletal disorders, osteoarthritis, polymyalgia rheumatica, rheumatoid arthritis, skin disorders, temporal arteritis, thyroid disorders

Antiphospholipid Antibody Syndrome

Antiphospholipid antibodies (APLA) syndrome is a rare and recently recognized immune system disorder associated with recurrent miscarriages and blood clots. Antiphospholid antibodies are abnormal proteins that sometimes react with certain phospholipids—substances that play a key role in blood coagulation—and interfere with the normal clotting process.

About 1 to 2 percent of the healthy adult population produces these antibodies, first identified in the 1950s, with no apparent problems. For a very small group of people, however, the antibodies are associated with various health problems and blood abnormalities. Only people who have detectable levels of antiphospholipid antibodies together with these problems are said to have APLA syndrome.

Who is likely to develop APLA syndrome?

Although the exact frequency of occurrence remains unknown, the syndrome appears to be more prevalent in women than in men. It can develop in otherwise healthy individuals (in which case it is called "primary APLA syndrome"), but is frequently associated with other health problems including lupus, rheumatoid arthritis, and scleroderma (see entries). This is related to the fact that somewhere between 30 and 50 percent of all patients with lupus, and a sizable number of patients with other autoimmune disease, have antiphospholipid antibodies.

Often people with both hemolytic anemia and thrombocytopenia (a condition known as Evans syndrome) also have antiphospholipid antibodies and are therefore more likely to have APLA syndrome.

Occasionally an infection or certain medications can also promote the development of the antibodies associated with APLA syndrome, as can certain medications, most commonly the antipsychotic drug chlorpromazine, but also the antiarrhythmic drugs procainamide and quinidine and the antiseizure drug dilantin.

A woman who tests positive for the antiphospholipid antibody but who has no symptoms will not necessarily develop blood clots or other APLA-related problems in the future, but she is at significantly higher risk than someone who does not test positive.

What are the symptoms?

People with APLA syndrome are likely to develop blood clots in various parts of the body, including the lungs (pulmonary embolism) and legs (deep venous thrombosis). Specific symptoms depend on just where these clots develop. For example, blood clots in the lungs may lead to high blood pressure in the blood vessels of the lung (pulmonary hypertension, a rare and potentially fatal condition). A clot in an artery supplying bone may ultimately destroy some of the bone.

Recurrent miscarriages are also common in women with APLA syndrome. These usually occur late in the first trimester (after 10 weeks) or into the second, although stillbirths can occur as well. Other pregnancy complications may include intrauterine growth retardation and preeclampsia, as well as clotting problems after delivery. Often the placenta is unusually small and filled with blood clots.

Other signs and symptoms associated with APLA syndrome are migraine headaches, Raynaud's phenomenon (temporary discoloration of fingers and toes after exposure to cold), vision disturbances, low platelet counts (thrombocytopenia), hemolytic anemia, and, rarely, kidney disease (see entries). A fine lacy rash often appears on the legs, especially after exposure to the cold.

More rarely, serious disorders such as stroke in relatively young people can be associated with APLA syndrome. In fact, about 1 in 5 people under the age of 40 who have strokes or heart attacks with no other risk factors turns out to have this syndrome. In a small number of people, diminished mental abilities—associated with tissue death (infarcts) in multiple areas of the brain—may develop unusually early in life, a condition known as early-onset dementia. Very rarely, and most often in people who have other autoimmune disorders, APLA syndrome may result in kidney failure and other life-threatening changes (multiorgan system failure).

How is the condition evaluated?

A clinician may suspect APLA syndrome in a woman who is having blood clotting problems or recurrent miscarriages and will perform blood tests to detect the presence of either of two different types of antiphospholipid antibodies—the anticardiolipin antibody and the lupus anticoagulant. At least one of these tests must be positive on at least two occasions more than three months apart to be considered valid. Tests for additional blood abnormalities associated with the condition (particularly low platelet counts) will also be performed. Other abnormal lab results, including false positive tests on the VDRL test for syphilis (see entry), increase the likelihood of APLA syndrome. The clinician uses the results from these tests, together with findings from a complete history and physical examination, to exclude other diseases with similar symptoms, including various clotting disorders.

How is APLA syndrome treated?

APLA syndrome usually requires lifetime treatment with anticoagulant medications such as aspirin and warfarin to prevent blood clots. If these are ineffective, the clinician may prescribe high-dose steroids and other drugs that suppress the immune system. In life-threatening situations a procedure called plasmapheresis, which temporarily removes antibodies from the blood, may also be used. Patients who smoke are urged to stop, since smoking is particularly dangerous in this condition as it increases the risk of stroke. Low platelet counts can be treated with steroids such as prednisone, the androgen danazol, high doses of immunoglobulins, or, if these are ineffective, removal of the speen (splenectomy).

During pregnancy, women with APLA syndrome are usually advised to take low doses of aspirin or aspirin and heparin to prevent miscarriage, although researchers still haven't determined whether taking aspirin or aspirin plus heparin is any more effective than taking nothing at all. Occasionally a solution of antibodies normally present in human blood (IVIG) may be administered intravenously as well.

Women who have high levels of anticardiolipin antibody or lupus anticoagulant but no symptoms of APLA syndrome are often advised to take low doses (81 mg per day) of aspirin, although whether or not this approach actually prevents blood clots remains to be proved. Many clinicians will also want to monitor carefully for any signs of blood clots or other problems that may develop.

Related entries

Anemia, circulatory disorders, headaches, kidney disorders, lupus, miscarriage, platelet disorders, Raynaud's disease, rheumatoid arthritis, scleroderma

Anxiety Disorders

Anxiety in common parlance is similar to worry. But the kind of anxiety that concerns physicians takes on large enough proportions to interfere with daily activities and is often accompanied by various physical symptoms.

One way to think of anxiety is to regard it as a fight-or-flight response gone awry. In this involuntary response—which developed in animals as a way to prepare themselves for danger—chemicals called catecholamines stimulate the central nervous system and produce increased alertness, quickened heart rate, and tensed muscles. In anxiety the physical and emotional reactions are identical, except that there is often no obvious or true danger—just the response itself.

Women with anxiety disorders may notice fluctuation of symptoms in conjunction with the menstrual cycle. Some women notice that symptoms worsen just before their menstrual period, although evidence so far is mixed. Some of these changes may be linked to premenstrual syndrome (see entry).

Types of anxiety disorders

Psychiatrists recognize several broad categories of anxiety disorders, including anxiety states (generalized anxiety disorder, panic attacks, and panic disorder), phobias, obsessive-compulsive disorder, and posttraumatic stress disorder.

Generalized anxiety disorder. Unlike the similar emotion of fear, generalized anxiety disorder often involves free-floating anxiety that does not seem to be tied to any particular situation or object. Often generalized anxiety is punctuated by more acute and short-lived panic attacks, but people with this disorder also have less intense, ongoing symptoms that continue apart from the attacks and are not the direct result of some well-defined irrational fear (phobia).

Panic attacks. These are brief, unexpected episodes of intense fear accompanied by various physical symptoms such as heart palpitations, shortness of breath, and dizziness. Panic attacks (see panic disorder) are not just everyday episodes of anxiety or nervousness but overwhelming physiological reactions to threat. In the case of panic attacks, however, the threat exists only in the mind of the individual. Often the attacks are brought on by some kind of extraordinary external stress, including loss of a job, a death in the family, a serious illness or surgery, a divorce, or childbirth.

More than 3 million people in the United States have had a panic attack at some point in their lives. Most people who experience panic attacks do not go on to develop panic disorders. Women are twice as likely as men to have them.

Social anxiety disorder. An extreme form of shyness that may afflict as many as 17 to 19 million Americans (many of them undiagnosed), social anxiety disorder is characterized by phobias (also called phobias of function) that are evoked by the presence of other people. Symptoms can often be traced back to early childhood, although the peak age of onset is between 11 and 15. People with social anxiety disorder are deeply afraid of embarrassing or humiliating themselves in public and therefore avoid social situations as much as possible. Among the more common phobias are fear of blushing (erythrophobia), fear of eating in front of other people, fear of using public restrooms, and fear of speaking in public.

Phobias. Phobias (see entry) consist of irrational, persistent fear and avoidance of an object, image, or situation. They differ from free-floating anxiety in that they are focused on a specific thing or circumstance such as cats, spiders, crowds, airplane travel, elevators, or confinement. Many of the things feared by people with phobias do have genuinely dangerous aspects, but statistically, the odds of being harmed by them are extremely small. People with phobias nevertheless fear these relatively harmless things to such an extent that they are compelled to avoid them or avoid even thinking about them—even though they are often able to admit that this compulsion is irrational. The need to avoid the object or circumstance of fear is often incapacitating and undermines the ability to lead a normal life. Phobias occur more frequently in women than in men, often in the aftermath of a panic attack.

Panic disorder. After a person has experienced a panic attack, she may develop a phobia about having another attack and will avoid situations or places associated with the initial attack. A woman who has had a panic attack while in a supermarket, for example, may no longer be able to shop for groceries, while a woman who panicked once while behind the wheel of a car may believe that she will die if she tries driving again. The combination of this "fear of fear" and recurring panic attacks is called panic disorder (see entry). Panic disorder may seriously interfere with a woman's work and family life, especially with her ability to function independently.

Obsessive-compulsive disorder (OCD). This anxiety disorder is characterized by persistent and repetitive thoughts (obsessions) or actions (compulsions) that appear senseless or destructive—even to the person with OCD—but are extremely difficult to resist. People with this disorder, which is somewhat more prevalent in women than in men, find themselves absorbed by various mental images or rituals—such as meticulously washing their hands dozens of times a day or checking again and again to make sure that a door is locked or the oven is off. The diagnosis of obsessive-compulsive disorder (see entry) is made when repetitive thoughts or actions occupy so much time that they interfere with normal functioning or cause significant distress.

Posttraumatic stress disorder. This anxiety disorder develops after a trauma overwhelms normal biological and psychological defense mechanisms. Characterized by intense and alternating feelings of vulnerability and rage, it can develop in people who have experienced military combat, sexual abuse, earthquakes, floods, fires, accidents, burns, kidnapping, torture, or concentration camps. It can also develop in those who have witnessed violence even though they have not been directly victimized. Common symptoms include flashbacks, nightmares, and hypervigilance.

Probably the most common sources of posttraumatic stress disorder (see entry), and certainly the most common sources in women, are rape, incest, and domestic abuse. All of these traumatic events have the potential to "victimize" a person and produce a sense of helplessness, loss of control, and even the threat of annihilation.

What causes anxiety disorders?

Many mental health professionals believe that all anxiety disorders can be traced back to traumatic or stressful experiences earlier in life which have been unconsciously repressed and then reemerge in the form of anxiety. Sometimes an immediate emotional stress—such as a serious illness, a death, or a divorce—may precipitate an anxiety disorder. There is also growing evidence that a person's biochemistry and genetic makeup play a role, particularly in the origins of panic attacks.

Who is likely to develop an anxiety disorder?

Generalized anxiety affects about twice as many women as men. About a third of all people who have it eventually recover, although men seem to have a somewhat better recovery rate than women.

Panic disorder usually develops in young adults, although no one is immune. There may be a genetic component involved as well, since panic disorder seems to run in families. Women who suffer from panic disorder before or during pregnancy may find that attacks become more frequent or severe after the baby is born. The attacks characteristically worsen within the first 2 or 3 weeks after delivery, often escalating to several panic attacks a day. It is not uncommon for postpartum depression to develop around the same time.

As many of 50 percent of people with OCD report having experienced symptoms before age 15. It is not uncommon for people with depression or anxiety or eating disorders to have symptoms of OCD as well. Pregnancy has the potential to worsen symptoms in women who have OCD before they conceive a baby. In other women, pregnancy may trigger symptoms of OCD where none existed before. After delivery some women seem to develop OCD as a form of postpartum psychiatric disorder (see entry).

Most long-term phobias (other than social phobias) begin in early adulthood. Agoraphobia, for example—literally, "fear of the marketplace," that is, fear of venturing outside the safe confines of one's home—usually begins between the ages of 18 and 35. As many as a third of all people with panic disorders eventually develop agoraphobia, and many also develop irrational fears of specific events or situations (such as crossing bridges) that they think may provoke a panic attack. Phobias of all types are more common in women than in men.

Posttraumatic stress disorder can develop in any person—and may be almost inevitable after certain particularly traumatic experiences—but it occurs most frequently in people who are psychologically or physiologically vulnerable, have suffered physical injury (especially to the head) during the trauma, or who lack social support systems. For this reason children and the elderly are the most frequent victims. Children are particularly vulnerable because neither their physiological nor their psychological functions are fully developed, and both are therefore more likely to be permanently damaged.

What are the symptoms?

Common symptoms of anxiety may occur in any of the anxiety states—generalized anxiety disorder, panic attacks, or panic disorder. In addition to feeling worried or nervous out of proportion to any actual danger, people with anxiety disorders often experience a vague sense of dread about the future and seem to be jumpy, irritable, and impatient. They may also suffer from insomnia and depression.

A variety of physical symptoms may occur, including heart palpitations, trembling, shaking, sweating, shortness of breath, "butterflies" in the stomach, "frog" in the throat, goose bumps, flushing, dry mouth, dizziness, and sharp or squeezing pains in the chest. Heartburn, belching, flatulence, and alternating diarrhea and constipation are also common. Chronic tension can lead to aches and pain in the muscles or joints, as well as headaches, particularly in the upper part of the head. Sleep problems may lead to chronic fatigue, which can jeopardize personal relationships and work performance. Substance abuse is another common problem among people with anxiety disorders, probably because drugs may be seen as a source of relief.

How are these conditions evaluated?

Anxiety disorders are diagnosed in large part by excluding other psychiatric and medical conditions that involve similar symptoms. Although anxiety itself is a symptom of nearly all psychiatric conditions, including depression and full-blown psychosis (loss of touch with reality), most of these disorders have other identifying features that differentiate them.

More difficult is the task of differentiating anxiety disorders from somatization disorder, in which *physical* complaints cannot be traced to any specific physical defect (see psychosomatic disorders). In addition to sharing a number of symptoms—including palpitations, diarrhea, flushing, and sweating—these two disorders overlap in many ways, not the least of which is the fact that anxiety seems to increase a person's sensitivity to bodily sensations and decrease her tolerance for pain.

Anxiety disorders are sometimes confused with physical disorders such as hyperthyroidism. And the heart palpitations characteristic of panic attacks in particular have more than once been misinterpreted by the patient as a heart attack. Usually the correct diagnosis can be made after the completion of appropriate physical and laboratory tests and detailed questioning about the patient's history of depression, anxiety, and any current or previous stressors, including physical and sexual abuse.

How are anxiety disorders treated?

Anxiety disorders are treated with medications called antianxiety drugs (see entry). But because drugs only relieve the symptoms of anxiety without eradicating its underlying cause, they are generally most valuable when used in conjunction with psychotherapy (see entry), especially cognitive-behavioral therapy (CBT).

The most effective forms of psychotherapy for anxiety disorders seem to combine behavior modification with cognitive restructuring, in which maladaptive and fearful thoughts are replaced with more realistic thoughts. Relaxation techniques (including meditation and hypnosis) can teach a person how to gain control over normally involuntary reactions (see alternative therapies). A new treatment for many anxiety disorders involves the concept of mindfulness, which teaches women to notice that they have anxiety and fear but to accept and recognize that the feeling will pass without their acting on it.

Treatment of OCD includes antidepressants or other drug therapy, often in combination with cognitive or other forms of behavioral psychotherapy. Phobias respond to behavioral therapy, together with occasional use of medications. The treatment of posttraumatic stress disorder usually involves behavior modification and cognitive or relationally oriented psychotherapy.

Related entries

Antianxiety drugs, antidepressants, depression, domestic abuse, obsessive-compulsive disorder, panic disorder, personality disorders, phobias, posttraumatic stress disorder, premenstrual syndrome, psychosomatic disorders, psychotherapy, sexual abuse and incest, social anxiety disorder, stress, substance abuse

Aortic Stenosis

In aortic stenosis the valve that separates the heart from the aorta—the main artery leaving the heart—narrows. As a result, the heart has to pump harder to keep the blood flowing

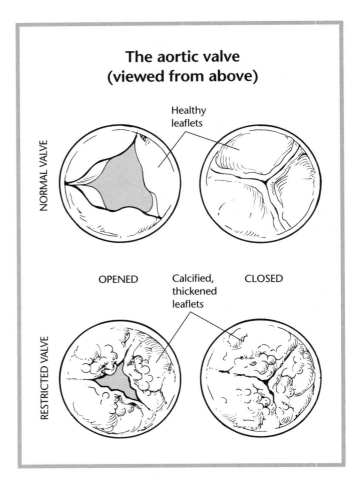

The aortic valve (viewed from above)

NORMAL VALVE

Healthy leaflets

RESTRICTED VALVE

OPENED   Calcified, thickened leaflets   CLOSED

through the valve, and the left ventricle (lower chamber) of the heart eventually becomes thickened and enlarged from its overexertion.

One of several forms of valvular heart disease, aortic stenosis is usually caused either by a congenital abnormality in the aortic valve or by age-related degeneration of the valve. This degeneration involves scarring and the buildup of calcium on the three flaps, or leaflets, of fibrous tissue that normally open and close the aortic valve (see illustration). This calcification, which restricts the size of the opening, tends to occur at an earlier age in women than in men.

Who is likely to develop aortic stenosis?

For reasons still unknown, as women age their valves calcify more quickly than men's. Thus, for the first 70 years of life, men are more likely than women to have aortic stenosis; after the age of 70, however, the condition is more common in women. In either sex symptoms are unlikely to appear before middle age. Occasionally, aortic valve problems (but not necessarily aortic stenosis per se) may occur in women who have had rheumatic heart disease—scarring of the heart valves following infection. This is particularly true in women who have immigrated to the United States from Southeast Asia, South America, or Central America, regions of the world where rheumatic fever, a rare complication of strep infections, is more prevalent.

What are the symptoms?

Because a narrowed aortic valve makes it difficult for the heart to pump blood through the valve and out to the body, various vital organs—not the least of which are the brain and the heart itself—become deprived of oxygen. The symptoms of aortic stenosis reflect this deprivation. For example, when the heart is deprived of blood, chest pain (angina) may result. When the brain is not getting enough oxygen, dizziness or fainting may result. Breathlessness is another common symptom—the body's reaction to its sense that not enough oxygen is reaching life-sustaining organs.

All of these symptoms tend to be most obvious during exercise, when oxygen demands are the highest, but as the condition worsens, they may occur even during rest.

How is the condition evaluated?

A clinician begins by listening to the heart with a stethoscope. If a characteristic murmur is heard, further tests will be done to differentiate aortic stenosis from several less serious conditions. These tests may include a chest x-ray to check for calcification on the valve and the overall size of the heart. An echocardiogram (ultrasound) will be done to inspect the narrowness of the valve. If aortic stenosis seems likely and symptoms are severe, a more invasive procedure, cardiac catheterization, may be necessary to measure how severe the narrowing is. This procedure involves threading a flexible tube (catheter) from the leg into the blood vessels of the heart and then passing a dye through the tube to show the extent of blockage (see coronary artery disease).

How is aortic stenosis treated?

If aortic stenosis is relatively minor, no treatment may be necessary. Most clinicians do recommend avoiding strenuous physical activity and suggest having regular physical examinations and echocardiograms to follow the progression of the condition.

If the valve is more significantly obstructed, or if symptoms have begun to appear, there are medications that can help temporarily. But surgery to replace or reconstruct the valve is the definitive treatment. Without it, people with serious aortic stenosis generally can expect to live only 2 or 3 additional years. Dilating the valve in a procedure using an expanding balloon (see coronary artery disease) does not seem to be as effective as valve surgery in ensuring a longer and more active life.

Abnormal blood flow around a diseased valve allows any tiny clumps of bacteria that may be present to infect the valve more readily. The result can be endocarditis—infection and inflammation of the membrane that covers the interior of the heart. To prevent this, people with aortic stenosis should use antibiotics before dental and certain surgical procedures, and should make sure their dentist is aware of their condition.

Related entries

Angina pectoris, antibiotics, chest pain, coronary artery disease, heart disease, mitral valve prolapse, stroke

Arrhythmia

Abnormalities in the rhythm of the heart are called arrhythmias. They can range in severity from the incidental skipped beat to life-threatening emergencies. If palpitations or other kinds of heart irregularity are noted—and are not easily attributed to strenuous exercise, drinking too much coffee, or emotional upset—a physician should be consulted to rule out a possibly serious medical cause. The good news is that while some arrhythmias can be cause for worry, advances in treating them mean that the prognosis is good in most cases.

The heart's chemical-electrical system regulates the action of its chambers, allowing blood to be pumped efficiently to meet the body's needs. The signal starts in the "pacemaker" area of the heart, the sino-atrial node, or S-A node (see illustration). The S-A node sends out a regular electrical signal, about once a second, prompting other cells in the heart to contract and push blood into the ventricles. At another node, the atrio-ventricular or A-V node, the flow of blood is stopped for a moment, allowing the ventricles to fill with blood, to be pumped on and delivered to the lungs and the rest of the body.

Arrhythmias occur when the signal is interrupted some-

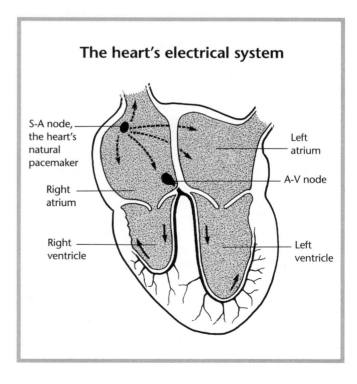

The heart's electrical system

S-A node, the heart's natural pacemaker

Left atrium

Right atrium

A-V node

Right ventricle

Left ventricle

where along this path. Coronary artery disease can reduce the blood supply and lead to the "electrical death" associated with heart attacks. Arrhythmias can also occur when the heart tissue is stretched (as in heart failure), when electrolytes such as potassium in the blood become imbalanced, and when stress or excitement raises the epinephrine levels in the blood. A number of substances (caffeine, alcohol, cocaine) can also cause arrhythmias.

Types of arrhythmias

There are many types, but most fall into the following 6 patterns.

Premature contractions. A thump in the chest is caused by a premature signal arising somewhere in the heart. The chambers contract earlier than normal, breaking step with the regular heartbeat. Infrequent premature contractions are common and do not require treatment; they can be brought on by anxiety or simply by smoking or overindulging in caffeine. They can also occur without any discernible triggering event.

Paroxysmal atrial tachycardia (PAT). Abnormal conduction pathways in the atria cause a fast, regular, often pounding heartbeat accompanied by a feeling of lightheadedness. Common in young, otherwise healthy adults, PAT usually can be treated with lifestyle modification (such as eliminating the use of caffeine, nicotine, and other stimulants and avoiding strenuous exertion) and if necessary with antiarrhythmic drugs.

Ventricular tachycardia (VT). Like PAT, ventricular tachycardia can be characterized by attacks of rapid heartbeat and dizziness, sometimes with chest pain. It can also be silent, and can cause fainting. The patient often describes "a feeling that something bad is going to happen." VT is far more serious than PAT, since it can degenerate into a fatal ventricular fibrillation (see below). This type of arrhythmia almost always occurs together with other serious heart disease. Immediate medical attention is essential.

Atrial fibrillation (AF). Random, chaotic electrical impulses in the atria cause the chambers of the heart to pump inefficiently. The pulse is rapid and irregular. This type of arrhythmia is usually seen in patients with heart disease, although it can occur in otherwise healthy people. If blood clots develop in the heart as a result of AF and break away to travel through the aorta, the consequence can sometimes be a stroke (see entry).

Ventricular fibrillation (VF). This pattern occurs when electrical activity in the ventricles becomes chaotic. The heart muscle tissue does not beat in a coordinated manner. Instead there is a series of localized twitching or writhing movements and no true pumping action. After a few minutes all heart ac-

tivity ceases. VF is frequently the cause of sudden death in patients with heart disease.

Bradycardia. "Brady-" means slow, and "bradycardia" simply means a slow heart beat, strictly defined as a rate slower than 60 beats per minute (bpm). Problems do not usually occur until the heart rate falls below 40 bpm. Many healthy people, especially athletes, have heartbeats well below 60 bpm. But since a slow heart rate can signal inefficient heart action and possible oxygen deprivation to tissues and organs, a visit to the doctor can rule out bradycardia caused by a malfunctioning S-A node or a problem with the A-V node known as a heart block. Certain drugs can also cause bradycardia, particularly in the elderly.

Who is likely to develop arrhythmia?

People with underlying heart disease—particularly coronary artery disease—are more likely to develop arrhythmias. Other factors associated with an increased risk are an enlarged heart for any reason, pregnancy, mitral valve prolapse, and an overactive thyroid gland (see hyperthyroidism). Arrhythmias are also more likely—and can be fatal—in women with severe anorexia nervosa, an eating disorder in which people, usually young women, deliberately starve themselves.

What are the symptoms?

An arrhythmia is often signaled by a racing or pounding heart, especially when the episode begins suddenly in the absence of exertion or emotional upset. The medical term for a racing heartbeat or a single skipped beat is palpitation. Arrhythmias are mostly experienced as palpitations, but because of the reduced supply of oxygen to the brain, they can also be experienced as episodes of fatigue, faintness, or blackout.

How is the condition evaluated?

Once an arrhythmia is suspected, the physician's initial goal is to determine the nature of the irregular heartbeat by ordering an electrocardiogram, or ECG. Because arrhythmias come and go and often elude detection during a visit to the doctor, a lightweight miniaturized electrocardiograph, the Holter monitor, may have to be worn on the belt for 24 hours. This device provides a record that can be analyzed by computer. Devices are also available to monitor heart signals for about a month and submit them to the clinician over the telephone—an ideal way to determine the cause of intermittent palpitations. Very complex rhythm problems may call for electrophysiological testing (in which tiny electrodes are threaded through the veins and planted directly in the heart). This procedure requires hospital admission and is performed by cardiologists with specialized training in this area.

How is arrhythmia treated?

Most arrhythmias requiring a doctor's attention can be treated with drugs called antiarrhythmics, such as digoxin, tocainide, flecainide, propafenone, and amiodarone. Propranolol (a beta blocker) and verapamil (a calcium-channel blocker) are frequently used as well. All of these drugs work by correcting the electrical imbalances that cause the irregular heartbeat.

Permanent pacemakers can correct the slow heartbeat caused by a heart block by overriding the heart's S-A node to initiate regular contractions of the ventricles. A pacemaker is a device about 3 inches square that is implanted under the skin, usually just below the collarbone. It consists of a battery and one or two leads whose tips are positioned in the right side of the heart. Some pacemakers last up to 15 years before having to be replaced.

In the case of ventricular fibrillation, a device similar to a pacemaker called an implantable defibrillator can be used to shock the heart back into normal rhythm. While a pacemaker delivers a mild electric shock, however, implantable defibrillators deliver a powerful burst of electricity, sometimes to the point of pain, to stop life-threatening fibrillation. A defibrillator can prolong the life of many patients with significant heart dysfunction and ventricular arrhythmia by shocking the heart back into a normal rhythm when it detects rhythms that might result in ventricular fibrillation.

How can arrhythmia be prevented?

The best prevention for some arrhythmia is to reduce one's risk factors for coronary artery disease (see entry). Since coffee, alcohol, and cigarettes, as well as extremely low calorie diets, can cause some types of arrhythmias, lifestyle changes in these areas may also be in order.

Recent research suggests that while stress and strong emotions can contribute to an episode of arrhythmia, emotions alone probably do not have a direct cause-and-effect relationship on the incidence of life-threatening rhythm disturbances. Out of every 10 people seen for such an episode, the study suggested, 8 had not experienced any extraordinary emotion, positive or negative, in the 24 hours before their arrhythmia. When there was a link between emotion and arrhythmia, anger was a more likely trigger than fear or grief.

Far more likely to trigger an episode of arrhythmia was extreme fatigue. It seems likely that emotional distress, in conjunction with other factors such as fatigue, may make the heart more susceptible to a sudden spasm in an artery or to a spontaneous abnormality in the action of the heart. But emotions alone do not trigger the arrhythmia. This is comforting news for patients and their families after the diagnosis of heart disease and during recuperation from a heart-related illness. There is no need for family members to "walk on eggshells" or for patients to give up an active life with all its attendant emotions.

Related entries

Angina pectoris, anorexia nervosa and bulimia nervosa, circulatory disorders, coronary artery disease, heart disease, hyperthyroidism, mitral valve prolapse, stress

Arthritis

Arthritis is a general term for a number of different conditions that involve swollen, painful, or stiff joints. The word comes from the Greek words *arthron* for "joint" and *itis* for "inflammation." Joints are the areas in the body connecting bones. Each is cushioned in a layer of connective tissue called cartilage and encased by a fibrous capsule that contains a lubricating substance called synovial fluid. Symptoms arise when various processes such as disease, mechanical wear and tear, or infection cause the synovial tissues to become swollen or inflamed (see illustration). Over time joints can become scarred and deformed.

Types of arthritis

Some forms of arthritis frequently experienced by women include osteoarthritis, rheumatoid arthritis, lupus arthritis, temporomandibular joint syndrome (TMJ), psoriatic arthritis, infectious arthritis, drug-induced arthritis, and, less commonly, gout.

Osteoarthritis. The painful joints characteristic of osteoarthritis (see entry) are due primarily to gradual loss of cartilage rather than inflammation. Cartilage, which normally protects the ends of bones from rubbing against one another, can break down because of physical injury, mechanical stress, or some underlying metabolic abnormality. As a result, bones begin to grate against one another, producing pain and further degeneration. Over time the bones may thicken and additional bone may grow along the sides, producing lumps (bone spurs).

Osteoarthritis tends to occur in joints most exposed to weight-bearing and stress, especially the knees, hips, spine, thumb, joints of the hands, and big toe. One form of osteoarthritis, erosive osteoarthritis of the hands, affects up to 70 percent of women at some point in their lives.

Rheumatoid arthritis. This chronic, progressive disease involves inflammation of the connective tissue, particularly the membranes that line the joints. Inflamed joints are painful, swollen, and warm to the touch. Wrists and knuckles are most commonly affected, but the disease often progresses to the elbows, shoulders, jaw, hips, knees, ankles, and feet. Eventually joints may become permanently deformed.

People with rheumatoid arthritis find that their joints are particularly stiff and achy for over an hour after waking in the morning or after inactivity of any sort. Symptoms usually develop slowly over weeks to months, and tend to come and go with varying severity. Rheumatoid arthritis (see entry) afflicts about 4 percent of women in the United States.

Lupus. This chronic autoimmune disease may involve inflammation not just in the joints but also in the blood ves-

Two common types of arthritis

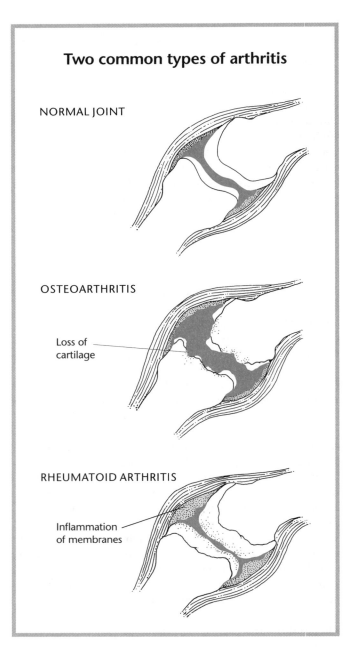

NORMAL JOINT

OSTEOARTHRITIS

Loss of cartilage

RHEUMATOID ARTHRITIS

Inflammation of membranes

most of them women, probably experience some degree of TMJ at some time in their lives. Temporomandibular joint syndrome (see entry) develops in 1 of 5 people with rheumatoid arthritis and is also common in people who have suffered from whiplash, trauma to the face, or emotional stress that leads them to grind their teeth (bruxism) or clench their jaw, particularly during sleep. People with osteoarthritis may experience some of the symptoms of TMJ (such as clicking or snapping jaw sounds) but tend not to have any associated pain.

Psoriatic arthritis. Women with psoriasis (a common skin disease in which areas of skin develop scaly red patches covered with silvery scales; see skin disorders) are more likely than men to develop psoriatic arthritis. In this condition, joints become painful and swollen, particularly the fingers, toes, knees, or elbows. Like most forms of arthritis, this condition is chronic, that is, it persists over a long period of time. In a small percentage of patients the arthritis can occur before the skin symptoms.

Infectious arthritis. This nonchronic form of arthritis can occur when an infectious agent spreads to a joint through the bloodstream or enters the joint directly through an open wound. In other cases, the antibodies that are directed against an infectious organism can cause immune complexes to deposit in the joint and cause arthritis.

Microorganisms that can produce infectious arthritis include those that cause Lyme disease (see entry), tuberculosis, boils, strep throat, gonorrhea, influenza, measles (rubella), mumps, bacterial endocarditis (inflammation of the membrane surrounding the interior of the heart), and hepatitis (inflammation of the liver). Joint pain and inflammation may be accompanied by fever, chills, or weakness. Although most forms of infectious arthritis are equally common in both sexes, gonococcal arthritis and rubella-related arthritis appear more often in women than in men.

Chemically induced arthritis. Joint pain and stiffness can also result from taking certain medications. These include Accutane (used to treat acne), procainamide (used to treat heart arrhythmias), and hydralazine (used to treat hypertension). Procainamide and hydralazine are often the culprits in a disorder known as drug-induced lupus.

How is the condition evaluated?

A clinician can often diagnose arthritic conditions from a patient's history and specific symptoms. A physical examination of joints and certain blood tests can be useful in distinguishing the various arthritic conditions. Fluid surrounding the joint can be removed with a needle and studied in a laboratory. Sometimes x-rays may be done as well to determine or monitor the extent of joint damage. If infectious arthritis resulting from gonorrhea is suspected, a culture may be taken from the cervix for analysis.

sels, heart, lungs, brain, and kidneys. Other symptoms include rashes and fevers after exposure to sunlight; the classic "butterfly" rash across the nose and cheeks; mouth and vaginal sores; chest pain and coughing; headaches; fatigue; disturbances of the central nervous system, including seizures and depression; abdominal pain; and Raynaud's phenomenon, a condition in which fingers turn white and blue after exposure to cold.

Temporomandibular joint syndrome. TMJ is a common disorder of the joint that connects either side of the jawbone to the skull. Between a quarter and a half of all Americans,

Joint stiffness and swelling that come on suddenly need to be evaluated promptly for infection because untreated joint infection can lead to permanent joint damage.

How is arthritis treated?

Treatment depends on the specific process underlying the symptoms. Most forms of chronic inflammatory arthritis are treated with antiinflammatory drugs (see entry), including aspirin, nonsteroidal antiinflammatory drugs (NSAIDS), and COX-2 inhibitors. Many name-brand "arthritis" pills are simply repackaged (and more expensive) forms of regular aspirin and NSAIDs. Chronic arthritis such as rheumatoid arthritis, lupus, and psoriatic arthritis may require stronger medications such as corticosteroids, disease-modifying agents such as methotrexate and hydroxychloroquine, immunosuppressive agents such as leflunomide (Arava), or the "anti-TNF" medications etanercept (Enbrel) and infliximab (Remicade).

Taking aspirin with food can help reduce stomach irritation. For certain types of inflammatory arthritis, if aspirin is ineffective, a doctor may prescribe NSAIDs, and in some cases corticosteroids (another form of antiinflammatory drug). Some patients need to be on long-term therapy with NSAIDs, but anyone taking these drugs for months or years should be under a physician's care to watch for side effects. In some cases a medication called misoprostol (Cytotec) can be taken together with NSAIDs to prevent gastritis and ulcers. Newer antiinflammatory drugs, the COX-2 inhibitors, have less potential for causing gastritis, although they are no more effective for the relief of arthritis pain.

Occasionally a person with arthritis will require hospitalization and surgery so that fluid and damaged tissues can be removed or the cartilage lining the joint can be smoothed. If necessary, the entire joint, such as a hip or knee, can be replaced with a prosthesis (see arthroplasty).

Other forms of treatment include resting the affected joint, immobilizing it with a lightweight splint, and starting individualized physical therapy to improve body alignment and strengthen supporting muscles. Nonstrenuous exercises such as gentle swimming which allow full range of motion to the joints can be helpful, but the specific exercises depend on the nature and location of the arthritis. For some people physical therapy and supervised exercises will provide sufficient relief without the use of any medications.

Some women also find that hot baths, heating pads, or hot water bottles placed on affected joints can relieve pain and swelling. At present there is no evidence that special diets or "miracle cures" such as copper bracelets have any effect on arthritis symptoms.

Related entries

Antiinflammatory drugs, arthroplasty, autoimmune disorders, carpal tunnel syndrome, knee pain, lupus, osteoarthritis, osteoporosis, rheumatoid arthritis, temporomandibular joint syndrome

Arthroplasty

Arthroplasty is a surgical procedure in which a joint (the connection point between bones) is re-formed or replaced. The decision to have joint surgery is based largely on how much pain and limitation of activity a person is experiencing. For example, if joint pain interferes with sleep and if other forms of treatment are not effective, the patient and her physician should probably consider surgery. Also taken into account is the woman's overall health, ability to tolerate the surgery, and willingness to cooperate with a physical therapist during the critical rehabilitation period afterward.

How is arthroplasty performed?

Arthroplasty can involve simple smoothing of the cartilage that lines the joint or a full-scale replacement of the joint with a metallic prosthesis (artificial device) on one side and a plastic prosthesis on the other. The prostheses are sometimes cemented onto the bone. Arthroplasty is usually performed on the hips or knees of people with severe osteoarthritis or rheumatoid arthritis (see illustration p. 62).

In a hip arthroplasty a steel ball on a stem and a polyethylene cup are glued with an acrylic cement onto the top of the femur (thigh bone) and cup of the pelvis, respectively. Some artificial joints are covered with a material that allows bone tissue to grow into it over time. A hybrid procedure is sometimes performed in which the femoral stem alone is cemented.

What happens after the surgery?

The surgery is usually done under general or spinal anesthesia and takes several hours. Hospitalization for several days afterward is required. Generally during this time patients are given medications to prevent blood clots from forming. Physical therapy is an important part of treatment, usually for several months. Afterwards many people who have had hip replacements find that they are able to walk once again and that pain has disappeared. Most patients return to a full, active life. Because of recent improvements in the technology of joint replacement, only 10 to 15 percent of patients now require repair or replacement 10 to 15 years after the initial surgery.

What are the risks and complications?

The outcome of joint replacement surgery is generally excellent. But all surgery entails risks from adverse reactions to general anesthesia, bleeding, and scarring. The major risk of arthroplasty is infection in the joint, and risks increase with each operation. In some patients artificial joints have to be replaced or repaired eventually.

Related entries

Arthritis, carpal tunnel syndrome, knee pain, osteoarthritis, osteoporosis, rheumatoid arthritis

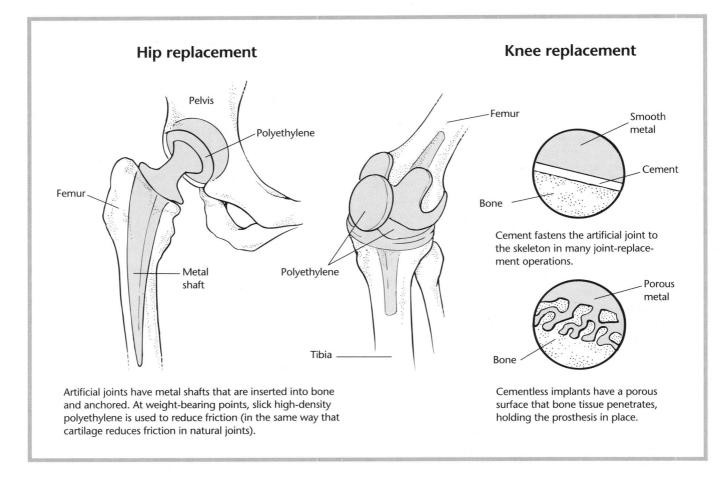

Hip replacement

Pelvis

Polyethylene

Femur

Metal shaft

Polyethylene

Artificial joints have metal shafts that are inserted into bone and anchored. At weight-bearing points, slick high-density polyethylene is used to reduce friction (in the same way that cartilage reduces friction in natural joints).

Knee replacement

Femur

Smooth metal

Cement

Bone

Cement fastens the artificial joint to the skeleton in many joint-replacement operations.

Porous metal

Bone

Tibia

Cementless implants have a porous surface that bone tissue penetrates, holding the prosthesis in place.

Artificial Sweeteners

For decades sugar, particularly refined white sugar, has had a bad name. A host of problems have been attributed to it over the years, including tooth decay, hyperactivity, mood disorders, premenstrual syndrome, yeast infections, and even some forms of cancer. Many of these attributions are overstated if not patently false, and there is no reason for most healthy people to fear the effects of moderate amounts of sugar in their diet. The only disease conclusively linked to sugar is tooth decay, and even here problems arise only when the sugar is consumed frequently or when it is contained in foods that cling to the teeth.

There is no denying, however, that sugar adds calories to the diet, and for people trying to lose weight, sugar can contribute to obesity. For them, as well as for people with diabetes (whose bodies metabolize sugar abnormally), artificial sweeteners may be a desirable way to enjoy otherwise forbidden foods. Chewing artificially sweetened gum may help prevent tooth decay or even retard the spread of preexisting caries.

Are artificial sweeteners effective?

Artificial sweeteners are heavily used in the United States, particularly by women. They can be found in diet soft drinks and many dietetic foods, and are sold for home consumption in supermarkets. Restaurant tables frequently include little packets of artificial sweetener alongside the regular sugar.

It is therefore surprising that so little concrete evidence exists showing that artificial sweeteners actually help people lose weight. A small study of healthy people of normal weight in France did indicate that eating aspartame-laced (or other low-calorie) food at breakfast led to an overall reduction in the number of calories consumed during the day. But in general there is no reason to think that drinking a diet soda or eating artificially sweetened pudding is going to fool the body into thinking it has reached its daily quota of calories. For the most part, artificial sweeteners simply allow people watching their weight to indulge in foods and drinks they would otherwise have to avoid.

The downside of artificial sweeteners is that dieters using them may develop a false sense of security and end up overindulging in some other food. For example, a woman who has a diet soft drink at lunch may feel entitled to an extra slice of pizza or a huge dessert, which more than compensates for any "saved" calories.

Are artificial sweeteners safe?

Despite valiant efforts to prove otherwise, there do not seem to be any particular dangers associated with aspartame (Nutrasweet, Equal), which today is one of the most widely used artificial sweeteners in the United States. Composed of two naturally occurring amino acids (one slightly modified), aspartame is 180 times as sweet as sugar (sucrose), so that the amount equivalent to 1 teaspoonful of sugar contains only 0.1 calorie. Aspartame destabilizes rather easily at high temperatures, however, or after long storage—as anyone knows who has tasted an old Diet Coke.

Early scares linking aspartame to brain tumors appear to be unfounded, and current concerns about potential neurological problems and behavioral disorders occurring in susceptible individuals remain purely anecdotal or theoretical. The only people who must scrupulously avoid aspartame are those with the hereditary disorder phenylketonuria (PKU), which makes them unable to metabolize phenylalanine, a product of the breakdown of aspartame. Some women with interstitial cystitis (see entry) find that aspartame worsens their symptoms, especially the urgency and frequency of urination. The long-term safety of aspartame for pregnant women has never been determined.

Another artificial sweetener, saccharin, is still on the U.S. market, despite efforts to ban it in the late 1960s. The saccharin scare was based on studies linking high levels of saccharin consumption to bladder cancer in laboratory animals. Subsequent epidemiologic studies failed to confirm this link in human beings, however, and saccharin was eventually given a special exemption from the Delaney clause, a federal law that generally bans from the U.S. market all substances known to cause cancer in any species.

Many scientists now believe that saccharin—which is 500 times sweeter than sugar—is generally safe for human consumption. But because the effects on young children are unknown, many experts recommend that it be avoided by children as well as by pregnant and breastfeeding women. The effects of heavy lifetime use of saccharin are also not known, though the same can be said for aspartame.

Yet a third artificial sweetener, acesulfame potassium (Sunette), has recently been introduced into the U.S. market in powder and tablet form. More stable than aspartame, acesulfame potassium is 200 times sweeter than sugar and contains no calories. Although some animal studies indicate that it may have certain toxic effects, the Food and Drug Administration maintains that there is no evidence of toxic effects in humans.

Related entries

Breastfeeding, diabetes, nutrition, obesity, pesticides and organic foods, premenstrual syndrome, urinary tract infections, weight tables, yeast infections

Asthma

Asthma is a chronic airway disease that involves episodic attacks of breathing difficulty, wheezing, coughing, or tightness in the chest. Just what triggers these attacks varies from one person to another, but allergies probably account for the majority of symptoms in people with susceptible airways. Other influences can include cold air, respiratory infections (including colds), smoke and environmental pollutants, sudden changes in temperature or humidity, and strenuous exercise. Only rarely is asthma attributed to emotional or psychological distress, although for many years this was considered one of the prime triggers.

During an asthma attack the muscles tighten around the tubes inside and leading to the lungs (the bronchi), and the lining of the tubes becomes swollen and inflamed. Often thick mucus accumulates in the airways as well (see illustration). In all cases airflow is restricted, and emptying the lungs of air becomes particularly difficult. These attacks can last anywhere from several minutes to several days. Although severely restricted airflow can be life-threatening, in most cases the attacks are mild or moderate. In fact, by avoiding triggers and using appropriate medications, most people with asthma can lead active, healthy lives.

Asthma has become increasingly common in early childhood, affecting as many as 10 percent of all children, probably because of a rise in both outdoor and indoor pollution. Up to the age of 10, boys are twice as likely as girls to have asthma, but by the preteen years the numbers even out. By age 20, as well as throughout the remainder of life, women are about 3 times more likely than men to be diagnosed with asthma. They are also more likely to be hospitalized for asthma and to die of an attack.

Some of the differences in diagnoses are undoubtedly attributable to the greater propensity of women to seek medical attention for any condition. The differences may also be related to the fact that asthma in men is often misdiagnosed as some other respiratory condition, such as chronic obstructive lung disease or emphysema (see breathing disorders). Even so, there is now intriguing evidence that at least some of the explanation for women's susceptibility lies in hormonal differences. About a third of women of reproductive age with asthma note an increase in symptoms just prior to their menstrual period. Also, women frequently have conditions (such as arthritis, menstrual cramps, and headaches) that lead them to use aspirin and other antiinflammatory drugs, which in rare cases may trigger asthma attacks. In addition, women may be exposed more frequently than men to certain inhaled allergens, such as the mites that grow in house dust and other indoor pollutants. Despite the many strides made in sharing household duties, a woman allergic to dust mites still is much more likely to be the one who does the vacuuming than a man with similar susceptibilities.

Clogged airways during an asthma attack

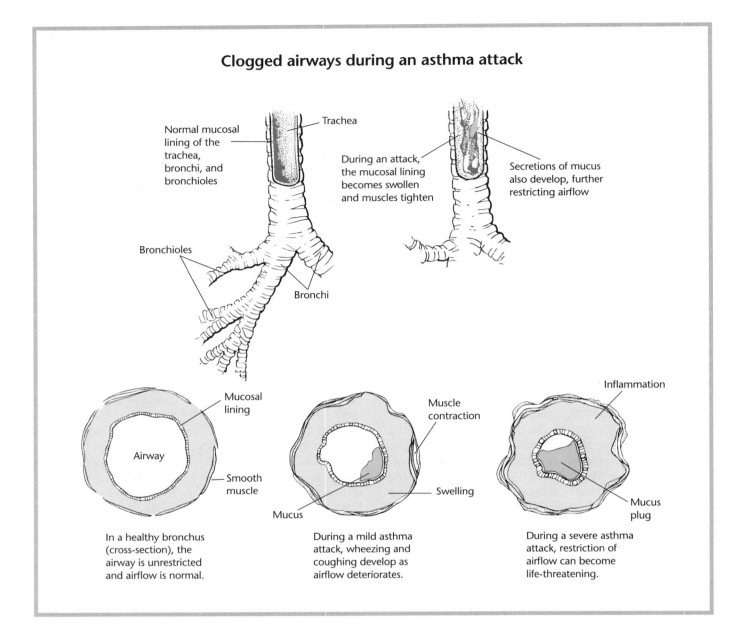

Normal mucosal lining of the trachea, bronchi, and bronchioles

Trachea

During an attack, the mucosal lining becomes swollen and muscles tighten

Secretions of mucus also develop, further restricting airflow

Bronchioles

Bronchi

Mucosal lining

Airway

Smooth muscle

Muscle contraction

Inflammation

Mucus

Swelling

Mucus plug

In a healthy bronchus (cross-section), the airway is unrestricted and airflow is normal.

During a mild asthma attack, wheezing and coughing develop as airflow deteriorates.

During a severe asthma attack, restriction of airflow can become life-threatening.

There is no evidence that asthma attacks become more severe or more frequent during pregnancy, but asthma can pose particular problems for a woman expecting a baby. This is because restricted airflow to the mother can potentially deprive the fetus of oxygen. During pregnancy many women who do not have asthma notice changes in breathing patterns or difficulty breathing because the growing uterus changes the shape of the chest cavity. In pregnant women with asthma, these body changes can make asthma attacks more difficult to control than usual. Still, most women with asthma can expect to stay healthy and have healthy babies if they continue to take their medications under the supervision of a clinician who is aware of their pregnancy.

Who is likely to develop asthma?

The susceptibility to asthma seems to be inherited, although asthma is not necessarily a lifelong condition and can appear at any point in life. In fact, it is not at all uncommon for asthma to appear in women in mid-life or later. People with allergies are particularly likely to develop it at some point. Among the allergens that trigger attacks in people with susceptible airways are dust mites, molds, pollens, animal dander, and certain foods. As much as 8 percent of the population is also allergic to food additives called sulfites (whitening agents), and they may experience an almost immediate asthma attack after eating foods containing these chemicals. Sulfites are often found in dried fruits and vegetables, wine, beer, potatoes, maraschino cherries, dehydrated seafood soups, baking mixes, shrimp, fruit drinks, and certain soft drinks.

Susceptible people exposed to large amounts of smoke (whether from cigarettes or woodburning stoves), gasoline fumes, fresh paint, and other environmental pollutants may have frequent attacks of asthma.

What are the symptoms?

The classic symptoms of an asthma attack are wheezing (noisy breathing), coughing (especially at night), tightness in the chest, shortness of breath, and labored breathing. Symptoms may begin upon exposure to the offending trigger or may develop slowly over many hours. Often attacks develop in the middle of the night. In some people asthma may take the form of a persistent cough alone, with obvious breathing problems occurring only if the cough goes untreated.

How is the condition evaluated?

Usually asthma is diagnosed by a clinician only after several attacks have occurred. Various tests—including pulmonary function tests—can help differentiate asthma from other respiratory diseases. Once asthma has been diagnosed, the clinician may suggest seeing an allergist, who can do skin tests to learn if there are any identifiable allergens underlying the attacks. The clinician may also suggest keeping a diary to help determine if the attacks can be linked to any particular substances or situations.

Many people with asthma also use a simple portable plastic device called a peak flow meter to help monitor and predict asthma attacks. By breathing into this device after inhaling deeply, the user can determine how much air is escaping from her lungs. On days when the reading is considerably lower than normal, a patient can start or increase medication to prevent an impending attack.

How is asthma treated?

Active asthma attacks are usually treated with a short-acting bronchodilator, such as albuterol (Proventil, Ventolin), which opens the airways by relaxing the smooth muscle around the bronchial tubes. In more severe attacks, these medications may be supplemented with corticosteroids such as prednisolone or prednisone, in an inhaled or oral form, to reduce the inflammation that is part of asthma attacks (see antiinflammatory drugs). Because it takes at least 6 hours for corticosteroids to take effect even if inhaled, bronchodilators are used to provide immediate relief of symptoms.

Once the attack is under control, the physician may prescribe maintenance medications, such as cromolyn (Intal), which reduce the chances that the airways will become inflamed. Corticosteroids are usually continued on a maintenance basis, in the inhalable form; long-term treatment with oral steroids is avoided if possible because they are associated with adverse side effects, including an increased risk of cataracts and glaucoma. A new and increasingly popular set of al-

ternatives to corticosteroids—with fewer side effects—are the leukotriene esterase inhibitors such as zafirlukast (Accolate) and montelukast sodium (Singulair), which work by directly attacking the immediate cause of asthma—that is, by keeping airways relaxed and uninflamed. These drugs, taken in tablet form on a daily basis, cannot be used to control an asthma attack already in progress.

Many asthma medications are available in aerosol form and can be inhaled into the lungs in specific amounts through a device called a metered-dose inhaler (see illustration). This inhaler can also be placed into a tube called a spacer, which makes inhalation a little less complicated and is particularly useful to children and older adults. The aerosol inhalers fit inside a purse and should be carried at all times to stave off emergency attacks. Bronchodilators are also available in a solution for use in an electric nebulizer, which produces a mist that the patient breathes through a hand-held inhaler attached by tubing to the machine. The mist may provide added relief at home during prolonged attacks. Bronchodilators can also be taken internally (e.g., as tablets or syrups) if necessary. Although some asthma medications are available over the counter, the condition should first be evaluated by a clinician.

Most asthma drugs are considered safe for use during preg-

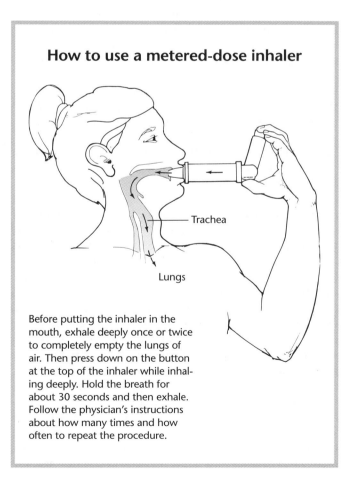

How to use a metered-dose inhaler

Trachea

Lungs

Before putting the inhaler in the mouth, exhale deeply once or twice to completely empty the lungs of air. Then press down on the button at the top of the inhaler while inhaling deeply. Hold the breath for about 30 seconds and then exhale. Follow the physician's instructions about how many times and how often to repeat the procedure.

nancy. If antibiotics are prescribed to treat the upper respiratory infections that can trigger asthma, tetracycline or sulfa drugs should be avoided because of adverse effects on the fetus (see antibiotics). Corticosteroids used in inhaled form are preferred over oral forms during pregnancy, since relatively little of the drug can reach the fetus through this route. But because severe asthma attacks can be life-threatening to the pregnant woman and so potentially damaging to the fetus, systemic steroids are considered an appropriate tradeoff for pregnant women with severe asthma, even though their safety for the fetus has not yet been proved or disproved.

In the past, people with known allergies received desensitization shots to reduce susceptibility to allergens. Today, however, allergists often advocate eliminating or reducing exposure to the allergen as a first course of action, partly because desensitization shots must be taken quite frequently, are not always effective (especially for adults), and are uncomfortable, risky, and expensive.

Anyone with asthma needs to be under the regular care of a clinician. This is because it often takes a good deal of trial and error before the right combination of medications and preventive steps can be determined.

How can asthma be prevented?

Although the underlying physical cause of asthma cannot be prevented, minimizing the frequency of asthma attacks boils down to eliminating or reducing exposure to anything known to trigger them. This is not always easy and is sometimes impossible, in which case the only recourse is heavy reliance on medications. The many asthma attacks that develop for no apparent reason obviously cannot be prevented either. Anyone who suspects certain allergens or environmental sources can try one or more of the following tactics.

See an allergist to have allergy tests. This is an obvious first step to help determine just what substances should be avoided if at all possible.

Minimize dust and other household allergens. Ordinary household dust contains many different materials that trigger asthma attacks, including the feces of dust mites and cockroaches, pet dander, and microscopic fabric fibers. Frequent dusting and vacuuming can minimize dust exposure over the long run, but often these well-intentioned efforts only stir some of the lighter-weight particles into the air, where they are readily inhaled. For this reason, someone other than the allergic person should be assigned these dust-busting tasks—and the allergic person should stay out of the room for at least half an hour after cleaning.

An alternative is to invest in a double-filtered vacuum cleaner or, better yet, a so-called high-efficiency particulate-arresting (HEPA) vacuum cleaner. HEPA air cleaners are a good investment for the bedroom, if not the whole house, because so much time is spent in that room during sleep. Many allergists also recommend more extreme measures such as ripping out carpeting, eliminating all stuffed and upholstered furniture, and removing books and dust-catching knickknacks, but not all people are willing or able to take these steps (nor do they necessarily help). Perhaps a more practical alternative is to cover the affected person's mattress and pillowcase with airtight rubber covers, wipe these down with water on a weekly basis, wash bedding frequently in very hot water, and keep the bedroom in particular as dust-free as possible. If there is a forced-air heating system in the home (which disperses dust even more than other heating systems), it should be equipped with an effective air filter to trap offending particles.

Various steps can be taken against specific allergens found in dust. If dust mites are the problem, for example, agents lethal to the mites, called acaricides, can be applied to carpeting—although these are probably not safe for use in the home of a pregnant woman. A cockroach problem may be reduced by having the house or apartment fumigated regularly by an exterminator. As for animal dander, the best solution is clearly to avoid owning a dog, cat, or other furry pet and to avoid long stays in homes inhabited by these animals. If this is impossible, having someone who is not allergic wash the pet on a weekly basis can be a significant help.

Avoid molds and pollens. Because many of these substances are prevalent only during certain seasons, the best tactic—for those unable to exile themselves temporarily to another climate—may be to stay indoors as much as possible, preferably in a home, car, or office with air-conditioned or filtered air. At all times of the year, shampoos and skin creams should be checked to make sure they do not contain extracts of cottonseed, flaxseed, or other natural substances that are sometimes allergenic. Those who are allergic to mold and dust mites in particular may want to invest in a dehumidifier, since humidity above 20 percent encourages the growth of these organisms. Adding a few drops of chlorine bleach to cut flower arrangements and changing the water daily can also help prevent mold. Also, because soil and water can foster the growth of molds, it is a good idea to keep indoor plants to a minimum. If there is a humidifier in the home, it needs to be cleaned regularly to prevent the growth of molds and other allergens.

Exercise with care. Even though exercise often triggers asthma attacks, there is no reason why people with asthma should have to forgo an activity so important to health and well-being. In fact, regular exercise that develops lung capacity is generally recommended. Just what steps need to be taken to keep exercise safe, however, will vary with the individual.

If exercise itself triggers attacks, it is often sufficient to inhale a bronchodilator before beginning the exercise. If cold or rapid temperature changes trigger attacks, it is best to restrict exercise to places with warm, humidified air (such as swimming pools or gymnasiums). If it is necessary to walk in the cold air, problems can be reduced by wearing a warm scarf or mask around the mouth and nose and breathing through the nose in order to warm, filter, and humidify the air before it reaches the lungs. If pollen plays a role as well as exercise, it makes sense to exercise indoors during allergy season.

Be wary of aspirin and other antiinflammatory drugs. Because many drugs used to reduce pain seem to promote asthma attacks, anyone with asthma should use these drugs with caution until she is certain they do not pose a problem for her. Aspirin (acetylsalicylic acid), which is sold under a variety of brand names, is a common culprit. Other analgesics that often cause problems are ibuprofen (Advil, Nuprin, Motrin, Rufen) and other nonsteroidal antiinflammatory drugs (NSAIDs).

Treat heartburn. Sometimes wheezing and coughing are due to underlying gastroesophageal reflux disease (GERD), more commonly known as heartburn (see entry). For this reason, asthma attacks may dissipate once the heartburn problem has cleared up. Here it is important to note that as many of 75 percent of patients with cough due to GERD do not have symptoms of acid reflux or "heartburn," so if a chronic cough isn't responding to standard asthma treatments, it's worth consulting a clinician about the possibility of GERD.

Avoid smoke and other pollutants. Anyone with asthma should cut out cigarettes and steer clear of other people's smoke—whether it is secondhand smoke from a cigarette or smoke from a woodstove, burning leaves, or an industrial chimney. It is also advisable to stay inside during pollution or ozone alerts in urban areas and to avoid breathing fumes from fresh paint, turpentine, insecticides, deodorants, chlorine, cleaning fluid, and other irritants.

Eliminate foods that cause problems. If the cause is a single food such as peanuts, the problem is relatively easy to avoid. It can be quite an ordeal, however, when the allergy is to eggs, milk, or flour—ingredients that are often hidden in processed foods or foods prepared in restaurants. Anyone who reacts to sulfites needs to be particularly careful in restaurants and should routinely check all labels on packaged foods eaten at home. The Food and Drug Administration (FDA) has banned the use of these agents on fresh fruits and vegetables and made it mandatory for manufacturers to include a notice on labels if "detectable amounts" of sulfites are present in a food product.

Consider getting a flu shot. If asthma is triggered by respiratory infections, it is a good idea to have a flu shot as well as a pneumonia vaccination every year. Other household members might also consider getting flu shots to minimize the chances that they will bring an infection home. If at all possible, contact with people who have viral infections (including colds) should be avoided.

Related entries

Antibiotics, antiinflammatory drugs, breathing disorders, colds, smoking

Autoimmune Disorders

Autoimmune disorders occur when the body produces antibodies or lymphocytes (T cells) that attack its own tissues. Although everyone has a certain number of these "autoantibodies," the numbers are usually too small to cause concern. When these autoantibodies proliferate, internal organ damage can occur and produce a number of diseases, many of which are particularly common in women.

Also intriguing is the suggestion that stress may interfere with immune function. Not only have many people linked stress to a *depressed* immune response—perhaps making people more susceptible to numerous diseases—but also there is some evidence suggesting that stress may *activate* autoantibodies and predispose people to other types of autoimmune disorders.

It is important to remember that our understanding of the interaction among the immune system, the reproductive system, and disease is still evolving. All of these connections, while fascinating, need considerably more exploration.

Female:male ratios in autoimmune diseases

Hashimoto's disease/hypothyroiditis	50:1
Systemic lupus erythematosus	9:1
Sjögren syndrome	9:1
Antiphospholipid syndrome	9:1
Primary biliary cirrhosis	9:1
Mixed connective tissue disease	8:1
Chronic active hepatitis	8:1
Graves' disease/hyperthyroiditis	7:1
Rheumatoid arthritis	4:1
Scleroderma	3:1
Myasthenia gravis	2:1
Multiple sclerosis	2:1
Chronic idiopathic thrombocytopenic purpura	2:1

Source: American Autoimmune Related Diseases Association

Types of autoimmune disorders

The following are some of the many disorders suspected by at least some researchers of being caused by an overactive immune system.

Lupus. This chronic autoimmune disease afflicts 8 to 10 times as many women as men. It may involve inflammation of the joints, blood vessels, heart, lungs, brain, and kidneys. A rash or "mask" over the nose and cheeks in the shape of a butterfly frequently appears in people with lupus (see entry).

The symptoms of the disease are variable and may include painful, swollen joints, particularly in the fingers and wrists; rashes and fevers after exposure to sunlight; inflammation of the membranes around the heart and lungs that can result in chest pain and coughing; fatigue; disturbances of the central nervous system, including headaches and seizures; abdominal pain; and Raynaud's phenomenon, a condition in which fingers turn white and blue after exposure to cold.

Many people with lupus have mild symptoms and require no treatment. Serious complications can result, however, in more advanced cases, including kidney disorders, joint deformity, depression, internal bleeding, reduced resistance to infection, and heart and respiratory problems. Most of the serious complications occur as the result of kidney disease, infection, and heart disease. Kidney disorders occur in about 50 to 70 percent of people with lupus and account for many of the complications and deaths from this disease, although severe kidney disease is much rarer. Complications tend to appear more frequently in African American women with lupus than in other women.

Celiac disease/gluten sensitivity. Celiac disease is an inherited disorder in which the body is sensitive to gluten, the protein contained in wheat, rye, and barley products (see bowel disorders). If this condition is untreated, the body cannot absorb vitamins and minerals from food, potentially resulting in anemia and malnutrition. Symptoms of celiac disease include diarrhea, weight loss, and bloating. Keeping gluten out of the diet is the best way to prevent these symptoms, although on occasion systemic steroids may be necessary.

Hashimoto's thyroiditis. This is an autoimmune disease in which an abnormal antibody destroys the thyroid gland, leading to underproduction of thyroid hormone (hypothyroidism; see entry). Hashimoto's disease is 3 to 5 times more common in women than in men. It can sometimes be acquired later in life after damage to the thyroid gland by radiation therapy.

Graves' disease. In this autoimmune disorder an abnormal antibody stimulates the thyroid to secrete excessive amounts of thyroid hormone. Graves disease is the most common cause of hyperthyroidism (see entry). Symptoms include increased appetite accompanied by weight loss, heat intolerance, insomnia, sweating, hand tremors, heart palpitations, enlarged thyroid gland (a goiter), shortness of breath, mood swings, muscle weakness, bowel disorders such as frequent bowel movements and diarrhea, hyperactivity (or, in elderly patients, apathy), and, though rarely, anorexia and vomiting. Bulging eyes, sometimes severe enough to impair vision, are characteristic. In addition, women often have irregular menstrual periods and fertility problems, including frequent miscarriages. Osteoporosis may develop because thyroid hormone can directly reduce bone density.

Myasthenia gravis. This rare autoimmune disorder occurs most often in women of reproductive age. It is characterized by episodes of muscular weakness; the most common symptoms are drooping eyelids and double vision. Symptoms usually occur following exercise or exertion and improve with rest. Many people with myasthenia gravis (see entry) also go through periods when it is difficult to speak, chew, or even swallow, and they may occasionally have weakness in the arms or legs. If the respiratory muscles are affected, breathing may become difficult as well—a situation that obviously calls for immediate medical attention.

Multiple sclerosis. This often crippling disease of the central nervous system occurs when the fatty protective coating (myelin) that surrounds nerves in the brain and spinal cord is lost and replaced by hardened plaques and scar tissue. Once it is lost, the transmission of messages between the brain and the body is slowed or even blocked completely. The result can be loss of coordination, problems with balance, vision disturbances, bowel or bladder incontinence, and a large number of other symptoms that come and go unpredictably.

Women are almost twice as likely as men to develop multiple sclerosis (see entry). The cause of the disease remains a mystery, but one school of thought is that the body's immune system destroys its own myelin and myelin-making cells. Indeed, people with MS do seem to have abnormally high concentrations of immune cells in their central nervous system. Other researchers contend that these immune dysfunctions may be traceable to some slow-acting virus acquired early in life, which decades later begins to damage either the immune system generally or the myelin directly.

Rheumatoid arthritis. RA is a chronic, progressive disease that involves inflammation of the connective tissue, particularly the membranes that line the joints. The disease causes red, swollen, and painful joints and can also affect internal organs such as the heart, lungs, kidneys, and eyes. Rheumatoid arthritis (see entry) afflicts about 4 percent of women in the United States. Its origins remain unclear, but there is some evidence suggesting that it may be due to an autoimmune reaction in which the body attacks some of its own tissues. Viral infection may also be involved in setting off the disease.

Polymyalgia rheumatica. This connective tissue disorder, which affects people over the age of 50, causes sore muscles and joints, particularly in the neck, shoulders, lower back, and thighs. Unlike the condition polymyositis (see below), polymyalgia rheumatica involves no muscle atrophy or weakness. Other symptoms can include fever, lack of appetite, weight loss, anemia, and apathy. Polymyalgia rheumatica (see entry) generally clears up by itself after a couple of years and is easily treatable. But 15 to 20 percent of people with this disorder also have a more serious condition called temporal arteritis.

Temporal arteritis. This vascular disorder (which affects women more often than men and is mostly seen in older women) involves inflammation of the large blood vessels throughout the body but particularly the temporal region and upper aorta. Some researchers think it may be due to an autoimmune reaction which causes inflammation and destruction of arteries. As a result blood supply is blocked to certain parts of the body, particularly the head and neck. Symptoms include headaches, visual disturbances, jaw achiness, fever, and malaise. Without prompt diagnosis and treatment, temporal arteritis (see entry) can lead to irreversible blindness in one or both eyes.

Polymyositis. Polymyositis is a connective tissue disorder in which muscles become inflamed and weakened. It affects women about twice as often as men. Although the condition has no known cause, there is some speculation that it may be due to autoimmune reactions. Symptoms of polymyositis (see entry) include progressive weakness in hip, shoulder, neck, pelvic, or throat muscles; pain and swelling in the joints; and skin rashes on the eyelids, chest, and hands. There may also be fever, weight loss, and difficulty swallowing. Raynaud's phenomenon—a condition in which fingers or toes turn white and blue after emotional stress or exposure to cold—sometimes occurs, especially when other connective tissue disorders are present as well. When areas of skin become inflamed, this condition is called dermatomyositis.

Chronic fatigue syndrome. CFS is characterized by debilitating fatigue as well as numerous accompanying physical and psychological symptoms. People with this syndrome appear to have an overactive immune system that is chronically waging battle against microorganisms and cells of the individual's own body that are in fact not a threat. This immunological disorder may turn out to be due to some complex relationship between psychological, environmental, and physical factors in susceptible people. For reasons still not understood, chronic fatigue syndrome (see entry) occurs about twice as often in women as in men.

Sjögren syndrome. This common but often misdiagnosed inflammatory disorder occurs when white blood cells (lymphocytes) infiltrate the tear ducts and salivary glands and impair the secretion of saliva and tears. Sjögren syndrome (see entry) can also involve inflammation of other organs such as the kidneys, thyroid, heart, and pancreas. The cause remains unknown, but it is suspected to be an autoimmune disorder. It can be associated with other autoimmune diseases such as rheumatoid arthritis.

Diabetes. Diabetes mellitus comprises a group of disorders characterized by high levels of glucose (sugar) in the blood. All of them result from problems with insulin, a hormone normally produced by the pancreas which removes excess glucose from the blood and causes it to be stored in body cells. Some researchers speculate that diabetes (see entry) may be an autoimmune disorder.

Scleroderma. In this rare condition, which appears about 4 times as frequently in women as in men, affected skin becomes permanently tight, shiny, and hardened. Internal organs may be involved as well, especially the kidneys, lungs, and heart. In some women scleroderma (see entry) causes disturbing cosmetic changes or reduced limb function. Its cause remains unknown, but scleroderma appears to be an autoimmune disorder which triggers overproduction of collagen, causing fibrosis (thickening) in multiple organs. In the CREST syndrome, a more limited form of scleroderma, the skin of the hands and the face is involved, and Raynaud's phenomenon, growths of tiny blood vessels on the face and hands, and difficulty swallowing often develop.

How are these conditions evaluated?

The physician who suspects an autoimmune disorder will complete a detailed history and physical, followed by specific blood tests. The tests assess "auto-antibodies," that is, antibodies produced by the body that attack one's own tissues. Examples include ANA (antinuclear antibody) or anti-double-stranded DNA (for lupus). Other tests may assess function of the target organ, such as TSH to assess indirectly the function of the thyroid gland.

How are autoimmune disorders treated?

Depending on the disease, treatment is focused on first alleviating symptoms and then treating the specific condition. Which medications are used will depend on the patient's particular constellation of symptoms and the organs involved.

Related entries

Anemia, chronic fatigue syndrome, diabetes, estrogen, fatigue, hyperthyroidism, hypothyroidism, infertility, lupus, menstrual cycle, multiple sclerosis, myasthenia gravis, platelet disorders, polymyalgia rheumatica, polymyositis and dermatomyositis, pregnancy, rheumatoid arthritis, scleroderma, Sjögren syndrome, stress, temporal arteritis

Back Pain

Over 80 percent of all Americans can expect to have back pain at some point during their lifetime. Many of them will experience considerable discomfort, disability, and even temporary immobilization. The indirect costs of back pain—which include doctor visits, lost time from work, and disability payments—are estimated to exceed $20 billion each year. On the plus side, the vast majority (up to 90 percent) of back pain disappears on its own within a few days no matter what a person does. This is no guarantee that the pain will not return later—as the many people who suffer from recurrent back pain will be the first to point out.

The backbone itself consists of 24 separate bones (called vertebrae) flexibly hinged together from the base of the skull down through the tailbone and held together by a network of muscles and ligaments. Cushioning the space between each vertebra and the next is a spongy, jelly-filled disk surrounded by a tough, fibrous coating (see illustration). In addition to supporting the weight of the body, the backbone also houses the spinal cord, which runs through the spaces between the vertebrae and serves as the main pathway for the central nervous system. From the spinal cord emerge many different nerve roots, which transmit messages between the brain and every other part of the body. The potential for danger in this complex structure is clearly enormous: a back injury can not only impede movement and weight-bearing ability but also, depending on the location, result in either pain or loss of sensation and paralysis.

Low back pain in particular is quite common in women. Some of this pain is associated with reproductive functions. For example, for many women back pain is a regular part of the monthly menstrual cycle, often occurring during or just before menstruation. A large number of women also develop lower back pain during pregnancy, as well as during childbirth itself. And some women with endometriosis (see entry) develop severe back pain both before and during menstruation.

Other conditions common in women—such as osteoarthritis and osteoporosis (see entries)—frequently involve some degree of back pain. Some women with osteoarthritis develop a kind of spinal stiffness known as spondylosis (also called degenerative joint disease or osteoarthritis of the spine). This disorder develops when disks wear out (owing to mechanical wear and tear or simple aging), with the result that the spaces between vertebrae narrow and are often filled in with bony spurs (osteophytes).

Although back pain can occasionally be due to an infection, a tumor (such as metastasized breast cancer), or an abscess, it is most commonly caused by mechanical pressure on the back resulting from heavy lifting or repetitive strain, or it can simply be a result of aging. Lower back pain in particular is often divided into three basic categories: strains and spasms, herniated disk syndromes, and lumbar spinal stenosis. In the first of these, a movement as simple as a sneeze, sudden twist, or stretch can pull or tear the muscles of the back, resulting in muscle spasms, strain, and pain.

In the case of a herniated disk—also known as a prolapsed, ruptured, or slipped disk—one of the disks cushioning the vertebrae ruptures, and some of the jellylike substance oozes out and presses on a spinal nerve. This often causes a kind of shooting pain called sciatica which radiates through the back of the thigh and down the outer part of the leg (see illustration).

In lumbar spinal stenosis, an overgrowth of bone and other tissue into the spinal canal compresses spinal nerves, resulting in pain, numbness, weakness, and often a feeling of heaviness in the legs, especially after walking.

Who is likely to develop back pain?

Backache is common in people who are obese, as well as in those with poor posture. Strains and spasms are the most common source of back pain among people in their 20s and 30s, and seem to be particularly prevalent in those who work in occupations that involve lifting or exposure to vibration. Although generally more common in men (probably because of work-related strains), mechanical back pain is a common development in the later months of pregnancy and in the first few months after delivery, when weight and body mechanics are not normal and there is extra stress on the back from lifting and carrying the baby.

Herniated disk syndrome most frequently begins in people in their 30s and 40s, with men and women affected about

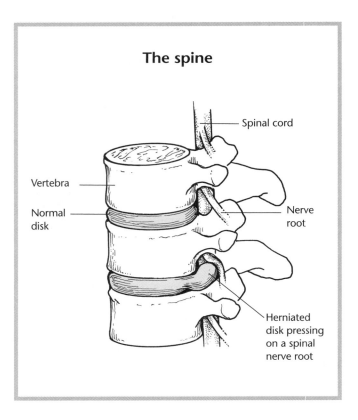

The spine

Spinal cord

Vertebra

Normal disk

Nerve root

Herniated disk pressing on a spinal nerve root

Sciatic pain

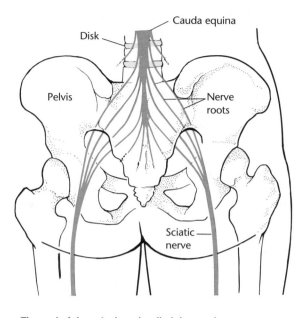

Disk

Cauda equina

Pelvis

Nerve roots

Sciatic nerve

Cauda equina

Vertebra

Lumbar nerve root

Normal disk

Herniated disk compressing a nerve root

The end of the spinal cord, called the *cauda equina,* branches into nerve roots along the lower backbone. Four of these roots thread through the pelvis and merge to form the sciatic nerves that extend down each leg.

In the most common form of sciatica, a ruptured (herniated) disk squeezes a sciatic nerve root against the backbone, causing inflammation and pain.

equally. By contrast, lumbar spinal stenosis seems somewhat more common in women, usually later in life. People who have already had problems with herniated disks also seem to be more susceptible to osteoarthritis of the spine.

What are the symptoms?

Whether attributable to strains, disk problems, or compressed nerves, most mechanical back pain involves a kind of deep aching in the lower spine which may or may not radiate into the buttocks or thighs (usually one side is affected more than the other). Sometimes there may be generalized stiffness as well.

With a herniated disk, shooting pain down the buttocks, thigh, and leg often occurs; it may be present during walking but may also occur after coughing, sneezing, or straining. Sometimes people with a herniated disk have problems with urinary incontinence or, if the disk injury is particularly low in the spine, other kinds of bladder problems and constipation.

Often people with lumbar spinal stenosis have pain, numbness, cramps, or weakness in the buttocks, legs, and feet, especially when they are walking or standing upright. Bending over often relieves the pain, which leads many people with stenosis to stoop.

How is the condition evaluated?

Because most back pain clears up on its own, it is often not necessary to have it evaluated at all. But if symptoms persist for more than a few weeks—or if they are seriously interfering with life, or growing significantly worse, or if a new and seemingly unrelated problem has developed out of the blue—it is probably prudent to consult a clinician for an evaluation and advice.

The evaluation involves first and foremost a careful history (description of the timing and nature of symptoms) and physical examination. Often the patient will be asked to raise and lower her legs from various positions so that the clinician can assess muscle strength as well as sensory and reflex abilities. Occasionally an imaging procedure (such as a CT scan, MRI scan, or, less commonly, a myelogram) may be done if a herniated disk or spinal stenosis is suspected. X-rays of the back are sometimes appropriate (although they tend to be overused) to check for structural problems or diseases of the backbone.

The clinician will also want to distinguish mechanical back pain from rarer, more life-threatening causes of lower back pain such as spinal tumors and infections. This may require certain blood and urine tests, and possibly tests of the arteries in the lower legs to distinguish spinal stenosis from vascular problems (see circulatory disorders). Cancers involving the spine are most likely in people over the age of 50 and in people with a previous history of cancer elsewhere in the body, unexplained weight loss, or back pain that does not resolve after a month. If the pain does not disappear after conservative therapy, and there are other symptoms not related to the back, such as fever, spinal infection is a possibility.

How is back pain treated?

Although back pain is a nagging, debilitating problem for many people, it is encouraging to know that—even without a clear diagnosis, and certainly without surgery or other invasive treatment—approximately 50 percent of mechanical back pain improves after one week, and 90 percent after one month. Even 90 percent of people with sciatica can expect their symptoms to improve after about 6 months, and fewer than 5 percent will go on to have surgery. Spinal stenosis, however, often slowly worsens with time as the underlying degenerative disease in the spine (osteoarthritis) progresses.

No matter what the ultimate cause of the pain, there are a number of simple self-help measures that often provide relief. Chief among these are antiinflammatory drugs (including aspirin), muscle relaxants, and mild exercise to strengthen supporting muscles. A short period of bed rest—1 or 2 days—is helpful for some people. Nonetheless, guidelines issued by the U.S. Department of Health and Human Services caution against bed rest that exceeds 4 days because it can weaken muscles. After 3 or 4 days, when acute pain is improving, many people find considerable relief from low-stress exercises such as biking, walking, and swimming. After a couple of weeks, conditioning exercises that strengthen the trunk can be started. The exercise that helps one person's aching back may end up aggravating another's, however. For this reason, people with back pain should consult a physician or physical therapist before beginning any exercise program—and should expect a period of trial and error before helpful exercises are found.

Some people find that frequent applications of moist heat and gentle massage to the affected area can relieve symptoms, at least temporarily. Sleeping on a firm mattress (or inserting a board beneath a mattress) is a good idea, and when pain is most severe it may help to spend some time lying on the back with legs bent and feet flat on the mattress (or floor), so that the natural curve of the lower back is flattened. If the pain is located in one definable area, corticosteroid injections can provide relief. Sometimes wearing a corset around the lower back—though awkward—may relieve the pain and pressure associated with lumbar spinal stenosis. Other people find that using special chairs and other back support devices provides considerable relief for chronic backaches.

There is no scientific evidence that treatments such as traction, ultrasound, biofeedback, acupuncture, or nerve stimulation provide measurable benefits for back pain. But evidence does suggest that chiropractic manipulation can significantly speed recovery in patients with acute low back pain (see alternative therapies). A study of patients treated for low back pain by primary care physicians, chiropractors, and orthopedic surgeons found that all recovered at the same rate, but chiropractic treatment significantly increased patients' satisfaction with their care (as well as doubling the cost). If initial treatment by a chiropractor does not help, however, U.S. Department of Health and Human Services guidelines recommend that a patient be rechecked by a physician.

If more conservative measures fail, surgery may be the answer for some people—particularly those with severe pain from disk problems. The government guidelines recommend surgery only after the problem has persisted for at least 3 months, unless there is evidence of serious spinal disease.

Surgery often takes the form of laminectomy, an operation in which a surgeon removes the part of the disk or bone that is compressing a nerve. This surgery frequently provides short-term relief, although it has little effect over the long term. As many as 17 percent of patients in one study required a second operation after 4 years, and 30 percent continued to have severe pain. Surgery seems to be more effective when there are no coexisting health problems (including depression and other mental illnesses), and it seems to work better for those who are bothered more by leg pain than by back pain, who have some distinct physical abnormality apparent during an imaging study, and who are not involved in a workers' compensation suit or other litigation that might make an individual more acutely aware of her symptoms.

Women seem to fare worse after surgery than men, according to some studies, perhaps in part because their condition tends to be more severe than men's by the time the decision is made to operate. The delay may reflect women's preference to avoid back surgery as long as possible, or, alternatively, it may represent unequal access to surgical care.

Another strategy for pain relief that can be carried out without making a surgical incision is called percutaneous diskectomy. In this procedure, the surgeon sucks disk material from between the vertebrae using a large probe inserted through the skin. Another nonsurgical alternative involves the injection of chymopapain, an enzyme derived from papaya trees. By dissolving the jellylike substance inside the cushioning disk, chymopapain relieves pressure on adjacent nerves and often eliminates pain. Fears about possible complications associated with these injections, as well as a substantial amount of skepticism on the part of physicians, has led to the abandonment of chymopapain injections by many clinicians in this country. And neither of these procedures will work if the nerve compression is due to something other than disk problems.

How can back pain be prevented?

Many experts believe that some back problems can be prevented—at least to some degree—by developing good habits of standing, sitting, lifting, and sleeping. Maintaining good posture whenever possible is one frequently advocated way to keep back pain from beginning in the first place. Also, people who work at sedentary jobs or spend long periods of time

Some back stretching and strengthening exercises

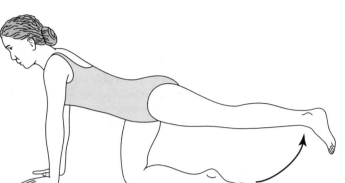

Raise one leg behind, with the knee slightly flexed. Do not arch the neck or back. Repeat 20 times on each side daily.

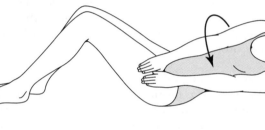

Starting with the back flat on the floor, raise the head and shoulders, rotating to one side as the shoulder blades clear the floor. Repeat 20 times each side daily.

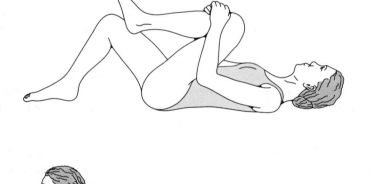

Pull the knee in to the chest until a comfortable stretch is felt in the lower back and buttocks. Repeat 20 times each knee daily.

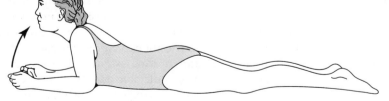

Raise up on the elbows as high as possible, keeping the hips on the floor. Repeat 20 times daily.

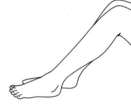

driving should try to take routine breaks to shift position and stretch muscles. Heavy objects should always be hoisted by bending the knees and using the muscles of the thigh rather than the back to lift the load gradually. Whenever possible, people prone to back trouble should avoid carrying heavy objects.

As for sleeping, the best position seems to be lying on the side with knees drawn up somewhat. A person who prefers to sleep on her back should put a pillow underneath her knees and neck. Sleeping on one's stomach should be avoided altogether unless the abdomen is supported by a pillow. Losing weight can reduce the chances of developing back problems, as can wearing low or flat-heeled shoes.

Finally, back pain later in life may be preventable by adopting a short, daily exercise program that increases flexibility of the back and strengthens the shoulder and abdominal muscles (see illustrations). This is especially important for young women with scoliosis (curvature of the spine), which frequently entails both upper and lower back pain. Women who experience low back pain during pregnancy are at higher risk of back pain later in life, and for these women, too, preventive exercises are particularly important.

Related entries

Alternative therapies, circulatory disorders, endometriosis, menstrual cramps, musculoskeletal disorders, obesity, osteoarthritis, osteoporosis, scoliosis

Bacterial Vaginosis

Bacterial vaginosis is the most common form of vaginitis in the United States today. It has gone under various names over the years, including nonspecific vaginitis and gardnerella vaginitis (which itself was formerly known as hemophilus vaginitis or corynebacterium vaginitis, depending on the current name used to describe the organism thought to cause the disease). When it became clear that the *Gardnerella* bacterium was not the only one responsible for this condition, the name was changed to bacterial vaginosis. It is now thought to result from an overgrowth of any of a number of different types of anaerobic bacteria (that is, bacteria that do not require oxygen to live).

There is some conflicting evidence that bacterial vaginosis may be associated with an increased risk of pelvic inflammatory disease, premature labor, and various complications of pregnancy.

Who is likely to develop bacterial vaginosis?

Bacterial vaginosis develops when the microorganisms that normally live in the vagina and protect it from harmful bacteria are disturbed. Many investigators think that the bacteria associated with bacterial vaginosis can be sexually transmitted, though these microorganisms are also often found in the vaginas of women who have never been sexually active.

What are the symptoms?

The bacteria that cause bacterial vaginosis break down compounds of amino acids in the body to produce chemicals called amines. These produce a thin, creamy white or grayish vaginal discharge that can smell fishy. A woman will find that the smell is especially noticeable after washing with soap or having sexual intercourse, for the amines are released into the air whenever they are mixed with alkaline substances such as semen or soap. The vulva and vaginal walls may itch, burn, or become inflamed, but some women with bacterial vaginosis have no irritation whatsoever. In some women, symptoms may fluctuate with the menstrual cycle.

How is the condition evaluated?

The most reliable indicators are "clue cells"—cells from the vagina covered with bacteria—which appear when vaginal discharge is smeared on a slide and examined under a microscope. Clinicians look for other signs of bacterial vaginosis such as an increased amount of vaginal secretion and a decrease in the acidity level of the vagina. Another sign is a fishy odor which develops after some of the vaginal secretions are mixed with a drop of potassium hydroxide, an alkaline substance.

How is bacterial vaginosis treated?

The traditional treatment has been 500 mg of the drug metronidazole (Flagyl or Protostat), taken 2 or 3 times daily for 7 days. This treatment is almost always effective, although it may be accompanied by side effects including nausea, headache, diarrhea, and a metallic taste in the mouth. Alcoholic beverages should be avoided by anyone taking metronidazole, since this combination of drugs can produce abdominal cramps, nausea, vomiting, headaches, and skin flushing.

There is now evidence that metronidazole is effective in larger doses over a shorter period of time (possibly even in a single dose). Another option is metronidazole in the form of a vaginal gel (Metro-Gel). This seems to be just as effective as tablets, with many fewer side effects.

Some women are concerned about using oral metronidazole because it has been shown to cause cancer in mice and rats. To date, however, it has never been linked to cancer in human beings. But because this drug crosses the placenta and can also pass into breast milk, it is considered unsafe for use during the first trimester of pregnancy or during breastfeeding. An equally effective, though more expensive, alternative for pregnant and nursing women, as well as other women who experience intolerable side effects with metronidazole, is the antibiotic clindamycin (Cleocin), available as a cream to be inserted directly into the vagina and as tablets for oral use.

Most clinicians think that bacterial vaginosis can be transmitted sexually. For this reason when a woman has recurrent infections (a common occurrence), her male partner should be treated with oral Flagyl even if he has no symptoms, and condoms should be used (or abstinence practiced) during treatment.

Related entries

Antibiotics, safer sex, vaginitis, yeast infections

Biopsy

A biopsy is the removal of a sample of living tissue for examination under a microscope. There are many different types of biopsy, and they vary considerably in complexity, technique, and amount and type of pain and anesthesia involved.

Skin biopsy. This is one of the quickest, simplest, and most common kinds of biopsy. It involves cutting out the area of skin in question. If the entire abnormality and a bit of surrounding normal tissue are removed, a skin biopsy can often constitute complete treatment as well.

Needle biopsy. This biopsy uses a fine, hollow needle to draw off or edge out fluid and tissue for analysis. Overlying skin is usually desensitized with a topical or local anesthetic. Imaging techniques such as CT scans and ultrasound make it possible for needle biopsies safely and precisely to reach sites well below the surface of the skin.

Surgical biopsy. When a suspicious lump or growth is relatively large, yields equivocal results, or is located too deep within the body for easy or controlled access with a needle, it is usually removed surgically with a scalpel or with the aid of an endoscopic instrument inserted gently into a body cavity.

Punch biopsy. One common form of surgical biopsy used in diagnosing cancer of the vulva, vagina, or cervix is the punch biopsy. This technique involves punching out a sample of tissue with an instrument that resembles a paper punch. Often several punches are necessary, in which case the procedure is called a multiple punch biopsy. Punch biopsies can usually be done without general anesthesia or hospitalization.

The tissue obtained in a biopsy is sliced into thin sections and placed on glass slides, where it is preserved with chemicals and stained with dyes or other contrast agents. These slides are then studied under a microscope by a pathologist. Results are usually available within about 48 hours.

More immediate results can be obtained by examining a tissue sample, called a frozen section, in which a section of tissue is rapidly frozen and stained. The advantage of this procedure is that fast results allow a malignant growth or other abnormality to be removed if necessary while the pa-

tient is still under anesthesia, thus avoiding a second operation. A disadvantage to a frozen section is that the results may lack accuracy, so some clinicians may suggest waiting a few days to consider the results of a biopsy rather than have the biopsy and treatment in one procedure. This can allay the anxiety, too, of undergoing general anesthesia without knowing whether or not another procedure will be performed, and it gives the patient time to discuss the pros and cons of treatment options with her clinician. For many cancers there is little to be lost in waiting a few days or weeks before treatment begins.

Why are biopsies performed?

Although the term biopsy often connotes a search for cancer, biopsies are actually performed to evaluate and diagnose a number of other conditions as well. These include various causes of infertility, anemia, and chronic hepatitis (inflammation of the liver), as well as inflammations of the arteries (see temporal arteritis).

Many unnecessary fears and fantasies about biopsies can be assuaged merely by asking the clinician what the exact purpose of the procedure is. Before scheduling a biopsy, a clinician should tell a patient whether hospitalization will be

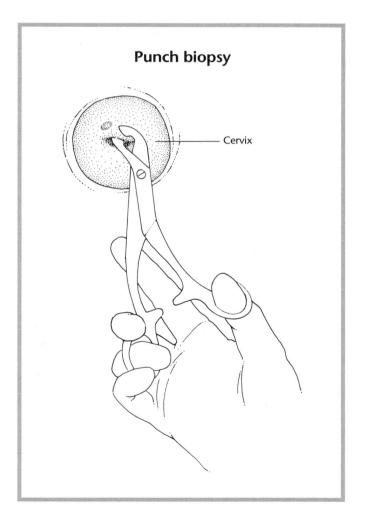

Punch biopsy

Cervix

required or whether the procedure can be performed in the office or at an outpatient surgical facility. The clinician should indicate whether local or general anesthesia will be necessary and if the patient can have any choice in the matter. Finally, a woman can ask about the pros and cons of doing a frozen section and the accuracy of such procedures in the experience of that particular clinician or hospital.

Types of biopsies performed only in women

Cervical biopsy. If a visual examination or a Pap test of the cervix reveals an abnormality, a punch biopsy may be done to remove a tissue sample from one or more locations (see illustration). This is also sometimes done as a follow-up in women who have already been treated for early cervical cancer or for precancerous cell changes in the cervix. Cervical biopsy can usually be done in a clinician's office without anesthesia. Some women experience mild cramping during the biopsy itself and vaginal spotting afterwards.

If the abnormality seems to extend beyond the tip of the cervix, another biopsy called an endocervical curettage may be necessary. In this type of biopsy, which can also be performed as an outpatient procedure, the clinician uses a curette, a thin metal instrument with a spoon-shaped tip, to scrape tissue from the cervical lining. Most women experience mild cramping during this process. There is also a small risk of infection following the procedure.

Colposcopy (see entry)—a technique for examining potentially abnormal areas of the cervix and vagina using a mounted, binocular-like instrument called a colposcope—has made the punch biopsy acceptable for most types of abnormal cervical cells. Sometimes, however, the result of a punch biopsy may contradict findings from a Pap test, or the abnormal area cannot be seen clearly with the colposcope. In such cases, cone biopsies are necessary.

Also known as a cold knife biopsy or conization, a cone biopsy can both diagnose and treat cervical abnormalities. This procedure involves the surgical removal of a cone-shaped wedge of tissue from the lower cervix (see illustration). The surrounding area is then sutured (stitched) or cauterized. Often the cone biopsy removes the suspicious cells (dysplasia) and therefore is itself a cure. If the dysplasia is recurrent or if the clinician finds evidence of pre-invasive cancer in the outer surface of the cervix (carcinoma in situ), hysterectomy may be recommended—particularly if the woman no longer wishes to bear children. If there is evidence of invasive cancer that is confined to the cervix, or cancer has progressed beyond the cervix, additional surgery or radiation therapy may also be considered.

Cone biopsy is relatively expensive and is performed under general or regional anesthesia. About 1 woman in 100 who have a cone biopsy has vaginal bleeding, which can begin up to 2 weeks after the biopsy. A small percentage also experience a narrowed or blocked cervical canal or loss of cervical glands, which in turn may affect fertility by inhibiting the

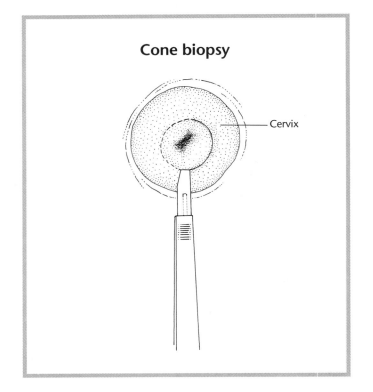

Cone biopsy

Cervix

passage of sperm. Perforation of the uterus and infection are also occasional complications.

Another rare complication during a subsequent pregnancy is cervical incompetence, which occurs if too much tissue has been removed. If untreated, cervical incompetence can increase the odds of miscarriage or premature labor. Also, cone biopsies cause temporary changes in cervical cells which make Pap tests difficult to interpret accurately for 3 or 4 months. For all these reasons, cone biopsies have lost favor in recent years, except in unusual circumstances.

Electrosurgical loop excision (see entry) can often be a simpler alternative to surgical cone biopsy. The procedure (also known as LEEP, which stands for Loop Electrosurgical Excision Procedure) uses a thin wire loop containing a low-voltage, high-frequency electric current to scoop out abnormal tissue from the cervix. As with cone biopsy, tissue can then be examined under a microscope to see if it contains any cancerous cells. LEEP can be performed on an outpatient basis with only a local anesthetic.

Endometrial biopsy. An endometrial biopsy, also called a uterine biopsy, involves the removal of tissue from the uterine lining—the endometrium. It is done to evaluate abnormal vaginal bleeding—to see if it may be caused by conditions such as endometrial cancer, endometrial hyperplasia, or endometrial polyps—and some forms of infertility.

It is accomplished by aspirating or scraping tissue from the uterine lining with a thin instrument which has been inserted into the uterus through the cervix (see illustration). If the tissue is aspirated with a suction device, the procedure is sometimes referred to as a vacuum aspiration (see entry). Usually the biopsy can be done in a clinician's office without anesthesia. Cramping, sometimes severe, may occur for the short time required to remove the tissue.

Vulvar biopsy. A biopsy of the vulva (a woman's external genitalia) is done if there is any lesion or abnormal growth that requires tissue for diagnosis. Usually this can be accomplished in the clinician's office with a small punch biopsy, and only local anesthesia is required. Alternatively, a larger surgical biopsy with either scissors or a scalpel may be needed to cut out deeper tissue.

Because the vulva is richly supplied with blood vessels, bleeding is a common complication of vulvar biopsies. To prevent this, the biopsied area may be treated with either silver nitrate sticks or a paste of ferrous sulfate. Larger areas may require some stitches. In the 7 to 10 days it takes the wound to heal, pain can be relieved by applying a local anesthetic. To avoid infection, regular cleansing and good basic hygiene are essential. A clinician should be contacted immediately if any unusual pain, redness, or swelling develops.

Breast biopsy. A breast biopsy may be done to check for breast cancer after a lump or mass is detected by a clinical exam or mammogram. If a clinician finds the lump or mass during a routine examination, or if the woman finds it herself during a breast self-examination, a mammogram will often

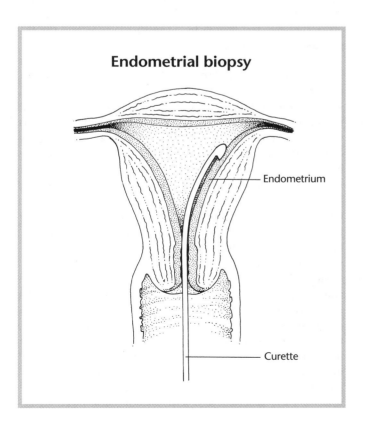

Endometrial biopsy

Endometrium

Curette

be done to make sure there are no other abnormalities in either breast.

Sometimes the first test performed is a needle aspiration, which can be done in a clinician's office with a local anesthetic applied to the overlying skin. In this procedure fluid is removed from the mass and examined under a microscope for abnormal cells. A particularly mobile mass may require several attempts before sufficient fluid can be withdrawn. If the mass is a cyst (and not cancerous), it will often collapse permanently after the fluid is removed (see breast lumps, benign). If the mass does not collapse, if it appears to be solid, or if laboratory analysis of the fluid is ambiguous, a surgical biopsy will be necessary. The suspicious area, along with surrounding tissue, can be removed by making a small cut in the breast. To prevent blood loss, the surgeon must suture or cauterize surrounding blood vessels. Sutures may also be necessary to close the incision itself.

This incisional biopsy of the breast is usually performed in a day surgery setting, often with only local anesthesia. Not so many years ago the standard breast biopsy was done in the hospital under general anesthesia, and a frozen section was analyzed on the spot so that the surgeon could remove the breast immediately if there were signs of cancer. Now that lumpectomy, rather than mastectomy, is often the treatment of choice, this procedure is no longer necessary, and the expense, inconvenience, and anguish often associated with hospital biopsies—and the anxiety of not knowing if one will wake up without a breast—can be avoided. If the woman has a particularly large or extensive lump, the clinician may recommend hospitalization and general anesthesia for the biopsy. The procedure may also require that a thin rubber drain be placed in the wound for a few days.

An alternative to the incisional biopsy that is particularly valuable in diagnosing very small lumps or lumps that cannot be felt is the stereotactic biopsy. In this approach, a radiologist uses a computer and special mammogram x-ray films to target the site of the lump more precisely. Before a stereotactic biopsy, the skin is cleansed and anesthetized. The radiologist then inserts a sterile biopsy needle, and x-rays of the breast are taken to confirm the site of the lump. The entire procedure from start to finish generally takes about an hour, including only about ten minutes of needle insertion (needles generally must be inserted three to five times to obtain enough tissue for analysis). Because the incision is so small, it can be covered with a Band-Aid, and normal activities can usually be resumed immediately.

After the biopsy the clinician will give instructions about how to change dressings over the wound, as well as advice about any restrictions on activity during healing. Even women who have undergone only a needle aspiration or needle biopsy may find that they have some uncomfortable bruising around the area where the needle or scalpel was inserted. Mild painkillers such as Tylenol can often provide relief. Aspirin-containing products should be avoided since they can sometimes increase bleeding.

Related entries

Anesthesia, breast cancer, breast lumps (benign), cervical cancer, cryosurgery, endometrial cancer, hysterectomy, laser surgery, mammography, Pap test, vacuum aspiration, vulvar cancer

Birth Control

In the best possible world, there would be a method of birth control that is not only safe and effective but also easily obtainable, convenient, unobtrusive, reversible, and affordable. Despite years of effort, no such ideal contraceptive has as yet been devised. A wide variety of methods are available today, but none meets all of these criteria, and choosing a method

How safe are the options?

Birth control method	Risk of death in any given year
Hormonal contraceptives	
Nonsmoker	1 in 63,000
Smoker	1 in 16,000
Barrier methods	0
Condoms, diaphragm, cervical cap, or sponge	
Intrauterine devices	1 in 100,000
Sterilization	
Tubal ligation (via laparoscopy)	1 in 67,000
Hysterectomy	1 in 1,600
Vasectomy	1 in 300,000
Natural birth control methods	0
Withdrawal, abstinence, fertility observation	
Abortion	
Illegal	1 in 3,000
Legal	
Before 9 weeks	1 in 500,000
Between 9 and 12 weeks	1 in 67,000
Between 13 and 16 weeks	1 in 23,000
After 16 weeks	1 in 8,700
Pregnancy and childbirth	1 in 14,300

of contraception continues to be a complicated process inevitably involving some degree of compromise.

Among the trade-offs a woman must consider are the method's effectiveness, ease of use, cost, and potential side effects and risks. Many women also consider the role contraceptives might play in reducing the chance of acquiring sexually transmitted diseases (including AIDS) and pelvic inflammatory disease (PID). Others might take into account the fact that a woman's life expectancy is inversely proportional to the number of pregnancies she has. Each woman must balance all of these factors against her personal situation—her overall health, lifestyle, personality, sexual habits, body image, financial situation, home responsibilities, future childbearing plans, and religious and cultural beliefs.

In addition, she must consider that a method which served her well at one point in her life may no longer be suitable later on. For example, the best method for an unmarried teenager who has sexual intercourse intermittently may be very different from that suitable for a young married woman who wants to become pregnant after a year or so, and very different, too, from that of an older woman who definitely does not want to bear any children in the future.

On the plus side, whatever method of birth control is chosen by a sexually active woman, the risks of illness and death resulting from the method itself are far less than those resulting from pregnancy and childbirth (see chart). The only exceptions are among women over 35 who take oral contraceptives and also smoke cigarettes, and, possibly, women who have a hysterectomy. This does not mean that a woman can disregard the possible disadvantages or side effects of any given method, but it does help put into perspective the fear of making the "wrong" choice.

Some women discover in their 30s or 40s, after they stop using birth control, that their fertility has drastically declined owing to natural causes, and that pregnancy is impossible without the assistance of fertility drugs. For women who wish to become pregnant, this discovery can constitute a crisis. Other women come to view their infertility as an asset, especially if they have completed their family. Natural infertility can allow a couple to have a spontaneous sex life without the bother of birth control devices or the risk of pregnancy. Sometimes, however, a woman who became pregnant while taking fertility drugs finds that her natural fertility has returned in the year or so following the birth of a child. This discovery is sometimes made (to either her delight or dismay) when she realizes that she is pregnant again.

Methods of birth control can be roughly divided into several categories: ‣ hormonal contraception (pills, injections, implants, and patches); ‣ barrier methods (condoms, diaphragms, and cervical caps); ‣ spermicides (used with or without other methods); ‣ intrauterine devices (IUDs); ‣ sterilization (tubal ligation and vasectomy); and ‣ "natural" methods (withdrawal or periodic abstinence, with or without fertility observation). When contraception fails, as it sometimes does in practice (see chart), women also have the op-

How effective are the options?

Birth control method	Theoretical effectiveness (%)	Typical effectiveness (%)
Oral contraceptives		
Combined pill	99+	97+
Progestin alone	99+	97+
Other hormonal contraceptives		
Implants (Norplant)	99+	99+
Injections (Depo-Provera)	99+	99+
Patch (Ortho-Evra)	99+	99+
Ring (NuvaRing)	99+	99+
Condoms		
Male without spermicide	98+	88+
Female	98+	88+
Other barrier methods		
Diaphragm with spermicide	94+	82+
Cervical cap	94+	82+
Spermicide alone	97+	79+
Intrauterine devices		
Copper T 380A	99+	99+
Mirena	99+	99+
Sterilization		
Tubal ligation	99+	99+
Vasectomy	99+	99+
Natural birth control		
Periodic abstinence	94+	80+
Withdrawal	96+	82+
No method	15+	15+

tion of terminating the pregnancy (see abortion, nonsurgical abortion, and vacuum aspiration).

Time-honored but ineffective methods of birth control include breastfeeding, douching, and the woman's refraining from orgasm. Breastfeeding does reduce fertility in some women some of the time, but it cannot be counted on as a method of birth control. Douching is even less effective, and female orgasm has no impact one way or the other on the likelihood of conception during intercourse.

Hormonal contraception

With these birth control methods, hormones—given in the form of pills, injections, patches, or implants—interfere with normal ovulation, conception, or implantation. Side effects sometimes include menstrual irregularities, headaches, acne, breast tenderness, weight changes, excess hair growth or hair loss, nausea, and depression. Yet for many women the benefits of hormonal contraception (see entry) far outweigh the disadvantages.

Oral contraceptives. The birth control pill is the most popular method of contraception in the Western world today. In the past, most of the dangers associated with oral contraceptives were due to the high doses of estrogen contained in earlier versions of the pill and were limited to women over the age of 35 who also smoked cigarettes. New and safer formula-

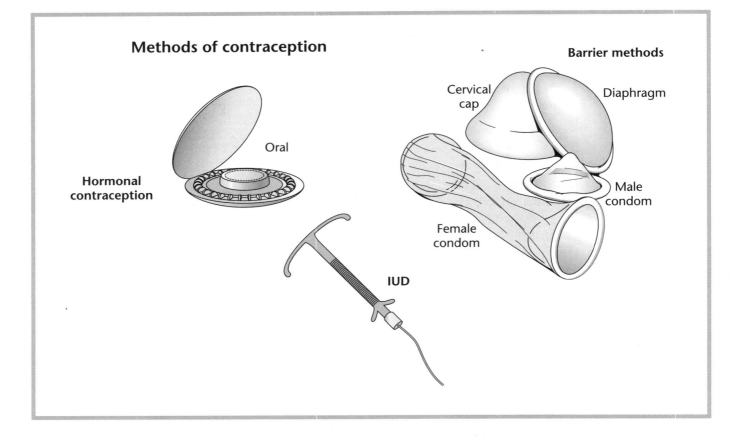

Methods of contraception

Hormonal contraception

Oral

IUD

Barrier methods

Cervical cap

Diaphragm

Female condom

Male condom

tions afford a highly effective and reasonably safe method of birth control for most nonsmoking women up to about menopause.

The pill has other advantages for women. It seems to reduce the chances of developing ovarian and uterine cancers, and it may help protect against benign breast tumors. It also seems to provide a significant degree of protection against pelvic inflammatory disease (PID)—which can cause severe pelvic and abdominal pain as well as infertility—and may help increase bone density when taken by women nearing menopause. Finally, for some women regular use of the pill reduces menstrual cramps and decreases heavy menstrual bleeding. But others experience side effects from oral contraceptives (see entry) which have kept investigators searching for new means of delivery.

Hormone injections. Considered to be an extremely safe and effective method of contraception, the injectable progestin Depo-Provera may circumvent some of the side effects of oral birth control pills since it does not contain estrogen. Moreover, because it is injected by a clinician into a woman's buttocks or upper arm every 3 months, it does not require the woman to think about birth control every day.

Depo-Provera works by preventing ovulation. When taken as scheduled, it is over 99 percent effective, and the contra-ceptive effects are fully reversible once the hormone is eliminated from the body.

Vaginal rings. Approved by the Food and Drug Administration in 2001, the Nuvaring is a flexible plastic ring that steadily emits low levels of hormones. The ring is inserted into the vagina by women at home and is left in place for 3 weeks each month, then removed for one week during menstruation.

One major advantage of the Nuvaring is that it requires no daily motivation for use, and it seems to control the menstrual cycle better than oral contraceptives. About 1 in 4 users, however, continues to have spotting even after the ring-free week, and some women complain that the ring can be felt—and may even fall out—during sexual intercourse.

Contraceptive patch. Another relatively new hormonal form of contraception, Ortho Evra, was approved by the FDA in 2001. It is a medicated adhesive patch that releases hormones into the body after weekly application to the buttocks, upper arm, or upper torso. It is 99 percent effective, although the failure rate is slightly higher in women weighing over 198 pounds.

Ortho Evra has considerable advantages over birth control pills in that it needs to be thought about only once a week. It is also much less likely to result in mid-cycle vaginal bleeding. Other adverse effects, however, are similar to those that occur with other forms of hormonal contraception.

The morning-after pill. In many cases it is possible to prevent conception from occurring even after unprotected intercourse has taken place. In the most effective method, a version of an oral contraceptive is taken in higher than normal doses within 72 hours after unprotected intercourse. Such agents probably prevent conception or implantation by interfering with normal ovulation, slowing the movement of the egg through the fallopian tube, or altering the uterine lining so that implantation is less likely to occur (see hormonal contraception). One method still being investigated involves taking a single dose of the antiprogesterone mifepristone (the "abortion pill" RU-486; see nonsurgical abortion) in the early luteal (second) phase of the menstrual cycle.

It is impossible to measure the efficacy of morning-after pills precisely, simply because no one knows for sure if conception would have occurred if the pills had never been taken in the first place. Still, by most estimates, taking these pills probably reduces the risk of pregnancy after unprotected intercourse by 90 to 95 percent.

Male hormonal contraception. Despite many years of effort, the prospects for finding a safe, effective male contraceptive pill still remain bleak. One of the basic problems is that the mechanisms that lead to sperm production are closely linked to those that control sex drive and potency. Moreover, the motivation in most men to use contraception or risk its side effects is not comparable to most women's. This means that even if an effective male contraceptive became available, women would be able to rely on it only in the closest and most trusting of relationships.

Barrier methods

Diaphragms, cervical caps, and sponges, as well as male and female condoms, physically prevent sperm from gaining access to the woman's reproductive system and fertilizing the egg. When used with spermicides, barrier methods are among the safest and least expensive methods of contraception available, and they may also help reduce a woman's risk of acquiring certain sexually transmitted diseases, pelvic inflammatory disease, and possibly even cervical cancer.

Still, barrier methods have a relatively high failure rate if not used consistently and correctly. They also require a fair amount of regular effort on the part of the woman, as well as cooperation on the part of her partner.

Diaphragm. A round rubber dome that fits inside the vagina and covers the cervix, the diaphragm is meant to be used with a spermicidal cream or jelly. The role of the diaphragm is essentially to hold in place the spermicide, which provides the major share of the contraceptive effect. Some couples are bothered by the feel, taste, or smell of the spermicide, though sometimes this problem can be solved by switching brands or choosing one of the tasteless, odorless versions now available.

Used consistently and correctly, the diaphragm has a failure rate of about 6 percent, but the typical failure rate is closer to 18 percent (see diaphragms and cervical caps). To reduce the risk of pregnancy, some couples use a condom as well as a diaphragm during the most fertile days of the menstrual cycle (around mid-cycle, that is, the time of ovulation).

Cervical cap. A cervical cap is a thimble-like rubber device that is fitted by a clinician to provide an airtight seal over the cervix. Whereas a diaphragm covers the cervix and part of the vaginal walls around it, the much smaller cervical cap fits directly onto the cervix and is held on by suction. The cervical cap requires less spermicide than a diaphragm and can be left in place for a longer period of time. Even the small amount of spermicide used may be enough to help prevent (but not guarantee against) the spread of certain sexually transmitted diseases. The cervical cap can be inserted up to 40 hours before vagina-penis contact. After intercourse, the cap should be left in place at least 6 to 8 hours, which gives the spermicide enough time to kill all the sperm. Although the expected failure rate for the cervical cap is only about 6 percent, the typical failure rate is about 18 percent.

Sponge. Removed from the market in 1995 because of manufacturing problems, the contraceptive sponge has been recently reintroduced. Made of polyurethane and permeated with the spermicide nonoxynol-9, the sponge is inserted into the vagina up to 24 hours before intercourse and appears to work by inactivating sperm with the spermicide, blocking the opening to the cervix, and absorbing and trapping sperm. After being left in the vagina at least 6 to 8 hours after intercourse, the sponge is removed by grasping a ribbon-like loop and then discarded. When used correctly, the sponge has a failure rate of about 10 percent, but the typical failure rate is closer to 15 percent.

Male condom. Also called a rubber, prophylactic, or safe, a male condom is a sheath worn over a man's erect penis to catch sperm and keep them from entering the woman's vagina. In addition to being a relatively effective means of contraception when used correctly, condoms (see entry) help prevent the spread of AIDS and other sexually transmitted diseases. There is some evidence that condom use may lower a woman's risk of developing cervical cancer.

Used alone, the condom has an expected failure rate of 2 percent and a typical failure rate of 12 percent, primarily because it can break or slip off the penis during withdrawal. Many couples reduce this rate to nearly zero by combining the condom with spermicidal foam, cream, or jelly—particularly at times of the month when the woman is most fertile.

Female condom. The female condom (also known as the vaginal pouch) is a relatively new nonprescription barrier method of contraception on the U.S. market. Sold under the brand names Reality and Femidom, it probably offers the same degree of protection against AIDS and other sexually transmitted diseases as the male condom—without requiring the same degree of participation and cooperation on the part of the male partner. In addition, the female condom is less likely to slip or burst.

The female condom consists of a prelubricated sheet of polyurethane which has a small flexible ring closing the center portion and a larger flexible ring encircling the outer edge. To insert the condom into the vagina, one squeezes the inner ring and pushes it back and up into the vagina until it covers the cervix. The ring is then released, and either partner checks to make sure the condom is properly placed—in which case the inner ring will be covering the cervix, the polyurethane sheet itself will be covering the vaginal walls, and the outer ring will remain visible just outside the vaginal lips.

The condom should be inserted before any penis-vagina contact occurs and carefully removed after ejaculation. After a single act of intercourse, it must be replaced with another one before there is any subsequent penis-vagina contact. The female condom appears to be just about as effective as the diaphragm and cervical cap.

Spermicides

Spermicidal foams, creams, films, and jellies are chemicals that are placed into the vagina close to the cervix before sexual intercourse in order to kill sperm. Creams and jellies come in plastic tubes together with a plastic applicator. They are differentiated primarily by color and consistency: creams are white and somewhat less gloppy than jellies, which are clear. Foams come in aerosol cans along with an applicator and look and feel a lot like shaving cream. Spermicides are also available as suppositories (such as the Encare Oval, Semicid, and Intercept) and films (VCF) which are inserted directly into the vagina.

Spermicides (see entry) are often used together with barrier methods of contraception such as diaphragms, cervical caps, and condoms. They may be used as a backup method of contraception during the first few months in which a woman is using oral, injectable, or implanted contraceptives or an intrauterine device.

At present it does not appear that the spermicides on the U.S. market pose any potential dangers other than an occasional allergic reaction. Using spermicides also does not appear to reduce a woman's fertility, and conception can be attempted as soon as she stops using them. A few years back there were some fears that spermicides might increase the risk of certain birth defects, but the data on which these fears were based have since been discredited.

Intrauterine devices (IUDs)

An intrauterine device (see entry) is a small object inserted by a clinician into the uterus to prevent pregnancy. Just how it accomplishes this is a matter of controversy. IUDs come in a variety of shapes and sizes, and some contain substances—such as copper or progesterone—that increase their efficacy while permitting the size of the actual device to be reduced (and thus reducing the risk of complications).

In the 1970s a number of women developed pelvic inflammatory disease and sometimes fatal septic abortions (infected miscarriages) after using the IUD known as the Dalkon Shield. The increased risk turned out to be related to the multiple filaments in this particular IUD's string, which increased the risk of infection. Today there are two types of IUDs available in the United States. The IUD is a very effective means of contraception, with an expected failure rate of about 1 to 2 percent (depending on the type) and a typical failure rate of about 3 percent. Nevertheless, menstrual cramps and excessive menstrual bleeding—or associated anemia—lead a sizable number of women to have their IUDs removed during the first year, although the newer levenogesterol-releasing IUD actually leads to fewer and lighter periods. IUDs also appear to increase the risk of developing pelvic inflammatory disease, particularly in the first few months of use and in women with multiple sexual partners. For this reason most clinicians will not insert an IUD in a woman who has not yet completed her family or who is not in a stable monogamous relationship.

In rare instances an IUD will perforate the uterine wall—a serious but sometimes unnoticeable problem that is also most common during the early months of use. Although an IUD does not directly reduce a woman's chances of becoming pregnant in the future, many of the complications that sometimes result can indeed render a woman infertile or sterile, either because conception is more difficult or because a hysterectomy becomes necessary.

Sterilization

Sterilization can be performed on both men and women, and in either case is more than 99 percent effective in preventing pregnancy. It is regarded as a permanent means of birth control, although it is sometimes possible to reverse a sterilization procedure with microsurgical techniques. No one who chooses to be sterilized should count on reversal as a realistic option, however.

Tubal ligation. The most common sterilization procedure for women is tubal ligation (see entry), in which the fallopian tubes are cut or banded so that sperm cannot reach any egg that is released by the ovary. As soon as the surgery is complete, a woman can regard herself as infertile and does not need to use any other form of birth control. Hysterectomy (see entry)—the removal of the uterus—is another procedure that results in female sterilization, although it is not generally done for the express purpose of contraception.

Vasectomy. In men sterilization involves a procedure called vasectomy, in which the spermatic tubes (vas deferens) are tied off so that the ejaculate becomes sperm-free (see illustration). Vasectomy is a much simpler—and safer—procedure than tubal ligation.

Natural birth control methods

Withdrawal and periodic abstinence are the two natural birth control methods (see entry) practiced most frequently. Sometimes they are assisted by fertility observation, in the form of charting basal body temperature and monitoring cervical mucus. The only health risk associated with natural birth control techniques (aside from the fact that they offer no protection from sexually transmitted diseases) is pregnancy if the method fails.

Withdrawal. Also known as coitus interruptus, this is a widely used method of contraception in which the man removes his penis from the woman's vagina before ejaculation occurs. The effectiveness of the method requires good timing, enormous self-control on the part of the man (and trust in that self-control on the part of the woman), and, probably, good luck.

Despite these limitations, the efficacy of withdrawal seems to be just about the same as that of most barrier methods of contraception: the lowest expected failure rate is 4 percent, with a more typical failure rate of 18 percent.

Periodic abstinence. This term includes a number of subtly different practices including those known as natural birth control, fertility observation, and the rhythm method. All require no artificial devices to prevent conception but instead rely on timing acts of sexual intercourse so that they do not occur during the most fertile part of the menstrual cycle.

Because ovulation does not always follow a calendar-based schedule, even in women with the most "regular" of menstrual cycles, most women and couples who use this form of contraception must rely on some sort of fertility observation. The two most commonly practiced methods are measuring basal body temperature (BBT) and monitoring cervical mucus (see natural birth control methods). Some women use ovulation detection kits, which are sold over the counter.

Many women combine fertility observation with barrier methods of birth control during the time of the month when they are fertile. In this combination method of birth control, no devices are necessary during the times of the month when the woman is not fertile, and no abstinence is necessary during the times of the month when she is fertile. This cuts down on some of the frustration many couples feel with strictly practiced periodic abstinence.

Options available outside the United States—and on the horizon

Various other contraceptive options, some of them already available in other countries, may soon be available in the United States as well. In Germany, for example, women can use handheld computers that indicate days on which they are most likely to conceive; a similar computer may soon be on the market in the United States, although its current price (around $200) may be prohibitive for many potential users. An injectable progestin that inhibits ovulation and lasts for two months (norethindrone enanthate, or NET-EN) is approved for contraception in many other countries, as is a one-capsule implanted contraceptive called Implanon that is easier to insert and remove than the hormonal implants currently approved for use in this country.

Efforts are currently under way to obtain sales approval for some of these products in the United States. Meanwhile, the Population Council is trying to develop an implant for males that would suppress sperm production.

Related entries

Abortion, acquired immune deficiency syndrome, cervical cancer, condoms, diaphragms and cervical caps, douching, hormonal contraception, infertility, intrauterine devices, lubricants, menstrual cycle, menstrual cycle disorders, natural birth control methods, nonsurgical abortion, oral contraceptives, pelvic inflammatory disease, pregnancy testing, safer sex, sexual dysfunction, sexual response, sexually transmitted diseases, spermicides, toxic shock syndrome, tubal ligation, vacuum aspiration, vaginal bleeding (abnormal)

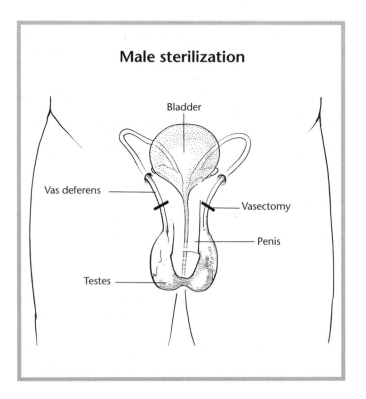

Male sterilization

Bladder

Vas deferens

Vasectomy

Penis

Testes

Blood Tests

Blood can be tested to diagnose or rule out a vast number of defects or disorders. The many tests available include procedures to analyze blood type (O, A, B, or AB), detect the presence of the Rh factor, and measure antibodies that indicate exposure to many infectious diseases, including rubella, acquired immune deficiency syndrome (AIDS), and hepatitis. Other blood tests can indicate the presence or absence of hundreds of disorders, including anemia, cancer, diabetes, hypoglycemia, leukemia, liver disease, kidney damage, syphilis, lupus, polymyositis, rheumatoid arthritis, temporal arteritis, and thyroid disorders.

The blood consists of two components, a pale yellow liquid called plasma and several types of cells that circulate within this liquid: red blood cells (erythrocytes), white blood cells (leukocytes), and platelets (thrombocytes). Blood tests that are performed to measure or evaluate the circulating cells are called hematologic tests. Tests that are performed to measure the contents of the plasma are called blood chemistry tests. Some of the more commonly performed blood tests are described below.

Complete blood count

The complete blood count (CBC)—the most commonly performed blood test—measures the amount of each type of blood cell per unit volume of blood. It also measures the amount of hemoglobin (the oxygen-carrying component of blood), the hematocrit (the percentage of red blood cells in the sample), and the white cell differential (the number of each kind of white blood cell), and includes a description of the size and shape of the red blood cells. The CBC can indicate the possible presence and nature of conditions including anemia, nutritional deficiencies, leukemia and other bone marrow disorders, thrombocytopenia (low platelet count), and various infections.

Erythrocyte sedimentation rate

The erythrocyte sedimentation rate (also called the ESR or sed rate) is a measure of the rate at which red blood cells separate out and settle to the bottom of a test tube. The ESR is not a very specific test, in that a high rate does not necessarily indicate that anything at all is wrong and is not a specific sign of any particular disease. Even so, a high rate (over 100) is often associated with a variety of disorders and infections, including active arthritis, anemia, inflammatory bowel disease, temporal arteritis, polymyalgia rheumatica, and several different cancers.

Coagulation tests

Coagulation tests measure how well the blood clots (thickens). Some of the most common coagulation tests are partial thromboplastin time (PTT) and prothrombin time, which measure the function of two different sets of clot-promoting factors. Coagulation tests are done to detect the presence of various clotting and liver disorders or to monitor the dosage of anticoagulant (blood-thinning) medications.

Glucose

Blood glucose tests measure the level of the sugar glucose in a given volume of blood serum. An abnormally high glucose level can indicate diabetes mellitus; an abnormally low level can indicate hypoglycemia, a term that means nothing more than low blood sugar. Because small variations in blood sugar levels frequently turn out to be meaningless or hard to interpret, people who have a modest elevation often need a more sensitive test to detect elevated blood sugar, a glucose tolerance test.

Blood urea nitrogen (BUN)

Urea nitrogen is a product of protein breakdown in the body. Normally it is excreted by the kidneys, but various kidney disorders can cause the level of urea nitrogen in the blood (the BUN) to rise to abnormal levels. High BUN levels can also be a sign of dehydration.

Creatinine

Creatinine is a breakdown product of phosphate, an important component of energy-containing molecules in the body. Like BUN levels, an elevated level of creatinine in the blood can be a sign of diminished kidney function, either because the ability to filter and remove waste products is impaired or because blood flow to the kidneys is blocked.

Blood enzyme tests

Enzymes are proteins that serve as catalysts in various biochemical reactions. When organs such as the heart, liver, and pancreas are damaged, some of the enzymes they contain may leak into the blood. For example, an elevated level of the enzyme alkaline phosphatase can signal a problem in the liver, bile ducts, or bone. An elevated level of the enzyme amylase, which facilitates starch metabolism, may occur if the salivary glands or pancreas becomes inflamed. If the level of one or more of the transaminase (aminotransferase) enzymes rises, the problem may be liver disease or, less frequently, muscle inflammation.

Bilirubin

Bilirubin is a yellowish liquid waste product that is formed when the liver breaks down old red blood cells. If the blood contains elevated levels of this substance, it is possible that red blood cells are being destroyed in excessive amounts (as in hemolytic anemia). Alternatively, there may be some dysfunction of the liver (including hepatitis; see entry) or obstruction of the bile ducts (such as gallstones; see entry) which interferes with the normal transport of bilirubin into the small intestine and causes it to accumulate in the blood. Some people have a harmless inherited anomaly (termed Gilbert syndrome) that leads to excessive levels of bilirubin in the blood.

Calcium and phosphorus

Abnormal levels of calcium or phosphorus in the blood can indicate a number of different disorders. An elevated level of calcium, for example, may signal some forms of cancer, an overactive parathyroid gland, hyperthyroidism, or an excessive intake of, or sensitivity to, vitamin D.

Electrolytes

Electrolytes are ions (charged molecules), including sodium, potassium, chloride, and bicarbonate. People with liver, kidney, or heart disease, as well as people taking diuretic drugs, often have abnormal electrolytes. Abnormally high levels of potassium, for example, can be a sign of kidney disease or an underfunctioning adrenal gland. If the levels are abnormally low, the problem may be caused by cirrhosis of the liver, malnutrition, vomiting, diuretic drugs, an overactive adrenal gland, or various metabolic disturbances. An eating disorder such as bulimia can also lead to electrolyte disturbances.

Uric acid

Uric acid is the final breakdown product of nucleic acids, the genetic building blocks that make up DNA and RNA. Although high levels of uric acid in the blood are not dangerous in and of themselves, they often occur in people who have certain risk factors for atherosclerosis and heart disease such as high cholesterol levels, hypertension, and obesity. In addition, some people with high uric acid levels develop kidney stones or gout, which is caused by the accumulation in the joints of tiny sodium urate crystals (made from sodium and uric acid).

Cholesterol

Cholesterol (see entry), which is manufactured by the liver, is an essential component of cell walls and building blocks of hormones. In the bloodstream it is wrapped in protein "packages" called lipoproteins. These come in three forms: low-density lipoprotein (LDL), very low density lipoprotein (VLDL), and high-density lipoprotein (HDL). High levels of LDLs, which generally correspond to high total cholesterol levels, are a risk factor for atherosclerosis, coronary artery disease, vascular disease (see circulatory disorders), and stroke, particularly in men. In contrast, high levels of HDLs, particularly in women, seem to be linked to a reduced risk of coronary artery disease. High levels of cholesterol in the blood can also occur in certain metabolic diseases.

Triglycerides

Triglycerides are fat molecules found in blood serum that are often measured along with cholesterol after an overnight fast. While the link between elevated triglyceride levels and the risk of heart disease and atherosclerosis is less clear than that for cholesterol, excessively elevated triglyceride levels (a condition called hypertriglyceridemia) have been linked to inflammation of the pancreas. In addition, women who are obese or diabetic, or who are taking supplemental estrogen (in the form of oral contraceptives or estrogen replacement therapy, for example), often have elevated levels of triglycerides.

Albumin and globulin

Abnormal levels of proteins carried in the blood can indicate problems in immune defenses, metabolism, or the transport of nutrients. Albumin and globulin are two of the most frequently measured of these proteins. An excessively low level of albumin may mean that the liver is failing to produce enough of this protein or that there are kidney or intestinal disorders that are causing albumin to be lost in excessive amounts. An excessively high level of globulin, in contrast, is sometimes a sign of inflammation, although abnormal levels of this protein can occur in perfectly healthy people.

Serologic test for syphilis (STS)

In many states this test is routinely performed as a requirement for a marriage license. Of the numerous tests for syphilis currently available, the ones most commonly used are the VDRL (Venereal Disease Research Laboratory) test and the RPR (rapid plasma reagin) test. These tests are positive if the antigen they contain reacts with an antibody called reagin antibody, which appears in the blood of people with syphilis. These tests are relatively quick and inexpensive, but they can give a positive result when the person has one of several other conditions (including acute infectious hepatitis) which can elevate levels of the reagin antibody. This means that a person with a positive VDRL or RPR needs to have a second, more sensitive (but also more expensive) test to confirm the diagnosis. The most commonly used of these are the FTA-ABS (fluorescent treponemal antibody absorption) test and the TPI (*T. pallidum* immobilization) test. Both of these tests use antibodies that react only with the specific microorganism that causes syphilis.

Thyroid studies

When a thyroid disorder is suspected, the blood serum can be tested for the levels of various hormones secreted by the thyroid gland. Most commonly a test is done to measure levels of thyroid stimulating hormone (TSH). Low concentrations of this hormone can be a sign of hypothyroidism, whereas high levels may indicate hyperthyroidism.

Blood tests during pregnancy

Good prenatal care includes blood tests for a number of different conditions that can affect the outcome of the pregnancy. Among the tests most commonly performed are tests for anemia, sexually transmitted diseases, hepatitis, HIV, and rubella (German measles). Some of these may be repeated several times during the pregnancy. In addition, many clinicians routinely do an alpha-fetoprotein (AFP) test at about 16 weeks' gestation to check for neural tube defects in the fetus and a blood glucose test at about 28 weeks to check for gestational diabetes in the mother.

What are the risks and complications?

Although most blood tests are reasonably accurate, every medical test yields a certain percentage of false positives—that is, tests that indicate a problem where none actually exists. They also yield a certain percentage of false negatives—tests that indicate there is not a problem when, in fact, there is one. In addition, a small chance of human or computer error—a mixed-up sample, a misread slide, a misprinted data sheet—always exists. Although many steps are taken to minimize these possibilities, clinicians routinely repeat blood tests that yield an abnormal result—especially if the person shows no obvious signs of a disorder—or perform additional tests to clarify an abnormal result. Similarly, a blood test may be repeated if a person continues to show clear signs of a disorder but had a single negative blood test.

Sometimes an abnormal blood test turns out to mean absolutely nothing. The individual, for whatever reason, just happens to have a lab value that differs from the average range for the population. Also, some values are based on populations of very sick people, and no one really knows if these values would change if vast numbers of healthy people were tested. As relatively obscure blood tests are more widely performed in healthy populations (or, as some would have it, incorporated into routine physicals), there is the potential for needless anxiety as healthy people are led to believe that they may be suffering from some grave abnormality.

This is an additional problem—at least potentially—for women. Normal values of various substances in the blood are sometimes based on studies of men and thus do not necessarily reflect what is normal for women. Even when the values are based on studies of both sexes, they may not reflect differences that occur in women of a particular age, ethnic group, or reproductive status. The normal range of levels of various substances for premenstrual women or women who are breastfeeding, for example, may conceivably differ from a population value obtained by testing a pool of healthy white men.

We already know that pregnancy can have a profound effect on some aspects of the blood count. The concentration of hemoglobin in the blood falls markedly during pregnancy because of a disproportionate rise in the ratio of plasma volume to red blood cell mass. As a result, women in the second and third trimesters of pregnancy are expected to have hematocrits that fall below the range considered normal in women who are not pregnant. In addition, the mean volume of red blood cells increases during pregnancy, and nearly half of all pregnant women have elevated white blood cell counts or some "abnormality" of the white blood cells.

Clinicians are aware of these changes during pregnancy and so evaluate blood tests in pregnant women according to a different set of norms. Problems can arise, however, when pregnant women begin to be widely screened for something that has been studied only in nonpregnant populations. For example, only recently have clinicians routinely begun to measure platelet levels as part of basic prenatal blood testing. The result was that some apparently healthy pregnant women were found to have abnormally low levels. Some of these women turned out to have diseases or disorders that accounted for these levels, of course, but others were found to have no obvious problems. The explanation came only later, when studies showed that about 8 percent of healthy pregnant women develop abnormally low platelet counts. These counts return to normal after delivery and have no apparent repercussions for the health of either the mother or the baby. It is possible, therefore, that the normal range of platelet levels shifts to some extent during pregnancy but that this is not yet accounted for in tables of normal values. Pregnant women whose platelet values are interpreted according to the standard values are thus still sometimes subjected to unnecessary laboratory tests and physical examinations, and to substantial anxiety.

Presumably, as more research attention is paid specifically to women's health in all stages of the life cycle, "normal" will take on a new, and more useful, meaning for women and their health care providers.

Related entries

Alpha-fetoprotein screening, anemia, anorexia nervosa and bulimia nervosa, arthritis, autoimmune disorders, cholesterol, diabetes, hepatitis, kidney disorders, obesity, platelet disorders, prenatal care, Rh disease, rheumatoid arthritis, rubella, sexually transmitted diseases, stress, stroke, syphilis, temporal arteritis, thyroid disorders

Body Image

Body image is a person's inner perception of her own physical appearance. This image may or may not correspond to objective reality. It is perfectly possible—and quite common—for women within normal weight ranges to perceive themselves as grossly obese; this is a particularly severe problem in women who have anorexia nervosa and bulimia nervosa. It is also quite possible for a woman who has unexceptional features to believe that her nose is too big or her lips are too thin. Study after study indicates that American women tend to be dissatisfied with their looks, rating themselves too ugly, too plain, too old, too pimply, too fat, too hairy, too tall, and so on. By contrast, men in general tend to be much more satisfied with their bodies, even when objective measurements indicate that they might not meet certain standards of perfection. Women's dissatisfaction with their bodies probably stems from unrealistic cultural ideals about what women's bodies should look like, including the notorious Barbie doll and other ubiquitous media images promoting one particular type of idealized woman.

It is often said that women are much more sensitive than men to certain aspects of their physical selves in general, perhaps because their daily lives are touched by bodily functions such as menstrual cycles, pregnancy, and childbirth, not to mention the natural functions of children and other people in their care. Whatever the explanation, it is undeniable that in women a poor body image can become an obsession so strong that it takes precedence over all other aspects of life. A poor body image is not merely a problem of women who are concerned about their sexual attractiveness but seems to be closely tied to women's overall sense of self-esteem and well-being.

Women who have a severe preoccupation with an imagined or slight defect in appearance may even suffer from body dysmorphic disorder (BDD), an increasingly recognized condition that can lead them to drop out of school, avoid leaving home, or even attempt suicide. Women with BDD have a skewed perception of their physical features in the same way that women with anorexia nervosa, an eating disorder, have a skewed perception of their weight and size. Researchers still don't know what causes BDD, although many suspect that it stems from a combination of biological, psychological, and sociocultural factors.

A chronic dissatisfaction with physical appearance can be related to all sorts of health problems in women. Women with a negative body image are prone to develop anorexia, bulimia, or obesity, for example. In addition, many women who are unhappy with their physical selves often experience sexual dysfunction, since sexual arousal depends to a large extent on feeling attractive and desirable. And finally, a number of the products and services women purchase to improve or alter their appearance—from shoes to cosmetics to liposuction—can lead to physical problems in their own right.

Body image and culture

Women throughout history and in many cultures have been subjected to a myriad of mutilations in the name of physical attractiveness—including foot binding and skin stretching. In modern America, women's chronic dissatisfaction with their bodies has fed a vast industry consisting of products and services that ostensibly improve a woman's appearance—and, implicitly or explicitly, her sex appeal. The consumer culture survives in part by creating solutions to physical problems that women may otherwise never be aware they have. The problem of vaginal "freshness" (or lack thereof), for example, was created by the manufacturers of feminine hygiene sprays.

Many of these products and services come at a cost to the body as well as the wallet. Feminists as far back as the nineteenth century have pointed out the damage women do to their bodies by binding their waists or breasts in tight foundation garments or cramming their feet into stylish footwear. Diet pills can lead to addiction, and some liquid diet products have caused serious heart problems and even death. Many cosmetics and fragrances can irritate the skin or provoke allergic reactions. Plastic surgery to alter facial features, to lift, reduce, or enlarge breasts, or even to suck the fat out of the abdomen and thighs carries health risks along with cosmetic benefits.

Not all of the problems women have with body image can be blamed on commercial advertisers. Some of women's compulsive behavior regarding appearance can be justified as a reasonable reaction to realities built into the world around them. Study after study seems to confirm that—like it or not—looks play a larger part in a heterosexual female's sexual attractiveness than in a heterosexual male's. For adolescent girls, in particular, popularity is related to peer assessment of physical attractiveness and appearance. For men, by contrast, power and wealth seem to be the more crucial attributes when it comes to wooing the other sex. Whether this difference is biological or cultural (or even attributable in part to the consumer culture) is a topic of hot debate, but whatever the explanation, for the time being it appears to be a fact of life.

A woman's attractiveness can have an effect on her grades in school and her employability after she is out in the working world. Sometimes these effects are unspoken or even unconscious. It just happens that the better-looking people (according to our society's standards of beauty) seem to get the better grades or to get hired for the job. Sometimes the effects are overt—as when an employer requires that all female workers wear makeup or skirts or meet a specific weight requirement. Some of these requirements are being overturned in courts of law.

In short, women are judged by stricter standards than are men when it comes to looks. This makes it particularly difficult for American women to accept their bodies as they are. Acceptance is even harder for women with obvious physical disabilities, since they face constant reminders that they do not measure up to the cultural ideal.

Body image and weight

Although true obesity is associated with certain serious medical conditions (such as hypertension, diabetes, and coronary artery disease), the thinness to which many women aspire has much more to do with fashion than with health. Because of concerns about the health effects of overweight, a fear and loathing of body fat (and by extension, in some circles, dietary fat) has pervaded certain segments of our society. These feelings probably have more to do with a fear of losing control than with legitimate concerns about health.

As a result of our culture's obsession with thinness, both overweight men and overweight women are subjected to job discrimination, name-calling by strangers, and ridicule when they exercise or show signs of sexuality. But overweight women in particular are made to feel as though their weight and their worth as a human being were one and the same.

A study from the Harvard School of Public Health and the Harvard Medical School showed that obese young adults of both sexes, but particularly women, are less likely to marry than thinner people and can expect to earn less money with the same job qualifications. Overweight women are also subjected to much harsher character judgments than are overweight men and are frequently given unsolicited advice about cultivating their willpower. They are likely to be treated as if they were somehow morally deficient for being overweight.

Afraid of being judged, some of these women only nibble on "acceptable" low-calorie foods when they eat in front of other people, and then make up the difference by eating higher-calorie foods in secret. Because self-esteem is so closely linked to body image in women, overweight women frequently shrink into the background—both literally by slumping and figuratively by remaining quiet and withdrawn. Alternatively, they cultivate a strong wit or self-mocking persona as a defense. They may also develop a number of stress-related disorders (irritable bowel syndrome, headaches, back pain) because of the pressure they feel just getting through each day without being humiliated.

Even women who fall within a normal weight range become obsessed with the bathroom scale. There are perfectly healthy women who cannot get out of bed before they plan precisely what they are going to allow themselves to eat that day, nor can they get from one meal to the next without feeling guilty about every excess calorie they have consumed. This obsession with weight rather than health has led millions of women to develop a pattern of yo-yo (up and down) dieting and, in some cases, eating disorders that can be life-threatening.

Body image in adolescence

The rapid physical changes of puberty make both boys and girls feel self-conscious and awkward about their bodies. In the preteen and early adolescent years, girls whose bodies are not maturing at the "average" rate tend to have a particularly negative body image and low self-esteem. The girl who has her growth spurt earlier than her classmates or who starts developing breasts before the others generally feels self-conscious. So does the girl who is shorter or less well developed than her peers.

It is normal for both boys and girls nearing puberty to gain weight just before undergoing the growth spurt, and girls who do not gain sufficient weight and body fat often fail to start menstruating on schedule. Nonetheless, because girls and young women feel that they need to be thin, many preteen and adolescent girls go on low-calorie or starvation diets, thus depriving themselves of nutrients essential for normal development.

In middle adolescence (usually the high school years), many girls begin to feel more comfortable with their new body image, but some do not. If a girl feels that her appearance does not correspond to accepted notions of femininity, or if she is confused about her sexual orientation (see entry), negative feelings about her body may persist. Other members of a teenager's family play an important role in the development of a young woman's body image. Parents who make their daughter feel that she is physically attractive and who accept her newly acquired sexuality can contribute greatly to her self-esteem. Many psychologists argue that encouragement from the father can be particularly important in helping a girl establish a positive sense of herself as a woman. Her mother can also help by providing information about normal physical changes and by serving as a role model of a person comfortable in her own body.

Body image in the reproductive years

For many women pregnancy enhances body image by making them feel that their body is working properly—even if they never before measured up to other physical standards of femininity. These women feel joy as they watch their waistline expand and their breasts swell. For other women the physical changes of pregnancy destroy a positive body image that rested on maintaining a trim waistline, clear skin, and small nipples.

After childbirth some women may have trouble adjusting to their fuller or altered figure or to stretchmarks or scars left from a cesarean section. Others begin to dislike their body as they struggle to lose the excess pounds gained during pregnancy or discover that leaking milk and engorged breasts make them feel as though they have no control over their own body.

Traumatic events associated with reproduction such as miscarriage, stillbirth, or genetic defects can be devastating to a woman's body image. These events leave some women feeling inadequate in what they consider their most basic biological role. A woman who has had a miscarriage or stillbirth may feel that there is something fundamentally wrong with her body because it cannot carry a healthy pregnancy to term or because it produced a nonviable embryo or fetus. A woman who has conceived a genetically defective child may feel guilty for carrying a genetic disease or feel angry at other women who are pregnant or who have healthy children. The associated problems with self-esteem often lead to sexual dysfunction and other marital difficulties.

Many women in their 30s who have postponed having children discover that they have an infertility problem which precludes their becoming pregnant. Still other women reach their late 30s without finding a partner with whom to have a child. In both of these situations women may begin to develop a negative body image, as they see signs of aging in a body that has not fulfilled its reproductive potential.

Although negative feelings such as these are unwarranted, many women who have reproductive difficulties find that they are haunted by them even as they fight them intellectually. Sometimes it can be useful to talk with a genetic counselor, psychotherapist, or other clinician who can help the woman assess herself more objectively, reduce her sense of grief and guilt, and put this particular problem into the context of her life as a whole. Many women find it helpful to talk with other women (individually or in support groups) who have experienced similar disappointments.

Body image and aging

Among all women, from full-time homemakers to full-time professionals, we tend to associate sexual attractiveness, particularly female attractiveness, with youth. The result is that many women find it particularly difficult to "grow old gracefully." Women whose self-esteem was once based on conforming to accepted standards of beauty often find that they do not know how to behave when people respond to them on another level. It is not uncommon for women nearing or past menopause to try (usually in vain) to rid themselves of the excess weight that comes with age, to dress themselves in garments more suited to a younger woman, to dye their hair, to bury their faces under camouflaging makeup, or to invest in a face lift or tummy tuck.

For some women, these efforts may help maintain a positive body image, if only temporarily. Many other women begin to feel better about their bodies only when they come to accept the inevitable and learn to appreciate—even if not everyone else can—aspects of themselves they may have overlooked earlier in life.

Related entries

Anorexia nervosa and bulimia nervosa, body odors, cosmetic dentistry, cosmetic surgery, dieting, face lifts, foot care, hair care, hair dyes, lipectomy and liposuction, nail care, obesity, psychotherapy, sexual dysfunction, sexual orientation, sexual response, skin care and cosmetics, skin disorders, social anxiety disorder, stress, substance abuse, weight tables, wrinkles

Body Odors

Many body parts—the sweat glands in the underarm and genital regions, the feet, and the mouth, in particular—produce secretions that result in distinctive odors. These odors are generally due not to the secretions themselves but to the naturally occurring bacteria that metabolize the secretions into aromatic by-products.

In many parts of the animal kingdom body odor plays an important role in sexuality. From insects to primates, attracting a mate depends to a large extent on giving off the right smell. In recent years there has been a great deal of discussion of pheromones—airborne chemicals emitted by animals which help regulate many social behaviors, including mating. Although there is some evidence that human secretions may also contain pheromone-like substances or other sexual attractants, it is clear that cultural factors override whatever subtle and perhaps unconscious power these chemicals may have over us. An odor that is attractive or irrelevant to one person may be offensive or unbearable to another.

Just how we respond to body odors, while partly a matter of personal sensitivity, is determined largely by our upbringing. There are plenty of people who have come to appreciate—or at least tolerate—their own natural odors as well as those of others. For women who do choose to mask or minimize body odors, a number of different options exist, most of which can be accomplished with minimal cost and effort.

Underarm odor

Underarm odor is the result of sweat, or perspiration, which is produced by the sweat glands underneath the skin (see skin care and cosmetics). Sweat glands are most active when the body is overheated because as the sweat evaporates into the air, the skin cools off to some extent. One type of sweat gland abundant in the underarm area, the apocrine glands, also secretes perspiration when a person is excited, scared, or sexually aroused. After puberty the sweat secreted from these glands can stain clothing and, when metabolized by bacteria, emits a strong odor.

Most people are able to minimize underarm sweating and odor by washing with lukewarm water and mild soap at least once a day—and more frequently in hot, humid weather or after intense exercise. Some women find that washing with an antibacterial soap or applying a topical antibiotic to the armpit can also reduce odor.

Antiperspirant sprays, creams, or roll-ons reduce the amount of perspiration, and deodorants (which are often combined with antiperspirants) can cover up odor with a more pleasant fragrance. Some women prefer to use perfumes or colognes under their arms in lieu of deodorants. All of these products can irritate the skin if used immediately after shaving the armpits, however. As for shaving itself, while it plays no role in reducing the amount of perspiration, it can prevent the accumulation of pungent sweat in the hair.

If these measures are inadequate, stronger antiperspirants (such as Drysol) are available by prescription. In severe cases the sweat glands can be surgically removed from the armpits.

Genital odor

Apocrine sweat glands also account for most of the sweating and odor in the genital region. Usually daily washing can keep this odor from becoming unpleasant, although pantyhose or underwear made of synthetic fabrics can increase sweating in the groin and thus the possibility of odor.

More drastic measures to mask genital odor are usually unnecessary. Vaginal douching—the forcing of water containing some kind of cleanser or deodorant into the vagina—can increase the risk of vaginal yeast infections by upsetting the normal balance of good and bad bacteria in the vagina. In addition, certain deodorants and other chemicals contained in over-the-counter feminine hygiene products can irritate vaginal tissue or cause allergic reactions in susceptible women. Those who feel they must douche after sexual intercourse or menstruation should limit the frequency and should stick to plain water or a very dilute solution of white vinegar in water.

If vaginal odor changes suddenly—particularly if it smells fishy or foul—a clinician should be consulted to see if the problem may be caused by vaginitis or a sexually transmitted disease.

Bad breath

Bad breath—also known as halitosis—is a foul or unpleasant odor from the mouth. Most of the time it is due to some factor in the mouth itself—either inadequate hygiene, decaying teeth, untreated gum disease, recent mouth wounds or surgery, dentures, or smoking tobacco. An infection in a location near the mouth—such as the tonsils, sinuses, or nose—can also produce bad breath.

Often the problem is caused simply by infrequent eating or drinking, since swallowing and chewing tend to circulate and cleanse the saliva. This is why people often wake up with what the mouthwash commercials call "morning breath." A whole night without eating or drinking leaves the tongue, cheeks, and gums coated with dead cells and decomposing matter.

Eating certain aromatic foods—most notably onions and garlic—or drinking alcohol can result in bad breath, even hours later. This is because after the food or drink is ingested and broken down in the digestive organs, it is sent through the bloodstream to the lungs, where the aromatic chemicals associated with it are expelled together with the breath.

For most of these problems the solution involves brushing and flossing after every meal and regular dental care. If the tongue is coated, it should be brushed gently as well. It is also helpful to rinse the mouth out with water many times throughout the day. Although mouthwashes and mints can sometimes mask the odor, their effects tend to disappear after an hour or so. People with particularly troublesome halitosis might want to try using these products every 2 to 4 hours, at least until they have eliminated the true cause of the problem.

People who brush their teeth frequently during the day should take special care to use a soft toothbrush and to brush gently. Vigorous frequent brushing can injure the gums and cause them to recede—a bigger health problem, in the long run, than occasional bad breath.

Bad breath can also be caused by a systemic disease. For example, people with kidney failure may have breath smelling of urine, people with ketoacidosis associated with diabetes may have fruity-smelling breath, and people with liver failure may have fishy-smelling breath. In rare instances, lung infections or impaired motility of the stomach can cause bad breath as well. In all of these cases the key to correcting the halitosis lies in treating the underlying disorder.

Foot odor

Feet contain densely packed eccrine glands, the kind of sweat gland that secretes perspiration when the surrounding area is overheated. When feet are trapped inside shoes—particularly shoes made of synthetic, "nonbreathable" materials—they tend to sweat. In some people this sweat takes on a particularly offensive odor.

To minimize this problem, when possible wear open-toed shoes or sandals, expose feet to the open air, wear absorbent cotton socks, and wash socks or stockings after every use. Feet and toes should be cleansed thoroughly with lukewarm water and a mild soap each day. Some people may find that they need to use foot deodorants or antiperspirants to minimize odor and sweating.

Related entries

Cosmetic safety, dentures/bridges/implants, diabetes, douching, foot care, gum disease, kidney disorders, skin care and cosmetics, vaginitis

Bowel Disorders

The bowels include both the small intestine and the colon or large intestine. In the United States, Canada, and northern Europe, women are more likely than men to seek the advice of a physician about changes in bowel function. Problems can include a change in the frequency of stool; a change in consistency or ease in elimination of the stool; gas, cramping, or pain; or even a general impression that bowel movements are somehow abnormal—although determining just what is normal can be quite difficult, since bowel function varies considerably from one person to the next.

Whether female hormones have some specific effect on bowel function remains unclear. Many women report consistent variations in bowel function during or around the time of menstruation, in pregnancy, and following a hysterectomy. These reports have stimulated clinical and basic research on the effect of changing levels of estrogen and progesterone on normal gastrointestinal physiology and bowel function. Findings so far have been controversial. Women with normal menstrual periods, for example, often report constipation or diarrhea that seems to fluctuate with the menstrual cycle. These reports are usually based on subjective impressions, however, and have not been confirmed in prospective studies. Similarly, although a few studies indicate that it may take longer for waste products to move through the intestines during the second half (luteal phase) of the menstrual cycle, other studies show no change in function throughout the menstrual period or even between men and women.

We do know that certain types of bowel disorders are more commonly reported in women than in men. These are irritable bowel syndrome (IBS), functional bowel disorder (a vaguely defined form of IBS), and intractable constipation. Whether women are more prone to developing these conditions because of their physiology or because of certain cultural patterns in the use of the health care system has not yet been determined.

Irritable bowel syndrome. The exact definition of IBS varies from one doctor to another, but the condition is generally

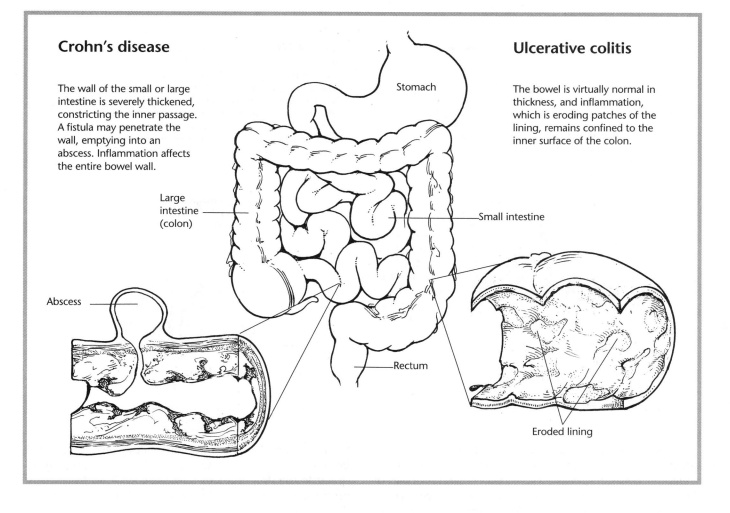

Crohn's disease

The wall of the small or large intestine is severely thickened, constricting the inner passage. A fistula may penetrate the wall, emptying into an abscess. Inflammation affects the entire bowel wall.

Ulcerative colitis

The bowel is virtually normal in thickness, and inflammation, which is eroding patches of the lining, remains confined to the inner surface of the colon.

Stomach

Large intestine (colon)

Small intestine

Abscess

Rectum

Eroded lining

characterized by long-standing crampy abdominal pain and some combination of constipation and diarrhea. Bowel movements may contain mucus and are frequently either loose and watery or else resemble pellets, small balls, or ribbons. People with IBS commonly feel bloated and pass excessive gas, and many complain of indigestion and heartburn. If only some of these symptoms occur, many doctors prefer to diagnose the condition as functional bowel syndrome, although other doctors use this term interchangeably with irritable bowel syndrome (see entry).

Constipation. Constipation (see entry) is usually defined as difficulty passing stools at least 3 times a week, or as bowel movements that occur less than once per week. Abdominal pain and bloating commonly occur as well. Constipation develops when weakened muscular contractions in the colon slow the movement of waste products as they approach the rectum and anus. Occurring twice as commonly in women as in men, constipation can be due to irregular or inadequate diet, too little water in the diet, lack of exercise, resisting the urge to defecate, reliance on laxatives, and use of other medications such as oral contraceptives, codeine, and some drugs

used to treat heart disease, depression, hypertension, and indigestion.

Diverticular disease. Diverticula—outpouchings in the colon—are present in 20 to 25 percent of all people over age 50. Sometimes these become infected or rupture, resulting in diverticulitis—which is less common in women than in men. Symptoms include unremitting pain—most often on the lower left side but sometimes on the lower right (suggesting appendicitis) or just above the pubic area. Usually there is a fever and possibly blood in the stool, lack of appetite, nausea, and vomiting. Sometimes there may be abdominal distension or crampiness (see diverticular disease).

Ulcerative colitis. This is a serious form of inflammatory bowel disease (IBD) common in young adults of both sexes. It is a chronic condition characterized by attacks of blood- or pus-tinged diarrhea (see illustration). The attacks can be sudden and severe, but they may also be separated by long, symptom-free periods. Other symptoms of ulcerative colitis may include malaise, fever, and lack of appetite. Arthritis and skin lesions occasionally occur.

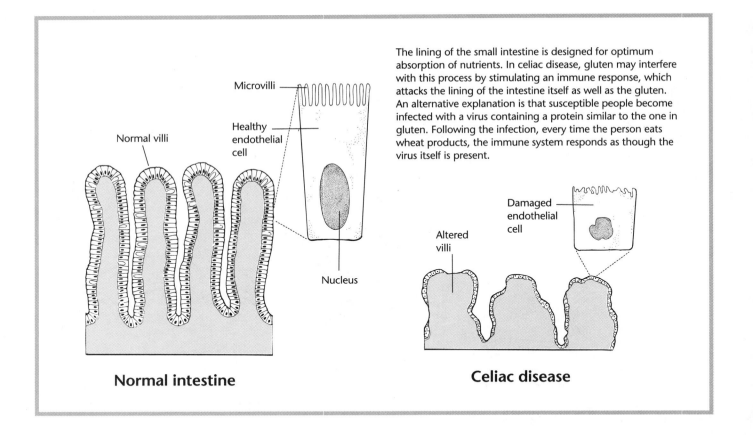

The lining of the small intestine is designed for optimum absorption of nutrients. In celiac disease, gluten may interfere with this process by stimulating an immune response, which attacks the lining of the intestine itself as well as the gluten. An alternative explanation is that susceptible people become infected with a virus containing a protein similar to the one in gluten. Following the infection, every time the person eats wheat products, the immune system responds as though the virus itself is present.

Normal intestine

Celiac disease

Although ulcerative colitis is often first treated with anti-inflammatory drugs and sometimes dietary changes, if the symptoms persist it may become necessary to remove part of the colon. One reason this may be done is to prevent colon cancer, since having ulcerative colitis for many years seems to increase the risk of developing this cancer later in life.

Crohn's disease. Yet another form of inflammatory bowel disease that can cause lower abdominal pain is Crohn's disease (also known as regional enteritis or ileitis). Unlike ulcerative colitis, this disease involves inflammation of any part of the digestive tract from the mouth to the anus (see illustration). Although relatively rare, it is most likely to affect young adults (under age 40) of either sex. In addition to episodes of lower abdominal pain or cramping, there may be chronic and sometimes debilitating diarrhea, low-grade fever, lack of appetite, and weight loss. Joint pains or skin rashes may also occur. Occasionally, fistulas (holes) and fissures (cracks) may form around the rectum and anus, and there may be some intestinal bleeding.

Besides considering these symptoms, a clinician will diagnose Crohn's disease based on the results of tests such as a barium x-ray of the digestive tract and a colonoscopy (a visual inspection of the colon with the aid of a flexible tube inserted through the rectum).

Treatment varies with the extent of the disease and specific symptoms, and can range from simple antidiarrheal pills to various forms of surgery, including colostomy (see entry). Of-

ten antiinflammatory medications and dietary changes will be recommended. If these don't help, symptoms may respond to the drug infliximab (Remicade). This drug was recently approved by the U.S. Food and Drug Administration for the short-term treatment of moderately to severely active Crohn's disease that does not respond to standard therapies, as well as for the treatment of open, draining fistulas.

Celiac disease. The lining of the small intestine is covered with fingerlike projections (villi) that extend into the space within the bowel (see illustration). Each villus is covered with endothelial cells, and the surfaces of the endothelial cells are covered with microvilli that maximize contact with nutrients. In a person with celiac disease, gluten (a protein contained in wheat and wheat products) is toxic to the villi, endothelial cells, and microvilli, with the result that the intestine cannot absorb food properly. Symptoms of celiac disease include diarrhea, weight loss, and bloating. The main treatment is a gluten-free diet; sometimes systemic steroids are necessary if symptoms are not controlled by diet. Although celiac disease was once thought to be relatively rare, new studies suggest that as many as 1 in 150 to 200 people in Europe and the United States may have this condition.

Arteriosclerosis of the bowel. Occasionally arteriosclerosis (or hardening of the arteries) of the bowel can cause crampy pain in the middle of the lower abdomen. Other symptoms, which are most common after eating, may include bloody stools. Arteriosclerosis of the bowel is most likely in people over the age of 60 who also have arteriosclerosis of the heart, brain, kidney, or legs. If a clinician suspects this condition, a special x-ray test called angiography will be done to evaluate circulation in the abdominal area.

Polyps. Colon polyps are usually detected when they produce visible blood in the stool, or when they cause a stool test, done for routine screening purposes, to show a positive result for "occult" (hidden) blood (see screening). Even when they are causing no symptoms, polyps should be evaluated after detection, since a small proportion will become cancerous (see illustration).

Two types of polyps may be found in the bowel. The most common type—termed hyperplastic polyps—probably carry no risk of becoming malignant. The second type, called villous and tubular adenomas, do carry a risk of becoming cancerous, and this risk increases as they grow. Most polyps can be removed during colonoscopy. Since development of new polyps is common, yearly tests of stool for occult blood should be performed and colonoscopy repeated if a positive test or any visible bleeding occurs.

Colon cancer. If abdominal pain or cramping is accompanied by rectal bleeding or a persistent change in bowel habits, a clinician should be consulted about the possibility of colon cancer (see entry). Other symptoms may be unexplained weight loss or anemia.

How are these conditions evaluated?

A woman's description of her symptoms is one of the most helpful pieces of information a clinician uses in diagnosing bowel disorders. Also helpful is a physical examination, including a rectal examination. Blood will be tested for signs of infection, chronic inflammation, or anemia.

Sometimes tests such as a sigmoidoscopy, colonoscopy, or barium enema of the colon may be done to rule out colon cancer, polyps, or other abnormalities of the intestines. Sigmoidoscopy involves examining the lower part of the colon with a bendable lighted tube called a flexible proctosigmoidoscope. No sedation or anesthesia is needed; the procedure causes, at most, mild discomfort and takes only about 15 minutes. Colonoscopy is a more extensive procedure in which the upper part of the colon is examined as well (see illustration). The patient receives light intravenous sedation

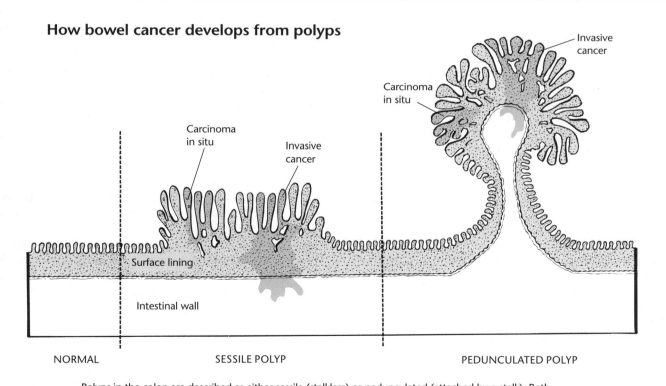

How bowel cancer develops from polyps

Carcinoma in situ

Invasive cancer

Carcinoma in situ

Invasive cancer

Surface lining

Intestinal wall

NORMAL   SESSILE POLYP   PEDUNCULATED POLYP

Polyps in the colon are described as either sessile (stalkless) or pedunculated (attached by a stalk). Both types of polyp can develop into invasive cancer. In its early stage (carcinoma in situ), cancer in a polyp remains within the surface lining of the intestine and does not have access to blood or lymph vessels. Once the cancer invades the intestinal wall below the lining, blood and lymph vessels can pick up cancerous cells and carry them away to distant parts of the body. When this occurs, the cancer has metastasized (spread) and may be life-threatening.

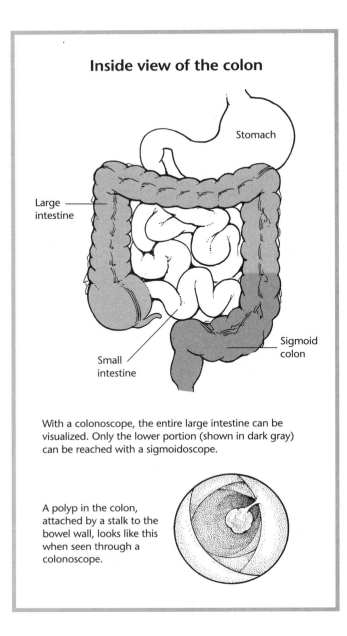

Inside view of the colon

Stomach

Large intestine

Small intestine

Sigmoid colon

With a colonoscope, the entire large intestine can be visualized. Only the lower portion (shown in dark gray) can be reached with a sigmoidoscope.

A polyp in the colon, attached by a stalk to the bowel wall, looks like this when seen through a colonoscope.

during the procedure, which takes between 30 minutes and an hour. A barium enema helps outline the structure of the gastrointestinal tract so that it can be examined by x-ray. In preparation for these procedures, enemas or laxatives are used to clean out the colon.

Although not all colon cancers will lead to blood in the stool, the test for hidden (occult) blood in the feces remains one of the easiest, least expensive, and most convenient means of detecting otherwise unrecognized cancers.

Related entries
Colon and rectal cancer, colostomy, constipation, diverticular disease, hemorrhoids, irritable bowel syndrome, laxatives, peptic ulcer disease, stress

Breast Cancer

Breast cancer is probably the most deeply feared disease among American women. It is their most prevalent form of cancer and, after lung cancer, the most lethal—striking 182,000 American women each year and killing approximately 40,200. Equally distressing for many is the fact that the cause remains unknown, as well as the prospect of the traditional "cure"—losing a breast.

These fears are not baseless, but with early detection most women who have this disease will not die from it. And women today have many more options for treatment than previous generations of women—including, often, the option of saving most of the breast. Thus, in the last decade the meaning of having cancer, for many women, has changed from facing an immediate risk of death and disfigurement to enduring some combination of surgery, chemotherapy, or radiation, and living with the worry that the disease may recur.

Has breast cancer become epidemic?
The incidence of breast cancer began to rise steadily in the United States around 1940 and increased sharply starting about 1980. In North America (and most populations studied worldwide), breast cancer rates are now twice as high as in 1940 and are increasing by approximately 1 to 2 percent per year. The rates of breast cancer are slightly lower in African American and Hispanic women than in white women.

Worldwide, the variation in breast cancer incidence is striking. The highest rates occur in Europe, New Zealand, Canada, the United States, and Israel, while the lowest rates occur in Asia and Latin America. These differences cannot be accounted for by genetic differences alone, since women who move from low-incidence countries (such as Japan) to higher-incidence countries (such as the United States) appear to have an increasing risk of breast cancer with each generation. That is why many researchers suspect that lifestyle changes and/or environmental exposures may play a role in promoting breast cancer.

On the plus side, in the past several years the worldwide trend of increasing death rates from breast cancer appears to have reversed in several countries, including the United States, the United Kingdom, Canada, Austria, and Sweden. This reversal may be due to more widespread screening (mammography), as well as increased use of effective chemotherapy and radiation therapy.

Most of the increase in the incidence of breast cancer in the United States has been among women over 50, even though it is younger women who seem to fear breast cancer the most. Only 5 percent of breast cancers occur in women under 40, and 25 percent occur in women under 50. A major reason why death rates from breast cancer have risen in older women is that mortality from other causes has declined. Since women are living longer in general, the number surviving long enough to develop breast cancer is rising. Nevertheless, as much as half of the increasing incidence in women of all ages appears to be due to other, still incompletely understood factors.

The gradual increase in breast cancer from 1940 to 1980 was probably a result of lifestyle changes, such as improved nutrition (which increases a woman's lifetime exposure to estrogen, by allowing menarche to start earlier), delayed childbearing, and possibly exposure to environmental toxins. A recent study suggests that the reduced amount of time spent breastfeeding infants in developed nations may play a major role in explaining the high rates of breast cancer in these parts of the world. These factors, as well as others that have not been identified, may actually have caused more breast cancers to develop. But the steep rise in the number of cases of cancer diagnosed since 1980 has been attributed largely to improved early detection with mammography.

This screening technique began picking up cases of breast cancer that previously would have gone undetected until they were much more advanced and less controllable. Between 1989 and 1992, death rates from breast cancer in American women fell 5 percent overall, with mortality for women in their 30s, 40s, and 50s decreasing as much as 9 percent—the largest short-term decline since 1950, according to the National Cancer Institute. Although African American women are less likely than white women to be diagnosed with breast cancer, they are more likely to die from the disease, possibly because their cancers are less likely to be detected at an early stage.

What is breast cancer?

The breasts, or mammary glands, consist of fat pads inside of which is a branching system of ducts. These ducts are designed to ferry milk from the milk-producing lobules to the nipples. Breast cancer develops as the result of malignant changes in the cells lining the ducts or the lobules.

The first abnormalities that occur are not themselves cancer but are simply an overgrowth of normal cells in the ducts or lobules (see illustration). These conditions are called intraductal hyperplasia and lobular hyperplasia. If these extra cells seem a bit odd-looking when examined under the microscope, the condition is called atypical hyperplasia. Atypical hyperplasia does not cause lumps and cannot be detected by breast examination or by mammogram. When it is discovered in the ducts or lobules, it is usually by accident, in the course of biopsying a suspicious lump.

If cells lining the ducts or lobules become odder still and start to clog them, the condition is called carcinoma in situ. Ductal carcinoma in situ and lobular carcinoma in situ by definition remain confined to the ducts or lobules, but they can sometimes be detected by mammogram, and in rare instances may produce a lump that can be felt. If the abnormal cells break away from these parts of the breast to infiltrate adjoining cells, the condition is called invasive cancer. It is at this point that a discrete malignant lump starts to grow.

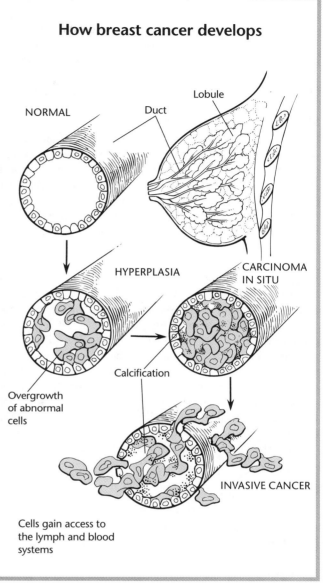

How breast cancer develops

NORMAL
Duct
Lobule

HYPERPLASIA
Overgrowth of abnormal cells

CARCINOMA IN SITU
Calcification

INVASIVE CANCER
Cells gain access to the lymph and blood systems

If cancerous cells escape the confines of the breast altogether and travel through the lymph system or bloodstream into more distant parts of the body—particularly the lungs, liver, and bones—we say that the breast cancer has metastasized. Cancer in the breast itself does not kill anybody, because the breasts are not vital organs. But when breast cancer cells start to grow in other organs essential for survival and begin to disrupt the normal function of those organs, breast cancer becomes a life-threatening disease.

Most researchers now believe that cells start to escape from the breast through the lymph system and bloodstream during the earliest stages of invasive cancer, even before a lump can be felt or detected on a mammogram. What keeps these cells from invading other organs is the body's own immune system, which destroys them. Eventually, however, as a breast cancer grows, the immune system cannot keep up with the vast numbers of cancer cells leaving the breast. At that point surgery and possibly radiation (to remove the source of the cells in the breast), and in most cases systemic chemotherapy or hormonal therapy (to assist the immune system in controlling the growth of cancer cells that have already spread throughout the body), must be undertaken.

Stages of breast cancer

Breast cancers differ according to a variety of characteristics in addition to location. For this reason the story of what happened to one woman with breast cancer is not necessarily applicable to another. To help distinguish among breast cancers, clinicians frequently use a system known as the international TNM staging system—with T standing for tumor size, N for the number of lymph nodes involved, and M for the presence of metastases in distant parts of the body.

Stage 0 breast cancer. A cancer at stage 0 is confined to the duct or lobule of the breast and is called, respectively, ductal carcinoma in situ (DCIS; see illustration) or lobular carcinoma in situ (LCIS). These "precancers" have not yet invaded the surrounding breast tissue and may never do so.

Some researchers contend that ductal and lobular carcinoma in situ should be regarded not as cancer at all but rather as an advanced form of hyperplasia, or abnormal cell overgrowth. Still, women with either type of in situ carcinoma have a 20 to 25 percent lifetime risk of developing future invasive cancer, and for that reason the question of just how to treat them is one of the most controversial in breast cancer therapy.

Stage 1 breast cancer. This consists of a small lump (less than or equal to about three-quarters of an inch in diameter) which has invaded the breast beyond the ducts or lobules but has not yet spread to lymph nodes or other parts of the body. The 5-year survival rate for women with stage 1 cancer is approximately 95 percent.

Stage 2 breast cancer. There is no concrete sign of distant metastases for stage 2 cancers, either, but a slightly larger tumor size or enlarged lymph nodes (see illustration) indicate that more trouble may be imminent. The 5-year survival rate is 80 percent for women with stage 2 cancer.

Stage 3 breast cancer. In this stage the cancer is larger than 2 inches in diameter or has invaded the chest wall or surrounding skin. Lymph nodes are enlarged, but tests and scans of the bones, liver, and lungs show no concrete cancer on these organs. The 5-year survival rate for women with stage 3 breast cancer drops to 50 percent, however, which suggests that undetected cancer is already lurking in distant organs in many of these women.

Stage 4 breast cancer. At this stage the cancer is definitely detectable in other organs and is considered incurable. Even so, 10 percent of women with stage 4 breast cancer will be alive 5 years later.

By far the best predictor of survival is the extent of lymph node involvement—which signals the extent to which the cancer has spread to more distant sites. But other factors can be useful in assessing the virulence of a tumor, including tumor size, extent of cell differentiation (the more the better), growth rate of the tumor, and the tumor's responsiveness to estrogen. Tumors that are stimulated by estrogen (called estrogen-receptor positive tumors, or ER+) can sometimes be slowed down by hormonal therapy.

What are the symptoms?

The classic symptom of breast cancer is a lump in the breast, but many lumps are not cancerous. They are the result of normal hormonal changes or trauma to the breast (see breast lumps, benign). Although half of all breast lumps in postmenopausal women (and three-quarters of all breast lumps in women over the age of 70) are malignant, the younger a woman is, the more likely it is that her breast lump is benign. Pain in the breast is also highly unlikely to signal breast cancer; only 6 percent of women with breast cancer have breast pain as a symptom.

If a lump is cancerous, it is generally difficult to move under the skin and often feels rock-hard with irregular edges. There is no sure way to distinguish a malignant from a benign lump by touch alone, however. For this reason, any woman who notices a change in her breasts—such as a lump or thickening, clear or bloody discharge, change in contours, dimpling of skin, redness, or retracted nipple—should consult a clinician (see breast self-examination).

How is the condition evaluated?

In the past some breast lumps were found during a routine physical examination, but most were discovered by the woman or her partner during the course of dressing, bathing, or lovemaking. Today an increasing number of lumps and other abnormalities are first discovered as a result of a mammogram. Ultrasound breast examination may also be used to differentiate solid masses from fluid-filled cysts (unlikely to be cancerous) and to detect cysts in women with dense breast tissue and normal mammograms. Radiologists also sometimes use computer-aided detection to double-check suspicious areas and look for subtle signs of breast cancer: microcalcifications (clusters of bright white specks) and dense regions of radiating lines that indicate possible cancer.

When a lump has been identified, the clinician will probably want to biopsy it right away—that is, to examine cells from the lump under a microscope. The results of the biopsy, together with information gathered from physical examinations and diagnostic tests (ordered if the biopsy is positive), help the clinician determine the cancer's stage of growth and the most appropriate course of therapy.

Either during the biopsy (see entry) or in a separate operation the surgeon may remove several lymph nodes to help as-

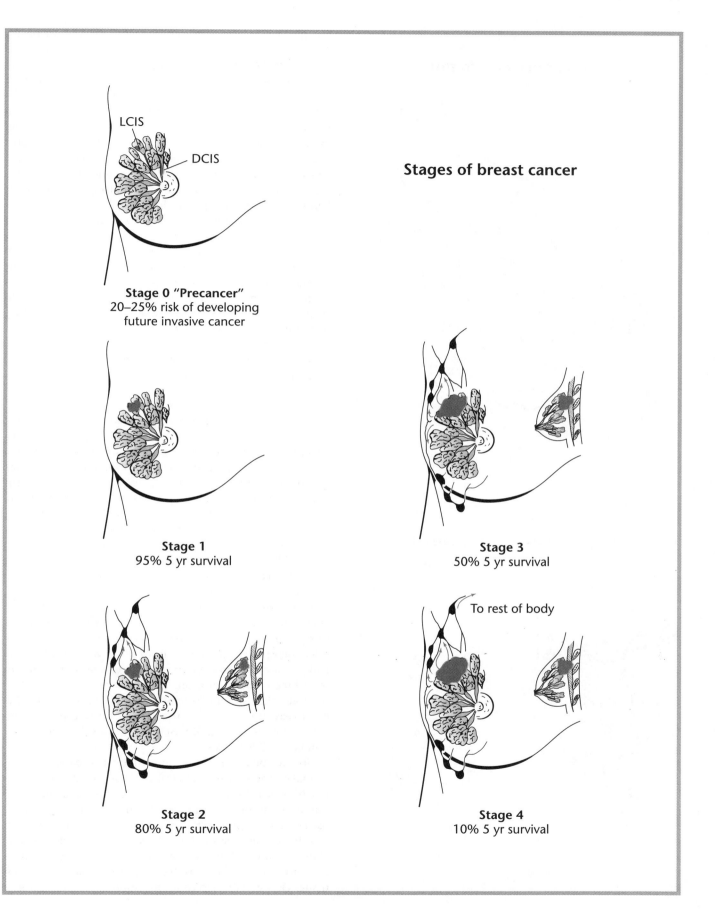

LCIS

DCIS

Stages of breast cancer

Stage 0 "Precancer"
20–25% risk of developing
future invasive cancer

Stage 1
95% 5 yr survival

Stage 3
50% 5 yr survival

Stage 2
80% 5 yr survival

To rest of body

Stage 4
10% 5 yr survival

Ductal carcinoma in situ

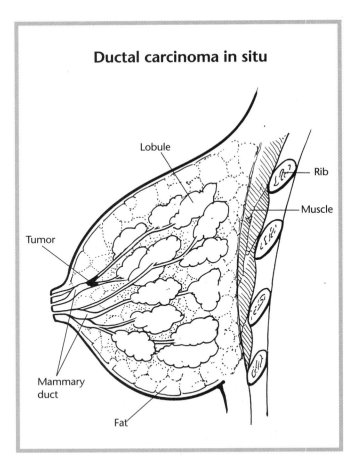

Lymph nodes near the breast

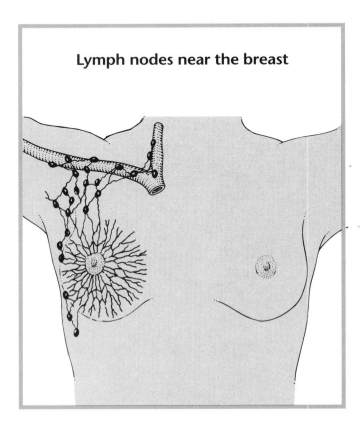

sess the chances that a cancer has spread beyond the breast. Although the absence of cancer cells in the lymph nodes is no guarantee that the cancer has not metastasized to other organs—as was once believed—it does mean that the chances are comparatively low.

If there is a reasonable possibility that the cancer has already invaded other organs, a liver function test, an abdominal CT scan, a chest x-ray, and a bone scan may also be done. A bone scan, which is performed in the nuclear medicine department of a hospital, involves the injection of a small amount of radioactive contrast material into a vein of the hand or arm. After the patient has waited 2 or 3 hours for the dye to spread throughout the skeletal system (drinking lots of water to help eliminate the remainder through the urine), a radiologist takes pictures of the entire skeleton with a special camera. An uneven pattern of radiation distributed by the contrast material indicates some problem in the bone. Because the chance of metastatic spread is low in women with small tumors and little or no lymph node involvement, they do not usually need to undergo these tests.

Ductal carcinoma in situ and lobular carcinoma in situ are discovered sometimes through routine mammography and sometimes when a suspicious lump is biopsied.

How is breast cancer treated?

Breast cancer is treated with surgery, radiation therapy, chemotherapy, and hormonal therapy. The particular combination of these therapies that is right for one type of cancer or one woman may be completely inappropriate for another. Among the many factors to be considered—in addition to the size, nature, and stage of the cancer—are the woman's menopausal status, age, and overall health, and the potential side effects, cost, convenience, and time commitment entailed by the treatment. Because the relative advantages of treatments may not be clear-cut, a woman with breast cancer should be prepared to take an active role with her physician in deciding which course to follow.

A diagnosis of breast cancer is almost never a medical emergency. Breast cancer is relatively slow-growing as cancers go, and there is no harm in taking a few weeks to consider the options carefully, talk to other women who have had breast cancer treatments, and get two or more opinions from breast cancer surgeons before making any final decisions at a time when a woman is often emotionally vulnerable. To ease this process, more and more breast cancer centers are offering women multidisciplinary consultations with a number of different specialists.

Most women with breast cancer have two basic decisions to make. The first is a surgical decision and involves how much tissue is to be removed—just the cancerous lump itself (lumpectomy, or, if a segment of the breast must be removed, partial mastectomy), or the whole breast (total mastectomy).

If the woman elects to have the lump alone removed, radiation therapy will be recommended in most cases to eliminate any errant cancer cells that may lurk in remaining breast tissue. Occasionally a second operation is required prior to radiation therapy to ensure that the entire cancer has been excised and to remove lymph nodes for examination. If the entire breast is removed, the woman has the option of having the breast surgically reconstructed (see breast reconstruction), wearing a prosthesis (which gives the illusion of a breast under clothing), or simply living with her new form as it is.

The second major decision a woman, working with her health care team, needs to make is what kind of systemic therapy (if any) is to be used to eradicate cancer cells that may already have spread to more distant parts of the body. These options include chemotherapy and hormonal therapy.

Surgical options. The goal of surgery today is to remove the original tumor from the breast so that it cannot send cancer cells to distant organs. Although it is common for a surgeon to remove some of the surrounding lymph nodes as well, this is done for the sake of assessing the stage of the cancer, since finding cancerous cells in the lymph nodes means the chances are greater that metastasis has already occurred. The idea that removing the adjacent lymph nodes can actually stem the spread of breast cancer has been discarded. The more lymph nodes removed, too, the greater a woman's risk of developing a lymphedema (see entry), a condition that occurs when lymphatic fluid pools in the layer of fat just under the skin and in other interstitial tissues, resulting in swelling and inflammation.

To avoid removing lymph nodes unnecessarily, many surgeons today are using a process called sentinel lymph node mapping. In this procedure, a dye is injected before surgery at the site of the tumor and traced during surgery to the first lymph node to take up the dye. This so-called "sentinel" node is then removed and analyzed for signs of cancer. If this node shows signs of the cancer, other lymph nodes are usually removed for analysis as well. If no signs of cancer can be found in the sentinel node, however, the chance that other lymph nodes are involved is very low, and full removal can usually be avoided. Whether or not this newer approach will ultimately save just as many lives remains to be seen.

For most women (the majority of whom have stage 1 or stage 2 cancers), 5-year survival rates from breast cancer are the same no matter which of the two main types of surgical procedure, lumpectomy or mastectomy, is done. A woman's decision about which type of surgery to have must take into account each procedure's degree of disfigurement, side effects, and associated treatments (such as follow-up radiation), along with the peace of mind that may come from removing as much of the cancer-stricken breast as possible. Before making the decision, she should review carefully the pros and cons of each operation (see mastectomy), and get a second opinion from another breast cancer surgeon.

The traditional treatment for lobular carcinoma in situ and ductal carcinoma in situ was mastectomy—and in the case of lobular carcinoma a double mastectomy, for if the condition was found in one breast, the risk of developing cancer in the other breast was high. Because abnormal cells do not form a discrete lump in carcinoma in situ and are therefore hard to localize, any surgery short of total mastectomy leaves some chance that an invasive cancer will develop. Many physicians today nevertheless recommend a watch-and-wait approach, carefully following the condition with good screening mammography. In the case of ductal carcinoma in situ, women may also be able to avoid a mastectomy by opting for a lumpectomy plus radiation, particularly when the tumors are small and low-grade. Nevertheless, any woman with either lobular carcinoma in situ or ductal carcinoma should understand that anything short of a mastectomy will involve some risk of recurrence and that some recurrences could be invasive forms of cancer. Ultimately, the decision is a personal one and needs to be made by weighing maximum peace of mind against the advantages of saving the breast or breasts but with a small risk of life-threatening consequences.

Radiation therapy. Any woman who chooses to remove only the cancerous lump should follow the surgery with radiation therapy (see entry). Radiation destroys cancer cells that may be present in the remaining breast tissue. Five-year recurrence rates after lumpectomy without radiation therapy are around 40 percent, whereas with radiation therapy they drop to around 10 percent.

Radiation is sometimes also given after a total mastectomy to eradicate cancerous cells that may still be in adjoining tissues. In the case of advanced incurable cancers, radiation therapy may be used to shrink tumors in the hope of alleviating pain, pressure, or bleeding.

Sometimes irradiation with external x-ray beams is supplemented with a newer form of radiation therapy, in which slender flexible tubes of radioactive material are implanted into the breast. These deliver radiation directly to the cancerous site without damaging surrounding tissues.

Uncomfortable side effects from radiation therapy can include initial nausea or loss of appetite, swelling and redness of the breast (which can last for months after treatment is over), fatigue, muscle pain, and sun sensitivity. Long-term side effects may include lung and heart problems, as well as cosmetic disfigurement. Radiation treatments, each lasting a few minutes, are required 5 days a week for approximately 6 weeks in most cases.

Chemotherapy. If cancer cells are present in the lymph nodes—or if other tests indicate a high probability that the cancer has spread, even when tests of the lymph nodes are negative—various options are available to help eradicate cancer elsewhere in the body. Chief among them are chemotherapy and hormonal therapy. The hope is that giving these treatments early enough in the course of the disease will slow the spread or prevent it from starting in the first place. For this reason there is a trend toward offering systemic therapies to women in even the earlier stages of the disease, although there is still no precise method for selecting the subgroup of women with very small tumors and no signs of metastases in the lymph nodes who will ultimately benefit.

Chemotherapy involves the administration, for up to 6 months, of drugs that interfere with the growth of cells—particularly cancer cells. It is often recommended for premenopausal women who have signs of cancer in their lymph nodes (that is, lymph node–positive women) and is generally started after surgery has been completed. Chemotherapy is also often effective for postmenopausal women under the age of 60, though success rates are somewhat lower. More and more cancer specialists now feel that chemotherapy should be tried in younger women who have negative lymph nodes—that is, no signs of cancer in their lymph nodes—if they have other signs of high risk such as a tumor that is bigger than an inch in diameter or one that is not estrogen-dependent.

The "classic" chemotherapy is called CMF, after the first letters of the three drugs involved: cyclophosphamide, methotrexate, and 5-fluorouracil. The side effects of this treatment can be unpleasant but are relatively mild as chemotherapy goes. This course of drugs usually causes nausea together with moderate hair loss. Other side effects include weight gain, mucous membrane inflammation, tearing of the eye, and conjunctivitis. In addition, the older a woman is, the more likely chemotherapy is to induce an early menopause: this seems to occur in 40 percent of women under 40 and 90 percent of women over 40.

Another combination of drugs commonly used to treat breast cancer is CA, which combines the drug Adriamycin (doxorubicin) with higher does of cyclophosphamide. CA is more toxic than CMF, and that is precisely why it may be more effective; that is, it may be better at killing growing cells, including cells in the body that are not cancerous. Among common side effects of CA therapy are nausea and complete hair loss. Large accumulations of Adriamycin in the body can eventually damage the heart. This combination is given in only 4 treatments over the course of 3 months and seems to be just as effective as 12 treatments with CMF over the course of 6 months.

The Food and Drug Administration has approved Taxol (paclitaxel) as a supplementary treatment for certain breast cancer patients following treatment with doxorubicin-containing combination chemotherapy. Recent studies showing little benefit from the addition of Taxol, however, have prompted debate among cancer specialists about its role.

Hormonal therapies. For postmenopausal women over the age of 50, hormonal therapy is often recommended, either alone or in combination with chemotherapy. By altering the cancer's response to hormones (particularly estrogen), hormonal therapy—which is much less toxic than chemotherapy—is particularly effective in slowing the growth of ER+ tumors (tumors that are responsive to estrogen), and new studies suggest that it may actually help premenopausal women with ER+ tumors as well. The most commonly used hormone treatment is the antiestrogen drug tamoxifen. Tamoxifen (Nolvadex) belongs to a class of drugs called selective estrogen receptor modulators, or SERMS, which work by competing with natural estrogen for estrogen receptors on cancer-prone molecules and therefore preventing the estrogen from promoting cancer. Most women are now given tamoxifen for 5 years, but studies are under way to determine the optimal length of therapy.

Women aged 50 to 69 may want to consider combining tamoxifen treatments with chemotherapy, since there is now good evidence that for women in this age group the combination is more effective in decreasing recurrence than tamoxifen alone, although it seems to have no effect on overall survival. Tamoxifen does not appear to be as beneficial when given to premenopausal women.

New studies suggest that surgically removing both ovaries—the chief sources of estrogen—in premenopausal women decreases breast cancer recurrence and mortality to rates comparable to those achieved with chemotherapy. Using drugs called GnRH agonists to suppress ovarian function is also effective in this population of women. Studies are under way to see if combining ovary removal (or suppression) with chemotherapy may be more effective than chemotherapy alone. Recent evidence suggests that combining tamoxifen treatment with lumpectomy and radiation can prevent recurrence in women with ductal carcinoma in situ. And in the National Surgical Adjuvant Breast and Bowel Project (NSABP) Breast Cancer Prevention Trial, tamoxifen decreased breast cancer incidence in women with lobular carcinoma by 56 percent.

Short-term side effects of tamoxifen can include hot flashes and a mucus-like vaginal discharge. Not enough is known about long-term effects, although, on the plus side, we already know that tamoxifen does not act as a pure antiestrogen. In parts of the body other than the breast, it actually seems to mimic estrogen rather than countering its effects. For example, like estrogen replacement therapy, taking tamoxifen seems to increase bone density and raise HDL cholesterol levels, thus possibly helping to protect a woman against osteoporosis and cardiovascular disease.

Tamoxifen increases the risk of endometrial (uterine) cancer and, to a small extent, the risk of developing blood clots and cataracts (a clouding of the lens of the eye), but most women find that the protection against breast cancer recurrence more than compensates for these relatively small risks. It is important for women taking tamoxifen to consult a physician promptly if any abnormal vaginal bleeding occurs.

Follow-up care of a woman with early-stage breast cancer. After a lumpectomy, a clinician will want to watch for a recurrence of the cancer. Usually this will involve a follow-up mammogram 6 months after the completion of radiation therapy. In addition, a physical examination should be done every 3 months during the first year, every 4 months in the second, and every 6 months after that. The clinician will play close attention to symptoms such as dry cough, chest pain, bone pain, or shortness of breath during exercise, any of which may be a sign that the cancer has spread to the lungs or bones. Blood tests for bone or liver dysfunction will also be done every 6 months, and some oncologists also check for elevations of certain tumor markers in the blood which can be an early sign that the cancer has recurred. Routine chest x-rays and bone scans are no longer considered to be useful parts of follow-up care.

Treating stage 4 disease. If the cancer has already spread beyond the breast (that is, if it is classified as stage 4), surgery is often pointless and unnecessarily painful unless the tumor is very large. Removing the original tumor or even the breast itself can do nothing to stop the cancer in the bones, lungs, liver, or other distant sites. Thus, the goal of treatment in most stage 4 breast cancers is alleviating as many symptoms as possible.

In some cases chemotherapy or hormonal therapy may be able to slow the spread of cancer throughout the body. Because hormonal therapy usually has fewer side effects than chemotherapy, it is often the treatment of choice for postmenopausal women with stage 4 cancer if the original cancer was estrogen receptor–positive. Premenopausal women with stage 4 cancer have traditionally been treated by having their ovaries removed, though some studies suggest that administering tamoxifen may be just as effective. Other possibilities are drugs called LHRH (luteinizing hormone releasing hormone) agonists, which lower estrogen levels by shutting down ovarian function.

It usually takes about 2 months for the body to respond to hormonal therapy, and the response lasts about a year or two. As a second line of therapy after the initial treatment stops working (and sometimes as a first line of therapy), a clinician may try drugs called aromatase inhibitors—anastrozole (Arimidex), letrozole (Femara), or exemesatane (Aromasin)—that block the conversion of androgens to estrogen in fat tissue, including breast tissue. Occasionally the progestin megestrol (Megace), an estrogen inhibitor, may be used, particularly in women who have lost weight or who need an appetite stimulant. Meanwhile, studies are under way to see if antiprogestin drugs (such as RU-486, most famous as the "abortion drug") may be yet another option.

If a stage 4 breast cancer is ER−, or if the disease is no longer responding to hormonal therapy, chemotherapy may be tried. And because it works a lot faster than hormonal therapy, chemotherapy may also be used in ER+ cancers if some vital organ is in imminent danger. Chemotherapy begins to shrink tumors within a couple of weeks and can provide considerable pain relief and an improved quality of life for women with stage 4 cancer. Women whose cancer has spread to the bone usually receive bisphosphonate pamidronate, which can relieve bone pain and prevent fractures.

One promising new drug, Herceptin (trastuzamab), was recently approved for use in combination with Taxol (paclitaxel) to treat certain stage 4 cancers. This monoclonal antibody was designed to attack the 25 to 30 percent of breast cancers that produce a specific protein called HER2 or HER2/neu. Another new drug, Xeloda (capecitabine), shows considerable promise in treating stage 4 breast cancer that hasn't responded to or has become resistant to conventional chemotherapy. In contrast to many other chemotherapeutic drugs, Xeloda causes only minimal hair loss and bone marrow depression, although side effects such as diarrhea, nausea, mouth sores, and pain and swelling of the hands and feet may still occur. Xeloda is taken orally rather than intravenously.

New drugs now in clinical trials that may someday be used to treat stage 4 breast cancer include angiogenesis inhibitors and tyrosine kinase inhibitors, as well as several vaccines.

Most remissions are only temporary, and the average patient with stage 4 cancer responds to chemotherapy for only 6 to 8 months and lives only 1.5 to 2 years after therapy begins. Although investigators are constantly trying different drugs and combinations of drugs, there are still no signs of a real cure on the horizon.

Psychological support. No matter what the cancer stage, support from friends, family, and clinicians can all be important parts of treatment. Various organizations (such as Reach to Recovery and ENCORE) send former breast cancer patients to the homes of women who have been diagnosed recently or are undergoing treatment, to listen and offer personal advice. Study after study shows that support from understanding people can alleviate a great deal of the fear, anxiety, depression, low self-esteem, damaged body image, and sexual dysfunction that often accompany a diagnosis of breast cancer and its treatment.

Many women find that joining a support group consisting of women who have undergone a similar experience is particularly valuable, and there is some intriguing evidence that women who belong to such support groups have a lower mortality rate from the disease, perhaps because of the supplementary emotional support itself or because of enhanced self-care encouraged by the group. Other women find psychotherapy (especially cognitive therapy) extremely helpful, and psychotropic drugs may allow a woman to cope better with the sometimes devastating psychological pressures of having breast cancer.

Who is likely to develop breast cancer?

Women often hear that their lifetime risk of developing breast cancer has increased from 1 in 9 a decade ago to 1 in 8. This change in statistical "risk" is not what it seems, however. It can be attributed to the fact that cancers in women over the age of 85 were recently added to the database. Thus, the 1 in 8 figure assumes that women will live to age 110, and it includes women who will develop cancer after the age of 75. Only 1 woman out of 40 is expected to die of breast cancer before reaching age 75.

Women frequently misconstrue the much-cited 1 in 8 lifetime risk factor to mean that 1 out of any 8 American women in a room has or will get breast cancer. What it really means is that, at the time of birth, a baby girl has a 1 in 8 chance of developing breast cancer at some point during her life. Risks are far lower that the average middle-aged woman will develop breast cancer in the coming year—or even at any given future date. Only 1 in 1,000 women in their 40s will be diagnosed as having breast cancer within the next year (see chart on page 97), and only 1 out of every 500 women in their 50s will receive such a diagnosis (assuming that a woman does not have some additional risk factor for breast cancer). Approximately 1 out of 25 40-year-old women will develop breast cancer by the age of 60, and about 1 of every 10 can expect to develop it by age 80 (see chart). The risk of dying of breast cancer before age 75 is only 2.5 percent.

A new model for predicting an individual woman's risk of developing breast cancer over the next five years and over her lifetime—the "Gail model"—now makes calculating breast cancer risk almost as simple as determining cholesterol levels. Knowing risk can not only be reassuring—particularly to a woman who believes herself to be at unusually high risk because her mother or another close relative had breast cancer—but also help clinicians evaluate the pros and cons of various risk-reduction strategies. In this model a woman's chance of developing breast cancer is estimated according to numerous risk factors determined by the Breast Cancer Detection and Demonstration Project, a long-term study of 275,000 women in the United States. A woman and her clinician can compare her specific relative risks to risks of women of the same age with different risk factors. (See chart).

It is important to note, though, that relative risk figures have not yet been sufficiently tested in non-Caucasian women. In addition, women often misinterpret these figures as their risk of developing breast cancer over a lifetime instead of their risks relative to a woman of the same age without the same risk factors. For example, consider a 40-year-old woman who, without any risk factors, has a 1 in 66 chance of developing breast cancer over the next 10 years. A 40-year-old woman who has a relative risk of 1.3 for developing breast cancer over the next 10 years elevates this risk only to 1 in 48 (the product of multiplying 1 in 66 by a factor of 1.3); she does not have the much more alarming risk of 1 in 7, which she'd get by multiplying 1.3 by her *lifetime* risk of developing breast cancer (1 in 8).

None of this should suggest that breast cancer is not a seri-ous or frightening disease. However one juggles the statistics, the fact remains that many women develop breast cancer, and many of them will eventually die from it. For this reason, some experts argue that breast cancer should be regarded as a chronic disease that is often lived with for decades but rarely eradicated.

Because there are still no definitive answers, each individual woman should try to find out as much as possible about the trade-offs so she can take an active role in preventing, detecting, and, if necessary, treating this disease.

A woman's chances of developing breast cancer vary with her age, ethnic group, menstrual and reproductive history, and family history of breast cancer. The greatest risk factor is having a mother or sister with breast cancer, particularly if that relative developed the cancer before menopause or in both breasts. Investigators have isolated two specific "breast cancer genes" (BRCA1 and BRCA2). Normally these genes seem to work by suppressing tumor development. Most women are born with two healthy copies of these genes, having received one copy from each parent, so that even if one becomes damaged in the course of a lifetime, the second copy can still keep cell growth in check. About 5 percent of the population, however, seems to have inherited a defective version of one or the other of these genes, so that any damage to the healthy gene triggers cancerous changes in breast tissue. BRCA1 and BRCA2 also seem to be linked to an increased risk of ovarian, colon, and possibly other cancers. Recent evidence suggests, however, that these genes do not predict risk in any simple way: it now appears that each of the breast cancer genes is subject to hundreds of different mutations, each of which is associated with a different degree of risk. And the same genetic defect may express itself more strongly in some families than in others.

These breast cancer genes—perhaps together with some other as yet unlocated breast cancer genes—may account for certain inherited forms of breast cancer. A woman who carries a breast cancer gene (which can be detected by a blood test) has a particularly high risk of developing the disease, and this risk increases as she ages.

Still, less than 10 percent of all breast cancer is thought to be inherited, and no more than 5 percent comes from a de-

Percent of women who will develop breast cancer, by age				
Current age	+10 years	+20 years	+30 years	Eventually
20	0.05	0.5	2	13
30	0.5	2	4.5	13
40	1.5	4	7.5	13
50	3	6	9.5	12
60	4	7	9	10
Source: National Cancer Institute				

fect in a single gene—which means that the breast cancer gene is not of particular value in predicting the majority of breast cancers. (It may nevertheless shed a great deal of light on how breast cancer develops in general, since damage to this gene probably promotes breast cancer even in women without a family history of breast cancer, the only difference being that this kind of damage can't be passed on to subsequent generations.)

Thus, having a first-degree relative who had breast cancer does not necessarily mean that a woman has inherited a breast cancer gene. It is very possible, for example, that the woman's mother or sister acquired breast cancer for the same nongenetic reasons as 95 percent of all women with breast cancer, and not because of some inherited genetic defect. If a female relative had breast cancer that developed after menopause or in only one breast, the odds are even lower that a defective gene is involved. Breast cancer in a male relative, however, makes it more likely that the family does carry a genetic defect.

Having had cancer in one breast greatly increases the risk that cancer will develop in the other breast. Also, women who are discovered (usually by accident) to have atypical hyperplasia are at increased risk and need to be evaluated frequently for breast cancer. This risk falls off with time, and if no breast cancer has developed within 10 years, having atypical hyperplasia does not add significantly to one's risk of developing breast cancer, compared with the risk for other women one's age. Furthermore, it is now clear that breast lumpiness (sometimes called fibrocystic disease) and benign breast lumps such as cysts and fibroadenomas do not put women at increased risk for breast cancer.

Women living in North America and Europe have a higher rate of breast cancer than those living elsewhere in the world, although when women of different national origins immigrate to the United States, their rate of breast cancer becomes similar. In recent years the incidence of breast cancer has been increasing in South America, Australia, and Asia.

The risk of acquiring breast cancer by the age of 75 is slightly higher for white American women than for African American women, and both have a higher risk than either Asian American or Hispanic American women. African American women are more than twice as likely as white women to die of breast cancer once they are diagnosed, however, largely because their disease often reaches a more advanced stage before it is treated, but to some extent also because their tumors may be more aggressive.

Women who have been exposed to high levels of estrogen over their lifetime—such as those who had an early menarche or a late menopause and those who have never given birth—seem to have a marked increase in breast cancer rates. But most women who used birth control pills (which contain low doses of estrogen) do not appear to have a higher than average risk of breast cancer. Women who take oral contraceptive pills for more than 12 years or who take high-estrogen pills in their mid-teens, may have an increased risk over the next two decades.

As for estrogen replacement therapy (ERT), evidence from the Women's Health Initiative indicates that long-term ERT moderately elevates the risk of breast cancer when the hormone progestin is added to estrogen. What this means is that a 60-year-old woman who had never taken hormones after menopause would have a 2 in 100 chance of developing breast cancer in the next 5 years; but if she had used hormones for at least 5 years, she would have a 3 in 100 chance of developing breast cancer in the next 5 years.

There may also be a slightly increased risk of breast cancer in women who took the drug diethylstilbestrol (DES) while pregnant. Daughters of these women are not known to be at increased risk for breast cancer, however.

During pregnancy, estrogen and progesterone reach high levels, causing cells in breast tissue to differentiate into new forms. This makes the cells ultimately more resistant to the stimulative effects of estrogen, and therefore lowers a woman's lifetime risk of breast cancer. But over the short run, pregnancy slightly increases the risk of breast cancer, perhaps because the rising estrogen levels may temporarily stimulate any premalignant cells lurking in the breast. Having a baby raises a woman's risk of developing breast cancer during the first 15 years after delivery, but after that her risks are lower than those of women who have never had children. If she has a second pregnancy, her risk rises again but to a lesser extent because the protective effects of the first pregnancy seem already to have set in.

Women who have their babies before age 30 have a lower likelihood of breast cancer than women who have their babies after 30 (possibly because there are likely to be fewer premalignant cells lurking in the breasts of younger women to be stimulated by estrogen during pregnancy, or, as a new study suggests, because the fetal growth-regulating protein alpha-fetoprotein may inhibit the growth of breast cancer cells). But women who have their babies after 30 still have a lower likelihood of breast cancer than women who have never had children. The longer the time between menarche (the first menstrual period) and the first full-term pregnancy, the higher the risk of future breast cancer. In fact, having a full-term pregnancy early in life (before the age of 15) decreases the relative risk of breast cancer to approximately 0.4. This particular benefit clearly does not outweigh the considerable disadvantages of teenage pregnancy, but it does lend credence to the connection between the menstrual cycle and breast cancer risk.

Mounting evidence suggests that breastfeeding one's babies may provide a protective effect against developing breast cancer—and may indeed be a more significant factor than any other known in determining an individual woman's risk. One study suggests that women who breastfeed for as little as 4 to 6 months over a lifetime (not necessarily just one baby) reduce their risk of developing breast cancer by at least 20 percent. The greatest decrease in risk (as much as 50 percent) occurred in women who started breastfeeding before the age of 20 and nursed for at least 6 months. And a recent study of women in rural China by Yale University researchers found that women who breastfed their babies for two years or longer reduced their risk of breast cancer (both before and after menopause) by 50 percent. This study confirms several similar studies in China and the United States. Another major recent study suggests that the greatest reductions in risk are found in women who bear numerous children and breastfeed each one of them for two or more years—not a pattern likely to be emulated in developed countries, or even desirable in them, but intriguing nonetheless.

The link between lifetime exposure to estrogen and breast cancer may help explain some of the increased incidence of breast cancer in developed nations, where better nutrition leads to earlier menarche and where women tend to delay childbearing.

Exposure to ionizing radiation earlier in life can also increase a woman's odds of developing breast cancer at some point, particularly if the exposure occurred when the woman was under 25 years of age. For this reason a woman who was treated with mantle radiation for Hodgkin's disease when she was under 25 should begin annual mammograms eight years after the radiation therapy, even if she is still under 40 (the age when most women are advised to begin having regular mammograms). The risk associated with radiation used to treat and screen for breast cancer is generally considered to be acceptably small. The risk of developing breast cancer in the other breast after radiation therapy and lumpectomy to treat primary cancer in one breast is raised by a factor of only 1.33 over a 10-year span. And perhaps no more than 1 case of breast cancer per year per 1 million women screened can be attributed to radiation exposure from screening mammograms. This risk, already regarded as negligible, will probably decrease even further as technology moves from film screen mammography to digital mammography.

It is important to remember, however, that fully three-quarters of all breast cancers cannot be linked to any of these risk factors. There is some limited evidence that exposure to environmental toxins—particularly pesticides—or possibly even to electromagnetic fields may increase the risk of breast cancer and might explain some of the rising incidence in developed countries. Pesticides such as DDT, polychlorinated biphenyls (PCBs), and polybrominated biphenyls (PBBs) are known carcinogens which act somewhat similarly to estrogen in the body, and they have been found in unusually large amounts in the tissues of women with breast cancer. More studies need to be done before these or any other toxic substances can be conclusively linked to breast cancer.

It already seems clear that exposure to high levels of ionizing radiation increases the risk, particularly if the exposure occurred while a woman was in her teens or 20s. The amount delivered in a mammogram or during radiation treatments for breast cancer, however, is not considered large enough to pose a significant problem.

Finally, evidence from the Nurses' Health Study suggests that heavy consumption of alcohol over many years increases the risk of dying from breast cancer.

How can breast cancer be prevented?

The risks associated with lifestyle and environment have led investigators to suspect—and hope—that at least some of the risk for breast cancer can be reduced. The goal is to find specific factors linked to breast cancer that can be eliminated or reduced by modifying the way we live. During the 1980s dietary fat was a leading contender, but subsequent studies have undermined much of the evidence—although a sizable number of people are still convinced that fat will eventually be proven to play a role. The Nurses' Health Study, involving nearly 90,000 nurses aged 34–59 who were followed up for 8 years, found no link between dietary fat intake and breast cancer.

In recent years preventing breast cancer has become as much a political as a scientific issue. Concerned that not enough research dollars were being devoted to breast cancer—and that interest was disproportionately focused on treatment rather than on causes and prevention—many women's groups have become active in demanding better studies and more federal research funding. As these groups have pointed out repeatedly, cancer research had focused on treatment ever since 1971, when President Nixon launched the National Cancer Act. No major studies on preventing breast cancer were approved by the National Institutes of Health (NIH) until the 1980s, and even a decade later studies of the links between breast cancer and diet or breast cancer and pesticides were few and far between.

One result of this outcry was the founding in 1991 of the National Breast Cancer Coalition (NBCC), a federation of nearly 2,000 support and advocacy groups. A year later this coalition, along with other groups, lobbied Congress to double the amount of money spent on breast cancer research. With a declaration by the NIH that women's health needed more attention, the result was an increase in the national budget for breast cancer research from $90 million to $420 million.

The fruits of all these studies are still years down the line. In the meantime, some women may feel they are doing their best to prevent breast cancer by eating low-fat diets, buying organic produce, or staying away from sources of electromagnetic radiation such as electric blankets or microwave ovens, but these behaviors are based at best on unproved (and sometimes disproved) hunches about what might cause breast cancer. Women of childbearing age might also consider bucking cultural attitudes and breastfeeding babies for as long as it is possible and comfortable. Further studies also need to be done to determine the role of a soybean-rich diet, which has been increasingly linked to a lower risk of breast (as well as colon and, in men, prostate) cancers—perhaps because soybeans contain significant amounts of estrogen-like compounds called isoflavones or phytoestrogens that may inhibit cancer growth.

Two tactics that may reduce the risk of breast cancer in some women—and have other proven health benefits in all women—are getting regular exercise and avoiding excessive alcohol consumption. A recent study showed that women who exercised regularly during adolescence had a significantly lower subsequent risk of breast cancer compared with those who were sedentary. The effect of exercise in older women is not known. Studies of the relationship between alcohol and breast cancer have shown an increased risk of cancer in women who have more than 3 alcoholic drinks per week. Women especially concerned about breast cancer might consider limiting their alcohol intake to this level.

For women at extremely high risk, prophylactic mastectomies (removing seemingly healthy breasts to prevent cancer from developing at some later time) are sometimes performed, although this approach is controversial and its effectiveness has not been proven. Many women with strong family histories of breast cancer are so overwhelmed by fear that they choose to take this drastic step in their 20s or 30s even though they show no signs of malignancy. Just because a woman has a sister or mother with breast cancer does not necessarily mean that she will develop breast cancer. Recent evidence suggests, however, that removing both breasts can reduce the incidence of breast cancer by about 90 percent in women with a high risk of developing breast cancer (based on family history) and that it may be preferable to living with uncertainty for some young women at very high risk—for example, young women who have more than one first-degree relative (mother, sisters, aunts) with breast cancer, together with a personal history of atypical hyperplasia.

With the discovery of the BRCA1 and BRCA2 genes, unnecessary prophylactic mastectomies should become much less common, since it now may be possible for a woman to determine her risk much more accurately with a simple blood test. Recent studies also suggest that women carrying a mutation in the BRCA1 gene can cut breast cancer risk significantly by having both ovaries removed, a procedure called a bilateral prophylactic oophorectomy.

The new knowledge of the breast cancer gene, like much of our newly acquired genetic information, does not come without a price. This is largely because our ability to predict disease still far outpaces our ability to treat it. Knowing that a woman or girl is likely to develop breast disease later in life is undoubtedly going to have some effect on her insurability and employability. And, unconsciously or not, it will also affect her self-image and the attitudes of friends and family toward her.

Nonsurgical (though still rather drastic) alternatives for women at very high risk may include injections of substances that can stop hormone production by the ovaries, or administration of tamoxifen to block the effects of a woman's own estrogen before cancer can develop. The U.S. Food and Drug Administration (FDA) has already approved tamoxifen for use by women aged 35 and older who are at high risk for breast cancer. Taking tamoxifen can cut the risk of developing cancer by 50 percent in women at high risk for breast cancer, possibly including women with cancer-promoting mutations of the BRCA1 and BRCA2 genes.

In addition, a large-scale clinical trial called STAR (Study of Tamoxifen and Raloxifene) was begun in early 1999 to compare the effectiveness and long-term safety of the osteoporosis prevention drug Evista (raloxifene) with that of tamoxifen in a similar group of women. Raloxifene is another antiestrogenic drug (or SERM) that works by blocking cancer-promoting natural estrogen from hooking into cancer-prone molecules. Its advantage over tamoxifen is that it does not stimulate the uterus, and therefore does not increase the risk of developing endometrial (uterine) cancer. The National Cancer Institute of Canada is conducting a related study on the preventive effects of yet another antiestrogenic drug, idoxifene, on both breast cancer and osteoporotic fractures.

Whatever these studies ultimately reveal, for the vast majority of women, the chief means of preventing breast cancer still lies in early detection, whether by a health care clinician, through mammography (see entry), or by breast self-examination (see entry). Controversy swirls around the efficacy of these procedures, but most health care professionals recommend them as a woman's best chance for preventing breast cancer.

Related entries

Biopsy, body image, breast lumps (benign), breast reconstruction, breast self-examination, chemotherapy, estrogen, hair loss, lumpectomy, lymphedema, mammography, mastectomy, ovary removal, pesticides and organic foods, psychotherapy, radiation therapy, sexual dysfunction

Breast Implants and Enlargement

Over a million women in the United States have silicone or saline breast implants, most of which were placed for the purpose of enlarging their breasts. Some women choose to have implants because they are unhappy with their breast size, while others want to enlarge breasts that have shrunk after childbearing or to enlarge one breast that is smaller than the other. It is important to recognize that this kind of surgery—as opposed to breast reconstruction (see entry), which is sometimes performed in cancer patients after mastectomy—is designed to improve the appearance of otherwise healthy breasts.

The implant itself is a plastic pouch made of a combination of carbon, hydrogen, oxygen, and silicon and filled with either silicone gel or a saline (saltwater) solution. Although there has been considerable controversy surrounding the safety of silicone gel–filled breast implants, a number of recent studies suggest that earlier fears about health risks are mostly unwarranted. Nonetheless, only saline-filled implants are currently approved for cosmetic uses.

The key to satisfaction after cosmetic surgery is to have a realistic understanding of the procedure beforehand and a reasonable set of expectations about what it can deliver. Plastic surgeons may have "before" and "after" pictures to show prospective patients so they will have some idea of how the surgery can change appearance. Any woman considering breast enlargement should beware of the surgeon who shows only beautiful women or stunning results. Appearance after surgery can vary considerably, so it is more helpful to see the usual result. That way, a woman will not be disappointed in her appearance if the surgery does not turn her into a men's magazine model. Of course, a woman may also be pleasantly surprised to see how good she looks.

Since breast enlargement surgery is almost always performed for cosmetic reasons, its costs are not covered by insurance. The patient will be responsible for the surgeon's fee, hospital and anesthesia expenses, and the cost of the implant itself. If there are complications after surgery, these may or may not be covered by insurance. Women should be prepared to pay hidden costs as well, such as time lost from work or child care expenses during recuperation. These financial considerations clearly put breast enlargement surgery out of the reach of many women.

How are these procedures performed?

During the surgery for breast enlargement, a pocket is created for the implant through a small incision. The incision can be located in the crease under the breast, around the areola, or in the armpit. The implant is inserted through this incision and placed behind the breast tissue to push it forward, thereby enlarging the breast. Usually the implant is placed behind the pectoralis muscle in the chest wall (see illustration). Since the breast tissue itself is pushed forward, much of it remains accessible to physical examination and mammography. Additional incisions for a breast lift may be required if the breast is especially saggy. Implants alone will not correct significant sag.

What happens after the surgery?

Breast enlargement is often a day surgery procedure, even though general anesthesia may be required. A woman can expect her breasts to be sore and swollen for a week or so, and often black and blue, though excessive bruising, swelling, pain, redness, or firmness is abnormal. Some surgeons use drains to help decrease blood accumulation and discoloration. Vigorous physical activities will be restricted for several weeks while healing takes place. Some surgeons suggest using a special brassiere for a period of time after surgery.

The breasts should become softer during the first several

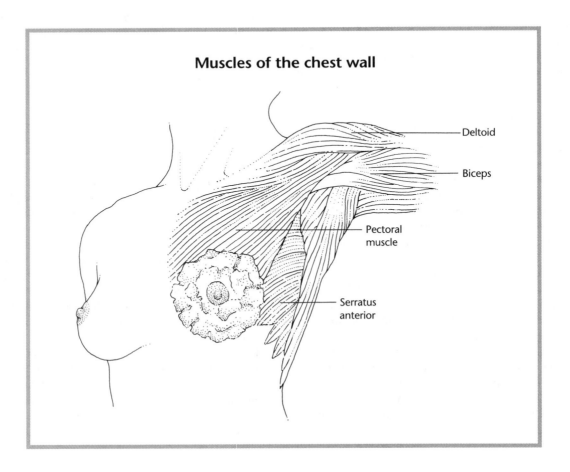

Muscles of the chest wall

Deltoid

Biceps

Pectoral muscle

Serratus anterior

months after surgery, although they may always remain firmer than natural breasts. Sensory changes that occur with the surgery tend to be temporary but may become permanent. In some cases these changes might affect sexual response to breast stimulation during the healing process or even thereafter. Massage may be recommended to enhance breast softness or to help sensory changes resolve more quickly. Enlargement surgery, after everything has healed, should not interfere with exercise or breastfeeding.

What are the risks and complications?

In qualified hands, breast enlargement surgery is a safe procedure with a low complication rate. It is essential, however, to seek a surgeon who is certified by the American Board of Plastic Surgeons.

Anyone considering breast enlargement needs to understand clearly what the surgery involves. There are certain potential complications connected with any type of surgery, while other complications are specific to surgery using implants.

All surgery requires some kind of anesthesia. A woman undergoing elective surgery should make sure that the anesthesia team and the operative facility are appropriately credentialed.

Bleeding is also a risk with almost any operation. During breast enlargement surgery a number of small blood vessels are exposed. If one of these vessels begins to bleed after the operation, it may cause a local accumulation of blood under the tissues. Such bleeding, called hematoma formation, is rare. It is also not life-threatening, though a second operation for drainage may be required.

All types of breast enlargement surgery require incisions, and all incisions leave scars, though some surgical techniques leave smaller or less conspicuous scars than others. Certain skin types, too, are more prone to developing particularly prominent scars. Scarring depends on an individual's genetic healing tendencies, not just on the skill of the surgeon. It is a good idea to discuss scarring in detail with the surgeon before making any final decisions.

The more complicated process of using natural tissues is not generally recommended for cosmetic breast enlargement; these operations rely solely on the use of artificial material. Infections, while uncommon during elective operations, can be a particular problem when artificial materials are involved. Once an infection settles around an implant, it is hard to get rid of. Usually an infected implant has to be removed in order for the infection to be controlled. The implant can be replaced at a later time after the infection has cleared up. Antibiotics are given around the time of surgery to minimize the chances of infection, and meticulous attention is paid to maintaining sterile conditions.

Also, no artificial material should be considered permanent: the human lifespan is longer than the useful life of most products made by human hands. If one lives long enough, sooner or later the implant shell will lose its strength and integrity. When this happens, the material inside the implant pouch will leak out. With saline implants, a hole or a tear in the pouch will allow all the saline inside to leak out (like water from a water balloon) and the implant will deflate. This is not dangerous, but it certainly could be inconvenient and embarrassing. If the implant deflates, it must be replaced, requiring additional surgery, though nothing as extensive as the original operation. In the past, saline implants had a significantly higher leakage rate than did silicone, but this problem seems to be less frequent with current versions.

Although silicone gel–filled implants are no longer used for cosmetic breast enlargement, they were quite common in the past, and many women still have them in place. A tear or rupture in a silicone gel implant causes the gel to escape from the shell. But since silicone gel is thick and does not migrate very rapidly, it is often not evident that a silicone gel implant is leaking. Small leaks can sometimes be felt as lumps in the breast as the body surrounds the gel with scar tissue. Any lump, however, needs to be taken seriously even if a woman has implants in place. A lump may be a silicone leak, but it could also be a breast cancer.

Concerns about whether leakage and breakdown of the implants containing silicone gel can lead to certain autoimmune or connective tissue diseases have largely been laid to rest by numerous scientific studies, although one large study did find a slight increase in self-reported connective tissue disease in women with silicone implants. Even so, because juries in several well-publicized cases awarded damages to women who claimed that breast implants led to autoimmune disorders—diseases that occur when the body produces antibodies that attack its own tissues—the Food and Drug Administration in 1992 banned further placement of silicone implants until their safety could be reviewed. The ban was subsequently modified to allow these implants to be used for breast reconstruction after mastectomy. The FDA ultimately judged silicone implants to be safe.

Because implants are foreign objects, the body reacts to them by walling them off with scar tissue. Scar tissue has a natural tendency to contract. If the scar tissue contracts excessively, the soft implant will become compressed into a firm ball that may shift in its pocket on the chest wall. This process is called capsule formation or capsular contracture. Implants are less likely to develop capsules if they are placed under the chest wall muscle, if they are saline filled, and if they have a textured surface. A new antibiotic solution that may help reduce or eliminate capsular contracture is under investigation.

Women who have the older silicone gel–filled implants in place experience capsule formation more frequently. Symptoms include firmness, tenderness, tightness, and even pain. Excessive capsule formation can also signal the leakage of silicone gel from the implant. A plastic surgeon experienced with implants can help identify specific problems. Often a mammogram combined with an ultrasound or an MRI will be required to identify leaks or ruptures. Even if an implant is not leaking or ruptured, the firmness of a capsule may be bothersome. To treat the capsules, surgery is currently recommended to remove the capsule around the implant and re-place the implant with a different kind. Squeezing the breast to rupture the capsule is not recommended, since this can actually damage the implant.

Although the capsules may make the breast feel firm or hard, they should not result in distinct masses or nodules. Any woman who feels a distinct mass in her breast should have a biopsy to eliminate the possibility of cancer. Having implants in place does not either increase or decrease a woman's chances of developing breast cancer, but it is important for a woman to undergo screening mammography and physical examination as appropriate for her age. Special mammogram views allow more of the breast tissue to be seen in cases where some of it is obscured by an implant. Investigations are under way to see if magnetic resonance imaging (MRI) may be a more sensitive screening method for women with implants.

Breast biopsies—either needle biopsies or surgical ones—are possible even with implants in place. There is a certain risk of damaging the implant with any biopsy technique, but the consequences of missing an early breast cancer are much more serious. It is desirable to have the biopsy done at a facility that is familiar with implants. If a cancer is detected, the treatment options include mastectomy or lumpectomy followed by radiation therapy. Implants do not react well to radiation, however, and there is a high incidence of complications (especially severe capsule formation and healing problems) when implants are exposed to radiation. A woman facing cancer treatment who wants to keep as much of her breast as possible should consider implant removal. Others might prefer a complete mastectomy with either immediate or delayed breast reconstruction. Breast cancer can be treated adequately in women with implants, but the pros and cons of the different types of treatment need to be weighed.

Related entries

Anesthesia, biopsy, body image, breast cancer, breast reconstruction, keloid scarring, lumpectomy, mammography, mastectomy, radiation therapy

Breast Lumps (Benign)

Breast lumps and breast lumpiness are not the same thing. Breast "lumpiness" consists of many little lumps (cysts) and strands of fibrous tissue in both breasts, and it is considered normal. Sometimes this condition is called fibrocystic disease, but it is not a disease at all. A breast lump, by contrast, stands out from general lumpiness as something distinctly different. It may be the size of a pea, a marble, a grape, or even a lemon, and it is clearly dominant, compared with any "background" lumpiness. (Women who do not have lumpy breasts can also develop a breast lump, of course.)

There are four types of breast lumps, three of which are virtually harmless. The fourth is a malignant lump, that is, cancer. The vast majority of breast lumps in premenopausal women are benign (noncancerous), but even so, a woman who detects a discrete lump in her breast should see a doctor as soon as possible for a diagnosis. Among postmenopausal women who are not taking estrogen replacement therapy (which can stimulate the development of benign lumps), 50 percent of breast lumps are benign, and the other half are malignant.

Types of benign breast lumps

Cysts. Most lumps in the breasts of premenopausal women are either cysts or fibroadenomas, and most of these are caused by fluctuating levels of ovarian hormones. Cysts are fluid-filled sacs of various sizes (see illustration). They usually feel soft and can be moved under the skin. Sometimes cysts produce a diffuse, dull pain in the affected breast, generally near the armpit.

Most cysts are filled with a yellow, brown, or green watery fluid, but a blocked milk-secreting duct in a woman nursing a baby can sometimes produce a milk-filled cyst called a galactocele.

Fibroadenomas. Fibroadenomas are noncancerous tumors composed of connective tissue and other cells that have multiplied faster than normal (see illustration). Unlike malignant tumors, they tend to have regular borders, be freely movable, and feel firm but not rock hard. Most are the size of a marble, but giant fibroadenomas can become as large as a lemon.

Pseudolumps. Pseudolumps are all the other masses in a breast that a clinician will want to evaluate. These may turn out to be just exaggerated lumpiness, but they are distinct enough from surrounding tissues to make a woman (and her clinician) want to check them out. When a doctor says a woman has "fibrocystic changes," she probably just has pseudolumps.

Other sources of pseudolumps (besides general lumpiness) may be scarring from previous surgery or some other trauma to the breast. They can also be caused by "fat necrosis"—death of a clump of fat cells owing to some injury or surgery. A pseudolump may be caused by an abscess (a collection of pus), in which case the woman would have a fever as well as a red, swollen, and painful breast (see mastitis). Mastitis occurs when bacteria from the skin or from a nursing baby's mouth enter the breast through dry cracks in the nipples. If the resulting infection is not treated promptly with antibiotics, an abscess sometimes develops.

Who is likely to develop benign breast lumps?

Cysts appear most often in women in their 30s, 40s, and 50s, and increase as menopause approaches. They rarely occur in young women or in women past menopause. Fibroadenomas are more common in teenagers and women in their 20s, al-

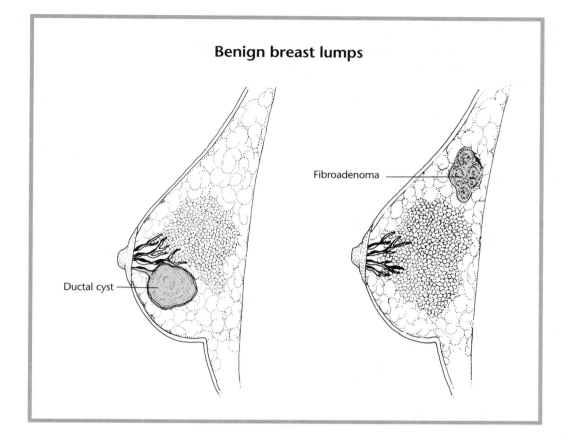

Benign breast lumps

Fibroadenoma

Ductal cyst

though they can develop in any premenopausal woman and in postmenopausal women who are taking estrogen replacement therapy. (If they are found in an older woman who is not taking ERT, usually they have been there for decades and simply went undetected.)

Relatively few women develop benign breast lumps after menopause: 1 out of every 2 lumps found in postmenopausal women turn out to be cancerous, as compared with 1 in 12 in premenopausal women.

How is the condition evaluated?

Every woman who detects a new lump in her breast should be evaluated by a physician. The doctor will discuss with her whether an ultrasound or a mammogram is appropriate to exclude the possibility of cancer. Physical examination alone is not sufficiently reliable to diagnose a breast lump, but some lumps can be evaluated without a mammogram or ultrasound.

For example, the quickest and least expensive test that can distinguish a cyst from cancer is fine-needle aspiration. In this test a needle syringe is inserted into the lump, and if greenish fluid can be aspirated, the physician knows that the lump is a cyst. Aspiration can be done in a surgeon's office, using a local anesthetic to numb the skin where the needle is inserted. Some clinicians send the fluid from a cyst to the lab for confirmation that it contains no cancerous cells, but others consider this step unnecessary. It is important, however,

to have a repeat examination in 1 to 2 months to make sure the cyst has not recurred, as this may signal the possibility of cancer.

If a cyst is discovered through a routine mammogram and diagnosed by ultrasound, and if it is not causing any discomfort, a woman may choose simply to leave it alone. But many physicians believe that all breast cysts should be aspirated to prevent them from obscuring underlying cancer by interfering with the breast exam. If a cyst is causing pain, aspiration can usually alleviate it.

A clinician experienced in evaluating breast lumps can be fairly confident in diagnosing a fibroadenoma through physical examination alone. But the only way to be sure is to do a needle biopsy and send the cells to the lab for confirmation. If the biopsy is negative, and if a follow-up mammogram or ultrasound is also negative for malignancy, the woman may choose to leave the lump alone.

Mammography is not a desirable diagnostic option for women who are pregnant, breastfeeding, or under 30 years of age (a time when breast tissue is too dense for a reliable mammogram). Ultrasonography is sometimes helpful in distinguishing a cyst or fibroadenoma from a malignant mass in a young woman and is often the first test done in women under 30.

Fibroadenomas are thought to be harmless in themselves. The only danger in leaving them alone is the possibility that a malignant cancer has somehow been missed. Because of this, clinicians usually recommend that middle-aged or older women have lumps that are thought to be fibroadenomas removed. This allows the clinician to biopsy the tissue to be absolutely sure that the lump is not cancer, while eliminating the condition at the same time. In younger women, for whom the chances of breast cancer are much lower, removing the lump may still be a good idea because fibroadenomas can become quite large during pregnancy and lactation, when removal can be complicated.

Women who develop multiple lumps over time will need to have each lump evaluated as it arises. After several negative biopsies, a woman and her doctor should discuss how to approach future lumps. In a very young woman with a low risk of having breast cancer, the physician may decide to evaluate a lump during one or two menstrual cycles before biopsying it for malignancy.

How are benign breast lumps treated?

Many women decide they can live with breast lumps once breast cancer has been ruled out. But others will want to have their cysts aspirated and their fibroadenomas removed for confirmation and peace of mind, not to mention comfort in some cases. The surgical procedure used to remove lumps is called lumpectomy (see entry).

Breast abscesses should be drained by a breast surgeon, as should galactoceles. Antibiotics may be prescribed for abscesses to treat the infection. No treatment is required for the lumps left by breast trauma.

Related entries

Biopsy, breast cancer, breast pain, lumpectomy, mammography, mastitis, menstrual cycle, ultrasound

Breast Pain

Breast pain (mastalgia) or tenderness is a common symptom and most frequently occurs as part of normal changes in the breast during the menstrual cycle.

Who is likely to develop breast pain?

Women from age 35 through menopause in particular often develop benign breast lumps or cysts in their breasts before their monthly menstrual periods. Diffuse and dull pain is common, with both breasts generally affected. Noncyclic pain (most often experienced by women with "lumpy" breasts; see breast lumps, benign) tends to occur in one breast only and can be sharp and stabbing. It generally occurs in women in their 40s. Women who have just started taking oral contraceptives or estrogen replacement therapy also sometimes experience breast pain, but this usually disappears within a few months.

In pregnant women breasts often become painful, tender, or tingly as early as a week or two after conception. In nursing mothers, breast pain can result from the engorgement with milk that sometimes occurs when the baby's need for milk is not coordinated with the mother's production. This often happens in the early stages of breastfeeding or during weaning. Nursing itself can produce cracked and sore nipples; limiting lactation time or rubbing the breasts with lanolin can often help relieve the pain. Blocked milk ducts can also produce red and tender lumps. These may be relieved by nursing the baby more frequently on the affected side. Occasionally a blocked milk gland will produce a painful cyst called a galactocele, which can be drained by a breast surgeon.

Nursing mothers may also develop mastitis, a breast infection that occurs when bacteria from the baby's mouth or surrounding skin enters the breast through cracks in the nipple. Women with mastitis will generally have chills, fever, and malaise in addition to breast pain; these can be treated with antibiotics. If there is also a palpable (easily felt) lump, however, the mastitis has probably produced an abscess (a collection of pus) under the skin, which will have to be drained by a surgeon.

Lymph node enlargement can accompany mastitis and should not be confused with breast cancer. The enlargement should go away as soon as the infection is cured.

How is breast pain treated?

Women who suffer from breast pain may want to keep a record of symptoms and menstrual periods to see if the pain is cyclic or noncyclic, that is, to see if lumps and pain worsen at particular times in the menstrual cycle. If the problem is cyclic, hormonal therapy such as oral contraceptives are sometimes helpful. There have been no convincing studies that eliminating caffeine intake helps relieve breast lumps or pain. Mild analgesics such as acetaminophen (Tylenol) or ibuprofen (Motrin) can help reduce discomfort, as can breast support from a good bra. Some women find that taking vitamin E relieves breast pain as well. An herbal remedy, evening primrose oil, in a dose of 1 or 2 capsules twice a day, has been reported to reduce breast pain in half of all women with cyclic pain. It is thought to work by reducing inflammation through its effects on inflammation-causing prostaglandins—similar to the action of anti-inflammatory drugs such as ibuprofen.

If any breast pain is associated with a small lump that does not go away, a woman should be checked for malignancies. Usually a normal clinical examination and a mammogram will reassure a woman that her breast pain has some other cause: only 6 percent of all women with breast cancer have breast pain.

Related entries

Breast cancer, breast lumps (benign), breastfeeding, estrogen replacement therapy, mammography, mastitis, menstrual cycle, oral contraceptives, pregnancy

Breast Reconstruction

Breast reconstruction is most commonly performed to restore the size and shape of the breast after a mastectomy for breast cancer. Reconstruction can be carried out for many other reasons as well. For example, an injury may result in a misshapen breast, especially if it occurs during childhood or early development. Malformations may also occur as part of the developmental process itself, not becoming evident until adolescence.

Approximately 180,000 women develop breast cancer each year, and a certain percentage of them will require the removal of part or all of the breast to treat the disease. Restoring the appearance to as natural a state as possible is the goal of breast reconstruction. The operation may be done at the same time as the cancer surgery or at a later date. Many factors influence the decision about timing. Although it was once feared that reconstruction would interfere with subsequent cancer treatment or detection, it is now well established that reconstruction is safe for the vast majority of women who are otherwise in good health. A need for postoperative chemotherapy or even radiation does not rule out reconstruction. A woman facing breast cancer surgery should discuss the pros and cons of both immediate and delayed reconstruction with a surgeon experienced in the most up-to-date procedures.

It may also be useful for a woman who is considering breast reconstruction to speak directly with someone who has gone through the surgery already, preferably someone whose situation is similar. A reconstructive surgeon, oncologist, or breast surgeon may be able to put prospective patients in touch with women who have had various types of reconstructive surgery. Support groups are also available as resources for women considering reconstruction.

The reconstructive surgeon should be able to show pictures that give an idea of what the different procedures can accomplish. Women are wise to be wary of a surgeon who shows only perfect results. Even the very best surgeons do not achieve a beautiful reconstruction every time. The pictures should give a general idea of what the operation delivers in the average patient.

Many women worry that seeking reconstruction is frivolous or vain. Nothing could be further from the truth. A number of psychological studies have affirmed the relationship of reconstruction to the restoration of a healthy body image and self-esteem. This does not mean that reconstruction is necessary for a woman to feel good about herself. But if reconstruction feels right, this is a normal and healthy inclination, not vanity.

Many health insurance plans provide coverage for reconstructive procedures. Each type of insurance in each state is different, though. A woman needs to explore her individual insurance situation before making her final decision about breast reconstruction surgery.

How is the procedure performed?

Breast reconstruction can be performed using the patient's own tissues, artificial materials, or some combination of the two. As a general principle, using one's own tissues will yield a more natural result but will require more surgery. Artificial materials do not require as much surgery, but often give a result that will not look as natural for many body types. A woman should balance the advantages and disadvantages of each technique before making her decision.

The easiest kind of surgery to do, but the one that "fits" the fewest number of women, uses a simple saline-filled implant to reconstruct the shape of the breast. A pocket is created for the implant under the pectoral muscle on the chest wall (see illustration). This muscle is readily visible when the breast is removed during a mastectomy. If reconstruction is to be done at the same time, the pocket is formed under the muscle, and the leftover skin is sewn up as a fine straight line across the chest. If reconstruction is to be done at a later time, the old mastectomy incision will be reopened to provide access to the pectoral muscle.

Using an implant for reconstruction, however, will form a breast that is shaped like an implant: rounded and quite upright. This shape often will not match the other breast, which may be more teardrop-shaped, with a certain degree of droop. And implant reconstruction can form only small breasts, since the pectoral muscle can be stretched only a little bit at any one time.

To form a medium-sized or large reconstructed breast, a process called tissue expansion must be used. This technique relies on the fact that skin and muscle can be stretched considerably if the stretching takes place gradually. To reconstruct a breast through tissue expansion, two steps are necessary. First, a stretching device is placed under the pectoral muscle, in the same spot where an implant would go if the implant-only technique were being used. This device, called a tissue expander, has a valve in it that allows it to be inflated gradually, over a period of time, like a balloon under the skin and muscle. In this way, as the tissues overlying the expander are stretched, a progressively larger pocket is created. When a sufficient amount of expansion has been achieved, the expander is replaced with an implant of comparable size. This requires a second surgical step, though it is a fairly small operation since most of the work has been done by the stretching process itself. Nonetheless, it takes several months to get to the end of this process—or longer if chemotherapy is required. Expanding the tissue expander is not painful and is done quickly in the doctor's office. The process should not interfere with normal activities.

This technique, though it allows a larger breast to be formed, still has limits. Using an implant means that the reconstructed breast will still be implant-shaped. Sometimes the other breast can be reshaped to look more like the reconstructed one. A breast lift, breast enlargement, or breast reduction on the natural side may help attain a match, but each of these procedures has its own set of risks that must be

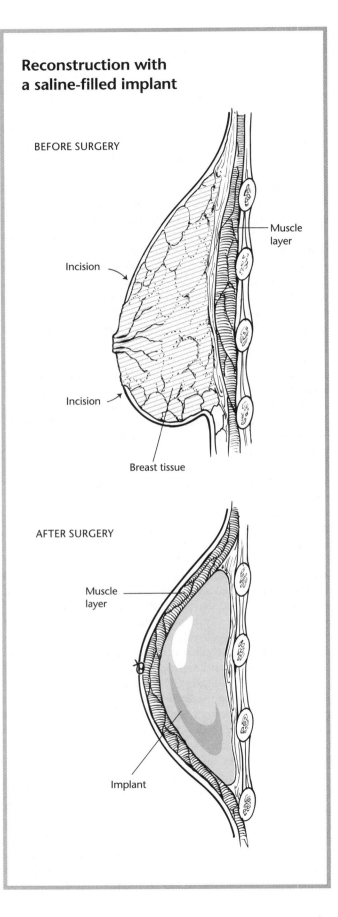

Reconstruction with a saline-filled implant

BEFORE SURGERY

Muscle layer

Incision

Incision

Breast tissue

AFTER SURGERY

Muscle layer

Implant

considered (see breast implants and enlargement; breast reduction).

Matching the natural side is often easier to accomplish if the woman's own tissues are used instead of implants alone. Skin, fat, and muscle moved from other parts of the body can be molded into a shape that more closely resembles the opposite side. Natural tissues should all age similarly, too, so the resemblance between the reconstruction and the other side will continue over time.

Tissues taken from the abdomen provide a good source for breast reconstruction. The skin and fat around the abdomen can be shifted to the breast region and shaped to match a natural breast. To provide the circulation for these living tissues, there must be a blood supply. The blood vessel supplying the skin and fat around the belly button comes down to the abdominal area through one of the muscles on the abdominal wall. With this blood vessel still connected to its source under the rib cage, the skin and fat around the belly button are moved to the breast area with circulation intact. Then the area where the tissues came from is simply sewn back together as in a "tummy tuck" (see lipectomy and liposuction). In fact, this technique for breast reconstruction was in part inspired by a patient who wanted a tummy tuck and who had had a previous mastectomy.

Although using abdominal tissues for reconstruction often yields the most natural result, the necessary surgery is extensive and is not right for everyone. Women with diabetes, circulation disorders, other serious medical problems, previous abdominal surgery, or other risk factors may not be candidates for the operation.

Natural tissues are also available for reconstruction by using a muscle from the back. This operation works on a similar principle: skin, fat, and muscle on the back are all supplied by a common blood vessel. Leaving this vessel connected at its origin in the armpit allows all the tissues it feeds to be freed up and shifted from the back to the front of the chest. The tissues can then be shaped to make a breast.

The back muscle has a healthy blood supply that allows it to be employed in situations where the abdominal muscle circulation may be inadequate. This technique leaves a scar on the back that can be hidden under clothes. Although it means moving a muscle from its normal location in the back, there are other muscles around the shoulder blade that can take over almost all of its function. The majority of women do not notice any change in strength or flexibility after the healing is completed. Unlike the abdomen, however, which often provides a substantial amount of natural tissue for reconstruction, the back is usually not as generous. As a rule the natural tissues of the back have to be supplemented by some type of artificial material, either an implant or an expander. The more natural tissue available, the more natural the result will be.

Advanced techniques also exist that allow tissues to be disconnected from their original blood supply and reattached to vessels in the breast area. These procedures are called free flaps, as opposed to the connected procedures, which are called pedicle flaps. Free flaps can remove tissues from the abdomen, buttock, or thigh and reattach their small blood vessels to other small blood vessels in the armpit, rib cage, or neck. Once circulation is reestablished, the tissues that have been moved are shaped to form a reconstructed breast.

These techniques have the advantage of taking donations from parts of the body where women often have unwanted fat. The shape of these "donor" areas is changed, though, and can look unusual. The advantage of getting rid of extra skin and fat must also be balanced against the complexity of these operations. If the blood vessels in the donor tissue do not stay open after they are connected, the tissues lose their circulation. More surgery may be required to reestablish circulation; if circulation cannot be restored, the tissues will die and the reconstruction will fail. Since these operations are so technically difficult, it is essential to seek out a surgeon with extensive experience in these specialized microsurgical skills.

After the shape of the breast has been restored, the nipple and areola can be reconstructed. The projecting part of the nipple can be rebuilt by dividing the other nipple, or by transplanting part of the earlobe, though the most common procedure is to wrap skin flaps around themselves on the breast itself. After the projecting nipple has healed, a tattoo gun is used to embed natural pigments in the surrounding skin.

The same techniques used to reconstruct a breast that has been lost to cancer can be adapted to other reconstructive situations. For example, abnormalities in the shape of the breast caused by lumpectomy or radiation therapy (see entries) can be corrected through reconstructive surgery, allowing the woman to feel more comfortable with her overall appearance and body image. Sometimes the side effects of radiation cause skin stiffness, breast firmness, breast pain, or even open areas that will not heal. Removing the damaged tissue and replacing it with natural tissue from the back or the abdomen can make the woman more comfortable while improving the way the breast looks.

Reconstruction can also be employed when the shape of the breast is distorted for some other reason besides cancer. An injury to the growing breast may cause the traumatized area to develop inadequately. In children, burns or deep wounds to the breast or nipple area are of particular concern. As the child develops, she may observe a concavity, a depression, or a total lack of shape to the injured area. Developmental abnormalities can also occur without any injury at all. Sometimes the breast bud, the precursor of the mature breast that is formed in the womb, does not contain all the tissue it needs to shape the breast fully during development. The child will then notice, with the onset of puberty, that one breast fails to grow or grows in an abnormal shape, while the other breast may grow normally or even overgrow. These abnormalities are especially stressful during early adolescence. Reconstructing these locally damaged areas often does not involve as much surgery as a total reconstruction after mastectomy, and can yield a very natural result.

What happens after surgery?

The healing process after breast reconstruction depends on the type of surgery. If the reconstruction has been done at the same time as a mastectomy for breast cancer, recovery after the surgery will be integrated into the overall treatment for the breast cancer.

If reconstruction is carried out after mastectomy, or if it is performed for a condition that does not involve malignancy, the plastic surgeon will coordinate most of the recovery process. In general, operations that use only artificial material involve less surgery and therefore less recovery. But though reconstructions using one's own tissues are more extensive surgeries, this should not dissuade someone who is in good health from selecting them. The recuperation time varies: a patient with an implant or a tissue expander may be back to work at a nonstrenuous job in a week, while a woman who has an abdominal flap reconstruction will take longer to get over the surgery itself and will be considerably more limited in physical activities while the healing process goes on. When recovery from either of these operations is completed, however, the woman should be able to return to virtually all activities that she participated in before the surgery.

If a reconstruction has been performed after cancer surgery, it is essential that the woman be followed closely for any return of the disease. The need for surveillance is no different than if there had been no reconstruction. Studies have demonstrated that cancer is no more likely to recur after reconstruction than after no reconstruction, and women with reconstruction have the same long-term survival as women without. Most important, there is no evidence that reconstruction prevents the detection of any new cancers. Recurrences are most likely to be found in the skin left over on the chest after a mastectomy. Cancer does not come back within the reconstructed tissue itself, since this tissue is different from breast tissue. But even though mammograms may not be needed on the reconstructed side, the opposite breast is still at risk for developing a cancer. Regular mammograms, physical examinations, and breast self-examinations on the natural side should be combined with a doctor's examination and self-exam on the reconstructed side.

What are the risks and complications?

All reconstructive surgery is major surgery, usually involving general anesthesia. Risks of any type of major surgery include problems related to anesthesia, bleeding, infection, and medical complications. All these occur at a very low rate in women who are otherwise healthy.

For reconstructions using artificial materials, the same types of implants are used as in breast enlargement, and the same types of potential problems can occur (see breast implants and enlargement). Implants may deflate, become overly firm, or become infected, and they do not afford the most natural shape. Furthermore, implants do not tolerate radiation well. Implant or expander reconstruction may not be suitable if there has been previous radiation to the breast or if radiation is anticipated after surgery.

Silicone gel–filled implants are available for reconstruction by certain surgeons who are participating in clinical study of the product. If a silicone gel–filled implant seems advantageous, a woman must seek out one of the centers where the clinical trials are being conducted. The researchers will provide an extensive review of the risks and benefits. Most commonly, though, saline-filled devices are used in reconstruction.

The use of natural tissues may allow the woman to avoid artificial materials. But these operations leave scars on the abdomen or the back, where the tissues came from, as well as deep scarring in the muscle beds that are used. Deep scar tissue can cause stiffness after surgery which may take a long time to stretch out. Loss of a muscle will also introduce stiffness, sometimes calling for physical therapy to speed up the recovery process. Numbness will also occur over the area where the tissues were taken from; this too will improve over time as the nerves regenerate. Numbness in the new breast may be permanent, though women tend not to notice it during daily activities.

Minor problems with healing happen occasionally and do not usually interfere with the reconstruction itself. The skin left after a mastectomy is especially vulnerable to healing delays. Fluid accumulation may also occur at the site of the reconstruction or at the site where the donor tissues came from. Drainage tubes are left in place after surgery to remove excess fluid, though after the drains are removed, the fluid may reaccumulate and have to be drained in the surgeon's office.

Related entries

Anesthesia, biopsy, body image, breast cancer, breast implants and enlargement, breast lumps (benign), breast reduction, breast self-examination, chemotherapy, keloid scarring, lumpectomy, mammography, mastectomy, radiation therapy

Breast Reduction

Breast reduction is a form of plastic surgery to decrease the size of one or both breasts. Many women choose to have it done because the size of their breasts has detrimental effects on their health, their emotional well-being, and their lifestyle. Not only can pendulous breasts interfere with athletic activity or serve as a source of social anguish (particularly for adolescents), but also they can leave women with breathing problems, poor posture, chronic back and shoulder aches, neck pain, skin rashes under the breasts, and deep grooves in their shoulders from brassiere straps.

Breast reduction may also be helpful for large-breasted women who face a mastectomy on one side. Even if a woman is planning to have breast reconstruction (see entry), making the remaining breast smaller and more upright may help the surgeon achieve a more symmetrical and comfortable result.

Insurance policies will sometimes cover breast reduction surgery if it is done to relieve these sorts of physical symptoms. Breast reduction (reduction mammoplasty) may also be chosen as cosmetic surgery by women without symptoms who think their breasts are too large or who have trouble fitting into certain styles of clothing. It is far too arduous a procedure, however, to be undertaken without a thorough weighing of the risks and benefits.

How is the procedure performed?

Considered a form of major surgery, breast reduction is technically more complicated than breast enlargement surgery (see breast implants and enlargement). There are many different ways to reduce the size of the breasts, although most can be assigned to one of two general categories.

In the first category of surgery, the original nipple and areola remain attached to the breast through a thin stalk of breast tissue. After the excess tissue is removed, the nipple and areola are relocated to a higher position on the breast. In the second category, the nipple and areola (the darkened ring encircling the nipple) are severed from the breast and excess tissue is removed from the lower part of the breast. The nipple and areola are then replaced with a skin graft.

The specific type of surgery chosen will depend on many factors: the woman's present size and shape, how much smaller she wants to be, her general state of health, whether she intends to breastfeed in the future, and the surgeon's experience with the pros and cons of each procedure. Whatever the specific procedure used, breast reduction usually takes 3 or 4 hours and is done under general anesthesia in a hospital.

Related to breast reduction surgery is an operation done to uplift sagging breasts. Called mastoplexy, this form of surgery is technically less demanding, takes less time, and has fewer potential complications than other forms of breast reduction surgery. It usually leaves the same scars as breast reduction, however: one around the areola, a vertical one from the areola down to the fold beneath the breast, and one that is hidden in the fold itself.

Natural forces may undo the results of mastoplexy over time, and some women choose to have the operation repeated. Even with breast reduction surgery, breasts tend to become somewhat more pendulous as scar tissue matures and softens.

What happens after surgery?

After the surgery the woman usually stays in the hospital at least overnight, although small reductions and breast lifts can be done safely on an outpatient basis. Stitches often are under the skin; those closing skin remain in place for 10 to 14 days, and drains may be necessary for a few days after the surgery. Recovery usually takes several weeks, and most surgeons advise against any strenuous arm activity in the first 3 weeks. Vigorous aerobic exercise should be avoided for at least 6 to 8 weeks after surgery.

What are the risks and complications?

Like any form of major surgery, breast reduction carries a small risk of complications, including adverse reactions to anesthesia, infection, and bleeding. There is also the possibility of abnormal scarring, which can make the results much less satisfactory than one might have imagined.

All women can expect to have scars on their breasts following the surgery, and these scars tend to be much more conspicuous than those resulting from breast enlargement surgery. Over time, as the scars mature, they become less noticeable, but women considering breast reduction must be aware that they are making a trade-off between the problem of breast size and the problem of visible scars.

Most types of breast reduction involve an incision—and leave a scar—in the shape of an inverted T, with the horizontal stroke of the T in the fold under the breast. Large, irregular keloid scars, though very uncommon, develop in some women. The risk of abnormal scarring should be discussed with the surgeon before the surgery is undertaken. Pictures of a variety of scars may be shown to prospective patients to help them visualize the range of possible results.

The forms of breast reduction that involve a grafted nipple and areola eliminate any future nipple sensitivity. Women who retain their own nipple and areola often find that these areas are particularly sensitive for some time after the operation as nerves grow back. Women who have had their natural nipple and areola detached will not be able to breastfeed in the future. Even women whose nipples remain attached may be unable to breastfeed because the tissue rearrangement can interfere with the normal function of the mammary ducts.

Women should continue to practice breast self-exam after reduction surgery. New lumps, if found soon afterward, are usually scar tissue, but any lump that persists should be investigated. Women over 30 should have a mammogram before surgery and again 6 months afterward. The postoperative mammogram establishes a new "baseline" against which all future mammograms are compared. Breast reduction does not increase the likelihood that cancer will develop, and the scars do not make detection more difficult if the radiologist has experience with patients who have had breast surgery. At the time of the surgery itself, all tissue removed from the breast should be sent to the pathology lab for analysis, so that any early signs of cancer can be detected.

Related entries

Breast implants and enlargement, breast reconstruction, breastfeeding, cosmetic surgery, keloid scarring

Breast Self-Examination

Breast self-examination (BSE) is a regular inspection by a woman for abnormalities in her breasts. Although physicians generally agree that women should examine their breasts on a monthly basis to help detect breast lumps (and thus potential cancer at an early stage), it is controversial whether self-examination alone or together with screening mammogra-

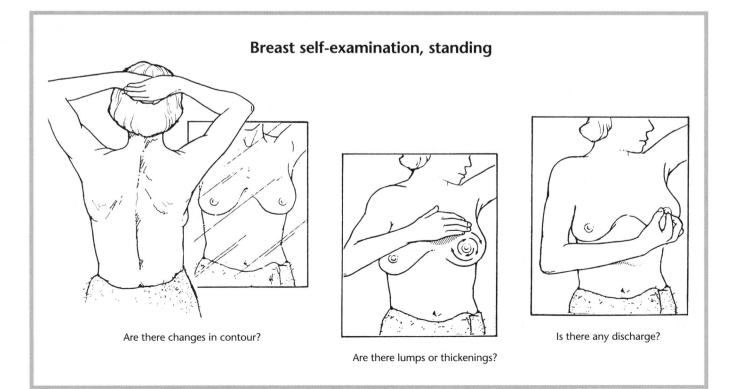

Breast self-examination, standing

Are there changes in contour?

Are there lumps or thickenings?

Is there any discharge?

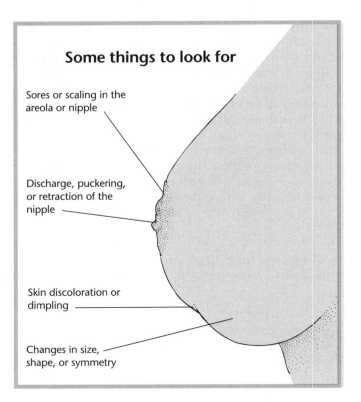

Some things to look for

Sores or scaling in the areola or nipple

Discharge, puckering, or retraction of the nipple

Skin discoloration or dimpling

Changes in size, shape, or symmetry

phy can actually reduce deaths from breast cancer. Decade-long experiments involving hundreds of women in the Soviet Union and China have shown no differences in either death rates or stage of diagnosis of breast cancer between women taught to perform careful BSE and those who do not perform it.

On an individual basis, though, if a woman is found to have a cancerous lump, early detection and treatment increase her chances for remission and potential cure. It is important not to rely on mammography alone to identify lumps because not all early abnormalities show up on the mammogram.

How is a breast self-examination performed?

Breast self-examination should ideally be done once a month, although an occasional exam is better than none. Consistent timing of the exams increases a woman's ability to identify a new abnormality. Many women find BSE easier to do after their clinician has demonstrated it to them; some clinicians also offer a pamphlet or videotape detailing effective techniques.

The best time to do a BSE for a premenopausal woman is right after the monthly menstrual period, when breasts are usually least lumpy and tender. Women who no longer menstruate, menstruate irregularly, or are pregnant can select a specific date to perform the exam each month. A thorough BSE begins with an inspection in the mirror in which breasts are checked for any changes from previous appearance (see illustration). These can include changes in shape, size, or symmetry; skin discoloration or dimpling; sores or scaling in the

areola or nipple; and discharge or puckering of the nipple (see illustration). Raising the hands above the head helps to reveal changes in contour, and placing hands on hips with shoulders forward will help show any dimpling.

Breasts should next be felt for lumps, thickenings, or any other changes from previous exams—all of which should be reported to a clinician. This is usually best accomplished standing in the shower or bath when the breasts are wet and soapy. To examine the right breast, the woman should raise her right arm above her head and gently use the left hand, fingers flat and pressed together tightly, to make a tiny circling motion into the very top of the breast (women with large breasts may find it easier to use two hands for each breast, with one hand supporting the underside of the breast and pressing up toward the other hand). Then fingers should slide slightly clockwise while repeating the tiny circling motion. This process should be continued clockwise until the entire outside of the breast has been examined.

It is particularly important to check the area between the nipple and armpit. The process should be continued in gradually smaller circles until the entire breast, including the nipple and areola, has been examined and then repeated for the left breast. Nipples should be gently squeezed to see if there is any discharge. It is a good idea to repeat this process while lying down with the raised arm tucked behind the head (see illustration). Some women find it helps to place a small pillow or folded towel under the shoulder on the side being examined.

Many women avoid doing BSEs because they fear finding a lump, but in reality most breast lumps and abnormalities turn out to be noncancerous, especially those found in premenopausal women. Women should keep in mind that the primary goal of BSE is knowing the topography of their breasts—not looking for cancer. This knowledge can be use-

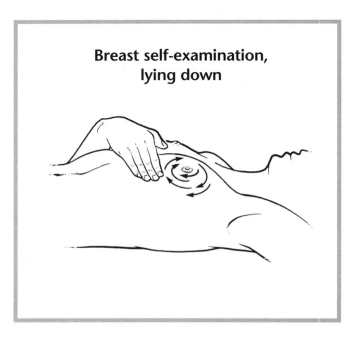

Breast self-examination, lying down

ful if a clinician subsequently detects a suspicious area. If a woman does detect a lump herself, it is important to have a clinician evaluate it.

Related entries

Biopsy, breast cancer, breast lumps (benign), mammography

Breastfeeding

Breastfeeding is the suckling of an infant from the human breast. Not only is breast milk considered the ideal form of nourishment for the newborn, but breastfeeding (also known as lactation or nursing) has many other benefits as well for both the mother and baby.

Why is breastfeeding a good choice for most mothers?

- Breastfeeding supplies the newborn with antibodies from the mother that give a natural immunity to most common childhood infections and decreases the chance of allergic reactions.

- After delivery, suckling a newborn stimulates the mother's pituitary gland to produce hormones that help the uterus contract back to its normal size.

- Breastfed babies are less likely to become obese because overfeeding is less likely than with bottle-feeding.

- Women who breastfeed often find it easier to lose excess pregnancy weight.

- Breastfeeding is much less expensive than bottle-feeding.

- Breastfeeding is often more convenient than bottle-feeding because it does not involve mixing formulas, heating bottles, sterilizing equipment, and carrying supplies from one place to another.

- Breastfeeding seems to encourage better mouth and tooth development in the baby.

- One study suggests that women who breastfeed for as little as 4 to 6 months—over a lifetime, that is, not necessarily with one baby—reduce their risk of developing breast cancer by at least 20 percent. The greatest decrease in risk (as much as 50 percent) occurred in women who started breastfeeding before the age of 20 and nursed for at least 6 months.

Many proponents of breastfeeding also contend that it makes "bonding" (attachment) between mother and infant easier to achieve, although few would dispute that mothers who bottle-feed are capable of bonding with their babies just as ef-

fectively if they hold them close and cuddle them during feedings.

Breastfeeding can usually be accomplished successfully with a premature baby or with twins or triplets if the mother is patient and determined. It is even possible to reestablish milk production in women who have had to stop nursing temporarily because of an illness. In some communities there are milk banks which store and distribute milk to infants whose own mothers are unable to nurse them.

Nursing does not permanently change the shape of the breasts, and there is no evidence that the size or shape of a woman's breasts or nipples affects the quality or quantity of her breast milk. Women who have had breast reduction, reconstruction, or implants, however, may not be able to breastfeed in some cases. The particular type of surgery performed determines whether breastfeeding is possible, so the matter should be discussed with one's surgeon (see breast implants and enlargement; breast reconstruction; breast reduction).

Breastfeeding does not necessarily have to tie the mother down, as so many women fear. What may at first seem an inconvenient or impossible task need not be if certain adaptations are made in the "classic" breastfeeding scenario—that is, breastfeeding an infant exclusively for at least 4 to 6 months. One alternative, for example, is to breastfeed primarily but to have the father or child care provider give the baby a bottle of formula or pumped breast milk at night or at other times when the mother may not want to be or cannot be the only caregiver. Milk can be manually expressed from the breast and refrigerated or frozen until it is needed.

Another alternative is to breastfeed for a short period of time (say, the first 6 weeks) and then switch to bottle-feeding, perhaps after maternity leave is over. One caveat about mixing bottles and breastfeeding is that babies use a different kind of sucking motion when they feed from a bottle, and this sometimes makes them unwilling to accept the breast. This problem may be avoided by introducing a bottle after the first 6 weeks (after the baby has had a chance to master the more complicated nursing suckle) but before the baby becomes too set in its nursing ways to accept a bottle. Another possibility is to limit substitute bottles to no more than one a day. A woman who breastfeeds more on one day than others, however, should try expressing or pumping milk at regular intervals during the times she is not nursing to avoid losing her milk supply or developing painful breast engorgement.

Although nursing a baby may delay or even prevent the return of ovulation and menstruation after childbirth, it cannot be considered a reliable method of contraception. Not only is it possible to conceive while breastfeeding, but also breastfeeding can be continued throughout a subsequent pregnancy so that both an older child and a newborn can be nursed at the same time if the mother wishes to do so. There is some evidence, however, that nursing a baby during a subsequent pregnancy may rob the growing fetus of necessary nutrients such as calcium, despite its benefits to the older child.

When is breastfeeding not appropriate?

For all its benefits, breastfeeding is not ideal for every woman or every baby. For example, some women may have medical problems that preclude nursing. These include women who are using medications that may pass into the breast milk and harm the baby, or women with certain infections (including AIDS, chicken pox, or active tuberculosis) which can be spread to a baby through the breast milk. Although most drugs pass into breast milk at such low levels that their effect on the baby is negligible, breastfeeding women who are using a medication should always check with a clinician to make sure that it is safe for use during lactation. Breastfeeding may also not be desirable for women who have certain obligations—such as a job that requires frequent travel—which make breastfeeding excessively complicated or inconvenient.

Breastfeeding may be inappropriate, too, for women who simply dislike the idea or find the process embarrassing. Many fears and concerns can be traced back to the late nineteenth and early twentieth centuries, when affluent women hired wet nurses to feed their infants because it was erroneously believed that sexual intercourse would "sour" a woman's milk. In the 1940s, when commercial infant formula made it possible for women to bottle-feed babies, breastfeeding continued to be associated with the poor and uneducated classes who did not have the means to afford more "scientific" methods. The association of the breast with sexual symbolism rather than infant nourishment since the 1950s—and the dissociation of sexual behavior from reproduction through the widespread use of contraception, particularly birth control pills, since the 1960s—undoubtedly contributed further to the movement away from breastfeeding.

Despite efforts beginning in the 1950s by La Leche League and others to change women's attitudes about breastfeeding, many women today prefer not to breastfeed in public; yet finding a secluded room in which to nurse a baby is not always convenient. Some states and localities have passed laws that uphold a woman's right to breastfeed in public places (such as shopping malls), but many women still feel that baring their breasts in such a place would be unacceptable—either to others or to themselves.

A woman who has negative feelings about breastfeeding should not feel guilty if she decides to bottle-feed. Not only would the associated stress and anxiety probably make breastfeeding difficult or impossible anyway, but also a bottle-fed baby today can be well nourished and happy.

A woman who does decide not to nurse her baby may experience several days of pain until the milk subsides after the delivery. Although in the past various hormones (including diethylstilbestrol, or DES, bromocriptine, and estrogen or estrogen-testosterone combinations) were administered to women to stop lactation, it turned out that most of these either were ineffective or had dangerous side effects. It is now known that the only safe and effective way to stop the breasts from producing milk is to keep a baby from suckling. This usually takes from 3 to 6 days, but in some women may take as long as a week or two. In the meantime, many women find that ice packs, mild painkillers, and a tight brassiere or breast binder can provide some relief.

How can a woman know that her baby is getting enough milk?

Many women who breastfeed are concerned because they have no way to measure just how much milk the baby is getting. There is really no need to worry. Breastfeeding works through a tightly coordinated feedback system in which the milk supply increases or decreases according to a baby's needs. The more a baby suckles, the greater the milk supply. That is why a baby may want to suckle at hourly intervals during a growth spurt, but then will soon settle back into a more widely spaced pattern once the frequent sucking has bolstered the milk supply. It is also why most breastfeeding authorities recommend breastfeeding babies "on demand"—that is, whenever they seem to be hungry, whether that is every 4 hours or every hour—rather than on some predetermined schedule.

If women aware of this supply-demand mechanism are still worried about their baby's getting enough milk, they can rest assured that a baby who is gaining weight to the pediatrician's satisfaction or who wets at least 6 to 8 diapers a day is getting plenty of nutrition. In rare cases a woman may have such a small amount of glandular (as opposed to fatty) breast tissue that she produces deficient quantities of milk. Termed low-milk syndrome, this problem is easily detectable if the baby is examined by a clinician 3 or 4 days after birth—a practice increasingly recommended by pediatricians. If the baby is not of adequate weight, the clinician will discuss with the mother ways to supplement the baby's nutrition.

Breastfeeding can be begun as soon as a baby (and, in the case of cesarean delivery, the mother) is stable—often within the first hour after delivery. In the first few days of nursing the only nourishment the infant will be getting is colostrum, a yellowish fluid full of antibodies, vitamin A, nitrogen, and minerals. For this reason many hospitals were once in the habit of "supplementing" a newborn's feedings with bottles of formula, but most breastfeeding authorities frown on this practice. Not only is colostrum sufficient nutrition for the newborn, but also the ease with which milk can be sucked from a bottle interferes with an infant's willingness to master the otherwise natural technique necessary to compress the milk ducts with the tongue and draw milk into the mouth. If a baby satisfied by formula refuses to suck at the breast, the mother's milk production will not increase as it normally would.

About 3 to 5 days postpartum the mother's milk supply will begin to come in. The method of delivery (whether vaginal or c-section) makes no difference in this timing. When the baby suckles, the pituitary gland in the brain releases a hormone called prolactin, which stimulates the milk glands to produce milk. It also releases another hormone called oxytocin, which produces the letdown reflex—a forcing of the milk through the breasts which some women experience as a tingling or tightening sensation. Oxytocin release can also be stimulated by a baby's cry—or sometimes even the thought of the baby—and the result is milk leaking from the breasts, sometimes at inopportune moments. This is why many lactating women wear absorbent nursing pads inside a nursing bra. Usually the letdown reflex becomes less noticeable and inappropriate after the early weeks of breastfeeding.

For the first 24 hours of feeding, newborns generally need to nurse for only about 3 to 5 minutes on each breast. This is long enough to stimulate milk production and short enough to help prevent the sore nipples which often plague nursing mothers. As the baby continues to nurse, the nipples will become toughened, and the baby will be able to nurse for longer periods of time. Another possibility (however painful) is to nurse frequently from the beginning, since this seems to prevent the breasts from becoming sore or engorged in the first place. Whichever method is tried, the baby will eventually need to nurse for about 10 to 15 minutes at each breast, although there is great variation from baby to baby.

Some of this time is for comfort, since the majority of the milk probably is depleted in the first 5 or 10 minutes. Women are sometimes told to switch the baby to the other breast after about 10 minutes in order to avoid engorgement (painful swelling) in the unused breast. If the baby is not willing to cooperate in this plan, another way to avoid the problem is to remember the breast last fed on and then start the baby on the alternate breast at the next feeding.

Women who have had a c-section may continue to need pain medication for a few days after the delivery. Although some of it crosses into breast milk, the amounts are believed to be little enough to pose no risk to the baby. Usually pain medications are needed right after nursing, since the uterine contractions caused by breastfeeding may increase the mother's discomfort. This schedule minimizes the amount of painkiller that is in the milk supply when the baby nurses. Sometimes a woman who has had a c-section finds that holding the baby in the traditional position is uncomfortable. She may want to try other positions, including the "football hold" (see illustration in cesarean section).

What are the risks and complications?

When the milk first comes in, it is not uncommon for the breasts to become engorged—that is, swollen, hard, and sore. Often the breasts become so full that the nipple flattens out into the areola. Many women find that engorged breasts are uncomfortably tender or painful and that it is hard to nurse, but nothing works better than nursing to alleviate the pain. Soon the breasts will respond more accurately to the baby's needs, and engorgement will cease to be a problem. In the meantime, the best solution may be to have the baby suck for a short period of time (as long as can be tolerated) or, if that is not possible, manually express a tiny bit of the milk to soften the areola and make the nipple easier to latch on to. Between feedings the breasts should be supported firmly, and hot or cold compresses or mild analgesics can be used to relieve any pain.

Some women who breastfeed find that their nipples become sore or cracked. This usually occurs when the skin around the nipple is left wet for too long or because the baby fails to latch on properly. It may help to expose the nipples to air or sunlight, rub lanolin on them, or express a small amount of milk and rub it into the nipples. If there is a painful crack, however, it may be better to have the baby nurse on the other side for a couple of days. In the meantime, a small bit of milk can be expressed from the sore nipple to prevent engorgement. Another possibility is to put a nipple shield over the affected nipple to protect the sore while the baby sucks.

To prevent future soreness or cracking, it is important to change wet nursing pads frequently, wash breasts in water only, and pat them dry with a soft towel or allow them to dry in the open air. Also, a baby who has fallen asleep at the breast should never be pulled away abruptly but eased off gradually by inserting a finger into the mouth to break the suction.

If an isolated part of the breast itself feels sore, there may be a plugged milk duct. This can be the result of engorgement, infrequent nursing, restrictive clothing, or an inadequate letdown reflex. Sometimes massaging the sore area will help unblock the duct, as will applying a hot compress or increasing nursing on the affected side. If a sore breast is accompanied by a fever or flulike ache, however, the problem may be mastitis (a breast infection; see mastitis). If this seems a possibility, a clinician should be contacted as soon as possible so that antibiotics can be prescribed.

Related entries

Anesthesia, birth control, breast implants and enlargement, breast reconstruction, breast reduction, cesarean section, childbirth, mastitis, postpartum issues

Breathing Disorders

Breathlessness, wheezing, coughing, or painful breathing can be symptoms of a number of common disorders. These include asthma, pneumonia, pleurisy, pulmonary embolism, pulmonary edema, anemia, and chronic obstructive lung disease. Painful breathing (and short, shallow breaths) can also be caused by a cracked or bruised rib or a strained muscle (see chest pain).

Disorders that cause breathing difficulties

Asthma. The classic symptoms of asthma (see entry) are wheezing (noisy breathing), coughing, tightness in the chest, shortness of breath, and labored breathing. During an attack the muscles tighten around the tubes of the lungs (the bronchii), and the lining inside the tubes becomes swollen and inflamed. This process is called bronchospasm. Airflow is restricted, and often thick mucus accumulates in the airways. In a severe attack breathing becomes rapid and shallow, heartbeat quickens, and the skin becomes bluish. Often asthma attacks can develop after exposure to allergens, cold air, or exercise, and can last for a few minutes to several days. Although severely restricted airflow can be life-threatening, in most cases asthma attacks are mild or moderate and can be readily managed with medications.

Pneumonia. If a woman has a persistent productive or pus-containing cough, accompanied by a fever and often a dull chest pain, the problem may be lung inflammation or infection, that is, pneumonia. Most bacterial pneumonias cause a productive cough with chest pain, but so-called atypical pneumonia (including "walking pneumonia," which is caused by the mycoplasma organism) results in a dry, hacking cough. A physical examination and sometimes a chest x-ray are needed to differentiate pneumonia from bronchitis, a less serious respiratory infection limited to the bronchial tubes and not involving the lungs.

Pleurisy. This condition, which seems to occur more often in women than in men, results from inflammation of the two-layered membranes surrounding the lungs and chest cavity (the pleura; see illustration). It can produce a sharp chest pain that worsens after coughing or inhaling, as the layers

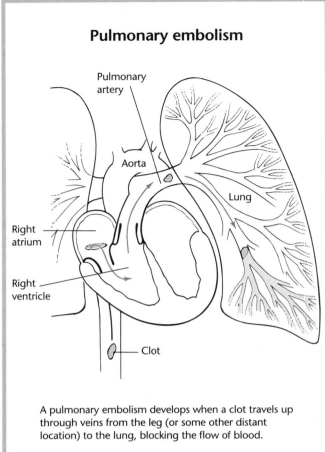

Pulmonary embolism

A pulmonary embolism develops when a clot travels up through veins from the leg (or some other distant location) to the lung, blocking the flow of blood.

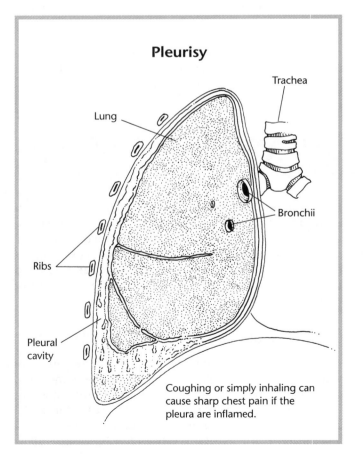

Pleurisy

Coughing or simply inhaling can cause sharp chest pain if the pleura are inflamed.

rub together. Consequently, people with pleurisy often take short, shallow breaths. The pain may also be felt in the shoulders, neck, or abdomen and can often be relieved temporarily by pressing on the painful area of the chest. When pleurisy is caused by a viral infection, it will clear up on its own after a few days.

Pulmonary embolism. In this condition a blood clot from elsewhere in the body lodges in one of the pulmonary arteries and blocks blood flow to the lungs, depriving the lung tissue of blood and thereby damaging it (see illustration). In addition to causing pleurisy, a pulmonary embolism can lead to shortness of breath, rapid breathing, accelerated heart rate, or bloody sputum. Severe or recurrent pulmonary embolism can result in shock or even death, so this condition requires immediate medical attention.

The risk of developing a pulmonary embolism is increased slightly in women who use oral contraceptives and either smoke or have hypertension, but estrogen replacement therapy after menopause does not seem to increase the risk. Other risk factors include pregnancy or recent pregnancy, recent pelvic or orthopedic surgery, prolonged bed rest, a history of phlebitis (see circulatory disorders), blood that clots

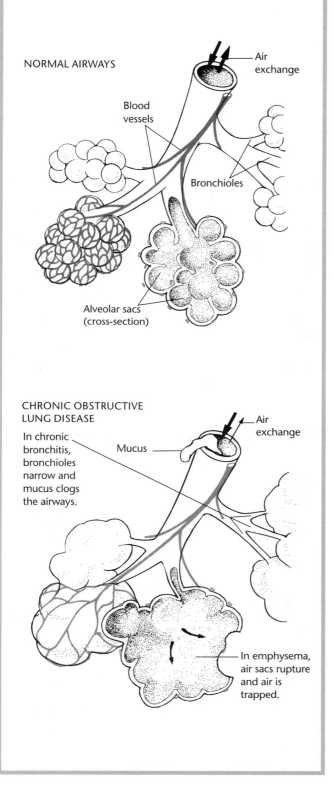

How chronic obstructive lung disease (COLD) affects breathing

NORMAL AIRWAYS

Air exchange

Blood vessels

Bronchioles

Alveolar sacs (cross-section)

CHRONIC OBSTRUCTIVE LUNG DISEASE

In chronic bronchitis, bronchioles narrow and mucus clogs the airways.

Mucus

Air exchange

In emphysema, air sacs rupture and air is trapped.

too readily, cancer, and lupus (see entry). When pulmonary embolism is diagnosed or strongly suspected, hospitalization is necessary for close observation and treatment, since the condition can lead to life-threatening complications.

Pulmonary edema. If the pumping from the left side of the heart is inefficient owing to congestive heart failure (see entry), blood will back up into the lungs, leading them to become congested with fluid. The result is a condition called pulmonary edema, which is generally characterized by breathlessness. Often people with mild congestive heart failure become short of breath mainly with exertion. In later stages breathlessness is present even when the person is lying down or sitting.

Chronic obstructive lung disease. Emphysema and bronchitis are examples of chronic obstructive lung disease (COLD), and women smokers of any age are more than 10 times as likely as nonsmoking women to die of these conditions. Healthy lungs contain millions of alveoli—air sacs in which oxygen is exchanged for carbon dioxide, through a fine web of blood vessels (see illustration). In people with emphysema, these air sacs rupture, blood vessels are lost, and stale air is trapped in the lungs. When chronic bronchitis is also present, the bronchioles narrow and are clogged by mucus.

Sleep apnea. People with this disorder have 30 or more periods during the night in which they stop breathing for up to 10 seconds or so. While it is most common in overweight males, women become increasingly prone to this disorder after they reach menopause. Usually sleep apnea (see entry on sleep disorders) results when a flap of muscle or other flabby structure in the upper airway partially blocks the flow of air. Occasionally it may also develop when the respiratory muscles stop working temporarily, possibly because something is interfering with breathing signals from the brain. Whatever the cause, sleep apnea leads levels of carbon dioxide in the blood to rise, stimulating the brain to increase air intake and ultimately resulting in loud snoring, violent grunting, and wild gasping. Severe sleep apnea can result in not only excessive daytime sleepiness the next day, but also irritability, shortened attention span, slowed thinking, and reduced short-term memory. In addition, it can trigger cardiac arrhythmias or even heart attacks, especially in people who have coronary artery disease. Risk of death is even higher during an apneic episode if the person is using alcohol or sleep medications.

How are these conditions evaluated?

To diagnose the cause of a breathing disorder, the clinician will ask the woman for a description of her symptoms and will do a thorough physical examination, which should include a careful check of the lungs, heart, chest wall, and ribs. Various tests—including pulmonary function tests—and possibly a chest x-ray can help distinguish among the many respiratory diseases that can cause breathlessness, coughing or wheezing, and pain. A clinician who suspects congestive heart failure may conduct tests of heart structure and function. If sleep apnea is suspected, brain waves and breathing patterns during sleep should be measured at a sleep disorders center.

How are breathing disorders treated?

Treatment of breathing disorders depends on the specific condition. Mild or moderate asthma can be readily managed with medications (see asthma). Bacterial or atypical pneumonia requires antibiotics, and cough medicines are often prescribed as well, especially if the cough is interrupting sleep or causing pain. The pain of pleurisy is usually relieved with nonsteroidal antiinflammatory drugs (NSAIDs), although occasionally additional pain medication is necessary.

In the case of pulmonary embolism, anticoagulation therapy—thinning the blood—is used to prevent extension of the blood clot and to allow time for the body's own mechanisms to stabilize and dissolve it. Anticoagulation with intravenous heparin is started in the hospital, and warfarin (Coumadin), an oral anticoagulant, is continued for 3 to 6 months at home.

Treatment of COLD is based on limiting further lung damage (by quitting smoking), maximizing airflow with medications, treating infections at an early stage, and improving lung function with supervised exercise. Supplemental oxygen is also helpful for many patients with severe COLD. Sleep apnea can be treated with a combination of lifestyle changes (including weight loss), mechanical devices to promote airflow during sleep, and, if necessary, surgery.

Related entries

Asthma, chest pain, colds, congestive heart failure, lung cancer, sleep disorders

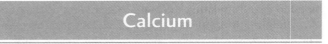

Calcium

Calcium is an essential mineral that plays an important role in the development of bones and teeth. Because there is evidence that inadequate levels of calcium throughout life may contribute to the development of osteoporosis (see entry), in recent years women in particular have become heavy consumers of calcium supplements, as well as of many food and beverage products fortified with calcium. Osteoporosis aside, many intriguing new studies are elevating calcium to "superstar" status as a nutrient. In one recent study, for example, calcium-enriched diets lowered blood pressure in African American teenagers. In another study, calcium-rich foods appeared to help prevent colon cancer. Yet other studies have linked diets high in calcium to lower overall levels of body fat and slowed weight gain in young women.

Current federal guidelines state that premenopausal adult women need at least 1,000 mg of calcium per day, while adolescent, pregnant, and breastfeeding women need 1,200 mg per day. Postmenopausal women not taking estrogen replacement therapy require 1,500 mg per day, while those who are taking ERT can continue at 1,000 mg per day.

RDA's

Most American women do not get even the recommended dietary allowance (RDA) of calcium (800 to 1,000 mg per day) established by the National Research Council. As women get older, calcium intake is likely to drop even more, partly because of a decrease in dietary intake of calcium and partly because of a decreased ability to absorb the calcium that is ingested. The typical postmenopausal American woman gets only about 400 to 500 mg per day.

What are the best sources of calcium?

Although calcium is readily available in milk and dairy products, as well as in dark leafy vegetables such as spinach, broccoli, kale, and collard greens (see chart), it is best absorbed from low-fat and nonfat milk and milk products. One simple way to boost calcium intake without adding fat is to spike foods such as coffee, soups, stews, sauces, gravies, dips, muffins, mashed potatoes, and meatloaf with nonfat milk powder. Another possibility is to check the supermarket for foods with extra calcium added, including orange juice, cereal, and bread.

Because most women—especially those who are lactose intolerant or who dislike milk—do not get adequate calcium from diet alone, many clinicians advise taking calcium sup-

Good sources of calcium in the diet		
Food	**Serving size**	**Mg of calcium**
Sardines	3 oz	372
Milk, skim	1 cup	300
Milk, buttermilk	1 cup	296
Milk, whole	1 cup	290
Cheese		
Cheddar	1 oz	210
American	1 slice	195
Mozzarella	1 oz	163
Turnip greens	⅔ cup cooked	184
Salmon	3 oz	167
Custard	½ cup	161
Tofu	3 oz	128
Ice cream	½ cup	99
Shrimp	3 oz	98
Spinach	½ cup cooked	88
Broccoli	½ cup cooked	68
Green beans	½ cup cooked	62

plements. Calcium carbonate (which is also contained in antacid tablets such as Tums) was traditionally the form recommended because it tends to be less expensive and better tolerated than other forms and was thought to be more readily absorbed. And, indeed, taking calcium carbonate with food—particularly milk—improves absorption considerably. New evidence suggests, however, that the calcium in calcium citrate (Citracal) is absorbed 2.5 times more readily than in the form of calcium carbonate. The maximum amount of calcium that can be absorbed at one time is about 500 mg, so women who need to take supplements in larger amounts should divide the dose into 2 doses daily.

Consuming vast quantities of calcium—or any other single vitamin or mineral—without attention to other factors often does not lead to the desired result (in this case, prevention of osteoporosis) and in some cases can be counterproductive. For example, diets high in protein, fat, sodium, caffeine, and phosphorus (which is found in meats, fish, poultry, carbonated drinks, and many processed foods) may increase the excretion of calcium in urine or interfere with its absorption in the intestine. Other minerals such as copper, fluoride, manganese, and zinc may also have some effect on calcium metabolism, although the evidence is still scanty.

No matter how much calcium is taken, it will not be absorbed adequately by the intestine without enough vitamin D. Premenopausal women need to have at least 200 IU (international units) of vitamin D per day (assuming they are getting 1,000 mg per day of calcium), and postmenopausal women should be getting 400 to 800 IUs per day, especially during the winter months when they may not be getting much sunlight exposure. Older women need additional vitamin D, partly because the aging intestine becomes less able to absorb vitamin D and also because as women grow older they are more likely to be poorly nourished or to be chronically ill or housebound. Many foods are now fortified with vitamin D, enough so that most people who are eating a diet rich in calcium are probably also getting enough vitamin D. Just drinking two glasses of milk a day, for example, provides 400 IU of vitamin D.

An ordinary multivitamin pill can usually fill any woman's need for vitamin D, since most contain 400 IU of the vitamin. No one should take more than 800 IU of vitamin D per day, because higher doses can increase calcium in the blood or urine to toxic levels.

Given the intricate interrelationship of nutrients in the body, calcium and vitamin supplements are no substitute for a balanced diet in promoting overall good health.

What are the risks and complications?

Women with a personal or family history of kidney stones containing calcium should consult their clinician before taking any calcium supplements. Women should also check with their clinician to make sure that certain medications they are taking (such as thyroid hormone, lithium, and some steroids, anticonvulsants, chemotherapy, and antacids) are not interfering with calcium stores or absorption.

Too much calcium (over 3,000 mg a day) can interfere with the absorption of zinc and iron, impair metabolism of vitamin K, and even leach calcium from the bones. Excess calcium intake can also cause nausea, diarrhea, and hardening (calcification) of the soft tissue.

Earlier studies suggested that many calcium supplements contained lead levels in excess of the Food and Drug Administration limit. More recent studies, however, suggest that none contain lead at levels even close to the maximum daily allowed intake (6 micrograms), and most authorities maintain that the benefits of getting enough calcium far outweigh the risks presented by a minuscule amount of lead. Even so, the safest approach is probably to avoid bonemeal, which appears to be the worst offender. Tablet or liquid forms of calcium with the USP (United States Pharmacopeia) seal of approval are a safer choice.

Related entries
Iron, kidney disorders, nutrition, osteoporosis, vitamins, zinc

Carpal Tunnel Syndrome

Carpal tunnel syndrome is a painful but treatable condition of the hands and wrists. It results from the compression of the median nerve, which runs through a narrow passageway (the carpal tunnel) in the wrists, to carry messages between the brain and the thumb, index finger, middle finger, and inner half of the ring finger (see illustration). Bound by bones and ligaments, the carpal tunnel can compress or pinch the median nerve if the tissues surrounding it become swollen.

Who is likely to develop carpal tunnel syndrome?
Occurring in about 1 out of every 1,000 people, carpal tunnel syndrome is particularly common in women 50 to 70 years old. It is also common in people who perform forceful, repetitive hand movements, particularly those that involve bending the wrist. These include typists, checkout clerks, factory workers, carpenters, upholsterers, meat packers, violinists, and waitresses, as well as people who knit, crochet, hook rugs, paint, do woodwork, or garden.

Carpal tunnel syndrome is more likely to occur in people who have other conditions that increase pressure within the carpal tunnel. These include rheumatoid arthritis and pregnancy. Carpal tunnel syndrome can also develop in people with diabetes and hypothyroidism (see entries).

What are the symptoms?
In the early stages of carpal tunnel syndrome the first three fingers occasionally feel numb or tingle. Symptoms often become worse at night. Over time they may progress to a burning, aching sensation in these fingers, as well as a painful numbness in the palm. Pain sometimes shoots from the wrist up into forearm or down into the palm or fingers. Typically

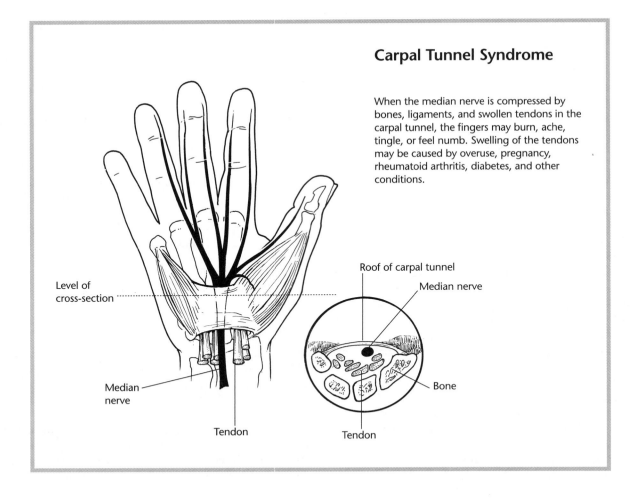

Carpal Tunnel Syndrome

When the median nerve is compressed by bones, ligaments, and swollen tendons in the carpal tunnel, the fingers may burn, ache, tingle, or feel numb. Swelling of the tendons may be caused by overuse, pregnancy, rheumatoid arthritis, diabetes, and other conditions.

Level of cross-section

Roof of carpal tunnel

Median nerve

Median nerve

Bone

Tendon

Tendon

symptoms are severe enough to interrupt deep sleep but can be relieved by shaking or rubbing the hand or hanging the arm over the side of the bed. In more severe cases, affected fingers may become permanently numb, and muscle atrophy may make the thumb difficult to move. Symptoms can occur in one or both hands.

How is the condition evaluated?

The initial evaluation can usually be performed by a primary care physician. Pain that results from pressing or tapping the inside of the wrist or holding the wrist in a flexed position for about a minute may suggest carpal tunnel syndrome. The gold standard for diagnosing the syndrome, however, is a nerve conduction test to determine if electrical signals are slowed by a compressed median nerve.

Performed on an outpatient basis, this test is similar to an electromyelogram (EMG). It involves taping to the skin two electrodes, each of which is connected to a machine that detects and records electrical activity. After a mild shock is applied to the arm, this machine measures the speed and nature of electrical impulses as they pass through the underlying nerve. Because this test involves a fair amount of discomfort, it is often reserved for cases in which the clinician suspects subtle weakness and is considering surgery.

How is carpal tunnel syndrome treated?

Most people with mild or moderate symptoms of carpal tunnel syndrome can obtain lasting relief by modifying work and recreational activities and by wearing wrist splints at night to rest the joint. An occupational therapist can often help the patient assess working conditions (such as computer keyboards) to minimize the symptoms. Splints may also be worn during the day if they do not interfere with work or daily living. Antiinflammatory drugs may relieve some of the pain by reducing swelling.

If symptoms persist, injections of corticosteroids (modified adrenal hormones such as cortisone) into the carpal tunnel may be tried. While generally safe and effective, these injections may provide only transient relief to people who have severe or constant symptoms. For these people surgery may be necessary to decompress the median nerve.

Called carpal tunnel release, this relatively simple outpatient surgical procedure involves cutting the ligament that binds the carpal tunnel. It often provides immediate relief, leaving only a small scar on the inside of the wrist. It is usually done under local anesthesia. Sensory function generally returns within months, although there may be some tenderness for a while at the incision site and at the base of the thumb and fingers. In some people this operation is ineffective and carpal tunnel syndrome recurs. For reasons not yet understood, people with work-related carpal tunnel syndrome appear to have a slightly longer recovery time and less overall success with this procedure.

Related entries

Arthritis, diabetes, hypothyroidism, occupational hazards, pregnancy, rheumatoid arthritis

Cataracts

Cataracts are the blurring or clouding of the lens of the eye, a structure behind the pupil which helps focus light onto the retina. Thought to result from chemical changes within the lens, cataracts interfere with the transmission of light and—because they often develop in both eyes—result in the gradual loss of vision. Indeed, cataracts are one of the leading causes of blindness in the world. On the positive side, modern surgical techniques allow vision to be restored if the cataract is the principal reason for blurred vision.

Who is likely to develop cataracts?

Cataracts are usually associated with the aging eye, and in fact are extremely common in people over the age of 60. This is probably because the body's ability to repair damaged proteins within the lens is limited. But cataracts can also occur at any age in people with certain medical conditions (such as diabetes and various endocrine imbalances), as well as in those taking certain medications (such as corticosteroids for inflammatory conditions) for a long period of time or in those with certain eye disorders or injuries. Excess exposure to ultraviolet radiation from the sun over the years can also make cataracts more likely to develop, as may cigarette smoking. A person may even be born with cataracts or may develop them in early childhood, probably for genetic reasons.

What are the symptoms?

The chief symptom of cataracts is blurred or hazy vision. Often this is accompanied by sensitivity to light or difficulty seeing at night. Vision can also be particularly difficult in bright light and glare, when the cataract scatters light in the same way that ice on a windshield does. Often people with cataracts will start to see a clear halo encircling lights, or will notice that they can read without the bifocals they required before (this "second sight" phenomenon—which eventually disappears—is known as nuclear sclerosis). These changes usually develop gradually.

How is the condition evaluated?

The symptoms of visual blurring associated with cataracts can signal or mimic a number of other eye conditions (including eye inflammation, glaucoma, and retinal holes and detachment), so anyone experiencing them should be examined by an ophthalmologist (a medical doctor specializing in the care of the eyes).

After a thorough and painless examination showing the presence of a cataract, the physician can consider whether treatment is needed. This decision will rest not just on the presence of the cataract but also on the person's visual needs.

How are cataracts treated?

Although attempts have been made to stabilize cataracts with drops, ointments, and drugs (including aspirin), the only known effective treatment is surgical removal of the defective lens and replacement with an artificial plastic lens (see illustration). A day surgery procedure, this operation involves removing the lens through an incision in the outer edge of the cornea. If both eyes have cataracts that significantly impair vision, surgery is done on separate occasions, with the more severely affected eye repaired first. The procedure takes less than an hour and is usually painless when done with mild se-

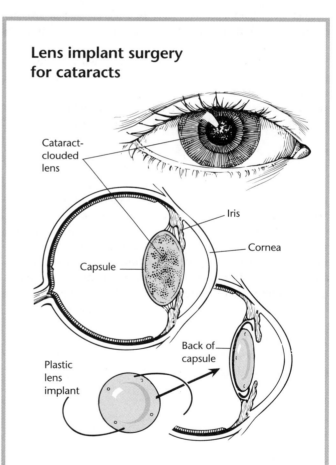

Lens implant surgery for cataracts

Cataract-clouded lens

Iris

Cornea

Capsule

Back of capsule

Plastic lens implant

The cross-section shows a cataract-clouded lens, which the surgeon removes and replaces with a plastic implant. The model shown is supported by the back wall of the lens capsule and by tension on two fine springs that protrude from its sides.

dation and local anesthesia. Afterward there is no significant pain in most cases; slight discomfort, if present, clears in a day or two.

Although ophthalmologists used to ask cataract patients to wait for surgery until a cataract had had a chance to "ripen," this is no longer necessary, given the safety and effectiveness of modern techniques. Still, any surgical procedure carries a small degree of risk, so most eye doctors suggest having the surgery at the point when the cataracts begin to interfere significantly with life. A person who has a precise visual need— say, a musician who needs to read music or a night shift worker who must drive home in the dark—will probably opt for surgery earlier than someone less reliant on sharp vision. Until surgery takes place, however, a person with cataracts should have an eye doctor monitor them on a regular basis.

After surgery over 95 percent of patients find that their vision is improved (unless they have additional eye disorders such as macular degeneration). Most will still require glasses for reading, however, since the artificial lens cannot "accommodate" to near distances. In rare cases, special glasses or extended wear contact lenses may be used in lieu of the implanted lens, but in most cases the implant is vastly more convenient and effective.

There are few, but real, risks associated with cataract surgery and implants; anyone considering cataract surgery should discuss the relative risks and benefits of both surgery and implants with her ophthalmologist, taking into account any other eye conditions and her overall health.

How can cataracts be prevented?

There is no known way to prevent cataracts, which are in most cases probably an inevitable by-product of aging. Wearing good sunglasses to prevent excessive ultraviolet exposure to the eyes, however, may be a reasonable way to prevent additional damage. If one has diabetes, tight control of glucose is important in the prevention of cataracts. Although some studies have suggested that diets high in vitamin C, and possibly vitamin E, lower the incidence of cataracts, more studies need to be done to prove that taking these vitamins can actually prevent cataracts from forming.

Related entries

Antiinflammatory drugs, diabetes, dry eye, eye care, glaucoma, macular degeneration, retinal detachment

Cervical Cancer and Dysplasia

The cervix is the neck of the uterus, which opens into the vagina. Cancer of the cervix is the third most common malignancy of the female genital tract (after endometrial and ovarian cancer). In the United States approximately 13,100 new cases are diagnosed each year, and 4,100 women die annually from this disease, which is second only to breast cancer as a documented case of cancer death among women. But with the widespread use of the Pap test as a screening tool, early detection and successful cure of this disease have become increasingly common.

The disease develops gradually, starting with abnormal cell changes called dysplasia (also called low-grade squamous intraepithelial lesions, or SIL). These abnormal cells are found most often in women between the ages of 25 and 35 but can occur in women of any age. They sometimes revert to normal cells. Nevertheless, these cell changes are considered a precancerous condition. In time (sometimes a full decade), some precancerous cells may develop into a localized forerunner of cancer, called carcinoma in situ, which affects the outer surface of the cervix.

If untreated, this cancer may eventually invade deeper tissues of the cervix or other organs (invasive carcinoma), including the vagina, pelvic ligaments and sidewall, bladder, and rectum; in more advanced cases it can spread through the bloodstream and lymph system to the lungs, liver, or bone.

Many researchers now believe that over 90 percent of all cervical dysplasias are linked to infection with the sexually transmitted human papilloma virus (HPV), which is also linked to visible genital warts (see entry). Some studies indicate that a whopping 15 to 30 percent of sexually active teenage women are infected with this virus, many of them with strains that have been linked to cervical cancer. A recent three-year survey at Rutgers University found that a full 60 percent of female students had been infected with the HPV, although only 1 percent of all infections lead to premalignant or malignant diseases.

Who is likely to develop cervical dysplasia and cancer?

Women of any age and ethnic group can develop cervical cancer, but African American women are twice as likely as white women to die of it. Hispanic and Native American women, along with African American women, have a higher incidence of this disease, as do women in Caribbean and Latin American countries. Lack of access to health care probably accounts for a large part of the difference.

Risk factors for cervical cancer in all populations include having multiple sexual partners, early age of first sexual intercourse, a prior history of sexually transmitted diseases, and cigarette smoking. The human papilloma virus, which is sexually transmitted and can cause changes in the cells of the cervix as well as visible genital warts (see entry), has been linked to cancer of the cervix; a history of this infection is a risk factor for cervical cancer. Infection with the human immunodeficiency virus (HIV), also sexually transmitted, increases the risk of abnormal cell changes (atypical cells or dysplasia) in the cervix, persistence of dysplasia, and eventual cancer.

Some studies have suggested a possible link between oral contraceptives and cervical cancer. Other studies have linked an increased risk with a deficiency of vitamins A and C in the diet. There is no convincing evidence that emotional stress,

Diagnosing cervical cancer under the microscope

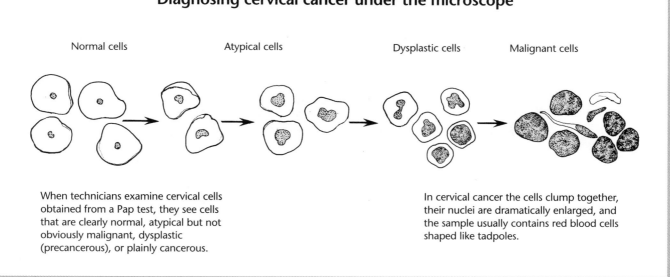

Normal cells   Atypical cells   Dysplastic cells   Malignant cells

When technicians examine cervical cells obtained from a Pap test, they see cells that are clearly normal, atypical but not obviously malignant, dysplastic (precancerous), or plainly cancerous.

In cervical cancer the cells clump together, their nuclei are dramatically enlarged, and the sample usually contains red blood cells shaped like tadpoles.

environmental pollutants, or estrogen replacement therapy is associated with cervical cancer.

What are the symptoms?

Cervical dysplasia and localized cervical cancer usually involve no symptoms whatsoever. Abnormal vaginal bleeding is often the first clue that the cancer may have spread beyond the outer portion of the cervix (invasive disease). Some women may notice this bleeding after intercourse or between menstrual periods. Others may have abnormally heavy menstrual periods. There may also be a pink-tinged or foul-smelling vaginal discharge. As the disease becomes more advanced, other symptoms may develop, including leg, back, or pelvic pain, painful urination, and swelling of the legs.

How are these conditions evaluated?

Both cervical dysplasia and cervical cancer are usually first diagnosed on the basis of an abnormal Pap test (see entry). This test, performed during a routine pelvic examination, allows examination of cell types from the cervix. These cells are classified as normal, atypical, dysplasia (either low grade or high-grade or carcinoma in situ—CIS), or some stage of cancer (see illustration). If the cells are classified as atypical (which is not the same as dysplasia), the Pap test is generally repeated in a few months. Atypical cells may come back labeled as ASCUS (pronounced *ask*-us), an acronym that stands for atypical squamous cells of undetermined significance. Many Pap tests that are atypical initially are normal at follow-up. Some clinicians may want to test for the presence of high-risk strains of HPV in women with ASCUS as well.

At present, the American College of Obstetrics and Gynecology recommends that a persistent abnormality of the cervix or any high-grade dysplastic change be evaluated with a colposcopy, a procedure in which the cervix is visually inspected with the aid of a special type of illuminated microscope called a colposcope. Atypical cells in the initial Pap test of a woman who has tested positive for HIV warrant an immediate colposcopy as well, as does a positive test for high-risk subtypes of HPV in a woman with ASCUS. This procedure usually causes about the same level of discomfort as a regular pelvic exam and can be done in the physician's office. If there is a visible abnormality of the cervix, a small piece of tissue will be removed from the cervix and examined under a microscope for dysplastic or cancerous changes ("punch biopsy"). This procedure sometimes produces a brief cramping or stinging sensation, and there may be some vaginal spotting for a day or two afterwards.

If the abnormality seems to extend beyond the tip of the cervix, another biopsy called an endocervical curettage may be necessary. In this type of biopsy, which can also be performed as an outpatient procedure, the clinician uses a curette, a thin metal instrument with a spoon-shaped tip, to scrape tissue from the cervical lining. Mild cramping is common, and there is a small risk of infection following the procedure.

If the results of the punch biopsy contradict the results of the Pap test, a cone biopsy may be necessary. Also known as a cold knife biopsy or conization, this procedure can both diagnose and treat cervical abnormalities. In a cone biopsy a cone-shaped wedge of tissue from the lower cervix is removed, and the surrounding area is then sutured (stitched) or cauterized (closed with heat). Often the cone biopsy removes the dysplastic cells and therefore is itself a cure. A common alternative to this procedure, which accomplishes the same ends, is the electrosurgical loop excision procedure (LEEP; see below).

If a diagnosis of cervical cancer is made, the physician will next "stage" the disease to see how advanced it is. A com-

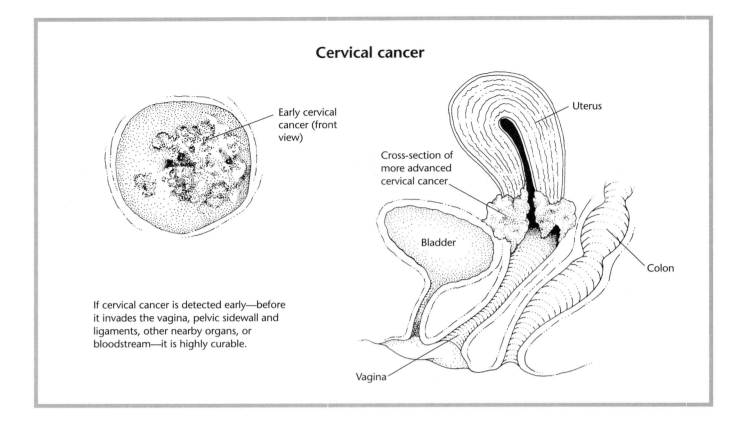

Cervical cancer

Early cervical cancer (front view)

Cross-section of more advanced cervical cancer

Uterus

Bladder

Colon

Vagina

If cervical cancer is detected early—before it invades the vagina, pelvic sidewall and ligaments, other nearby organs, or bloodstream—it is highly curable.

plete history and physical exam will be necessary, as well as routine blood testing, a chest x-ray, intravenous pyelogram (an x-ray of the kidneys and bladder), and a barium enema. Other tests such as a lymphangiogram, bone scan, CT scan, or MRI may also be used to help plan appropriate treatment.

The smaller the tumor size and the earlier the stage, the greater the chances of successful recovery. When cervical changes are treated while they are still precancerous, survival and cure rates are almost 100 percent.

How is cervical dysplasia treated?

If the biopsy confirms dysplastic changes, a woman should discuss treatment options with her clinician. One possibility may be simply to watch cervical changes carefully with frequent Pap tests and colposcopies to see if the cells revert to normal. Because as many as 60 percent of low-grade dysplasias may revert to normal without treatment, this option may be reasonable for women who receive regular health examinations. Even so, many women (and their clinicians) prefer to have the abnormal cells removed, given that a substantial proportion of dysplasias will become more severe or even cancerous over time (and some associated with HIV infection may progress unusually quickly). In addition, all high-grade dysplasias should be treated. Dysplastic cells can be removed through one of several techniques, all of which can be done on an outpatient basis. These techniques include cryosurgery, laser surgery, electrosurgical loop excision (LEEP), and, less commonly, cone biopsy.

Cryosurgery, a technique in which liquid nitrogen is used to destroy abnormal tissue, is best used to treat the mild or moderate dysplasia affecting a small area of the cervix. It is generally done in a doctor's office, takes only a few minutes, and requires no anesthesia. After inserting a speculum into the vagina, the doctor touches the affected area with a metal-tipped cryoprobe that is cooled by a compressed gas. This sometimes produces a sensation of cold or mild cramping. After the frozen tissue is sloughed off, a scab will form and is eventually replaced by new tissue.

Another option is laser surgery using a carbon dioxide laser to vaporize abnormal tissue and seal off blood vessels without requiring an incision. Laser surgery generally involves less pain, bleeding, healing time, and risk of infection or other complications than other forms of surgery. Particularly useful for destroying large lesions, laser surgery can be done on an outpatient basis with either local or general anesthesia.

Electrosurgical loop excision procedure (LEEP) is an increasingly popular option and is better suited for treating more extensive dysplasia than cryotherapy. The tissue removed can then be examined under a microscope to see if it contains dysplastic or even cancerous cells. The obvious advantage over both cryosurgery and laser surgery is that diagnosis and treatment of dysplasia can be accomplished with a single procedure. LEEP can be done in a physician's office or outpatient clinic and requires only local anesthesia.

Rarely, a physician may use a procedure called cone biopsy (see previous section) to remove dysplastic cells. Because this procedure is relatively expensive, and because it is a minor surgical procedure that can result in complications and may require general or regional anesthesia, it has become less popular in recent years. Cone biopsy is also more likely than other treatments to interfere with future childbearing capability, and, like the LEEP procedure, it may cause temporary changes in the cervix that make Pap tests difficult to interpret accurately for 3 or 4 months. It may be necessary, however, if the dysplastic cells extend too deeply into the cervical canal for other methods, including laser surgery, to reach.

A still experimental approach that may be used to treat dysplastic changes involves applying topical "immune response mediators" such as imiquimod (Aldara, a drug already used to treat genital warts) to the cervix itself. The aim in this approach, which is undergoing clinical trials, is to deactivate the HPV and prevent it from promoting cancerous cell changes.

All of these procedures usually preserve the ability to bear children. Hysterectomy (removal of the uterus, including the cervix) is occasionally recommended as a last-resort treatment for recurrent dysplasia, but it is rarely recommended for young women, many of whom may want to bear children later in life.

After any surgical treatment for dysplasia there may be some cramping, tenderness, bleeding, or vaginal discharge. To minimize pain and risk of infection while the cervix is healing, tampons and sexual intercourse should be avoided for several weeks.

Even if all dysplastic cells are removed by one of these techniques, it is important to continue checking for abnormalities on a regular basis. Human papilloma virus can be difficult to eradicate and, in about 10 to 20 percent of women, can lurk in perfectly normal cells for years, potentially infecting future sex partners and causing subsequent changes in the cervix. That is why after any treatment for cervical dysplasia a woman should have frequent Pap tests for the next year or so—usually three months, six months, and one year after the surgery. If all of these Pap tests are normal, an annual Pap test and pelvic examination will usually suffice.

How is cervical cancer treated?

Treatment depends on the stage of the disease. Preinvasive disease is not cancer and can be locally excised with techniques such as cryosurgery, laser surgery, or electrosurgical loop excision (see entries). All of these procedures usually allow childbearing in the future, if a woman so desires. After the procedures there may be some cramping, tenderness, bleeding, or vaginal discharge. To minimize pain and risk of infection while the cervix is healing, women should avoid tampons and sexual intercourse for several weeks.

Treatment for early-stage cervical cancer (cancer that has not yet spread beyond the cervix) has changed dramatically in recent years. Although surgery to remove part or all of the uterus was traditionally considered to be the most effective treatment, it left women at risk for a recurrence if pelvic lymph nodes tested positive for metastatic cancer. Radiation therapy could prevent recurrence but seemed to have no effect on long-term survival and left women at risk for damage to the small intestine. It was generally considered desirable only for earlier stages of the disease when surgery was inappropriate—for example, if a woman was elderly or obese, or had a particularly large tumor or a coexisting medical illness. A breakthrough report in 1999, however, showed that supplementing radiation therapy with the chemotherapy drug cisplatin improves the chances of overall survival.

For women with more advanced stages of cervical cancer, radiation therapy is also the treatment of choice, generally supplemented with weekly chemotherapy. Chemotherapy alone, however, is successful for fewer than 1 in 5 women, and usually for only a short time. For that reason it is reserved for disease that has recurred after treatment or has spread beyond the pelvic region. It may also be useful in shrinking tumors so that they are more easily removed by surgery or controlled by radiation therapy.

Women should continue to have regular checkups and Pap tests after treatment has been completed.

On the horizon is an HPV vaccine that researchers hope will someday eradicate cervical cancer completely. Clinical trials are currently open for women with metastatic or recurrent disease.

How can cervical cancer be prevented?

Using a barrier method of birth control (a condom or diaphragm) may help reduce the risk of cervical cancer, perhaps by preventing the spread of sexually transmitted diseases. In addition, starting at age 18 or at the onset of sexual activity, all women should have a yearly Pap test and pelvic examination. The Pap test appears to be a highly effective screening tool for cervical cancer and has been credited with greatly reducing mortality from this disease and reducing the rate of invasive cancer in the past half century.

Although the exact timing of subsequent exams remains controversial, many doctors recommend that women who have no risk factors and have had 3 consecutive annual Pap tests that were normal can have the test repeated every 3 years. Women at high risk—for example, those with new or multiple sexual partners—should generally have annual exams. A woman whose mother used DES during pregnancy should discuss with her clinician having more frequent exams.

At what age to stop having Pap tests remains controversial. Studies of women over 65 show that as many as 60 percent have never had a Pap test at all. Because there is an increased risk of developing cervical cancer with increasing age, women over 65 who have never or rarely had a previous Pap test should ask their physician to perform one. Women who have had frequent negative Pap tests before age 65 benefit less from routine screening after 65.

Related entries

AIDS, biopsy, birth control, cryosurgery, diethylstilbestrol (DES), electrosurgical loop excision, genital warts, hysterectomy, laser surgery, Pap test, pelvic inflammatory disease, radiation therapy, safer sex, screening, sexual dysfunction, sexually transmitted diseases, smoking, vaginal bleeding (abnormal)

Cesarean Section

A cesarean section is a surgical procedure in which a fetus is removed from the uterus through a surgical opening. Once extremely dangerous operations performed only to save a baby's life at the cost of the mother's, c-sections today are safe and are done for a variety of reasons. These include breech presentation (feet or buttocks first), disproportion between the baby's head and the mother's pelvis (cephalopelvic disproportion), "fetal distress" (which is now called "nonreassuring fetal heart rate pattern" and is often due to a compressed umbilical cord), weak and ineffective contractions (uterine dysfunction), placental problems such as placenta abruptio and placenta previa (see vaginal bleeding during pregnancy), or, in rare situations, fetal complications related to health disorders in the mother such as diabetes, high blood pressure, heart trouble, or preeclampsia (a complication of pregnancy characterized by hypertension, protein in the urine, and fluid retention).

Cesareans now account for as many as 23 percent of all deliveries in the United States, in contrast with about 3 percent half a century ago. Many clinicians report that an increasing number of women are asking for c-sections even when they are not necessary. Part of the explanation for this increase is the fact that modern anesthetic, antiseptic, antibiotic, and blood transfusion techniques have made cesarean deliveries relatively safe as major surgical procedures go. Another factor (though actually a minor contributor) is the rise in the number of older women choosing to have babies. The older the mother, the greater the chances of complications that may require a c-section (see pregnancy over age 35). Also, sensitive fetal monitoring techniques during labor allow detection of problems in the baby that would have gone unnoticed years ago. And an increasing number of women, rejecting the idea that a vaginal delivery makes them better mothers, are electing to have c-sections to avoid labor pains, to control the time of delivery, or in the hope of preventing pelvic floor dysfunction.

It is undeniable that cesareans have saved the lives of many women who otherwise would have died from complications during childbirth. But many critics argue that cesarean sections are too often performed as "defensive medicine"—that is, to prevent the possibility of a malpractice suit—whenever there is the slightest chance of a complicated labor. In the majority of these cases, the critics say, the mother's life or health is not threatened, and the baby, though under some physical stress, would be born healthy if a vaginal birth were allowed to proceed. In addition, choosing to have a medi-

cally unwarranted c-section puts a woman at unnecessary risk for serious complications, including urinary tract infections, inflammation of the uterine wall, blood clots, hemorrhage, and even death.

How is the procedure performed?

Many cesarean sections are scheduled in advance of the delivery date because of some anticipated problem. Others occur on an emergency basis. In both cases the first step in the procedure is thoroughly washing the lower abdomen (possibly including shaving pubic hair if time permits). Usually an intravenous tube has already been inserted into a vein so that fluids and medications can be given later.

The woman is moved to the operating room, where anesthesia is administered. A catheter is inserted into the bladder after the anesthetic has taken effect. In a nonemergency cesarean either epidural or spinal anesthesia is used to numb the woman's body from the waist down while allowing her to remain conscious during the operation. If circumstances allow, she will be able to see and possibly even hold the baby as soon as it is born. Depending on the situation, emergency c-sections may require general anesthesia, however, which leaves the woman unconscious during the birth and groggy afterward. General anesthesia is usually not necessary if a woman already has an epidural in place during labor and then has to have an emergency c-section. Spinals are also used for many emergency c-sections.

Usually the birthing partner is allowed in the operating room during a cesarean section, though in emergency situations this is not always possible, and even in nonemergency deliveries the partner has to wait outside until the anesthetic has taken effect. If the woman is awake, a screen is usually placed between her upper and lower body so that she does not have to view her internal organs as the baby is lifted out (though squeamish birthing partners should know that they will probably see these organs if they watch the birth).

The surgical site is prepared with antiseptic and a sterile drape is placed around it. Once the anesthesia has taken effect, the surgeon makes an incision through the woman's abdominal wall. This incision can be either vertical (from just below the navel to just above the pubic bone) or horizontal (extending from side to side just above the pubic bone). The latter cut—sometimes called a bikini cut—leaves a less visible scar after the operation. In an emergency situation, however, the surgeon will usually opt for a vertical cut because it allows faster access to the distressed baby.

Regardless of which type of incision is made, there is a small risk in cesarean surgery, as in all abdominal surgery, that a keloid or other abnormal scar will develop. These scars may be thicker, wider, and more uneven in appearance than normal scars and tend to pucker. A woman usually cannot get rid of the scar by having a c-section with her next child, since keloids almost always recur. There are no special closure techniques, dressings, corsets, or injections to minimize keloids after a second c-section for a woman who developed them after her first.

The surgeon next makes a second cut into the uterus itself,

through which the baby will be delivered. This cut can also be either vertical or horizontal (transverse), regardless of the direction of the abdominal incision. If possible, most surgeons today choose to make a horizontal cut in the lower part of the uterus, since it heals quickly and has a lower rate of complications (such as blood loss and ruptured scars) during this and subsequent deliveries. In certain situations, such as a difficult fetal position or an unusually large head (hydrocephalus), the surgeon may opt to do a low vertical incision instead, which can sometimes cause more bleeding and other complications.

Another option is the classic cesarean incision, a vertical cut made higher in the body of the uterus. Though riskier than either vertical or horizontal cuts made lower in the uterus, classic incisions are still used in certain emergency situations because they provide the fastest, easiest access to the baby. They are often used, for example, if the placenta is near or blocking the cervix or if the baby is lying in a crosswise position.

Once baby and placenta have been removed from the uterus, the uterine incision and then the skin incision are sutured or clipped together. The entire procedure is usually completed in an hour or less.

What happens after surgery?

Soon afterward the catheter is removed from the bladder. The intravenous tube remains in place for another day or two, and fluids are given intravenously until the woman is ready to eat and drink on her own.

Women who have had a cesarean need to stay in the hospital longer than women who have given birth vaginally—an average of 4 days—and may experience significant discomfort as the anesthesia wears off and the incision begins to heal. Medication for pain relief is routinely administered for several days, sometimes through an epidural or intravenous catheter under the woman's control, or in pill form as needed. If taken right after breastfeeding, these fast-acting painkillers are at low levels in the milk during the next feeding, and in any case are not thought to be harmful to the baby.

Once she goes home, adjusting to life with a new baby can be somewhat more difficult for a woman who has had a c-section, since there are usually restrictions on lifting, climbing stairs, and driving for a few weeks after the surgery. Sometimes women who have had a cesarean find it painful to hold the baby across their abdomen while breastfeeding and have more success using the "football hold"—that is, positioning the baby under one arm at the side of the body so that it does not rest directly on the wound (see illustration).

What are the risks and complications?

Like any major surgical procedure, cesarean sections may result in hemorrhage (internal bleeding) requiring blood transfusion, or infection of the uterus or adjacent pelvic organs. Though rarely, a cesarean section may lead to decreased bowel function or blood clots in the pelvic organs, the legs, and occasionally the lungs. Women who have a cesarean sec-

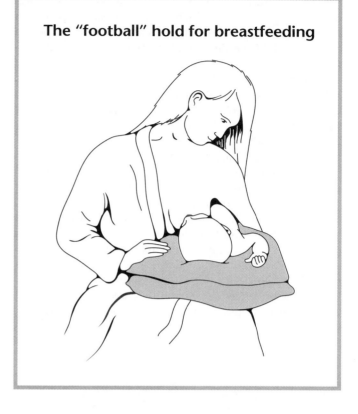

The "football" hold for breastfeeding

tion are 5 times more likely to die from complications of childbirth than women who have a vaginal delivery. But most women who die from c-sections had preexisting medical problems that raised their overall risks during childbirth and necessitated the cesarean in the first place.

How can cesarean sections be prevented?

No woman should regard having a c-section as a failure of maternity. But the increased risks to both mother and baby—and cost to the health care system—are sufficient justification for trying to minimize unnecessary cesareans. A woman might consider discussing this procedure with her clinician well in advance of the delivery date if possible, inquiring just how frequently he or she performs the procedure and under what circumstances.

Another way to minimize unnecessary cesareans is for women who have already had the procedure to consider the feasibility of vaginal delivery in subsequent pregnancies. Called vaginal birth after cesarean (VBAC), this option has become increasingly advocated in the United States over the past decade (and for much longer in other parts of the world). Contrary to earlier belief, it turns out that—in many cases—uterine scars from previous cesareans have very little chance of rupturing during subsequent deliveries. The chances are particularly small if a transverse cut was made in the uterus. Women interested in having a VBAC should consult their clinician about which type of incision was previously used. It is not always possible to judge the direction of the uterine incision from the scar outside the body, since surgeons sometimes follow a transverse abdominal incision with a vertical uterine incision. A classic (high vertical) incision in particular is fairly likely to rupture during a subsequent delivery, posing a risk of serious bleeding problems that can endanger both mother and baby.

Whatever the type of incision, any woman considering a VBAC should realize that she might have to opt for another cesarean should problems arise during delivery. Thus, she will need to give birth in a facility equipped to perform special monitoring as well as an emergency cesarean if necessary. Nevertheless, most healthy women (at least 60 percent) who attempt a VBAC after 1 or more previous cesareans are successful. This is particularly true for women whose cesareans were due to fetal distress or breech presentation rather than an underlying medical condition or an unusually narrow pelvis. Hospitals and birthing centers increasingly are offering classes geared specifically to women interested in VBAC.

Related entries

Anesthesia, breastfeeding, childbirth, diabetes, high blood pressure, preeclampsia, pregnancy over age 35, Rh disease, vaginal bleeding during pregnancy

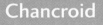

Chancroid

Chancroid is a sexually transmitted disease caused by the bacterium *Hemophilus ducreyi*. Most women with chancroid (also known as soft chancre) have no symptoms, but they are often unknowing carriers of the organism and can therefore perpetuate its spread if the condition remains untreated. Some researchers believe that people with active chancroid sores may be more susceptible to infection by HIV, the virus that causes acquired immune deficiency syndrome (AIDS).

Who is likely to develop chancroid?

It is most common among people who live in tropical climates, but it is becoming increasingly prevalent in North America. Chancroid can develop in anyone who has sexual or skin-to-skin contact with an infected person, even if that person has no symptoms.

What are the symptoms?

The majority of women infected with chancroid have no noticeable symptoms. If symptoms do develop, they usually involve a small, raised, painless or mildly tender sore surrounded by a reddish border that develops 3 to 7 days after initial infection, most often on the vulva, vagina, urethra, cervix, or inner thighs. In men, the sores most often appear on the penis or urethra. If the sore fills with pus, it will be painful and may rupture, resulting in an open, running sore with ragged edges which can easily be confused with a herpes lesion. Sometimes the sores run together to form one long, narrow ulcer.

Although chancroid sores generally heal spontaneously within days, the bacteria often invade nearby lymph glands in the groin. Within about a week of the initial infection, the glands become hard and swollen, sometimes fusing together into an abscess, or bubo, which is covered by shiny red overlying skin. If untreated, buboes can rise to the surface of the skin and rupture, producing pus and a large, open sore that is easily infected by other microorganisms.

How is the condition evaluated?

Because the bacterium that causes chancroid is difficult to culture, diagnosis often has to be based on the appearance of the chancre lesion and by ruling out other sexually transmitted diseases that can produce similar symptoms—particularly herpes, syphilis, and lymphogranuloma venereum (see chlamydia). This approach makes it difficult to diagnose chancroid in most women with the disease—who, since they do not have any symptoms, may never go in for testing in the first place.

How is chancroid treated?

Chancroid can usually be eradicated with antibiotics—most often erythromycin, azithromycin, or ciprofloxacin for a period of 1 to 7 days, depending on which drug is used. If any buboes are present, the clinician will probably aspirate the pus from them. After treatment it is important to return for follow-up exams over the next few months to make sure that the disease has been eradicated.

How can chancroid be prevented?

Preventing the spread of chancroid is similar to preventing the spread of other sexually transmitted diseases and essentially boils down to practicing safer sex, particularly using condoms. Because women can easily spread the disease unknowingly, it is especially important that they look for signs of chancroid in any sexual partners and avoid unprotected intercourse until an infected partner has been treated successfully.

Related entries

Acquired immune deficiency syndrome, antibiotics, chlamydia, condoms, herpes, safer sex, sexually transmitted diseases, syphilis

Chemotherapy

Chemotherapy is treatment that uses chemical agents to cure, prevent, or relieve disease or the symptoms of disease. The term is most commonly applied to treatment with anticancer drugs.

Chemotherapy is used in several different ways in the treatment of cancer: ▸ as a means to eradicate a tumor or cancer cells that have spread (metastasized), ▸ as a means to prevent the spread of a tumor in earlier stages, and ▸ as a means to prolong life or alleviate pain in the case of an incurable cancer. For many forms of cancer, chemotherapy has been dramatically effective in curing malignancies such as Hodgkin's disease, choriocarcinoma (which may result from a molar pregnancy; see entry), and childhood leukemia. For other forms of cancer such as breast cancer, chemotherapy can be very effective for controlling recurrences of disease and improving quality of life.

Deciding whether or not to embark on a course of chemotherapy means weighing all of the expected gains in life span or quality of life from the treatment—which vary considerably from drug to drug and from cancer to cancer— against the negative factors. It can be reassuring to talk to other people who have gone through chemotherapy to understand that the side effects were indeed temporary and to discuss ways to cope with chemotherapy and cancer in general.

Above all, a supportive relationship between the patient and her health care team is essential for dealing with the many unknowns, uncertainties, and side effects of cancer and chemotherapy.

How is chemotherapy performed?

Today there are approximately 50 anticancer drugs in use, both singly and in combination, and they are administered in pills, liquids, injections, or intravenous lines. In all cases these drugs work by interfering with a cancer cell's ability to grow and reproduce, either by killing the cell outright or by blocking the production of DNA (the cell's genetic material) and therefore preventing cell division.

What happens after the procedure?

Because anticancer drugs cure or control cancer by interfering with the growth and reproduction of rapidly growing cancer cells, there are side effects in parts of the body that depend on rapid growth of cells for healthy functioning. Cells in the bone marrow, the gastrointestinal tract, the reproductive system, and hair follicles are most disturbed by the side effects of anticancer drugs.

In the bone marrow, suppression of cell growth interferes with the production of blood cells. The result may be anemia (owing to a deficiency of red blood cells), bleeding problems (owing to a deficiency of platelets), or susceptibility to infection (owing to a deficiency of white blood cells). New drugs on the market can readily counterbalance some of these effects in many patients. These include granulocyte stimulating factor (GSF), which increases white blood cell production, and erythropoietin (Epogen), which increases red blood cell production. In the gastrointestinal tract, the most common immediate effects are nausea and vomiting, but again, some newer antiemetic treatments are quite effective in relieving these symptoms.

Women who receive chemotherapy often experience amenorrhea (a cessation of menstrual periods), sometimes permanently. Less permanent but upsetting to many women is hair loss. Hair may fall out gradually or all at once, but

after chemotherapy is stopped it usually grows back in a few months or so. Many chemotherapy patients wear a scarf, hat, or wig until their hair grows back. Fatigue and weight gain or loss are other common side effects of chemotherapy.

Although the physical effects of cancer treatment can be difficult to tolerate in the beginning, with the help of some newer medications and various nondrug techniques—including visualization (see alternative therapies)—they can be managed.

What are the risks and complications?

In rare instances certain chemotherapies can also cause serious damage to the heart, lungs, kidneys, or liver. Occasionally problems such as mouth ulcers, skin rashes, difficulty swallowing, diarrhea, and constipation may develop up to several weeks after the treatments.

Related entries

Alternative therapies, amenorrhea, anemia, antibiotics, breast cancer, cervical cancer, colon and rectal cancer, constipation, endometrial cancer, hair loss, melanoma, ovarian cancer, platelet disorders, radiation therapy, vaginal cancer, vulvar cancer

Chest Pain

Pain in the chest is often associated with heart attacks and other life-threatening events. But chest pain (see illustration) can also be a symptom of many other conditions, some of which are relatively minor. Each year approximately 200,000 new cases of chest pain not associated with significant coronary artery disease—that is, disease of the arteries that supply blood to the heart muscle—are identified in the United States.

Yet in many cases chest pain—especially in a woman over 50—does indeed signal a life-threatening condition which requires immediate medical attention. Because cardiovascular disease is still too often considered a "man's problem," however, women with chest pain are more likely than men to be dismissed (or to dismiss themselves) as having heartburn or psychological problems, although this is beginning to change, especially in large medical centers.

Any woman who experiences a heavy squeezing pain across her chest which lasts longer than 20 minutes should seek emergency care immediately. She may be having a life-threatening heart attack.

Problems in the heart

Ischemic chest pain. Chest pain in a woman over the age of 60 is likely to be caused by inadequate blood supply to the heart, and should be evaluated by a clinician (see angina

Some sources of chest pain

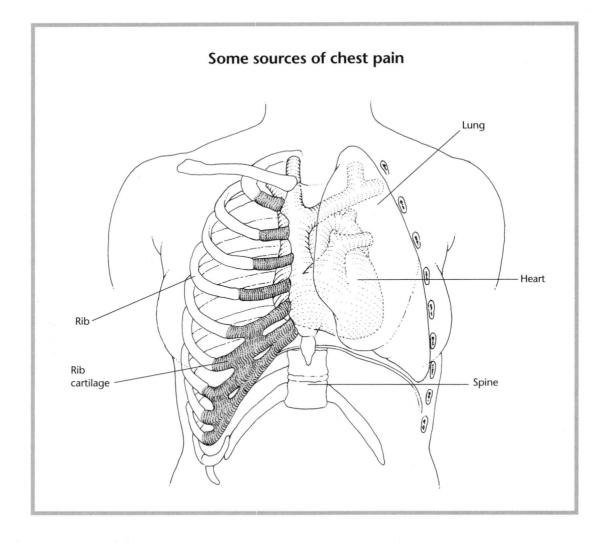

pectoris and coronary artery disease). A small minority of women with chest pain and normal coronary arteries may have a syndrome called "microvascular angina." Although this condition, which primarily affects women, involves certain heartbeat abnormalities, heart function is normal, and most patients have few problems.

Other heart abnormalities. In addition to coronary artery disease, other forms of heart disease (see entry) can cause chest pain. Hypertrophic cardiomyopathy (in which the left ventricle of the heart has become excessively thick and stiff and cannot adequately pump blood from the heart) can lead to chest pain as well as breathlessness, palpitations, lightheadedness, or fainting. Pericarditis (inflammation of the membranous sac surrounding the heart muscle), which is often due to a viral infection, can cause chest pain, too, as can various disorders of the heart valves such as mitral valve prolapse and aortic stenosis (see entries). An aneurysm (widening) in the aorta, the main artery carrying blood away from the heart, if it starts to tear, can cause severe chest pain similar to that of a heart attack except that it comes on very suddenly. The result may be a sharp fall

in blood pressure (shock), loss of consciousness, or even death.

Problems in the lungs

Pleurisy and pneumonia. Often the two-layered membranes surrounding the lungs and chest cavity (the pleura) become inflamed. This condition, called pleurisy, can produce a particularly sharp chest pain which worsens after coughing or inhalation of air as the layers rub together. As a result, people with pleurisy often find themselves taking short, shallow breaths. Pain from pleurisy, which seems to occur more often in women than in men, may also be felt in the shoulders, neck, or abdomen.

Pleurisy can be caused by pneumonia (which can itself produce a dull pain in the chest, even if there is no pleurisy) or, in some cases, by a life-threatening and often overlooked condition called pulmonary embolism. In this disorder a blood clot from elsewhere in the body lodges in one of the pulmonary arteries and blocks blood flow to the lungs, depriving the lung tissue of blood and thereby damaging it (see breathing disorders).

Problems of the muscles and bones

Muscle strain. Excessive coughing, unaccustomed exercise, and lifting heavy objects can lead to muscle strain in the chest. In contrast to pain caused by heart or lung disorders, the pain of muscle strain is made worse by moving the torso, arms, and ribs (whether during exercise or simple breathing) or by pressing the injured areas with a fingertip. Muscle strain usually disappears on its own after a few days of rest, accompanied by hot compresses and aspirin or acetaminophen to relieve the pain.

Costochondritis. Inflammation of the junctions between the ribs and the cartilage can develop after excessive coughing, unaccustomed exercise, lifting heavy objects, or bruising nearby muscles. This condition (called costochondritis) is 3 times more common in women than in men. Usually the pain takes the form of a dull, gnawing tenderness in the chest which lasts for hours or days, but occasionally it can be sharp and fleeting. Pressing on the front of the rib cage usually exacerbates the pain, as does bending, twisting, or other exercises that involve moving the ribs.

Usually symptoms of costochondritis disappear on their own if strenuous activities are avoided for a few days. In the meantime, aspirin or antiinflammatory drugs can be helpful. Like other relatively harmless sources of chest pain, however, suspected costochondritis in a woman over 50 should be evaluated by a clinician to rule out the possibility of heart disease.

Cracked or fractured ribs. Physical trauma can sometimes crack or fracture a rib. A cancer that has spread to the ribs from elsewhere in the body can also result in a rib fracture. In addition, a trivial injury, or even vigorous coughing, is enough to fracture ribs in women with severe osteoporosis. The result may be sharp pain that becomes worse with every inhalation of air. In contrast to pain traceable to the heart or lungs, pain from a rib fracture becomes worse when the torso is bent or twisted.

Fractured ribs usually heal without treatment, but a clinician should be consulted to determine whether the fracture was due to some serious but potentially treatable underlying disease.

Osteoarthritis of the spine. Sometimes arthritic deformities in the spine put pressure on nerves running from the backbone to the chest (see osteoarthritis). The result can be chest pain similar to that of angina. The difference is usually that the pain increases after prolonged sitting or reclining. Like the pain of angina, this pain may radiate to the jaws, arms, and neck and sometimes follows strenuous movement of the upper torso and arms.

Fibromyalgia. Fibromyalgia (see entry) is a disorder of the connective tissue which is 4 times more common in women than in men. It involves painful and stiff muscles, tendons, and ligaments, as well as fatigue and sleep disturbances. People with this disorder have a number of tender points—particular muscles and tendons that become painful when pressed. Often pressure on a tender point between the ribs and cartilage can result in chest pain.

Problems in the gastrointestinal tract

Heartburn. Heartburn (see entry), more technically known as gastroesophageal reflux disease (GERD), is a common problem with symptoms sometimes indistinguishable from those of angina or a heart attack. Heartburn accounts for 30 to 60 percent of chest pain in women with normal coronary arteries.

Finding out that chest pain is due to heartburn rather than heart disease can be a tremendous relief. It is important to remember, however, that some people have heart disease in addition to heartburn. The clue that makes heartburn alone the more likely diagnosis is that antacids relieve the chest pain. If pain occurs mainly while the person is lying down, is not aggravated by exertion, and is accompanied by difficulty swallowing, the chances are even greater that the symptoms can be traced to the esophagus. Nevertheless, any woman in a high-risk group for heart disease (and any woman over 50) should consult a clinician before concluding that her chest pain is due to heartburn alone.

Esophageal motility disorders. Another common gastrointestinal cause of chest pain occurs when there is some abnormality in the way food moves through the esophagus to the stomach. Normally food moves downward through a series of wavelike muscular squeezes known as peristalsis. In a fairly common condition known as nutcracker esophagus (also called hypertensive esophagus or supersqueezer), the peristaltic waves become unusually large and long-lasting, and the result can be severe chest pain.

Less frequently, chest pain may result when strong nonperistaltic contractions develop spontaneously in the esophagus (diffuse esophageal spasm), or when there is excessively high pressure on the sphincter muscle (hypertensive lower esophageal sphincter). Even more uncommon is achalasia, a condition in which there is no peristalsis whatsoever and the sphincter muscle fails to relax. As a result, the upper reaches of the esophagus dilate and produce chest pain.

Sometimes just learning that chest pain is due to the esophagus rather than the heart provides significant pain relief. As with heartburn, however, an esophageal motility disorder does not necessarily preclude the possibility of angina or another heart condition. Therefore, it is important for a woman over 50 to have a clinician rule out heart disease before her chest pain can be attributed to the esophagus.

Once it is established that the esophagus accounts for the pain, a clinician may prescribe drugs such as nitrates or calcium-channel blockers to relieve it. If pain is severe, an operation may be necessary to cut some of the muscular tissue in the esophagus. Occasionally, alternative therapy such as bio-feedback may also be helpful.

Irritable bowel syndrome. Chest pain can also be due to irritable bowel syndrome (see entry), a condition particularly common in women which is characterized by frequent abdominal pain and changes in bowel habits. Although most symptoms of IBS are thought to be caused by exaggerated contractions in the large intestine, they often seem to be accompanied by similar changes in the esophagus—which presumably accounts for the associated chest pain. In fact, it has been suggested that the name "irritable bowel" syndrome be changed to the more comprehensive "irritable gut" syndrome.

Peptic ulcer disease. Peptic ulcer disease (see entry) is a condition in which erosions develop in the inner lining of the stomach or part of the small intestine closest to the stomach. The result is a burning pain, sometimes described as occurring in the chest. Older women with arthritis and others who take aspirin or nonsteroidal antiinflammatory drugs (NSAIDs) on a regular basis are particularly likely to develop ulcers, as are women of all ages who smoke cigarettes. In addition, some women who use alcohol excessively may develop an inflammation of the stomach lining (gastritis) which can also result in chest pain.

Gallbladder disease. In rare instances women with gallbladder disease (see gallstones) may develop chest pain, particularly after eating fatty foods. This often spasmodic pain tends to occur on the upper right side of the abdomen and may extend to the right shoulder blade. It can last for several hours and then gradually subside.

Other physical causes

Menopausal changes. Some women going through menopause have symptoms of chest pain and palpitations. These symptoms may occur in conjunction with hot flashes and are often triggered by exercise or episodes of stress. Some researchers have speculated that the chest pain may have something to do with microvascular angina and with falling levels of the hormone estrogen (see angina pectoris).

Shingles. This common condition develops when the long-dormant herpes zoster virus that caused chicken pox many years before suddenly becomes reactivated. It most often occurs in people over the age of 50 and in people whose immune system is weakened. Sometimes the first sign of shingles is pain along one side of the chest. Only several days later, when a rash consisting of fluid-filled blisters erupts along the site of the pain, does it become clear that the problem is shingles (see entry). Both the pain and rash are usually gone within weeks, but about 10 percent of all people with shingles, and about 50 percent of those over the age of 60, develop chronic pain in the affected area.

Psychological factors

If a clinician cannot find an obvious physical explanation for chest pain and palpitations, psychological factors will probably be considered. Among the most common possibilities are panic disorder and other anxiety disorders, depression, psychosomatic disorders (particularly somatization disorder) with or without a history of domestic abuse, and substance abuse (particularly if it involves cocaine, alcohol, or benzodiazepines). If chest pain occurs together with breathlessness, another possibility is hyperventilation syndrome. People with this syndrome, the majority of whom are women, may experience stiffness in the arms and legs and numbness or a "pins and needles" sensation around the mouth, fingers, and toes.

How is chest pain evaluated?

Chest pain presents a great challenge to the clinician because the same symptom can result from such a wide array of possible sources. The pain of angina can be confused with the pain of indigestion; the tightening in the chest caused by stress can be confused with the tightening caused by a heart attack; or the symptoms of pericarditis can be confused with the symptoms of pleurisy. Complicating matters further is the fact that there is often more than one possible source of the chest pain.

Women have to be vigilant about getting a thorough evaluation, since some clinicians are still less inclined to check for heart conditions in women than in men, whatever the specific nature of the chest pain. Interestingly, some research suggests that women who present their complaints in a "businesslike" as opposed to a "histrionic" manner are more likely to be evaluated for heart disease.

The first step in evaluating chest pain is to rule out any sudden life-threatening conditions, such as unstable angina (see entry), heart attack, pulmonary embolism, pneumothorax (collapsed lung), ruptured aneurysm (a tear in the wall of the aorta, a major artery), or a perforating ulcer or tear of the esophagus. If any of these conditions seems likely, the woman may need to be hospitalized for further evaluation.

In the course of ruling out life-threatening conditions, the clinician will take a history which includes information about the timing, precise location, and nature of the chest pain and any associated symptoms. The clinician will want to know, for example, whether the pain radiates out from the chest; whether reclining, exercising, coughing, or moving the chest wall makes it worse; whether eating, taking antacids, holding the breath, or sitting up makes it better; and whether the pain is accompanied by breathlessness, difficulty swallowing, or edema (fluid retention).

Once a life-threatening condition has been ruled out, the clinician will also want to know whether the woman has completed menopause and will ask for details about her previous medical history, risk factors for heart disease, and dietary habits, as well as her use of alcohol, caffeine, anti-inflammatory drugs, and other medications. A woman who can provide information about any past sexual or domestic abuse, depression, anxiety, or other life stresses will also help ensure an accurate evaluation. Finally, the clinician will do a thorough physical examination, which should include a careful check of the lungs, heart, chest wall, and ribs.

Related entries

Abdominal pain, alcohol, angina pectoris, antibiotics, antiinflammatory drugs, anxiety disorders, aortic stenosis, breathing disorders, circulatory disorders, colds, coronary artery disease, depression, domestic abuse, fibromyalgia, gallstones, heart disease, heartburn, irritable bowel syndrome, menopause, mitral valve prolapse, musculoskeletal disorders, osteoarthritis, osteoporosis, panic disorder, peptic ulcer disease, physical examinations, psychosomatic disorders, rape, shingles, sleep disorders, smoking, stress, substance abuse

Childbirth

Childbirth involves both labor (the process of giving birth) and delivery (the birth itself). No one fully understands just what triggers labor, but it normally occurs spontaneously between 37 and 42 weeks after a pregnant woman's last menstrual period. On average, the entire process lasts about 12 to 14 hours for a first baby and somewhat less for subsequent deliveries. The many stories of 40-hour labors, however, as well as the stories of women who quickly and painlessly drop their babies on the kitchen floor, attest to the wide range of experiences included in this average.

What are the signs of labor?

There are several different signs that suggest that labor may be beginning. The rhythmic, recurring, bandlike tightening around the abdomen and lower back known as contractions are, of course, the classic signs. Some women find contractions excruciating, particularly as labor progresses, while others compare the pain to that of a bad backache or menstrual cramps.

Many women experience irregular and sometimes uncomfortable contractions (Braxton-Hicks contractions) during the latter part of their pregnancy and may find themselves reporting to the hospital only to be sent home with a diagnosis of "false labor." This is nothing to be embarrassed about, since it is sometimes difficult to distinguish real labor from false without examining the cervix.

In general, however, contractions can be assumed to signal real labor if they are regular, persist during walking or other

What to expect during childbirth		
First stage	**Changes in cervix and uterus**	**Physical symptoms**
Early (latent) phase	Cervix dilates to 4 or 5 cm, flattens and shortens.	Contractions are mild, gradually becoming more regular. Bloody "show" may occur.
Active (mild) phase	Cervix dilates from 4 to 8 cm, continues to flatten and shorten.	Contractions become stronger.
Transition Phase	Cervix dilates from 8 to 10 cm and flattens so much that it disappears.	Contractions come almost one on top of the other. Some women have nausea, vomiting, trembling, chills, or irritability.
Second stage	Begins when cervix is fully dilated and ends with delivery of baby. Uterine muscles push baby downward with help of abdominal muscles and diaphragm. Amniotic membranes rupture now, if not earlier.	Contractions slow. Pushing begins, and baby descends through birth canal.
Third stage	Placental separates from uterine wall and is expelled.	Contractions are closer together but may be less painful.

exercise, and increase in intensity, frequency, and duration as time goes on. The contractions of actual labor also tend to begin in the lower back and radiate around to the front, whereas Braxton-Hicks contractions are often felt in the abdomen alone. In addition, Braxton-Hicks contractions are more apt to occur late in the day, after physical exercise, or when the woman is particularly tired.

Another sign of impending labor is the passage of the thick mucus plug that has been blocking the cervical opening throughout pregnancy. This large clump of mucus is passed through the vagina as the cervix effaces and dilates in preparation for delivery, although many hours or even days can elapse between passage of the plug and the onset of labor. The plug may be clear, pinkish, or somewhat bloody (in which case it is known as "bloody show"). Continuous bright red bleeding in the third trimester of pregnancy, however, should be reported immediately to a clinician (see vaginal bleeding during pregnancy).

Rupture of the amniotic membranes (the "bag of waters") which have surrounded the baby can also signal the beginning of labor. This can occur either as a gush of fluid (as much as a quart or more) or a slow, steady trickle. A woman who thinks her membranes have ruptured should always call a clinician because, unless delivery occurs within the next 24 hours or so, there is a risk of infection to both mother and child. Usually labor will proceed by itself within the next several hours if she is near term, but if nothing happens after a day or so the clinician will probably want to induce labor with the drug pitocin.

For a first pregnancy, women are generally advised to call their clinician when contractions have been 5 to 7 minutes apart and 30 seconds long for 1 hour. In subsequent pregnancies contact should be made earlier, generally when contractions are 7 to 10 minutes apart. Again, however, since not all women follow the same standard progression, it makes sense to call a clinician whenever contractions are becoming unusually uncomfortable or when there are other signs of labor, even without contractions. Many clinicians advise women who think they are in labor and are planning to have a hospital delivery not to eat or drink, in case emergency anesthesia becomes necessary.

Most clinicians divide labor and childbirth into 3 stages (see chart). There is great variation, however, from woman to woman and from pregnancy to pregnancy in just how long each stage takes and what a woman feels as she passes through each one. Still, even without the strict time limits that are sometimes attached to the phases and then taken too literally, it is fair to say that all women who go through vaginal deliveries (as opposed to cesarean sections) pass through these 3 general stages.

What happens during labor and delivery?

In the first, and generally longest, stage of labor the cervix opens up (dilates) and thins out (effaces). These changes are brought on by the release of various hormones, as well as by uterine contractions, which many women find quite painful.

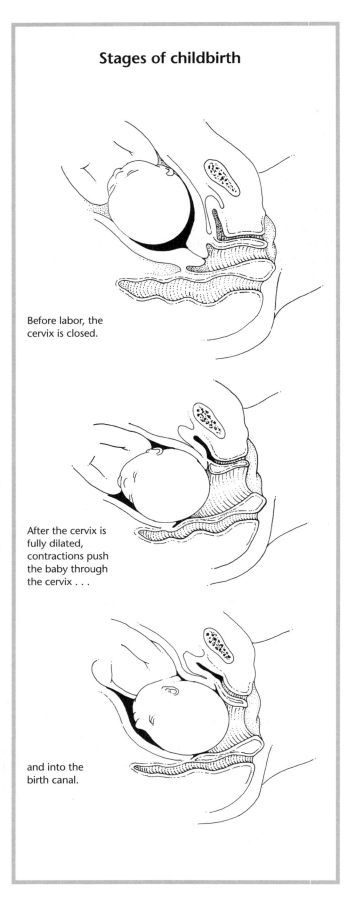

Stages of childbirth

Before labor, the cervix is closed.

After the cervix is fully dilated, contractions push the baby through the cervix . . .

and into the birth canal.

Effacement is measured in percentages, ranging from 0 percent (no effacement) to 100 percent (thinned out to the point of disappearing). Dilation is measured in terms of centimeters, ranging from 0 cm (no dilation) to 10 cm (fully dilated). When the cervix is 100 percent effaced and 10 cm dilated, the first stage of labor is said to be complete.

Many women choose to endure the discomfort of labor without the help of painkillers. Other women, even many who have prepared for the birth by taking birthing classes, discover that the contractions of labor are more than they wish to bear, and they ask for some sort of pain relief (see anesthesia).

Strong contractions continue into the second stage and help push the baby deeper into the mother's pelvis and through the birth canal, usually head first (see illustration). After the baby's birth, the third, and usually shortest, stage of labor involves the expulsion of the placenta from the uterus through the birth canal.

This scenario, while the most common, does not fit all women. Some wind up having an emergency cesarean section, while others decide on a c-section after 24 hours or more of unproductive, exhausting labor.

What happens after the delivery?

After delivery a nurse, midwife, or other clinician will often massage the mother's abdomen to help the uterus contract. This helps the uterus shrink back to its prepregnancy size and also helps prevent excessive bleeding (postpartum hemorrhage). For several days after the birth, periodic contractions may continue to occur on their own, as well as while the baby is breastfeeding (caused by the release of the hormone oxytocin). Some women experience these contractions as uncomfortable afterpains. Afterpains are often particularly severe after the birth of a second or subsequent baby, perhaps because the uterus has become more efficient at contracting.

It is now common practice for a healthy newborn to be placed immediately into the arms of the mother, where cuddling, stroking, and perhaps breastfeeding can begin as soon as possible. More and more hospitals have instituted rooming-in, a policy allowing newborns to sleep in the same room as their mother—and sometimes their father as well.

Related entries

Anesthesia, breastfeeding, cesarean section, postpartum issues, pregnancy, vaginal bleeding during pregnancy

Chlamydia

With 4 million cases diagnosed each year, chlamydia is today the most commonly occurring sexually transmitted disease in the United States. Although it is easily curable with antibiotics, this disease often produces no symptoms—particularly in women—and goes undiagnosed. As a result, chlamydia currently accounts for between a quarter and a half of all cases of pelvic inflammatory disease (PID), which in turn increases a woman's risks of infertility, pelvic adhesions (scarring), chronic pelvic pain, and ectopic pregnancy (see entry). Chlamydia also underlies about half of all cases of cervicitis (inflammation of the cervix; see vaginitis) and up to a fifth of all cases of urethritis (inflammation of the urethra, sometimes called nongonococcal urethritis, or NGU, if thought to be caused by a sexually transmitted microorganism).

If a pregnant woman becomes infected with chlamydia, the consequences for the newborn who passes through her birth canal can be quite serious. Between 35 and 50 percent of infants born to infected mothers develop a relatively minor conjunctivitis (inflammation of the membrane that lines the eyelids), while 25 percent develop a form of pneumonia severe enough to require hospitalization. From 8 to 12 percent of all pregnant women in this country are infected with chlamydia, and the percentage is as high as 30 percent among unwed pregnant teenagers living in inner cities.

Chlamydia is spread through sexual contact—vaginal, anal, and, less frequently, oral—with anyone infected with chlamydia bacteria, whether or not that person has any noticeable symptoms. The bacterium itself, known as *Chlamydia trachomatis,* is a rather unusual microorganism that exists in a number of different strains. The first three strains—A, B, and C—cause trachoma, a chronic conjunctivitis that is the leading cause of blindness in the world. Strains D through K are all transmitted sexually and account for the symptoms associated with chlamydia.

Three other strains of chlamydia—L1, L2, and L3—are also transmitted sexually but cause the symptoms of a different sexually transmitted disease (STD) known as lymphogranuloma venereum (LGV) or lymphogranuloma inguinale. LGV is most common in the developing countries of Asia, Africa, and South America, but in recent years a number of cases have been diagnosed in North America. Unlike chlamydia, LGV occurs 5 times more frequently in men than in women. Women infected with the L1, L2, or L3 bacteria rarely have any symptoms of disease.

Who is likely to develop chlamydia?

Women who are young, poor, sexually active, and do not use barrier forms of contraception are most likely to acquire a chlamydial infection. But any woman who is sexually intimate with an infected man has as much as a 75 percent chance of becoming infected herself, unless condoms are used consistently. (The odds of woman-to-woman infection are still unknown.)

What are the symptoms?

Most women with chlamydia have no symptoms at all. Many never even suspect that anything may be wrong until a male partner notices symptoms of urethritis such as burning during urination or a discharge from the urethra—and even this is not fail-safe, since some infected men never develop symptoms either.

When a woman develops symptoms, they are often easily confused with those of gonorrhea or of urinary tract infections caused by other bacteria. Among the most obvious symptoms are frequent painful urination, pus in the urine, increased vaginal discharge, lower abdominal pain, or bleeding after sexual intercourse, as well as irritation, redness, and swelling of the urethra or labia.

In rare cases a woman with chlamydia may also develop inflammation of the liver. In addition to abdominal pain in the upper righthand part of the abdominal region, other symptoms of this syndrome include fever, nausea, and pain that resembles a gallbladder attack (see gallstones). Occasionally chlamydial infection can spread from the genital region to the eye and produce redness and discharge.

Many women do not realize that they have a chlamydial infection until they develop symptoms of pelvic inflammatory disease. These symptoms include vaginal discharge, painful sexual intercourse, heavy menstrual bleeding, abdominal tenderness, and fever. There is evidence that chlamydia can also cause a symptomless form of PID, which can have serious consequences—infertility in particular—without any warning signs.

How is the condition evaluated?

Most authorities now recommend that all sexually active women, especially those with multiple sexual partners, be screened for chlamydia on a regular basis. The problem is that chlamydia can be difficult to diagnose, even when both a woman and her clinician are looking for it. It is also easily overlooked in a woman without symptoms, and those symptoms that do appear are too easily attributable to a number of other conditions, including gonorrhea, urinary tract infections, or even certain psychological problems. Very rarely women discover that they are infected with chlamydia when the *Chlamydia trachomatis* leaves telling marks on a Pap test.

In most cases merely examining the cervix during a pelvic examination will not reveal that anything is wrong, although sometimes the cervix may be red, swollen, or covered with a puslike discharge. If a clinician does suspect chlamydia, the first step in diagnosis may be a urinalysis (for NGU) and sampling of cervical mucus cells or discharge to screen for chlamydia and other diseases such as gonorrhea, since chlamydia so often coexists with other STDs. Because chlamydia is so common, it (or NGU) can sometimes be assumed if no other disease can account for the symptoms. Even if gonorrhea—or some other STD—is diagnosed, there is no guarantee that the woman does not have chlamydia as well, particularly since co-infection is common.

Rapid diagnostic techniques to isolate the chlamydia bacterium directly have largely replaced the complex culture techniques of the past. These new techniques involve an examination of pus or cervical discharge cells that have been swabbed from the cervix or other suspicious area. Since the chlamydia bacteria can live only inside human cells, special care must be taken in obtaining the sample of pus or a false-negative result will come back from the lab—that is, the sample will be bacteria-free even though the woman is infected. Tissue culture (growing the bacteria on a nutrient plate) is considered the most accurate of these tests, but it takes 48 to 72 hours, requires the expertise of trained laboratory personnel, and is expensive. The other tests—which involve techniques of molecular biology—are faster, easier, and cheaper. Even newer technologies now make it possible to diagnose chlamydia from a urine specimen or a self-administered vaginal swab. If the encouraging results from initial testing of these methods are corroborated, these tests may allow more widespread screening of both men and women in the future.

How is chlamydia treated?

Chlamydia is readily treated with antibiotics such as doxycycline, tetracycline, or erythromycin taken for 7 to 10 days. It is important to finish the entire course of medication to eradicate the infection and to prevent resistant bacteria from developing. If taken correctly, these drugs are usually effective, although occasionally they may miss bacteria lodged inside cells. For this reason it is important to have a clinician repeat the swab test to check for infection after the entire course of medication has been completed.

If these drugs cause stomach upset or other side effects, one type of fluoroquinolone antibiotic (ofloxacin) seems to be fairly effective in treating chlamydia, though some studies have shown a failure rate of up to 19 percent. Women who are pregnant and women who are under 18 should not use fluoroquinolone, since it can interfere with bone growth in a fetus or a teenager. Another alternative antibiotic—azithromycin (Zithromax)—seems to be effective in a short course of treatment and has to be taken only once a day.

If a pregnant woman needs to be treated for chlamydia, the drug of choice is erythromycin. Both fluoroquinolones and tetracycline are generally avoided during pregnancy, and there simply are not enough data about the effects of azithromycin during pregnancy to consider it safe.

No treatment for chlamydia can be considered complete until the woman's partner or partners have been treated as well—whether or not they have symptoms. If only the woman is treated, the disease will simply be passed back to her once medication has been stopped; there is no lifelong immunity to chlamydia or to other sexually transmitted diseases. Even after treatment is over, women should be on the lookout for any signs of PID so they can be treated as early as possible.

How can chlamydia be prevented?

Preventing the spread of chlamydia depends to some extent on following the safer sex practices that are part of preventing all STDs. Since most women with chlamydia are symptom-free, however, a vital part of prevention depends on the willingness of men to notify female partners when they find out they are infected. Both partners must avoid sexual relations until treatment has been completed.

Current tests for chlamydia are quite expensive and often yield false-negative results and an occasional false-positive result. Even so, routine screening of women at high risk—particularly young women with multiple sexual partners or those with other STDs or PID—can play an important role in prevention. The Centers for Disease Control and Prevention (CDC) recommends annual screening for chlamydia for all sexually active females under 20 years of age and all women 20 and older with one or more risk factors for chlamydia (particularly new or multiple sex partners and lack of barrier contraception). They also recommend annual testing for all pregnant women and all women with infection of the cervix.

To prevent chlamydial infection of babies, many hospitals now routinely instill erythromycin drops—instead of the 1 percent silver nitrate drops commonly used to prevent the spread of gonorrhea—into the eyes of all newborns. This prevents conjunctivitis, but the bacteria can still enter the nose and throat, thus leaving infants born to infected mothers susceptible to chlamydial pneumonia.

Related entries

Adhesions, antibiotics, condoms, ectopic pregnancy, gonorrhea, infertility, Pap test, pelvic inflammatory disease, safer sex, sexually transmitted diseases, urinary tract infections, vaginitis

Cholesterol

Cholesterol is an odorless, white, powdery chemical manufactured by the liver and used to make essential body substances such as cell walls and hormones. It is part of every animal cell and is found in all foods that come from animals. In the bloodstream (which transports cholesterol throughout the body), it is wrapped in protein "packages" called lipoproteins, which come in several forms. The lipoprotein that has been of greatest concern to investigators is low-density lipoprotein (LDL; sometimes referred to as "bad" cholesterol). This protein contains a high percentage of cholesterol relative to protein, and when LDL levels in the blood are high, cells lining the inside of the arteries transport LDL and its cholesterol load into the artery wall, setting the stage for atherosclerosis.

In atherosclerosis, scar tissue and fatty deposits build up in the walls of arteries throughout the body (see illustration). Eventually a clot can form on the surface of these obstructions, abruptly blocking the flow of blood in the already narrowed artery. If the blocked artery supplies blood to the heart, the result is a heart attack. If the artery supplies blood to the brain, the result may be a stroke.

Numerous studies in middle-aged men have linked high LDL levels in the blood to an increased risk of heart attacks, stroke, and other vascular diseases. They have also established that lowering LDL cholesterol in the blood reduces the risk of developing (and dying from) coronary artery disease (CAD). For years researchers have wondered whether these conclusions were equally valid for premenopausal women, who, because of the hormone estrogen, seem to metabolize cholesterol differently. It now appears that there are some important distinctions between men and women when it comes to cholesterol. For example, in women high levels of LDL in the blood seem not to be the best predictor of the risk of dying from cardiovascular disease and stroke, as they are in men. Rather, it is the level of HDL (high-density lipoprotein); that is, women with higher levels of HDL seem to have less coronary artery disease. This "good" cholesterol contains a high percentage of protein relative to cholesterol and is believed to take cholesterol *away* from cells and transport it back to the liver for processing or removal.

Also, in women, having high triglyceride levels *combined with* low levels of HDL appears to be the most potent predictor of risk for CAD. Triglycerides are other lipids (fatlike substances) in the blood that are packaged in a third type of lipoprotein called VLDLs (very low density lipoproteins). Triglycerides seem to be less important as a predictor of risk in men.

Most people's blood cholesterol levels are relatively constant regardless of how much actual cholesterol they eat, since a feedback mechanism slows synthesis of cholesterol in the liver whenever dietary levels are high. But for the 1 person in 5 with a faulty mechanism for cholesterol control, changing cholesterol in the diet is the first line of defense against high blood levels of LDL. And since it is hard to know just which people have a defect in this mechanism, everyone has been advised by the National Institutes of Health (NIH) to limit dietary cholesterol to under 300 mg per day.

Today most people are aware that fats and oils, rather than cholesterol itself, are the major components of the diet that can raise LDL cholesterol to dangerous levels. Saturated fats, which come from animal tissues and some kinds of vegetable oils, in particular stimulate production of LDL relative to HDL. Because of the large toll taken by heart disease in the United States—and despite uncertainties about the meaning of high or low cholesterol levels in women (not to mention in the elderly of both sexes and in children)—the National Cholesterol Education Panel (NCEP) of the NIH has recommended that all people keep their intake of dietary fats and oils low.

More and better data may one day refine the NCEP's dietary and blood cholesterol recommendations for particular groups. It is known, for example, that estrogen alters the way women convert dietary cholesterol and fats into blood cholesterol, and this may help explain why premenopausal women (and those postmenopausal women who are taking estrogen replacement therapy) have a relatively low inci-

From cholesterol to coronary artery disease

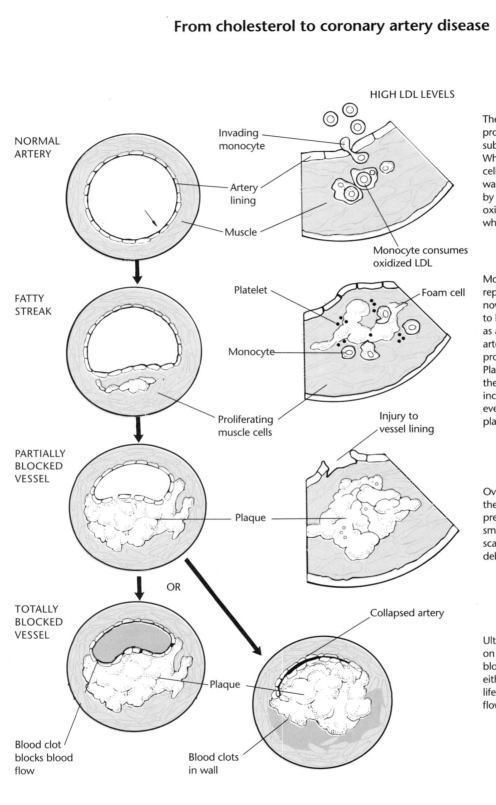

HIGH LDL LEVELS

NORMAL ARTERY

Invading monocyte

Artery lining

Muscle

Monocyte consumes oxidized LDL

The cells lining healthy arteries protect them from damaging substances in the bloodstream. When LDL levels are high, these cells transport LDL into the artery wall, where—no longer protected by antioxidants in the blood—it oxidizes (a chemical process in which oxygen is added to LDL).

FATTY STREAK

Platelet

Foam cell

Monocyte

Proliferating muscle cells

Monocytes (white blood cells that repair injured tissue) consume the now-toxic (oxidized) LDL and swell to become foam cells. These appear as a fatty streak on the surface of the artery wall. In response, muscle cells proliferate, making the wall thicker. Platelets (blood-clotting elements in the blood) make growth factors that increase the thickening, which eventually becomes artherosclerotic plaque.

PARTIALLY BLOCKED VESSEL

Plaque

Injury to vessel lining

Over decades, further injury to the artery lining from high blood pressure, toxic gases in cigarette smoke, or other factors causes scarring and the accumulation of debris, further narrowing the artery.

OR

TOTALLY BLOCKED VESSEL

Collapsed artery

Plaque

Blood clot blocks blood flow

Blood clots in wall

Ultimately, a blood clot can form on the surface of the plaque or blood can leak into its core. In either event, the result can be a life-threatening blockage of blood flow to a vital artery.

dence of coronary artery disease, regardless of what they eat. But for the time being, the NCEP recommends that women and men of all ages strive for low blood cholesterol, and if necessary adjust their diet to accomplish that goal. Avoiding fried foods and eating skinless poultry, fish, shellfish, lean red meats, and low-fat dairy products, as well as ample portions of fruits and vegetables, breads and grains, and dried beans, are the first steps usually recommended.

Phytoestrogens—estrogen-like substances found in soybeans, chickpeas, and other beans—may also play a role in improving cholesterol levels and arterial function in women. Although evidence is still too preliminary to allow definitive dietary recommendations, increasing support for this possibility is coming from the Women's Ischemia Syndrome Evaluation (WISE), a 4-year, $8–10 million study of 1,000 women aimed at developing better techniques for diagnosing heart disease in women. One WISE-supported nationwide study conducted by researchers at Cedars-Sinai Medical Center in Los Angeles found that increased phytoestrogen levels in women were associated with higher HDL cholesterol levels as well as lower total cholesterol, LDL cholesterol, and triglycerides—all established factors in decreasing the risk of heart disease. Additional studies are under way to determine if eating foods high in phytoestrogens, and/or taking supplements, might improve cholesterol levels in women.

How is blood cholesterol evaluated?

The current NCEP screening guidelines recommend that all adults over the age of 20 have total cholesterol and HDL levels measured once every 5 years (total cholesterol is the combination of LDL and HDL). Since most of the total in both men and women consists of LDL, a high total cholesterol level generally indicates a high LDL level. Many doctors prefer to check levels at least twice, and to make sure that the two results are reasonably consonant, before drawing definitive conclusions. This is because cholesterol testing can be inaccurate, with wide discrepancies sometimes occurring between levels measured on different days or by different laboratories. Most often, if the first test shows high levels, a second will be done after a 12-hour fast. Generally more accurate results come from tests done on blood drawn from a vein in the arm as opposed to blood drawn from a finger.

The NCEP considers a total cholesterol of 200 mg/dL or less in the initial screening as desirable, 200 to 239 mg/dL as borderline high risk, and over 240 as high risk. Anyone who falls into the borderline-high or high-risk categories, as well as people in the low-risk category but who have HDL levels under 35 mg/dL, should have a more specific lipoprotein analysis to determine actual levels of LDL. This more specific test is performed after fasting for 9 to 12 hours, with two measurements taken from 1 to 8 weeks apart. Triglycerides are measured along with lipoproteins. If triglyceride levels are too high, the LDL measurement is considered inaccurate. The NCEP recommends this more detailed test as the initial screening procedure in people who already know they have coronary artery disease and in women with diabetes.

For people without preexisting coronary artery disease, LDL levels under 130 mg/dL are considered desirable, 130 mg/dL to 159 mg/dL are considered to be borderline high risk, and over 160 mg/dL is high risk. The NCEP recommends dietary changes for people in the high-risk group, as well as for people in the borderline-high group who also have two or more additional risk factors for coronary artery disease. These might include premature menopause, having a family history of early coronary artery disease, smoking, having high blood pressure, and being obese or diabetic. (Diabetes in women erases any protection against coronary artery disease they get from being female, and in fact puts them in the highest-risk group.) These people should also have a complete physical examination, history, and laboratory tests to determine if some other condition (such as a hereditary disorder, hypothyroidism, or kidney disorder) may underlie the high lipid levels. If so, the NCEP dietary guidelines should be followed in addition to whatever other treatment is appropriate.

For people with preexisting coronary artery disease or diabetes, the NCEP recommends starting dietary therapy if LDL levels are between 100 and 130 mg/dL, and drug therapy if LDL is 130 mg/dL or higher.

How is high cholesterol treated?

Dietary therapy. For people whose total blood cholesterol levels are too high, the NCEP recommends a 2-step dietary plan. In step 1, the diet should contain no more than 8 to 10 percent of calories from saturated fat, no more than 18 to 20 percent from other fats, and no more than 300 milligrams of cholesterol per day. In step 2, the daily diet should contain less than 7 percent of calories from saturated fat and less than 200 mg from cholesterol. For people trying to obliterate preexisting arterial plaque, an even more rigorous diet consisting of under 10 percent of calories from fat and 5 to 10 mg of cholesterol per day is recommended—a diet which few people are able to follow.

Overweight people are advised to lose weight, since this not only lowers LDL and triglyceride levels but also reduces hypertension, another risk factor for coronary artery disease. Combining weight reduction with physical exercise (and cooking with olive oil, a monounsaturate, which seems to have a beneficial effect on coronary risk) is also generally believed to decrease LDLs and triglycerides and increase HDLs.

Reducing saturated fat and cholesterol intake may lower HDL as well as LDL levels in women—and HDLs are thought to be important in protecting women from coronary artery disease. Adding regular exercise to the "heart-healthy" diet, however, seems to counter this reduction, bringing the HDLs back to the same level where they were before the beginning of the diet and exercise regime. Although lowering LDLs is supposed to be beneficial for everyone, the fact that HDL levels are better predictors of a woman's risk of coronary artery disease leaves in question the overall benefit of a diet that might lower HDL at the same time that it lowers LDL. Still,

Maximum daily intake of total fat and saturated fat for healthy women of normal weight		
Daily calories	Total grams of fat (should not exceed 30% of total calories)	Total grams of saturated fat (should not exceed 10% of total calories)
1800	60	20
2000	67	22
2200	73	24
2500	83	28
Source: American Heart Association		

at present, in light of the great uncertainty, most doctors recommend that women generally follow the NCEP guidelines—with special attention to HDL levels.

As with all recommendations about cholesterol, however, women should take dietary guidelines with a grain of salt. For one thing, current beliefs about the exact effect of specific dietary fats on cholesterol levels are in a state of flux and are bound to change as better information accumulates. New data keep pouring in, making it clear that original proclamations about good and bad foods were far too simplistic. No longer are all saturated fats considered alike. For example, though 3 of the 4 types of saturated fat do appear to raise total blood cholesterol levels, the type found in beef and chocolate (called stearic acid) is now considered neutral. Similarly, while monounsaturated fats (such as those in olive oil) have been touted as desirable alternatives to saturated fats, it appears that one structural form of monounsaturates (found in margarine and many packaged snack foods) actually increases the risk of coronary artery disease in women.

Although polyunsaturated fats such as those found in fish oils may decrease the blood's ability to clot and therefore decrease the risk of heart attacks and stroke, they are also easily incorporated into LDLs and may make them more susceptible to oxidation, which promotes atherosclerosis. A few studies have suggested an increased risk of cancer from a diet that contains more than 10 percent polyunsaturated fats, while others have suggested that polyunsaturates can lower HDL levels as well as LDL levels—and this is not desirable. The American Heart Association advises limiting polyunsaturated fats to 10 percent of caloric intake.

Significantly altering blood cholesterol levels through diet alone can require considerable effort and change in lifestyle. The success of a given diet varies with the individual, but the average person can anticipate that following the NCEP guidelines will reduce LDL and total cholesterol by 10 to 15 percent. This means that a person who starts out with a to-

tal cholesterol count of 300 can reasonably expect to lower it to only about 260 by diet alone. A person who starts with a total cholesterol level of 220 can expect to lower it to about 195.

It usually takes at least 6 months, with nutritional consultation, for LDL levels to fall. If they fail to fall after this amount of time, drug therapy may be necessary.

Drug therapy. Because low levels of HDL may be an important risk factor for coronary artery disease in women, many clinicians recommend drug therapy both to reduce LDL and to increase HDL if dietary therapy is ineffective. Unless there is a family history of high cholesterol or additional risk factors for CAD, however, drugs are generally not prescribed as the first line of therapy for premenopausal women. In addition, there is still no general agreement about the best treatment for women who have normal LDLs, low HDLs, and borderline-high to high triglyceride levels. At the moment many experts suggest that such patients should try to increase physical activity and, when appropriate, reduce weight.

There are 5 main categories of cholesterol-lowering drugs: bile acid sequestrants, "statins," nicotinic acid, fibric acid derivatives, and probucol.

The bile acid sequestrants—which include cholestyramine (Questran) and colestipol (Colestid)—are usually prescribed for people with high LDL levels. They work by lowering these levels and slightly increasing HDL levels. Side effects can include constipation, abdominal pain, nausea, and bloating.

The "statins" (such as lovastatin and atorvastatin, sold under the trade names Mevacor and Lipitor) also work by lowering LDL levels and slightly increasing HDLs, but they are in rare cases associated with a different set of side effects—including hepatitis and muscle inflammation. They are not given to pregnant women or women considering pregnancy because of the risk of birth defects.

People with high LDL and triglyceride levels and low HDL levels may be prescribed nicotinic acid (niacin), which lowers LDLs and triglycerides and raises HDLs. Niacin is a naturally occurring vitamin found in many foods, but at therapeutic doses it can occasionally result in side effects, including hepatitis, gout, hyperglycemia, ulcer formation, insomnia, various skin disorders, and certain heart arrhythmias (irregular heartbeat). Taking an aspirin half an hour before a dose of niacin and taking it with meals can lessen unpleasant flushing.

Another category of drugs, fibric acid derivatives such as clofibrate (Atromid) and gemfibrozil (Lopid), lowers triglycerides, raises HDLs, and either raises or lowers LDLs. Side effects may include gallstones, hepatitis, high LDL levels, decreased sex drive, muscle inflammation, heart arrhythmias, increased appetite, abdominal pain, and nausea.

The fifth category of lipid-lowering drugs consists of the drug probucol (Lorelco), which is generally prescribed to people with an inherited form of high cholesterol. Besides lowering both LDL and HDL levels, probucol functions as a potent

Foods that raise or lower cholesterol

Raises blood cholesterol	Sources	Examples
Dietary cholesterol	Foods from animals	Meats, egg yolks, dairy products, organ meats (heart, kidney, etc.), fish, and poultry
Saturated fats	Foods from animals	Whole milk, cream, ice cream, whole-milk cheeses, butter, lard, and meats
	Certain plant oils	Palm, palm kernel and coconut oils, cocoa butter
Trans-fats	Partially hydrogenated vegetable oils	Cookies, crackers, cakes, French fries, friend onion rings, donuts
Lowers blood cholesterol	**Sources**	**Examples**
Polunsaturated fats	Certain plant oils	Safflower, sesame, soy, corn and sunflower-seed oils, nuts, and seeds
Monunsaturated fats	Certain plant oils	Olive, canola and peanut oil, avocados

Source: American Heart Association

antioxidant—that is, it prevents oxidation, which is thought to prompt LDLs to promote atherosclerosis. Side effects can include altered heart rhythms, low HDL levels, diarrhea, bloating, nausea, and abdominal pain.

Any of the lipid-lowering drugs can reduce blood cholesterol levels by as much as 30 percent within 6 weeks. Anyone taking cholesterol-lowering medications should have blood lipid levels checked regularly.

Related entries

Circulatory disorders, coronary artery disease, diabetes, estrogen replacement therapy, exercise, heart disease, high blood pressure, nutrition, obesity, smoking, stroke

Chorionic Villi Sampling

Chorionic villi sampling is a prenatal test that allows screening for a genetically abnormal fetus as early as 9 to 12 weeks of gestation. Chorionic villi are microscopic fingerlike projections that surround the chorion—the outermost membrane of the fertilized egg which will develop into the placenta. Be-

cause the villi come from the same fertilized egg as the fetus, their cells have the same genetic makeup.

How is the test performed?

In CVS, a catheter (a small, hollow, flexible plastic tube) is guided into the chorionic tissue either via the cervix (transcervical; see illustration) or through the abdomen (transabdominal). Which approach is taken generally depends on where the placenta is implanting into the uterus. An ultrasound picture helps ensure proper placement of the catheter, which withdraws some of the chorionic villi, cells of which are then grown in a special culture and prepared for analysis of chromosomes through a procedure called karyotyping.

Unlike amniocentesis, CVS cannot evaluate the components of the amniotic fluid such as alpha fetoprotein to determine the presence of neural tube defects. It usually takes about a week or two for results, although preliminary reports may be available within a few days.

How accurate, reliable, and safe is the procedure?

Complications of CVS can include bleeding, rupture of membranes, and infection, which in turn may lead to miscarriage. After the procedure it is normal to have some bleeding, spotting, or minor cramping, but if bleeding is more than in a

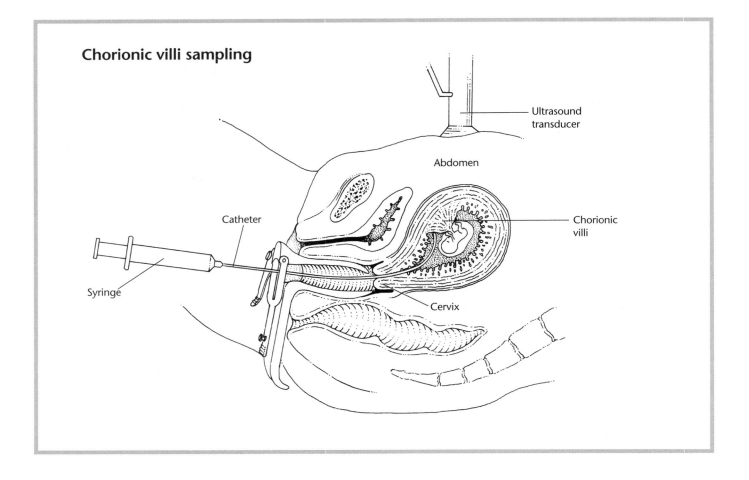

Chorionic villi sampling

Ultrasound transducer

Abdomen

Chorionic villi

Catheter

Cervix

Syringe

normal menstrual period or cramping is intense, a clinician should be contacted.

When the procedure is performed by an experienced doctor or technician, the risk to the fetus is usually minimal and probably not significantly higher than that of amniocentesis. There is conflicting evidence, however, about whether CVS can lead to malformations of the limbs, mouth, and jaw. One large-scale study estimated that 1 in 3,000 tests results in a child born with missing or underdeveloped fingers or toes—as opposed to the normal rate of 1 in 18,500.

For these reasons, and because many centers still have little experience with CVS, obstetricians and genetic counselors currently recommend CVS only to women with extremely high risks of carrying a genetically abnormal fetus (such as those who have already borne such a child or who are carriers for genetic diseases such as Tay-Sachs or sickle cell anemia). Women who have previously had an abnormal amniocentesis and who underwent a second trimester abortion often opt for a CVS for emotional reasons—even if, statistically speaking, they have a relatively low chance of having a second abnormal fetus.

Related entries

Abortion, alpha-fetoprotein screening, amniocentesis, genetic counseling, miscarriage, preconception counseling, ultrasound

Chronic Fatigue Syndrome

Chronic fatigue syndrome, or CFS, is difficult to diagnose, and its causes are unknown. It is characterized by debilitating fatigue as well as numerous accompanying physical and psychological symptoms.

Until recently, many people with this condition (also known as chronic fatigue immune dysfunction syndrome, or CFIDS) would go from doctor to doctor anxiously searching for a diagnosis, at the same time hearing from friends, family members, and co-workers that their symptoms were "all in their head." People with CFS often found themselves ineligible for insurance or disability benefits because their illness did not fit into any recognized disease category.

For a while investigators hoped to find one specific virus that would account for the illness, which at various times has been called chronic Epstein-Barr virus syndrome, chronic mono syndrome, and yuppie flu. Yet none of these turned out to explain all of the cases. Researchers are now investigating various theories linking CFS to immune dysfunction; imbalances of hypothalamic, pituitary, or adrenal hormones; disturbed regulation of blood pressure and pulse; and nutritional deficiencies. The possibility also exists that CFS may be a condition resulting from any of these factors, or a combination of them. Even though no specific biological cause had been found, in 1988 the Centers for Disease Control in Atlanta recognized chronic fatigue syndrome as an official medical condition.

Because it has no known cause, and because symptoms are shared by so many other diseases, chronic fatigue syndrome is still easily confused with many disorders involving fatigue. Lack of a clear definition has also made this syndrome difficult to study in any consistent way. Indeed, some investigators now suspect that not all people with chronic fatigue syndrome have precisely the same disorder, but rather that there are a number of related "chronic fatigue syndromes." These syndromes (some of which may turn out to be identical to others) include neurasthenia (profound weakness and fatigue), myalgic encephalomyelitis (brain and muscle inflammation), postviral fatigue syndrome, fibromyalgia (see entry), and chronic mononucleosis (see mononucleosis).

Whether chronic fatigue syndrome turns out to be one condition or several, there is now increasing evidence—though by no means conclusive—that it is an organic disorder, that is, one caused by a physical or physiological defect. People with this syndrome appear to have an overactive immune system that is chronically waging war against microorganisms and cells of the individual's own body which are in fact not a threat (see autoimmune disorders). This syndrome may turn out to be due to some complex relationship between psychological, environmental, and physical factors in susceptible people.

For reasons still not understood, chronic fatigue syndrome occurs about twice as often in women as in men. Part of the explanation may lie in the fact that women are particularly susceptible to disorders involving the immune system, such as multiple sclerosis, lupus, and inflammation of the thyroid gland (all of which can be confused with CFS). Women are also more likely to report suffering from fatigue in general than are men.

Who is likely to develop chronic fatigue syndrome?

Chronic fatigue syndrome most often affects young adults, but it can occur at any age. It has not been linked exclusively to any one infectious agent, and it may be triggered by an illness involving one of many microorganisms, including the Epstein-Barr virus, influenza virus, parvovirus, and the Lyme disease spirochete. Between 60 and 80 percent of people with this syndrome have long-standing allergic disorders, in contrast to only 20 percent of the general population. In addition, about 1 out of 3 people with chronic fatigue syndrome has a history of psychiatric disorders that occurred before the onset of the syndrome.

What are the symptoms?

Chronic fatigue syndrome typically begins abruptly with a flulike illness. This is followed by a debilitating fatigue that cannot be relieved through rest or sleep and usually worsens after types of exercise that, previously, the person would have tolerated without difficulty. In addition, people with this syndrome have a number of other chronic or recurring symptoms. These may include low-grade fever, chills, sore throat, muscle soreness, headaches, joint pain, swollen lymph nodes, and sleep disturbances. Exercise generally exacerbates these symptoms as well as the fatigue. Night sweats occur in nearly half of all people with chronic fatigue syndrome.

Depression is also an extremely common symptom, although there is much debate about whether it is a consequence of chronic fatigue syndrome or a reaction to the debilitating fatigue. Whatever the explanation, some people with chronic fatigue syndrome find that the depression becomes the most debilitating part of their illness, although it can often be successfully treated with medication and psychotherapy.

How is the condition evaluated?

Along with its recognition of chronic fatigue syndrome, the CDC established specific criteria necessary for the diagnosis of this previously elusive condition. First, the fatigue must have arisen recently and be debilitating enough to have severely interfered with the activities of work and daily living for at least 6 months. Second, the numerous other psychiatric, organic, and lifestyle disorders that may account for this fatigue must be eliminated by a physician. This can be accomplished by the clinician's taking a thorough history, doing a physical examination, and performing appropriate laboratory tests.

Once these two conditions have been met, the clinician trying to diagnose chronic fatigue syndrome will look for 4 or more of the following symptoms, which have been present for 6 or more months: ‣ sore throat, ‣ painful lymph nodes in the neck or armpits, ‣ general weakness, ‣ muscle pain or discomfort, ‣ prolonged fatigue after previously tolerated exercise, ‣ generalized headaches that differ from those the patient may have had earlier, ‣ pain that moves from joint to joint without swelling or redness, ‣ sleep disturbance (either extreme sleepiness or insomnia), and ‣ impaired memory. Also present may be ‣ fever or chills, and any of various mental or neurological disturbances, including ‣ intolerance of light, ‣ transient blind spots, ‣ irritability, ‣ confusion, ‣ difficulty thinking or concentrating, and ‣ depression.

How is chronic fatigue syndrome treated?

Like many conditions that are hard to diagnose and that have no effective cure, chronic fatigue syndrome is ripe for exploitation. People with this syndrome need to beware of "quack" and other unproven remedies that may be touted as quick fixes by both "alternative" and so-called mainstream healers (who, while conventionally trained M.D.s, may offer costly and questionable treatments). Among these commonly suggested remedies for chronic fatigue syndrome are gamma globulin injections (which may have a transient benefit), B12 injections, extensive laboratory tests, and magnesium supplements. Some popular books advocate homeopathy, bodywork, nutritional therapy, and meditation. Although many of these approaches, particularly those involving mind/body manipulations, are harmless and may help relieve symptoms, the danger is that people who have never been formally diagnosed as having CFS and who actually have a different, potentially life-threatening disorder may pursue these alternative therapies instead of getting a thorough physical examination and appropriate treatment. Before pursuing an alternative approach, it therefore makes sense to see a conventional physician to make sure that CFS is indeed the source of the symptoms.

What may also work, at least for some patients, is taking tricyclic antidepressant medications (such as amitriptyline or doxepin) in doses much lower than those used to treat depression. Even here, conclusive studies still need to be done, but there is mounting anecdotal evidence that these drugs may improve the quality of sleep in people with chronic fatigue syndrome, as well as relieve tiredness, muscle and joint pain, and cognitive problems. One reason why doctors have been willing to try these drugs at all is that they have already been proved effective in treating a similar condition, fibromyalgia. Anyone taking tricyclic antidepressants to treat chronic fatigue syndrome should be aware that for the first week she may actually feel more tired in the morning than before.

If depression is a symptom, low doses of the antidepressants Prozac (fluoxetine) or Zoloft (sertraline) at bedtime have also helped some patients for whom tricyclic antidepressants do not seem to work. Other antidepressants as well as psychotherapy may help relieve the depression, although they rarely have any effect on the remaining symptoms. A few studies have also shown a modest improvement in symptoms with low doses of oral hydrocortisone.

Most physicians now encourage people with chronic fatigue syndrome to be as active as possible but to avoid activities that involve intensive physical or emotional stress. Nearly all doctors experienced in treating this disorder recommend limbering exercises, but many advise more caution when it comes to aerobic exercises. The best guide is to start all new exercise regimens and other physical activities gradually, curtailing any activity that leads to a relapse of symptoms.

People with chronic fatigue syndrome should be aware of the growing numbers of support groups and hotlines that provide moral support. Many issue publications that describe new research findings and offer advice about coping at home and at work with a debilitating illness. They may also make referrals to doctors with experience in treating chronic fatigue syndrome.

Related entries
Alternative therapies, autoimmune disorders, depression, fatigue, fibromyalgia, headaches, insomnia, mononucleosis, psychosomatic disorders, psychotherapy, stress, thyroid disorders

Circulatory Disorders

Circulatory disorders occur when blood flow in the arteries and veins is somehow restricted. Blood circulates throughout the body inside a connected series of blood vessels (see illustration). Beginning in the right side of the heart, blood is pumped into the lungs, where it picks up oxygen and then returns through the left side of the heart into a large blood vessel called the aorta. From the aorta the oxygen-rich blood enters thick muscular tubes called arteries, which eventually branch into smaller arterioles and finally into the even smaller capillaries, which supply tissues in all parts of the body with oxygen. The oxygen-depleted blood then returns to the heart for recirculation through tiny venules and then thicker veins, passing through the liver and kidney along the way, where carbon dioxide and other waste products are removed.

Because some vascular disorders common in women may involve no symptoms, researchers do not know the true incidence of these disorders in women. They do know, however, that women generally develop circulatory disorders at later ages than men do.

Disorders of the arteries

Atherosclerosis. When circulation in the arteries is impaired, the cause is most frequently fatty deposits which clog the vessels and eventually develop into plaque. Under the age of 60, men are generally more likely than women to develop this condition. But women under 60 who have diabetes or high blood pressure seem to be at higher risk than their male counterparts, and having a close relative with atherosclerosis also increases the odds that a woman will develop this problem. In both sexes, smoking cigarettes raises the risk of developing atherosclerosis.

In a normal artery, blood is confined to the lumen (the central channel through which blood flows) by a smooth lining of flattened cells tightly joined to one another (see illustration). When kept in good repair, this lining (called the endothelium) permits blood to flow without clotting. Surrounding the lining is a thin sheath of muscle cells which contracts and relaxes to control the diameter of the artery and thus helps regulate the rate at which blood flows through it.

Over time the endothelium may become damaged. The cause may simply be wear and tear from excessively turbulent flow of blood in a particular area, such as a branch or sharp bend in an artery, where blood strikes against the vessel wall with great force. Or it may be caused by high blood pressure or toxic gases in cigarette smoke. Whatever the cause, once the lining is damaged, cholesterol, monocytes, platelets, blood, proliferating muscle cells, scar tissue, and other debris accumulate in the artery wall and create a combination of fat and muscle called plaque (see cholesterol). Plaque

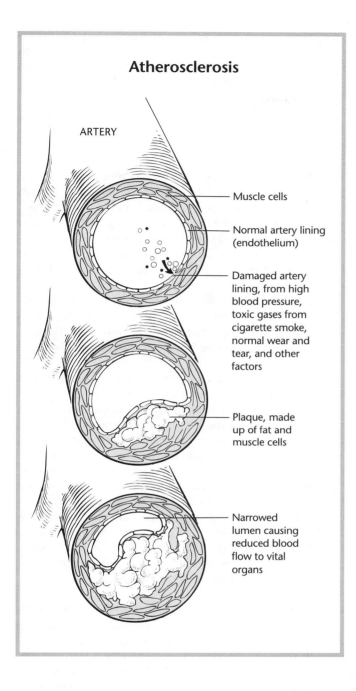

Atherosclerosis

ARTERY

Muscle cells

Normal artery lining (endothelium)

Damaged artery lining, from high blood pressure, toxic gases from cigarette smoke, normal wear and tear, and other factors

Plaque, made up of fat and muscle cells

Narrowed lumen causing reduced blood flow to vital organs

thickens the artery wall and narrows the lumen. Eventually, if a clot forms on the surface of the plaque, the flow of blood in the narrowed artery may be completely blocked.

If the blocked artery supplies blood to the heart, the result is chest pain (angina) and perhaps a heart attack. If the artery supplies blood to the brain, the result may be a stroke. If the narrowed artery supplies the legs, claudication (calf pain with exertion) may occur. Narrowing of arteries from plaque can also set the stage for an arterial embolism.

Arterial embolism. An embolism is a fragment of tissue (such as a blood clot or piece of plaque) that travels from the arteries in the heart or some other location and lodges in a distant artery. If not treated promptly (with surgery or anticoagulant medications), an arterial embolism in the arm or leg can lead to tissue death in the organs that the artery would normally supply with blood. If it lodges in an artery supplying oxygen to the brain, it can lead to stroke (see entry).

A blood clot that lodges in one of the pulmonary arteries blocks blood flow to the lungs, depriving them of oxygen and therefore damaging them. Pleurisy (pain when taking a deep breath) often develops, as well as shortness of breath, rapid breathing, accelerated heart rate, or (rarely) bloody sputum. A pulmonary embolism can result in shock or even death and requires immediate medical attention.

Hypertension. Blood pressure is the amount of pressure exerted by the blood against the walls of the arteries. It is affected by many factors, such as the pumping power of the heart, the resistance (elasticity and smoothness) of the arteries, and the functioning of the kidneys. Consistently high blood pressure (see entry)—called hypertension—is considered a major cause of stroke and coronary artery disease.

Damage to the arteries of the brain, eyes, heart, and kidneys from chronically high blood pressure can lead to debilitating and life-threatening complications. For example, hypertension can constrict the arterioles (the smallest and thinnest of the arteries). The result can be an enlarged heart, since the heart muscle expands as it works more vigorously to pump blood into these vessels. Eventually the walls of an enlarged heart become thickened and stiff and can no longer pump blood effectively (see congestive heart failure). Damage to other arteries can lead to strokes, kidney disease, heart attacks, congestive heart failure, mental changes, and bleeding in the retina of the eye.

Among the many known and suspected causes of hypertension are smoking, obesity, diabetes, sodium (in susceptible people), stress, and family history.

Aortic aneurysm. Especially in people with hypertension, atherosclerosis may cause the wall of the aorta to become weakened and balloon out as blood pulses through it. An aortic aneurysm usually enlarges slowly over a number of years, and there may be no symptoms until blood seeps through the walls of the blood vessel. Eventually the aorta may rupture, resulting in loss of consciousness, shock, or even death.

Temporal arteritis. Among the arterial disorders particularly common in elderly women is temporal arteritis (see entry). In this disease large blood vessels throughout the body become inflamed. The cause is unknown, but some researchers think it may be due to an autoimmune reaction which somehow thickens arteries. As a result blood supply is blocked to certain parts of the body, particularly in the head and neck. Temporal arteritis occurs more frequently in women than in men, and if untreated can lead to irreversible blindness.

Other nonatherosclerotic disorders of the arteries. In Raynaud's phenomenon (see entry) fingers or toes turn temporarily white and blue after exposure to cold or sometimes after emotional stress. In fibromuscular dysplasia (also called fibromuscular hyperplasia), which predominantly affects middle-aged women, the artery supplying blood to the kidney may be narrowed. Although there may be no symptoms, fibromuscular dysplasia can result in hypertension (a condition called renal artery stenosis) or stroke.

How are these conditions evaluated?

If an arterial disorder is suspected, the first order of business is ruling out any sudden life-threatening conditions, such as heart attack, pulmonary embolism, aortic aneurysm, or stroke. If any of these conditions seems likely, the woman may need to be hospitalized for further evaluation.

In the course of ruling out life-threatening conditions, the clinician will take a history which includes information about the timing, precise location, and nature of any pain and associated symptoms, such as breathlessness, abdominal complaints, or swelling. When diagnosing an arterial disorder, a clinician may also measure blood pressure in localized areas by using a pneumatic cuff and a flow sensor (see high blood pressure).

Numerous noninvasive tests are now available to distinguish the nature of an arterial disorder as well as the extent of the disease. Magnetic resonance imaging (MRI) and magnetic resonance angiography (MRA) have largely eliminated the need for angiography, a procedure that involves injecting a contrast dye into the arteries before an x-ray is taken (see coronary artery disease). If imaging tests reveal a blockage, however, angiography remains the gold standard for precisely delineating the extent and location of the obstruction.

How are arterial disorders treated?

When the peripheral arteries (especially those supplying the legs and feet) become clogged with plaque, the feet and toes may become numb, painful, or ulcerated. Eliminating or treating some of the risk factors for atherosclerosis, getting regular exercise, and adopting a careful watch-and-wait approach may be enough to control some of these symptoms, with painkillers used in the meantime.

When cramps develop in the calves and feet during exercise and resolve with rest, the condition is called intermittent claudication. It may sometimes be avoided by using a vasodilator—a kind of drug that improves blood flow—called pentoxifylline (Trental). If atherosclerosis progresses, however, tissues may become starved for blood, causing pain in the legs and feet even at rest. In the most extreme cases the tissues eventually turn black and die, a condition known as gangrene. Occasionally gangrenous tissues need to be amputated.

Sometimes an arterial embolism in the arm or leg can be removed with suction embolectomy, a procedure in which the surgeon inserts a suction-tipped catheter into the artery and pulls out the clot. A pulmonary embolism can usually be treated with anticoagulation therapy (see coronary artery disease). Mild hypertension is initially treated with lifestyle changes, but more severe or unresponsive elevations require

medication. An aortic aneurysm, if discovered early, can be repaired surgically. Temporal arteritis is initially treated with high doses of a corticosteroid (an antiinflammatory drug derived from adrenal hormones), usually prednisone.

Disorders of the veins

There are two basic circulatory disorders of the veins: thromboembolic disease and chronic venous insufficiency.

Thromboembolic disease. Also called phlebitis or venous thrombosis, this disorder occurs when a blood clot or clots form in a vein of an extremity (usually in the leg or the pelvis) and produce redness, pain, and swelling in the overlying skin. If a vein lying just under the skin is involved, this condition is rarely serious and may be treated by elevating the limb, applying heat, and taking antiinflammatory medications for a few weeks.

If a vein lying deeper under the surface is affected, the condition may be life-threatening, mainly because of the danger of a potentially fatal pulmonary embolism—a condition in which the clot breaks free from the vein and lodges in the lungs.

These acute episodes tend to be equally common in men and women, but certain circumstances unique to women increase their odds of developing thromboembolic disease in general. Chief among these is taking birth control pills, even the low-dose estrogen oral contraceptives, especially among smokers. This may be because estrogen seems to prompt the formation of various factors in the blood that promote clotting. Among the other risk factors that predispose women to thromboembolic disease are surgery, especially operations on the reproductive organs or urinary tract, or hip replacements; cancer; pregnancy and childbirth; infection, including infection following childbirth; and accidents and other trauma. Sometimes just sitting for prolonged periods of time is enough to induce superficial thrombophlebitis.

Chronic venous insufficiency. As many as half of all people with thromboembolic disease that involves deep veins will also go on to develop some degree of chronic venous insufficiency, the second basic form of circulatory disorder involving the veins. More often, however, this condition develops without any history of thromboembolic disease. It is usually due to malfunction in the valves of the veins. Often the legs feel full, achy, tired, or swollen—particularly at the end of the day. Eventually, if the condition worsens, eczema, ulcerations, and a brown mottled color of the lower leg and ankles may appear.

Chronic venous insufficiency, which occurs more frequently in women than in men, can be subdivided into three forms: varicose veins (see entry), superficial venous incompetence, and deep venous incompetence.

How are these conditions evaluated?

Circulatory disorders of the veins can usually be differentiated from one another—and from arterial disorders—by visual inspection, ultrasound, and tests to measure blood flow.

Sometimes a venogram—the venous counterpart to the arteriogram—may be done as well to delineate the state of valves in the veins.

How are they treated?

For acute thromboembolic disease, hospitalization is often necessary. The leg will be elevated, and an anticoagulant drug (such as heparin), as well as drugs to dissolve clots, may be administered intravenously. Later another anticoagulant such as warfarin (Coumadin) may be taken orally for 3 to 6 months to prevent the clot from recurring.

For all forms of chronic venous insufficiency, compression stockings (either lightweight support hose for mild symptoms or heavier elastic stockings for more severe ones) can be used to restrict swelling. These are more effective than below-the-knee support stockings; women using them should put them on every morning before walking around.

If there are enlarged, tortuous portions of the vein, ulcerations, or other skin changes, surgery may be necessary. In the case of varicose veins, which generally involve the superficial veins, this may involve either sclerotherapy or laser surgery (see entries). Occasionally the veins may also be surgically removed or stripped, particularly if the disease extends all the way from the ankle to the groin. Stripping is not an option if blood clots have developed in the deep veins, because of the possibility of disabling swelling. In this case the only recourse is therapy to relieve the symptoms.

Related entries

Antiinflammatory drugs, chest pain, coronary artery disease, diabetes, estrogen replacement therapy, headaches, heart disease, high blood pressure, laser surgery, Raynaud's phenomenon, sclerotherapy, stroke, temporal arteritis, varicose veins

Coffee

Breast cancer, osteoporosis, cardiovascular disease, cancer: for years coffee—or the stimulant in it, caffeine—has been suspected of causing these and numerous other disorders. Even earlier, health crusaders blamed coffee for various crimes, including stunting growth and corrupting the morality of youth. All the while coffee has remained a popular, nearly ubiquitous beverage. Although many Americans have cut down their consumption for fear of health hazards, the recent growth of specialty coffee bars across the country attests to the continuing allure of the bean. To the relief of those who enjoy sampling exotic blends or simply starting the day with a cup of instant Maxwell House, coffee has retained a relatively unblemished record despite all the outcry.

Of the numerous studies done so far, nearly all have serious flaws. Some, for example, have involved giving excessively high doses of caffeine to animals that do not have the same caffeine tolerance as humans. Other studies have included mainly or only men and thus are not necessarily applicable to women. Still others have not clearly differentiated the effects of caffeine from the effects of coffee per se. And many large-scale, well-designed studies have yielded results that contradict those of equally large-scale, well-designed studies.

None of this means that coffee or caffeine gets off scot-free. There are indeed some preliminary findings which suggest that coffee—both caffeinated and decaffeinated—may pose a risk to human health. But judgment must still be reserved. For the time being, it looks as though people can continue to enjoy their coffee—at least in moderation.

What are the effects of caffeine?

Some of the ills attributed to coffee are not necessarily due to the caffeine it contains. The controversial studies linking coffee consumption to heart disease, for example, have included both caffeinated and decaffeinated coffee. Similarly, in the case of heartburn, both types tend to relax the esophageal sphincter muscle, causing food to reflux from the stomach back into the esophagus.

Some of the health problems that have been attributed to coffee consumption may instead be due to other potentially harmful habits that tend to be more common in coffee drinkers—such as cigarette smoking, lack of exercise, or consuming a higher than average amount of fat or alcohol in the diet.

All the same, caffeine is a mild stimulant drug that definitely has some clear-cut effects on the human body, including causing full-fledged drug addiction. In low doses it tends to induce feelings of alertness, well-being, and euphoria, and these effects last for several hours after ingestion. Still, as few as 2 cups of coffee can induce insomnia in some people, even if consumed as much as 6 hours before bedtime. Caffeine also may increase levels of the stress hormone adrenalin in the body.

At higher doses caffeine can lead to periods of inexhaustibility, as well as rambling speech and thought and rapid heartbeat—all symptoms that can sometimes be mistaken for panic attacks or the manic episodes of manic-depressive disorder. People can become addicted to caffeine and experience symptoms of withdrawal—including insomnia, neck cramps, headaches, nervousness, and mild depression—when they stop using it.

In pregnant women and in people with liver disease the effects tend to be longer-lasting, while in smokers they tend to be more brief. Also, contrary to popular mythology, caffeine works to exacerbate the effects of alcohol, so that a person who tries to counteract a drinking binge with a pot of coffee will end up with even slower reflexes and more sleeplessness.

A number of studies have suggested that caffeine may have a specific effect on women. One study of 841 female college students linked caffeine to symptoms of premenstrual syndrome (see entry). Women who think this might apply to them should make sure to avoid menstrual cramp medications (such as Midol) that contain caffeine.

Caffeine readily crosses the placenta, and there is some controversial evidence suggesting that drinking more than about 2 cups of coffee a day during pregnancy may slightly increase the risk of miscarriage. Thus, for the time being, pregnant women may want to keep coffee consumption down to an average of about a cup a day, just to be safe. There is, however, no conclusive evidence at this point associating coffee drinking or caffeine with any known birth defect or growth retardation in the fetus.

Coffee is not the only culprit when it comes to caffeine (see chart). Plenty of other beverages—as well as various medications for insomnia, appetite control, and headaches—are sources of the stimulant, although, when it comes to beverages, coffee is indeed the most common source. The full-bodied specialty coffees that have become so popular in this country have less caffeine per brewed cup than the coffee sold in cans at supermarkets. This is because specialty coffees (as well as the coffee sold by franchises such as Dunkin' Donuts) are made from arabica beans rather than the robusta beans used in grocery store brands, and arabica beans contain less caffeine. In addition, the process of dark roasting to which specialty coffee is subjected burns off some of the caffeine.

What are the links between coffee and disease?

The evidence linking coffee or caffeine to cardiovascular disease remains unconvincing. A few studies have suggested that caffeine, at least in certain doses, may have some effect on blood cholesterol levels or on temporary rises in blood pressure. And some studies have suggested that drinking more than 3 or 4 cups of coffee a day may moderately increase the risk of having a heart attack—at least in men. But other equally impressive studies have shown no such associations, so for now there is no reason to believe that moderate coffee consumption puts people at risk for cardiovascular disease.

The evidence implicating coffee consumption in pancreatic cancer or colon or rectal cancer is equally shaky. Moreover, contrary to common perception, there is no convincing evidence that drinking coffee increases the risk of breast cancer or that it promotes the formation of noncancerous breast lumps. Some limited evidence has suggested that coffee may increase the risk of bladder cancer, but no one knows just how much coffee consumption should be considered a problem.

As for osteoporosis, it is not known if coffee drinking alone (apart from other habits, such as smoking) increases the risk of bone fracture. High levels of caffeine do seem to deplete the body's stores of calcium, and thus may promote bone loss. By consuming a glass of milk a day—or otherwise upping calcium intake—a woman who drinks coffee in moderation can easily counteract this effect.

Is decaffeinated coffee better for us?

Many people opt for decaffeinated coffee either because they want to get some sleep or because they fear the effects of

How much caffeine?	
Commercial brand coffee (6–8 oz)	**Mg of caffeine**
Instant	65–100
Percolated	80–135
Filtered	115–175
Drip brewed	154–210
Decaffeinated	1–5
Specialty coffee (Arabica beans; 6–8 oz)	81–100
Tea (6–8 oz)	
Instant	35–70
Brewed	28–154
Iced	39–44
Cola beverages (8 oz)	24–31
Chocolate	
Dark semisweet (1 oz)	5–35
Milk chocolate (1 oz)	1–15
Chocolate cake (1 slice)	20–30
Cocoa (8 oz)	3–32
Chocolate milk (8 oz)	2–7
Drugs (1 dose)	
Anacin	33
Aqua-Ban (diuretic)	200
Dexatrim (appetite suppressant)	200
Dristan	30
Empirin	33
Excedrin	64–65
Midol	33
No-Doz	100–130
Prolamine	140
Vanquish	33

caffeine on their health. The decaffeination process involves immersing green coffee beans in warm to hot water, which helps bring the caffeine to the surface of the beans. It is extracted with a chemical solvent (such as methylene chloride), and the beans are then rinsed, dried, and roasted. This process removes 97 to 99 percent of the caffeine in coffee beans. This does not mean that the resulting coffee still contains 1 to 3 percent caffeine. Rather, it means that if a regular cup of coffee contains 100 mg of caffeine, a decaffeinated version of the same coffee would contain only

1 to 3 mg—an amount unlikely to have much of a stimulant effect.

In recent years concerns have been expressed over the residual solvent that may be left on the beans from conventional decaffeination methods. The U.S. Food and Drug Administration (FDA) has set the safe limit for methylene chloride in brewed coffee at 10 parts per million, and coffee brewed according to conventional methods has to meet this standard. Most specialty coffee producers go even further to eliminate methylene chloride by using direct contact decaffeination or water processing. In direct contact decaffeination, coffee is roasted at about 400°F for about 15 minutes. Since methylene chloride boils at 114°, this is more than enough time for virtually all traces of the solvent to disappear. In water processing decaffeination (also called Swiss water processing), no chemical solvents are used at all. Instead, caffeine is removed with hot water and steam and then filtered through activated charcoal. Both of these processes tend to be rather time-consuming and expensive.

Related entries

Alcohol, breast lumps (benign), diuretics, headaches, premenstrual syndrome, smoking

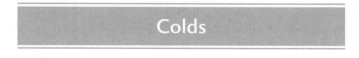

Colds

The common cold is an acute, self-limited upper respiratory infection caused by a virus. It is the fourth most common reason for office visits to physicians in the United States and the most frequent cause of work and school absences. Adults average 3 colds per year.

Most colds can be easily treated without consulting a physician. The important thing to know is when a "cold" is not a cold—that is, when symptoms may signal a more serious problem that requires medical attention.

What causes colds and other respiratory infections?

The common cold is caused by a wide variety of viruses that are virtually indistinguishable clinically. The great number of cold-producing viruses (more than 200) makes it unlikely that a vaccine against colds could be effective.

The flu is another common respiratory infection, caused mainly by various strains of the influenza virus which tend to change slightly from year to year.

Other infections that may mimic colds or develop as complications of colds are caused by bacteria rather than by viruses. These include sinusitis (infection of the sinuses—the air-filled spaces above, behind, and below the eyes) and otitis media (infection of the middle ear). Infections of the throat (pharyngitis), the large airways to the lung (bronchitis), and the lung tissue itself (pneumonia) may be caused by either viruses or bacteria (see breathing disorders).

Studies from the British Cold Virus Research Unit, a famous research group that has recruited hundreds of volunteers willing to be infected with the cold virus in the interests of medical science, show that exposure to cold, damp, and drafts does not increase the risk of catching a cold. Cold viruses do have natural seasonal peaks in the early fall, midwinter, and late spring, however. In winter, crowding indoors further increases the chance of infection.

Cold viruses appear to be transmitted mainly by direct physical contact. People with colds often unconsciously touch their noses; and since the cold virus can survive up to 4 hours on hands, any hand-to-hand contact the person has with others can pass the cold along. Most cold viruses are not transmitted easily through the air, although viruses that cause flu are readily spread this way.

Who is likely to develop colds and other respiratory infections?

Children's noses are the main reservoir of the rhinovirus, the most common culprit in colds. Preschoolers average 6 to 10 colds a year. As people age they get fewer colds, partly because of immunity and partly because contact with children decreases. For women, however, this may not be the case. Mothers tend to catch colds from their children at a higher rate than fathers do, and grandparents who care for young children are at high risk as well.

What are the symptoms?

The symptoms of the common cold are all too familiar: a runny or congested nose, sneezing, sore throat, cough, and hoarseness. Fever, if present, is usually mild. Symptoms typically last for up to a week but can sometimes persist for 2 weeks.

Women and men tend to respond differently to cold symptoms, according to studies from the British Cold Virus Research Unit. Men as a group rate their cold symptoms much more severely than women, even though women tend to have symptoms objectively judged (by a presumably impartial male researcher) to be worse than those in the men. (Other studies involving different types of illnesses that affect men and women alike have also shown that women tend to make less of their symptoms than men do.)

The symptoms of flu are systemic, including general malaise, headache, muscle aches, and fever. Local symptoms such as a sore throat and runny nose sometimes occur as well. People with flu usually feel sick for 1 to 2 weeks, but full recovery can take up to 4 weeks.

The congestion associated with a cold sometimes causes a feeling of pressure or blockage in the ears. If bacterial infection develops in fluid trapped in the middle ear, the result may be a severe earache. If sinusitis develops, symptoms will include facial pain, fever, and greenish nasal secretions. Pharyngitis caused by bacteria (typically streptococcus, the culprit in "strep throat") produces a sore throat together with fever of 100°F or more and swollen glands in the neck. The symptoms of bronchitis and pneumonia—cough, fever, and greenish sputum—are often indistinguishable from one another.

How are colds and other respiratory infections evaluated?

Knowing when to treat oneself and when to call the doctor is the most important part of managing colds and other respiratory infections. If it is not clear, most clinicians welcome the chance to assess symptoms by telephone before an office visit is scheduled.

In general, a physician should be consulted if typical cold symptoms last for more than 3 weeks or are recurrent; the latter suggests the possibility of allergy. Since otitis media and sinusitis are bacterial infections that need antibiotics for speedy resolution, a woman with earache or facial pain with or without greenish nasal discharge should contact a clinician.

A cough together with greenish or blood-streaked sputum, chest pain, wheezing, shortness of breath, or prolonged or high fever can indicate pneumonia. Only a physical examination by a clinician (and in some cases a chest x-ray) can distinguish pneumonia from bronchitis. A sore throat needs medical attention if it is accompanied by a fever, swollen glands, marked pain, or difficulty swallowing. Women who are elderly, who smoke, or who have a history of asthma or chronic obstructive lung disease should contact a physician to evaluate any upper respiratory symptoms (see asthma; breathing disorders).

To evaluate an upper respiratory infection, a clinician will elicit the history of the symptoms and examine the throat, nose, ears, and lungs. In some cases a throat culture, chest x-ray, or blood test may be necessary.

How are colds and other respiratory infections treated?

Over-the-counter cold remedies are a big business, to the tune of $2 billion a year. Most of the medications sold for treating colds are effective and safe, and they need not be costly if trendy combination products are avoided. Drug manufacturers heavily promote "shotgun" remedies designed to relieve multiple symptoms. These formulas cost much more than single-ingredient preparations and increase the likelihood of side effects.

For the nasal congestion of the typical cold, decongestants are the first line of treatment. Nasal sprays—such as oxymetalozine (Afrin) or phenylephrine (Dristan, Neosynephrine)—are more effective than oral decongestants such as pseudoephedrine (Sudafed). Nasal decongestants must be used for no more than 3 to 5 days, however, because longer use increases the likelihood of rebound nasal congestion (caused by inflammation of the nasal passages) after stopping the drug. Oral decongestants can be safely combined with nasal sprays and can be taken for a longer period, up to a few weeks. The preparations listed above can be safely used by people with controlled high blood pressure and thyroid disorders. Over-the-counter antihistamines such as chlorpheniramine are sometimes helpful for sneezing and runny noses, although they can cause drowsiness.

Aspirin, acetaminophen (Tylenol), or ibuprofen (Advil, Nuprin, Motrin IB) will soothe the body aches, headaches, and fever that accompany many upper respiratory infections. A cough suppressant such as dextromethorphan (Robitussin DM, Benylin DM) can allow needed sleep and can break the cycle of cough-irritation-cough that prolongs some cases of bronchitis. A cough that occurs over and over for hours and cannot be controlled with cough suppressants—or any increasing difficulty in breathing that leads to wheezing—needs medical evaluation for possible asthma, which can develop out of the blue in some people with respiratory infections. A warm salt-water gargle temporarily reduces discomfort from a sore throat; use of a humidifier, along with simply resting the voice, can alleviate hoarseness.

A nonmedical way of lessening the misery of a cold is eating chicken soup, which helps the body clear nasal mucus, according to data from scientific studies (as well as the experience of grandmothers). Steam and cool mist promote clearance of secretions as well. Vitamin C, however, which has been studied in a number of scientific trials, produces no consistent improvement in cold symptoms.

A widely publicized study in 1996 showed that zinc gluconate lozenges reduced the duration and severity of cold symptoms. This finding led to a major upsurge in the popularity of zinc lozenges of all sorts. Even so, the research community still questions the potency of zinc as a treatment or preventive measure for the common cold, mainly because numerous studies suggest that zinc may have no effect on the course of a cold whatsoever—and in some cases may even weaken immune status. Some researchers believe that the zinc in some of these products may become inactivated by flavoring agents; others believe that zinc simply has no effect on the common cold or on the immune system. Nevertheless, some clinicians do recommend taking zinc in the first 24 to 48 hours after a first sniffle to help reduce the duration of symptoms, perhaps because zinc somehow interferes with the attachment of cold virus particles to the lining of the nose.

Generally, antibiotics have no role in treating colds or other viral respiratory infections. An exception is the form of flu caused by influenza A virus, for which antiviral antibiotics can reduce the severity of illness in frail elderly people and in adults with serious chronic illnesses. Antibiotics, in combination with symptomatic remedies, *are* needed to treat some cases of pharyngitis, sinusitis, otitis media, bronchitis, and pneumonia.

How can colds and respiratory infections be prevented?

Since colds seem to be spread primarily by hand-to-hand transmission, washing hands frequently and avoiding contact with cold sufferers offer the best path to prevention. A person suffering from a cold can reduce the chance of passing it along by using tissues rather than handkerchiefs, keeping the hands away from the nose as much as possible, and washing hands often. Smoking does not increase the likelihood of catching the common cold, but it impairs the body's mechanisms for clearing infection and increases the likelihood of bronchitis and other complications. Any smoker who acquires a cold or upper respiratory infection should consider using it as an opportunity to quit for good.

Each fall, flu vaccine against that year's common strains has traditionally been recommended for healthy persons over age 65 and for people of any age who have chronic respiratory diseases or other serious ailments. But even in healthy working adults, recent studies have shown that flu vaccine can reduce episodes of upper respiratory infection by 25 percent and sick leave from work by 40 percent. These studies suggest that giving flu vaccine to healthy adults makes good health sense for individuals and is also cost-effective.

Many people take high-dose supplements of vitamin C in the belief that it will prevent colds, if not cure them, but the scientific studies conducted thus far have not been able to detect any preventive benefit.

Related entries
Antibiotics, asthma, breathing disorders, immunizations, smoking

Colon and Rectal Cancer

Cancer of the colon, or large intestine (see illustration), and the rectum—collectively called colorectal cancer or sometimes simply colon cancer—is one of the most common forms of cancer in the United States. It afflicts approximately 130,200 Americans a year, of whom about 55,000 will die, and it is currently the third leading cause of cancer death for women in this country (after lung and breast cancers). Since 1950, however, death rates have been dropping, particularly among women.

Although little is understood about why colorectal cancer affects men and women differently, the contrasts are striking. According to an investigation at the National Institutes of Health (NIH), only 15 out of 100,000 women with colorectal cancer died in 1990, down from 25 out of 100,000 in 1950. In men the decline in death rate was much more subtle, falling only from 26 to 22 out of 100,000 over the same period of time. Furthermore, between 1950 and 1984 the number of women diagnosed with colorectal cancers remained steady, while the number of men increased. After 1985, however, the incidence began to decline in both sexes. Other studies have shown that older men and women in particular may be susceptible to different kinds of colorectal cancer: whereas older men appear more likely to develop rectal cancer and cancer

of the left side of the colon, right-side colon cancer seems unusually prevalent in older women.

Some investigators think that differences in diet and exercise habits may be part of the explanation. Higher levels of fiber in the diet, a lower consumption of alcohol, greater consumption of aspirin and other nonsteroidal antiinflammatory drugs (NSAIDs), and a greater benefit from physical activity and body mass have all been suggested as contributing to women's greater degree of protection. There is also some speculation that hormones produced during a woman's childbearing years—and interactions of these hormones with the foods she eats—may continue to affect a woman's risk of colorectal cancer later in life. Recent studies have shown a decreased risk of colon cancer in women who use postmenopausal estrogen replacement therapy. Although some studies suggest that having children or bearing a child at a young age may decrease a woman's risk—as has been suggested in studies of breast cancer risk—the evidence so far has been inconsistent. These kinds of links are currently under active investigation.

One reason why gender differences have been hard to explain is that there is still a lot of uncertainty about what causes colorectal cancer in the first place despite the fact that more is understood about this cancer than any other common cancer. For years there has been considerable speculation about dietary factors such as high-fat, high-calorie, low-fiber diets. The fact that the incidence of colorectal cancer is much lower in countries such as Japan, where the diet is much lower in fat than in the United States, has led a number of investigators to target fats as a possible culprit. Furthermore, evidence from the large Nurses' Health Study (which followed 90,000 nurses for 6 years) firmly identified animal fats—especially from red meat—as a risk factor for colorectal cancer in women. Women who ate beef, pork, or lamb as entrées on a daily basis had a risk of colon cancer 2.5 times higher than that of women who ate red meat less than once a month.

Although suggestive, this kind of retrospective evidence alone is not enough to implicate red meat or fat: it remains possible that women who ate a lot of red meat may also have had other characteristics (such as certain lifestyle habits or even genetic backgrounds) that predisposed them to develop cancer. The answer will come only after more studies are done to see if making dietary changes alone can lower the incidence of colorectal cancer among otherwise similar groups of people.

Colorectal cancer is often curable by surgery if it is detected and treated early enough. People who have their cancer removed before it has spread (metastasized) beyond the colon or rectum have an 80 to 90 percent chance of being alive 5 years after diagnosis. Once spread has occurred, this 5-year survival rate falls to under 50 percent.

Who is likely to develop colorectal cancer?
Colorectal cancer can run in families. About 1 in 5 of these cancers can be traced to a predisposing gene. African Ameri-

Warning signs for colorectal cancer

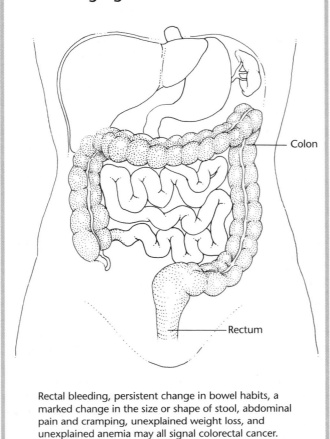

Colon

Rectum

Rectal bleeding, persistent change in bowel habits, a marked change in the size or shape of stool, abdominal pain and cramping, unexplained weight loss, and unexplained anemia may all signal colorectal cancer.

cans are at somewhat higher risk of developing and dying from this disease than are people of other ethnic backgrounds.

Most colon cancers develop from polyps, specifically the type called adenomas or adenomatous polyps. The progression from adenomatous polyp to cancer probably takes at least 10 years in most people. Having a prior history of ulcerative colitis (see bowel disorders) also increases the risk of developing cancer. Having a close family member (parent, sibling, or child) with these conditions—or who had colorectal cancer—also raises the risk.

What are the symptoms?

Most colon cancers cause no symptoms until they are quite advanced. Rectal bleeding (of any color) is the most typical early warning sign of colorectal cancer. Although in most cases such bleeding is the sign of a much less serious condition (such as hemorrhoids), it is vital to have the possibility of cancer eliminated. Other symptoms of colorectal cancer—such as a change in bowel habit or a marked change in the size or shape of stool—are frequent occurrences for most peo-

ple and thus can easily go unnoticed. Occasionally, people with colorectal cancer may have additional symptoms such as abdominal pain and cramping or unexplained weight loss.

How is the condition evaluated?

Even though odds are high that rectal bleeding is caused by hemorrhoids or some other benign condition, anyone with noticeable blood in the stool should be evaluated for colorectal cancer. A clinician may also want to evaluate a patient who has otherwise unexplained anemia (which may result from unnoticed internal bleeding). A clinician may also want to check for colorectal cancer following a positive screening test, which should be done as part of a yearly examination in people over the age of 50.

Screening often involves a stool test for occult (hidden) blood. Although not all cancers will produce blood in the stool, this screening test remains one of the easiest, least expensive, and most convenient means of detecting otherwise unrecognized cancers. To perform the occult blood test, which is prepared by the patient at home and later interpreted by a clinician or laboratory technician, the patient spreads small specimens of feces on a chemically treated test card with an applicator stick and then returns the card to the clinician. Several drops of a peroxide solution are added to the test areas. If these areas contain unusually large amounts of blood (normal loss is about half a teaspoonful a day), the paper underneath will turn blue within about 30 seconds. Usually 3 separate bowel movements are tested on 3 separate cards. Since each of these cards has 2 test spaces—one for a sample of the stool interior and the other for its surface—a total of 6 stool samples are tested in all.

To increase the reliability of these occult blood tests, the clinician may recommend certain dietary and drug restrictions for the few days before stool is collected. For example, avoiding red meat, turnips, horseradish, and excess iron can reduce the chances of false-positive readings, as can avoiding aspirin and other antiinflammatory drugs. Vitamin C pills can cause false-negative results—which could lead to a cancer being missed—and therefore should not be taken in the days before the test.

A positive stool test does not necessarily indicate colorectal cancer (see illustration). About 95 percent of people with positive tests ultimately turn out to have other reasons for the bleeding, including intestinal polyps, hemorrhoids, Crohn's disease (a form of inflammatory bowel disease), or diverticula—or no known disorder. If any of the stool samples tested for occult blood is positive—or if the other screening tests suggest problems—more extensive testing may be necessary.

The initial tests used to diagnose colorectal cancer include a manual rectal examination (which can reveal "reachable" cancers and remove stool samples for testing), sigmoidoscopy (in which a flexible lighted tube is inserted into the rectum and the lower part of the large intestine), a special colon x-ray called a barium enema, and colonoscopy (an inspection of the entire colon with a lighted flexible tube inserted through the rectum). Such tests allow the clinician to visual-

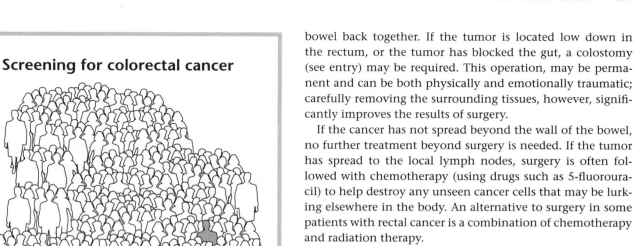

Screening for colorectal cancer

380 negative
(1 false negative)

400 screened

19 no cancer

1 cancer detected

20 positive

If 400 people over age 40 are screened for colorectal cancer using tests to detect occult blood in the stool, no bleeding will be detected in 380 people (1 of whom will actually have cancer; this is a false negative result). Of the 20 who have a positive result, 19 will turn out not to have cancer but rather to have other causes of bleeding. One person out of the original 400 people screened will have a cancer detected with this screening method.

ize the intestine and rectum and to evaluate both appearance and function. They also allow diagnosis of other conditions that may account for the symptoms. A colonoscopy also permits the clinician to take tissue samples for evaluation under a microscope (biopsy). Some of these tests are costly and uncomfortable, and, in the case of colonoscopy, carry a slight risk of perforating the colon. An increasing number of experts nevertheless believe that the value of these tests in preventing deaths from colorectal cancer more than compensates for these shortcomings.

How is colorectal cancer treated?
If colorectal cancer has not yet spread, it is usually removed surgically. Often this requires simply cutting out the segment of bowel that includes the tumor and then stitching the

bowel back together. If the tumor is located low down in the rectum, or the tumor has blocked the gut, a colostomy (see entry) may be required. This operation, may be permanent and can be both physically and emotionally traumatic; carefully removing the surrounding tissues, however, significantly improves the results of surgery.

If the cancer has not spread beyond the wall of the bowel, no further treatment beyond surgery is needed. If the tumor has spread to the local lymph nodes, surgery is often followed with chemotherapy (using drugs such as 5-fluorouracil) to help destroy any unseen cancer cells that may be lurking elsewhere in the body. An alternative to surgery in some patients with rectal cancer is a combination of chemotherapy and radiation therapy.

Surgery may also be an option in more advanced cancers, but usually only to prevent or treat bowel obstruction or bleeding. Once the cancer has spread beyond the colon and rectum, the treatment of choice is chemotherapy (5-fluorouracil, irinolecon, or oxaliplatin) to shrink the tumor and reduce any symptoms that may interfere with quality of life.

How can colorectal cancer be prevented?
There is mounting evidence that regular screening in people over the age of 50 can reduce deaths from colorectal cancer. In practice, screening for colorectal cancer is usually individualized according to the patient's willingness to undergo sigmoidoscopy or colonoscopy. Experts agree that, at a minimum, people over age 50 should have a stool occult blood test (3 specimens collected at home) every year. In addition, most recommend a sigmoidoscopy every 5 years or colonoscopy every 10 years.

Those at high risk—including people with a close family member who has had colon cancer or adenomatous polyps or a personal history of adenomatous polyps or ulcerative colitis—should be screened at an earlier age and at more frequent intervals. Colonoscopy is the preferred screening method for high-risk individuals since the entire colon can be examined and any polyps removed. Removal of polyps detected by screening dramatically reduces the likelihood of dying from colorectal cancer.

There is some evidence that the odds of developing colorectal cancer can be lowered with certain nutritional and lifestyle practices—particularly by eating a diet rich in high-fiber foods such as fruits, vegetables, whole grains, and legumes. Although two recent studies in the *New England Journal of Medicine* failed to find any link between low-fat, high-fiber diets and lowered colon cancer risk, most experts still recommend this diet—regarded as healthy in general—as a means of cancer prevention. Boosting exercise levels also may help reduce risk, as may limiting the amount of alcohol one drinks. In both the Nurses' Health Study of 16,000 women and the Health Professionals' Follow-Up Study of 9,500 men, people who consumed more than 2 drinks (30 grams) of alcohol a day seemed to be at increased risk for colon cancer.

Although the evidence about fat and colon cancer is still preliminary, cutting down on fats "just in case" is probably a good idea, since—if nothing else—it will decrease the odds of coronary artery disease. Anyone considering a very low fat diet for the sake of preventing colorectal cancer, however, should first consult a clinician to evaluate the impact of this decision on her overall health—and to come up with strategies to prevent nutrient deficiencies.

Just why fruits and vegetables in particular are so helpful remains unclear, although their high levels of fiber and antioxidants probably have something to do with it. High levels of the vitamin folic acid (folate) in citrus fruit and green vegetables may also play a role by helping to prevent adenomatous polyps in the colon. Some researchers have speculated that folic acid activates methylation, a chemical process that seems to turn on certain tumor-suppressing genes that retard the uncontrolled cell growth that characterizes cancer. Alcohol, in contrast, may inhibit methylation, therefore indirectly encouraging the growth of these polyps in the colon, and ultimately cancer.

Folic acid supplements have also been shown to help prevent colon cancer in people with ulcerative colitis. But there is still not enough information about the role of folic acid to justify supplements in otherwise healthy people. For everyone else, following the National Cancer Institute's recommendations that adults eat at least 5 servings of fruits and vegetables daily is probably sufficient.

Mounting evidence does suggest that aspirin reduces the risk of colon and rectal cancer in women (as well as men). The Nurses' Health Study has shown that women who took 4 to 6 aspirins a week for 10 years reduced their risk by almost half. If this kind of cancer is a particular concern, a woman may want to consider taking a regular-strength aspirin daily if she has no other reasons (such as gastritis, ulcers, or asthma) to avoid it. Estrogen replacement therapy has also been linked to a lower incidence of colon cancer, but more research is needed to establish its role in the prevention of this disease.

Related entries

Anemia, antiinflammatory drugs, biopsy, bowel disorders, chemotherapy, colostomy, constipation, diverticular disease, exercise, hemorrhoids, irritable bowel syndrome, laser surgery, nutrition, radiation therapy, sexual dysfunction, vitamins

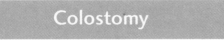

Colostomy

Colostomy is a surgical procedure used to treat certain bowel disorders. It is most commonly performed to treat severe inflammatory bowel disease—particularly Crohn's disease (see bowel disorders)—and certain colon and rectal cancers (see entry). Colostomy is necessary when the diseased portion of the colon cannot be removed in a way that allows the re-

maining colon simply to be sewn back together, retaining the normal pathway for elimination of solid wastes.

How is the procedure performed?

The surgeon removes the diseased section of colon and reroutes the intestine through an opening (stoma) in the abdominal wall so that feces can be collected in a plastic or rubber pouch (also called a colostomy bag or appliance). This pouch is worn tightly over the opening in the body and, since wastes can no longer be eliminated voluntarily, must be emptied regularly.

What happens after the surgery?

For women who have a colostomy to treat inflammatory bowel disease, the surgery often means an end to disabling symptoms and a return to more normal life. And for those who have colorectal cancer, surgery often provides a complete cure for disease that is otherwise life-threatening. Still, despite those benefits, having a colostomy is traumatic physically and emotionally. Not only must patients live with a constant and cumbersome reminder of their surgery and possible disease, but also merely readjusting to a new routine takes considerable time and effort. In the first 2 months or so after the operation, strenuous activities, driving, and sexual activity must be restricted or avoided, according to the surgeon's instructions. Eventually, most of these activities can be resumed. Permanent changes may be necessary in the diet to help control the consistency of the stool.

Sexual dysfunction often develops in both men and women who have had a colostomy, with problems ranging from lack of desire to pain during intercourse. Although some of these problems are due to physical changes related to the position of the stoma, others result from an altered body image or from simple awkwardness or embarrassment about resuming sexual intimacy. Sometimes these problems can be resolved by discussing them with an understanding partner or by trying other sexual positions that may be more comfortable. If sexual dysfunction persists for more than a few months, professional help may be advisable.

Pregnancy and childbearing are both possible in women who have had a colostomy—assuming they are in good health otherwise—and many can deliver vaginally. If possible, it is wise to give the body a year or two to recover after the colostomy surgery before becoming pregnant. Many obstetricians also recommend having no more than 2 pregnancies after a colostomy.

Suggestions about how to cope with the many changes and obstacles that colostomy entails—as well as emotional support—can often be provided by self-help groups consisting of other people who have had this surgery.

What are the risks and complications?

Like all major surgery, colostomy carries the risk of adverse reactions to anesthesia, bleeding (possibly requiring transfusion), infection, blood clots, damage to other organs, abnormal scarring, internal adhesions, and a small chance of death.

Related entries

Body image, bowel disorders, colon and rectal cancer, psychotherapy, sexual dysfunction

Colposcopy

Colposcopy is a technique for examining potentially abnormal areas of the cervix and vagina using a mounted, binocular-like instrument called a colposcope. Colposcopies are generally done after an abnormal Pap test has come back from the lab. Occasionally colposcopy may also be done to help identify reasons for abnormal bleeding or pain during intercourse, or to examine sores on the vulva. Women whose mothers took the drug DES while pregnant with them should have regular colposcopic examinations.

When cancer or precancerous changes are suspected, colposcopy combined with a biopsy (tissue sample) can sometimes be used instead of riskier, more expensive surgical procedures such as cone biopsies. Biopsies done during a colposcopic examination are particularly accurate because the colposcope enlarges tissue by 5 to 30 times and illuminates the areas most prone to cancerous changes.

How is the procedure performed?

Usually done in a doctor's office, the procedure takes about 20 minutes. The clinician begins by inserting a speculum into the vagina, washing the vagina with acetic acid (a concentrated form of vinegar), and then aiming the colposcope toward the vagina. Because the colposcope is positioned outside the body, most women feel little if any discomfort, although some find the prolonged speculum exam unpleasant.

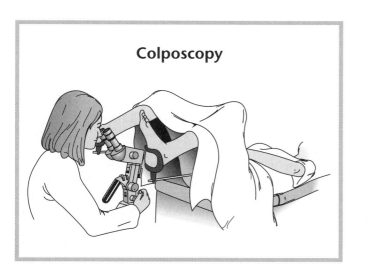

Colposcopy

What are the risks and complications?

There are no risks or complications associated with colposcopy itself. If a biopsy is performed, minor bleeding or infection can occur.

Related entries

Biopsy, diethylstilbestrol (DES), pain during sexual intercourse, Pap test, vulvar disorders

Computerized Axial Tomography (CT) Scans

A computed axial tomography scan—CT scan or CAT scan for short—is a sophisticated x-ray technique that has greatly improved diagnosis of many different disorders since its introduction in the mid-1970s. Because CT scans can provide a much better image of soft tissues and bones than conventional x-rays, they are particularly useful in evaluating tumors, infections, and injuries.

How is the procedure performed?

In this technique the patient is placed in a doughnut-shaped scanning device in which an ultrathin x-ray beam ro-

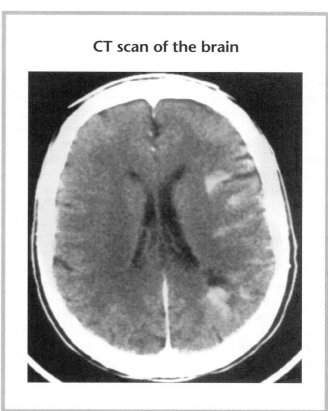

CT scan of the brain

tates around the patient. Detectors measure the absorption of x-rays with each rotation, and a scanner computer produces images that appear as cross-sectional slices of the body. The computer can also stack all the slices to permit parts of the image to be viewed in longitudinal and other planes as well as to allow the production of three-dimensional pictures.

CT scans can be done on an outpatient basis and are painless, although some examinations require contrast materials (dyes) to be injected into the bloodstream via an intravenous needle. Modern scanners require only 30 to 60 seconds to scan a portion of the body.

What are the risks and complications?

Although radiation exposure from a CT scan is greater than that for most x-rays, it is not known to pose any immediate or long-term health risk. Of more concern is the possibility of an allergic reaction to the contrast material which is sometimes administered intravenously during a CT scan to enhance the ability to detect abnormalities. For that reason, any history of previous reactions to contrast material should be mentioned to the radiologist.

Related entries

Magnetic resonance imaging, mammography, stroke, ultrasound

Condoms

Condoms, like diaphragms and cervical caps, are a barrier method of birth control. A male condom is a sheath worn over a man's erect penis to catch sperm and keep them from entering the woman's vagina. Although usually made of a latex rubber material, condoms made of "skin" (usually lamb membrane and polyurethane) are also available. Skin condoms tend to be less effective than latex, and are more expensive. Condoms should also be placed on dildos or other sex toys if they are used by more than one person.

In addition to being a relatively safe and effective means of contraception, male condoms made of latex (also called rubbers, prophylactics, or safes) are often used to prevent the spread of AIDS and other sexually transmitted diseases. Condoms made of animal membrane are porous to viruses and do not provide adequate protection from HIV. There is some evidence that a male partner's condom use may lower a woman's risk of developing cervical cancer. The same degree of protection from sexually transmitted diseases is provided by female condoms (also called vaginal pouches), a relatively new nonprescription contraceptive device that lines the vagina and covers the cervix.

Male condoms

These condoms, which are sold without prescription, are unrolled over an erect penis (see illustration) just before penis-vagina contact, with at least half an inch of space left at the end to catch the ejaculate. Some condoms are prelubricated (ideally with a spermicide—a cream, gel, or foam that kills sperm and, possibly, infectious organisms), or can be lubricated after the condom is on the penis with a spermicide or water-based lubricant (such as K-Y jelly). This can ease insertion and reduce the chances of tearing, although lubrication also increases the chance that the condom will slip off during intercourse.

After intercourse, one partner must hold the end of the condom tightly over the man's penis to make sure that the condom remains in place until the penis is withdrawn from the vagina. If the condom accidentally bursts or slips off, spermicide should be inserted into the vagina promptly. If this sort of "accident" happens to a woman who thinks she is nearing ovulation, she might consider discussing morning-after contraception with her clinician (see hormonal contraception).

Used alone, the male condom has an expected failure rate of 2 percent and a typical failure rate of 12 percent—that is, 12 percent of women who rely on male condoms to prevent pregnancy will nevertheless become pregnant within the year. Many couples reduce this rate to nearly zero by combining the condom with some other form of contraception such as a spermicidal foam, cream, or jelly—particularly at times of the month when the woman is most fertile. Using the condom with a water-based lubricant can also reduce the possibility of condom breakage.

Condoms are readily available without prescription at most pharmacies and supermarkets and can easily be carried by either a man or a woman until they are needed. They can usually be stored for up to 5 years before use, but people who store them in a back-pocket wallet should be aware that heat from the body (or anywhere else) can cause the latex to deteriorate well within that period of time.

Although placing the condom on the penis can interfere with the spontaneity of sex, some couples find this is less of a problem if the woman puts the condom on the man as part of foreplay. Condoms are also a much less messy form of contraception than most barrier methods, which require inserting spermicide into the vagina.

Condoms vary in price considerably, depending on the brand, features (such as ribbing, color, and lubrication), and quantity (generally the more purchased at once, the cheaper the unit price). In general, a package of 3 condoms costs about $3 or so.

Condoms are not associated with any serious side effects. Some men complain that condoms interfere with sensation, and some women dislike the feeling of the rubber against their vaginal walls or find the friction irritating. Using lubrication can sometimes make this less of a problem, but it is important not to use Vaseline or other oil-based lubricants,

How to use a male condom

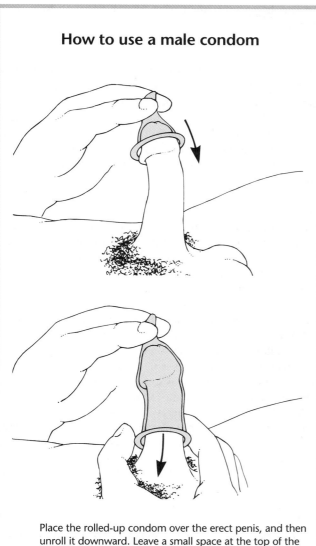

Place the rolled-up condom over the erect penis, and then unroll it downward. Leave a small space at the top of the condom to hold the man's semen after ejaculation.

which can cause the latex to deteriorate. Condom use has no effect on future fertility. A couple who want to have a baby can simply stop using condoms.

Female condoms

The female condom (also known as the vaginal pouch) is a nonprescription barrier method of contraception relatively new to the U.S. market. Sold under the brand names Reality and Femidom, the female condom probably also offers the same degree of protection against AIDS and other sexually transmitted diseases as does the male condom—without requiring the same degree of participation and cooperation on the part of the male partner. In addition, the female condom is less likely to slip or burst during intercourse than is the male condom.

The female condom consists of a prelubricated sheet of polyurethane with a small flexible ring around the center portion and a larger flexible ring encircling the outer edge (see illustration). To insert the condom, a woman squeezes the inner ring and pushes it back and up into the vagina until it covers the cervix. The ring is then released, and either partner checks to make sure the condom is properly placed—in which case the inner ring will be covering the cervix, the polyurethane sheet itself will be covering the vaginal walls, and the outer ring will remain visible just outside the vaginal lips.

The condom should be inserted before any penis-vagina contact and carefully removed after ejaculation. After a single act of intercourse, the female condom must be replaced with another one before there is any subsequent penis-vagina contact.

The female condom appears to be just about as effective as a diaphragm or cervical cap. That is, it has about a 6 percent theoretical failure rate (reflecting use under ideal conditions) and an 18 percent typical failure rate (reflecting usual conditions of use, including the possibility of human error). Because the female condom can be inserted well before sexual activity begins, it is less likely to interfere with spontaneity than is the male condom, which has to be placed on an erect penis. The condom itself is easily obtained without a prescription or visit to a clinic and can be carried unobtrusively until needed. Like all barrier methods of contraception, however, the female condom has to be used at every instance of penis-vagina contact.

There are no known side effects associated with the female condom, although some women, and some men, are bothered by the fit and feel of the device or find the outside ring bothersome. There is no reason to think that using the female condom will have any effect on a woman's ability to become pregnant in the future; she need only stop using the condom.

Related entries

Abortion, acquired immune deficiency syndrome, birth control, diaphragms and cervical caps, douching, hormonal contraception, intrauterine devices, lubricants, natural birth control methods, nonsurgical abortion, oral contraceptives, pregnancy testing, safer sex, sexual response, sexually transmitted diseases, tubal ligation, vacuum aspiration

Congestive Heart Failure

Congestive heart failure occurs when the heart fails to pump blood adequately, causing blood to back up in the veins that return blood to the heart. As a result, tissues throughout the body are deprived of oxygen which is normally transported by the blood. Backed-up blood causes fluid to collect in various parts of the body such as the lungs, lower legs, ankles, and liver.

Congestive heart failure can result from a variety of underlying problems, including mechanical problems of the heart valves, previous heart attacks, heart rhythm disturbances, damaged heart muscle, or long-standing high blood pressure. In women it is less likely to be associated with coronary artery disease than in men. Instead, it tends to involve problems in different parts of the pumping mechanism.

There are two phases to the pumping action of the heart: the "squeeze" (systole), when the heart muscle contracts, pumping blood through the arteries; and the "relaxation" (diastole), when the muscle relaxes and the heart fills with blood, ready to begin a new pumping cycle. The type of congestive heart failure caused by coronary artery disease ("systolic heart failure"—the type most common in men) occurs because damaged heart muscle loses its ability to "squeeze." In women, problems with the relaxation phase are more common ("diastolic heart failure"). The heart muscle becomes stiffer or thickened and does not allow the heart to fill with blood. The most common cause is long-standing high blood pressure; the heart muscle enlarges and stiffens because it is forced to pump against high pressure in the arteries.

Who is likely to develop congestive heart failure?

In both sexes, hypertension greatly increases the risk of developing congestive heart failure. Women with diabetes are also at particularly high risk because they are more prone to coronary artery disease, which causes scarring of heart muscle and loss of "squeeze." Congestive heart failure occurs more frequently in men than in women and strikes women at a later age, but women who develop it are much more likely to die from the disease.

What are the symptoms?

The main symptoms of congestive heart failure are breathlessness, fatigue, weakness, and swelling (edema). Which of these symptoms occurs depends on which part of the heart is failing. If the pumping from the left side of the heart is inefficient, blood will back up into the lungs, leading them to become congested with fluid. The result is a condition called pulmonary edema, which is generally characterized by breathlessness. Often people with mild congestive heart failure become short of breath mainly with exertion. In later stages breathlessness is present even when the person is lying down or sitting.

If the right side of the heart is failing, backed-up blood congests the liver and the legs, resulting in swelling in the lower legs and ankles and liver malfunction. If blood flow to the kidneys is reduced, excess fluids will accumulate in tissues throughout the body, leading to more generalized edema. Swelling throughout the body, as well as breathlessness, will also occur if both sides of the heart are failing, which is often the case. In addition, inadequate blood flow to muscles leads to fatigue and weakness.

How is the condition evaluated?

A clinician who suspects congestive heart failure will listen to the heart and lungs with a stethoscope and then conduct a number of tests of heart structure and function. These tests may include an electrocardiogram (ECG) to check for abnormalities in the heart's rate or rhythm and an echocardiogram to examine the heart's pumping action, as well as a chest x-ray. Various blood and urine tests will be done to evaluate kidney function.

How is congestive heart failure treated?

There is no specific cure for most cases of congestive heart failure, but various steps can be taken to help people with this condition achieve a relatively normal life. Traditionally treatment has consisted of a combination of rest (to take some of the strain off the heart and other organs), salt-restricted diet (to reduce swelling), certain heart medications (such as digoxin) to increase the heart's pumping capacity, and others (such as ACE inhibitors) to reduce the resistance to blood flow. In some cases surgery to repair or replace damaged heart muscle or valves is necessary. For the most severe cases heart transplantation is sometimes considered.

It now appears that some of the drugs commonly prescribed for congestive heart failure—including diuretics (which increase the output of salt and water by the kidneys, thereby decreasing the volume of blood and lowering blood pressure), digitalis (which increases the force of the heart's pumping action), and vasodilators (which widen the arteries and decrease resistance)—may not work for some women whose congestive heart failure is caused by the inability of the heart to fill adequately with blood. Other types of medications, particularly beta blockers and calcium-channel blockers, may also be used to treat this kind of congestive heart failure (see high blood pressure).

The outlook for people with congestive heart failure varies depending on the underlying condition. When an abnormal heart rhythm is the cause and can be treated, heart failure is unlikely to recur. Heart failure caused by long-standing high blood pressure or by minor damage to the heart from a heart attack can often be successfully treated with medication. When the heart muscle has been extensively damaged by a single large heart attack or multiple small attacks, the outlook is less encouraging; the patient's activity is likely to be drastically limited. Finally, global damage of the entire heart muscle from an infection, often caused by a virus, has the worst outlook: this condition, which can occur in relatively young people, may be successfully treated only with a heart transplant.

Related entries

Aortic stenosis, circulatory disorders, coronary artery disease, diabetes, diuretics, edema, fatigue, heart disease, high blood pressure

Constipation

The popular wisdom that a daily bowel movement is a key to good health causes many people excessive worry and wasted effort because habits of elimination vary considerably from one individual to the next. It is often normal to have a bowel movement as frequently as 3 times a day or as infrequently as 3 times a week. A bothersome change in bowel patterns that cannot be alleviated with the occasional use of mild laxatives, however, may require medical attention.

Constipation is usually defined as difficulty passing stools at least 3 times a week, or as bowel movements that occur less than once per week. Abdominal pain and bloating commonly occur as well. Constipation develops when weakened muscular contractions in the colon (also called the bowel or the large intestine) slow the movement of waste products as they approach the rectum and anus (see illustration). Occurring twice as commonly in women as in men, constipation can be due to many factors, among them irregular or inadequate diet, too little water in the diet, lack of exercise, resisting the urge to defecate, and excessive reliance on laxatives. It can also be caused by taking certain medications. These include oral contraceptives, codeine, and some of the drugs used to treat heart disease, depression, hypertension, and indigestion.

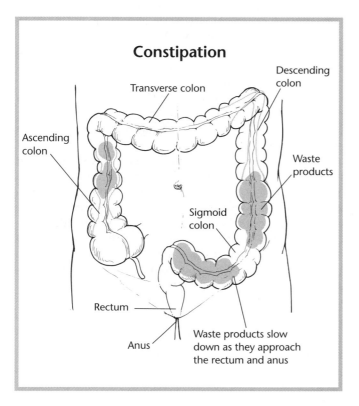

Constipation

Transverse colon

Descending colon

Ascending colon

Waste products

Sigmoid colon

Rectum

Anus

Waste products slow down as they approach the rectum and anus

Who is likely to develop constipation?

Constipation is often a problem for people who have other medical conditions such as hypothyroidism and various gastrointestinal disorders, including irritable bowel syndrome, diverticular disease, and, less commonly, colon cancer (see entries). For unknown reasons, severe constipation that is not caused by a known medical disorder occurs predominantly in young women of reproductive age. Hysterectomy may also increase the incidence of constipation in a small subset of women.

Constipation is often cited as a frequent problem during pregnancy, but many studies indicate that most pregnant women actually experience no change in bowel function. Some evidence even suggests that when there is an effect, it is more often an increase rather than a decrease in frequency. The discrepancy may be due to improved eating habits on the part of some of the women who have been studied, which may have reversed any tendency toward constipation. In any case, there is still no question that some women who previously had normal bowel function do develop constipation during pregnancy. This may be because pregnancy hormones relax intestinal muscles or because the enlarging uterus puts pressure on the colon. In addition, taking prenatal vitamins, which contain high levels of iron, may exacerbate constipation.

How is the condition evaluated?

A doctor evaluating a patient with constipation will first want to make sure that it is not caused by some serious underlying medical condition. In some cases a serious cause of constipation can be ruled out on the basis of the patient's symptoms and a physical examination. Occasionally the sigmoid colon (the lower part of the large intestine) will be examined with a bendable lighted tube called a flexible proctosigmoidoscope to look for abnormalities. The lining of the rectum and colon may also be studied with a special type of x-ray that provides images after infusion of a metallic element called barium, which helps outline the structure of the gastrointestinal tract. Sometimes a doctor may assess the movement of the intestine by measuring the amount of time it takes for radiopaque markers to travel from mouth to anus.

How is constipation treated?

The first line of treatment for constipation involves eating high-fiber foods to stimulate muscle activity in the colon, drinking plenty of fluids, and exercising regularly. Good sources of fiber include fresh fruits and vegetables, bran, prunes, raisins, figs, dates, whole grains, and nuts. Because certain sources of fiber may produce bloating in some people, it is often necessary to experiment with different diets. It may also help to use a bulk stool softener ("natural laxative"), which works by absorbing water in the colon. These products include psyllium (Metamucil, Konsyle, Effersyllium), methylcellulose (Citrucel), calcium polycarbophil (Fibercon), and pectin.

Using other laxatives for a short time can be helpful, but

regular use (more often than a couple of times a month) can increase constipation and lead to dependence. Among the more mild laxatives are mineral oil (such as Haley's M-O) and nonabsorbable sugars such as lactulose, sorbitol, and glycerin. These should be tried before resorting to harsher laxatives such as milk of magnesia, magnesium citrate, castor oil, bisacodyl (Dulcolax), senna, or cascara, which work by irritating the lining of the intestine or by stimulating intestinal contractions.

If the bowel is allowed to fill up and become distended (stretched out of its normal shape) for 2 weeks or so, the nerves that stimulate evacuation may temporarily lose their ability to function properly, and stool may start to "leak" out of the rectum involuntarily. This problem of constipation combined with leakage will continue to get worse unless oral laxatives and suppositories are used to clear the bowel. A woman who has these symptoms should see her clinician for an evaluation. Strong laxatives may be prescribed for a week or so to keep the bowel unobstructed while the nerves and muscles recover their normal shape and function, and milder laxatives may be needed for several weeks thereafter.

Constipation during pregnancy can usually be relieved by eating more high-fiber foods and drinking more fluids. It is also safe to add up to 40 grams (a little more than an ounce) of a bulk stool softener per day, or, if constipation persists, the nonabsorbable sugars. Other laxative use should be limited because of the risk of dependence. Laxatives to avoid are those that contain saline (such as milk of magnesia), which can cause the woman to retain salt; castor oil, which may start uterine contractions; and cascara, which may cause diarrhea in the newborn. Although many women attribute some of their constipation to the iron in prenatal vitamins, the vitamins should be continued if at all possible, at a lower dose if necessary.

How can constipation be prevented?

Constipation can sometimes be prevented in the same way it is treated—by eating a high-fiber diet, drinking 6 to 8 glasses of water daily, getting regular exercise, and following the urge to defecate. Enemas should be avoided, as they can actually promote constipation. In women who find defecation painful following childbirth, using a bulk stool softener can help prevent constipation (and possibly hemorrhoids) from developing.

Related entries

Bowel disorders, colon and rectal cancer, diverticular disease, exercise, hemorrhoids, iron, irritable bowel syndrome, laxatives, nutrition

Contact Lenses

Contact lenses are prosthetic devices that fit over the cornea of the eye, thus helping to refocus the rays of light on the retina. Like eyeglasses, they can be used to correct visual defects such as nearsightedness, farsightedness, and astigmatism (see eye care) and are made to fit an individual prescription. An estimated 20 million Americans today wear contact lenses.

There are two basic types of contact lenses available: hard and soft. Hard lenses come in two forms: regular and gas permeable. Soft lenses are available as regular soft, extended wear, and disposable lenses. Each of these types involves specific advantages and disadvantages, generally involving cost, comfort, and convenience.

Who should consider wearing contact lenses?

Although frequently associated with vanity, contact lenses also have some real practical and even medical benefits. People who participate in sports often find contacts more convenient (and durable) than eyeglasses, while those who rely on their eyesight for work enjoy the greater field of vision provided by contact lenses. Contacts are also better suited than eyeglasses to correcting certain eye conditions (such as corneal scarring and keratoconus, a rare hereditary disease).

Contacts, however, are often a bad choice for people who have conditions such as rheumatoid arthritis of the hands or otherwise impaired coordination, and for people with the condition called dry eye (see entry). People who need bifocals—which correct for both near and far distances—may have difficulty with contact lenses alone, but this problem can be solved if the person is willing to wear half glasses for reading. Bifocal contact lenses are available, but learning to use them can be difficult. For some people, a satisfactory approach may be to correct one eye for distant vision and the other for near vision with two different lenses. This eliminates the need for glasses, but the drawback is limited depth perception, which may make stairs and other uneven terrain somewhat treacherous.

A woman who is considering contact lenses—or who is having problems with her current lenses—should speak with an ophthalmologist (a physician specially trained in the diagnosis and treatment of eye diseases) about currently available options. An ophthalmologist not only will provide up-to-date and accurate information but also will perform a thorough eye examination to determine if the woman has other eye problems and to make sure just which—if any—lenses are appropriate. Above all, a proper fit and correct cleaning and care are essential to the use of all contact lenses.

Hard lenses

Hard lenses, the oldest form of contact lens, are the least expensive over time, the easiest to care for, and the most durable of all contacts currently available. They also provide the sharpest vision, especially if any astigmatism is present.

But it takes longer to adjust to hard lenses than to soft ones, and many people are never able to use them comfortably. Hard lenses also tend to dry out and slip off the cornea onto the white of the eye (sclera)—which is not dangerous but can be irritating and inconvenient. There is some fear that wearing hard contacts over the long term may result in corneal warping or abnormal growth of blood vessels (owing to oxygen deprivation), although most ophthalmologists believe that they are perfectly safe to wear so long as they are fitted properly and are comfortable, and provided the eyes are checked periodically for signs of intolerance.

Hard lenses are placed onto the cornea after being rubbed with a commercial "wetting solution." Most are made of a material called polymethylmethacrylate (PMMA) and can be tinted in various shades to make them easier to locate should they slip in the eye or (as occasionally happens) onto the floor (these shades have no effect on eye color or the visual perception of color). They can be worn for up to 18 hours a day after the initial adjustment period, and need to be soaked each night in a special solution, which can be bought premixed at most pharmacies. Although they should be rubbed between the fingers with special cleaning solutions on a regular basis, care is generally minimal so long as basic rules of hygiene are followed.

Hard contacts should not be worn during sleep, for more than a brief period, or they may adhere to the eyelid. And because they can produce corneal swelling and abrasion, they should be removed at the first sign of pain or other eye irritation. They should also be removed if blurred vision or light sensitivity ever occurs. These can be signs of oxygen deprivation in the eye.

Gas permeable hard lenses

Somewhat easier on the eye are the gas permeable hard lenses, which allow oxygen and carbon dioxide to pass more freely between the contact lens and the cornea. Made of various plastics (such as cellulose acetate butyrate, pure silicone, or polymers of silicone and PMMA), these lenses are slightly more flexible than conventional hard lenses. Consequently, they allow for better flow of tears across the surface of the eye and transmit heat more readily. At the same time, they are just as durable as regular hard contacts and provide vision just as sharp. All of these properties tend to make gas permeable lenses more comfortable than regular hard lenses.

On the minus side, the gas permeable lenses are a bit more expensive than regular hard contacts and also require somewhat greater care (for example, they may need to be cleaned with special solutions).

Soft lenses

For many people, soft contact lenses have been a godsend, making comfortable contact lens wear possible for the first time. Composed of semifluid materials such as hydroxyethyl-methacrylate (HUMA), these contacts are somewhat larger than hard ones. Special toric soft lenses can be used to correct astigmatism (caused by an irregularly shaped cornea).

For the aesthetically minded, there are also soft contacts available in shades that can tint the eye to any desired color or can disguise certain defects of the cornea, iris, and pupil. Because soft lenses have become so popular, they are often readily obtainable, which can be a plus if, for example, a lens is lost or destroyed while one is traveling.

Because soft lenses are more fragile than hard ones, however, they are also more apt to be damaged in the first place—and replacement can be costly. Also, soft lenses may not provide quite as sharp a visual correction as hard lenses, and they are significantly more expensive to fit and replace. They require much more meticulous and frequent care, too, although in recent years the procedures have become considerably streamlined. Now it is usually possible to clean the lenses with special antiseptic and rinsing solutions made for soft lenses rather than by boiling them each night.

Even so, if not cleaned properly (and, according to some eye doctors, perhaps even if they are), soft lenses may predispose the eye to infection or ulcers—which, if left untreated, can result in corneal scarring and loss of vision. In susceptible people the cleaning solutions have been known to produce allergic reactions in the eyes and on the hands and fingers used to handle the lenses. The preservative thimerosal in particular is a common source of eye irritation and hand rashes. Such reactions may be avoided, however, by using an enzyme cleaner weekly (neutralized with a disinfectant) and using newer solutions which do not require preservatives or which use hypoallergenic preservatives. If the eyes ever become red or painful, contact lenses should be removed at once and an eye doctor promptly consulted.

Continuous wear lenses

Continuous wear contact lenses (also called extended wear lenses) are a form of soft lens that can be worn round-the-clock for up to 4 weeks at a time. Originally used by patients who had undergone cataract surgery, they are now more frequently the choice of people who simply do not want the bother of removing and cleaning lenses every single night.

Many ophthalmologists caution that continuous wear lenses tend to be abused by wearers who do not clean them regularly or who wear them beyond advisable limits. This makes the risk of infection much higher than with conventional soft lenses, predisposing the eye to a condition called infectious keratitis (ulcerative keratitis)—an infection caused by bacteria, fungi, or protozoa which leads to ulcers on the cornea.

Deposits of tear film on these lenses can be difficult to remove and increase the possibility of infection and allergic reactions. Many people are also allergic to preservatives in the cleaning and disinfecting solutions, or simply find that the cleaning and disinfecting process is inconvenient and time-consuming. Because they are unusually thin, continuous wear lenses tend to be particularly fragile. They should never be worn by people with corneal conditions such as dry eye or blepharitis (infection of the eyelid). Anyone considering extended wear lenses must have a thorough eye examination first to rule out any problems that may preclude use.

Disposable lenses

Many people find that these "throwaway" lenses are the solution to the cleaning problems often associated with other soft lenses. Disposable contact lenses are worn continuously for a week or two and then are simply tossed out and replaced by fresh lenses. The convenience of this approach is obvious, but the expense can be considerable (approximately $95 for a 3-month supply of lenses, plus the cost of office visits), although this has to be balanced against the expense of the cleaning and disinfecting solutions used with conventional lenses. There is a great temptation to abuse the convenience (and save a little money) by using the lenses longer than recommended. This is truly a penny-wise, pound-foolish practice, since it can result in serious eye infection and injury.

Related entries

Cataracts, dry eye, eye care, glaucoma, macular degeneration, retinal detachment, rheumatoid arthritis

Coronary Artery Disease

Coronary artery disease is a form of heart disease caused by obstructions in the arteries that supply the heart with blood. Although CAD is the number-one killer of both men and women in this country, on average it tends to affect women about 10 or 15 years later in life. This difference is thought to be due to the protective effect of the hormone estrogen in premenopausal women, which seems somehow to stall the progression of atherosclerosis—the process in which fat and cholesterol are deposited in the arteries (see circulatory disorders).

Coronary artery disease is actually a continuum of atherosclerotic conditions, the most mild of which may involve no symptoms. As atherosclerosis progresses, however, scar tissue and other debris are deposited inside the muscular wall of the coronary arteries—the main arteries that supply the heart muscle with blood (see illustration). This can result in angina, a kind of chest pain that often follows exercise or emotional stress. When one or more coronary arteries are seriously narrowed, a heart attack (myocardial infarction) may result.

During a heart attack, cells in part of the heart cease functioning because they are so severely deprived of blood. Unless the blocked artery is opened promptly, this injury will be permanent and, depending on the extent of muscle death and its location, may be fatal. If the heart attack has been precipitated by a blood clot that has lodged in the narrowed artery, as is often the case, it is called coronary thrombosis.

Who is likely to develop coronary artery disease?

Women do not have to worry about one of the major risk factors for coronary artery disease: maleness. The mere fact of being a man increases the odds of developing CAD by a factor of 3.5. Some of this female advantage may be attributable to differences in blood cholesterol levels between men and premenopausal women. The fact that a woman's risk of developing CAD increases greatly after menopause—when blood cholesterol levels take on a more male pattern—lends credence to this possibility.

The biggest risk factor for CAD in women is age. The older a woman is, the greater are her chances of developing atherosclerosis and thus CAD. By the age of 70, in fact, women have just about the same chance of developing CAD as men their age. Ethnicity also plays a role. The rate of CAD is highest in African American men, followed by white men, African American women, and white women. Rates of CAD in Hispanics and people of Asian descent are somewhat lower for both sexes, although data are limited and conflicting. Some of these differences may be related to anatomical or functional differences between the sexes or between ethnic groups, but others may be related to lack of appropriate referral and treatment for older women and minorities (see heart disease).

Many of the same factors that increase a man's chances of developing CAD—including hypertension, diabetes, cigarette smoking, cholesterol levels, family history of heart attack before the age of 60, obesity, and a sedentary lifestyle—also increase a woman's risk. The limited studies that have been done so far, however, suggest that some of these factors affect women differently from men.

Diabetes. Although both men and women with diabetes mellitus are at increased risk of developing CAD, the risk is actually higher for women with diabetes. In fact, this risk is so high (twice that of women who do not have diabetes) that it outweighs any female advantage in avoiding heart disease.

Cholesterol. The significance of various blood cholesterol and lipid levels also varies between the sexes. In women, having low levels of HDL (high-density lipoprotein) cholesterol and high triglycerides may increase the odds of developing CAD, whereas in men high levels of LDL (low-density lipoprotein) cholesterol seem to be more problematic. High levels of triglycerides (a kind of fat molecule) appear to be a risk factor for coronary artery disease in women but not in men (see cholesterol).

Sedentary lifestyle. Whether women are more sedentary than men—and thus at particularly high risk for CAD—remains questionable. Lack of exercise increases the risk of

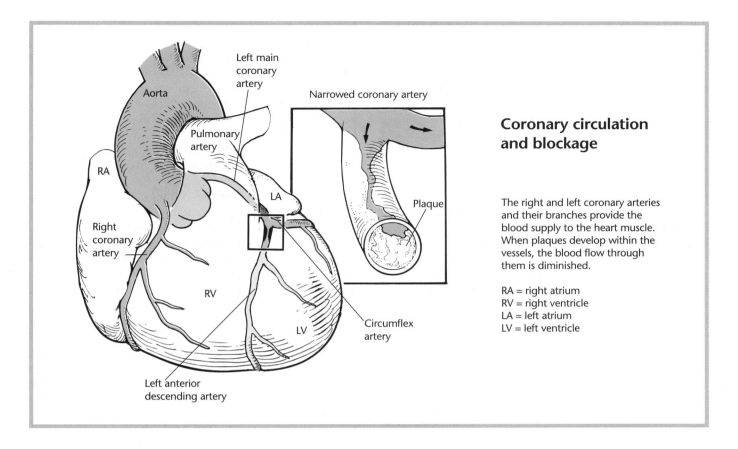

Coronary circulation and blockage

The right and left coronary arteries and their branches provide the blood supply to the heart muscle. When plaques develop within the vessels, the blood flow through them is diminished.

RA = right atrium
RV = right ventricle
LA = left atrium
LV = left ventricle

(Diagram labels: Aorta; Left main coronary artery; Pulmonary artery; RA; Right coronary artery; LA; RV; LV; Circumflex artery; Left anterior descending artery; Narrowed coronary artery; Plaque)

CAD in both sexes, and physical activity levels decrease with age, but it is not clear that women actually get less exercise than men. This is because questionnaires typically used to measure physical activity were developed primarily for men and may overlook the amount of energy that women expend doing housework, caring for children, gardening, and engaging in other nonsport activities. Nevertheless, it is increasingly clear that, however they compare to men, many women are not getting enough exercise. One recent survey, for example, revealed that over 70 percent of U.S. women are underactive, with even lower rates of activity in black and Hispanic women and women of lower socioeconomic status.

Smoking. Middle-aged women who smoke are at greater risk for heart attacks than middle-aged men with similar risk factors. A full 50 percent of heart attacks in women can be attributed to tobacco. As a result, public health officials fear that the recent increase in smoking among young women could seriously increase the amount of coronary artery disease among women in the future.

Obesity. Although obesity is also considered to be a risk factor for CAD in men, this is only because men who are obese tend to have other risk factors for CAD at the same time (such as high blood pressure). In women the mere fact of being obese increases the chances of developing CAD, even in the absence of other factors. Women who have a relatively high waist-to-hip measurement ratio in particular appear to be at increased risk.

Family history. Women with a close relative who experienced a heart attack at a relatively young age—under 55 in males or under age 65 in females—are also at increased risk for coronary artery disease.

C-reactive protein and homocysteine. Regardless of cholesterol levels, women who have high levels of c-reactive protein and/or homocysteine in their blood appear to be at increased risk of CAD as well. At the same time, women who consume relatively large amounts of vitamins B_6 and folate, both of which can decrease homocysteine levels, appear to have lower rates of CAD.

Risk factors unique to women. Women who have had their ovaries removed before natural menopause are at increased risk for developing coronary artery disease. Hysterectomy (the removal of the uterus) does not increase the risks, so long as at least one ovary is retained. Natural menopause, in and of itself, does not increase the risks of CAD either, but it does take away the protective effect of estrogen. Consequently, after menopause the risk of CAD goes up as women age. One might say that it is aging that causes CAD, not menopause; estrogen just delays the aging of the cardiovascular system until later in life.

As for the use of oral contraceptives, recent data indicate that there is no increased risk of CAD in women under 30 or in nonsmoking women over 30—unless these women have other cardiac risk factors. Earlier findings associating birth control pills with heart attacks were based on studies using pills with much higher doses of estrogen and progesterone than those commonly prescribed today. Women over the age of 35 who smoke and use birth control pills, however, are at increased risk for heart attacks.

Women of low socioeconomic status seem to be at increased risk for CAD. In fact, the rate of CAD is 3 times higher for women in blue-collar occupations than for women in white-collar positions. The stress many women experience balancing roles as worker, wife, mother, housekeeper, and caretaker of elderly parents may also indirectly contribute to other risk factors such as smoking, hypertension, and obesity. Some studies have suggested that working women who have an unsupportive supervisor, limited job mobility, or suppressed hostility appear to be at increased risk for developing CAD. Depression may play a role as well; while it is a risk factor for heart disease in both men and women, women are twice as likely to suffer from depression as men.

What are the symptoms?

The symptoms of coronary artery disease range from none at all to angina to heart attack to sudden cardiac death (the instantaneous cessation of heartbeat). Just which symptoms appear depends on the degree of damage in the coronary arteries, as well as on the person's sex.

For many men the first symptom of CAD is a heart attack, but women are more likely to develop the chest pains of angina as their first symptom. And when women do have heart attacks, they are more likely than men to have pain, nausea, breathing difficulties, and fatigue in addition to chest pain. Although men with CAD are more likely than women to experience sudden cardiac death, CAD still accounts for about one-third of deaths from heart disease in women. Two-thirds of these sudden cardiac deaths among women occur without any earlier symptoms of CAD.

How is the condition evaluated?

The three methods most commonly used today to evaluate coronary artery disease are exercise stress testing, perfusion imaging, and coronary angiography.

Exercise stress test. This test, also called exercise electrocardiography or exercise tolerance test (ETT), is used to evaluate the availability of blood to the heart during the stress of exercise. Electrodes attached to wires are pasted onto the arms, legs, and chest, and the heart's electrical activity is measured by a machine while the person walks or jogs on a treadmill.

In most medical centers women with symptoms of heart disease such as chest pain are much less likely than men with similar symptoms to receive a stress electrocardiogram, and when they are given stress tests, their hearts seem to respond differently to exercise than men's and give different readings. Too often women who show signs of CAD on an exercise stress test turn out to have perfectly normal arteries, while women who show no signs of CAD on the test turn out to have blocked arteries. This high rate of false positives and false negatives may be traced in part to the fact that, until quite recently, exercise stress testing was developed and validated primarily on men. The fact that women are less likely to be able to do all the physical tasks required by the test may also help explain some of the false negatives.

Perfusion imaging. This test combines a stress test with a scan of blood flow to the heart; it is often done in conjunction with an exercise ECG or when a resting ECG is abnormal. It involves injecting a small amount of radioactive material into a vein and then using a scanner to detect emitted radiation. The amount of radiation emitted reflects the amount of blood that has reached various parts of the heart muscle.

Women undergo perfusion imaging much less often than men, and their lower tolerance for exercise leads to a high number of false negatives in women who do have thallium stress testing. One solution for women unable to exercise is to use drugs called pharmacologic stressors, which dilate the blood vessels as though the women were actually exercising. Technological improvements, including ECG-gated imaging, newer radioactive agents, and single-photon emission computed tomographic (SPECT) scanning, are all improving the accuracy of diagnoses, however.

Stress tests are designed to stratify risk: they tell the clinician who is likely to have significant (and possibly dangerous) CAD. The results of the tests often indicate whether medicine or surgery should be the next step. If the stress tests are equivocal or ominous, catheterization will be used to assess the exact degree of blockage, and from that the decision can be made whether to do angioplasty or coronary bypass surgery.

Coronary angiography. The most accurate tool to evaluate a woman suspected of having CAD is coronary angiography, also known as cardiac catheterization. In this procedure a catheter (hollow tube) is guided into a coronary artery and then an opaque contrast agent is injected through it to make the blood visible on a moving x-ray image (see illustration). The result is a detailed picture of blood flow to the heart as well as a depiction of any blockages in the arteries. Before a patient undergoes any type of surgery for coronary artery disease, a coronary catheterization must be performed.

Abundant studies suggest that women with abnormal ECGs, typical angina, and risk factors for CAD are much less likely than men to be referred for this test. In addition, because women who do undergo cardiac catheterization tend to be older and sicker than their male counterparts, they are also more likely to experience complications, heart rhythm abnormalities, and hemorrhage (internal bleeding). But women are no more likely than men undergoing this proce-

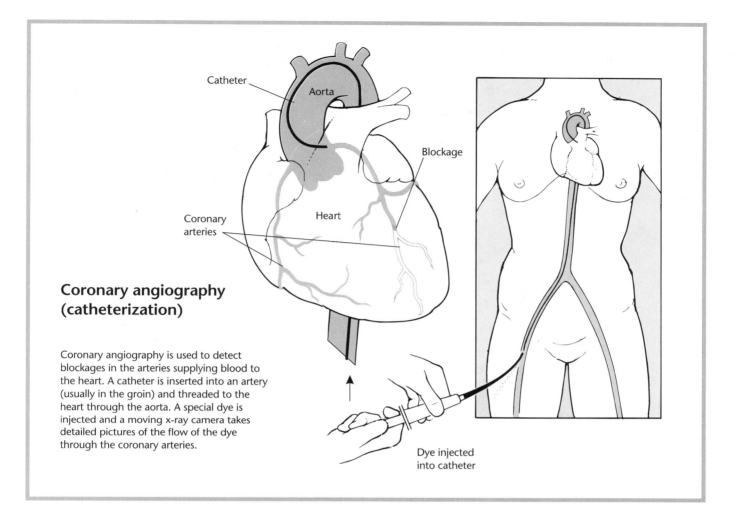

Coronary angiography (catheterization)

Coronary angiography is used to detect blockages in the arteries supplying blood to the heart. A catheter is inserted into an artery (usually in the groin) and threaded to the heart through the aorta. A special dye is injected and a moving x-ray camera takes detailed pictures of the flow of the dye through the coronary arteries.

dure to experience heart attacks, strokes, vascular complications, or allergic reactions.

Even though the likelihood of serious CAD is lower in women than in men overall, if a woman has symptoms and risk factors, her physician should take an aggressive approach to her evaluation, including ordering stress tests and possibly catheterization when circumstances warrant it.

Echocardiography. Interpreting alternative noninvasive tests can also be challenging in women. Echocardiography is a safe, noninvasive test that uses sound waves from the heart to generate an image that corresponds to the direction and velocity of the blood flow when the heart is working hard (stressed). This test, which is particularly useful in detecting blockage in a single blood vessel, is sometimes called "stress echo" because exercise and/or drugs (such as dobutamine) are used to stimulate the heart to beat quickly and strongly before the test. Nevertheless, women are more likely than men to get false-positive or uninterpretable results on these tests because they often have poor exercise capacity or because those tested often have a relatively low probability of disease. Investigations sponsored by the National Institutes

of Health (NIH) are currently under way to determine whether other noninvasive tests—including CT scans, magnetic resonance imaging, and PET scans—may be useful in diagnosing coronary artery disease in women.

How is CAD treated?

Coronary artery disease can be treated with either medication or surgery, together with an effort to control or eliminate risk factors such as high blood pressure and behaviors such as smoking. Just which approach is chosen depends on the patient's age, her general health, and the severity of heart-related symptoms. But in the case of both drugs and surgery, the results are both better studied and better understood in men than in women. Until quite recently clinical trials involving these treatments routinely excluded women, mainly because they were restricted to people under the age of 75, and in women CAD is more likely to occur at a later age.

Cholesterol-lowering therapy. Even before coronary artery disease produces any symptoms, a clinician may prescribe a cholesterol-lowering medication to a woman with high levels

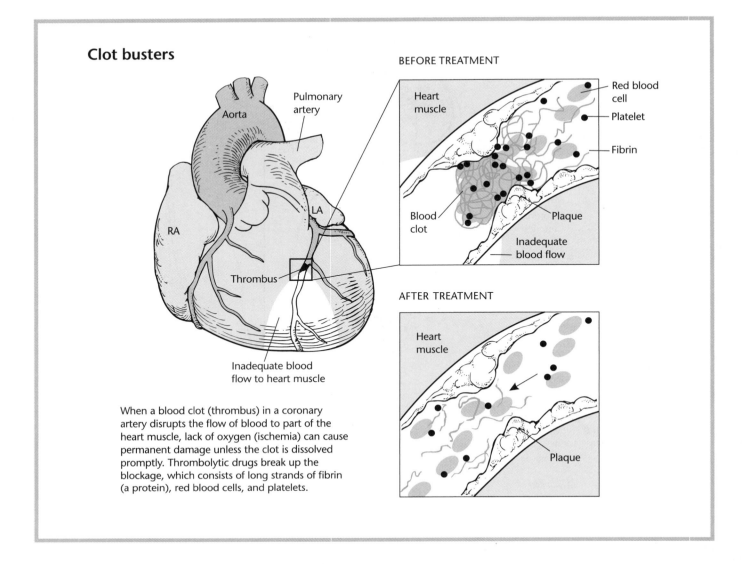

Clot busters

Aorta

Pulmonary artery

LA

RA

Thrombus

Inadequate blood flow to heart muscle

When a blood clot (thrombus) in a coronary artery disrupts the flow of blood to part of the heart muscle, lack of oxygen (ischemia) can cause permanent damage unless the clot is dissolved promptly. Thrombolytic drugs break up the blockage, which consists of long strands of fibrin (a protein), red blood cells, and platelets.

BEFORE TREATMENT

Heart muscle

Red blood cell

Platelet

Fibrin

Blood clot

Plaque

Inadequate blood flow

AFTER TREATMENT

Heart muscle

Plaque

of cholesterol, particularly if she is postmenopausal or has other risk factors for heart disease. There are 5 main categories of cholesterol-lowering drugs: bile acid sequestrants, "statins," nicotinic acid, fibric acid derivatives, and probucol. These drugs work by lowering levels of LDL (the "bad" cholesterol) and triglyceride, by raising levels of HDLs (the "good" cholesterol), or both. These drugs can lower blood cholesterol levels by as much as 30 percent within 6 weeks. Because cholesterol-lowering drugs may affect liver function, however, anyone taking them should have a blood test periodically to check liver enzymes (see entry on cholesterol).

Nitrates. Nitrates (nitroglycerin, Isordil, Ismo) are thought to increase blood flow to the heart by dilating coronary arteries. When used to treat an attack of angina (chest pain), a nitrate tablet is held under the tongue until it dissolves. Other forms can be swallowed for longer-lasting protection against chest pain. Nitrate ointments can also be rubbed directly into the chest or arm, or, for slower release, applied as a patch soaked with nitrate and covered with adhesive plastic; over time,

however, nitrate patches lose their effectiveness. The few studies that have been done on women with angina indicate that nitrates may not be as effective in reducing either the frequency or the intensity of symptoms as in men.

Beta blockers. These drugs work by lowering the heart's demand for blood. Normally the heartbeat is stimulated by chemical messengers sent through the nerves to sites in the heart called beta adrenergic receptors. In a person with CAD, blocked coronary arteries diminish blood supply to the heart, and the nerves respond by sending out plenty of this chemical messenger. The heart beats faster and requires a faster blood flow, but the blocked arteries still cannot respond. The result is the pain of angina.

Beta-blocking drugs relieve this pain by slipping into the sites that would otherwise be filled by the chemical messengers, thus keeping the heart from beating faster and thereby allowing more time for the coronary arteries to fill. Beta blockers can also help reduce the risk of death after a heart attack. Many physicians, however, are still not prescribing these and other relatively inexpensive drugs as often as they should to certain elderly patients, including those who are female, African American, and/or poor.

Beta blockers also slip into beta receptors in other parts of the body, sometimes producing uncomfortable side effects such as breathing difficulties, depression, and fatigue. Propranolol (Inderal), an older beta blocker, may cause such unwanted effects. Some of the side effects can be avoided with the newer beta blockers (called cardioselective beta blockers), which enter only beta receptors in the heart. Atenolol (Tenormin) is a widely used cardioselective beta blocker.

Calcium-channel blockers. These medications keep the arteries from going into spasm and temporarily restricting the flow of blood. Coronary artery spasms are a particularly common cause of chest pain in women. They seem to be switched on by the mineral calcium, which is dissolved in the blood and body fluids and enters channels that begin outside the wall of the blood vessels. Calcium-channel blockers fill these channels, thus preventing the entrance of calcium into the vessel and any resulting spasm (see angina pectoris).

Various calcium-channel blockers are available, including verapamil (Calan), diltiazem (Cardizem, Tiazac), and nifedipine (Procardia), each of which varies somewhat in its efficacy against different aspects of CAD. Often it is necessary to try more than one of these drugs before the optimal one is found.

Thrombolytic therapy. If CAD has progressed to the point of a heart attack, drugs that dissolve clots may be employed. This is called thrombolytic therapy (see illustration).

For a clot-busting drug to work, it has to be administered within a few hours of the attack. Two recently approved clot-busting drugs, lanoteplase and tenecteplase, can be given in a quick, single shot during a heart attack, making it easier than ever to meet this deadline. Because these drugs can potentially be used even before a patient reaches the hospital, they may allow the early treatment that can make a huge difference in the amount of heart damage and chances of survival. Even so, thrombolytic therapy of any sort seems to produce less benefit in terms of survival for women than for men, and it more frequently causes serious bleeding complications in women. Part of the explanation may be that we still do not understand very well how weight, age, and sex affect the optimal dose of a clot-busting drug.

Heart attacks in women are usually more severe when they first occur than in men, and women are more likely to have additional health problems, in large part because they are older on average than men who have heart attacks. All of these factors may make them less appropriate candidates for thrombolytic therapy. The decision as to which therapy is optimal must be made by the individual patient and her physician.

Aspirin, another form of thrombolytic therapy, has become a mainstay in the treatment of CAD. Technically aspirin does not break up existing clots, but it does stop them

Conventional balloon angioplasty

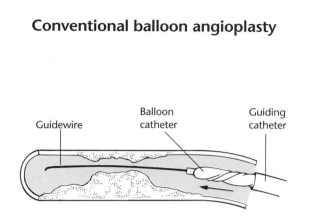

A guiding catheter is positioned in the opening of the coronary artery and a thin, flexible guidewire is pushed down the vessel and through the narrowed artery. The balloon catheter is then advanced over this guidewire.

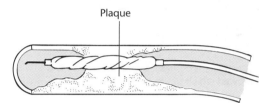

The balloon catheter is positioned next to the atherosclerotic plaque.

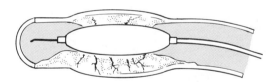

The balloon is inflated, stretching and cracking the plaque.

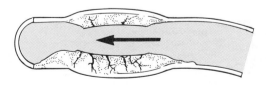

When the balloon is withdrawn, blood flow is reestablished through the widened vessel.

Coronary stent

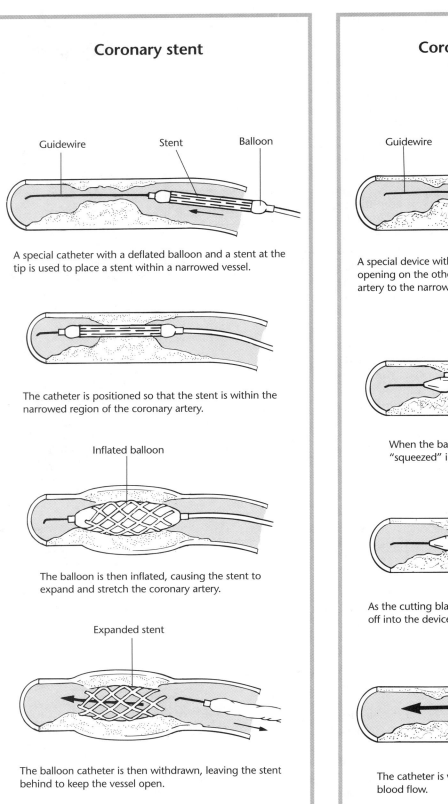

Guidewire   Stent   Balloon

A special catheter with a deflated balloon and a stent at the tip is used to place a stent within a narrowed vessel.

The catheter is positioned so that the stent is within the narrowed region of the coronary artery.

Inflated balloon

The balloon is then inflated, causing the stent to expand and stretch the coronary artery.

Expanded stent

The balloon catheter is then withdrawn, leaving the stent behind to keep the vessel open.

Coronary atherectomy

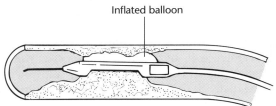

Guidewire   Deflated balloon   Atherectomy device   Cutter

A special device with a deflated balloon on one side and an opening on the other is pushed over a wire down the coronary artery to the narrowing.

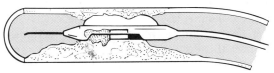

Inflated balloon

When the balloon is inflated, part of the plaque is "squeezed" into the opening of the device.

As the cutting blade is rotated, pieces of plaque are shaved off into the device.

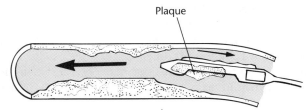

Plaque

The catheter is withdrawn, leaving a larger opening for blood flow.

from increasing in size. For this reason aspirin is given immediately to any person suspected of having a heart attack in progress. It is also given to people with known CAD to reduce the chances of future heart attacks and stroke. Aspirin seems to be equally effective in men and women. Several studies suggest, however, that women—as well as African Americans and the poor—are less likely to receive aspirin and other inexpensive therapies than other patients with similar conditions.

Balloon angioplasty. In this surgical procedure the physician inserts a thin catheter with a balloon at the end into the affected artery and pushes it into the blocked area. As the balloon is expanded, it pushes the obstruction aside and opens up a passage for blood flow. Conventional balloon angioplasty (along with its more recent relatives coronary stent, and atherectomy; see illustrations) has been performed commonly on women and is now accepted as a standard procedure for unclogging blocked coronary arteries. It is especially effective in treating relatively short areas of blockage or when used in people under 65 years of age or who have had symptoms for only a short time. Balloon angioplasty is often preferred over thrombolytic therapy for heart attacks in medical centers with the facilities to perform the procedure quickly.

Balloon angioplasty can occasionally result in serious complications. These include a torn artery or the formation of a blood clot which, if not corrected immediately, can cause a heart attack rather than prevent one. These complications are very rare when the procedure is performed by an experienced cardiologist. Of more concern is the fact that arteries will narrow again within a year in 1 out of 3 patients who undergo conventional balloon angioplasty, and that may necessitate a repeat procedure or even a more complex procedure such as coronary bypass surgery (see below).

Despite the fact that men who receive balloon angioplasty usually have more advanced CAD than women, women who have this procedure experience a lower rate of success at clearing the obstruction and relieving chest pain. Originally it was thought that these differences might be due to the smaller size of women's arteries, so cardiologists tried using a smaller balloon. This modification has made very little difference. Now cardiologists believe that women's relatively greater age and coexisting health problems account for their higher risk of complications.

Even so, balloon angioplasty is still a good option for many women, particularly because the long-term outcome for men and women is similar, except that chest pain tends to recur more often in women. And when the procedure is successful at opening women's arteries, their blood vessels are less likely than men's to become blocked again.

Coronary bypass surgery. In this operation a short piece of vein or other graft material from the thigh or the internal mammary artery (IMA) from the chest is grafted onto a narrowed coronary artery to reroute blood around a blockage (see illustration). There is abundant evidence that this sur-

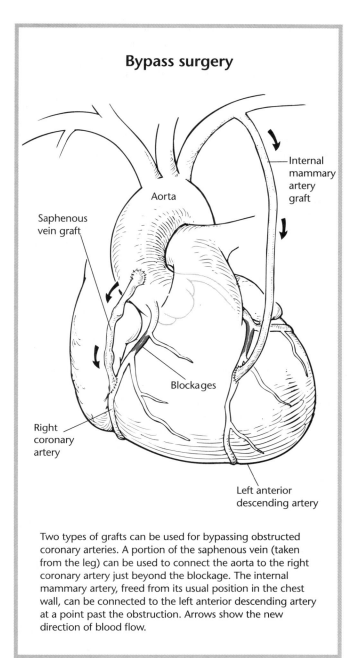

Bypass surgery

Two types of grafts can be used for bypassing obstructed coronary arteries. A portion of the saphenous vein (taken from the leg) can be used to connect the aorta to the right coronary artery just beyond the blockage. The internal mammary artery, freed from its usual position in the chest wall, can be connected to the left anterior descending artery at a point past the obstruction. Arrows show the new direction of blood flow.

gery is effective in relieving anginal pain that has not responded to medications, as well as for CAD in 3 arteries or in the left main coronary artery. About half of all people who have had this procedure remain free of pain 5 years after the surgery.

Even so, bypass surgery is not something to be undertaken lightly. It cannot prevent atherosclerosis from developing in the new grafts. In fact, some studies indicate that as many as 4 out of 5 people who have had bypass surgery develop life-threatening blockages in the graft within 10 years of surgery. The IMA seems less prone to subsequent blockages than a vein from the thigh; since this artery is increasingly being used, the problem may become less significant (although IMA bypasses are technically more difficult to perform).

There is still no consensus about whether bypass surgery actually lengthens life expectancy—except in the case of severe obstruction, in which bypass surgery can mean the difference between life and death. Although both sexes are equally likely to be alive 5 to 10 years after bypass surgery, women are about twice as likely as men to die during or soon after the operation. This may be due in part to differences in body and blood vessel size in women, as well as to the fact that many women undergoing bypass surgery are older, have advanced disease, or have other serious health problems such as diabetes, hypertension, or congestive heart failure. More often than not, too, a woman having bypass surgery is in an emergency situation, and mortality rates therefore tend to be higher. Also, many of the studies of mortality in women were done when techniques of bypass surgery were less advanced than they are today. Using the internal mammary artery and routine antiplatelet therapy to prevent blood clotting has reduced mortality rates in both sexes.

All of these factors may help explain why women with symptoms of CAD may be less likely than men to be offered coronary bypass surgery, although they do not explain why African Americans of both sexes are less likely to undergo coronary artery bypass procedures for CAD than are whites. Yet, given the high cost of bypass surgery—not to mention the relatively high risk of complications and the risk of death from these complications (which vary from doctor to doctor and from hospital to hospital)—not having this surgery, or any other surgery, is not necessarily a bad thing. The consensus is that women with mild or moderate angina run no particular risk from delaying surgical procedures for CAD until they have first tried relieving their symptoms with drugs, diet, and exercise.

How can coronary artery disease be prevented?

Coronary artery disease is the product of a number of variables (see chart), some of which (such as family history) cannot be controlled. It is nonetheless possible to lower the risk of CAD by changing certain habits that may precipitate risk factors. Giving up cigarettes, for example (or, better yet, never starting to smoke them), cuts the risk of mortality from CAD in half. More than 60 percent of heart attacks in women under the age of 50 can be attributed to cigarette smoking, and women who stop smoking after a heart attack have a longer life expectancy than women who continue to smoke.

For women with high blood pressure, controlling blood pressure lowers risk of future CAD substantially. As for improving blood fat and cholesterol levels, it is becoming clear that the benefits in women are similar to those in men, although recent studies have suggested that there is some benefit in raising the relative proportion of high-density lipoprotein (HDL) to low-density lipoprotein (LDL) cholesterol and lowering triglycerides (see cholesterol). Usually clinicians advise women to begin by increasing exercise and eating a relatively low fat diet, and, if necessary, to use medications to control high blood cholesterol or lipid levels.

Major risk factors for CAD in women

Factors that increase risk:

- Age >55 or premature menopause
- Diabetes
- Family history of sudden death before age 55 years, premature coronary heart disease, or heart attack
- Current cigarette smoking
- High blood pressure (>140/90 mm/Hg, or taking blood pressure medication)
- LDL cholesterol >160

Factors that decrease risk:

- HDL cholesterol >60

Despite some well-publicized studies on both sides of the question, the effects of moderate amounts of alcohol on blood lipid levels remains controversial. Compared with nondrinkers, women who consume 3 to 9 drinks a week appear to have a somewhat lower risk of heart disease, probably because alcohol seems to elevate levels of HDL cholesterol. The same effect appears to occur in men as well. This potential benefit has to be weighed against the well-known risks of alcohol consumption in women, which include alcohol dependence and liver damage (see alcohol), as well as the potentially increased risk of breast cancer.

There is growing evidence that weight loss is an effective strategy against CAD. The link between obesity and CAD in women has been well established. But even a weight gain of 10 to 20 pounds in a middle-aged woman increases her future risk of coronary disease, according to some recent studies. Women who are overweight and have other risk factors for CAD should work with a clinician to find a safe and effective means of weight control.

Women (as well as men) who have Type I (insulin-dependent) diabetes (see entry) may be able to decrease their risk of heart disease by controlling their blood sugar level and using intensive insulin therapy. Whether this "tight control" is equally effective in people with Type II diabetes is a question that requires further investigation.

Some evidence suggests that daily use of small dosages of aspirin (1 regular strength or baby aspirin per day) in women over 50 can reduce the chances of having a heart attack. For patients who have had a heart attack, many clinicians recommend using aspirin and beta blockers to reduce the risk of a second heart attack. This therapy, widely prescribed for men, should be promoted for women as well.

Specific dietary practices may also help prevent CAD as well, especially when combined with regular physical activity, maintenance of a healthy body weight, and avoidance of smoking. Evidence continues to accumulate that using non-hydrogenated unsaturated fats as the predominant form of fat in the diet and whole grains as the main form of carbohydrates, and eating abundant fruits and vegetables and adequate omega-3 fatty acids (found in fatty fish and oils such as canola and soybean), can provide significant protection against heart disease.

Related entries

Alcohol, angina pectoris, arrhythmia, cholesterol, circulatory disorders, congestive heart failure, diabetes, dieting, estrogen replacement therapy, exercise, heart disease, high blood pressure, nutrition, obesity, smoking, varicose veins, weight tables

Cosmetic Dentistry

Cosmetic dentistry encompasses a variety of techniques designed to improve the appearance of teeth. Sometimes called aesthetic restorative dentistry, this field has been growing by leaps and bounds in recent years, yielding numerous new procedures and materials that make it easier and safer than ever before to straighten misaligned teeth, fill gaps and cracks, and even whiten stains. Increasingly, dental offices are equipped with digital cameras and sophisticated graphics software that allow a patient to assess a proposed cosmetic procedure in advance by creating images of reshaped, repositioned, and/or whitened teeth.

Some of these techniques have distinct health benefits—such as improving nutrition or helping to prevent gum disease—and most are invaluable in boosting self-esteem, body image, and (for people in certain professions) even employability.

These benefits carry a hefty price tag, however, which often must be paid out-of-pocket by the patient (unless the teeth problems can be proved detrimental to one's physical health). As a result, many of cosmetic dentistry's most impressive innovations are not used as much as they might be. Moreover, it may be years before we can state with certainty the strengths, weaknesses, and limitations of many of these offerings. The rapid-fire pace at which materials and techniques keep appearing means that the newer procedures in particular still need to be undertaken with a certain degree of caution.

Among the various techniques and devices now available to alter the appearance of the mouth and teeth are crowns, bonding, veneers, and bleaching; orthodontia (see entry); and dentures, bridges, and implants (see entry). Among these, only bonding, veneers, and bleaching are usually classified as cosmetic because they are most often done primarily for aesthetic reasons (when less expensive alternatives may be available to solve the purely physical problems). But health and aesthetics are not mutually exclusive. Many so-called cosmetic procedures also have distinct health benefits. Conversely, aesthetics are often an important consideration in procedures primarily done for reasons of dental health. Witness adult orthodontia—which is not generally considered cosmetic dentistry but is done just as much (if not more) because of concerns about appearance. People who choose to use implants in lieu of dentures or bridges to replace their missing teeth are generally motivated to pay the considerable difference in price for reasons of aesthetics, comfort, and convenience.

Deciding which of the many available dental techniques is most appropriate to solve a cosmetic problem depends not only on the nature of the defect (crooked or discolored teeth, bite problems, cracks, gaps, and so on) but also on a woman's cosmetic standards, the overall health of her teeth and gums, and, of course, her personal finances. Most women can achieve perfectly respectable results with the most conservative of today's cosmetic techniques—that is, crowns, bleaching, and direct bonding. If teeth are badly damaged or discolored, however, or if longer-lasting restorations are needed, more extensive techniques may make sense. People who have little money but a lot of time may be able to afford the more expensive procedures by having the work done at a dental school.

Just which kind of dentist performs these procedures varies from one practice to another. Many dentists commonly perform at least some cosmetic dentistry procedures, while others refer patients to specialists, particularly for more involved procedures such as dental implants. Among the dental specialists who may be consulted are oral surgeons (who treat diseases and defects of the jaw, face, and mouth), prosthodontists (who manufacture and fit artificial devices for defective or missing teeth), orthodontists (who correct misaligned teeth and bite problems), and periodontists (who treat gum disease).

Tooth bleaching

Dentists have been actively trying to bleach teeth since the mid-nineteenth century to remove unsightly stains and restore natural color. Until recently, however, most of these attempts were inordinately expensive, dangerous, ineffective, or all of the above. There has been a marked resurgence of interest in tooth bleaching lately, largely because of the advent of what appear to be fairly simple, safe, and effective home-bleaching techniques. Although today's methods are still rather costly, the embarrassment caused by tooth discoloration can be so distressing that many people consider the price more than justified.

Teeth can become stained by substances such as tobacco, coffee, tea, and berries, as well as by deposits of tartar (calculus). Internal discolorations can also result from certain illnesses and from exposure to excess fluoride. Sometimes an injury to the mouth will produce a single darkened tooth. A person whose mother took the antibiotic tetracycline during pregnancy may also have particularly noticeable yellow, brown, or purple discolorations. This type of stain is notoriously difficult to remove. Most dental insurance policies will not pay for tooth bleaching, though they may cover the bleaching of tetracycline-stained teeth. Tetracycline-stained teeth can be lightened with extensive bleaching but can rarely be thoroughly whitened; irregular lines and splotches remain visible even after treatment.

There are two principal means of tooth bleaching that are recommended today: home bleaching and office bleaching. Both of these techniques, which must be done under the supervision of a dentist, involve hydrogen peroxide (or carbamide peroxide, which breaks down into hydrogen peroxide and urea). The peroxide is thought to work through a chemical process known as oxidation, which either removes some of the unattached organic matter from the tooth without dissolving the protective enamel or changes the discolored portion of the tooth to a colorless form.

Home bleaching. Also called passive bleaching or dentist-prescribed home bleaching, this is today the most popular means of removing stains from one or more teeth. The whole procedure costs about $200–$500, depending on the dentist and region of the country.

The patient must first visit a dentist and have an impression made of the teeth, from which a special rubberlike Mylar tray (carrier) will be built to fit over the teeth. This customized tray is then taken home, together with a bleaching kit that consists of several small syringes and some bleaching gel. Certain bleaching kits instruct patients to put a small amount of gel into the tray and to cover the teeth to be bleached with the tray while they sleep. Other brands are used for 1 to 2 hours twice a day or as little as a half hour per day, depending on the tooth's initial shade and the degree of whiteness ultimately desired. Because the gel is very viscous and the tray is custom-fit, only a minuscule amount of gel is swallowed or even reaches the gums.

If home bleaching is done according to directions, it is usually quite effective within about 2 to 3 weeks. Since teeth tend to darken with time, most dentists recommend bleaching the teeth to a slightly lighter shade than is ultimately desired.

Office bleaching. Because office bleaching involves stronger concentrations of peroxide, it generally works much faster than home bleaching. But good results require anywhere between 2 and 10 weekly appointments, so the cost for office bleaching can be considerably higher. And because stronger concentrations of bleaching agent are used, the chances of temporary tissue irritation are somewhat higher than with home bleaching. For all of these reasons, office bleaching is rarely done now that home bleaching has become widely available.

Like home bleaching, the office procedure is usually painless and requires no anesthesia. It can sometimes be a bit uncomfortable, largely because a rubber dental dam (the same kind of latex square used in root canal operations) is placed over the necks of the teeth to be bleached to protect the gums from caustic chemicals. Once the dam is in place, a protective gel is rubbed over the gums, and the bleaching agent is painted onto the teeth. Each bleaching session generally takes about 45 minutes. Office bleachings may need to be touched up about once a year.

Some patients prefer to have their teeth bleached with an even newer, and faster, technique that involves using a laser beam ("power bleaching") to activate a high concentration of hydrogen peroxide applied to the teeth. The precision and speed of this approach—which requires only a single two- to three-hour office visit—is understandably appealing. Nevertheless, whether this procedure whitens teeth even more than regular gel treatment is a matter of considerable controversy. In addition, many dentists still do not use this procedure because the cost (as much as $1,000 or more) is hard to justify, given the availability of effective and long-lasting, less costly alternatives.

Over-the-counter bleaching kits. A third means of bleaching—involving the use of various bleaches sold without prescription at many drug stores—is generally considered only marginally effective at best. Some of these kits work like the dentist-prescribed systems, except that the mouthpiece (tray) is not custom-made. Others require a three-step process that involves a tooth-cleansing rinse, a peroxide rinse, and a polishing cream. Despite television ads to the contrary, studies so far suggest that these kits do not work—and even raise some concern that they may possibly damage tooth enamel.

Without a custom-fitted mouthpiece the bleaching agent in these kits is more likely to spill over onto sensitive gum tissue. In addition, using over-the-counter kits inevitably reduces the odds that teeth will be professionally evaluated before treatment begins. As a result people are apt to attempt bleaching without first learning the reason for the discoloration (so recurrence of the problem is much more likely) and without ever getting a baseline ("before") picture of the teeth (so there is nothing to measure success against). Over-the-counter kits also preclude the kind of monitoring and instruction that can help minimize the risks of treatment.

How safe is bleaching? With the exception of pregnant and breastfeeding women, who should probably avoid bleaching teeth until more is known about the effects, adults who want to (and can afford to) whiten their teeth should feel comfortable with either form of dentist-supervised bleaching. If directions are followed, side effects are rare, although some people may experience temporary gum irritation or some tooth sensitivity to hot and cold. There is still some concern, however, that bleaching agents may erode enamel from the teeth, permeate a "leak" in a filling and harm a tooth's nerve, damage materials used for restorations, or irritate surrounding gums to the point of permanent damage. So far, however, the various small studies indicating such problems have been contradicted by equally small studies indicating just the opposite. Until better data are available, the safest course of action is probably to use bleaching cautiously.

There is also fear that bleaches have the potential for misuse and abuse, since some people may start using them repeatedly in an endless quest for whiter teeth. Such fears have some justification, but the same can be said for other supposedly "safe" dental products such as fluoride-containing toothpastes or rinses and alcohol-containing mouthwashes. Ensuring the absolute safety of any procedure is difficult, and ultimately the risks of bleaching have to be viewed in the light of risks of other, more accepted dental procedures such as crowns and ceramic inlays (extensive fillings). Many of these other procedures also carry a small degree of risk but are usually accepted unquestioningly, the assumption being that the benefits of the procedures far outweigh the risks. Indeed, because these procedures are so well accepted, few people even consider that there may be any risk at all. The same argument can be made for tooth bleaching, at least given the limited knowledge of risks currently available.

Crowns

Crowns are coverings for teeth that are severely decayed, chipped, damaged, discolored, or misaligned. Crowns (or caps) are also sometimes necessary after a root canal operation or to cover a cracked (fractured) tooth that cannot be repaired with a regular filling. Sometimes damaged teeth can be repaired with another cosmetic technique called bonding (see below), but if a molar—which is subject to high levels of wear and abrasion—or badly fractured or decayed tooth is involved, a crown will probably be necessary.

Two separate office visits are usually required to fit and place a crown. In the first visit the dentist removes any decay that may be present and shapes the tooth into a base for the crown. An impression is made of this base and is sent to a laboratory so that a custom-made crown can be manufactured out of gold, porcelain, or porcelain fused to metal. A temporary crown is placed over the tooth stump. On the next visit (usually about 2 weeks later), the dentist removes the temporary crown and cements the custom-made crown over the original tooth. If the tooth is severely damaged, a metal post may be inserted for additional support. Often local anesthesia is used during these procedures.

This elaborate procedure can be cut to under 15 minutes, however, if the dental office is equipped with a new system that makes the impression, temporary crown, and second office visit unnecessary. The dentist simply "scans" the tooth with a cameralike device that then sends a "picture" of the tooth to a milling machine in another room. This machine cuts the restoration out of solid ceramic, and within minutes the crown or inlay is ready for placement. This technology is still inconsistently reliable, however, and is not yet widely used.

Crowns last between 5 and 15 years, depending on how well the teeth are cared for and the material used. Because food and plaque can easily be trapped around the gumline and adjacent teeth, it is important to brush and floss along the edges of the crown. Should a crown ever fall out, the material should be saved (outside of the mouth) and the dentist called immediately for an appointment. In the meantime, the teeth should be brushed and flossed as usual.

Bonding

Bonding can involve any of a number of procedures in which tooth-colored, puttylike materials (called composite resins) are applied to the teeth to repair chips, cracks, and gaps. Often done to improve appearance, this procedure is also a way to repair and protect broken teeth. In people with gum disease, for example, composite resins may be applied to the tooth roots, which are sometimes exposed as the gums recede. These roots are covered by dentin, a softer material than the enamel that covers the rest of the tooth and thus are particularly susceptible to decay, as well as unusually sensitive to extremes of temperature.

Composite resins can also be used to fill small cavities in decayed teeth. This is particularly desirable in front teeth, since the resins, being tooth-colored, are much less conspicuous than other fillings. Composite resins are less durable than fillings and inlays made of silver amalgam (an alloy of mercury, silver, copper, and other metals), gold, or porcelain, however, and tend to stain.

Bonding is usually a simple procedure that can be accomplished in a single visit and rarely requires anesthesia or drilling. The dentist first treats the tooth's surface with a special acidic "etching" solution to promote adhesion. Resins are then blended to match the tooth's natural color, applied to the teeth, and contoured into shape. The resins are then dried and hardened under a bonding light for 20 to 60 seconds, after which they are smoothed and polished. Some dentists prefer to do the polishing as part of a second, follow-up appointment.

Some dietary changes and other changes will be necessary to keep the bonding material from chipping and staining. Most dentists recommend avoiding cigarettes, coffee, tea, and berries—all of which are likely to stain the resin. Highly acid foods and alcohol should also be avoided, since they can damage the resins. In addition, chewing on ice, popcorn kernels, hard candy, and the like—or using the teeth as tools—can put excess pressure on bonding material and lead to cracks.

Despite the most valiant efforts, however, some periodic chipping may occur after about 3 to 5 years because bonding material is simply not as strong as natural tooth enamel. In such cases, the composite resins will have to be replaced.

Veneers

An offshoot of tooth bonding, veneers are another option for women whose teeth are permanently stained or discolored, who have small gaps between the front teeth, or whose teeth are poorly shaped or misaligned. Made from acrylic, composite resins, or porcelain, veneers are custom-made shells that adhere to the surface of teeth in much the same way that false fingernails adhere to the nails. They are more expensive than bonding and are generally used for more severe problems, so long as the supporting tooth structure is healthy and free of decay.

Like the composite resins used for tooth bonding, veneers are affixed directly to the tooth, usually without any need for anesthesia. Two separate visits are necessary. The first appointment involves preparing the tooth for the veneer by removing a small amount of enamel. An impression of the tooth is made and sent to a dental laboratory, where a veneer will be produced to match the tooth's shape and color. The patient returns to the office once this veneer is ready. A mild etching solution (such as phosphoric or hydrofluoric acid) is applied to the front of the tooth to roughen its surface and facilitate adhesion. Then the veneer is placed on the tooth, held in position with composite resins, and hardened with a bonding light.

With the help of special video cameras and computers, it is now possible to have a veneer made and fitted all in a single sitting—without the need for additional appointments or tooth impressions. Nonetheless, for most dentists—and patients—the trade-offs involved are not worth the convenience: not only are there still certain problems with the fit of these computer-fabricated veneers, but also the cost can be exorbitant.

Although veneers sometimes fracture, chip, peel, slip, or discolor, they can be repaired. Good oral hygiene and regular dental visits minimize the chances of staining and cracking. This includes avoiding activities that put excess pressure on the veneer—such as fingernail chewing or chomping on ice cubes—as well as eschewing cigarettes and heavily pigmented foods such as coffee, tea, red wine, and berries. The latter precautions may be less important with the newer porcelain (cast ceramic) veneers, which have properties quite similar to those of natural tooth enamel in terms of looks, durability, and stain resistance. On the minus side, veneers made of porcelain also tend to be quite costly and can take an unusually long time to manufacture.

Related entries

Antibiotics, body image, coffee, dentures/bridges/implants, gum disease, nutrition, orthodontia

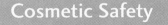

Cosmetic Safety

Despite the tendency among Americans to assume that any well-advertised product must have been tested for safety and effectiveness, the cosmetics industry is only loosely regulated by the Food and Drug Administration (FDA), and there is still little correlation between the price and the performance of cosmetics.

Still, some self-regulation by the cosmetics industry has reduced the credibility of companies that tout magic ingredients such as royal queen bee jelly, turtle oil, shark oil, pigskin

extracts, chick embryo extract, or horse blood serum. Most of the products currently on the market seem to be reasonably safe. Whether they make some objectively measurable difference or not, cosmetics can make women feel pampered and beautiful, and only the individual woman can determine if the boost to self-esteem in itself justifies the price.

Cosmetics versus drugs

The FDA defines a cosmetic as a product "intended to be rubbed, poured, sprinkled, sprayed on, introduced into, or otherwise applied to the human body or any part thereof for cleansing, beautifying, promoting attractiveness, or altering appearance." Under this definition, manufacturers of cosmetics are allowed to claim that their cosmetics do just about anything, so long as they do not claim that they affect the "structure or function of the human body" (in which case the product is treated as a drug).

This does not mean that manufacturers can put anything they wish into a cosmetic. They are prohibited from using specific toxins—in particular, biothional, chloroform, halogenated salicylanilides, hexachlorophene, mercury compounds (except as preservatives in eye makeup), methylene chloride, and vinyl chloride and zirconium salts (in aerosol products).

Many cosmetics do include substances such as hormones and vitamins which, in other preparations, most certainly affect the structure or function of the body. But so long as a product is labeled a cosmetic, the manufacturer is under no obligation to substantiate claims for what these vitamins and hormones can do. And though labels must contain a list of ingredients in the order of prevalence, the average consumer may find many of the chemical names indecipherable.

Although the FDA currently requires nonprescription cosmetics containing estrogens to state that they do not include sufficient hormone to rejuvenate the skin, there is good evidence that these products do have enough of the hormone to produce feminizing effects such as premature breast development in young girls or abnormal vaginal bleeding in women past menopause.

And though it is true that vitamins A, D, E, K, and some in the B complex group are necessary in the diet to help maintain healthy skin and hair, this does not mean that directly applying these vitamins to the skin or hair will have the same effect. That is why the FDA currently requires vitamins to be listed by chemical name only in the list of ingredients. They argue, along with many dermatologists, that the likelihood of vitamins' penetrating the epidermis or the outer cuticle of hair is extremely small. Some manufacturers claim that they have evidence to the contrary, but they are in something of a catch-22 situation: if it turns out that vitamins actually can penetrate skin, the FDA would have to classify products containing them as drugs.

Cosmetics testing

Some manufacturers routinely conduct premarketing tests to evaluate the safety of their products, a practice that has led to a great deal of outrage about animal testing. The Cosmetic Toiletry and Fragrance Association, the industry's major trade group, also sponsors the Cosmetic Ingredient Review, a safety evaluation of cosmetic ingredients conducted by a panel of scientists.

If a cosmetic already on the market is suspected of causing allergic reactions, manufacturers are generally willing to provide clinicians with samples for individual testing—even though the offending ingredient may not be revealed unless an individual has an adverse reaction. Many manufacturers even report manufacturing and formulation information and any identifiable problems to a voluntary databank at the FDA. This databank is incomplete and often out of date or inaccurate, but it at least allows the government to accumulate some baseline information about the relative safety of certain categories of cosmetics. Federal law provides that any cosmetic which leads to an adverse skin reaction can be returned for a full refund.

Cosmetics and cancer

Currently, no convincing evidence has associated cosmetics with any form of cancer, in spite of the fact that some products do contain low levels of known carcinogens. Examples are nitrosamines, which can cause liver cancer in mice and which seem to contaminate certain cosmetics at very low levels. Although these chemicals are absorbed through the skin, they have not been linked to liver cancer or any other type of cancer in humans who use these preparations. Another carcinogenic contaminant of cosmetics, 1,4-dioxane, is so volatile that it probably evaporates before it has a chance to penetrate the skin.

Skin irritations

There is substantial underreporting of the adverse effects of cosmetics—if only because no formal mechanism is in place to collect consumer complaints. For this reason it makes sense to watch out for problems commonly associated with cosmetics. This is particularly true for fair-skinned, fair-haired, blue-eyed women, who seem especially prone to skin reactions, as well as women with acne and other troublesome skin conditions or allergies. Most skin reactions seem to occur with facial makeup and hair products, particularly those containing fragrances, preservatives, and lanolin. It also makes sense to discard mascara (however pricey) after 4 to 6 months to minimize the chance of bacterial contamination, which can cause eye irritation or infection.

Many dermatologists feel that some ingredients in makeup—such as lanolin and D and C red dyes, which are often used in blush—may clog facial pores, altering skin growth and encouraging the development of acne. Others disagree. Rashes and redness that occur almost immediately after contact with a cosmetic are usually due to direct irritation by some chemical in the product. If a rash develops only after the product has been used a second or subsequent time, it is more likely to be due to sensitization, an allergic reaction that occurs when the body develops an immune reaction to some chemical in the product. Other rashes may develop only after skin covered with the cosmetic is exposed to the sun. This process is known as photosensitization.

The term "sensitive skin" is usually used to describe skin that burns or tingles or develops a rash when certain cosmetics are used. Skin that has been damaged or inflamed, either by the environment or by physical injury, is said to be compromised. Various surveys of cosmetic users have shown that 50 to 75 percent believe they have sensitive skin. Any woman who thinks she has sensitive or compromised skin should use only products labeled hypoallergenic. Hypoallergenic products are those with a lower rate of associated allergic reactions than other cosmetics in the same category. Other terms used to describe hypoallergenic products are "allergy-tested," "noncomedogenic," "preservative-free," "fragrance-free," "PABA-free," "clinically tested," "nonirritating," "nonsensitizing," "irritant-free," and "safe for sensitive skin." None of these terms is a guarantee that a woman with sensitive skin can use these cosmetics with impunity, however. It always makes sense to test products on a small, inconspicuous area—such as the crook of the elbow—before attempting any widespread application. A dermatologist may need to be consulted if a woman continues to have problems finding cosmetics that she can use safely.

Related entries

Acne, body image, body odors, cosmetic surgery, dermabrasion and chemical peels, eyelid surgery, face lifts, hair care, hair dyes, nail care, skin care and cosmetics, skin disorders, wrinkles

Cosmetic Surgery

Cosmetic surgery is surgery done to change a person's appearance for aesthetic rather than medical reasons—although there may also be medical benefits. It involves the techniques of plastic surgery, a field of medicine in which surgery is used to repair or rebuild damaged or abnormal tissues.

Among the most common plastic surgical operations done for cosmetic reasons are face lifts (rhytidectomy); nose jobs (rhinoplasty); breast enlargement, reconstruction, or reduction surgery (mammoplasty); and fat removal (lipectomy and liposuction). There are also procedures available to correct wrinkled eyelids or the bulges under the eyes (blepharoplasty), pin back the ears (otoplasty), strengthen the chinline (mentoplasty), alter the jawline (mandibuloplasty and maxilloplasty), remove wrinkles (rhytidoplasty), augment the cheekbones (malarplasty), and smooth over old pockmarks and acne scars (dermabrasion).

Women considering cosmetic plastic surgery should first arrange for a consultation with a plastic surgeon to discuss which surgery, if any, may be appropriate, as well as the limitations of the surgery, its potential risks, and its costs. At the same appointment the surgeon will ask the woman about her medical history and current physical condition. "Before" photographs will be taken either at this time or at some subsequent visit before the operation, and a computerized image of the body part in question may be manipulated to suggest the end result. Of course, the idealized picture on a computer screen does not necessarily reflect the real end result, which is ultimately a product of the surgeon's skill and the individual patient's physical makeup.

A reputable surgeon will clearly delineate the risks and benefits of each procedure and make a conscientious effort to nip unrealistic expectations in the bud. Women should be extremely wary of any surgeons who promise 100 percent success and satisfaction or who do not fully disclose the range of potential complications.

Some medical doctors who perform cosmetic surgery have not been specifically trained in this subspecialty. One way to find a skilled surgeon is to get names from other women who have had a similar operation and have been pleased with the results. Often a primary care physician can suggest a competent surgeon with particular expertise in the type of cosmetic surgery a woman desires. To ensure that the surgeon has been trained in both general and plastic surgery and is properly accredited, check with the American Board of Plastic Surgery. It is equally important to check the accreditation (by the American Association for Accreditation of Ambulatory Surgery) of the facility in which surgery will be performed, especially because so many cosmetic surgeons now perform surgery in their own suite of offices or "minihospitals."

How is cosmetic surgery performed?

Women often assume that their form can be changed drastically by cosmetic surgery. Surgery, though, involves natural processes of healing, scarring, and swelling. The surgeon tries to harness these processes to bring about the desired result, but there will naturally be some imprecision. Although these techniques can often make a dramatic difference in a woman's appearance, anyone expecting perfection is bound to be disappointed. It is important that a woman understand how her surgeon is planning to deal with the components of the human form—skin, fat, and muscle—in the context of the specific procedure that is appropriate for her. Most forms of cosmetic surgery involve the removal of excess skin and underlying tissue, coupled with tightening and smoothing of the remaining skin. Some procedures involve implants, skin grafts, or reshaping of bone as well.

Cosmetic surgery may be done on an outpatient basis or in the hospital, depending on the nature of the operation and the personal preferences of both the surgeon and the patient. Many procedures require general anesthesia, and some require hospitalization after surgery.

Because cosmetic surgery is an elective procedure, most insurance companies are not willing to pay for any part of the operation. Exceptions may occur, however, if the procedure is done to alleviate some physical symptom. For example, some policies will cover part of a rhinoplasty if it is done to correct a breathing problem, or may pay for breast reduction surgery if pendulous breasts are producing severe back pain or shoulder pain.

What are the risks and complications?

Despite the adjective "cosmetic," cosmetic surgery is still surgery. Skin is cut open, sensitive nerves and blood vessels are manipulated, and anesthetics are used. Risks follow accordingly. Of course, women who choose this form of surgery are often in better overall health than people undergoing surgery for debilitating physical problems. But this does not mean that there will be no pain, discomfort, and temporary incapacitation, nor does it eliminate the risk of infection, bleeding, nerve damage, or complications of anesthesia.

In addition, although cosmetic surgeons make every effort to leave inconspicuous scars, some people simply scar more visibly than others and may end up with unsightly keloid scars in the site of the surgery. Any woman who has developed a keloid scar following any other surgery or wound should be very cautious about undergoing cosmetic surgery. Plastic surgeons are often willing to show potential patients photographs of abnormal scarring to inform them about this particular risk (see keloid scarring).

To minimize the chance of complications, women should always tell the plastic surgeon about any previous or current health problems—particularly diabetes, high blood pressure, asthma, allergies, mental illness, kidney disorders, heart disease, medication use, or substance abuse—as well as any past bleeding or anesthesia-related problems during surgery and any previous abnormal scarring. Cigarettes, alcohol, and certain medications (including aspirin, antihistamines, and estrogens) can increase the risk of bleeding problems or other complications and should be discontinued prior to surgery. Smoking should be discontinued for as long as possible prior to surgery.

What happens after surgery?

Most people have some stiffness for several days after the operation, and in many procedures swelling and bruising will be noticeable for 2 or 3 weeks, prompting many women to avoid social engagements or work for that period of time. In most cases recovery is complete within 1 to 6 months.

It is unrealistic to expect cosmetic surgery to correct miraculously all the emotional and psychological problems that may have gone into the decision to have the surgery in the first place. A woman who has suffered for years with a specific defect may indeed find that her self-esteem and self-confidence are greatly improved after surgery. But no cosmetic change is going to fix a bad marriage, ease the pain of divorce, or protect a woman from the aging process indefinitely. No one should have cosmetic surgery immediately following a family or personal crisis, since stress can actually slow down the recovery after surgery and may affect the decision to have surgery in the first place.

For many women, too, deep disappointment occurs when the physical results fall short of expectations. Many a woman has entered the operating room unrealistically hoping for perfection, only to go home to find that she does not look the way she expected to look. Computer "after" images can be particularly deceiving. There is a small but real chance that a woman will end up less satisfied with her new appearance than with her original one. And, of course, results of cosmetic surgery do not last forever; although surgery can be repeated, there is a limit to the number of times skin can be trimmed and stretched with aesthetically pleasing results.

Related entries

Anesthesia, body image, breast implants and enlargement, breast reconstruction, breast reduction, dermabrasion and chemical peels, eyelid surgery, face lifts, keloid scarring, lipectomy and liposuction, otoplasty, rhinoplasty, skin care and cosmetics

Cryosurgery

Cryosurgery is a technique in which liquid nitrogen is used to destroy tissue by freezing it. It is used most often to treat mild to moderate cervical dysplasia (abnormal cell growth), a form of precancerous cell changes that can develop into cervical cancer if left untreated (see cervical cancer). Cryosurgery (also called cryotherapy) is also sometimes used to treat benign (noncancerous) growths on the cervix such as polyps, endometriosis involving the cervix or vagina, and genital warts, a form of sexually transmitted disease (see entries).

Cryosurgery is frequently used by dermatologists to treat actinic keratoses (precancerous conditions caused by the sun) and warts, among other things.

How is the procedure performed?

Usually done in a doctor's office, cryosurgery requires no anesthesia and takes only a few minutes. After inserting a speculum into the vagina, the doctor touches the affected area with a metal-tipped cryoprobe which is cooled by a compressed gas. This sometimes produces a sensation of cold or mild cramping. After the frozen tissue is sloughed off, a scab will form and is eventually replaced by new tissue.

What happens after surgery?

After surgery some women may have a watery vaginal discharge for up to 3 weeks and should not have sexual intercourse or use tampons during this time. A follow-up Pap test should be scheduled for 3 months after cryosurgery for dysplasia. Until the cervix heals (which takes about 3 months), a Pap test may falsely reveal abnormal cells. In a few women, scarring after cryosurgery can make future Pap tests difficult to interpret.

What are the risks and complications?

Although cryosurgery occasionally leads to bleeding, infection, or in rare cases infertility from scarring, it is still a much less risky (and less painful) procedure than electrocautery, which was formerly used to treat the same conditions and is still sometimes used by clinicians who do not have access to cryosurgery equipment. If available and affordable, laser surgery or electrosurgical loop excision (LEEP) may be used as alternatives to cryosurgery in the treatment of certain conditions, and may be especially advantageous in treating large abnormal areas.

Women considering these procedures should discuss the options with a clinician. Often the clinician's personal preferences and level of experience with a given technique has more bearing on surgical outcome than the technique itself.

Related entries

Cervical cancer, electrocautery, electrosurgical loop excision, endometriosis, genital warts, laser surgery, Pap test, polyps, skin disorders

Cushing Syndrome

Cushing syndrome is a disorder caused by excess levels of glucocorticoids, hormones that regulate metabolism. Glucocorticoids are produced by the adrenal glands. These glands lie on top of the kidneys and consist of two parts: an inner core (medulla) and an outer layer (cortex). Controlled primarily by signals sent from the pituitary gland, the adrenal cortex produces 2 types of hormones called corticosteroids: sex hormones (androgens and estrogens in both men and women) and glucocorticoids (which regulate metabolism and also have antiinflammatory effects).

The most common cause of Cushing syndrome is the long-term use of steroids, often prescribed for asthma and rheumatoid arthritis.

Who is likely to develop Cushing syndrome?

When Dr. Harvey Cushing, a renowned American surgeon, first identified this disorder, he attributed the excess of glucocorticoids to a noncancerous pituitary tumor called an adenoma. Today this particular problem is called Cushing *disease* and occurs most often in women of childbearing age.

Cushing *syndrome* may result from a variety of conditions associated with increased production of glucocorticoids from the adrenal glands. Taking steroids (such as Prednisone) is the most frequent cause of Cushing syndrome. A tumor of the adrenal glands themselves (which may or may not be cancerous) or a cancerous lung tumor may also produce this disorder.

What are the symptoms?

Cushing syndrome includes a gradual rounding and reddening of the face; the development of a "buffalo hump" of fat between and above the shoulder blades; stretchmarks on the skin, especially the abdomen; fatigue and muscle weakness; water retention; delayed wound healing; and a tendency to bruise easily.

In women with Cushing syndrome, menstrual periods stop or become irregular, excess body hair starts to grow (a condition called hirsutism), the voice deepens or becomes hoarse, and acne appears or worsens. These symptoms are due partly to the virilizing properties of glucocorticoids and partly to the excess production of androgens (a condition called hyperandrogenism) which often occurs in Cushing syndrome.

Cushing syndrome predisposes women to serious diseases such as hypertension, osteoporosis—loss of bone density, especially in spinal and pelvic bones, which can lead to fractures—arteriosclerosis and heart attacks, peptic ulcer disease, and diabetes. It may also produce sleep disorders, mood swings, depression, manic depression, and other psychiatric disturbances.

How is the condition evaluated?

To diagnose Cushing syndrome a physician will first consider the combination of symptoms and history of steroid use. If a woman is taking a corticosteroid drug to treat some other condition, diagnosis is fairly simple. Otherwise, determining the cause of Cushing syndrome involves further tests, many of which can be done in an outpatient setting.

Specialized blood and urine tests can check for high levels of glucocorticoids. Levels of adrenocorticotropin (ACTH, the pituitary hormone that stimulates the adrenals to produce glucocorticoids) may also be tested directly. An initial screening test called the dexamethasone suppression test (or low-dose DST) can determine whether Cushing syndrome is present. The drug dexamethasone is given orally the night before the test, and then the level of glucocorticoids in the blood plasma is measured the next morning. Normally dexamethasone suppresses glucocorticoid levels; but if this does not happen, a more extensive (and reliable) dexamethasone test (high-dose DST) will be done, in which the drug is taken orally every 6 hours for 2 days and plasma hormone levels are monitored accordingly. If the results of this test are also abnormal, further testing is performed to determine whether the underlying problem stems from the adrenal gland, the pituitary gland, or (rarely) a hormone-producing tumor in another organ. This testing can include additional blood and urine studies and a CT scan or MRI.

How is Cushing syndrome treated?

If Cushing syndrome results from excessive doses of steroid medication, treatment consists of gradually stopping use or decreasing the dosage of these drugs. It is crucial, however, not to stop using steroids without consulting a physician, because sudden termination can lead to acute adrenal failure. Also, for up to a year after steroid medication has stopped, any kind of injury, infection, or surgery can put undue stress on the adrenal glands' function and lead to a dangerous underproduction of adrenal hormones. This can result in symptoms of adrenal insufficiency such as severe vomiting, diarrhea, dehydration, loss of consciousness, and possibly death. Any woman who uses or has recently stopped using artificial steroids should therefore think seriously about carrying some form of identification (a necklace, bracelet, or card) in case she requires emergency treatment, and she should certainly inform all physicians who may be treating her of her status.

If symptoms are caused by a tumor of the pituitary (in which case the diagnosis is Cushing *disease*), treatment usually involves removal of the tumor by an experienced surgeon and possibly irradiation of the pituitary gland as well. Sometimes an endocrinologist will prescribe drugs that can inhibit the production of glucocorticoids.

Adrenal tumors can be removed surgically. If one adrenal gland is removed as well, the woman will need to take pills that replace glucocorticoids for 6 to 12 months. If both are removed, lifelong cortisone treatment is required. Sometimes long-term cortisone therapy is also needed after the removal of an adrenal tumor.

How can Cushing syndrome be prevented?

Cushing syndrome cannot be prevented, although the chances of developing it can be reduced if steroids are prescribed at the minimum effective dosage for the treatment of other illnesses.

Related entries

Acne, amenorrhea, antiinflammatory drugs, asthma, autoimmune disorders, depression, diabetes, edema, fatigue, hirsutism, hyperandrogenism, manic-depressive disorder, obesity, osteoporosis, rheumatoid arthritis, sleep disorders

Cystocele, Urethrocele, and Rectocele

A cystocele is a condition in which the bladder bulges into the front of the vagina. Also called a fallen or dropped bladder, it occurs when the pelvic muscles that normally hold the bladder away from the vagina are weakened. Weakened pelvic muscles can also cause the urethra to bulge into the vagina, leading to a condition called a urethrocele, which often occurs together with a cystocele. In a rectocele, the rectal wall bulges into the back of the vagina, again because of weakened pelvic muscles.

Who is likely to develop these conditions?

Cystoceles, rectoceles, and urethroceles (see illustration) most commonly occur after childbirth and are usually caused by the stretching of the pelvic muscles that support the va-

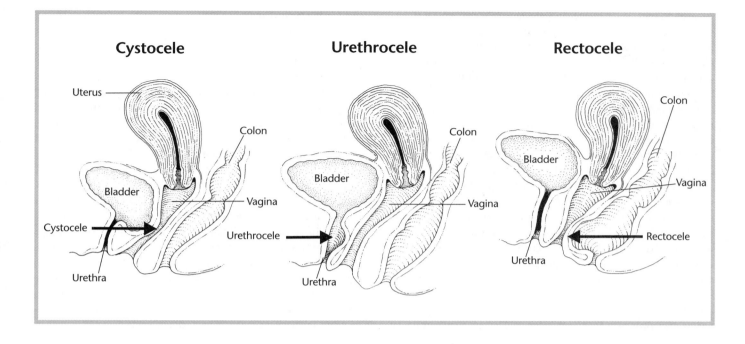

gina, rectum, and bladder. Symptoms may develop only after menopause, when loss of estrogen further weakens supporting tissues. Stretched and weakened muscles are particularly common if a woman has given birth to very large babies or has had many pregnancies or long, difficult labors. Another condition that results from weak muscles, and often accompanies these three, is a prolapsed uterus (see entry), in which the uterus drops down into the vagina.

What are the symptoms?

Women with a cystocele, rectocele, or urethrocele may notice pressure or aching in the vagina, as well as difficulty with urinating and with penetration during sexual intercourse. Stress incontinence, a condition in which urine leaks out when a woman laughs or coughs, is another common symptom. Cystoceles seem to predispose women to urinary tract infections, with symptoms such as burning during urination and an urgent need to urinate frequently. Rectoceles can cause a feeling of pressure or discomfort during a bowel movement, as well as constipation.

How are these conditions evaluated?

A clinician can easily detect a cystocele, urethrocele, or rectocele during a routine pelvic examination.

How are cystoceles, urethroceles, and rectoceles treated?

Minor symptoms of all three conditions may be relieved by practicing Kegel exercises (see entry), which involve alternately contracting and relaxing the pelvic floor muscles. For postmenopausal women, estrogen replacement therapy is often recommended to help reverse some of the atrophy of the pelvic support tissues.

If the discomfort is severe or if frequent urination or uri-

nary incontinence interferes with daily activities, a cystocele or urethrocele can be corrected with surgery in which the bladder is pushed upward and sewn into position. If this procedure fails to correct incontinence, the surgeon may try a different procedure in which the angle of the bladder opening is altered through an abdominal incision. Because these forms of surgery can be painful and may involve a lengthy recovery period, alternate treatments for incontinence (such as medications that promote urinary retention, or insertion of a vaginal pessary) may be tried first.

If symptoms of a rectocele are severe, this condition can also be corrected by surgery. The surgeon makes an incision along the back wall of the vagina, pushes the rectum back and up, and sews it into its normal position.

Related entries

Estrogen replacement therapy, incontinence, Kegel exercises, menopause, prolapsed uterus, urinary tract infections

Dentures, Bridges, and Implants

Until recently it was the rare individual who made it beyond middle age without losing most, if not all, of her teeth— mainly because of advanced gum disease (see entry). Recent improvements in oral hygiene now allow many more Americans to keep more of their teeth for a lifetime, but tooth loss remains a sizable problem.

Anyone who loses her teeth (or even one permanent tooth) should seriously consider a prompt replacement—and not only for the sake of appearance. Each tooth plays a role in keeping the other teeth in line, so that a single missing tooth can ultimately alter the bite (the way the top and bottom teeth meet) and sometimes even make chewing and speaking difficult. If back teeth are lost, the whole character of the face may change as adjacent teeth shift to fill vacant spaces, producing pouches on the sides of the jaw, sunken cheeks, taut and thin lips, and an upwardly jutting chin. Missing teeth can also predispose the mouth to decay and disease.

The three principal solutions to the problem of missing teeth—dentures, bridges, and implants—all have their advantages and disadvantages. A number of different factors should be reviewed in consultation with a dentist or dental specialist, including aesthetics, convenience, comfort, functionality, cost, and hygiene, as well as the health of the teeth and gums and the amount of remaining underlying bone.

Dentures

Often the only alternative to toothlessness until quite recently, dentures are removable sets of artificial teeth. If all the teeth are missing (or need to be extracted), dentures consist of a full set of teeth in a plastic frame that covers the gums as well as part of the upper palate. If a few healthy teeth remain, they are specially prepared to provide stability and support for a special kind of denture (called an overdenture) designed to fit right on top of the remaining teeth. Sometimes a root canal will be performed first to remove the nerve supplying the remaining teeth. People who wear overdentures need to have their roots cleaned every 6 months or so, just as if the teeth were still intact.

People who are missing just a few teeth but whose gums are too weak to support a fixed bridge (see below)—or who find the cost too high—can also have a partial denture made. In this device the artificial teeth are attached to a metal or plastic base with clips at the end. This entire device then fits into the space where the tooth (or teeth) is missing. People who cannot wear regular dentures or whose dentures are loose and uncomfortable may want to consider implant-supported dentures (see below). These provide more stability and allow wearers to eat a greater variety of foods than do traditional dentures.

It usually takes 4 or 5 visits to the dentist to have dentures properly made and fitted, and several follow-up appointments for minor adjustments. In the initial visits worn teeth may have to be extracted and impressions made of the toothless gums. It is often necessary to wait some time between these two steps, since gums can change their shape as they heal from the extractions. Women concerned about being toothless in the interim can sometimes have "immediate dentures" ready and waiting as soon as the teeth are removed. If the jaw changes shape as it heals, however, proper fit can be problematic.

Because artificial teeth wear down eventually and underlying bone and gums shrink with age, dentures usually must be replaced at some point. The time can range from 1 year to

over 5 years and depends on a number of factors, some of which cannot be controlled very much by the denture wearer (such as the materials used and the overall health of the jaw). What denture wearers can do to increase the longevity of the denture is to pay careful attention to fit and maintenance. Dentures that fit well should not require any adhesive to stay snugly and securely in the gums and—after the initial period of adjustment—should rest comfortably in the mouth. In the first few weeks, however, it is normal for dentures to feel loose or bulky, for the tongue to feel crowded, and to experience some soreness while chewing.

Some people also find that they salivate more in the early weeks, and some even feel nauseated. All of these adjustment problems are usually overcome once the muscles of the cheek and lip have time to adjust. In the meantime, it often helps to eat soft foods and to chew with the back teeth as much as possible to help train the gums and to keep the dentures from tipping sideways. Soon it will be possible to go back to a more normal diet, although certain permanent changes in eating habits may be necessary—such as slicing whole apples or removing corn kernels from the cob. If dentures feel loose or uncomfortable, or if the lips and cheeks feel sore after the initial adjustment period, a visit to the dentist or prosthodontist is in order.

Dentures have to be checked periodically for fit and to make sure that there are no problems with bone loss (which may occur because of reduced chewing pressure in the jaw) or mouth sores. Bone loss in the jaw is accelerated by aging, lost teeth, and ill-fitting dentures. Signs of problems include loose lower dentures, mouth pain, and inflamed gums. Sometimes bone loss can be corrected with metallic supports implanted in the bone or operations to build up tissues in the gum or jaw.

Good oral hygiene is extremely important for wearers of both full and partial dentures to keep the devices free of food particles and plaque. These devices should be rinsed thoroughly with water after meals and removed each night to give the gums a rest. At night the dentures need to be rinsed again and gently brushed with a denture cleanser and a denture brush or soft-bristled toothbrush. The denture cleanser should be rinsed off completely to prevent gum irritation. To avoid warping, full dentures should be stored in water overnight (sometimes together with a denture cleaning agent), though partial dentures with a metal base should not be soaked in cleaning agents for more than about 15 minutes. To help maintain gum strength, the exposed gums should be stimulated with a brush, cloth, or finger massage. Any remaining natural teeth should still be brushed and flossed as usual.

Bridges

Bridges are artificial teeth that are permanently attached to adjoining natural teeth. They can be used to replace up to 4 adjacent front teeth or up to 2 adjacent side teeth in people whose remaining teeth are still healthy and who have adequate gum and root support. Because they are fixed permanently in the mouth, bridges are often more appealing than partial dentures, though partial dentures may still make more sense for people who are likely to lose additional teeth (because of gum disease, for example) or who are on a fixed budget. Not only are these considerably less expensive than bridges, but also they can be more easily altered if necessary to accommodate additional false teeth. A 3-tooth porcelain-to-metal bridge can cost in the range of $2,000 to $3,000 or more.

It usually takes 2 or 3 visits to the dentist to have a bridge installed. In one common style, called a fixed bridge, the artificial teeth are attached to a metal framework with artificial crowns (caps) at either end. These crowns are placed over natural teeth (abutments) on either side of the gap after the teeth have been filed down to accommodate them. In another common style of bridge, called a bonded (or Maryland) bridge, the adjoining natural teeth simply serve as anchors that support metal wings fastened to one or more artificial teeth, bridging the gap between them. In this style of bridge there is no need to file adjoining teeth. A third type of bridge—known as an implant-supported bridge (see below)—may be used by people who cannot wear regular dentures or whose dentures are loose and uncomfortable, as well as in people who want to avoid having adjoining teeth filed to hold a regular fixed bridge.

Whatever type of bridge is used, recovery from the installation is generally rapid, and no changes need to be made in eating habits or diet.

Keeping bridges clean can be challenging because these devices are fixed in the mouth. Although they themselves cannot become decayed, they easily trap food and plaque, which can promote decay and gum disease elsewhere in the mouth. People who wear bridges therefore need to be scrupulous about brushing and flossing after each meal. Because flossing in particular can be cumbersome, dentists sometimes provide a special floss threader or interdental cleaner to make it easier to clean between the teeth.

Implants

Implants are artificial tooth supports anchored permanently in the jaw by natural bone. When attached to artificial crowns, bridges, or dentures, they can replace a single tooth, multiple teeth, or an entire set of upper or lower teeth respectively.

The idea of implants (also known as osseointegration) can be traced back to the work of the Swedish investigator Per-Ingvar Brånemark, who in the 1950s discovered that titanium implants could be structurally integrated into living bone without being damaged or permanently inflaming the soft tissue. Brånemark is credited with finding ways to implant foreign objects into the gums while still protecting them from excessive heat (as would be produced by a high-speed drill, for example), infection, or inadequate support by surrounding bone.

Because they are convenient, comfortable, and permanent, implants are often a welcome alternative for people who cannot tolerate conventional dentures—whether for emotional or physical reasons. An added plus is that by allowing chew-

ing pressure that nearly mimics that of natural teeth, they help prevent the bone in the jaw from deteriorating. However appealing they may be in theory, though, implants are by no means a realistic choice for everyone with a missing tooth or teeth. For one thing, they can work only in people with healthy gums and enough bone to support them (although various bone augmentation procedures may sometimes be used to restore normal contour using bone from the chin, jawbone, or other places). Not everyone with missing teeth is willing to commit to the scrupulous oral hygiene required for successful implant use. Nor is everyone willing to undergo the lengthy process required to have an implant placed, which takes something on the order of 3 to 9 months to complete. Usually one or more surgical procedures are necessary—done either in the specialist's office, outpatient clinic, or hospital—with monthly checkups in the interim.

Finally, implants are unaffordable to many otherwise willing and able candidates: even patients with good dental insurance often discover that their plan will cover only conventional dentures to replace missing teeth, the argument being that these are the cheapest solution to the problem. It may be possible to have at least some of the surgical costs of implants covered by medical insurance if there are underlying health problems, and some insurers now cover the prosthetic part (crowns) of the implant procedure. In general, implants themselves cost about the same as bridges, since the added price of the implantation procedure itself is relatively minor (unless hospitalization is necessary).

The implantation procedure (see illustration) is usually performed by a dental specialist, most commonly a periodontist (who specializes in treating gum disease) and sometimes by an oral surgeon (who treats diseases and defects of the jaw, face, and mouth). A single-tooth implant can sometimes be done with only a local anesthetic; multiple implants usually require a local anesthetic with supplemental sedation or, rarely, general anesthesia. The specialist first makes an incision over the implant site, drills the bone with a low-trauma instrument, and screws or presses a metal fixture into the jawbone. There are three main types of supporting fixtures; the choice depends both on the number of teeth to be replaced and on the amount of supportive bone underlying the gums. The root form (or cylinder), which requires the most underlying bone, involves screwlike anchors that are set into the bone. If there is some degree of bone loss, a blade (or plate) fixture may be used instead, especially if there are still some natural teeth remaining in the jaw, but this procedure is rarely used. Finally, when bone loss is so extensive that inserted fixtures would impinge on underlying nerves, a frame can be molded to the surface of the bone and implanted under the covering membrane. This is known as a subperiosteal fixture.

Once the fixtures are in place, the implantation site is covered and left alone for several months until bone grows around it. (Meanwhile, the patient can have conventional dentures readjusted to replace the missing teeth temporarily.) Once the fixture is integrated into natural bone, the top of

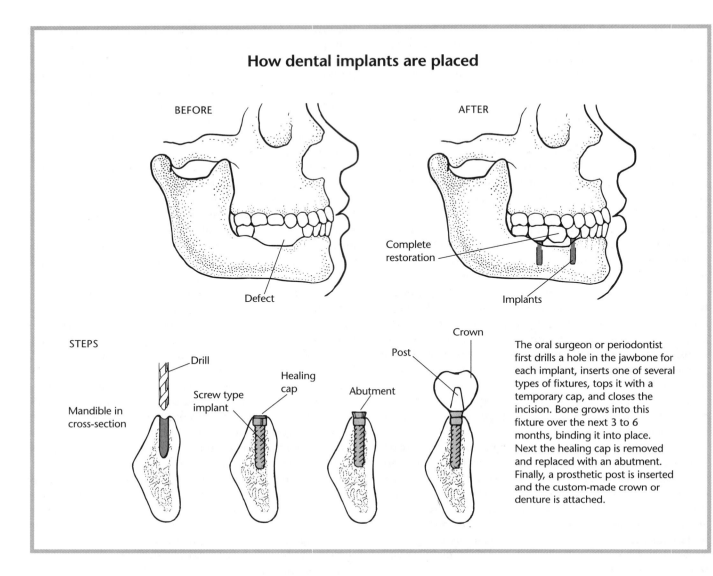

How dental implants are placed

BEFORE

AFTER

Defect

Complete restoration

Implants

STEPS

Mandible in cross-section

Drill

Screw type implant

Healing cap

Abutment

Post

Crown

The oral surgeon or periodontist first drills a hole in the jawbone for each implant, inserts one of several types of fixtures, tops it with a temporary cap, and closes the incision. Bone grows into this fixture over the next 3 to 6 months, binding it into place. Next the healing cap is removed and replaced with an abutment. Finally, a prosthetic post is inserted and the custom-made crown or denture is attached.

the fixture is exposed and—if this has not been done in the original surgery—small holes are punched in the gum tissue that covers it. Then a knoblike abutment which passes through the soft gum tissue is attached to the end of the fixture. About a week or two later, the dentist makes a cast of the jaw so that artificial teeth can be customized to fit on top of the abutments. These artificial teeth are screwed or snapped into place.

During the 1- to 2-week recovery period after the initial implantation, gums may be bruised or swollen, sometimes to the point where prescription painkillers may be required. Eating soft foods or resorting to a liquid diet may be necessary until the gums have had a chance to heal. Many dentists also prescribe antibiotics to prevent infection. People with a lowered resistance to infection—such as those being treated with steroids—are at increased risk of complications.

Caring for implants is much the same as caring for a bridge—and requires scrupulous brushing and flossing to remove food and plaque. Using a small, tapered toothbrush is often helpful in cleaning hard-to-reach areas, and a special interdental cleaner may make flossing considerably easier.

Related entries
Anesthesia, antibiotics, cosmetic dentistry, gum disease, orthodontia, Sjögren syndrome

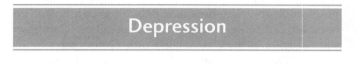

Depression

Depression encompasses a wide variety of emotional and mental states, ranging from sadness and low self-esteem to disabling apathy and suicidal behavior. It may develop in reaction to some outside event, such as the death of a loved one, or it may have no apparent cause. The former is called reactive depression and the latter clinical depression.

Psychiatrists further divide depression into types depending primarily on the severity and nature of symptoms. In women the most prevalent types of depression are dysthymia (once called depressive neurosis) and major depression. Dysthymia usually begins during childhood or adolescence and is characterized by sadness, negative attitude, and low self-esteem. Major depression involves similar but much more severe, sometimes intolerable symptoms. It usually begins in the late 20s but may occur at any age. A related mood disorder is manic-depressive disorder (see entry), which is marked by cycles of mania and depression.

At the molecular level depression is thought to be caused by inadequate numbers of neurotransmitters in the brain. This disturbance can result from numerous physical illnesses, as well as reactions to certain medications, including beta blockers, diet pills, tranquilizers, oral contraceptives, and alcohol. Some people are particularly vulnerable to depression for genetic reasons; the disorder is more likely to occur in people whose parents or siblings have a history of depression.

But there are other risk factors for depression that do not readily lend themselves to a biological explanation: a history of sexual or physical abuse, marital discord, or having children under the age of 5 at home, as well as living in poverty or in an urban environment, to name a few. In a given individual the ultimate explanation for depression may be a constellation of interrelated factors—sociocultural as well as biological. Being a member of a stigmatized group (a minority or a lesbian, for example) may increase a woman's risk for depression.

What are the symptoms?

Everybody is sad or blue now and then because of job loss, death of a loved one, a failed romance, and the like. Clinical depression occurs when this sadness lasts longer than it should or when it is intense enough to interfere with normal functioning. Depressed people feel persistent numbness, helplessness, hopelessness, worthlessness, and guilt. They generally lose interest in life, work, and other activities previously found pleasurable, including sex. Life may feel so gloomy or meaningless that suicide seems the only solution—and is sometimes attempted. For others, particularly adolescents, the apparent solution may come in the form of alcohol and substance abuse, which can lead to further depression.

Many people with depression have trouble thinking, concentrating, remembering, responding, and making decisions, and some experience hallucinations or delusions, as well as anxiety and psychosomatic disorders (see entries). They also commonly have physical symptoms such as appetite changes, weight loss or gain, dizziness, headaches, inexplicable weeping or sad facial expressions, sleeping too much or sleeping too little (insomnia), early morning awakening, and fatigue. Depression frequently coexists with hostility and irritability. This can be directed toward the source of the problematic relationship (such as the spouse) or deflected toward others (such as the children).

Who is likely to develop depression?

Depression appears at least twice as often in American women as in American men. It afflicts at least 1 woman in 10 at any given time; and as many as 1 woman in 3 may become clinically depressed at some point during her lifetime, in contrast to about 1 man in 9.

Why women are so prone to depression is the subject of many theories and much active investigation. Some feminist psychologists believe that the interpersonal and relationship issues may be more relevant than the biological ones in understanding women's depression. Proponents of this "psychosocial" approach regard depression as a reaction to certain stressful developments throughout the life span—mainly involving work, family, and health changes.

According to this view, women tend to interpret the world in terms of personal relationships, whereas men rely more on abstract laws and rules. From an early age women generally seek to cultivate and maintain their connections with others, but their lifelong quest for intimacy is viewed as a weakness in a culture that values self-sufficiency and independence. The discrepancy between the behavior of most women and the values of the culture leads to a loss of self-esteem, a feeling of "just not being good enough."

Moreover, because of a power imbalance between the sexes, this argument goes, it is hard for a woman to establish and maintain connections with others while preserving her inner or "true" self. In many women the inner self is "silenced" for the sake of preserving relationships. Often physical or emotional abuse forces this silence on women, but many women also end up silencing themselves. The high price they pay for "saving" their relationships in this way is depression.

Depression may occur because women feel they cannot be themselves in their relationships and must conform to someone else's idea of what a good woman, partner, or mother should be. Even when they accept the standard, many women become depressed when they discover that they are simply unable to live up to it. Throughout the life span, according to this theory, the priority that women give to maintaining personal connections can lead to stresses that precipitate depression. Whether they work inside or outside the home, whether they choose to have children or not, whether they choose men or other women as partners, women still find that their relationships are the primary source of both meaning in their lives and depression.

Depression in premenopausal women. Major depression is most common in women between 18 and 44, with the late 20s being the average age at which it begins. For those who marry in their early 20s, marital discord often peaks at about this time (roughly 7 years into a marriage), and unhappily married women (as well as lesbians in unhappy relationships) show more clinical depression than unmarried women or women who are satisfied with their partners. Having and caring for young children, also common in this age group, only increases the risk of depression. Many studies suggest that couples with young children feel more stress and pressure than any other family group. Research also shows that in cultures where there is greater access to child care and support for child rearing, rates of depression in women are lower.

One of the possible connections between depression, marriage, and children may be that women feel overwhelmed by, and often experience conflict over, family responsibility. Even as more husbands take on additional obligations in the home, women continue to bear the greater burden of time and emotional strain for child care and housework. Juggling long commutes, inadequate child care, unequal domestic responsibilities, sleep deprivation, care for sick children, homework, and a full-time job can drain life of joy and turn it into little more than a series of self-denying duties.

Despite all these stresses on the working mother, there is a slightly greater risk of depression in women who are at home full-time with young children. Considerable research shows that women report being happier at work than at home, whereas the reverse is true for men. This is probably because working women have greater access to social support, and work provides an alternative source of pride, gratification, and self-esteem. Housework is a notoriously lonely and repetitious activity which brings little external reward. Mothers do not get a raise for keeping cupboards neat or getting up at 3 A.M. to coerce a screaming toddler into swallowing a dropperful of medicine. For many women the self-sacrifice and tiring, repetitive tasks of child care dilute its intrinsic challenges and rewards.

Infertility problems in their late 20s and 30s also start many women down the road to depression. Attempts to conceive a child often involve costly and invasive medical procedures, and the uncertainty, or failure, associated with infertility can shake the foundations of a couple's relationship—especially if the woman feels the stigma of infertility more strongly than her partner or if either partner raises issues of guilt or blame. Conceiving and rearing children can be especially stressful for lesbian women (see sexual orientation). Women of childbearing age are also subject to postpartum depression (see entry on postpartum psychiatric disorders), which can last for over a year after the birth of a baby.

Divorce, though it affects every age group, is particularly likely to underlie depression in premenopausal women. Divorce is most likely to occur during the early years of a marriage, in childless marriages, among those who marry young, and among people who come from families with unhappy marriages. To a woman in her late 20s or 30s who has children, divorce may raise the specter of poverty and economic hardship, as well as fears for the welfare of her children. To a woman in a childless marriage, divorce may seem to slam the door on the possibility of ever having a family of her own.

Depression in the 40s and 50s. Many women who become depressed at menopause have suffered from depression previously or have other life problems that can account for the depression. Menopause itself does not increase a woman's risk for depression, but women who have many physical symptoms at menopause do experience more transient de-

pressive symptoms than those who go through menopause with hardly a hot flash or sleepless night.

What is more common in women in their 40s and 50s is a mild melancholy over impending health changes. For the first time in their lives women may find themselves dealing with high blood pressure or struggling with unwanted weight gain. Menopausal symptoms, sometimes troubling in themselves, may be a reminder of these other changes. The physical symptoms of menopause seem to be worse in women with depression and in women who did not know what to expect from menopause. Menopause may also intensify feelings of loss among both heterosexual and lesbian women who were unable to conceive children, or who chose not to have children earlier in their life.

Women in their 40s and 50s are more likely than women in other age groups to have teenage children. Intense emotional outbursts from adolescents are upsetting and can lead to discord between parents. Divorce in this age group is often precipitated by a husband's extramarital affairs, which can be particularly threatening to a woman who is no longer young. Depression at this time of life (in either sex) may relate to facing mortality and the finitude of life. A woman in particular may dwell on the failing health of her husband and the possibility of being widowed. Also during these decades many women take on the care of elderly parents, or are forced to place them in a nursing home. The stress, guilt, and grief that come from attending the slow death of a mother or father leave many middle-aged women depressed.

Depression in the elderly. Risk factors in this age group include stress, losses, maladaptive personality styles, and previous histories of psychiatric or physical illness. Depression is the most common psychological problem among older women.

Often older women are diagnosed for depression only when they are seen by a doctor for some other reason, usually a physical ailment. At times the depression itself may result in some physical problem without the woman's ever realizing that she is depressed (see psychosomatic disorders). Too often some of the mental symptoms of depression are mistaken for signs of senility or Alzheimer's disease.

By contrast, some women are treated for mild depression unnecessarily. One study found that although people between 60 and 74 had fewer life crises and less psychic distress than any other age group, they were more likely to be prescribed psychoactive medications. Forty-four percent of the women in this study had received a prescription for such a drug in the previous year, and 20 percent were taking these medications on a regular basis. This overmedication may be related to the fact that older people visit physicians more often than younger ones. Whatever the cause, it remains a concern because psychoactive drugs tend to have a higher rate of adverse effects in the elderly.

How is the condition evaluated?

Because patients often mask depression with a physical complaint, doctors can easily overlook it. Many people suffering from depression try to downplay their emotional symptoms, and even if a doctor does diagnose depression, many patients have trouble accepting the diagnosis. Women with depression are also particularly likely to suffer from somatic (bodily) symptoms, which often mask the psychological origin of their complaints.

Primary care providers who suspect depression use various tests and questions to evaluate it and distinguish major depression from dysthymia and other forms. Part of the evaluation involves determining if the patient has any underlying medical conditions or is taking any medications known to cause depression.

In addition, the primary care provider will want to determine if there is any risk of suicide. These findings will be taken very seriously. Any patient contemplating suicide will be sent for evaluation and treatment by a mental health professional, who will then decide whether hospitalization is necessary. Patients with depression who are abusing drugs or alcohol or who have symptoms of psychosis (such as hallucinations), a history of failed treatments, or severe symptoms will also be referred to a psychotherapist for further evaluation and treatment.

How is depression treated?

Depression is usually treated with some combination of psychotherapy and antidepressant medications. Short-term psychotherapy is particularly effective in treating reactive depression in women who have marital, family, or work-related stresses. It is also recommended for women with mild depression or dysthymia and for those who choose not to take medication.

Cognitive therapy (which can be short-term or longer) can help a patient change negative patterns of thinking, while other forms of behavior therapy (including assertiveness training) can help a patient change inappropriate behaviors.

Many women with depression can benefit from either family or marital counseling. A psychotherapist sensitive to women's issues can help the patient find ways to develop healthy, mature forms of interdependence that are free from compulsive caretaking and repression of the self.

Antidepressants (see entry)—drugs that elevate mood—are often prescribed in conjunction with psychotherapy and are effective in about 65 percent of people with depression. They are most appropriately used for patients with a family history of depression, who have had 3 or more previous episodes of depression, or who have severe symptoms.

Many psychotherapists emphasize that individuals with depression cannot be healed in isolation. Because the self is shaped by its relationships with others, it can only be reshaped through those relationships. Again and again, social support (which many depressed people shun) has been shown to be a buffer against depression.

Related entries

Alcohol, anorexia nervosa and bulimia nervosa, antidepressants, anxiety disorders, infertility, insomnia, manic-depressive disorder, menopause, personality disorders, psychosomatic disorders, psychotherapy, seasonal affective disorder, sexual assault, stress, substance abuse

Dermabrasion and Chemical Peels

Dermabrasion is a form of cosmetic surgery—although some would debate whether or not it involves actual surgery—in which the upper layers of skin are sanded away or abraded. Some of the same results can be achieved with chemical peels (chemosurgery), a technique in which acid is applied to the skin to erode the blemished area.

These procedures are usually used on the face to remove pitted acne scars or to smooth fine lines around the mouth. Dermabrasion can also eliminate large birthmarks and may even be effective in eliminating scars from injuries if they involve only the superficial layers of skin.

How are these procedures performed?

Appealing as it may sound to have blemishes and wrinkles wiped away, dermabrasion and chemical peels can be complicated processes. In dermabrasion the skin is subjected to the sanding power of a high-speed rotary drill, a tool with a rotating rubber tire at its end. The procedure is often quite painful and can take a great deal of time, depending on the depth to be drilled. Although some women are able to endure the ordeal by using only tranquilizers or by having their skin frozen with cold gas, the surgery is painful, and most prefer to use general or supplementary intravenous anesthesia.

In chemical peels the area to be treated is washed carefully, and the patient is heavily sedated. The surgeon or technician then applies some kind of acid (usually a solution of phenol or a fruit acid) to the skin and covers the area with strips of waterproof adhesive tape or Vaseline. The skin begins to sting as soon as the acid is applied, and pain often remains quite severe for the next day or so.

What happens after the procedure?

After dermabrasion the skin is red and exudes clear fluid, and may bleed for up to half an hour. After that time a nonadhesive dressing (such as Vaseline topped by gauze) is applied and removed the next day. Skin will stay red and tender for up to 6 weeks. Direct exposure to sunlight should be avoided during this period. A powerful sunscreen should be applied to the face daily, even in winter, for up to a year after the surgery. The use of makeup or certain cosmetic lotions can be irritating until healing is complete. Some surgeons recommend using fine soap granules to cleanse the face to prevent the formation of pinhead-sized white papules (milia) which sometimes develop after dermabrasion.

If new skin is red, abnormally pigmented, or scarred, it may be necessary to repeat the procedure (this can be done about 4 weeks later). Sometimes the procedure has to be repeated several times before deeply pitted scars are removed to satisfaction. Usually the new skin will be lighter or pinker than the original skin, so it is a good idea to have large areas (such as the entire face) treated rather than one small, conspicuous area.

A chemical peel tends to be more painful than dermabrasion. The tape or dressing is removed after 24 to 48 hours, and then an antibacterial powder is applied to the wound, which will be extremely red and sore. As with dermabrasion, skin can stay red for up to 6 months after a chemical peel, during which time it is essential to use sunblocks to protect the skin from damaging ultraviolet rays.

What are the risks and complications?

There is no guarantee that the procedure used will correct the problem to a woman's satisfaction. Furthermore, some people are genetically predisposed to developing raised scars. Occasionally scars or scar formation can be minimized by taking cortisone injections over a long period of time or applying pressure to the wounded area. Although there are surgical procedures that can reshape a scar so that it is less conspicuous, the scars that can form after dermabrasion or chemical peel may be hard to revise. Women who have developed the type of abnormal scarring called keloid scarring (see entry) as a result of a previous surgical procedure such as a cesarean section should be very wary of dermabrasion.

To maximize the safety and effectiveness of these procedures, it is wise to have them performed by a highly trained and experienced dermatologist or plastic surgeon under sterile conditions. Although some full-service beauty salons offer dermabrasion and chemical peels, these are effective only when the blemish involves the most superficial layer of skin (the epidermis). Dermabrasion is not appropriate for active acne or inflamed skin, and it can actually cause more harm than good if the scars are too deeply embedded in the skin, since drilling too deep into the skin simply results in additional scarring. Also, because estrogen can produce color changes in new skin, dermabrasion is not recommended for any woman taking estrogen replacement therapy or oral contraceptives. It is always a good idea to have the procedure tested on a small, inconspicuous patch of skin before making any kind of commitment to either dermabrasion or a chemical peel.

Related entries

Acne, anesthesia, cosmetic surgery, estrogen replacement therapy, skin care and cosmetics, skin disorders, wrinkles

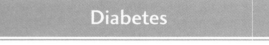

Diabetes

Diabetes mellitus is a group of disorders characterized by high levels of glucose (sugar) in the blood. All of them result

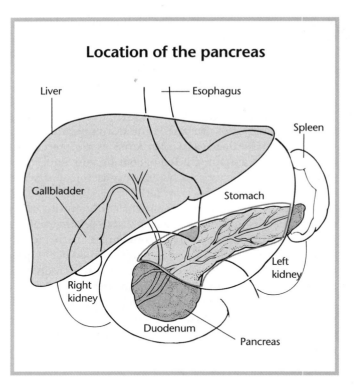

Location of the pancreas

Liver — Esophagus — Spleen — Gallbladder — Stomach — Right kidney — Left kidney — Duodenum — Pancreas

from problems with insulin, a hormone that removes glucose from the blood and causes it to be stored in body cells. Type 1 and Type 2 diabetes are the most common forms, but up to 3 percent of women who did not previously have (or know they had) diabetes may develop it during pregnancy (a condition called gestational diabetes).

In Type 1 diabetes (also called juvenile diabetes) the pancreas—a long, soft, irregularly shaped gland located behind the stomach (see illustration)—does not produce enough insulin. Most people with Type 1 diabetes require regular injections of insulin for life. Although boys and girls run an equal risk of developing Type 1 until about age 12, around the time of puberty the incidence in females begins to decrease in comparison to that in males. Up to age 30 approximately 25 percent more men than women develop Type 1 but later on the risk is about the same for men and women.

Most people who develop diabetes as adults have Type 2, a form in which the body requires greater than normal amounts of insulin to maintain normal blood glucose levels, probably because cells throughout the body do not respond appropriately to insulin (see illustration). Type 2 (formerly called adult-onset diabetes) typically begins after the age of 40, often in people who are overweight or obese, and in those with a family history of diabetes. In recent years, however, Type 2 diabetes has been increasing dramatically among children and adolescents. Whether men or women get Type 2 diabetes more often is still inresolved.

Gestational diabetes is a unique form of the disorder which occurs in pregnancy, probably as a result of hormones made by the placenta which alter the way insulin works. Although glucose levels usually return to normal after the baby is born, women who have gestational diabetes do run a higher than average risk of developing Type 2 diabetes later in life. Gestational diabetes most often occurs in pregnant women who are over the age of 30, who are obese, who have previously given birth to a very large (over 9 pounds) or stillborn baby, or who have a family history of diabetes.

People with either Type 1 or Type 2 diabetes have an increased risk over their lifetime for stroke, coronary artery disease, high levels of blood cholesterol, foot infections, an eye disorder called diabetic retinopathy which can lead to blindness, chronic kidney failure, and nerve damage in the hands and feet. Recent research has conclusively shown that normalizing blood glucose levels in Type 1 diabetics helps prevent these complications. Some studies suggest that this holds true for Type 2 diabetics as well.

The strategy for controlling blood glucose for Type 1 diabetics is to watch diet, maintain a regular exercise program, and adjust insulin dosages carefully according to frequent blood glucose measurements. A woman can check her own glucose level several times a day at home with a simple device called a glucometer. The patient takes a small lancet, pricks the end of a finger lightly, and puts a drop of blood on a strip of paper, which is placed into a small machine. After several seconds to a minute, the reading appears.

For the majority of women with diabetes (that is, those who have Type 2 diabetes), weight control is an especially important strategy for controlling blood glucose. For many, not all, women with Type 2 diabetes who are overweight, a return to normal body weight can bring blood glucose to normal levels. Maintaining a healthy body weight may even help prevent Type 2 diabetes from developing in the first place. If blood glucose cannot be controlled by attention to weight (through exercise and diet), insulin therapy or oral medications—for example, oral hypoglycemics and metformin (Glucophage), which makes the body more sensitive to insulin, or other drugs (Actos, Avandia) that decrease resistance to insulin—are the next step. In addition, health practices that make sense for everybody—such as getting adequate exercise, avoiding cigarettes, having regular checks of blood pressure and cholesterol levels, and preventing ingrown toenails, corns, and calluses on the feet—are particularly important for people with diabetes.

In certain women with diabetes the hormones of the menstrual cycle appear to influence control of glucose levels. Some women may require more insulin during the luteal phase (days 14 to 28) of the menstrual cycle, perhaps because the higher levels of progesterone produced at this time increase the body's resistance to insulin. And some women have noticed that they require less insulin once they reach menopause.

Recurrent yeast infections

Women with diabetes tend to have a disproportionate number of yeast infections. This is because the microorganism that causes these infections thrives in the presence of glucose, which often appears in the vaginal secretions and urine of women with diabetes. Before menopause, yeast infections are so common among all women that several yeast infections should not be a cause for panic. Recurrent or chronic yeast infections, however—especially in women who have other symptoms of diabetes such as frequent thirst and urination, fatigue, headache, dizziness, blurred vision, or weight loss despite increased appetite—warrant an evaluation, even in premenopausal women. If a yeast infection develops in a postmenopausal woman, the clinician should screen for diabetes.

Symptoms may be relieved with a topical vaginal antifungal treatment (available over the counter) or with stronger creams or oral medications (fluconazole) available by prescription. Oral therapy for yeast infections can interfere with oral glycemic medications, so women taking both of these drugs should be monitored closely. Improving control of her blood sugar level can markedly reduce the number of yeast infections a woman gets.

Urinary tract infections

Diabetic women seem to have 2 to 3 times more urinary tract infections (UTIs) than do nondiabetic women. Because women with diabetes are prone to serious kidney infection

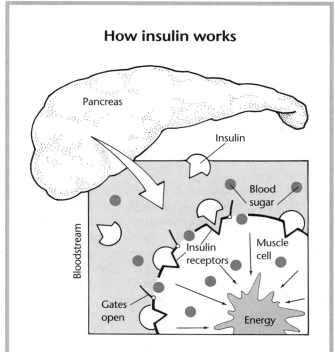

How insulin works

The pancreas secretes insulin into the bloodstream in response to a high level of blood sugar. The insulin molecules then bind to special insulin receptors on the surface of cells in muscles and other organs. The receptors signal the cell to allow sugar to enter, so that it can be available as a source of energy.

In people who are resistant to insulin, sugar has difficulty entering the cell even though insulin binds to the receptors.

(pyelonephritis), a woman with diabetes who suspects a UTI should contact her clinician for early evaluation and treatment. If an infection is diagnosed, doctors generally recommend a full 7 days of antibiotics for bladder infections (as opposed to the shorter-course therapy now frequently prescribed for nondiabetic women; see urinary tract infections).

A woman with diabetes who develops a kidney infection requires intravenous antibiotics. Symptoms of kidney infection in a woman with a urinary tract infection include fever, chills, and flank pain (pain over the back where the kidneys lie). When a woman with diabetes develops an infection of any sort, she may notice that her blood sugar level is difficult to control. She should consult her physician for help in monitoring it and making any necessary adjustments in her medications.

Cardiovascular disease

Compared with men of the same age, nondiabetic women seem to have a degree of protection from diseases of the heart and blood vessels until they reach menopause. Women with diabetes seem to lose this relative protection and at all ages are at increased risk of developing or dying from coronary artery disease, congestive heart failure (inefficient pumping of the heart), strokes, and peripheral vascular disease (see circulatory disorders). Cigarette smoking, hypertension, high cholesterol, and obesity all magnify these risks.

In some cases women with diabetes are at higher risk than men with diabetes of the same age. The risk of dying from heart disease, for example, is higher for diabetic women than for diabetic men, though both men and women with the disease have a higher risk of dying from these problems than do people in the general population. This is partly because their blood vessels are often extensively damaged and partly because their heart attacks may involve unusual symptoms that make them harder to detect.

Certain operations commonly performed on patients with heart disease may be especially risky for women with diabetes. For example, coronary artery bypass surgery (an operation in which part of a vein taken from the thigh or chest is used to "bypass" blocked arteries to the heart) tends to be less successful in women in general, possibly because they have smaller blood vessels than men or because they tend to be diagnosed later in the course of coronary artery disease. Some (but not all) studies now suggest that bypass surgery may be even less effective and riskier in women with diabetes. If this turns out to be true, it may have something to do with the nature of the fatty deposits in the arteries of women with diabetes.

Whether diabetic women develop more complications from "balloon surgery" or angioplasty than do nondiabetic women or diabetic men is not known. This is a procedure used to open narrowed or blocked coronary arteries by threading a balloon-tipped device through the arteries to the place of blockage and then inflating it (see coronary artery disease).

Estrogen replacement therapy (ERT; see entry), once recommended for many postmenopausal women, especially those with diabetes, is no longer considered useful for preventing heart disease in either diabetic or nondiabetic women.

Eating disorders

Up to 20 percent of women with Type 1 diabetes have some kind of eating disorder (see anorexia nervosa and bulimia nervosa). These disorders in turn predispose them to further complications with glucose control. One reason why eating disorders develop is that treatment of diabetes itself greatly emphasizes weight control, dietary habits, and food. Also, young women with Type 1 diabetes may suffer from the stress, poor self-esteem, and altered body image that can result from any chronic illness, and these contribute to the risk for eating disorders.

Women with Type 1 diabetes sometimes adopt a unique "purging" method: they either omit insulin or take an inadequate dose. Since insulin helps cells take up glucose, too little insulin means that the body will be deprived of calories. This practice can result in a vicious cycle: noting the poor control of glucose, a doctor will probably increase the dose of insulin. This leads to further weight gain in women who take the prescribed dose and thus to increased pressure to diet. At that point a young woman may decide on her own to cut back the insulin she takes, and this starts the cycle all over again.

A physician may suspect an eating disorder if there have been significant changes in weight, persistently poor control of blood sugar levels, and recurrent episodes of low blood sugar or ketoacidosis (a result of too little insulin which can lead to loss of consciousness). A psychiatrist can help confirm the diagnosis. Other than focusing more on controlling glucose levels, the treatment for eating disorders in women with diabetes is similar to that for nondiabetic women.

Contraception

Diabetes is associated with health risks to both mother and baby during pregnancy—particularly in an unplanned pregnancy, when glucose control may not be optimal. Therefore, contraception is a key concern for women with diabetes. Barrier methods such as a diaphragm or condoms are good choices because they do not involve hormones that can affect the control of diabetes. An intrauterine device (IUD) also has this advantage, as well as a higher efficacy rate. Failure rates appear to be the same (about 1 percent per year) with the copper IUD for both diabetics and nondiabetics; and according to recent studies, women with diabetes run no greater risk for infection, inflammation, bleeding, or other complications. An IUD is not an optimal contraceptive for women who plan to bear children, however.

The most controversial of the methods available today is the oral contraceptive pill. The pill is appealing because of its convenience and its low failure rate. It was once thought by some investigators that the doses of estrogen (even in the newer low-dose pills) might potentially worsen the heart, nerve, and eye problems that already plague many women with diabetes. Recent studies have shown no increase in the risk of eye or kidney complications in diabetic women on birth control pills. But the progesterone component of oral contraceptives has been associated with an increase in blood pressure and LDL cholesterol, as well as a decrease in HDL cholesterol—all risk factors for cardiovascular disease. As a result, oral contraceptives are generally recommended only for relatively young, nonsmoking diabetic women with normal blood pressure, normal lipid levels in their blood, and no evidence of small blood vessel damage—that is, women who are at low risk for cardiovascular disease.

Another issue with birth control pills is their effect on carbohydrate metabolism. The lower-progestin pills seem to have the least effect on daily insulin requirements, particularly those that contain a form of progestin called norethindrone (found, for example, in Necon) rather than a form called norgestrel (found, for example, in Triphasil or Levora). The progestin-only pill (the "minipill"), which has been found not to raise blood pressure or lipid levels, may be a safer alternative for diabetic women. There are no data on the use of Depo-Provera (medroxyprogesterone acetate).

A diabetic woman who has completed her family or who has circulatory or kidney damage might want to discuss the possibility of tubal ligation (sterilization) with her clinician. This will allow her to reduce as much as possible the chances of another pregnancy and its attendant risks.

Diabetic women who become pregnant

Babies of diabetic mothers whose glucose levels are not under tight control tend to be abnormally large—which can make delivery difficult—and often have oversized but immature organs. This is because high levels of glucose in the mother's blood freely cross the placenta, stimulating the baby to increase its production of insulin, a potent growth factor. In addition to having fatter babies, diabetic mothers with poor glucose control have an increased risk of excess amniotic fluid, miscarriage, premature delivery, and stillbirth, and their babies have a greater risk of low blood sugar, respiratory distress syndrome (which occurs when the baby's lungs are not fully developed), and serious congenital malformations. Even with the best control, pregnant women with diabetes run a risk for developing hypertension, preeclampsia, and eclampsia—complications of pregnancy that can lead to convulsions, unconsciousness, coma, and in rare cases death—4 times greater than that for nondiabetic women. They also have a higher than average risk of developing various infections during pregnancy, such as bladder (cystitis) and kidney (pyelonephritis) infections.

Pregnant women with diabetes are unquestionably "high-risk," but new knowledge about how to control diabetes has made pregnancy considerably safer than in the past. Proper monitoring and control of blood glucose levels both before and during pregnancy can significantly reduce the risk of these complications.

Any woman with diabetes who is considering becoming pregnant should seek counseling before she conceives (see preconception counseling). In the best-case scenario, the mother's diabetes should be brought under tight control before the pregnancy begins—with exercise, diet, and appropriate medications if necessary. Women who are taking oral hypoglycemics prior to pregnancy and who wish to become pregnant will be switched to insulin, and blood glucose levels will be monitored closely throughout the entire pregnancy. Many women with Type 2 diabetes who do not normally require insulin may need it during pregnancy. Furthermore, the need for insulin may vary during the course of the pregnancy. Pregnant women will be expected to test themselves at least 4 or 5 times a day. Daily home monitoring of blood glucose levels is vital to ensure that insulin doses are properly adjusted.

Throughout the pregnancy special tests may be required to help pick up problems as early as possible. For example, a test is often done to measure a substance called hemoglobin A1C in the mother's blood. Higher than normal levels of this substance indicate problems with glucose control. Pregnant women with diabetes are also advised to have alphafetoprotein screening (see entry) at 16 to 18 weeks and an ultrasound test during the first trimester and at 18 to 22 weeks. They should also be examined frequently for signs of eye and kidney damage both before and during the pregnancy, since these conditions often worsen in pregnant women with diabetes.

During the last trimester the baby's condition may be monitored with nonstress tests, ultrasound, and amniocentesis, in part to determine if the lungs are mature enough to allow cesarean section or induction of labor. One of these procedures is almost always attempted if the pregnancy goes beyond 38 weeks' gestation.

It was once thought that all pregnant women with diabetes needed to have a cesarean delivery, but today most pregnant women with diabetes deliver their babies safely through the vagina. Babies that appear too big for the birth canal or that develop fetal distress may need to be delivered by c-section, however.

Achieving tight control of diabetes during pregnancy requires extra effort by the woman (and her caregivers) throughout the pregnancy. The benefits, however—producing a healthy baby and avoiding complications of delivery—are well worth it.

Pregnant women who become diabetic

Between 1 and 3 percent of all women who were not previously diabetic develop diabetes during pregnancy. For this reason many clinicians now routinely screen all pregnant women for this condition between 24 and 28 weeks' gestation. The screening test involves drinking a flavored sugar solution and then having blood drawn an hour later so that glucose levels can be measured. If the results of the screening test are positive, a 3-hour oral glucose tolerance test will be performed.

As with any type of diabetes, gestational diabetes—if not kept under tight control—increases the risk of having a larger than normal baby and other potential complications. For this reason, special tests are often necessary to monitor the size of the fetus before delivery. Some women with gestational diabetes can control blood glucose levels by eating a special diet and monitoring blood glucose levels. Taking insulin twice a day may become necessary if the glucose is not well controlled through diet.

Some studies have shown that a woman with gestational diabetes has a 20 to 30 percent chance of developing Type 2 diabetes within 5 years after delivery. Because of this risk, it is a good idea to have one's blood glucose measured again several months after the baby is born to make sure that the level has returned to normal, and in some cases to have a glucose tolerance test. Women who are overweight or obese after the pregnancy ends can markedly decrease their risk of developing Type 2 diabetes later by adjusting their eating and exercise habits in order to lose weight (see weight tables).

Related entries

Alpha-fetoprotein screening, amniocentesis, anorexia nervosa and bulimia nervosa, antibiotics, birth control, cesarean section, cholesterol, circulatory disorders, congestive heart failure, coronary artery disease, dieting, eclampsia, estrogen replacement therapy, exercise, eye care, fatigue, foot care, high blood pressure, hypoglycemia, kidney disorders, nail care, nutrition, obesity, preconception counseling, preeclampsia, prenatal care, smoking, stress, stroke, tubal ligation, urinary tract infections, weight tables, yeast infections

Diaphragms, Cervical Caps, and Sponges

Like condoms, the diaphragm and the cervical cap are barrier methods of contraception—that is, methods that physically prevent sperm from gaining access to the woman's reproductive system and fertilizing an egg. Among the safest and least expensive methods of contraception available, barrier methods may also help reduce a woman's risk of acquiring certain sexually transmitted diseases, pelvic inflammatory disease, and possibly even cervical cancer. Barrier methods have a relatively high failure rate if not used consistently and correctly, however. They also often require consistent effort on the part of the woman, as well as cooperation on the part of her partner.

Diaphragms

A round rubber dome that fits inside the vagina and covers the cervix (see illustration), the diaphragm is meant to be used with a spermicidal cream or jelly. In fact, the role of the diaphragm is essentially to hold in place the spermicide (see entry)—which provides most of the contraceptive effect.

There are three basic kinds of diaphragms, differentiated according to the type of spring or rim on the dome: coil-spring, flat, or arcing. Each of these is available in a range of sizes and must be fitted by a clinician to tuck snugly under the pubic bone and cover the cervix entirely. If a woman gains or loses more than about 20 pounds or if she has just given birth or had a miscarriage or abortion, the diaphragm needs to be refitted.

The diaphragm can be inserted up to 6 hours before sexual intercourse. After that period the spermicide begins to lose its contraceptive effect. Before inserting the diaphragm, the woman fills the cup of the diaphragm with a teaspoon to a tablespoon of spermicidal cream or jelly (available without a prescription at pharmacies and some supermarkets). A bit of this spermicide should be smeared just inside or on the outer rim of the diaphragm. Then the diaphragm is squeezed together, inserted between the lips of the vagina (either by hand or, in the case of the flat-spring diaphragm, with a special applicator if preferred), and gently pushed back and up toward the cervix. This is usually most easily accomplished if the woman squats, lies on her back with her knees bent, or sits on the toilet. The sides of the diaphragm are then released so that the cup springs back into its original shape.

Properly placed, the diaphragm covers the entire cervix (which, felt through the rubber, feels a bit like the tip of the nose) and fits snugly back under the pubic bone. If the diaphragm slips, hurts, or feels at all uncomfortable, it needs to be checked or refitted by a clinician.

After intercourse, the diaphragm must be left in place for 6 to 8 hours—enough time for the spermicide to kill any remaining sperm—but should be left in the vagina no longer than 24 hours. If the couple has intercourse again, additional spermicide must be inserted into the vagina with a special applicator (sometimes included with the spermicide) with the diaphragm still in place. To remove the diaphragm, the woman reaches up toward the cervix, slips a finger or two just under the rim (being careful not to puncture the rubber with a fingernail), and pulls the device out of the vagina. The same positions used to insert the diaphragm usually work best for removing it. After removal, the diaphragm should be washed with mild soap and warm water, dusted with corn starch if desired, and placed away from light in its case. Before each insertion, it is a good idea to hold the diaphragm up to the light (or fill it with water) and check for holes or leaks. A diaphragm with even a pinprick of a hole needs to be replaced. The diaphragm can continue to be used during menstruation because the cup will catch the menstrual flow.

Used consistently and correctly, the diaphragm has a failure rate of only about 6 percent—that is, 6 out of every 100 women who use it can expect to become pregnant within a year. In reality, however, the typical failure rate is closer to 18 percent. To reduce the risk of pregnancy, some couples use a condom as well as a diaphragm during the most fertile

How to insert a diaphragm

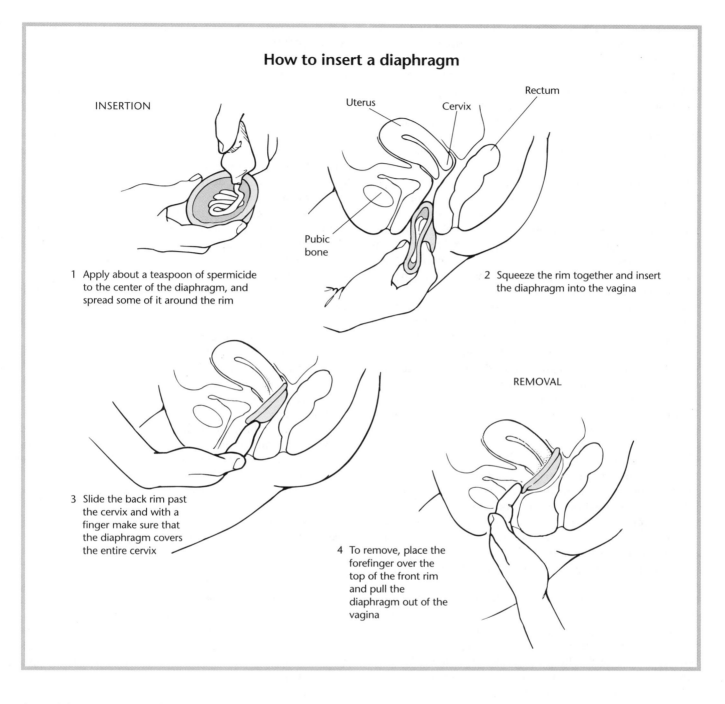

INSERTION

1 Apply about a teaspoon of spermicide to the center of the diaphragm, and spread some of it around the rim

Uterus Cervix Rectum

Pubic bone

2 Squeeze the rim together and insert the diaphragm into the vagina

3 Slide the back rim past the cervix and with a finger make sure that the diaphragm covers the entire cervix

REMOVAL

4 To remove, place the forefinger over the top of the front rim and pull the diaphragm out of the vagina

days of the menstrual cycle (just before ovulation and 2 days after).

A diaphragm is not a particularly convenient—or romantic—form of birth control in that it must be inserted and removed before and after each sexual encounter. Although this can become burdensome for couples who have sexual intercourse on a regular basis—and can disrupt spontaneity for any couple—many women make the best of the situation by incorporating diaphragm insertion into foreplay or simply by inserting the diaphragm every night before going to bed. Women who use the diaphragm also have to remember to have enough spermicidal cream or jelly on hand and to

bring their supplies with them whenever they are away from home.

Diaphragms, which are available only by prescription, generally cost around $20, but added to this is the cost of seeing a clinician for a fitting. Just how much a woman will pay for spermicide depends on how frequently she has intercourse. A 3.8-ounce tube of cream or jelly contains about 12 applications of spermicide and usually costs between $7 and $10.

The diaphragm is one of the safest forms of birth control available and has virtually no side effects. Occasionally a woman may find that a particular spermicidal cream or jelly irritates her vagina, in which case she can simply switch to another brand. There is also some evidence that diaphragm use may predispose women to recurrent urinary tract infections and yeast infections as well. Taking proper care of the diaphragm and removing it soon after the requisite 8 hours have passed can sometimes reduce the chances of developing these problems. Changing to another size or type (particularly a "wide-seal" diaphragm, which puts less pressure on the urethra) may also help.

A diaphragm that causes pain or cramping probably has not been fitted correctly. There are some women, however, who simply cannot use diaphragms. Whatever the size, their body just "spits out" the diaphragm. Among the problems that can preclude diaphragm use are severe uterine prolapse (fallen uterus), cystoceles, urethroceles, rectoceles, or vaginal fistulas (openings in the vagina), spina bifida, or some forms of scoliosis. Women who have a history of recurrent urinary tract infections or toxic shock syndrome are also generally not good candidates for a diaphragm.

Women who want to become pregnant simply need to stop using the diaphragm and can expect to be just as fertile as if they had never used this method of birth control in the first place. A few years back some now discredited evidence suggested that spermicides might be linked in some way to birth defects, and some clinicians advised women to use another form of birth control (such as a condom) for a month or so before attempting conception. This practice no longer appears to be necessary.

Cervical caps

Like the diaphragm, the cervical cap fits over the cervix to block sperm from entering the uterus and flowing up into the fallopian tubes (see illustration). Unlike the diaphragm, however, the cervical cap requires relatively little spermicide and can be left in place for a longer period of time. Even the small amount of spermicide used may be enough to help prevent (but not guarantee against) the spread of certain sexually transmitted diseases.

The cervical cap is a thimblelike rubber device that is fitted by a clinician to provide an airtight seal over the cervix. Whereas a diaphragm covers the cervix and part of the vaginal walls around it, the much smaller cervical cap fits directly onto the cervix and is held on by suction. The cervical cap can be inserted up to 40 hours before vagina-penis contact. Before insertion, about a third of the cap should be filled with spermicidal jelly or cream. After intercourse the cap should be left in place for at least 6 to 8 hours to give the spermicide enough time to kill all the sperm. Leaving the cap in place longer than 48 hours, however, may increase the risk of toxic shock syndrome (and possibly pregnancy), although evidence is still rather inconclusive. It is probably safest— if possible—to remove the cap daily, or at least every other day. In any case, the cap should definitely be removed regularly—or not used at all—during menstruation, since menstrual flow can break the airtight seal around the cervix. After the cap is removed, it should be washed with mild soap and warm water, rinsed, and dried.

If intercourse seems to dislodge the cap, or if it is uncomfortable, it needs to be rechecked by a clinician and probably refitted. During the first months of use, it is a good idea to check the fit right before sexual intercourse or to use some additional means of contraception (such as a condom) as a backup method. Although the expected failure rate for the cervical cap is only about 6 percent, the typical failure rate is about 18 percent.

A cervical cap is more convenient than the diaphragm because it can be inserted long before intercourse and because it can be left in place much longer. In addition, since the cap requires far less spermicide than does the diaphragm, it is generally less messy (and also causes less worry about running out of spermicide). But some women find the cervical cap harder to insert than a diaphragm, and others cannot be fit at all because of the shape of their cervix. Women who have had several babies are often harder to fit than women who have never had children.

A cervical cap costs about $30, plus the cost of the initial examination and fitting. The cost of spermicide will vary depending on how often the woman has intercourse, but is far less than when a diaphragm is used since the cap requires so little spermicide to be effective. A 3.8-ounce tube of spermicidal cream or jelly generally costs between $7 and $10.

Like all barrier methods of contraception, the cervical cap is relatively free of potential side effects. Some women may find that the cervical cap makes them more susceptible to urinary tract infections, however, or that their vagina is irritated by a certain brand of spermicide. Other women (or their partners) are bothered by odor, discharge, or discomfort associated with the cap. There is also some evidence of mildly abnormal Pap test results in about 4 percent of women who use this form of contraception.

Women who stop using the cervical cap can try to become pregnant immediately. Having used the cap seems to have no effect on a woman's future chances of conception.

Contraceptive sponge

Removed from the market in 1995 because of manufacturing problems, the contraceptive sponge has since been reintroduced. Made of polyurethane and permeated with the spermicide nonoxynol-9, the sponge is about 1.75 inches in diameter and half an inch thick. It is inserted into the vagina up to 24 hours before intercourse and appears to work by inactivating sperm with the spermicide, blocking the opening to the cervix, and absorbing and trapping sperm. After being left in the vagina at least 6 to 8 hours after intercourse, the sponge is removed by grasping a ribbon-like loop and then discarded.

Because it is readily available without a prescription, easy to use, and relatively safe and inexpensive, the contraceptive sponge appeals to many women who have only infrequent sex and don't want to bother with condoms or with messy spermicidal foams, jellies, and creams. When used correctly, the sponge has a failure rate of about 10 percent, but the typical failure rate is closer to 15 percent. Whether or not the spermicide in the sponge provides any protection against sexually transmitted diseases remains unclear.

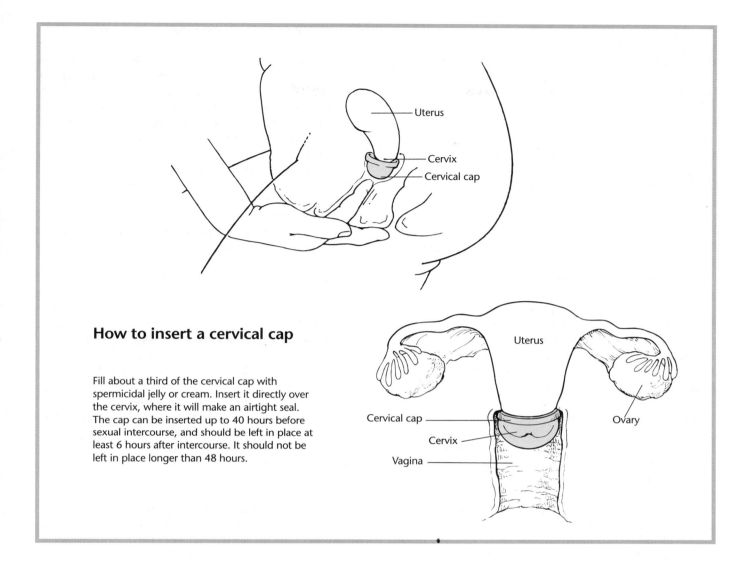

How to insert a cervical cap

Fill about a third of the cervical cap with spermicidal jelly or cream. Insert it directly over the cervix, where it will make an airtight seal. The cap can be inserted up to 40 hours before sexual intercourse, and should be left in place at least 6 hours after intercourse. It should not be left in place longer than 48 hours.

Related entries

Abortion, acquired immune deficiency syndrome, birth control, condoms, cystocele/urethrocele/rectocele, douching, hormonal contraception, intrauterine devices, lubricants, natural birth control methods, nonsurgical abortion, oral contraceptives, pregnancy testing, prolapsed uterus, safer sex, scoliosis, sexual response, sexually transmitted diseases, spermicides, tubal ligation, urinary tract infections, vacuum aspiration

Diethylstilbestrol (DES)

Diethylstilbestrol, more commonly known as DES, is a synthetic form of the hormone estrogen. From 1940 to 1970 it was widely prescribed to pregnant women (especially those with diabetes) under a variety of brand names to prevent miscarriage, stillbirth, premature labor, eclampsia, and other complications—despite the fact that there was never strong evidence that it actually made much of a difference. In the mid-1950s DES began to be associated with a number of serious birth defects and other disorders of the reproductive tract in the daughters of women who had taken it while pregnant. Nonetheless, DES continued to be prescribed in this country until about 1971, when the federal Food and Drug Administration (FDA) advised against using it during pregnancy. In 1979 the FDA banned the use of DES as a growth promoter in livestock. It was used into the 1980s in some European countries.

Until recently DES was sometimes prescribed in the United States to suppress lactation or to serve as a "morning-after" contraceptive. The only appropriate medical use for DES today, however, is to relieve the pain associated with breast and prostate cancer.

Who is likely to be affected by DES exposure?

At least 2 million American women were prescribed DES before 1971, with perhaps more than a million receiving the drug between 1945 and 1955 alone. Although peak exposure occurred in the 1950s, another 10,000 to 16,000 females born between 1960 and 1970 were exposed to DES during gestation. Nonetheless, estimates of the percentage of adult women today who were exposed before birth range from fewer than 1 percent to as many as 10 percent.

What are the effects of DES exposure?

DES taken during pregnancy readily crosses the placenta and can induce a number of carcinogenic (cancer-causing) and other long-term toxic effects in the fetus—many of which do not appear for years after birth. Probably the most common of these is a condition called vaginal adenosis, a kind of abnormal cell growth (dysplasia) in which the types of glandular cells normally found in the cervix develop in the vaginal walls.

Vaginal adenosis is estimated to affect between 35 and 90 percent of DES-exposed daughters. The wide variation in these numbers reflects methodological variations in the studies on which they were based—largely the fact that investigators used different definitions of adenosis, so that cells counted as abnormal in one study went under the heading of normal in another. Whatever the true numbers, there is no doubt that DES exposure in the uterus raises the odds of adenosis considerably, particularly in younger women. Risk is greatest among women whose mothers used DES before the 18th week of pregnancy.

Adenosis sometimes presages a form of cancer of glandular tissue called clear-cell adenocarcinoma, which in rare cases (1 in 1,000) may develop in the vagina or cervix of DES-exposed daughters. Extremely unusual in other women, adenocarcinoma is most common in women whose mothers used DES before the 12th week of pregnancy. Adenocarcinoma most frequently develops sometime between menarche (the first menstrual period) and the age of 24, although it has occurred in both older women and prepubertal girls. With early detection and treatment it is a highly curable form of cancer. Although the lesions of adenosis associated with potential adenocarcinoma can be removed surgically, burned off with electrocautery, or frozen off with cryosurgery, most clinicians think it preferable—and reasonably safe—to leave them in place and watch them regularly for signs of cancer.

Other abnormalities common in DES-exposed daughters are small transverse folds resembling hoods or collars (transverse fibrous ridges) in the vagina or cervix. Also fairly common are abnormalities in either the size or shape of the uterus, such as a T-shaped uterus or an unusually small uterine cavity. Such abnormalities may help explain why these women also have higher rates of miscarriage, ectopic pregnancy, stillbirths, and premature labor. (Evidence is still unclear as to whether fertility problems are also more common.) Although these risks justify classifying a pregnancy in a DES-exposed daughter as "high-risk," it is reassuring that 4 out of 5 DES-exposed women can expect to bear a healthy child.

For years investigators have suspected that women who took DES themselves may have an elevated risk of developing cancers of the breast and endometrium (lining of the uterus) later in life. The belief about endometrial cancer is largely extrapolated from the better-established link between these cancers and supplemental estrogens given as part of estrogen replacement therapy. Since DES is a form of estrogen, many investigators suspect that it may have similar effects on the uterus in women who took the hormone during their pregnancy. The evidence for endometrial cancer is still inconclusive, but studies show that DES mothers do have a modestly increased risk of developing breast cancer later in life.

Sons born to mothers who used DES are not immune to its effects, although the evidence about specific defects remains largely inconclusive. A number of genital and urinary abnormalities have been reported, but the only well-documented association is a higher than average risk of testicular cancer.

Finally, all of the physical effects associated with DES take their emotional toll as well, both in mothers who took the drug and in their offspring. Many women who took DES during pregnancy feel considerable guilt, anxiety, and anger. These feelings are generally even stronger if their children actually develop reproductive problems. Daughters who know that their mother took DES are also understandably fearful of potential dangers down the line. If they have specific defects, they may even feel angry about their fate or hostile toward their mother for exposing them, even unknowingly. At least one formal study, however, indicates that undergoing this experience together gives most mothers and daughters a common "enemy" and leaves them feeling closer than before.

How is the condition evaluated?

Any woman born between 1941 and 1971 should try to find out if her mother may have used DES. A woman who cannot get this information can have a special pelvic examination by a clinician experienced in screening for DES to see if she shows any signs of exposure. This examination may include a biopsy of cells from the vaginal walls and cervix and an inspection of these areas with a binocular-like instrument called a colposcope.

DES-exposed daughters should be sure to have yearly Pap tests, pelvic examinations, and colposcopy (when advised by their physician) beginning right after the time of their first menstrual period (menarche) or by age 14, whichever comes first. (DES sons should consult a urologist to be screened for genital abnormalities, preferably as soon as they have reached puberty.) In addition to these regular examinations, a clinician should be consulted if there is ever any unusual bleeding or discharge from the vagina.

Annual pelvic examinations and Pap tests are equally important in women who used DES themselves. Because of the association of DES use with breast cancer, having a yearly breast examination by a clinician is also recommended, as is a monthly breast self-examination and periodic mammography (see entry).

Most clinicians use a watch-and-wait approach for any noncancerous cell changes associated with DES exposure.

Regular follow-up is critical, though, because of the chance—however small—of developing clear-cell adenocarcinoma.

Related entries

Biopsy, birth control, breast cancer, cryosurgery, diabetes, eclampsia, electrocautery, endometrial cancer, estrogen replacement therapy, infertility, menarche, miscarriage, Pap test, pelvic examinations

Dieting

Strictly speaking, a diet is any eating plan. Hospitals offer various diets to patients, for example, depending on their medical needs, while an athlete may go on a high-carbohydrate diet to maximize stamina and a socially conscious individual may go on a vegetarian diet to maximize the planet's resources. Generally speaking, however, when women in our society talk about "dieting," they are referring almost exclusively to eating plans undertaken to lose weight.

Why do diets usually fail?

At any given time a hefty percentage of American women claim to be "dieting." But the vast majority of these diets fail—with many women ending up weighing more than they did when they began. Part of the problem is that many of the women who are dieting simply do not need to lose weight in the first place. Furthermore, women frequently set unrealistic goals for themselves, expecting to reach some ideal weight on a chart or, even more impossibly, hoping to achieve the pencil-thin figure of a model. Another problem is that many women are dieting not because they really want or need to but because, in a society that values slimness, they feel that they ought to. Diets based on the expectations of other people—that is, diets based on guilt or fear—are almost always doomed from the start.

Increasing evidence that each human being has a "set point" for body weight also helps explain why unnecessary dieting can be counterproductive. According to set point theory, the body's metabolism slows down as weight is lost (and increases as weight is gained). This phenomenon probably evolved as a strategy to help protect the human race in times of famine. As less food became available, less was needed for survival. The result in our society of abundance, however, is that losing weight often becomes an unending uphill bat-

	Very low fat	Moderate fat	Low carbohydrate
Examples	Ornish Diet Pritikin Diet	USDA Food Guide Pyramid NIH DASH Diet Weight Watchers Jenny Craig Nutri-System	Atkins Diet *The South Beach Diet* *Protein Power* *The Carbohydrate Addict's Diet*
% calories from carbohydrate	75	60	<20
% calories from fat	10	20–30	55
% calories from protein	10–15	15	30
Average total calories per day	1450	1450	1450
Comments	Vitamin B_{12} may need to be supplemented (Ornish)	Calculated to provide a deficit of 500–1000 calories per day without limiting required nutrients	High in saturated fat and cholesterol, low in fruits, vegetables, and fiber, low vitamin A, calcium, iron, and potassium

Popular diets

tle. Women for whom dieting has become a way of life may be dismayed to find that they rebound to a slightly higher weight after each diet effort. Furthermore, women who expect to maintain their new weight often discover that they will have to eat less and exercise more for the rest of their lives.

What makes a diet succeed?

A diet can be successful even if a person fails to reach some idealized weight goal. Individual circumstances—dieting history, age, ethnic heritage, physical limitations, medication use, psychological factors, and so on—ought to be taken into account so that realistic expectations and practical strategies can be formulated. There is now good evidence that the greatest health benefits from weight loss occur with the first 10 to 20 percent of excess body fat that is lost—which is the easiest weight to lose. This may be little consolation to the woman who is dieting for social or fashion reasons, but it should be encouraging to those who need to lose a few pounds for the sake of their health.

Setting realistic goals usually means aiming to lose no more than 10 percent of body weight. Thus, a 160-pound woman should aim to lose no more than 16 pounds. Then, if necessary, a new goal of another 10 percent can be set after the new weight has been maintained for a year. This 10 percent reduction in body weight will reduce the woman's risk for chronic diseases such as hypertension, coronary artery disease, diabetes, and degenerative arthritis, while still leaving her with a normal (not overly slowed) metabolic rate. Unless a woman weighs 20 percent more than the healthy ideal for her height (see weight tables), increasing exercise and activity levels and developing healthy eating habits usually makes more sense over the long run than weight loss diets per se.

In general, any valid weight control plan will emphasize gradual weight loss (a pound a week). Crash dieting or starvation, while often producing a gratifying weight (or, more accurately, water) loss over the first few days, only lowers the metabolic rate, which ultimately makes it harder to burn fat. Fasts and unbalanced diets often result in the loss of lean tissue and important nutrients. Over-the-counter liquid protein diets, supplemented with vitamins and minerals, are much safer, but they rarely produce long-term weight loss. As for high protein diets that have become increasingly popular in recent years (e.g., Atkins, the Zone, the Carbohydrate Addicts Diet, and SugarBusters), there is still little convincing evidence that these are more effective approaches to weight loss in the long term. Because these diets involve eating large amounts of protein and small amounts of carbohydrates, fiber, and many essential nutrients, they can result in significant short-term weight loss—hence the many advocates who swear by these diets. Most people, however, have great trouble sticking to low-carbohydrate diets over the long term, and as a result, most eventually gain back the weight. Even those people able to stick to these diets for long periods of time may increase their risk of coronary artery disease be-

cause these diets involve eating moderate to high levels of fat.

Because it takes about 3,500 calories to produce a single pound of fat, losing 20 pounds requires restricting caloric intake over time by a total of $20 \times 3,500 = 70,000$ calories. But calorie cutting alone does not ensure a safe or successful diet. Any safe and effective diet plan for an adult woman should be based on the Food Guide Pyramid (see nutrition), with emphasis on starches, fruits, and vegetables, and including low-fat or nonfat milk and yogurt to meet calcium needs. Intake of simple sugars and fats should be limited. Such a plan will call for eating several meals and snacks distributed throughout the day, a daily caloric consumption of at least 1,000 to 1,200 calories, adequate protein, and a fat intake limited to 25 percent of total calories. In a 1,200 to 1,500 calorie a day plan, this means eating no more than 27 to 33 grams of fat a day. In an 1,800 calorie diet, it means eating no more than 44 grams of fat. An easy way to estimate and keep track of fat intake is to use a fat gram counter book, read food labels, and record total fat intake in a food diary.

Increasing one's physical activity plays a major role in any successful weight loss program. Exercise sessions that last longer than 30 minutes are particularly helpful, since after this length of time the body starts burning body fat (in addition to carbohydrate sugars) for energy.

Whatever the plan, women tend to lose less weight than men do because they have a lower lean body mass. People who are less overweight to begin with, or older, also tend to lose weight with more difficulty.

Many women find group programs such as Weight Watchers helpful. These organizations provide education and diet advice, as well as peer support and encouragement. The best programs focus on making lifetime changes in nutritious food choices and exercise patterns, as well as reversing destructive attitudes about food and eating. They also rarely involve buying expensive "substitute" foods and vitamins. Often these groups offer behavior modification programs that can be helpful in changing abnormal eating patterns.

Although some researchers believe that there is clear and convincing evidence that modern appetite suppressant drugs (such as over-the-counter amphetamines and derivatives) are effective and safe, others argue that most people who try them lose only a small amount of weight, which is soon regained. They also argue that drugs can too easily become a substitute for education, exercise, and good nutrition, so ultimately maintaining the new weight becomes difficult. In addition, appetite suppressants can cause drug dependency and increase heart rate and blood pressure to dangerous levels in some women. "Starch blockers" and "fat blockers"—drugs that prevent the absorption of calories by the gut—sound appealing but in reality have too many side effects to be practical.

Some people find that hypnosis, acupuncture, and other alternative therapies help them control their appetite and change their eating habits. To date, scientific investigation has not established the safety and effectiveness of most of these approaches, but it may be worth discussing some of these possibilities with a clinician.

What about weight loss drugs?

Although some researchers believe that there is clear and convincing evidence that modern appetite suppressant drugs (such as over-the-counter amphetamines and derivatives) are effective and safe, others argue that most people who try them lose only a small amount of weight, which is soon regained. They also argue that drugs can too easily become a substitute for education, exercise, and good nutrition, so that ultimately maintaining the new weight becomes difficult. In addition, appetite suppressants can cause drug dependency and increase heart rate and blood pressure to dangerous levels in some users.

So-called "natural" products that promise effortless, quick, and safe weight loss can be dangerous as well, despite the common misconception that everything "natural" is inherently harmless. Herbal weight loss products (sometimes called "herbal fen-phens," in reference to the now banned prescription appetite suppressant) usually contain ephedra, a stimulant and appetite suppressant, often in combination with the antidepressive herb St. John's wort. Because ephedra has been linked to serious side effects, including nervousness, insomnia, headache, high blood pressure, irregular heartbeat, psychosis, heart attacks, and stroke, the U.S. Food and Drug Administration (FDA) is considering banning it or requiring a warning label on all products that contain it. Despite all the hype, too, other "natural" weight loss products—including those that feature amino acids or chromium picolinate—have never been proven either safe or effective and are probably a waste of money at best. Because these products are classified as "dietary supplements" in the United States, moreover, they are not required to undergo any standardized quality control procedure; thus, there is no guarantee that they contain what they claim to or that they are uncontaminated.

Other nonprescription products sometimes used to hasten weight loss are diuretics and laxatives, agents that speed emptying of the bladder and bowel, respectively. Neither can make any significant difference in long-term weight loss, and both put the body at risk of serious and sometimes even life-threatening mineral imbalances (see entries on diuretics and laxatives).

Despite considerable marketing hype, too, no prescription diet drug on the market today can substitute for good nutrition, healthy eating habits, and exercise, although such drugs may be of benefit to seriously obese women. New prescription "miracle" anti-obesity drugs continue to appear on a regular basis, often becoming wildly popular before researchers have time to explore their dangerous side effects or long-term effects. Worries about unproven dangers came to pass with the appetite suppressant fenfluramin (the "fen" in "fen-phen," sold under the trade names Redux and Pondimin), which was banned from the U.S. market in 1997 after studies suggested that it might cause heart valve defects in some users.

Anti-obesity drugs available today include phentermine (Apidex-P, Fastin, Ionamin), which is the still approved part of "fen-phen," and subutramine (Meridia). A more recent offering is orlistat (Xenical), a drug that works not by suppressing the appetite but by blocking the body's absorption of dietary fat. None of these drugs is a quick fix—and all come at a considerable cost. Whatever weight loss they bring cannot be maintained without concomitant changes in eating and exercise habits, and studies of their long-term safety or the effects of taking them together, as often happens, remain limited. These drugs are approved only for use by the truly obese. Even so, some of these drugs can easily be obtained by just about anyone (sometimes over the Internet).

Desperation for rapid, effortless weight loss leads many women to overlook the considerable expense, limitations, and side effects associated with all of these drugs. After taking the "hottest" of them, orlistat, for a full year, for example, users can expect to lose only 5 to 10 percent of their weight, and only if they also follow a reduced-calorie diet. In other words, even with orlistat and a strict diet, it would take an entire year for a 200-pound woman to get down to 190 or 180, and just as long for a 130-pound woman to shed an extra 5 or 10 pounds. During that year, daily vitamin supplements would be essential, too, because orlistat blocks absorption of fat-soluble vitamins (A, D, E, and K, and beta carotene) as well as fat. And many users will experience embarrassing and unpleasant side effects such as flatulence, bloating, diarrhea, and fecal incontinence, especially if dietary fat intake is not kept to a minimum.

What are the risks and complications?

Despite the health risks inherent in obesity, the very act of dieting can be risky for some women. Not only have decreased self-esteem and self-confidence been associated with chronic dieting, but also the desire for thinness, particularly in women, has been associated with a high prevalence of eating disorders such as anorexia nervosa, bulimia nervosa, and "binge eating disorder." Adult women dieters who have little weight to lose (less than 10 percent of their weight) may end up losing excessive lean body mass rather than unwanted fat.

On the plus side, it no longer appears that yo-yo dieting—cyclic weight loss and gain—poses any particular risks to health. Earlier and widely publicized reports of this belief were based on studies that failed to differentiate between people who lost weight voluntarily and those who lost it owing to illness.

Dieting can be particularly unwise in adolescence, a time of critical growth and development. Not only can caloric deprivation interfere with physical growth, but also an obsession with thinness and dieting can result in eating disorders or a lifetime of poor self-image. Increasing activity and making healthy food choices make much more sense for the mildly overweight adolescent. Although dieting may be appropriate in the case of a severe weight problem, this should be initiated only under the guidance of a clinician. As with all eating disorders, family therapy may be advisable in some cases as well.

Related entries
Alternative therapies, amenorrhea, anorexia nervosa and bulimia nervosa, antidepressants, artificial sweeteners, body image, cholesterol, exercise, iron, nutrition, obesity, vitamins, weight tables

Dilatation and Curettage

In this surgical procedure the cervix is widened, or dilated, and the lining of the uterus is scraped with a tool called a curette. Although simpler and less expensive procedures such as endometrial biopsy and vacuum aspiration are rapidly replacing the D&C as a diagnostic tool, the procedure is still commonly used to diagnose and treat a number of conditions in women.

In the past the D&C was the main procedure available to determine the cause of abnormal vaginal bleeding—for example, to diagnose uterine fibroids, endometrial polyps, and endometrial cancer. It is still sometimes performed for this reason today. More often, simpler methods such as endometrial biopsy (see biopsy) are used to diagnose bleeding. A D&C can help stop heavy bleeding resulting from endometrial hyperplasia (an overgrowth of the uterine lining) and to remove endometrial polyps (a condition in which thickening occurs in one spot rather than throughout the entire uterus).

A D&C is also used to remove pregnancy tissue from the uterus after miscarriage, childbirth, or incomplete abortion. This is done to stop bleeding and prevent infection that occurs when tissue is retained in the uterus. Finally, although it has generally been replaced by other methods such as vacuum aspiration, a related procedure (dilatation and extraction, or D&E) is still sometimes used to perform an abortion between 12 and 16 weeks of pregnancy.

How is the procedure performed?
Since the cervix must be dilated during a D&C, some form of anesthesia (see entry) is needed. The options include general anesthesia, regional anesthesia (either epidural, spinal, or caudal), or local anesthesia (sometimes with sedatives). Local anesthesia (such as a paracervical block) minimizes the risks and costs of other forms of anesthesia and sometimes allows the procedure to be done on an outpatient basis. Yet a local will still cause the woman to feel some cramping during the procedure. In addition, if a doctor needs to have a particularly accurate view of the pelvic organs, general anesthesia is preferable because it totally relaxes the pelvic muscles.

Once anesthesia has taken effect, the D&C takes only a few minutes to perform. With the woman lying in the same position as in a pelvic examination, the doctor first inserts a speculum to hold open the vaginal walls and then inserts a clamp called a tenaculum to hold the cervix steady. The angle of the cervix and depth of the uterus are determined by inserting a thin metal rod called a sound through the cervix and into the top (fundus) of the uterus.

Next the cervix is dilated (stretched), usually by inserting a progressively widening series of tapered metal rods into the cervical opening. In a dilatation and evacuation to terminate a pregnancy, sometimes the cervix is dilated less painfully by inserting laminaria (long rods of kelp) into the cervix 24 hours before the operation. Once the cervix is fully dilated, another thin metal instrument with a spoon-shaped end, called a curette, is inserted through the cervix into the uterus and used to gently scrape out some of the uterine lining (endometrium) and any polyps that may be present. Usually a small tissue sample scraped from the endometrium (or the cervical canal) is later analyzed for abnormal cells (see biopsy).

What happens after a D&C?
After the procedure many women have mild cramping and backache and pass small clots of blood for a day or so. Vaginal bleeding and staining may last for a couple of weeks. To prevent infection while the cervix is closing, sexual intercourse, douching, and tampons should all be avoided until bleeding has stopped.

What are the risks and complications?
Signs of infection that require immediate medical attention include fever, heavy bleeding, severe cramps, or a foul-smelling vaginal discharge. If promptly reported to a clinician, the infection can be treated with antibiotics before it becomes serious. A woman should also have a postoperative checkup about 2 weeks after the D&C.

Although complications are rare, a D&C is a surgical procedure and therefore involves certain risks, including the risks related to anesthesia. Other rare complications may include perforation of the uterus (a small puncture which often heals itself) or of the bladder or bowel by a surgical instrument.

Related entries
Abortion, anesthesia, biopsy, endometrial hyperplasia, hysteroscopy, infertility, miscarriage, pelvic examinations, polyps, uterine fibroids, vacuum aspiration, vaginal bleeding (abnormal)

Disabilities

While the definition of disability varies widely, in general the term describes any physical or mental impairment that substantially limits at least one major life activity—including walking, seeing, hearing, speaking, breathing, learning, working, and caring for oneself. According to this definition, an estimated 28 million women in the United States live with a physical, cognitive, psychiatric, and/or communication disability. Other surveys and studies, using slightly different definitions, come up with somewhat different figures, but there is no question that disabilities are pervasive, even among younger women. In fact, according to a subsample of the 1990 U.S. Census, nearly 1 in 5 Americans (19.4 percent) aged 15 and older has a disability.

Who is likely to have a disability?

Not surprisingly, the chance of developing a disability increases with age. Approximately 40 percent of women aged 65 and older have at least one functional limitation. Anyone, however, of any age or sex can have a disability, either temporary or permanent. Some are inherited, others result from accidents or disease, and many simply develop as part of the natural aging process.

Generally speaking, disabilities are more common in women than in men, but they vary in incidence by ethnic group. Rates are roughly similar among Native American, African American, and white women (all approximately 1 person in 5), with Asian Americans and women of Pacific Island origin significantly less likely to be affected (just over 1 in 10). Severe disabilities—defined as an inability to perform a functional activity such as self-care or working—are most prevalent in African American women (12.2 percent), followed by Native Americans (9.8 percent), whites (9.4 percent), and Hispanics (8.4 percent). And, as with milder disabilities, the rate of severe disability in women of Asian or Pacific Island origin (4.9 percent) is only about half that for the general population.

Women who experienced physical, sexual, or emotional abuse during childhood run an increased risk of developing disabilities that involve physical and mental dysfunction in adulthood. In some cases these disabilities may be related to other health problems common in women with a history of childhood abuse, including a higher rate of substance abuse, risky sexual behavior, eating disorders, and psychosomatic complaints—as well as a tendency to avoid medical care or disregard medical advice.

What disabilities are most common in women?

Disabilities, by their nature, come in a huge variety of forms. Many—including vision impairments, arthritis, and neurological diseases such as multiple sclerosis—are all more common in women than in men. Some of these disparities may be related to the fact that women generally live longer than men, and thus have more time to develop these age-related disabilities. In the case of arthritis at least, however, relative age does not appear to be a factor; for reasons still not understood, this condition just seems to affect women more than men.

What are the special health care needs of women with disabilities?

The health care system seems particularly ill equipped to deal with the needs of relatively young women (under age 65) with disabilities. These women are more likely than women in the general population to delay medical care for a wide variety of problems. This may be due in part to the relative difficulty of finding health insurance and other financial resources to pay for care. Mental health care, dental care, prescription drugs, and eyeglasses are particularly difficult to obtain for younger women with severe disabilities. Women in the workforce with disabilities not only earn less than women without disabilities but also earn less than working men with disabilities. Perhaps as a result, these women are at increased risk for depression and anxiety, and are twice as likely to smoke cigarettes as women their age who do not have disabilities.

African American and Hispanic women with disabilities have even higher rates of unemployment than other women with disabilities. Combined with cultural barriers, the financial problems that result from these discrepancies undoubtedly exacerbate the disability by further hindering access to medical care.

Women aged 65 and older with disabilities face additional problems, depending on the specific nature of the disability. Many women who develop hearing problems late in life become socially isolated—and, ultimately, angry and/or depressed—because they either refuse to acknowledge the problem or have trouble using a hearing aid for an extended period of time. And many age-related disabilities leave women with a debilitating sense of helplessness, again sparking feelings of depression and anger. Even women who have successfully handled one lifelong disability may feel overwhelmed when age-related disabilities develop. A woman who came to terms with her unpredictable epileptic seizures earlier in life, for example, may experience a renewed sense of helplessness if she begins to lose her vision in her 70s.

Whatever their age, women with disabilities often have to battle pervasive stereotypes that can interfere with the quality of health care they receive. Within the general population, women with disabilities are frequently viewed at best as courageous, if pitiable, victims and at worst as weak, helpless burdens. They are often assumed to be asexual or passively heterosexual as well. Clinicians are not necessarily immune to these stereotypes. Indeed, the very fact that a patient has a disability may make a practitioner feel uncomfortable and helpless, at least unconsciously. For many practitioners, a disability (even an inherited one, or one that requires no medical intervention) is a signal that the medical system has failed. These feelings may lead a practitioner to focus on the disability rather than on the patient as a whole human being, who obviously has issues that go beyond the disability itself.

As a result of these attitudes (which, in most cases, are unconscious), a clinician may sometimes leave out certain routine tests and screening procedures. If a clinician assumes that a woman with a disability is asexual or abstinent, for example, or if he or she focuses only on the disability and not on the patient as a whole person, he or she may decide not to bother offering her a Pap test—thus possibly missing an early-stage, and still treatable, cervical cancer. Similar assumptions may keep a clinician from asking about high-risk activities such as alcohol or tobacco use—despite mounting evidence that having a disability actually increases the risk for substance abuse. Neglect of these procedures may result in part from the well-intentioned but misguided notion that life with a disability must be so intolerable that people with disabilities should be permitted whatever little pleasure they can derive from smoking and drinking.

The result of these realities is that women with disabilities often choose one of two approaches to their health care. Either they delay or avoid care altogether, or else they learn to become advocates for themselves, directing their own health care whenever possible. Unfortunately, the latter approach has led some women with disabilities to be labeled "difficult" patients, although a growing understanding in the medical community of the needs of women with disabilities is slowly changing this situation.

Clinicians are increasingly aware that the most productive approach is to partner with a patient and consider her opinions about her own health and values. This means that clinicians and patients may sometimes have to reconcile differences of opinion about the relative desirability of a treatment. A woman with multiple sclerosis, for example, might disagree with her clinician about a medication that relieves one of her symptoms but has side effects that interfere with her vitality, mental health, and general physical well-being. Ideally, the clinician and patient will together weigh the pros and cons of alternative approaches by considering both the disability itself and the patient's assessment of her overall quality of life.

What are the special social and psychological health issues?

Having a disability can leave a person feeling helpless, frustrated, and out of control. Contrary to popular belief, however, having a disability does not in and of itself necessarily override the possibility of receiving happiness from all other aspects of life. In fact, most people with disabilities appear to be just about as satisfied with their lives as people in the general population. Those who are dissatisfied usually attribute their feelings to social and economic concerns that may stem from the disability—not the physical or mental limitations themselves.

The specific concerns vary widely, depending on the exact nature of the disability, but in general, many women with disabilities complain about limited opportunities for employment, education, recreation, health care, public services, and participation in community life. Negative attitudes on the part of prospective employers, lack of accessible buildings and public transportation, shortage of sign language interpreters, and general disregard for the special needs of the disabled all contribute to these complaints.

The same myths about disabilities that can undermine health care can also lead to feelings of depression, anger, and frustration. They may underlie a negative body image as well—a chronic dissatisfaction with the physical self that is associated with a myriad of other health problems (see body image).

Just how prevalent mental illness is among adults with learning disabilities or mental retardation is a matter of considerable debate. Many experts contend that psychiatric symptoms may go undiagnosed because of a common misperception that sadness, mood swings, or other symptoms of psychiatric disorders are an inevitable consequence of any kind of intellectual impairment. Still little understood are the effects of standard psychotropic drugs on people with learning disabilities and mental retardation.

Some women also resent and reject the notion that they are disabled at all. Many people who were born deaf (or who lost their hearing in infancy), for example, view themselves as members of a different but absolutely normal cultural minority with its own language and values.

What health services are available for women with disabilities?

Although in some sense the majority of people with serious health problems might be considered to have a disability, the medical community has only recently started addressing the needs of this diverse group of patients in any kind of systematic way. In the past, a small number of physicians specialized in treating particular groups of patients who lived in institutions.

Today, however, an increasing number of primary care clinicians have begun treating more patients with disabilities. One reason for this change is that many people with severe physical and/or mental disabilities live among the general population rather than in specialized institutions. In addition, as the general population ages, the percentage of people with disabilities has risen as well. At the same time, increasing numbers of managed care health plans—Medicaid and Medicare, as well as private insurance plans—now cover disabilities. And in spite of the fact that some people with disabilities either shun or have no access to health care services, people with disabilities still tend to use health services more than people in the general population—partly because lack of appropriate care in the past has led them to develop health problems in addition to the disability.

All these other factors aside, a key reason for the rise in health care services to the disabled is that most clinicians are now required by law to provide disability-accessible practices.

What legal protections are available?

The Americans with Disabilities Act (ADA), enacted in 1990, prohibits "professional offices of health care providers" from discriminating against patients with disabilities—something that physicians were legally free to do in the past. This act, as well as similar laws passed by certain states and municipalities, is intended to ensure that people with disabilities have the same access to medical facilities and services as people without disabilities.

The ADA requires medical offices to make reasonable modifications in their rules, policies, and practices to accommodate patients with disabilities. They may need to alter a policy prohibiting patients from bringing pets into the office, for example, to allow a visually impaired patient to bring her guide dog. Or they may have to modify policies regarding outsiders attending medical examinations if a woman with severe disabilities requires a personal care attendant to help lift, dress, or undress her. Other policies may have to be modified (without charge to the patient) to allow women with cognitive impairments more than the usual amount of time to communicate, or to provide an office assistant to explain procedures if the patient so desires. Braille materials, large-print materials, audio recordings, or computer diskettes may have to be used to improve communication with patients who are visually impaired. Sign language interpreters, or perhaps note-writing or printer facilities, may be required to aid women who are deaf or hard of hearing.

Some structural changes may also be necessary to make offices physically accessible to patients who have trouble with mobility. While specific requirements vary, in general there must be at least one accessible entrance to every health care facility. Often this is accomplished with some combination of specially designated parking spaces, curb cuts for wheelchairs, palpable markings on elevator control buttons, flashing alarm lights, widened doorways, special door hardware such as electronic push-buttons, and wheelchair-accessible examination rooms, restrooms, telephones, and water fountains. In some cases, waiting rooms need to be rearranged to accommodate wheelchairs as well. Clinicians are also required to provide sensitivity training for all staff regarding appropriate ways to interact with people with disabilities, and to offer information about procuring qualified sign language interpreters, to refer women to accessible mammogram facilities, and to identify accessible battered women's shelters.

Providers are not required to make any changes that would fundamentally alter their programs or services or pose undue financial or administrative burdens. In these cases it is acceptable to substitute a less expensive or burdensome accommodation or to seek funding for the accommodation from a source other than the patient.

The ADA does not require every single clinician to serve every woman for every health condition. But it does require that the criteria used to determine eligibility be the same for women with and without disabilities. If a physician with a busy practice decides not to accept any new patients, it is perfectly acceptable to refuse to treat a new patient with a disability. Similarly, it is fine for a clinician to refer a woman with a disability to another practitioner for some necessary treatment or service, but it is unacceptable to refer a patient to someone else solely on the basis of her disability. Certain rules, such as requiring a patient to have a driver's license in order to pay by check, would violate the law. In some cases, however, a person with a disability may be excluded from treatment if, on the basis of the best objective evidence, she is perceived to be a threat to the health or safety of others—and the threat cannot be mitigated or eliminated.

How can women with disabilities optimize preventive health care?

Physical examinations. Preventive care—including regular physical examinations (see entry)—is particularly important for women with disabilities because many disabilities put women at relatively high risk for other common health conditions. A thorough physical examination for any woman, with or without a disability, will include information about weight control and substance abuse, as well as a discussion about appropriate forms of exercise (see entry). In many cases, adopting an exercise program adapted to the woman's individual needs—perhaps with the help of a physiatrist, a physician who specializes in restoring function—can relieve pain and improve cardiovascular endurance, muscle strength, coordination, and flexibility.

Because women with disabilities seem unusually likely to experience domestic violence, clinicians will often include a confidential discussion about this issue with the patient alone—outside the presence of any caregiver, friend, or family member who accompanied her to the exam. If appropriate, the clinician will often be able to provide information about shelters accessible to women with disabilities.

Breast examinations. Women who have disabilities that hinder their manual dexterity or the range of motion in their arms may have difficulty performing self-examinations that can help detect breast lumps and thus potential cancer at an early stage. That is why regular mammograms and breast examinations by a clinician are particularly important for women with disabilities. The catch, however, is that disabilities can also make office examinations difficult if not impossible. Women who cannot stand or raise their arms and turn their bodies cannot be screened with standard mammography equipment. And many clinicians are not trained in performing optimal breast examinations for women with mobility impairments.

Many of these problems can be overcome by asking clinicians for a list of facilities with mammogram machines that are accessible to women with impaired mobility. The state public health department may also help identify such facilities.

Pelvic examinations. Regular pelvic examinations—and, in some cases, tests for sexually transmitted diseases—are as vital for a woman with disabilities as for her non-disabled counterparts. In fact, wheelchair users are particularly susceptible to vaginal infections because of poor ventilation and accumulation of moisture in the genital region. In addition, women with sensory impairments may not be able to feel pain associated with pelvic diseases, and women with visual disabilities may overlook lesions associated with various sexually transmitted diseases such as herpes, syphilis, or genital warts.

Too often, however, clinicians avoid doing pelvic examinations (see entry) on women with disabilities, partly because of the misconception that women with disabilities are sexually inactive, and partly because pelvic examinations can be painful, difficult, or even dangerous for women with certain disabilities. Often these obstacles can be overcome by using alternative positions for the examination or by providing patients with specially equipped examination tables (particularly ones equipped with handrails and adjustable boots that accommodate different leg positions). Patients with neurological conditions that prevent them from controlling their legs can often be helped by applying lidocaine gel (to relieve pain) and gently stretching the lower extremities while getting into position. Emptying the bladder and bowels before the examination can help minimize accidents in patients with neurological disabilities as well.

Sexuality, contraception, and pregnancy. Clearly, certain disabilities by nature interfere with a woman's sexuality—both her desire to have sex (libido) and her ability, physical and/or psychological, to enjoy it. What isn't as obvious is that, in many cases, treatment for various disabilities can also interfere with sexuality. For example, a number of medications—including diuretics, serotonin reuptake inhibitors (antidepressants), phenytoin, lithium, digoxin, reserpine, and naproxen—can interfere with sex drive.

A disability can also affect decisions about pregnancy and birth control. Pregnancy is clearly risky in women with certain disabilities, including multiple sclerosis, paralysis, and cerebral palsy. Birth control choices can be limited by a disability as well. On the one hand, oral contraception is often ill advised in women with problems such as diabetes, kidney failure, heart disease, circulatory disorders, or impaired muscle tone or mobility in the legs. Diaphragms and cervical caps may pose a problem for women with recurrent vaginal or bladder infections, weakened pelvic muscles, or limited manual dexterity. And intrauterine devices (IUDs) may be a poor choice for women who lack the manual dexterity to locate the string and determine if the device is in place, or who can't feel pain that would otherwise warn them about dislocation or infection.

These issues are often overlooked in the course of a physical examination. In fact, one study of people undergoing rehabilitation for spinal cord injuries found that women were twice as likely as their male counterparts to receive no sex education or counseling whatsoever. Undoubtedly this silence is the result of the widespread misconception that women with disabilities are asexual, or at least abstinent, combined with the lack of confidence that many women feel when it comes to asking questions about sexuality and contraception. That is why it is important for a sexually active woman with a disabilitiy to find a clinician who routinely asks nonjudgmental questions about sexual activity to all patients, regardless of disability status.

Related entries
Body image, domestic abuse, eating disorders, exercise, pelvic examinations, physical examinations, psychosomatic disorders, sexual abuse and incest, substance abuse

Dissociative Identity Disorder

Dissociative identity disorder (DID), (formerly multiple personality disorder) is a psychiatric condition in which the person's identity is split between two or more alternating personalities. Often people with this disorder have problems establishing intimacy with other people and have histories of intense, stormy, unstable relationships. These same difficulties in close relationships also make them particularly vulnerable to victimization by lovers, family, and caregivers.

Who is likely to develop DID?
Standard textbooks of psychiatry classify dissociative identity disorder (DID) as a form of conversion disorder—a psychosomatic disorder (see entry) which involves a loss or alteration of some physical function that seems to have a physical cause but is actually caused by an identifiable psychological conflict or need. There is accumulating evidence, however, that DID is more appropriately understood as a variant of posttraumatic stress disorder (see entry) following abuse or other trauma.

One study, for example, showed that virtually all people with dissociative identity disorder had experienced some kind of childhood trauma, including incest or witnessing the violent death of a close friend or relative. A background of childhood trauma also predisposes people to developing borderline personality disorder and severe depression, both of which often occur with dissociative identity disorder. The vast majority of people with DID are women.

What are the symptoms?
Usually people with dissociative identity disorder have a primary personality and at least one secondary personality. Typically the primary personality is conventional, conservative, moralistic, sickly, and "good," while the secondary personality (or one of the secondary personalities) is uninhibited, playful, irresponsible, healthy, and "bad." There may be many other personalities as well, always including one personality who knows about all of the others. Whereas the primary personality tends not to be aware of the secondary personality, the secondary personality not only knows about the primary but frequently ridicules it or undermines it. The primary personality may, however, hear voices telling it to behave in ways it considers inappropriate.

There is often a variety of other symptoms as well. The primary personality may have a number of psychosomatic complaints such as headaches, mysterious aches and pains, and gastrointestinal problems. Other symptoms associated with hysteria—such as paralysis that does not seem to be linked to a physical disorder—are also common. These symptoms disappear when the secondary personality takes over.

How is the condition evaluated?
Dissociative identity disorder is often extremely difficult to diagnose. This is partly because the symptoms can be so var-

ied and often suggest other mental disorders. It is also because people tend to deny the diagnosis of dissociative identity disorder once they receive it. Whatever the explanation, it takes an average of 6 years for a person with this disorder to receive an accurate diagnosis after entering the mental health care system. Frequently women with dissociative identity disorder are misdiagnosed as having schizophrenia (see entry), conversion disorder, or somatization disorder.

How is dissociative identity disorder treated?

Dissociative identity disorder is generally treated with long-term psychotherapy, with the goal for the patient of integrating disparate personalities and of being able to tolerate and accept the negative emotions (for example, rage and vulnerability) which were originally splintered into separate entities because the woman could not bear them. If the source of the disorder turns out to be an earlier traumatic experience, the psychotherapeutic process should resemble that for treating posttraumatic stress disorder.

Related entries

Depression, domestic abuse, personality disorders, posttraumatic stress disorder, psychosomatic disorders, psychotherapy, schizophrenia, sexual abuse and incest

Diuretics

Diuretics—also called water pills—are drugs that increase the amount of urine excreted by the kidneys and, as a result, decrease the body's water and salt content.

Diuretics are often the drug of choice in treating high blood pressure. They are commonly used to treat mild congestive heart failure as well as certain disorders of the circulatory system and liver which lead to excess fluid retention. Diuretics are sometimes taken to relieve the bloating that can accompany premenstrual syndrome or menstruation. Used as prescribed, diuretics are generally safe.

The use of diuretics in pregnancy, once a common defense against fluid retention and preeclampsia (see entry), is no longer recommended, since it can be dangerous to both mother and child.

What are the risks and complications?

People with eating disorders or substance abuse disorders often abuse diuretics in the attempt to lose weight quickly or to wash out traces of drugs in their urine. Though not physically addictive, diuretics can cause a psychological addiction which reinforces the desire to lose weight or the craving for other substances.

Increased frequency of urination can be a disturbing side effect for anyone who has problems with incontinence. Also, an overdose of diuretics has the potential to cause various mineral imbalances, which, if uncorrected, can produce fluid

depletion, heart arrhythmias, shock, or, in very rare circumstances, death.

A depletion of potassium is one of the most common side effects of taking diuretics, especially if combined with a vigilant low-salt diet (as is commonly advocated in the treatment of hypertension). This problem is usually easily remedied with potassium supplements, and possibly by adding potassium-rich foods such as tomatoes, oranges, raisins, and bananas to the diet—although the dietary changes necessary to overcome potassium loss from diuretics may be unrealistic. It is a good idea for people using diuretics on a daily basis to have their blood potassium levels monitored regularly. Some diuretics can increase levels of cholesterol or sugar in the blood, which can be problematic for people with heart disease or diabetes.

Various herbal remedies are often advocated as risk-free alternatives to diuretic medications. Some of these, though never scientifically studied for effectiveness, may be worth trying to see if they relieve relatively minor conditions such as premenstrual bloating. Celery, asparagus, cucumbers, and parsley are claimed by some self-help advocates to have diuretic effects, and eating them is safe even for more serious disorders so long as this does not preclude regular consultations with a clinician to make sure other treatment is not required.

It is important to remember, however, that just because something is "natural" or "herbal" does not necessarily mean it cannot have potent and sometimes toxic effects on the body. Diuretic herbal teas, for example, should be used only in moderation until safe dosages have been determined. In addition, products marketed specifically as "herbal remedies" must be used with particular care because they are not subjected to rigorous inspection procedures for purity and potency as are official medicines.

Related entries

Alternative therapies, anorexia nervosa and bulimia nervosa, edema, incontinence, premenstrual syndrome, substance abuse

Diverticular Disease

Diverticular disease is a common cause of pelvic or abdominal pain. In its mildest form, known as diverticulosis, outpouchings called diverticula form in the colon. Usually found in the lower (sigmoid) portion (see illustration), these are thought to result from slow-moving stools which increase pressure within the colon. Diverticulosis has become increasingly common in industrialized Western countries over the past 75 years or so, and this has led many investigators to link it to the practice of milling, which removes much of the fiber content from flour. The lower a country's fiber intake, it appears, the higher its incidence of diverticular disease.

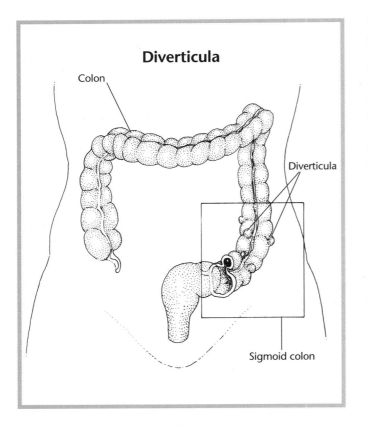

Diverticula

Colon

Diverticula

Sigmoid colon

Sometimes feces become lodged in the diverticula, making them susceptible to ulceration, abscess formation, and bacterial infection. If the diverticula become inflamed or rupture, the condition is called diverticulitis. The inflamed segment may stick to the bladder, small bowel, or nearby pelvic organs such as the vagina (particularly after a hysterectomy), and this can result in a fistula—or abnormal passageway—from one organ to the other. Perforated diverticula can spill pus or fecal material from the colon throughout the abdominal cavity, resulting in a serious condition called peritonitis, in which the lining of the abdominal cavity becomes inflamed or infected.

Who is likely to develop diverticular disease?

The incidence of diverticular disease increases with age. Between 30 and 40 percent of people over 50 have diverticula in their colons, usually without experiencing any symptoms. The percentages are higher with each additional decade of age.

What are the symptoms?

Most of the time diverticulosis involves no symptoms at all and may only be discovered after a barium enema is done to check for polyps, cancerous growths, or other abnormalities of the gastrointestinal tract. Some people do develop chronic or constant abdominal pain and changes in bowel habits, most frequently episodes of constipation. Alternatively, there may be periods of constipation that alternate with diarrhea and then with long stretches of normal bowel function.

These problems may worsen after eating and be relieved after a bowel movement or passing gas.

Symptoms most often develop if one of the diverticula becomes infected, resulting in diverticulitis. The classic symptoms of diverticulitis are abdominal pain, especially on the lower left side, and fever. Occasionally the pain may be felt instead just above the pubic area or on the lower right side, where it may be mistaken for appendicitis. There may be some blood in the stool, as well as nausea, vomiting, and lack of appetite. Although the pain may be mild at first, it can quickly become severe, especially if peritonitis has developed. If the bowel is obstructed, the abdomen can become distended and feel crampy. Some people also feel pain during urination if diverticula are sticking to the bladder.

How is the condition evaluated?

Although examinations of the gastrointestinal tract with tests such as a barium enema or colonoscopy can reveal diverticula, the mere presence of these outpouchings does not necessarily implicate them as the cause of the symptoms. Other common causes of abdominal and pelvic pain in women include irritable bowel syndrome, colon cancer, and ectopic pregnancy (see entries). These can be ruled out by one or more of a number of procedures for examining the gastrointestinal tract (such as a barium enema, colonoscopy, ultrasound, and sigmoidoscopy; see bowel disorders) and various blood tests.

How is diverticular disease treated?

Many physicians recommend no treatment at all for people with diverticulosis but no symptoms. Eating a low-fat, high-fiber diet—one that includes large amounts of grains, legumes, fresh fruits, and vegetables—is all the "treatment" that is required.

When symptoms of diverticulitis develop, treatment consists of antibiotics and "bowel rest"—a diet of clear liquids only, which gives the inflamed area a chance to heal. If a person becomes severely ill or has rectal bleeding, hospitalization is necessary. Treatment may include intravenous fluids and electrolytes, antibiotics to combat infection, blood transfusions, and a diet of clear liquids. Surgery may be needed to prevent life-threatening hemorrhage or widespread infection, especially if diverticula have ruptured.

Related entries

Bowel disorders, colon and rectal cancer, constipation, irritable bowel syndrome, nutrition

Domestic Abuse

Over 2 million women in the United States are battered by a family member each year, and over two-thirds of all violent attacks against women are committed by someone the victim knows. Women are 10 times more likely than men to be attacked by spouses, ex-spouses, partners, boyfriends, parents, or children. One in 3 women seeking emergency room care has a history of partner violence. One in 4 pregnant women is battered. One in 7 women visiting a doctor's office has a history of domestic abuse. Up to half of all murders in this country occur within the family. Battering is an all too frequent occurrence between lesbian partners as well.

Domestic abuse can be psychological or sexual as well as physical. Sexual abuse is any form of forced sex or sexual degradation by a family member. In psychological abuse, a jealous or possessive family member may threaten or intimidate a woman with words alone, forcing her to curtail all other relationships and thus restrict her sources of social support. Demeaning comments, constant criticism, or outbursts of temper directed at a woman on a regular basis are a form of psychological abuse. Regardless of which form it takes, all domestic abuse against women (along with rape, incest, and sexual harassment) is an act of violence in which the perpetrator asserts control or power, thereby victimizing a woman and limiting her personal freedom.

There are many reasons why women continue a relationship despite a history of abuse. Women often continue to love and forgive their abusive partner and cling to the frequent apologies and promises to reform. Sometimes the impulse to forgive reflects a woman's low self-esteem or an inability to express anger or aggression. It can also be bolstered by ties to the partner—through children or finances—that cannot easily be severed. Religious and cultural pressures, including traditional gender roles, may also be a factor.

Some women feel that it is their personal duty to help their "sick" partner or that abusive partners may do physical harm to themselves or others if abandoned. They may believe that if the partner would only overcome a drug or alcohol problem, the abuse would dissipate. Often a woman feels that she cannot leave an abusive relationship because she has no place to go and no way to support herself. She may think that if she leaves, her partner will find her and kill her and her children. Fear plays a major role in her decision to stay.

Who is likely to be a victim of domestic abuse?

Women who were themselves abused as children or witnessed domestic abuse between their parents are much more likely than others to end up as abused spouses later in life—and to abuse their own children. They are also more likely to be dependent on alcohol or other substances, or to have a relationship with a dependent partner.

Women between the ages of 18 and 24 are at the greatest risk of being abused by a partner, although domestic abuse can occur against women of any age. Commonly the male partner is underemployed or has a job that he feels is beneath his wife's occupational or educational level. Pregnant women are particularly likely to be victims of domestic abuse, and often at this time the violence is directed at the fetus. For example, kicks or blows to the abdominal area or breasts are common, as is sexual assault or increased demand for sexual

intercourse. In addition to threatening a woman's health and sometimes even her life, abuse during pregnancy increases the risk of miscarriage and delivering an infant of low birth weight.

What are the symptoms of domestic abuse?

In addition to the direct damage inflicted by physical blows, domestic abuse takes a severe toll on a battered woman's health, well-being, and self-esteem. Nearly half of the 206 females seeking help for gastrointestinal complaints in one study had a history of childhood sexual and physical abuse, and about half of them claimed that they were still experiencing some form of abuse. Among these women, the ones with a history of physical abuse were 4 times more likely to have diffuse pelvic pain, backaches, and shortness of breath. In other studies, researchers found that women with a history of abuse had undergone more surgeries during their lifetime than women without that history, and they were more likely to have been hospitalized—not just for trauma resulting from the abuse but also for suicide attempts, gynecological problems, and general observation for undefined disorders.

Women who have been physically or sexually abused have a higher than normal incidence of abdominal pain, irritable bowel syndrome, and functional bowel disease, and are more prone to headaches, insomnia, and fatigue. This does not necessarily mean that the abuse actually leads to the physical symptoms. There is a possibility that women who complain about physical symptoms also tend to speak up more about sexual abuse and violence, as well as a possibility that there is some emotional factor that increases a woman's chances of both developing such symptoms and entering into an abusive relationship. The precise link between abuse and physical symptoms has not been fully explored.

Studies of the psychological consequences of battering and victimization also remain in their infancy. Still, it is clear that women with a history of domestic abuse have substantially increased rates of psychological illness—particularly depression, eating disorders, alcoholism, and substance abuse. Typically, abused women have feelings of despair, helplessness, hopelessness, inadequacy, worthlessness, and fear. They are also more likely than other women to abuse family members physically or verbally or to abuse themselves through self-mutilation, self-starvation, or revictimization (returning to a partner only to experience further abuse). Those women who have been both physically and sexually abused are also more likely to experience sexual dysfunction, with loathing and disgust sometimes accompanying the thought of sexual relations.

Over a quarter of women who attempt suicide are victims of domestic violence, and some studies suggest that 40 percent of women in alcohol treatment programs started out as battered women. Abused women, including women who have been stalked as well as those who have been physically or psychologically assaulted, often show signs of posttraumatic stress disorder (see entry), a mental illness characterized by both psychological and physiological reactions. This disorder occurs when severe trauma overwhelms normal psychological and biological coping mechanisms.

Women who have been battered seem to have an increased rate of personality disorders (see entry), especially borderline personality disorder and antisocial personality disorder. Victimization is also associated with a high rate of psychosomatic disorders (see entry), such as conversion disorder, somatization disorder, and chronic pain syndrome (often involving pelvic pain).

How is the condition evaluated?

One study found that only about 1 in 5 doctors detected abuse in battered women, despite the fact that many of these women had visited them multiple times. In some cases these women had seen the doctor 6 or 7 times in one year. The problem is that domestic abuse can be exceedingly difficult for a clinician to spot. For one thing, battered women are often afraid, unable, or unwilling to acknowledge the source of their injuries—or may even deny them to themselves. Many battered women distrust the medical care system and have difficulty communicating with health care professionals. The abusers themselves may also prevent women from seeking medical attention, except perhaps for prenatal care or to have an induced abortion (especially after sexual abuse). Women who see themselves as saviors of their abusers often fear that acknowledging the abuse to a medical professional may result in the abuser's arrest and prosecution (as indeed, in some cases, it may, especially if the victim is a minor).

Clinicians are only now being trained to look for these problems and to take them seriously. If a woman comes into a doctor's office seeking help for a headache or fatigue, for example, it is not always immediately obvious that her real problem is forced intercourse or domestic abuse.

How do victims of domestic abuse get help?

Efforts by the women's movement and the victims of crime movement have helped diminish misperceptions about domestic abuse and made it easier for battered women to get help. There are now shelters and support groups for battered women and their families in many communities around the country. These groups can provide information about the legal rights of battered women and can advise them on child custody issues. Advocates from these programs can accompany a woman to court if necessary and help her attain temporary or permanent restraining orders against the abuser. Both state and federal victims of crime programs can help women recover any lost wages or uncovered medical or psychotherapy costs incurred while under care for abuse. Unfortunately, most abused women still do not use shelters. Many shelters are poorly equipped to care for women with severe medical problems, who are pregnant, who have a history of substance abuse, or who are in abusive same-sex relationships.

Increasing numbers of physicians are learning that victims of domestic abuse need more than treatment for their physical wounds, and, together with a nurse practitioner and so-cial worker, can assess a woman's risk of future injury, direct her to appropriate referral centers or a psychotherapist, and help her find a safe and supportive place to stay. They can also reinforce the idea that the woman is not alone and not to blame, and that assistance is available.

In the past the mental health community held that domestic abuse was a family matter and that family therapy was the only appropriate way to treat it. Now many authorities in this area think that this approach is too idealistic. Today it is generally agreed that if psychotherapy or any other kind of intervention is to be effective, the abuser must first be arrested.

Related entries

Alcohol, depression, miscarriage, pelvic pain, personality disorders, posttraumatic stress disorder, psychosomatic disorders, psychotherapy, sexual abuse and incest, sexual assault, sexual harassment, stress, substance abuse

Douching

Douching is a means of washing out the vagina by forcing water or some other fluid up into it. With the exception of douches prescribed by a clinician to treat certain vaginal infections, douching is never necessary for health. Baths and showers normally provide adequate vaginal cleanliness for women in good health.

Douching is the oldest—and probably the least effective—form of birth control. Although douching immediately after sexual intercourse to flush semen from the vagina may slightly decrease the chances of fertilization (and this is debatable), the fact is that sperm can reach the uterus and usually the fallopian tubes well before most women can get to the bathroom to douche. In fact, some of the sperm may actually be sped along toward the egg at the same time that other sperm are being washed away. Douching is similarly ineffective as a means of protection against sexually transmitted diseases. Nonetheless, a woman who wants to become pregnant should certainly avoid douching after intercourse.

Women who feel uncomfortable unless they douche after menstrual periods or sexual intercourse should use plain water or a very dilute solution of white vinegar in water.

What are the risks and complications?

The feminine hygiene products sold over the counter often contain deodorants and other chemicals that can irritate or inflame vaginal tissue or provoke allergic reactions in susceptible women. Douching can also force disease-causing microorganisms farther up into the reproductive system and upset the vagina's normal acidity, thereby increasing the risk of vaginitis.

Under no circumstances should douching be done at

any time during pregnancy or within 6 weeks after giving birth. Women should not douche within 2 weeks of a dilatation and curettage (D&C) or abortion, and they should not douche for 24 hours before a pelvic examination, since washing out natural vaginal secretions can make it difficult to diagnose vaginal infections.

Related entries
Birth control, natural birth control methods, sexually transmitted diseases, vaginitis

Dry Eye

Dry eye is the name for a group of conditions in which the tear film that normally lubricates and protects the eye is inadequate. A nagging problem for many women, dry eye only rarely progresses to the point of vision damage.

The tear film normally covers the cornea—the transparent layer of tissue on the outer surface of the eye which helps focus light. It consists of an inner mucous layer, a middle aqueous (watery) layer, and an outer lipid (oily) layer that keeps the watery layer from evaporating. A rather complex liquid structure, this film is susceptible to a number of problems which lead to its disruption, resulting in common eye complaints and even serious, blinding disease.

These problems become particularly prevalent as the eye ages. Age can bring on dysfunctions in the glands that secrete each of the three layers of tear film. Over time the mucous membrane of the tear film can break down so that it no longer adheres to the middle (watery) layer of tears. Problems with the outer two layers of the tear film can also expose the mucous layer to the air and ultimately cause it to deteriorate. For example, some eye specialists suspect that hormonal changes related to menopause may interfere with the normal functioning of the lacrimal gland, which secretes the middle (watery) layer of the tear film, and of other glands in the eyelid which secrete the lipid and mucous layers. Also contributing to dry eye in older people is the weakening of the eyelid muscles that normally open and close the eye. This can make the eyelid less efficient at squeezing away old tear film and replenishing it.

Who is likely to develop dry eye?
Although dry eye appears to be particularly common among menopausal and postmenopausal women, the ultimate cause of the problem remains somewhat mysterious. Breakdown in the tear film is sometimes attributed to a decrease in the hormone estrogen, but there is no available evidence backing this theory. In fact, some eye doctors have noted that women who take estrogen replacement therapy are no less likely to have symptoms than other women of the same age.

Occasionally, dry eye can occur in women who have had eyelid surgery (blepharoplasty). This is probably because the resculpted eyelids may be particularly tight and unable to close fully, thus exposing the tear film to drying air. Dry eye can also be a side effect of a number of different medications, including some eyedrops and ointments. It is also a common symptom of Sjögren syndrome, an autoimmune disorder that can affect the kidneys, blood vessels, and nervous system, as well as the tear glands.

Pregnant women also commonly have problems with dry eyes because of hormonal changes that decrease the production of tears. These changes generally begin about the 10th week of pregnancy and can last up to 6 months after the birth of the baby—when hormone levels have at last readjusted—or longer in breastfeeding women. Some pregnant women who wear hard contact lenses, which can be uncomfortable without adequate tear film, may have to rely on their eyeglasses for the duration of the pregnancy.

What are the symptoms?
Dry eye is characterized by persistently scratchy, red, swollen, hot, or otherwise irritated eyes which may feel as if they have a foreign body lodged in them. Sometimes dust or glaring lights may actually lead dry eyes to water profusely, but not with the normal tear film that would help lubrication.

How is the condition evaluated?
A clinician evaluating dry eye will want to rule out any easily remediable sources of the problem—such as prescription medications—and then check to see if there are any abnormalities in the tear film or the surface of the eye. Tests may be done to analyze the nature of the tear film, to estimate its volume, or to assess the time it takes to break up. Other tests may be done to check for debris in the film, to determine the thickness and quality of the lipid layer, or to assess the function of the glands that produce each layer of film. All of these tests are best done when the eye is free of eyedrops and the lids and lashes free of makeup.

How is dry eye treated?
Although treatment for dry eye depends to some extent on the underlying defect, symptoms can often be relieved with artificial tears. These are available in drop form without a prescription. In addition, if inflammation of the eyelids—called blepharitis—is also present, better eyelid hygiene and even antibiotic medications may help. Researchers are looking into the possibility of using certain biochemically active substances (such as enzyme activators or inhibitors) that help increase the production, preservation, or secretion of the natural tear film.

How can dry eye be prevented?
Some eye specialists believe that it may be possible to preserve the function of the tear-producing meibomian glands with weekly "lid scrubs." These involve carefully washing the lash line with a cotton swab or clean washcloth dipped in dilute baby shampoo and then rinsing with warm water. After-

ward, warm compresses should be placed on the lids to encourage gland secretion. This good "eye hygiene" may not be a bad idea and may indeed reduce the chance of eyelid infection, although it probably cannot prevent most cases of dry eye.

Related entries

Estrogen, estrogen replacement therapy, eye care, eyelid surgery, menopause, rheumatoid arthritis, Sjögren syndrome

Eclampsia

Eclampsia is a serious complication of pregnancy in which the pregnant woman develops convulsions, becomes unconscious, and lapses into a coma. Every year 3 in 100,000 pregnant women (0.003 percent) die from complications of eclampsia. These include strokes, bleeding disorders, liver failure, and kidney failure, as well as blindness and placenta abruptio (the premature separation of the placenta from the uterine wall). The risks to the fetus include premature birth, which may lead to respiratory distress and other potentially life-threatening conditions.

Who is likely to develop eclampsia?

Eclampsia is almost always preceded by preeclampsia (see entry)—characterized by high blood pressure, swelling, and protein in the urine—and it can often be prevented with monitoring. The cause of both preeclampsia and eclampsia is unknown. About 6 percent of pregnant women develop preeclampsia after the 20th week of pregnancy, and about 0.1 percent of all pregnant women go on to develop eclampsia.

Women at highest risk for preeclampsia include those who are having their first baby, who are under 20 or over 45 years of age, who are carrying two or more fetuses, who have high blood pressure, who have a history of preeclampsia in a previous pregnancy, or who have diabetes, a kidney disorder, or an autoimmune disease. But some women who have none of these risk factors nevertheless develop preeclampsia. The more severe the symptoms of preeclampsia, the greater the risk that the condition will progress to eclampsia.

What are the symptoms?

Seizures (convulsions) during pregnancy, labor, or delivery or after delivery are the chief symptoms of eclampsia. Although some women may have only one or two seizures, others may have many if the condition goes untreated. These seizures can be severe enough to cause unconsciousness or coma, or, in severe cases, death.

In about half of the women with eclampsia, seizures develop before delivery. Usually labor follows shortly thereafter and is often quite rapid. About a quarter of women with eclampsia do not start having seizures until labor or delivery begins, however. Sometimes convulsions start again the day after delivery. Another quarter of women with eclampsia do not develop any symptoms until after delivery is over. These usually occur during the first 24 hours after childbirth.

How is the condition evaluated?

A clinician will attribute convulsions and coma in a pregnant or postpartum woman to eclampsia if there is no explanation other than the prior existence of preeclampsia.

How is eclampsia treated?

Once convulsions begin, a woman with eclampsia is hospitalized and generally given magnesium sulfate or other anticonvulsants to control the convulsions. She may also receive antihypertensive medications to lower her blood pressure. If she has not yet had the baby, labor will usually be delayed (if possible) until symptoms are under control. Ultimately, however, the treatment for eclampsia is delivery of the baby.

After delivery the woman will be monitored closely to make sure symptoms do not recur. Because most seizures occur within 24 hours of delivery, she may be given magnesium sulfate for at least this long to prevent seizures. Meanwhile, fluid intake and output will be closely monitored.

Most complications of eclampsia can be managed with medication. Stroke, however, can have devastating and irreversible consequences.

How can eclampsia be prevented?

Eclampsia can often be prevented with early detection and treatment of preeclampsia. This in turn involves good prenatal care, including increasingly frequent checkups during the third trimester of pregnancy, as well as frequent checks of weight gain, blood pressure, and urine. If symptoms of preeclampsia develop, labor may have to be induced as soon as possible to prevent eclampsia, although some women may be able to get by for a few weeks with bed rest and frequent, careful monitoring.

There is no evidence that a protein-rich diet can help prevent preeclampsia or eclampsia, nor does taking strong sedative or anticonvulsive drugs seem warranted. It is controversial whether women who have had either preeclampsia or eclampsia are more predisposed than other women to develop hypertension later in life. It is probably prudent for women with a history of preeclampsia to have a yearly blood pressure evaluation.

Related entries

Diuretics, edema, high blood pressure, preeclampsia, prenatal care

Ectopic Pregnancy

Ectopic pregnancy—also called tubal pregnancy—occurs when the fertilized egg implants in some part of the body other than the uterus, usually one of the fallopian tubes (see illustration) but in rare cases the ovaries, abdominal cavity, or cervical canal instead. If the condition goes undetected, the fallopian tube or other body part usually tears or ruptures because it cannot accommodate the growing embryo. This can lead to severe internal bleeding and possible future fertility problems from scarring. If not treated promptly, an ectopic pregnancy can be life-threatening. For this reason, any woman of reproductive age who experiences sharp or constant one-sided pain in the lower abdomen or pelvis for more than a few hours or irregular bleeding or staining after a light or late menstrual period should obtain prompt medical attention.

Who is likely to have an ectopic pregnancy?

The incidence of ectopic pregnancy has risen in the past few decades. Although any woman in her reproductive years is at risk, ectopic pregnancy is more common in women whose fallopian tubes have been damaged as a result of endometriosis, pelvic inflammatory disease, pelvic adhesions, gonorrhea, ruptured appendix, ruptured ovarian cyst, tubal surgery, or previous ectopic pregnancy. These conditions produce scar tissue which may interfere with the passage of the fertilized egg into the uterus. Risk of ectopic pregnancy is also higher in women who conceive while taking oral contraceptives containing only progestin, and in women whose mothers took diethylstilbestrol (DES) during pregnancy. Women who have already had an ectopic pregnancy are at increased risk, too. In any subsequent pregnancies, these women may require extra checkups and tests.

What are the symptoms?

Some women with an ectopic pregnancy experience no symptoms until the tube ruptures. Some do not even realize that they are pregnant, since an ectopic pregnancy may not result in a positive pregnancy test. Usually, however, a woman with this condition will begin experiencing slight bleeding or pain approximately 6 to 8 weeks after conception (which is usually 4 to 6 weeks after a missed period) or earlier. Signs that the tube has ruptured or is about to rupture include sharp or constant pain in the lower abdomen, often on one side and sometimes accompanied by shoulder pain. Some women faint or black out because of severe blood loss.

How is the condition evaluated?

Ectopic pregnancy can be difficult to differentiate from conditions such as threatened miscarriage, infection of the fallopian tubes, the vaginal bleeding or spotting that many women experience during a successful pregnancy, or even appendicitis. If there is pain as well as bleeding in a pregnant woman, however, the cause is probably ectopic pregnancy or miscarriage. Bleeding will often be heavy in the case of miscarriage, whereas it is usually spotty in the case of ectopic pregnancy. Also, a woman having a miscarriage generally has cramping in her lower abdomen, whereas a woman with an ectopic pregnancy has sharper and constant one-sided pain, and, because of internal bleeding, can sometimes feel pain in

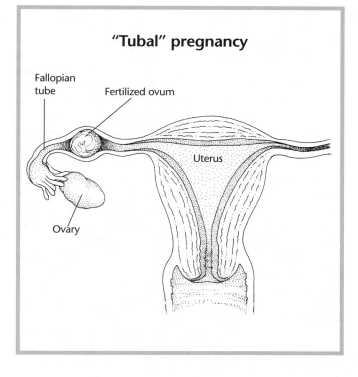

"Tubal" pregnancy

Fallopian tube

Fertilized ovum

Uterus

Ovary

the shoulder or near the diaphragm. Rapid pulse, low blood pressure, and a low blood count can also signal internal bleeding.

One way to determine an ectopic pregnancy is to measure the levels of the hormone human chorionic gonadotropin (hCG) in blood samples taken over a period of time to see how much they rise as the pregnancy progresses. A special kind of quantitative blood test called a radioimmunoassay can detect extremely low levels of this hormone (which is secreted by the developing placenta), even when hCG is not detectable in urine pregnancy tests. If levels of hCG in the blood do not rise by 66 percent to 100 percent after 48 hours, then an abnormal pregnancy (either ectopic or potential miscarriage) is suspected. Ultrasonography may also be performed. If no gestational sac can be detected within the uterus, ectopic pregnancy is the more likely diagnosis. Diagnosis can be particularly tricky in the first 4 weeks of pregnancy, when ultrasonography (which is generally quite sensitive) is still sometimes unable to detect the location of the embryo. A combination of ultrasound and blood tests (see pregnancy testing) can detect most cases.

How is ectopic pregnancy treated?

Treatment options vary, depending on the woman's age or desire to bear subsequent children, as well as the extent of damage and the presence of infection. Whatever the decision, action must be taken quickly to prevent life-threatening hemorrhage. Usually the developing fetus, placenta, and surrounding tissue can be removed through the incision made during a laparoscopy. Otherwise the practitioner will make a somewhat larger incision through the abdomen (see laparotomy).

Although the affected tube can sometimes be preserved, one that has already ruptured usually must be removed, which means that for subsequent pregnancies the woman will have to rely on the one remaining tube (although eggs can travel from the remaining ovary to the distant tube for fertilization). If one tube has already been removed, the loss of the second would prevent future pregnancies unless a woman was willing to use in vitro fertilization—a laboratory procedure in which eggs are extracted from the woman's ovaries, mixed with sperm, and then placed inside the uterus for implantation. The affected fallopian tube should be removed if it is damaged beyond repair, if the woman has had more than one ectopic pregnancy, or if she does not want any subsequent pregnancies. After any kind of surgery the woman will be followed up on a weekly basis until radioimmunoassay can no longer detect any hCG in the blood.

In some women in the early stages of an ectopic pregnancy, drug treatment may be an alternative to surgery and may increase the odds of successful future pregnancies. Methotrexate, a drug used to treat certain forms of cancer because it is toxic to growing cells, can sometimes be given by injection over a period of days to help dissolve the embryonic tissues. It can also be administered in the hospital over a shorter period of time or injected directly into the ectopic site during laparoscopy or under ultrasonic guidance. A physician can determine if drug treatment is appropriate for a particular ectopic pregnancy.

How can ectopic pregnancy be prevented?

The only precautions that a woman can take to try to prevent ectopic pregnancy are to avoid pelvic inflammatory disease (PID), which produces scar tissue in the fallopian tubes. PID is caused by chlamydia and other sexually transmitted diseases.

Related entries

Adhesions, diethylstilbestrol (DES), dilatation and curettage, infertility, laparoscopy, miscarriage, pelvic inflammatory disease, sexually transmitted diseases, vaginal bleeding (abnormal), vaginal bleeding during pregnancy

pregnancy, or earlier in hot weather. In both cases the exact cause of the edema is unknown, but it is generally attributed to changes in levels of estrogen and progesterone.

Substantial edema can be a symptom of more serious medical conditions. Although bloating is a common development in normal pregnancies, for example, if it is accompanied by rapid weight gain, it may signal preeclampsia. This complication of pregnancy can progress to life-threatening eclampsia if untreated. Severe edema can also be a symptom of serious heart, kidney, or liver disorders.

How is the condition evaluated?

Where the bloating occurs is sometimes a clue to the underlying problem. Swollen ankles, for example, are most commonly due to malfunction of the veins in the legs. This condition (termed venous insufficiency) is relatively benign. Less often, ankle swelling may be a sign of heart or circulatory disorders. Fluid that accumulates in the lungs (pulmonary edema) can be a complication of congestive heart failure, which requires immediate medical attention. A thorough physical examination, and whatever tests seem appropriate based on the physical examination and the patient's history, are the first steps a clinician will take to evaluate a woman whose primary complaint is swelling.

How is edema treated?

Edema will frequently disappear once the underlying medical condition is treated. Less severe swelling can often be relieved by restricting intake of salt, since sodium increases water retention in body tissues. Diuretics—water pills—may also provide relief because they decrease the body's water and salt content by increasing the amount of urine excreted. Support stockings or elastic stockings (sold in drugstores and medical supply stores) are also helpful for reducing ankle edema caused by venous insufficiency.

Related entries

Circulatory disorders, congestive heart failure, diuretics, eclampsia, heart disease, kidney disorders, preeclampsia, pregnancy, premenstrual syndrome

Edema

Edema—also called bloating or fluid retention—is the abnormal accumulation of fluid in body tissues. It can be a symptom of many conditions, some relatively benign.

Who is likely to develop edema?

Many women experience noticeable bloating in the abdomen and slight weight gain for 5 to 15 days before each menstrual period begins. Some pregnant women have mild swelling in the face, fingers, or ankles during the last trimester of

Electrocautery

Electrocautery is a technique used to destroy cells by applying heat to them. Formerly a common treatment for genital warts, precancerous lesions of the cervix (see cervical cancer), and cervicitis (see vaginitis), it is gradually being replaced by less risky and painful procedures such as cryosurgery, laser surgery, and electrosurgical loop excision (see entries). Electrocautery may still be used in the many centers where equipment for these other procedures is unavailable. It is also sometimes used to close the fallopian tubes in a tubal ligation, and is commonly performed in the operating room as part of many surgical procedures.

How is the procedure performed?
Electrocautery for genital warts or cervical lesions is usually performed in a doctor's office. After inserting a speculum into the vagina, the doctor applies the heated tip of a cautery probe to the affected area, killing the surface cells. The woman may feel moderate pain for a few seconds when the probe is applied.

What happens after surgery?
After surgery there may be a profuse watery discharge (and sometimes staining or bleeding) from the vagina for up to 3 weeks. Until the discharge has stopped, nothing should be inserted into the vagina. Sometimes the cervical canal may narrow temporarily owing to swelling.

What are the risks and complications?
In rare cases infection may result or, if too many cervical mucus glands have been damaged, infertility.

Related entries
Cervical cancer, cryosurgery, electrosurgical loop excision, genital warts, laser surgery, Pap test, tubal ligation, vaginitis

Electrosurgical Loop Excision

Electrosurgical loop excision is both a diagnostic and a therapeutic procedure for cervical abnormalities. It is also called loop electrosurgical excision procedure, or LEEP.

How is the procedure performed?
Under the guidance of a colposcope (a lighted magnifying instrument used to visualize cells within the vagina and cervix), a clinician quickly scoops abnormal tissue from the cervix with the aid of a thin wire loop that emits a low-voltage, high-frequency radio wave. The tissue can then be examined under a microscope to see if it contains cancerous cells. Usually this procedure removes any abnormal tissue at the same time. The obvious advantage over both electrocautery and laser surgery is that diagnosis and treatment of precancerous cells or early-stage cancer are accomplished with a single procedure. Electrosurgical loop excision can be done on an outpatient basis with only a local anesthetic.

What happens after the procedure?
After surgery there may be some discharge (and sometimes staining or bleeding) from the vagina for up to 3 weeks. In the month or so that it takes for the cervix to heal completely, women should avoid using tampons or having sexual intercourse.

What are the risks and complications?
Persistent bleeding and infections are rare complications of the procedure.

Related entries
Cervical cancer, electrocautery, laser surgery, Pap test

Endometrial Cancer

An endometrial cancer is a malignant growth on the lining of the uterus. It is the most common malignancy of the female genital tract in the United States, and 2 or 3 out of every 100 women are expected to develop it at some point in their lives. If detected and treated in an early stage, however, endometrial cancer is highly curable.

The tumor begins in the uterine lining, or endometrium (stage 1A; see illustration), and is detected in most women at this point. If undetected or untreated, however, it may invade the muscular wall of the uterus (stages 1B and 1C), the cervix (stage 2), the organs and structures surrounding the uterus (stage 3), and, eventually, the bladder, bowel, and more distant organs (stage 4). About 85 percent of women with stage 1 and 60 percent of women with stage 2 cancer can expect to survive 5 years after therapy, in contrast with 30 percent of women with stage 3 disease and 10 percent of women with stage 4.

Who is likely to develop endometrial cancer?
Although endometrial cancer usually develops after menopause, 20 percent of all endometrial cancer occurs in premenopausal women and 5 percent in women under age 40. The risk of developing it rises in any woman who has had prolonged exposure to excessive levels of the hormone estrogen relative to the hormone progesterone. Thus, women who had an early menarche or late menopause or who never bore children are at higher than average risk. So are women who have had long-term estrogen replacement therapy which was not combined with progesterone. For this reason, in the 1980s most doctors began prescribing lower doses of estrogen, usually in combination with progesterone, for women who chose estrogen replacement therapy.

Most of the cases in younger women occur in those who have infrequent or no periods and have symptoms of excessive androgens—hormones that cause masculine features such as excessive hair growth on the face, deepening of the voice, abnormal amounts of muscle mass, and so on. This is because persistent failure to ovulate, common in these conditions, can overstimulate the endometrium with estrogen, without any counterbalancing progesterone (which is normally produced after ovulation).

Estrogen exposure and consequent risk of endometrial cancer is also unusually high in women with liver disease, which

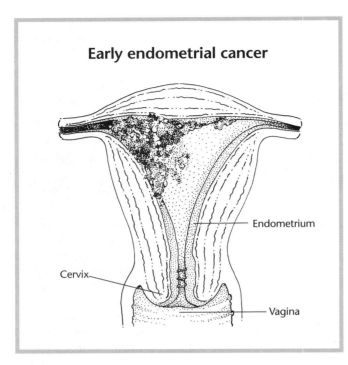

Early endometrial cancer

Endometrium

Cervix

Vagina

interferes with the normal destruction of excess estrogen, as well as in women who are obese, since fat cells boost the level of estrogen in the body. The risk of developing endometrial cancer triples for women who are 21 to 50 pounds overweight and increases 10 times for women more than 50 pounds overweight. Although women with hypertension and diabetes also seem to be at increased risk, this may be because many women with these conditions are obese.

Another high-risk group is women who have previously had ovarian cancer or breast cancer. In addition, women with a history of breast cancer who are taking the drug tamoxifen to reduce the chance of its recurrence are at increased risk for endometrial cancer.

Studies have shown that bearing many children or using oral contraceptives dramatically reduces the risk of developing this disease.

What are the symptoms?

The most common symptom of endometrial cancer is vaginal bleeding or spotting in a woman who has completed menopause. But in any woman, abnormal vaginal bleeding—whether bleeding between menstrual periods, spotting, or unusually heavy menstrual flow—may signal endometrial cancer, as well as various other conditions. Some women with endometrial cancer may also notice a watery vaginal discharge.

Only in more advanced stages of the disease is there generally any kind of pain or discomfort. But if the tumor has narrowed the neck of the cervix, where blood and pus can accumulate, pain is not uncommon.

How is the condition evaluated?

A clinician will suspect endometrial cancer in any postmenopausal woman with vaginal bleeding or in any premenopausal woman with several risk factors. In addition, if any endometrial cells (either atypical or normal) appear on a Pap test (which is taken from the cervix) from a postmenopausal woman, the clinician will suspect endometrial cancer, although other possibilities include endometrial hyperplasia (see entry) and uterine polyps (see polyps). Atypical glandular cells (AGUS) found in any routine Pap test may also lead a clinician to suspect these possibilities.

The clinician will first perform a thorough physical exam, including a pelvic exam, to assess uterine size, check for abnormal masses, and exclude any other sources of abnormal bleeding. Usually a Pap test will be done as well.

If the clinician still suspects endometrial cancer after these examinations, an endometrial biopsy is generally performed to examine the cells of the uterus. This procedure can be done in a doctor's office and, while occasionally uncomfortable, usually requires no anesthesia (see biopsy). Some women who continue to experience bleeding despite a negative biopsy may require a D&C (dilatation and curettage; see entry).

If cancerous cells are detected, a woman will probably be referred to a gynecological oncologist (a doctor who specializes in treating cancers of the reproductive organs). The gynecologic oncologist will want to "stage" the cancer so that treatment can be individualized. This involves an assessment of the woman's history and another physical and pelvic examination with special emphasis on possible sites of spread. Next the woman will be hospitalized for exploratory surgery, usually through a midline vertical incision.

How is endometrial cancer treated?

Once the stage of the cancer has been determined, the surgeon will perform a total hysterectomy as well as removal of both ovaries and fallopian tubes (see hysterectomy). Surrounding lymph nodes are also removed and are then examined (biopsied) for signs of cancer. The decision about postoperative treatment depends on the woman's risk for recurrence of disease, which in turn depends on the surgeon's findings. Following the hysterectomy, a woman with stage 1 disease may be given radiation therapy, depending on how large the tumor was and how far it had invaded the muscular wall of the uterus. If the disease is minimal (stage 1A or 1B), radiation is not needed.

Stage 2 disease is almost always treated with radiation after hysterectomy because of the risk that the cancer has spread to other nearby lymph nodes. Women with cancer at stage 3 undergo hysterectomy and then receive radiation therapy tailored to the tissues and structures near the uterus known to be diseased and to other sites at high risk for recurrence. This may require extensive abdominal radiation.

If the cancer has reached stage 4, or if an earlier stage of the cancer has recurred after radiation treatment, hormonal therapy or chemotherapy may be tried. One type of hormonal therapy calls for taking a form of progesterone. In 3 cases out of 10 it slows the growth of cancerous endometrial cells by counteracting the effects of estrogen, which normally stimulates the growth of these cells. (Because of this effect of estrogen, all women who have had endometrial cancer must avoid estrogen replacement therapy, even if they suffer from severe postmenopausal symptoms or osteoporosis.)

How can endometrial cancer be prevented?

There is currently no acceptable screening technique for endometrial cancer. The risks associated with both endometrial biopsy and D&C, which include infection, uterine perforation, and discomfort, are too great to justify routine use. Although Pap tests can sometimes detect cancerous cells of the endometrium, they often (in as many as 4 out of 5 cases) appear normal even in the presence of cancer. For these reasons the American College of Obstetricians and Gynecologists currently does not recommend routine screening of women for this disease and does not support routine biopsy of the endometrium prior to starting estrogen replacement therapy.

It may be possible for some women to reduce the risk of endometrial cancer by controlling obesity (which, in any case, has other benefits). But this is still speculative advice because it has never been established whether obesity itself predisposes women to the cancer or whether there is some underlying condition that predisposes women to both obesity and endometrial cancer. In premenopausal women, using oral contraception can also reduce the risk of endometrial cancer.

Women who have not had a hysterectomy and who are taking supplemental estrogens should be sure to take progesterone as well, since there is no increased risk of developing endometrial cancer if progesterone is added to the estrogen. Finally, any woman who experiences abnormal vaginal bleeding should seek medical attention so that endometrial cancer can either be ruled out or diagnosed as early as possible.

Related entries

Amenorrhea, biopsy, breast cancer, chemotherapy, dilatation and curettage, endometrial hyperplasia, estrogen replacement therapy, hyperandrogenism, hysterectomy, infrequent periods, menopause, menorrhagia, obesity, Pap test, radiation therapy, vaginal bleeding (abnormal)

Endometrial Hyperplasia

In this condition there is an overgrowth of the uterine lining, thought to result from the presence of excessive estrogen. Because this same hormonal imbalance also predisposes women to cancer of the uterine lining (endometrial cancer), hyperplasia is sometimes considered a precancerous condition, particularly in postmenopausal women or women approaching menopause. This risk is taken particularly seriously if the presence of cells labeled "adenomatous" or "atypical" is noted in a pathology report. In younger women, however, endometrial hyperplasia is almost always noncancerous, and even in older women it is usually easily treatable.

Who is likely to develop endometrial hyperplasia?

This condition most frequently occurs in women who are not exposed regularly to the hormone progesterone. In women who have not yet entered menopause, progesterone is normally produced after ovulation. Women nearing menopause (in whom ovulation is erratic) and postmenopausal women are prone to hyperplasia, as are some teenagers just past menarche who have not yet established a regular pattern of ovulation.

Endometrial hyperplasia may also occur in women who have used estrogen replacement therapy without supplementary progestins (progesteronelike substances). Hyperplasia can also occur in women with infertility, absent or infrequent periods caused by lack of ovulation, obesity, polycystic ovaries, or hyperandrogenism (see entry)—an excess of hormones that promote masculinization. All of these conditions have been associated with excessive exposure to estrogens.

What are the symptoms?

The most common symptom of endometrial hyperplasia is vaginal bleeding in a postmenopausal woman. For premenopausal women, any abnormal vaginal bleeding such as unusually heavy or prolonged menstrual periods or bleeding between periods may sometimes indicate hyperplasia.

How is the condition evaluated?

If a doctor suspects endometrial hyperplasia, the uterine cells will need to be examined in a laboratory. Cells are generally obtained through an endometrial biopsy, an office procedure that usually requires no anesthesia but may be uncomfortable (see biopsy). This procedure can help distinguish hyperplasia from endometrial cancer and from uterine polyps (a condition in which the thickening is in one spot rather than throughout the entire uterus).

Sometimes cells are obtained for biopsy via a vacuum aspiration or dilatation and curettage (D&C). In some instances these procedures can eliminate the hyperplasia at the same time by removing enough endometrial tissue to stop the abnormal bleeding.

How is endometrial hyperplasia treated?

Younger women with abnormal vaginal bleeding may be advised to take birth control pills containing both estrogen and progestin (combination pills) for a few months, even before a doctor does a biopsy to confirm hyperplasia as the cause of the problem or to help stop the bleeding. In a woman nearing or past menopause, progestin supplements can be given to reverse the tissue buildup and eliminate bleeding. If these efforts fail, however, the woman will usually need a hysterectomy.

How can endometrial hyperplasia be prevented?

In women who do not ovulate regularly, use of supplemental progestins reduces the risk of hyperplasia. Women with polycystic ovary syndrome or other forms of hyperandrogenism often take the birth control pill for this purpose. Postmenopausal women who take estrogen replacement therapy can reduce their risk of endometrial hyperplasia and cancer by taking progestins for about 12 days each month.

Related entries

Amenorrhea, biopsy, birth control, dilatation and curettage, endometrial cancer, estrogen replacement therapy, hyperandrogenism, hysterectomy, infertility, infrequent periods, menopause, menorrhagia, menstrual cycle disorders, obesity, polyps, vacuum aspiration, vaginal bleeding (abnormal)

Endometriosis

Endometriosis is a chronic and sometimes extremely painful disease in which tissue that normally lines the uterus appears to migrate to other parts of the body (see illustration). This tissue can grow on the ovaries, the lining of the abdominal cavity, uterine ligaments, fallopian tubes, bladder, or intestines, or in the space between the uterus and the rectum. In some women it travels as far as the lungs, brain, and legs.

Because they are made up of endometrial tissue, these growths respond to hormonal changes of the menstrual cycle by building up and then breaking down each month just as the endometrium does. The result is internal bleeding, inflammation, formation of blood-filled cysts and scar tissue (adhesions), and chronic pelvic pain. Endometriosis can also predispose women to ruptured ovarian cysts and ectopic pregnancies (see entries).

In addition, some women with endometriosis have problems with fertility. These may occur because pelvic adhesions hinder the ability of the fallopian tubes to "capture" an egg. A woman's chances of being infertile do not seem to be related to the degree of endometriosis, however. The same is true for other symptoms of endometriosis, such as painful menstrual cramps.

This lack of correlation between the extent of the disease and the severity of symptoms has led some investigators to speculate that there may be other processes involved in producing the symptoms of endometriosis. In the case of infertility these may include failure to release an egg, hormonal imbalances, and immunological disturbances. In the case of

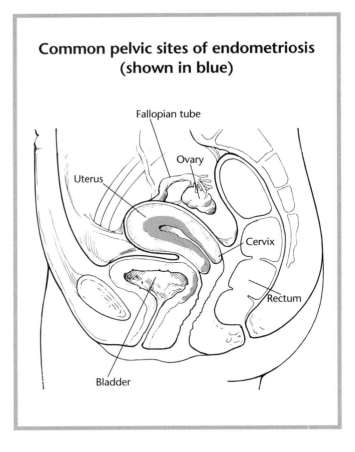

Common pelvic sites of endometriosis (shown in blue)

Fallopian tube

Ovary

Uterus

Cervix

Rectum

Bladder

painful menstrual cramps, the culprit may be elevated production of hormonelike substances called prostaglandins (even in women with mild disease) which cause uterine contractions and stimulate the intestines.

No one knows precisely what causes endometriosis, but there is increasing evidence that it may be related in some way to the immune system. Researchers have theorized that the disease may have something to do with the "reverse menstruation" now known to occur in as many as 90 percent of all women: menstrual fluid not only exits through the cervix and vagina but also travels up and out of the uterus through the fallopian tubes and spreads to other parts of the body (see illustration). Of course, the question remains why only a small portion of women who experience reverse menstruation develop the symptoms of endometriosis. The answer (which is still purely speculative) may be that they have a growth-promoting factor that stimulates the migrant tissue to implant on other organs and develop, or that they lack an immune response that normally would check its growth.

Other researchers believe that migrant endometrial tissue may spread through the blood vessels and lymph nodes, while others hypothesize that certain stimuli—such as infections or hormones—cause undifferentiated cells within the lining of the abdomen to develop into endometrial cells. More recently, a group of investigators has linked the environmental toxin dioxin to the endometriosis in rhesus monkeys. They hypothesize that some women may develop endometriosis after excessive exposure to dioxin or related pesticides in their diet or after inhaling airborne pollutants. Ultimately it may turn out that any, some, or none of these intriguing but as yet unproven theories plays a role in the development of endometriosis. Most researchers now believe that more than one factor is involved, and that no single theory can explain every case of endometriosis.

Who is likely to develop endometriosis?

Women with endometriosis continue to bear the stigma of having what was once known as "the career woman's disease." For many years endometriosis was thought to afflict primarily upwardly mobile working women in their late 20s and early 30s who somehow along the way had "neglected" to have children. These women were also assumed to be white, relatively affluent, and saddled with a nervous and anxious character to boot. The implication was that endometriosis was a preventable condition and that women were to blame for developing it.

These beliefs can be traced to the fact that affluent white working women without children were also most likely to seek (and be able to pay for) help for their symptoms. It now appears, however, that endometriosis does not discriminate on the basis of age, socioeconomic status, childbearing history, or ethnicity. Although the disease never begins before the first menstrual period and only rarely continues after menopause, it can occur in any woman of childbearing age.

Endometriosis tends to run in families. Having a first-degree female relative (mother or sister) with endometriosis increases by 7 times the risk of developing this disease. In addi-

tion, any condition that obstructs the outflow of menstrual fluid—such as scar tissue on the cervix as a result of treatment for cervical cancer or precancerous changes (dysplasia)—increases the likelihood of developing it.

What are the symptoms?

Early symptoms of endometriosis generally involve pelvic pain and cramps during the menstrual period. It is sometimes hard to tell if a woman with these symptoms is suffering from primary dysmenorrhea (cramps with no underlying disease) or secondary dysmenorrhea (pain caused by an underlying disorder, in this case endometriosis). Over time, however, other symptoms of endometriosis may develop, depending on where the endometrial tissue has implanted in the body. If the tissue has resulted in adhesions, or if there is an endometrioma (endometriosis within the ovaries, which forms a cyst), then the pelvic pain can occur throughout the entire cycle, not just during menstruation. In addition to menstrual cramps and pelvic pain, the most common symptoms are pain during sexual intercourse and infertility (see entries).

If the rectum or bladder is involved, bowel movements may be difficult or painful or blood may be passed with the urine (generally during the time of the menstrual cycle when the growths are largest or are bleeding). In rare instances, a woman may spit up blood during menstruation or develop chest pain or other problems of the lungs, back pain and leg weakness, vaginal bleeding after a hysterectomy, or symptoms of irritable bowel syndrome or bowel obstruction. Up to a third of women with endometriosis have no symptoms at all, however, and may discover that they have endometriosis only during an infertility evaluation.

How is the condition evaluated?

Because endometriosis has no characteristic symptoms or obvious physical signs, it is often confused with other conditions, including pelvic inflammatory disease, ectopic pregnancy, ovarian cysts, irritable bowel syndrome, and various cancers of the reproductive organs. Sometimes it is dismissed as simply painful (or even imaginary) menstrual cramps. There are certain suspicious findings that may appear during a pelvic examination, however—including pelvic nodules and tenderness, masses on the uterine ligaments, ovarian enlargement, pigmented and painful lesions on the back wall of the vagina, or a retroflexed (tipped back) uterus that is hard to move.

Coupled with a woman's complaints, these findings may warrant an exploratory laparoscopy, a procedure that allows the doctor to look directly inside the pelvic region and determine if there are any endometrial growths outside the uterus. Ultrasound is done first to look for other causes of pain, but only a laparoscopy can provide a definitive diagnosis of endometriosis. Yet even during a surgical exploration the lesions associated with endometriosis can be mistaken for those of other conditions. Someday it may be possible to diagnose endometriosis by looking for certain characteristic

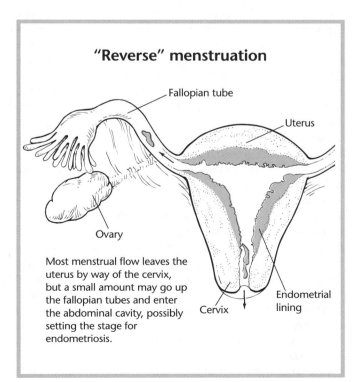

"Reverse" menstruation

Fallopian tube

Uterus

Ovary

Cervix

Endometrial lining

Most menstrual flow leaves the uterus by way of the cervix, but a small amount may go up the fallopian tubes and enter the abdominal cavity, possibly setting the stage for endometriosis.

proteins or antibodies in the blood. At present this technique is still in the experimental stages.

How is endometriosis treated?

Though potentially painful and sometimes disabling, endometriosis is neither malignant nor inevitably progressive. This means that having mild endometriosis does not sentence a woman to developing more severe symptoms. In fact, only between 25 and 40 percent of women with mild endometriosis go on to have severe disease. Even though no one knows how to predict which women these will be, many doctors advise against subjecting a woman to drug or surgical treatment if her only concern is fertility in the distant future.

Endometriosis is a chronic disorder whose severity can wax and wane. A woman diagnosed with endometriosis who wants to have a baby should bear in mind that conception can become more difficult if the disease progresses. During pregnancy, symptoms often subside, but they may recur after the baby is born.

For women who have severe or disabling symptoms, various drug and surgical treatments can provide about 18 to 24 months of pain relief. Because each option for treating endometriosis has certain associated drawbacks and side effects, each woman, together with her doctor, must weigh these against potential benefits. One important consideration is whether the goal is pain relief, enhancement of fertility, or both. Another consideration involves the side effects and temporary benefits of drugs and the cost and potential risks of surgery.

If surgery is a possibility, it is important to find out about the skill and experience of the surgeon in treating endometriosis. Not all surgeons have the experience and talent with a laparoscope to perform difficult techniques such as removing extensive adhesions or diseased segments of the bowel. Often it is difficult for a patient to obtain such information. Women may have to make several attempts and insist on seeing concrete figures about the number of patients operated on, the nature of the surgery, and the results. Primary care physicians can be a valuable resource in assessing a surgeon's experience.

Surgical treatments generally are longer lasting than drug treatments, have fewer side effects, and are the best option for a woman who wants to become pregnant right away. But they are relatively expensive and carry the same risks as any invasive procedure. The goal of surgery for endometriosis is to relieve pain by destroying or excising as much errant tissue as possible. If the woman wants to become pregnant, the surgeon must be particularly careful to avoid creating any new adhesions that could further interfere with conception.

These goals can be accomplished equally well with a variety of surgical techniques under the guidance of a laparoscope, including laser surgery, electrocautery, knife excision, or curettage (scraping). At the same time the surgeon can also perform other procedures to prevent future pain. For example, uterine ligaments can be shortened and then sewn against the abdominal wall away from adhesions. Further relief can come from cutting certain nerves in the lower back with a laser beam so that pain impulses can no longer be transmitted to the brain.

More radical abdominal surgery such as laparotomy may be necessary if there are extensive adhesions or endometriomas. Alternatively, if previous surgeries have failed, or if the woman no longer wishes to bear children, hysterectomy (removal of the uterus) and usually removal of the ovaries is an option. Although it may seem a definitive cure, occasionally women continue to have symptoms even after the ovaries and uterus have been removed—presumably because the migrant endometrial growths continue to bleed or because of preexisting scar tissue and cysts. Symptoms are more likely to recur after hysterectomy if the woman is taking estrogen replacement therapy (ERT).

If surgery is ineffective or if the woman prefers nonsurgical treatment, various prescription medications are available. These can also be used to reduce any implants that remain after surgery. Almost all the drugs prescribed for endometriosis work by inhibiting the menstrual cycle, which in turn inhibits pain from the monthly buildup and breakdown of endometrial tissue. For women who do not want to conceive a baby for the time being, oral contraceptives (combination pills with both estrogen and progesterone) are often the best option. This treatment is known as "pseudopregnancy" because it mimics the hormonal effects of pregnancy. If taken continuously without a monthly withdrawal period, oral contraceptives relieve pelvic pain and cramps in about 80 percent of women. They generally have only minimal side effects and can be taken for long periods of time.

Drugs called GnRH agonists (gonadotropin releasing hormone agonists) are an option if symptoms persist or recur after surgery or after continuous use of oral contraceptives. These drugs produce a state of false (but fully reversible) menopause. The pituitary gland starts secreting reduced levels of luteinizing hormone (LH) and follicle stimulating hormone (FSH), which in turn lowers the production of estrogen and interrupts the menstrual cycle (see entry). The Food and Drug Administration (FDA) has approved three GnRH agonists for the treatment of endometriosis: leuprolide acetate (Lupron), nafarelin acetate (Synarel), and goserelin acetate (Zoladex). These are taken, respectively, as daily or monthly injections, nasal sprays, or implants placed within the upper abdominal wall every 28 days.

While extremely effective in relieving pelvic pain, GnRH agonists also have frequent side effects associated with menopause such as hot flashes, irregular vaginal bleeding, and, less frequently, headaches, depression, insomnia, vaginal dryness, weight loss or gain, and hair loss. Also, because these drugs promote bone loss, they can be taken for only 6 months at a time, after which symptoms often reappear. It is possible that bone loss may be averted by taking estrogen and progestin supplements at the same time, so that GnRH agonists can be taken for a longer period, but this regimen still needs further study.

One large study indicates that the synthetic steroid dimetriose (Gestrinone) may be just as effective as the GnRH agonist leuprolide in relieving pain associated with endometriosis by inhibiting the release of hormones that stimulate the formation of endometrial tissue. Only 5 to 15 percent of patients stop therapy because of unwanted side effects (the most frequent ones being increased appetite, acne, and vaginal discharge). Treatment usually begins on the first day of the menstrual period and continues for six months. Most women can expect to stop menstruating while taking this drug.

Other drugs commonly prescribed to treat endometriosis include Danazol (a synthetic male hormone) and Provera (a synthetic progesterone). Both of these medications have significant side effects and cannot prevent symptoms from recurring once they are discontinued. Danazol, which was the first medication approved by the FDA for treating endometriosis, frequently leads to weight gain, edema, acne, breast atrophy, oily skin, hot flashes, muscle cramps, changes in sex drive, and fatigue. It also lowers levels of HDL cholesterol and raises levels of LDL cholesterol, thus potentially increasing the risk of coronary artery disease. Provera, too, often leads to breast tenderness, breakthrough bleeding (bleeding between menstrual periods), irritability, and depression. In addition, 4 out of 5 women gain anywhere from 5 to 30 pounds while taking this drug.

Preliminary studies on mifepristone (RU-486)—a drug more widely known for its ability to induce nonsurgical abortion—show that a dose as low as 50 mg a day can decrease the extent of endometriosis and associated pain. Side effects were found to be minimal and included flushing, reduced appetite, and fatigue. If these findings are confirmed by larger clinical studies, mifepristone may prove to be a safe and well-tolerated alternative for treating endometriosis.

Because neither drugs nor surgery can completely eradicate endometriosis, and because all current treatments have unpleasant risks and side effects, some doctors advise women with endometriosis to alternate drug and surgical therapy. With this approach a woman has a laparoscopy to evaluate and treat the disease every 4 years and is then exposed to the side effects of drug therapy every 4 years as well, starting 2 years after the initial laparoscopy. This process continues until natural menopause occurs. As improved surgical and drug regimens become available, it may be possible to lengthen the interval between treatments.

For more immediate pain relief, nonsteroidal antiinflammatory drugs (NSAIDs) may be helpful. Sometimes a clinician will prescribe mild narcotics as well, although care must be taken to avoid drug dependency. Alternative therapies—visualization, meditation, acupuncture, chiropractic, homeopathy, herbs, and nutritional therapy—are being evaluated by the Endometriosis Association.

Related entries

Adhesions, antiinflammatory drugs, electrocautery, estrogen replacement therapy, hysterectomy, infertility, laparoscopy, laparotomy, laser surgery, menopause, menstrual cramps, menstrual cycle, oral contraceptives, pain during sexual intercourse

Epilepsy

Epilepsy is not a single disease but a group of related disorders, all of which involve recurrent seizures. These seizures are caused by inappropriate electrical firing (discharging) of neurons in the brain, which leads to various abnormal behaviors. Because there are many different kinds of epileptic seizures—which can involve different parts of the brain and have very different behavioral manifestations—most clinicians and researchers prefer the term "seizure disorders" (or sometimes "the epilepsies"), even though the term epilepsy is still used in popular parlance.

Most seizure disorders can be classified into one of two types: generalized or partial. Generalized seizures involve abnormal electrical activity throughout the brain (see illustration). The most common forms of generalized seizures are grand mal seizures (the classic attacks involving loss of consciousness and convulsive movements of the arms, legs, and torso) and absence or petit mal seizures (which involve multiple brief—and often unnoticeable—lapses of consciousness).

Partial seizures either involve a limited area of the brain or begin in a specific area and only later spread throughout the brain. The most common kinds of partial seizures are temporal lobe seizures, which result in abnormal physical movements or repetitive acts. Other common partial seizures are called focal seizures, and involve numbness or jerking in one side of the face or other limited area of the body.

Anyone can have a seizure under certain conditions. Having a single seizure of any sort is not the same as having a seizure disorder (or epilepsy). A single seizure, twitch, or blackout can occur because of inadequate blood flow to the brain (from illness, heart disease, or holding one's breath, for example), high fever (especially in infants and young children), or head trauma of all sorts. People with seizure disorders, by contrast, have recurring seizures, and when their brain waves are studied in a laboratory with an electroencephalogram (EEG)—a procedure that records patterns of electrical activity in the brain—they usually show abnormal patterns characteristic of people with seizure disorders.

In susceptible people seizures can be provoked by drinking too much alcohol; withdrawing from alcohol or other drugs in people who are dependent; getting too little sleep; or undergoing physical stress as a result of infection, starvation, dehydration, exhaustion, or trauma. External stimuli ranging from flashing lights, noise, reading, and eating to sexual activity or even a specific thought or movement can sometimes provoke a seizure in some people. Women with epilepsy seem to be particularly susceptible to seizures around the time of menstruation.

The principal divisions of the brain

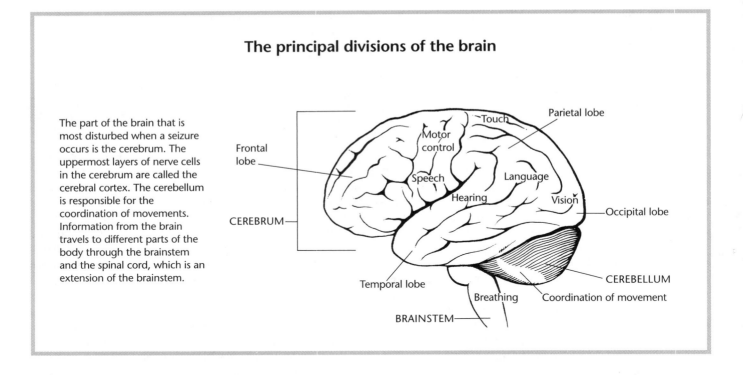

The part of the brain that is most disturbed when a seizure occurs is the cerebrum. The uppermost layers of nerve cells in the cerebrum are called the cerebral cortex. The cerebellum is responsible for the coordination of movements. Information from the brain travels to different parts of the body through the brainstem and the spinal cord, which is an extension of the brainstem.

About 4 percent of the population has some kind of seizure disorder (and 10 percent of the population will have a seizure at some time during their life). Despite advances in the understanding and treatment of epilepsy, many of these people are still discriminated against when it comes to finding jobs and obtaining health insurance. Potential employers and others sometimes falsely assume that people with epilepsy are mentally deficient or emotionally volatile—or even that they are malingerers who are consciously exploiting their illness.

Misperceptions about seizure disorders often leave people with epilepsy isolated from colleagues and neighbors, racked with feelings of guilt or shame, and insecure about their ability to support or nurture a family. Parents—or people considering becoming parents—may worry about the considerable anxiety their seizures could provoke in their children. Marital problems are common in couples when one partner has a seizure disorder, particularly if seizures are poorly controlled. Often the afflicted partner becomes so consumed with the illness—or the partner without the disorder becomes so overwhelmed with worry or resentment—that there is little emotional energy left for the relationship.

The fact is that most seizure disorders can be controlled with medications, and patients and their families can benefit greatly from the support provided by a therapist who has experience with this particular illness.

Who is likely to develop a seizure disorder?

Occasionally seizure disorders can be traced to some specific brain injury such as a stroke, an abscess, trauma to the brain from an accident, or—especially in older people—a tumor.

But many seizure disorders have no known cause and are labeled "idiopathic." This is particularly true in people whose first seizures occur in young adulthood. Idiopathic seizure disorders do sometimes run in families, however, which suggests an underlying genetic predisposition in a minority of cases.

Absence seizures (also called petit mal epilepsy) are almost exclusively a disease of children and adolescents. The condition usually begins between the ages of 6 and 12 and resolves on its own, or transforms into some other seizure disorder, in young adulthood. Many people with generalized seizures in childhood go on to develop temporal lobe seizures as well, with the first of these seizures often occurring during adolescence.

What are the symptoms?

Grand mal seizures (also called generalized tonic-clonic or convulsive seizures) usually begin with a loss of consciousness and muscular rigidity so that the person having the seizure falls to the ground. This is called the tonic phase, and it lasts about 15 seconds. In the clonic phase which follows, the person remains unconscious while her arms and legs jerk about violently. Sometimes there may be loss of bowel or bladder control. Afterward, many people feel groggy and disoriented, and have no memory of the seizure, although some later recall a brief sensation of total paralysis before losing consciousness. For a few minutes or hours they may experience amnesia and not recognize people they know. Grand mal seizures consume an enormous amount of energy and usually leave an individual exhausted.

In contrast, absence seizures can occur without bystanders

noticing anything amiss. These brief, sudden losses of consciousness—sometimes accompanied by a facial twitch, fluttering eyelids, or drooping head—can recur dozens of time a day. A focal seizure can sometimes be hard to differentiate from an absence seizure in that it also involves barely noticeable lapses of consciousness, although there may be sudden sucking, chewing, or swallowing motions. This disorder involves very different brain wave patterns, however—and requires very different treatment—because it stems from one damaged area of the brain, whereas absence seizures involve neurons all over the brain.

A temporal lobe seizure (sometimes called a complex partial or psychomotor seizure) usually originates in the temporal lobe of the brain, after which it may spread to other areas. These seizures are often preceded by an aura—an ominous sense that something bad is about to occur. This aura can take the form of an upset stomach, nausea, a need to defecate, sensory hallucinations, intense fear or anxiety, or even a sense of déjà vu or depersonalization. It is sometimes followed by a brief loss of consciousness and then some kind of simple repetitive movement such as lip smacking, spitting, or grimacing. The afflicted person often feels confused for minutes or even hours afterward, and remembers nothing of the seizure except the aura.

Sexual dysfunction is common in people with epilepsy—although whether this is due to the epilepsy itself or to the drugs used to treat it remains debatable. Both men and women with temporal lobe seizures often have diminished sex drive (libido).

Women with epilepsy run a risk of having a baby with a congenital defect, especially cleft lip and palate or heart defects, that is 2 to 3 times higher than normal. Researchers still are not sure if this higher risk occurs because of the seizure disorder itself or because of anticonvulsant medications taken during pregnancy (all of which are known to increase the risk of birth defects). Risk of complications during labor and delivery is also higher for women with epilepsy. Sons of women with idiopathic grand mal seizures are at a slightly increased risk of developing seizure disorders themselves. It is important to remember, however, that with close management by their obstetrician, most women with seizure disorders can have normal pregnancies and healthy babies. Any woman with a seizure disorder who is contemplating pregnancy should talk with her physician before changing her medication.

Death from any type of seizure is relatively rare, and when it occurs is largely attributable to the underlying cause of the seizure (such as a brain tumor or head trauma)—or to suicide. Among women with seizure disorders, mortality rates are essentially the same as those for the general population; among men with epilepsy they are higher.

How is the condition evaluated?

Diagnosing a seizure disorder—and differentiating one seizure disorder from another—requires an EEG. To produce this tracing of the brain waves, electrodes are pasted to many places on the scalp. These detect fluctuations in voltage in the part of the brain that is just underneath the electrode. The fluctuations from each electrode are transmitted to a voltage-sensitive needle that rests against a constantly moving sheet of paper. As the needles are deflected up and down with changes of voltage, the pattern of changes is recorded digitally. In most cases the EEG will help to establish that a seizure disorder exists, and in some cases it can suggest the underlying cause.

The procedure is painless, but sometimes patients are required to stay awake most of the night before so that they will be extremely tired. Fatigue is important to the test, for two reasons. Better recordings are obtained if the patient falls asleep during the test, and fatigue itself can make abnormalities show up in the tracing which might otherwise be masked. Sometimes during the waking part of the test strobe lights are flashed, or the patient will be asked to hyperventilate, to see if these stimuli provoke abnormal electrical activity in the brain.

Often other tests—such as blood tests, a CT scan, or MRI—are also done to see if the cause of the seizures can be determined.

How is epilepsy treated?

About 75 percent of seizure disorders can be effectively controlled with anticonvulsant medications. Which drug is chosen depends on the particular type of seizure disorder as well as the individual patient's responses to it. If the seizures stem from some underlying illness or other problem, successful treatment will involve eliminating that underlying cause. Medications commonly used to treat both grand mal and focal seizures include phenytoin (Dilantin), carbamazepine (Tegretol), and phenobarbital.

Women with epilepsy who are using birth control pills may have to choose an alternative method of contraception—particularly if they are taking Dilantin. Not only can phenytoin reduce the efficacy of birth control pills, but also birth control pills seem to increase menstrual irregularities and reduce seizure control in women taking phenytoin.

Therapy can be complicated during pregnancy. Although some antiseizure medications have been linked to birth defects, having seizures during a pregnancy can be harmful to both the mother and the fetus. And even if a woman is trying to keep seizures under control, problems with severe vomiting in the first trimester (see morning sickness) may make it hard to keep the medications down—and result in increased seizures. Women with epilepsy who are pregnant or considering pregnancy should discuss the risks and benefits of medication with their clinician. Medication withdrawal before pregnancy is often tried if the woman has been seizure-free for 2 years and has not had a grand mal seizure. Again, even if it is not possible to discontinue or change medications to reduce the risks, women with epilepsy can have healthy, normal children—even when they take their medications during pregnancy.

Many anticonvulsant drugs have a number of unpleasant

side effects, including restlessness, nausea, drowsiness, and decreased sex drive. These side effects are most frequent and severe in people over the age of 60. Also of great concern to many women are the cosmetic side effects associated with certain anticonvulsants—particularly rashes, skin darkening, and growth of dark, coarse hair on the face, arms, and legs (see hirsutism). Also, enlarged, tender gums (a condition called gingival hyperplasia; see gum disease) often result from taking Dilantin for many years. Some women are so bothered by these side effects that they stop taking the medication altogether. A better solution is to talk to a clinician about alternative therapies or—when none are feasible—launching a direct attack on the symptom itself (with electrolysis for hirsutism or careful dental care and gum surgery for gum disease if necessary).

Talking to a clinician is also the best course of action for dealing with the sexual problems that can result from seizure disorders and their treatment. Most of these problems are surmountable. The solution may require a change in medication (for either the seizure disorder or some other coexisting condition), frank communication with the sexual partner, or help from a sex therapist or specially trained physician or counselor. Family therapy can be particularly helpful in coping with epilepsy, regardless of which family member has the illness.

How can epilepsy be prevented?

Although there is no way to prevent most seizure disorders, susceptible individuals can minimize attacks by avoiding provocative situations and stimuli—such as excessive alcohol consumption, substance abuse, irregular hours, or overcommitment. Following the basic tenets of good health and hygiene to prevent unnecessary infection and exhaustion may also help.

Related entries

Acne, alcohol, birth control, gum disease, headaches, hirsutism, morning sickness, prenatal care, psychotherapy, sexual dysfunction, sleep disorders, stroke, substance abuse

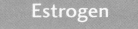

Estrogen

Estrogen is a generic term for the principal female sex hormone. It regulates the development of secondary sex characteristics in women, stimulates the growth of the uterine lining during the menstrual cycle, and helps maintain that lining during pregnancy, thus facilitating implantation of the ovum and fetal nutrition. Produced by the ovaries, adrenal glands (two glands that sit on top of the kidneys), and, during pregnancy, the placenta, estrogen comes in a variety of forms, including estradiol, estrone, and estriol. Fatty (adipose) tissue also converts some of the androgens (virilizing

hormones) produced by the adrenals into estrogen. The low levels of estrogen found in men are produced by the testes.

Supplemental estrogen

Both natural and synthetic forms of estrogen are administered for a variety of purposes, including the prevention of pregnancy (see birth control) and the treatment of menopausal symptoms (see estrogen replacement therapy). Supplemental estrogen can also be used to suppress lactation after childbirth in women who do not wish to breastfeed, and to treat certain forms of cancer. The amount of estrogen in different treatments varies dramatically. For example, the estrogens in birth control pills are roughly 10 times more potent than those used in estrogen replacement therapy after menopause.

Supplemental estrogen can produce a number of side effects, including breast swelling and tenderness, headaches, dizziness, nausea, vomiting, fluid retention, and abnormal vaginal bleeding. Whether these side effects become a problem depends to some extent on the form in which estrogen is given, the dose (for example, the morning-after pill causes more side effects than low-dose estrogen replacement therapy), and individual variations in women's reactions to estrogen. Those with a personal history or family history of blood clots, heart disease, hypertension, breast cancer, endometrial cancer, obesity, diabetes, and gallbladder disease should carefully discuss the pros and cons of supplemental estrogen with their physician, since some forms of supplemental estrogen can increase the risks associated with these disorders.

Related entries

Amenorrhea, birth control, breast cancer, circulatory disorders, diabetes, endometrial cancer, endometrial hyperplasia, estrogen replacement therapy, gallstones, high blood pressure, menopause, menstrual cycle, obesity, osteoporosis, vaginal bleeding (abnormal)

Estrogen Replacement Therapy

Before menopause, estrogen is secreted in large quantities by the ovaries, and in smaller quantities by the adrenal glands, which sit atop the kidneys. In addition, fatty (adipose) tissue converts some of the androgens (virilizing hormones) produced by the adrenals into estrogen. As menopause approaches, estrogen production by the ovaries tapers off, affecting many different tissues in the body, including the reproductive system, urinary tract, blood vessels, bones, breasts, skin, and parts of the brain. Taking estrogen at the time of menopause can reduce some of the negative effects of these changes.

Historically, estrogen replacement therapy (ERT) was initially popularized in the 1970s, when it was touted as a way for women to reverse the tide of aging and remain "feminine forever." Early enthusiasm for estrogen therapy was tempered by the discovery that it increased the risk of endometrial cancer, although this risk could be offset by taking estrogen together with a form of progesterone (called hormone replacement therapy, or HRT). Later, the use of estrogen therapy to prevent chronic conditions that occur more frequently after menopause, such as heart disease and osteoporosis, was advised by many medical authorities, based on the strength of the existing scientific evidence supporting the benefits of taking estrogen. These recommendations, which received enthusiastic support from the pharmaceutical companies, led to the use of ERT by about 40 percent of postmenopausal American women in 2000.

In 2002 the publication of startling results from the Women's Health Initiative, a controlled trial of hormone replacement for prevention of disease in women after menopause, caused doctors to make a drastic change in their recommendations. The study showed that, instead of preventing heart disease, hormone replacement therapy actually caused a slightly elevated risk of heart attack compared to placebo. To date there is no evidence that estrogen taken alone (without progesterone) increases the risk of heart disease; nevertheless, it does appear to increase the risk of breast cancer when taken for more than a few years. Because of the results of the Women's Health Initiative, currently estrogen replacement therapy (with or without progesterone) is viewed largely as a short-term treatment aimed at specific symptoms, not a long-term panacea for the prevention of chronic disease.

How is ERT administered?

The most commonly prescribed form of ERT in the United States involves mixtures of several forms of estrogen taken from the urine of pregnant mares. Called conjugated estrogens, these preparations are sold under various trade names, including Premarin. Natural forms of estrogen (manufactured in the laboratory), which are less potent than conjugated estrogens, are also sometimes used; these include estradiol (Estrace and Estraderm), estropipate (Ogen), and esterified estrogens (Estratab).

ERT can be administered in the form of pills or absorbed through the skin from transdermal patches (see illustration). Because hormones from patches (such as Estraderm) enter the bloodstream directly, they bypass the digestive system and are not immediately processed in the liver, where estrogen affects protein synthesis in both positive and negative ways. Estrogen in the liver seems to increase the proportion of the so-called good cholesterol, HDL, but it can also have adverse effects on the liver and may exacerbate high blood pressure.

Women who cannot use any of these systemic estrogens have the alternative of vaginal preparations, which are not generally considered a full-scale form of ERT but which can relieve symptoms of vaginal atrophy—the drying and thinning of tissues in the vaginal wall. Vaginal estrogen,

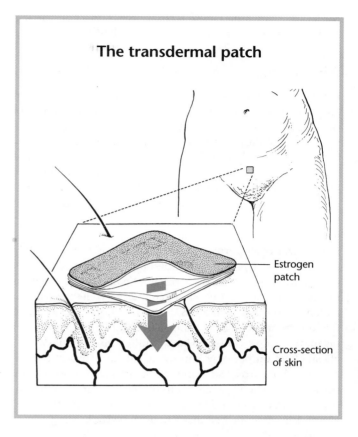

The transdermal patch

Estrogen patch

Cross-section of skin

which is available as a cream, contains conjugated estrogens (Premarin) or estradiol (Estrace). Usually women are instructed to use a half or full applicator daily for 3 weeks, after which time just half an applicator once or twice weekly usually suffices. There is also a vaginal estradiol tablet (Vagifem), which is inserted twice a week. A newer form of vaginal estrogen is the Estring, an estrogen-impregnated ring that a woman inserts in the vagina, much as she would insert a diaphragm. The ring remains in place for 3 months and is then replaced. It is generally not perceptible during intercourse, although occasionally it can be dislodged. Vaginal estrogen creams and tablets can theoretically cause some systemic effects from estrogen absorbed into the bloodstream, but these are usually minimal. The Estring results in no measurable effect on estrogen levels in the blood. For this reason it is sometimes prescribed for women who cannot take oral estrogen (for example, because of a history of breast cancer) but are troubled by vaginal atrophy.

Because the estrogen used for ERT is only about one-tenth as powerful as the estrogen used in oral contraceptives, the risks and benefits associated with birth control pills cannot necessarily be extended to ERT. In fact, several of the more serious risks and complications once associated with ERT were caused by doses of estrogen much higher than are now generally prescribed. Daily doses of conjugated estrogen used to be as high as 1.25 to 2.5 milligrams; today the standard dose is 0.3 to 0.625 mg. Usually taken daily, these dosages seem to confer the same protective effects as higher doses but are less likely to overstimulate breast and uterine tissues.

What are the benefits of ERT?

Relief of menopausal symptoms. There is no question that ERT is highly effective in easing many of the symptoms of menopause. Not only does it eliminate hot flashes and reverse vaginal atrophy and associated changes within weeks, but it can even help firm sagging pelvic muscles. There is also some evidence that daily estrogen treatment can improve mood in women who become mildly depressed at menopause. It has no proven effect on the aging of skin or hair loss.

Preventing osteoporosis. Also impressive is the well-established ability of ERT to slow the bone loss associated with osteoporosis. Osteoporosis (which literally means "porous bones") is a systemic and often debilitating skeletal disease in which the bones become less dense and more susceptible to fracture from even slight trauma (see illustration). Estrogen taken in low doses of 0.3 to 0.625 milligrams daily has a beneficial effect on bone by improving calcium absorption and retarding bone loss. Estrogen is most effective for preventing osteoporosis when it is started in the first 5 years after menopause, a time when bone loss is most rapid. The Women's Health Initiative showed that women who took estrogen plus progestin had one-third fewer hip fractures than untreated women, but the overall number of fractures prevented was small—about 1 less fracture per 2,000 women treated for 1 year.

Colon cancer. The Women's Health Initiative found that women who took estrogen and progestin had one-third fewer cancers of the colon and rectum than women who took no ERT. These results were consistent with the findings of earlier studies, including the Nurses' Health Study, conducted by researchers at Brigham and Women's Hospital and the Harvard Medical School in Boston. The mechanism by which estrogen might affect colon cancer risk is not well understood.

What are the risks and complications?

Heart disease. The effect of estrogen replacement therapy on heart disease has recently become controversial. A number of studies over the past few decades linked estrogen replacement therapy to lowered rates of heart disease. One of the most commonly cited of these studies, the Nurses' Health Study, involved 48,470 postmenopausal nurses who were followed for 10 years or more. Of these women, those who took no estrogen had a heart attack rate almost twice that of the women on estrogen replacement therapy. These findings were buttressed by a growing body of basic scientific research which demonstrated that estrogen had numerous effects on blood vessels and cholesterol levels, most of them favorable.

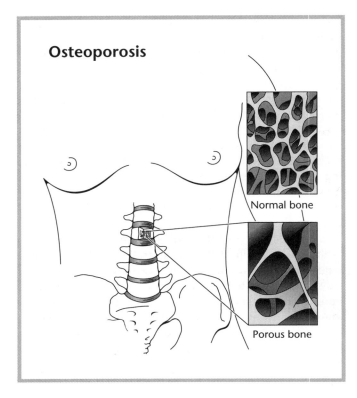

Osteoporosis

Normal bone

Porous bone

The controversy started to bubble up in the late 1990s, however, after controlled trials such as the HERS study (Heart and Estrogen/Progestin Replacement Study) showed that women who already had heart disease fared no better after starting hormone replacement therapy than those who took no estrogen. The controversy came to a boil when the results of the estrogen/progestin arm of the Women's Health Initiative were published in 2002. In that study, healthy postmenopausal women without known heart disease who took ERT were found to have slightly higher rates of heart attack compared with women who took no estrogen. Although the rate of heart attacks was low (7 additional cases per 10,000 women per year), this finding was enough to prompt a drastic reconsideration of the routine use of ERT to prevent heart disease.

Researchers speculate about a number of reasons for the discrepancies between older studies and the Women's Health Initiative results. Some possible explanations include differences in the age of the populations (the WHI included a larger proportion of older women, who are at higher risk for heart disease), differences in health habits and socioeconomic status, and differences in the doses and types of estrogens and progestins studied. Whatever the reason for the different results, women with risk factors for heart disease should think twice about using ERT. If they must use estrogen to control symptoms at menopause, they should use it at the lowest effective dose and for the minimum time possible. Whether any medications such as aspirin can effectively counter the slight increase in risk of heart disease associated with ERT is unknown.

Hypertension, stroke, blood clots, and migraine. Unlike the birth control pill, which uses higher doses of estrogen, estrogen replacement therapy does not usually affect blood pressure. It may slightly increase the risk of stroke, however. Although findings from studies on ERT and stroke risk are not entirely consistent, the Women's Health Initiative found that there were 8 more strokes per year in 10,000 women treated with estrogen than in a comparable untreated group.

It has been known for years that estrogen increases the risk of blood clots (also called thromboembolism). Blood clots that occur in the legs can be uncomfortable and occasionally lead to long-term problems with leg swelling. The real danger, however, is that the clot will develop in or travel to the lung, where it can be life-threatening. Blood clots occur about 2 to 3 times more often in women who take estrogen than in those who do not, but the overall risk is low: about 1 in 3,000 to 5,000 women per year.

As for the association between ERT and migraine headaches, the jury is still out. There is evidence linking both estrogens and progestins to migraines, plus some circumstantial evidence indicating that these hormones probably have something to do with who gets headaches and when. Even so, while some women find that ERT exacerbates their headaches, just as many others find that it either provides relief or causes no change at all. The best strategy is probably a little personal experimentation, with the understanding that if one hormone regimen makes migraines worse, it might be worth trying another one (such as a lower dose of estrogen or a transdermal patch) before abandoning the idea of ERT altogether.

Endometrial cancer. There seems to be no significant increase in endometrial cancer from ERT when estrogen is supplemented with progestins. For this reason progestins are now a routine part of ERT, except in women who no longer have a uterus (in which case endometrial changes are impossible). In women who have had a hysterectomy, clinicians usually recommend unopposed estrogen (that is, estrogen without progestin).

Adding progestin to ERT has its own set of disadvantages. Some progestins can partially offset any positive benefits to the heart provided by estrogen. Progestins can also produce transient bloating, breast tenderness, irritability, and (in higher doses) depressed mood. More distressing to many women is the resumption of monthly menstrual bleeding. The traditional way in which clinicians prescribe ERT includes low doses of medroxyprogesterone (Provera) taken for about 12 days each month. In 85 to 90 percent of women on this regime, monthly withdrawal bleeding begins as soon as the Provera is stopped. This monthly bleeding usually continues for a number of years after ERT is begun, but as the uterus ages, the bleeding eventually ceases.

Because many women are unwilling to tolerate having "periods" again after menopause, many clinicians prescribe progestins on a continuous daily basis. In the United States this usually involves taking 0.3 to 0.625 mg of conjugated estro-gen along with 2.5 mg of medroxyprogesterone acetate each day. But even this regime can lead to irregular spotting or bleeding in 30 to 50 percent of women for the first 6 months (this seems to be less of a problem in women well past menopause). Since abnormal spotting can be a symptom of uterine tissue abnormalities, such as hyperplasia or cancer, it can be difficult for a clinician to know whether to recommend an endometrial biopsy or "watchful waiting."

Breast cancer. Many studies in the past few decades have attempted to document an association between breast cancer and ERT. Although the results have not been completely consistent, most point to a modest increase in risk—about 30 percent—with use of estrogen for 5 years or more. For a 50-year-old woman, that translates roughly into an increase in lifetime risk from 10 percent to 13 percent. Most studies show what scientists call a dose-response effect: the risk increases with higher doses of estrogen and longer duration of use.

The Nurses' Health Study has shown that the risk of breast cancer in women who use estrogen alone is similar to that when estrogen is combined with progestins. Other studies have shown that the cancers developed in women using ERT seem to be slower-growing and more curable than other breast cancers—perhaps because ERT-associated cancers are biologically different. On the other hand, new data from the Women's Health Initiative suggest that the combination of progestin with estrogen poses a greater breast cancer risk than estrogen alone—in contrast to the protection against endometrial cancer that progestin confers.

Gallstones. ERT seems to put women at slightly increased risk of developing gallstones, probably because estrogen stimulates the liver to increase the amount of cholesterol in the bile. Using progestins in conjunction with estrogen does not seem to affect this risk.

Individual decision

Each woman's experience of menopause is different. For those whose quality of life suffers because of hot flashes or vaginal atrophy, estrogen therapy is still one of the most effective treatments. When used to treat such symptoms, however, the dose of estrogen should be the lowest that provides relief so as to minimize the likelihood of side effects. Treatment should be reevaluated at least annually, and ideally discontinued within a few years of menopause. The estrogen dosage should be tapered gradually, then stopped, so as to reduce the likelihood of "rebound" hot flashes.

Some women swear by estrogen replacement therapy for its supposed salutary effects on various aspects of health, including mood, memory, energy, sleep, and sexual functioning. Data from the Women's Health Initiative showed, however, that over a few years' time, women taking hormone replacement therapy fared no better than those taking placebo on most of those fronts. Women who have been taking estrogen for a while for these sorts of reasons should consider a trial period off estrogen, to see whether there are any noticeable changes.

On average, ERT offers benefits as well as risks. But of course, no one is average. Each individual has her own risk of developing heart disease or breast cancer, based on her own health and family history, as well as other factors. In addition, many of the judgments about the advisability of ERT are based on health risks for white women—and these may not apply to women of other races and backgrounds. Also, some women may find that they experience intolerable side effects when they use various forms of ERT.

For all of these reasons, each woman must consider her personal situation—not to mention her individual feelings about quality of life—and discuss these matters with her clinician before making a decision about ERT.

There are some women for whom ERT may simply be inappropriate. These include women who have had breast or uterine cancer or who currently have active liver disease. Women with a history of stroke, heart attacks, or circulatory disorders involving blood clots have also traditionally been counseled against ERT. Women with high levels of triglycerides in the blood or very high blood pressure should also weigh the pros and cons carefully with their physicians. These women need close monitoring after starting ERT to be sure that it does not exacerbate the underlying condition.

Finally, whatever her personal risk factors, every woman who is using ERT should have annual pelvic and breast examinations. She should also have a mammogram done when therapy is initiated and then at yearly intervals so long as ERT is continued. Women on unopposed estrogens who still have a uterus (for example, women who for whatever reason cannot tolerate the side effects of progestins) need to have yearly endometrial biopsies to check for cancerous or precancerous changes. These women may sometimes experience abnormal vaginal bleeding, including withdrawal bleeding (on the days when the estrogen is not taken) and irregular bleeding—which may but does not necessarily indicate a problem. Regular endometrial biopsies are generally unnecessary for women using a combination of estrogen and progestin unless they experience heavy, irregular, or prolonged bleeding (more than a normal menstrual period).

Related entries

Biopsy, breast cancer, coronary artery disease, depression, diethylstilbestrol (DES), endometrial cancer, endometrial hyperplasia, gallstones, headaches, heart disease, high blood pressure, hysterectomy, menopause, obesity, osteoporosis, pelvic examinations, smoking, stroke, vaginal atrophy, vaginal bleeding (abnormal)

Exercise

In the early years of the nineteenth century, many doctors warned that strenuous physical activity would destroy a woman's femininity and reproductive capacity. Middle- and upper-class female patients—that is, those who had a choice in the matter—took them at their word. Even well into the twentieth century, girls and women were subtly discouraged from participating in sports by similar beliefs, as well as overt lack of opportunity and funding for girls' athletics. Today, however, we know that regular exercise and physical fitness play a vital role in preventing certain disorders that afflict women, including coronary artery disease, diabetes, osteoporosis, constipation, sleep disorders, premenstrual syndrome, certain cancers (including breast and colon cancers), and fatigue. It is also becoming clear that regular exercise can relieve stress, help slow the effects of aging, and minimize the symptoms of other debilitating diseases such as arthritis, and that it is an essential part of any weight loss or weight maintenance program.

The nineteenth-century doctors were right in one respect, however: exercise can sometimes be too much of a good thing. Excessively strenuous exercise can alter a woman's ratio of body fat to lean muscle mass enough to produce menstrual irregularities or stop periods altogether. These symptoms are common in female athletes and performers, particularly those engaged in activities that emphasize leanness, such as gymnastics, dancing, and figure skating (although some women with extremely low body fat levels continue to menstruate regularly). Many women with eating disorders such as anorexia and bulimia also use exercise as a means of burning calories and have been known to jog themselves into a state of collapse. Although exercise-induced amenorrhea is reversible, it does seem to cause calcium to leach out of bones (particularly the lower spine) and promote bone thinning—which predisposes these women to osteoporosis later in life. (In extreme cases women have developed osteoporosis in their 20s and 30s.) This effect is probably due to the estrogen deprivation that results from strenuous exercise rather than the exercise itself, since postmenopausal women who exercise actually reduce their risk of osteoporosis. In other words, exercise up to a point makes bones stronger, but excessive exercise in premenopausal women—the kind of exercise inspired by the "no pain, no gain" philosophy—suppresses estrogen production and makes bones weaker.

Moderate physical activity—as simple as a daily brisk walk—is another matter for women of almost all ages and health conditions. Evidence from the Nurses' Health Study has linked this kind of exercise in women to a lowered risk of heart disease, stroke, Type 2 diabetes, osteoporosis, certain cancers, and many other chronic diseases. The 1996 Surgeon General's report, *Physical Activity and Health,* also showed that regular, moderate physical activity can not only help prevent heart disease, stroke, cancer, and diabetes but also reduce symptoms of depression, stress, and anxiety, as well as enhance the ability to meet daily physical demands.

Making exercise a daily habit—and an enjoyable one—is no mean feat, however. Poll after poll shows that although Americans claim to want more exercise, and many recognize its connection to improved health and appearance, they simply aren't finding ways to fit it into their lives. Many women in particular find it challenging, if not virtually impossible, to incorporate the exercise they know they ought to have into an already overpacked schedule of work and family responsibilities—which far too many women put before their own health and fitness. Other women give up the idea of regular exercise even before they try it because they assume it will simply involve more effort than they can muster. And many women, particularly those of middle age and older, simply feel uncomfortable or inexperienced taking up activities they were discouraged from participating in earlier in life.

Over a third of all women in the United States between the ages of 18 and 64 and nearly half of all women over 65 report getting no regular exercise at all. Fewer than half of all American women report exercising even three times a week. In all age groups, women say they exercise less often than do men, and African American, Hispanic, and Asian women exercise less than their white counterparts.

Add to this a notoriously unhealthy diet high in fat and calories, and it's no wonder that more than half of all Americans are overweight and a third, 32 million women and 26 million men, are obese—that is, they weigh at least 20 percent more than is recommended for their height. Approximately 300,000 deaths each year are attributed to a combination of inactivity and poor diet. That is why finding some way to fit in an extra 30 minutes of aerobic exercise each day, plus muscle-strengthening exercises twice a week, is a challenge worth meeting. Without continuing good health, after all, fulfilling all those other responsibilities will simply be that much more difficult.

Starting an exercise routine

Even without the other demands many women face, starting new habits is never easy. Making vague resolutions to lose weight or run more often, for example, is rarely effective. Neither is paying a large sum to join a health club and then never going because there never seems to be enough time, or purchasing an expensive piece of exercise equipment and using it as a clothes rack.

What can often be effective, however, is to start with a specific goal—such as firming up the abdominal muscles, working off the 10 extra pregnancy pounds, or fitting into a favorite dress—and then working out a very specific plan for meeting that goal. A realistic plan usually means a slow start—perhaps nothing more than getting into some exercise clothes on the first few days, or waking up 15 minutes early—and increase expectations over time. A realistic plan will include both incrementally more challenging exercises and exercises that can be accomplished without excessive exertion.

For most women, plans that involve hours of huffing and puffing are not only unrealistic and doomed to failure but also unnecessary; evidence continues to mount that vigorous sweating is not necessary, and for some women may even be counterproductive. Of course, women who enjoy more vigorous exercise can still benefit from it both physically and psychologically, and may achieve even greater benefits. But for more sedentary women, much more moderate activity is still perfectly adequate. Even better, if finding time is a problem, the good news is that short bouts of exercise—10 minutes here, 10 minutes there—appear to be just as effective as one long session. In other words, hopping on the exercise bike for 15 minutes while waiting for the dryer to finish, and then taking a brisk 15-minute walk with the dog later that day, are just as beneficial as sitting on the bike for a full half hour. It's also fine to fit the exercise around a regular activity—such as watching TV. A woman who watches an hour of television per day can simply use an exercise machine or do some weight-lifting while watching the same show. A woman who spends half an hour a day chatting with friends may be able to induce one or two of them to walk—and talk—with her instead of relying on the telephone. Making exercise a family activity—perhaps a game of tennis or a hike through a nature preserve with the kids—is another good way to get some exercise without sacrificing precious family time.

Once a goal and plan are set, keeping a daily record showing how well the goal is being met also helps keep many women on track. Part of the plan should be to keep the goals modest at first—perhaps 2 days a week of exercise, then gradually increasing. Some women find it helpful to write down their reactions to each day's progress or lack thereof. Others find it helpful to offer themselves little rewards or perks at the completion of each successful day or week—a new outfit, a membership in a health club, a professional massage, or even just a soak in the tub or a special cup of coffee.

It's also important to find an exercise that suits an individual's lifestyle and tastes if exercise is going to become a regular habit. Some women find exercising alone or at home more convenient and pleasurable, or they enjoy having some time with their thoughts during exercise. Other women just can't find the motivation or discipline to exercise unless they're part of a class. Some women may find it easier to get into an exercise routine if the exercise involves walking or talking with a friend. Without some creativity about the type and mix of exercises, as well as a realistic setting for the exercise, it's unlikely that any exercise plan will become a long-term habit.

Types of exercise

A complete fitness program for women generally includes 3 basic types of exercise (see illustration): ‣ flexibility exercises, ‣ aerobic exercises, and ‣ weight-bearing exercises. Women should not forget to take into account the amount of exercise they get as part of daily life. A woman whose job involves a great deal of walking or manual labor—or a young mother who spends half her day running up and down the stairs, vacuuming floors, and chasing after toddlers—will obviously have different supplementary exercise needs than a woman

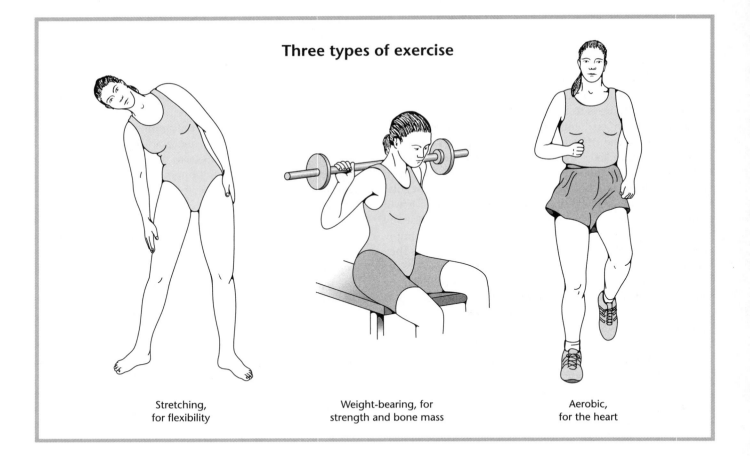

Three types of exercise

Stretching,
for flexibility

Weight-bearing, for
strength and bone mass

Aerobic,
for the heart

who drives to work, sits all day at a desk, and pays someone to clean her house.

Flexibility exercises. These emphasize stretching muscles and mobilizing joints, taking advantage of women's naturally looser joints and smaller muscles. Building flexibility is important for both sexes because it minimizes the risk of muscle strains and pulls during other exercises as well as during daily activities. Many exercises once considered "alternative"—including yoga, tai chi, and qi gong—can all improve both balance and flexibility.

Aerobic exercises. Also called endurance exercises, these significantly increase the heart rate and the body's demand for oxygen. They are believed to decrease the risk of coronary artery disease and high blood pressure by strengthening the heart and lungs, widening the blood vessels, improving the efficiency with which oxygen is delivered to body tissues, and boosting levels of high-density lipoprotein (HDL; see cholesterol). Examples of aerobic exercise include jogging, brisk walking, long-distance or uphill bicycling, swimming, walking on a treadmill or stair climber, and dancing.

Weight-bearing exercises. These exercises, performed against the force of gravity, increase bone mass and also improve overall agility and balance. New evidence also suggests that weight-bearing exercises can help raise resting metabolism, thereby making it easier to lose or maintain a healthy weight. Like aerobic exercise, weight-bearing exercises can also help improve emotional well-being, appearance, and self-esteem. These exercises include walking, hiking, jogging, stair climbing, jumping rope, weight training, dancing, and tennis.

When weight-bearing exercises include weight-lifting, they are called strength-training exercises. The Surgeon General's report *Physical Fitness and Health* recommends at least 2 strength-training exercises a week. These exercises should include at least 8 to 10 exercises that use the major muscle groups of the legs, trunk, and shoulders, with each exercise repeated at least 8 to 12 times. Even elderly women can benefit from these exercises in terms of building muscle and replacing bone.

Contrary to popular myth, strength-training exercises do not make muscles bulky, add unwanted weight, or increase blood pressure (except during the exercise itself).

Exercise over the life span

There are many different ways to incorporate these kinds of exercise into one's weekly routine. Specific routines may vary according to a woman's individual capacity, lifestyle, and interests as well as her stage of life and overall health. Whatever exercises are chosen, however, the plan currently believed to be most effective for virtually all healthy women involves about 30 minutes of moderate aerobic activity per day. This 30 minutes can be broken up into several shorter periods of 10 or 15 minutes each, depending on individual preferences and schedules. If at all possible, it's also a good idea to include a couple of short strength-training (weight-bearing) sessions per week, as well as some daily stretching exercises to maintain flexibility.

All women just beginning an exercise routine should start slowly and only gradually increase the frequency and length of sessions. Most physiologists recommend that women aim to reach about 75 to 85 percent of the average maximum heart rate for their age group during aerobic exercise. This rate can be calculated by subtracting the woman's age from 220. Thus, a 40-year-old woman has an average maximum heart rate of 180 (220 minus 40) beats per minute, and at peak condition her heart rate should equal 75 percent of that, or 135 beats per minute. Beginning exercisers should be satisfied reaching just 50 to 60 percent of their average maximum heart rate during workouts.

Adolescents. Celebrated female athletes, ubiquitous health clubs, and an increasing number of well-funded community sports teams and athletic facilities all make exercise attractive to many teenage girls today. Even so, most American adolescents are not getting enough exercise for optimal health. Not only does physical activity decline dramatically during adolescence, but also, according to the American Heart Association, daily enrollment in physical education classes has declined among high school students from 42 percent in 1991 to 25 percent in 1997. According to the American Heart Association, nearly half of Americans aged 12 to 21 do not exercise energetically even 3 times a week for 20 minutes, which is itself far less than the recommended 30 minutes of moderate weight-bearing exercise per day. And according to the Centers for Disease Control and Prevention (CDC), about 14 percent of young people in the National Youth Risk Behavior Survey reported no recent physical activity at all. Inactivity was more common among females (14 percent) than males (7 percent) and among black females (21 percent) than white females (12 percent).

These statistics are particularly distressing because regular exercise during the adolescent years can help maintain physical fitness, reduce stress, help control weight, reduce body fat, prevent numerous health disorders, and boost self-confidence. Adolescents who are athletes often have better self-esteem than those who do not participate in sports and are at lower risk for adolescent health hazards such as drug abuse and unplanned pregnancy. In addition, those who incorporate regular exercise into their lives during their teenage years are more likely to maintain a healthy lifestyle later in life.

Healthy premenopausal women. Making or keeping exercise a regular part of one's life can help women maintain muscle mass and bone strength, lose weight and keep it off, build joint strength and flexibility, and boost mood and energy levels. Most exercise physiologists recommend that women in this age group perform some form of continuous aerobic exercise daily, or nearly daily, for at least 30 minutes at a stretch. These should be preceded by about 5 minutes of warm-up flexibility exercises and followed by 5 or 10 minutes of cool-down exercises—such as deep breathing, walking, or stretching. It's not necessary to choose a single activity—2 days a week might involve swimming, 3 days brisk walks, and 2 playing tennis—but the goal should be to build the full 30 minutes of aerobic activity into each day.

In addition, premenopausal women (including adolescents) should try to incorporate some kind of weight-bearing exercise into their regular exercise routine—or, ideally, choose a form of aerobic exercise (such as brisk walking) that is also a weight-bearing exercise. Strength-training exercises should be done about twice a week and involve 8 to 12 lifts for each major muscle group. To prevent injury to joints and muscles, it is important to rest at least a day between each of these strength-training sessions.

Pregnant women. Pregnancy is usually not a good time to take up skiing or skydiving, but women who were already engaged in athletics can usually continue to enjoy them during pregnancy—with certain caveats such as not exercising to the point of exhaustion and avoiding sports that might cause falls. Women who previously engaged in swimming, jogging, tennis, dancing, or brisk walking can usually continue these activities, so long as they make sure to keep their pulse rate under 140 beats per minute (well-trained athletes may be able to go a little higher). Even women who have led sedentary lives before pregnancy generally find that a regular exercise program during pregnancy decreases fatigue and helps improve muscle tone and endurance, thus easing the physical stress of both pregnancy and childbirth.

Regular exercise during pregnancy can help prevent excess weight gain and make it easier to shed pounds afterward. There are many bending and stretching exercises designed especially to relieve backache, reduce tension, improve circulation, and strengthen abdominal muscles in pregnant women. Information about these exercises is available from clinicians as well as from almost any pregnancy book. In addition, local YWCAs, hospitals, and park districts often offer exercise classes designed specifically for pregnant and postpartum women.

The American College of Obstetricians and Gynecologists (ACOG) cautions pregnant women against deep knee bends, full sit-ups, double leg raises, and straight-leg toe touches because these exercises may injure tissues that connect the leg and back joints. After about 20 weeks of pregnancy, women should also avoid exercises that require lying on the back on the floor for more than a few minutes. ACOG also recommends that pregnant women avoid jerky, bouncy, or high-impact motions, that they exercise on a wooden floor or tightly carpeted surface to reduce shock and prevent slipping, and that they stand up gradually from a lying or sitting position to avoid dizziness and fainting. To prevent dehydration, pregnant women should drink plenty of water both before and after exercise, and they should stop exercising and consult a clinician if any unusual symptoms (such as pain, bleeding, rapid heartbeat, or dizziness) occur.

Postpartum and breastfeeding women. Once the baby is born, daily exercises can help restore muscle strength and return the body to its pre-pregnancy shape. They can also help minimize the fatigue so common to new mothers. Most women find that their strength and flexibility are significantly diminished in the first few days following delivery (tears and stitches do not help matters), but in most cases there is marked improvement from one day to the next. A clinician or pregnancy book can recommend several simple exercises appropriate for the weeks after childbirth, including Kegel exercises to restore vaginal tone, and leg slides, head lifts, curl-ups, and pelvic tilt exercises to strengthen abdominal muscles.

Women who did not exercise during pregnancy should start with easy exercises and only gradually add more difficult ones. Women who have had a cesarean section or postpartum complications should check with their clinician before beginning an exercise program. After the first few weeks, many women find that brisk walking or swimming is a good way to return to a regular exercise routine. Others find it helpful to join a postpartum or mother-baby exercise class.

Occasionally a baby may reject milk from the breasts of a mother who has recently exercised. This seems to be because the level of lactic acid in milk increases substantially after exercise. To avoid this problem, breastfeeding mothers may want to nurse the baby just before an exercise session or wait an hour or two afterward before feeding. Yet another alternative is to have a bottle of expressed milk ready and waiting in case the baby is hungry too soon after the mother exercises.

Postmenopausal women. Both aerobic and weight-bearing exercises continue to be important after the childbearing years have ended. New studies indicate that a regular aerobic routine can significantly increase aerobic capacity in women of all ages, and decrease the risks of coronary artery disease and noninsulin-dependent diabetes in middle-aged women. The benefits of exercise continue into the 70s, 80s, and beyond. Weight gain, joint stiffness, muscle atrophy, loss of balance and coordination, thinning bones, and decreased aerobic capacity—all of these problems and more were once thought to be inevitable accompaniments of aging. It now appears that as many as two-thirds of these debilities are attributable more to inactivity than to aging per se. A regular exercise program may be able to help even elderly women avert—and even reverse—many of these problems.

Some doctors caution that jogging may not be the ideal sport after menopause—although there is considerable controversy about this matter. Naysayers argue that frequent pounding of feet into the ground may cause joint problems in the spine and legs or promote osteoporosis-related fractures if the bones have already begun to thin. Whether or not this theory proves true, the benefits of weight-bearing exercise for the musculoskeletal system cannot be overemphasized for older women. The rate of bone loss greatly accelerates in the first years following menopause, increasing the risk of osteoporosis. Regular weight-bearing exercise can help reverse this loss, even for women who are not taking estrogen replacement therapy or supplemental calcium. There is some evidence that exercising just one part of the body can stimulate bone growth in other areas, possibly because the exercises stimulate the production of growth hormone. This is called crossover training.

Strength-training exercise in middle-aged and older women can also help increase muscle power and mass, even in women who are already aerobically conditioned. Weight machine workouts seem to help strengthen atrophied muscles and improve balance—at least temporarily—even in people in their 80s and 90s. Strength-training exercise can help even the oldest of women build muscle and replace bone, thereby helping to prevent osteoporosis.

What are the risks and complications?

Runner's highs aside, exercise is not always pleasant, and to be effective it has to involve a certain amount of discomfort. When exercise involves dizziness, sharp pain, pressure in the chest, or shortness of breath, serious injury is a possibility. The exercise should be stopped immediately, and a clinician should be consulted if symptoms continue.

Overall, women are no more likely than men to sustain injuries while engaged in sports. There is no evidence that blows to the breasts can cause breast cancer, nor is there any particular reason to stop athletic activities during menstruation. Women beyond the first trimester of pregnancy, however, should avoid sports in which they risk blows to the abdominal region. And women seem to be unusually prone to injuries of the ankles and knees, particularly shin splints (pain in the front of the lower leg) and pain in the front part of the knee.

Often proper clothing and equipment can avert injuries. For example, large-breasted women may want to consider wearing a sports bra designed to prevent chafing and give added support during exercise. Runners, walkers, and tennis players should use footwear designed especially for their sport to help avoid blisters, fungal infections, foot strain, and sprains. However comfortable they may feel, men's athletic shoes are not appropriate for most women since they are not made to accommodate the narrower heels and higher arches typical of women's feet.

Before beginning any active exercise program, a woman who has been sedentary should have a thorough physical examination. This is especially important for women over 45 and for those who have underlying medical disorders such as heart disease, diabetes, multiple sclerosis, anemia, hypertension, bursitis, backaches, and asthma. Once they have the go-ahead from their clinician, however, many women with these conditions find that a regular activity program provides considerable relief from both symptoms and side effects of treatment. It can also help alleviate the depression, anxiety, and/or fatigue that often accompany chronic illness.

Related entries

Amenorrhea, anorexia nervosa and bulimia nervosa, coronary artery disease, fatigue, Kegel exercises, knee pain, musculoskeletal disorders, obesity, osteoarthritis, osteoporosis, premenstrual syndrome, sleep disorders, stress

Eye Care

Generally the eyes require no special care beyond common sense. This includes making sure that there is adequate light for reading and doing other close tasks, wearing special protective goggles or eye gear when working with chemicals or when participating in contact sports, and protecting eyes from ultraviolet rays with sunglasses.

Probably the most common eye problems are refraction errors, which include nearsightedness and farsightedness (see entry). Other eye diseases and disorders are particularly common later in life and occur as the structures facilitating vision begin to deteriorate. Among the (often) age-related conditions are glaucoma (abnormally high pressure within the eyeball), cataracts (blurring or clouding of the lens of the eye), dry eye, macular degeneration (gradual deterioration of the central part of the retina), and retinal holes and detachment (tears in the retina that can lead to a peeling away of the retina from the back of the eye; see entries for these disorders).

Anyone over the age of 40 should have her eyes checked for glaucoma and macular degeneration about every 2 years—and every year in those over 50 or 60 or who are at high risk for these conditions. An ophthalmologist should also be consulted if symptoms such as difficulty seeing, blurred vision, floaters, flashing lights (especially "white" light or shadows, which may indicate a retinal detachment), red eye, eye pain, or chronic irritation ever arise.

Anyone with symptoms of retinal detachment requires immediate medical attention—either by an ophthalmologist or in the emergency room of a hospital—to prevent permanent loss of vision. Symptoms may include a shower of floaters, a sudden burst of flashing lights or sparks, or the perception of a dark curtain moving over a portion of the visual field.

Floaters are small light or dark specks, spots, strings, or squiggles that appear to be floating across or flitting through the visual field. They are easiest to perceive against a light background, such as a white wall or the sky. Floaters are caused by tiny clumps in the vitreous fluid (the gel-like substance between the lens and the retina) and become increasingly common with age, although they may become less conspicuous over time. In most cases, they represent nothing more than a nuisance and usually disappear quickly on their own. In rare cases a sudden burst or shower of floaters may

signal a more serious problem—such as hemorrhage or the age-related collapse of the vitreous gel—which in turn can lead to retinal holes and detachment. This is particularly true if the floaters are accompanied by blurred vision, the illusion of flashing lights, or shadows drifting across the field of vision. An ophthalmologist (eye physician) should be consulted immediately if these symptoms appear suddenly.

Finding an eye doctor

A good rule of thumb is to see an ophthalmologist—a medical doctor who has been specially trained in diagnosing and treating diseases of the eye—if there is any possibility of a disorder more serious than nearsightedness or farsightedness. The medical evaluation and procedures conducted by ophthalmologists are generally more extensive and precise than the diagnostic tests conducted by optometrists—who are not physicians but who have completed a specialized degree program. Furthermore, ophthalmologists can perform surgical procedures on the eye, which optometrists cannot. Although some states prohibit optometrists from diagnosing and treating eye diseases, that should not stop young, healthy women from consulting an optometrist for a routine eye examination and the prescription of contact lenses or eyeglasses.

Home care for the eyes

Many minor problems of the eye, in addition to floaters, resolve spontaneously and may require no medical attention. Red, bloodshot eyes, while often troublesome cosmetically, are usually a sign only of fatigue or eyestrain and disappear with a little rest. Red, painful eyes, by contrast, may indicate glaucoma, infection, or the presence of a foreign body and should be evaluated by an ophthalmologist. To reduce redness and increase comfort, vasoconstrictive drugs (such as tetrahydrozoline) can also be used. Although available without prescription, these drops should not be used habitually; overuse can lead to "rebound" redness.

Subconjunctival hemorrhages—red splotches of blood in the white of the eye—are another minor problem that can cause alarm. These hemorrhages have no associated pain or discomfort and are commonly caused by carrying heavy objects or straining. They clear on their own in a few days.

Many people occasionally find that one or both of their eyelids twitch involuntarily for a few seconds or even for several minutes. In most cases this occurrence (termed a fasciculation) is nothing more than an annoying muscle spasm which will disappear on its own, although it may recur frequently. There is some speculation that unusual stress or fatigue may make these spasms more likely. Time is usually the best cure for twitchy eyelids, although some people find that gently pressing or rubbing the eyelid or applying cracked ice to the lid or the side of the eye can help relieve the spasm.

Women are particularly likely to develop a severe eyelid spasm known as benign essential blepharospasm. In this chronic (long-lasting) condition of unknown cause, involuntary muscle contractions cause the eyelids to blink or squint abnormally. Sometimes this condition develops to the point

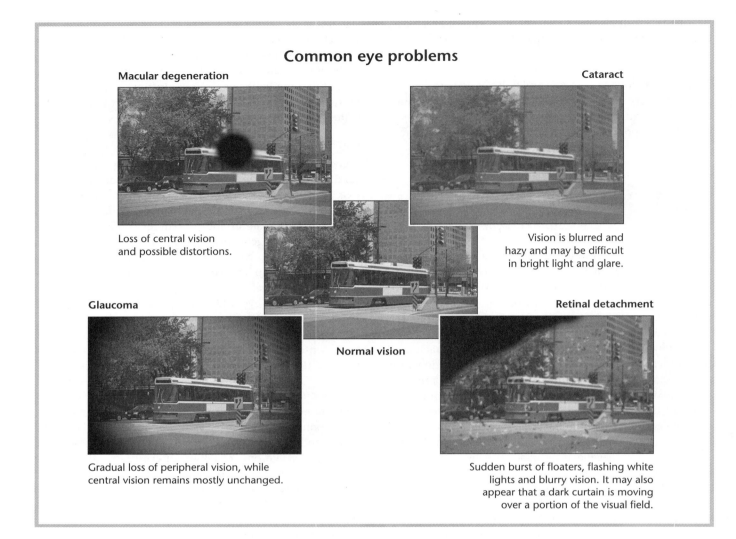

Common eye problems

Macular degeneration

Loss of central vision and possible distortions.

Cataract

Vision is blurred and hazy and may be difficult in bright light and glare.

Normal vision

Glaucoma

Gradual loss of peripheral vision, while central vision remains mostly unchanged.

Retinal detachment

Sudden burst of floaters, flashing white lights and blurry vision. It may also appear that a dark curtain is moving over a portion of the visual field.

of functional blindness, when the eyes can be opened only if the lid is lifted by hand. Benign essential blepharospasm is particularly common among women in their 50s and 60s. Investigators have had good initial results relieving this condition with injections of the botulism toxin. Twitchy eyelids that signal more serious diseases (such as multiple sclerosis) are almost always accompanied by additional symptoms.

Another common problem that rarely requires medical treatment is itchy eyelids—although it is important to avoid excessive rubbing or scratching of the eyes, which can induce even itchier patches of skin (lichen simplex chronicus). Here vasoconstrictive eyedrops containing antihistamines can be helpful—especially if the itchiness is allergy-related. Occasionally the itchiness may be traced to eye makeup, in which case switching to a hypoallergenic formulation—or cutting out cosmetics altogether—may be the answer.

Finally, a simple but crucial aspect of eye care—one that should be practiced even by those with the healthiest of eyes—involves protecting the eyes from damaging ultraviolet sunlight. This invisible, short-wavelength light can promote both cataracts and macular degeneration. The easiest way to accomplish this is to wear sunglasses all year long whenever one is out in bright sunshine. Ultraviolet light is especially (but not exclusively) damaging to eyes of lighter shades.

Selecting the right pair of sunglasses used to be somewhat complicated (and expensive) but today rarely poses much of a problem. Whatever their tint, most sunglasses sold currently in the United States shield the eyes from both types of ultraviolet light (UVA and UVB) known to cause eye damage—and they state this fact on the label. Only lenses with special reflective coatings protect against infrared radiation, which is being increasingly implicated as an additional source of eye damage. Polarized sunglasses may be effective in reducing glare and reflections.

Complete protection from ultraviolet light requires "wraparound" sunglasses which extend to the temples and keep light from seeping in through the sides. A reasonable alternative for women who consider this to be a fashion sacrifice is to choose relatively large lenses.

Related entries

Cataracts, contact lenses, diabetes, dry eye, eyelid surgery, glaucoma, macular degeneration, multiple sclerosis, nearsightedness and farsightedness, retinal detachment, temporal arteritis

Eyelid Surgery

An eyelid lift or eyelid alteration is a kind of cosmetic surgery done to correct bags or wrinkles on the eyelid or under the eyes. Puffy eyelids frequently run in families and can appear even in very young women. Over time this puffy area often becomes wrinkled as well. In addition, as women age they may develop wrinkles under the eyes even without puffiness. Eyelid surgery (blepharoplasty) can be used to correct any of these conditions, as well as to pull up a low-lying upper lid that sometimes interferes with peripheral vision.

How is the procedure performed?
Blepharoplasty may be done as part of a face lift or as a separate operation. When done by itself, it is an outpatient procedure; when combined with a face lift, an overnight stay in a hospital may be required. Although an eyelid lift can be performed under local anesthesia, women concerned about surgery performed so close to the eye may opt for some kind of supplementary sedation. Some surgeons also use protective plastic lenses to shield the eye during the operation.

Before beginning the procedure, the surgeon will mark planned incisions and skin that is to be removed. The face is cleaned and anesthesia is administered. Once the anesthetic has taken effect, the surgeon makes an incision or incisions so that excess fat can be trimmed away and fat pads removed. Surgeons generally try to make incisions that will leave scars that are as inconspicuous as possible. For example, cuts on the upper lid can be made along natural creases so that they will not be noticeable when the eye is open. Some surgeons make the incision inside the lid so that there will be no external scar at all. Incisions beneath the eye are often made just under the lower lid so that the lower eyelashes will cover the scar completely. Under-the-skin (subcuticular) stitches can minimize visible scarring even further.

Often the surgeon will use a colored solution to mark planned incisions before the operation so that the patient will know just what to expect.

What happens after the surgery?
After the operation a cold compress is applied to relieve pain and minimize swelling, and an antibiotic ointment is used to prevent infection. Stitches are removed within a few days, but the area around the eye will appear markedly bruised and swollen for 7 to 15 days. Most women feel uncomfortable going about daily life without dark glasses during the first couple of weeks. It can take several months before the last traces of swelling disappear.

What are the risks and complications?
Like all forms of surgery, blepharoplasty involves certain risks, including infection, excessive bleeding, reactions to anesthesia, and abnormal scarring. Eyelid surgery can interfere with the function of the tear ducts, at least temporarily. Occasionally the operation leaves the patient with a droopy lower lid. This usually corrects itself over time but may require additional surgery. In very rare cases blepharoplasty may result in a permanent loss of vision.

Related entries
Anesthesia, body image, cosmetic surgery, eye care, face lifts, keloid scarring, wrinkles

Face Lifts

A face lift is a surgical operation to tighten sagging skin and eliminate wrinkles, jowls, and sometimes double chins. The surgeon may also tighten the deep muscle layers of the face and remove excess fat from the face and neck with liposuction (see lipectomy and liposuction).

Although many surgeons prefer not to do face lifts on anyone under the age of 40 or 45, in certain appearance-conscious communities there has been a trend toward cosmetic surgery at younger and younger ages, with women in their 30s and even 20s opting for surgery. Given that the average patient may see signs of aging within 6 to 8 years, these younger patients may elect to go through a large number of operations in their remaining years of life.

How is the procedure performed?
Some surgeons like to perform face lifts using general anesthesia, although some use only local anesthesia combined with light sedation. In a simple face lift an incision is made on the side of the face, usually from the temple down one side of the ear and then up the back side of the ear. The surgeon then carefully separates the skin and subcutaneous fat from underlying muscles and removes excess fat and tissue. After the remaining skin is pulled back and up and stitched into place, the same procedure is repeated on the other side. More extensive correction requires work on deeper tissues and muscles. Each face lift should be customized to the patient's particular anatomy and concerns.

Creases between the eyebrows or wrinkles on the forehead require a forehead or coronal lift. In this procedure the surgeon makes another incision from ear to ear just under the hairline or across the top of the scalp. This elevates the hairline to some extent after surgery. To eliminate a double chin, a small incision must be made under the jaw. Here, too, the surgeon trims sagging skin and excess fat in surrounding areas and then stitches the tightened skin back into place. Newer technology using narrow lighted instruments called endoscopes may permit these procedures to be performed through much smaller incisions.

What happens after the surgery?

After surgery a drain may be inserted under the skin to remove blood and serum and thus minimize bruising and swelling. Often a dressing will be placed over the wound as well. Stiffness is common, especially around the sides of the neck, but any accompanying pain can be relieved with mild narcotics.

Many women also feel a temporary loss of sensitivity or odd itchy feelings in the healing skin. Stitches can usually be removed in a week or so, although it takes 2 to 3 weeks for bruising and swelling to decrease. The time required for full recovery is dependent on the woman's general health, the elasticity of her skin, the amount of stress in her life, and heredity, but in most cases it takes at least 1 to 2 months for the surgery to produce its optimal effect. The surgeon may want to make minor surgical corrections at about 6 months.

Many women emerge from face lifts feeling euphoric and reinvigorated, but unrealistic expectations have been the undoing of many a woman undergoing this operation. Nobody should expect a face lift to remove every wrinkle or tighten every hint of sagging skin. By the time most women have these operations (that is, by middle age), the skin has already begun to lose some of its natural elasticity, and underlying bones have begun to shrink. For this reason, no amount of tucking and trimming is going to restore the complexion and facial contour a woman may remember from her adolescent years.

Furthermore, face lifts do not last forever and cannot be regarded as a fountain of youth or as a way of conquering the aging process. Although it is possible to have repeat operations, there is a limit to the number of times these can be done before excessively tightened skin results in a permanent smile and awkwardly shaped facial features.

On the positive side, even if a face lift is never repeated, skin will generally be tighter and smoother than if the operation had never been performed in the first place. In addition, the effects of the face lift can often be extended by avoiding excess sun exposure, maintaining a constant weight, and limiting the intake of drugs, alcohol, and cigarettes—steps that can also help minimize wrinkling and other facial changes in the first place.

What are the risks and complications?

Like any form of surgery, face lifts can result in a number of complications, including infection, excessive bleeding, nerve injury, problems related to anesthesia, and abnormal scarring.

Plastic surgeons make every effort to leave inconspicuous scars, but some susceptible people end up with unsightly raised scars at the site of the surgery. Any woman who has developed a keloid scar following other surgery or a wound should be very cautious about undergoing a face lift. Plastic surgeons are often willing to show potential patients photo-graphs of abnormal scarring to help inform them about this particular risk.

There is also the risk, though small, of permanent facial paralysis if a part of the facial nerve is damaged during surgery. Muscular control of the face may be somewhat affected for a time if swelling temporarily compresses the nerve.

Some women find that their skin pigmentation has changed after healing. Another common complication of a face lift is the formation of a hematoma (a blood-filled swelling under the skin), which can lead to infection, tissue loss, unsightly scarring, or delayed healing. Hematoma formation may require another operation soon after surgery to drain the wound. Delays in healing and increased scarring are more frequent in smokers and women with certain medical conditions such as diabetes. Many surgeons believe that these women are not safe candidates for face lift surgery.

Related entries

Anesthesia, body image, cosmetic surgery, dermabrasion and chemical peels, eyelid surgery, keloid scarring, otoplasty, rhinoplasty, smoking, stress, wrinkles

Fallopian Tube Cancer

Cancer of the fallopian tube is rare. Although it may be linked to chronic pelvic inflammatory disease of the fallopian tube (salpingitis) or tuberculosis, the connection remains unclear. If untreated, the cancer can spread to adjacent organs such as the uterus or ovaries or invade more distant parts of the body through the lymphatic system. Chances of surviving for 5 years after treatment without a recurrence of the cancer are between 5 and 48 percent.

Who is likely to develop fallopian tube cancer?

The peak incidence occurs between the ages of 50 and 60.

What are the symptoms?

Usually women with this malignancy feel vague discomfort as the tumor presses on the bladder or rectum. Some women also may have a watery or bloody vaginal discharge.

How is the condition evaluated?

A pelvic examination may reveal a large pelvic mass or fluid accumulation. Since these findings can signal ovarian as well as fallopian tube cancer, a laparotomy or laparoscopy (see entries) is generally necessary to make the diagnosis.

How is fallopian tube cancer treated?

Treatment is usually identical to that for ovarian cancer, including a hysterectomy—removal of both tubes, both ovaries, the uterus and cervix, supporting ligaments, and sometimes pelvic lymph nodes. The tumor often spreads to the upper abdomen. At surgery, all of the tumor is removed if possible. Surgery is followed by chemotherapy.

Related entries

Chemotherapy, hysterectomy, laparoscopy, laparotomy, ovarian cancer, ovary removal, pelvic inflammatory disease, radiation therapy, vaginal bleeding (abnormal)

Fatigue

Fatigue is such a common problem that sometimes it seems a normal accompaniment of modern life. Some surveys indicate that 1 adult in 5 claims to "always feel tired," and nearly 15 million medical office visits per year in the United States are for the complaint of fatigue.

Statistics such as these are somewhat hard to interpret because different people use the term fatigue to mean different things: an unusual urge to sleep during the day, trouble finding the energy to start new tasks, difficulty concentrating, muscle weakness, or perfectly normal tiredness that can result after exercise or lack of sleep. Still other people use the term synonymously with chronic fatigue syndrome (see entry), a much less common condition that involves other physical symptoms besides fatigue.

Who is likely to complain of fatigue?

Most patients seeking care for fatigue are women, for reasons that remain elusive. Some investigators have speculated that some of this tiredness may be a physical reaction to the stresses of a woman's role in contemporary society. Proponents of this idea argue that women in Western culture are under particular stress from trying to balance home and work life while, at the same time, remaining subordinated and undervalued. Given these facts of life, coupled with the propensity of women to seek medical attention (and interpersonal support in general) more readily than men, the argument goes, it is no wonder that fatigue is reported more often in women.

Fatigue can also be a symptom of hundreds of actual diseases, ranging from psychiatric disorders to cancer and diabetes. Among the most common organic causes of fatigue in women are thyroid disease, various autoimmune disorders such as multiple sclerosis and lupus, allergies, and chronic fatigue syndrome (which increasing numbers of investigators now believe to be an organic illness, that is, one originating in a bodily organ). Fatigue is also a classic symptom of pregnancy, particularly in the first and third trimesters. Often, however, fatigue cannot be traced to either an organic or a psychiatric condition.

How is the condition evaluated?

A doctor evaluating fatigue will first try to determine if lifestyle factors—such as overwork, lack of sleep, or too little or too much exercise—may underlie the problem. Often fatigue may mask a more serious condition which the patient is either unaware of or unable to admit openly to the doctor—alcohol abuse, for example, or domestic violence (either past or present). A doctor evaluating fatigue will try to elucidate any underlying psychological as well as physical problems, since both depression and anxiety disorders often manifest themselves as fatigue.

The doctor will take a complete history, perform a physical examination, and order appropriate laboratory tests to see if the fatigue may be related to some organic disease.

How is fatigue treated?

Treatment varies according to the specific cause of the fatigue. Using caffeine, alcohol, or other drugs to "treat" fatigue can be counterproductive in the long run.

Related entries

Alcohol, anxiety disorders, autoimmune disorders, chronic fatigue syndrome, depression, insomnia, sexual abuse and incest, sleep disorders, stress, substance abuse, thyroid disorders

Fibromyalgia

This condition involves painful and stiff muscles, tendons, and ligaments, as well as fatigue and sleep disturbances. Although the exact prevalence is unknown (estimates range from 3 to 17 million Americans with fibromyalgia), most of the cases—approximately 80 percent—occur in women. Once regarded as having a psychological origin, fibromyalgia is now thought to be largely a physical problem that may be aggravated by stress or other emotional factors.

Who is likely to develop fibromyalgia?

Fibromyalgia (also called fibrositis, fibromyositis, or chronic muscle pain syndrome) is most likely to develop in middle-aged women, with 50 being the mean age of onset.

What are the symptoms?

The most common symptoms are diffuse aches and pains, particularly in the lower back, neck, shoulders, thorax, and thighs. People with fibromyalgia also have multiple "tender points"—particular muscles and tendons that become painful when pressed. Common spots include the neck, knee, or shoulder; just below and inside the elbow; and the hip joint (see illustration).

Symptoms of fibromyalgia usually last for years unless treated, although they sometimes disappear for several months at a time and then recur. Many people with fibromyalgia have difficulty sleeping and experience morning stiffness upon awakening (in more diffuse locations than generally occurs in inflammatory arthritis). Some people also

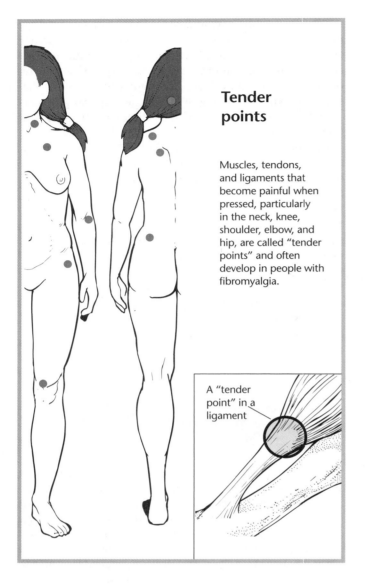

Tender points

Muscles, tendons, and ligaments that become painful when pressed, particularly in the neck, knee, shoulder, elbow, and hip, are called "tender points" and often develop in people with fibromyalgia.

A "tender point" in a ligament

disease, degenerative spinal disk disease, and osteoarthritis—and it often coexists with the latter condition in elderly patients.

If other causes of pain are excluded, if tender points are present, if diffuse pain has lasted for at least 3 months, and if the patient is experiencing profound fatigue, fibromyalgia may be diagnosed. Nonetheless, there is considerable controversy within the medical community about whether or not fibromyalgia is indeed a distinct condition, partly because there has been little scientific research so far. Indeed, it is entirely possible that the set of symptoms sometimes called fibromyalgia may often overlap other conditions that have similar symptoms. These can include chronic fatigue syndrome (CFS), multiple chemical sensitivities, and myofascial pain syndromes (MPS), which resembles fibromyalgia except that instead of tender points there are "trigger points" which produce pain in another area when pressed. Symptoms of MPS can be reduced by eliminating aggravating actions and by injecting a local anesthetic or vapocoolant spray such as ethyl chloride into trigger points and then passively stretching affected muscles.

How is fibromyalgia treated?

There is still no specific therapy for fibromyalgia. Taking tricylic antidepressants such as amitriptyline (Elavil) and the muscle relaxer cyclobenzaprine (Flexeril) seems to relieve sleep problems and pain in about a third of the people with this condition. They can also help alleviate the depression experienced by more than half of all people with fibromyalgia. A key component of treatment is aerobic conditioning, including low-impact exercises such as swimming or walking. Heat, massage, relaxation therapy, stress elimination, and improved posture can also help.

Taking an active role in treatment and understanding that fibromyalgia is not a progressive, crippling disease can also be important in controlling this condition. Various organizations that provide up-to-date information about the nature and treatment of fibromyalgia, as well as local support groups consisting of other people with the condition, can provide useful advice as well as emotional support.

Related entries

Antidepressants, autoimmune disorders, chronic fatigue syndrome, depression, fatigue, lupus, musculoskeletal disorders, polymyalgia rheumatica, polymyositis and dermatomyositis, rheumatoid arthritis, sleep disorders, stress

notice numbness, difficulty concentrating, headaches, anxiety, and symptoms of irritable bowel syndrome, while others sense swelling in their hands and feet that is not objectively detectable. Fatigue, tension, inactivity, overwork, and even changes in the weather or environment can aggravate any of the symptoms.

How is the condition evaluated?

Because there is no specific biochemical or anatomical defect associated with fibromyalgia, it can be diagnosed only after other causes of the symptoms have been eliminated. A doctor will take a thorough history and perform a physical examination, including a neurological examination. Various laboratory tests may be done to discover any sign of other connective tissue diseases such as rheumatoid arthritis, polymyositis, and lupus, as well as hypothyroidism. Fibromyalgia must also be distinguished from various other conditions that can lead to similar symptoms, including chronic Lyme

Foot Care

Feet are subject to a wide variety of woes, including aches, pains, sweating, odor, fungal infections, warts, ingrown toenails, corns, calluses, bunions, blisters, hammertoes, and

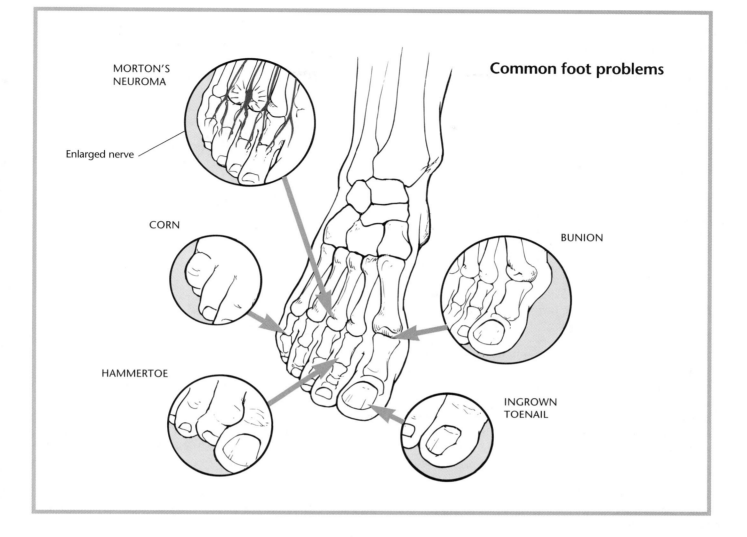

Common foot problems

MORTON'S NEUROMA

Enlarged nerve

CORN

HAMMERTOE

BUNION

INGROWN TOENAIL

neuromas. In both men and women some of these problems may result from sports-related injuries or systemic diseases. Foot ulcerations and even gangrene (death and blackening of body tissue) can occur in people with diabetes, while a painful big toe is a characteristic symptom of gout—an inflammatory joint disease involving high levels of uric acid which commonly afflicts men of all ages and women after menopause.

With these exceptions the vast majority of foot problems that women experience can be prevented—or at least postponed—by adhering to a few precepts of basic foot care: keep the feet clean and well ventilated (see skin care and cosmetics; body odors), keep toenails properly trimmed (see nail care; diabetes), exercise the feet with regular walking, and wear properly fitting, supportive, comfortable shoes.

Choosing footwear

When it comes to foot coverings, women have a lengthy record of foot abuse. Throughout history numerous attempts have been made to deform the female foot in the interest of heightening sexual attractiveness. The link between feet and eroticism has a neurological basis: the feet and toes are rich in nerves that respond to sexual excitement—which is why feet often point or toes curl during sexual arousal and why "footsie" is such a popular game. As countless psychologists, anthropologists, sociologists, and historians have observed, feet and their coverings have been linked to sexuality, sensuality, and fertility in various cultures since the beginnings of civilization. Myths and customs linking shoes to romance are abundant throughout the world—ranging from Cinderella's glass slipper, to the wedding custom of tying old shoes to the newlywed couple's car, to the practices of young Sicilian women who put shoes under their pillows to help them find a husband or French brides who keep their wedding shoes to ensure a lifetime of physical union. Women in rural Greece burn old shoes to retrieve lost lovers, while in several other countries the groom traditionally unties the bride's shoe at the wedding to suggest defloration.

From a psychosexual perspective, in which "foot care" includes cultivating the foot as an object of beauty and even of sexuality, the features of the modern female shoe—high heels (which alter posture, undermine balance, and make walking graceful), low-slung (revealing) sides, pointed toes, and a tight fit around the foot—can be easily explained. From a physical perspective, the shape of the modern female shoe, in turn, easily explains why women so frequently develop painful growths and deformities on the feet and toes (see illustration).

The ideal shoe from a health perspective is one that fits properly, cushions the foot without squeezing it excessively, and distributes weight comfortably onto both soles. That usually means a shoe with a rounded or boxy toe area and a modest heel at most.

Bunions

A bunion is a bony protrusion at the base of the big toe. It is usually caused by a minor foot disorder, called hallux valgus, which causes excessive flexibility in the metatarsal joint that joins the toes to the foot (*hallux* is Latin for "big toe," and *valgus* is Latin for "bowlegged"). In this condition, the joint of the big toe thrusts out beyond the normal border of the foot, and the tip of the toe thrusts inward and may overlap other toes. The resulting bump on the inner edge of the foot is called a bunion.

Although a predisposition to bunions is genetically determined, bunions are about 3 times more common in women than in men. Wearing high heels or narrow-toed shoes seems to encourage their development in people who are already genetically predisposed to them. Most bunions are only moderately uncomfortable, but the misshapen foot may make it difficult to find comfortable or acceptable-looking footwear.

Bunions sometimes become extremely painful and stiff when pressure on the joint leads to bursitis—an inflammation of the metatarsal joint's bursa, which is a small sac filled with lubricating fluid that normally serves to minimize friction in the joint. More pain and stiffness can result from the premature osteoarthritis that sometimes occurs in joints affected by bunions. Also, because the big toe thrusts out beyond the side of the foot, constant rubbing can result in a callus (a thickening of the skin) on top of the bunion.

Usually a bunion can be diagnosed through visual inspection. Occasionally a physician or podiatrist (foot specialist) may also want to take x-rays of the joint to confirm the diagnosis and to make sure that the symptoms are due to the bunion alone and not to some other condition.

Bunions can often be treated with self-help measures. These include choosing shoes with heels no higher than 1 inch and with a roomy toe box (see illustration); a toe box that is too narrow can promote bunions. Shoes should be selected on the basis of the way they feel on the feet rather than the stated size, which can vary enormously from manufacturer to manufacturer and even from shoe to shoe within the same line. It is also important to remember that shoes which fit perfectly in the store may cause problems if they are worn with constricting or overly thick socks or stockings. Also, feet tend to enlarge with age—or after pregnancy—so shoes that once fit well can become uncomfortable over time.

Already owned but imperfect shoes can sometimes be doc-

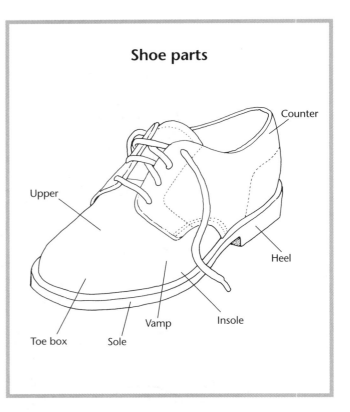

Shoe parts

Counter

Upper

Heel

Vamp

Insole

Toe box

Sole

tored with foam rubber inserts or other orthotic devices to make a bunion more comfortable. Some women find that covering the bunion with a commercially available felt pad cut to size (such as Dr. Scholl's pads) provides relief. If the bunion develops bursitis, it may be necessary to wear an old shoe with a hole cut through the side until the inflammation subsides. It can also help to rest the foot as much as possible, soak the bunion in warm water, and take nonsteroidal antiinflammatory drugs (NSAIDs) such as ibuprofen (Advil, Nuprin, Motrin) or naproxen (Aleve, Naprosyn).

Severe bunions may need to be drained by a clinician, or treated with a protective shield or arch support (mold) to redistribute pressure on the foot. Arch supports are commercially available in many pharmacies and shoe stores, but they are not as effective as full foot molds or protective shields made by a podiatrist using a plaster impression from the individual patient's foot.

In some cases, surgery called bunionectomy may be performed to realign the bones, remove excess bony tissue, and possibly insert an artificial joint. Performed under local anesthesia, this operation can be painful, and full recovery can take up to 6 months. In the meantime, it is usually necessary to wear a plaster cast, splints, or special surgical shoes.

Because bunions are due to a hereditary weakness of the toe joint, they are not entirely preventable. Still, any woman who thinks she is prone to this condition may be able to hold off serious problems, especially if she starts taking preventive steps while still in her teens or early 20s. By far the best means of preventing bunions is to wear shoes with ample room for the toes and to avoid high heels whenever possible. It also makes sense to wear athletic or walking shoes whenever there is a need to stand or walk for long periods of time.

Corns and calluses

Corns and calluses are thick, hardened patches of dead skin that result from repeated pressure or friction. Corns are smaller than calluses (under a quarter of an inch in length) and tend to occur on the toes. Calluses can be as long as an inch and are more likely to appear on the bottom of the foot, over a bunion, or on the fingertips.

It is the rare person who goes through life without ever developing a corn or callus, and women generally develop many more of them than men, particularly on the feet. In most cases they are little more than minor irritations. The exception is in people who have impaired circulation or sensation in the extremities, as happens with diseases such as diabetes. For these people corns and calluses easily become deeply ulcerated or infected.

Wearing shoes that rub or pinch is the most common cause of corns and calluses. Shoes with a triangular, pointed, or flat toe box that crowds the toes are primarily responsible for corns and calluses in women. In a properly fitting shoe, the heel should be wide enough so that force is distributed evenly, and no higher than an inch; high heels put extra pressure on the toes and the ball of the foot, causing corns and calluses.

Even with the best-fitting footwear, however, there seem to be some people who develop corns and calluses anyway. This can be because they have relatively little cushioning tissue between the bones and skin of their feet, because their toes turn inward as they walk (excessive pronation), or because they have conditions that promote increased pressure on the feet, such as high arches or arthritis.

Minor corns and calluses usually produce no symptoms other than unsightliness. Thick calluses, however, can cause a burning sensation during walking, and corns on the little toe often cause excruciating pain, particularly when shoes fit tightly.

Corns and calluses are usually evaluated easily from their appearance. Occasionally a clinician may want to do a more careful inspection to rule out similar-looking conditions such as plantar warts, foreign bodies, or problems caused by a blocked sweat duct.

After several weeks of wearing shoes that fit properly, women usually find that corns and calluses disappear on their own. Putting spongy rings around corns to prevent any direct pressure can help ease the pain in the meantime. The process can be speeded along by gently abrading dead skin with a pumice stone, towel, or emery board after the skin has been softened with soap and water. It may also help to rub the hardened skin with a mild skin lotion. Women with diabetes or other conditions that make them prone to infection should not try to remove any skin by themselves, and no one should use sharp tools or unprescribed medications on corns and calluses.

If self-help measures are inadequate, it may be necessary to consult a podiatrist or a physician who can remove the tissue with a scalpel or with chemicals. Corns and calluses caused by excessive pronation or conditions such as arthritis or high arches can be prevented only by correcting the underlying condition; in some of these cases orthotic devices or surgery may be attempted.

Hammertoes

In hammertoe the bones of one or more of the smaller toes curl downward into a clawlike position. This deformity may begin with a tight tendon, which prevents the toe from resting flat on the ground, or from muscle weakness or arthritis. But usually the cause is improperly fitting shoes. The toe next to the big toe is most often affected, sometimes in conjunction with a bunion that puts pressure on it. A toe box that is too short can aggravate hammertoes; a shoe that fits properly has a finger's width of room between the front of the shoe and the big toe and puckers slightly when the broadest part of the shoe is squeezed.

Initially a hammertoe is flexible, and any discomfort can be relieved by using a "toe pad" sold in drug stores. Switching to roomier shoes, with more space in the toe box, keeps the toes from bunching up. Exercises, as well as splints or other orthotic devices, may be recommended by a physician when pain is bothersome.

Over time hammertoes become harder to treat because they stiffen up. A small piece of bone may have to be surgically removed so that the toe can assume a normal position.

Morton's neuroma

When two toes rub together and irritate a nerve, the nerve may become enlarged and painful. If the vamp of a shoe is too constricting, it can produce neuromas. Sometimes instead of (or in addition to) pain there is burning, cramping, or numbness, which can be felt not just between the toes but in the ball of the foot. The pain feels like the pain of repeatedly stepping barefoot on a pebble.

Foot massage, roomier shoes, pads, and sometimes cortisone injections may help. If not, the growth can be surgically removed, although the nerve tissue may regrow and form another neuroma.

Heel Pain

Heel pain can often be traced to inflammation of the fibrous tissue under the foot—a condition known as plantar fasciitis. This condition is often due to improperly fitting shoes, but it can occur for no obvious reason as well. Pain—which is usually greatest early in the morning (or after staying off the foot for an extended period of time) and dissipates after walking around a bit—is most noticeable on the inner part of the sole directly in front of the heel. Stepping or pressing on the tender spot, or flexing the foot upwards, also tends to aggravate the pain.

Staying off the foot or cushioning the heel with a foam pad often provides relief. Inserting a special heel cup or shoe insert into all shoes frequently helps if these first efforts fail. Meanwhile, icing the heel after activity can relieve inflammation, as can taking nonsteroidal antiinflammatory drugs (such as ibuprofen). Many women find that exercising the foot—flexing it up and down and back and forth—before stepping onto the foot can alleviate pain as well.

If pain continues, special custom-fitted devices are available from podiatrists. If necessary, plantar fasciitis can be treated with ultrasound or injections of corticosteroid medications.

Occasionally bony projections (bone spurs) develop on the heel bone and can also cause severe heel pain. While these can be removed surgically, treating the pain in the same manner as plantar fasciitis is often sufficient to relieve symptoms. In fact, in many cases the pain attributed to bone spurs turns out to be due to coexisting plantar fasciitis.

Whatever its cause, heel pain can often be alleviated by wearing well-fitting shoes with cushioned soles or soft, well-cushioned socks, taking antiinflammatory medications, and alternately applying heat and cold to the affected area as needed.

Ingrown toenails

Ingrown toenails form when the edge of the nail tip—which grows faster than the center—curls under and grows into the soft nail bed underneath (see nail care). Wearing shoes with a toe box that is too tight, fungal infections, deformities of the foot or toes, and injuries caused by pounding from sports or aerobic exercise can all cause ingrown toenails. Wearing low-heeled, wide-toed shoes that fit properly helps prevent ingrown toenails, since these can keep toes from being pinched or from sliding into the front of the shoe.

Warm compresses and warm-water soaks can ease the swelling and pain of an ingrown toenail. If the surrounding skin becomes red and tender or develops a discharge, medical attention should be sought. Antibiotics and possibly minor surgery to remove a small bit of the nail may be required.

Related entries

Body image, body odors, diabetes, nail care, osteoarthritis, skin care and cosmetics

Galactorrhea

Galactorrhea is a condition in which a woman who has not recently been breastfeeding can express milk or a milky discharge from one or both breasts.

Who is likely to develop galactorrhea?

The most common cause is continued nipple stimulation after weaning, which often happens if a woman wants to see if she is still producing milk. By doing so, she keeps up the lev-

els of lactation hormones—particularly prolactin—and milk continues to be produced.

In women who have not recently weaned a baby, however, galactorrhea is usually a clue to some underlying hormonal problem. About 1 in 5 women with galactorrhea will turn out to have a noncancerous tumor of the pituitary gland (a prolactinoma). This tumor produces excess prolactin, leading to a condition called hyperprolactinemia. Galactorrhea can also result from a deficiency of thyroid hormone. Certain tranquilizers, antidepressants, and antihypertensives can also produce galactorrhea, as can oral contraceptives.

Less common causes include diseases of the central nervous system and hydatidiform moles—abnormal embryonic tissue which develops into a grapelike cluster of cells rather than a fetus.

Galactorrhea may occur as an isolated symptom, or may be associated with hormonal disturbances resulting in irregular menstrual periods or infertility.

How is the condition evaluated?

Any woman not currently breastfeeding who notices a spontaneous milky discharge should be checked for a pituitary gland tumor as well as for hypothyroidism. This can be done through blood tests that check the levels of prolactin and thyroid stimulating hormone. If prolactin levels are elevated, a magnetic resonance image (MRI) or computerized tomography (CT) scan will be done to check for a prolactinoma.

Galactorrhea must also be distinguished from other forms of breast discharge. Many adult females can express a yellowish or greenish discharge from both breasts. This is a normal response to nipple stimulation or repetitive nipple squeezing.

Also distinct from galactorrhea is the nipple discharge associated with breast cancer, which is almost always spontaneous and bloody, and usually occurs in the affected breast only. About 90 percent of the time, however, spontaneous bloody discharge from a nipple is associated with nonmalignant causes such as benign tumors of the milk ducts, dilation of the milk ducts, or benign breast lumps. To be safe, however, any woman with nipple discharge from one breast only, whether bloody or clear, should consult her physician, who may then suggest further workup.

How is galactorrhea treated?

Galactorrhea does not always require treatment. When treatment is needed (for example, to restore a normal menstrual cycle), it most often takes the form of a drug called bromocriptine. This drug lowers prolactin levels, which in turn eliminates the milky discharge. Bromocriptine treatment can also shrink tumors that may be causing the excess prolactin, sometimes making surgery unnecessary, or at least making very large tumors easier to remove. Nausea, nasal congestion, headache, dizziness, and constipation are frequent side effects of this drug, but they can be minimized by starting the drug at very low doses and taking it with food at bedtime. Dosage can then be raised incrementally at weekly intervals until prolactin is in the normal range.

Often tumors can be successfully removed without damaging the function of the pituitary gland. Occasionally radiation therapy may be necessary following surgery. Hypothyroidism and the associated galactorrhea can usually be treated with thyroid hormone supplements. Eliminating the responsible drug or underlying defect will alleviate galactorrhea that is due to other causes.

Related entries

Breast cancer, breast lumps (benign), estrogen replacement therapy, hyperprolactinemia, hypothyroidism, mammography, radiation therapy, thyroid disorders

Gallstones

Gallstones form in the gallbladder, a pear-shaped sac that lies in the upper right quadrant of the abdomen and primarily serves to store bile which has been produced in the liver. The gallbladder excretes the bile via the common bile duct into the duodenum (a portion of the small intestine), where it aids in the digestion of fats. Gallstones are crystalline structures that form in the gallbladder and sometimes migrate to block the bile duct as well. Approximately 1 in 10 American adults has 1 or more gallstones, ranging in size from that of a grain of sand to that of a golf ball (see illustration).

Gallstones are classified into three basic types. Cholesterol stones are composed largely of crystallized cholesterol, combined with small amounts of calcium salts. The other two types of gallstones—black pigment stones and brown pigment stones—are made of varying amounts of calcium salts and bilirubin (a breakdown product of red blood cells). In the United States 80 percent of all gallstones are cholesterol stones.

Many people have gallstones without ever knowing it, but others go on to develop serious complications. These can include inflammation of the gallbladder, bile duct, or pancreas, or, rarely, gallbladder cancer. The longer a person has had gallstones without symptoms, the lesser the chances of complications. Between 15 and 20 percent of people with gallstones go on to develop complications over the next 5 years. Even so, because complications can be quite serious, anyone who experiences what she thinks is a gallbladder attack should seek prompt medical attention.

Just what causes gallstones in some people and not in others is still not fully understood. But the fact that women are at least twice as likely as men to develop gallstones does shed some light on the process. There is now good evidence that the hormones that are found at higher levels in women than in men (estrogen and progesterone) somehow stimulate the synthesis and secretion of cholesterol. As a result, the bile stored in the liver becomes supersaturated with cholesterol, so that the bile acids can no longer keep crystals of choles-

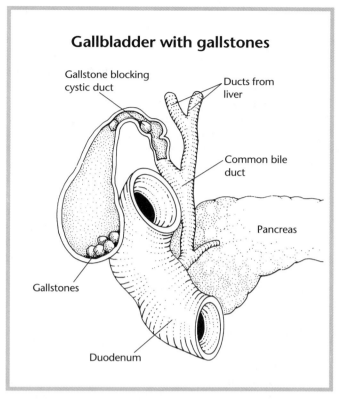

Gallbladder with gallstones

Gallstone blocking cystic duct

Ducts from liver

Common bile duct

Pancreas

Gallstones

Duodenum

terol from precipitating out. Once the bile becomes supersaturated with cholesterol, it often becomes more sluggish in clearing itself of cholesterol—thus further increasing the cholesterol levels in the gallbladder. At the same time, progesterone directly decreases the amount of bile emptied out of the gallbladder.

Who is likely to develop gallstones?

Women in general are at higher risk of developing gallstones than men because they are exposed to high levels of estrogens and progesterones at so many points in their life cycle—including puberty, pregnancy, and when taking birth control pills or postmenopausal estrogen replacement therapy. Not surprisingly, the more pregnancies a woman has had, the greater her chances of developing gallstones.

There is some evidence that estrogen replacement therapy does slightly increase the odds of developing gallstone disease. And even after estrogens are stopped, gallbladder problems often persist, since gallstones rarely dissolve or pass out of the body spontaneously. Estrogens taken via transdermal patches, however, are much less likely to result in gallbladder problems than estrogen taken orally.

Other factors that increase a woman's odds of developing gallstones are high triglyceride levels in the blood, obesity, and—paradoxically—rapid weight loss diets. These extremely low calorie diets (around 500 calories a day) impair the production of bile acids by the liver. As a result, there are not enough bile acids to dissolve the cholesterol in the bile, and gallstones quickly crystallize.

In both sexes, the odds of developing gallstones increase with age, although a woman's relative risk is higher when she is young (largely because of pregnancy). The younger a person is when gallstones develop, the more likely she is to have symptoms and complications. Complications of gallstones are also more common in people who have diabetes. Conditions that can slow down the secretion of bile by the gallbladder—including nerve damage from diabetes or a spinal cord injury, or a fat-restricted diet—can predispose people to gallbladder disease. And conditions such as anemia and cirrhosis of the liver, which increase the amount of bilirubin excreted into the bile, raise the odds of developing black pigment stones.

Finally, gallstones appear more often in certain ethnic groups. People of Native American—particularly Pima Indian—origin are at unusually high risk. Approximately 80 percent of older Pima Indian women have gallstone disease. Gallstones are much rarer in people of African or Asian descent, while the prevalence in European populations is somewhere in between.

What are the symptoms?

Gallstones cause symptoms only when they migrate into a duct. When the stones intermittently obstruct or pass through a duct (which they generally do no more than a few times a year), the result can be sudden, constant, intense abdominal pain that lasts from 30 minutes to several hours. Often the pain is felt more in the shoulder or back than in the abdomen itself. These "gallbladder attacks" are particularly common after meals and at night, and are more likely to occur in pregnant and postpartum women with gallstones than in people with gallstones in the general population.

There may be additional symptoms such as jaundice, high fever, or chills if complications have already arisen, but people almost always have symptoms of simple gallstones before complications begin to develop.

Nausea, diarrhea, constipation, bloating, heartburn, irregular bowel habits, and stomach upset are *not* symptoms of gallstones.

How is the condition evaluated?

If a patient believes she is having a gallstone attack, a clinician will first do a physical examination to look for signs of complications. If gallstones seem probable, various blood tests will be done to check levels of bilirubin and liver enzymes, and an abdominal ultrasound examination will be performed to check the size and number of stones. If no stones are located in the gallbladder itself, other tests may be done to see if there might be stones obstructing the bile duct. Occasionally scanning techniques such as radionuclide scanning (scintigraphy) or computerized tomography (CT) may be used to diagnose complications or assess stone density.

How are gallstones treated?

Gallstones can be treated in a variety of ways, ranging from surgery to drugs to "watchful waiting." "Watchful waiting," that is, observation of symptoms over time without active treatment, is a reasonable option for women whose gallstones are detected incidentally (usually by ultrasound performed for another reason). Since people with asymptomatic gallstones run only a 20 percent risk of having future episodes of gallstone pain or an infected gallbladder, the risks and side effects of surgery or drug therapy are usually not worth undertaking.

Some women with only a single gallbladder attack may also wish to watch and wait, since there is an 80 percent chance that symptoms will not recur over the next 5 years. A woman who is planning a pregnancy in the near future, however, will have higher odds of recurrence and should discuss treatment with her physician. For such women, as well as women with recurrent symptoms, the most definitive approach is surgical removal of the gallbladder. Technically called cholecystectomy, this procedure is one of the most common operations performed on women, with approximately 500,000 done each year in the United States. Until recently this was usually accomplished by opening up the abdomen, but it is now more and more frequently done via a laparoscopy—which involves a much smaller incision just above or below the navel (see illustration).

Hospitalization, pain, and recovery time are much shorter with laparoscopic surgery. Although injuries to the bile duct are a bit more common, the risks are minimal in the hands of an experienced surgeon. In about 5 percent of surgeries, complications such as bleeding problems make it necessary to resort to the more conventional operation.

If gallstones are clogging the bile ducts, they are often removed with the aid of an endoscope, an illuminated optical instrument that can reach into the duct. Sometimes surgical endoscopy is done in lieu of gallbladder removal in older women or in women for whom surgery would be too risky.

If gallstones are relatively small, or if there is only a single moderately sized stone, there may be less invasive options. One possibility is taking a drug called ursodiol (ursodeoxycholic acid), a naturally occurring bile acid that helps dissolve cholesterol. Ursodiol will work only if the stones are made of cholesterol and if the bile ducts are clear of stones (so that the drug can reach the gallstones in the first place). If these conditions are met, ursodiol therapy seems to work in about two-thirds of patients. Side effects—mainly diarrhea—are relatively rare. Ursodiol tablets can take up to 2 years to work, and over that time the size of the stones has to be regularly monitored by ultrasound.

Other drugs that dissolve cholesterol gallstones are under investigation. One of the most promising is a solvent called methyl tert-butyl ether. This substance can dissolve stones of any size and number if injected directly into the gallbladder under the guidance of ultrasound. Because methyl tert-butyl ether is also a powerful and flammable solvent, it can damage surrounding tissues; thus delivery of the material is difficult.

Recently it has become possible to couple drug therapy with a technique called lithotripsy. This technique uses high-energy shock waves from outside the body to fragment the

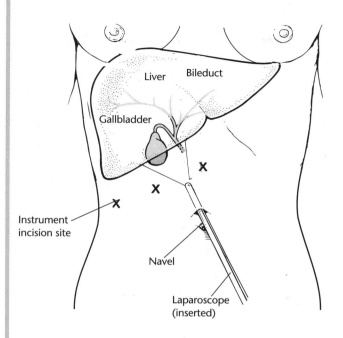

Instrument
incision site

Navel

Laparoscope
(inserted)

The view through the laparoscope is projected onto a video monitor. Two forceps hold the gallbladder in place as a third is used to place a clip on the cystic duct (which normally permits bile to enter and leave the gallbladder). Two other clips are placed on the cystic duct and on the artery to the gallbladder.

Removing the gallbladder with laparoscopy

The gallbladder rests against the underside of the liver. The laparoscope is inserted through a small incision just above the navel and pointed upward, toward the gallbladder. Three other small incisions (marked by Xs) are needed. Grasping instruments inserted through the two incisions on the patient's right are used to position the gallbladder during surgery. Operating instruments inserted through the third incision detach the gallbladder from the liver; apply clips to the artery, vein, and cystic duct; cut these structures; and finally drain the gallbladder, which can then be pulled out.

VIEW THROUGH SCOPE

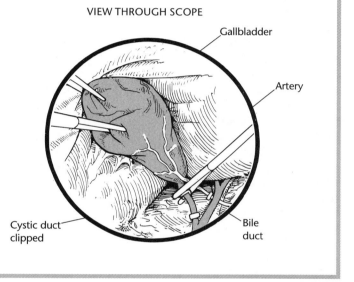

stones into pieces small enough to dissolve more readily or to pass through the bile duct and out of the body. The procedure usually requires only a day or two of hospitalization and, if successful, greatly speeds up the time it takes to relieve symptoms. After the gallstones are gone, ursodiol treatments must be continued for 3 months.

A drawback to drug therapy (and drug therapy combined with lithotripsy) is that gallstones often recur once the treatment is stopped. As many as half of all patients treated with these therapies can expect to have gallstone problems again within 5 years. Thus, it is necessary to have follow-up ultrasounds about every 6 months and to start using ursodiol as soon as any sign of gallstones, however small, appears.

If gallstones occur during pregnancy, clinicians will try to delay surgery until after the baby is born. Ursodiol is considered safe for use in pregnancy and is often the first-line treatment if other conditions for drug therapy are met. If symptoms are severe, or if there are complications, it is relatively safe to have an experienced surgeon remove gallstones from the bile ducts with an endoscope, so long as special steps are taken to protect the fetus from radiation. Conventional gall-

bladder surgery also seems to be safe during the first and third trimesters of pregnancy but may bring on premature labor if attempted during the second trimester.

Once the baby is born, all of the treatments for gallstones become much safer. At present there is no evidence that ursodiol is excreted in breast milk, although more studies on safety for a breastfeeding baby are needed.

How can gallstones be prevented?
People prone to developing gallstones can sometimes prevent them by taking supplementary capsules of ursodiol. This is a particularly good idea for anyone who must undergo a rapid weight loss diet, given the extremely high risk that gallstones will develop. An even better choice is to avoid crash dieting in the first place, since gradual weight loss is safer, more effective in the long run, and not associated with gallstone formation.

Related entries
Abdominal pain, dieting, laparoscopy, obesity, ultrasound

Genetic Counseling

Genetic counseling—offered for years to women at increased risk of carrying a congenitally abnormal fetus (see entry on prenatal genetic counseling)—has in recent years been expanded to people who are at risk for certain inherited adult-onset conditions, including forms of cancer, diabetes, cardiovascular disease, and degenerative neurologic conditions. It is generally done for either of two purposes: diagnosing a disease in someone who already has symptoms, and predicting the future in someone without symptoms. In the first case, the purpose of the testing is to help guide treatment decisions. For example, the family of a woman with dementia might want her tested for genes related to Alzheimer's disease, since a positive result would make it more likely that Alzheimer's is indeed the cause of the dementia. In that case, decisions about other diagnostic tests and treatment strategies—as well as plans for future care—could be adjusted accordingly.

The second use of genetic counseling is to identify health risks in people whose close family members have diseases that have been linked to identifiable genes. This is useful largely because knowledge of a genetic predisposition can encourage more vigilant screening for treatable diseases and may lead people to seek medical attention for symptoms that otherwise might escape notice. A woman who knows she carries the BRCA1 gene for breast cancer, for example, may choose to begin having regular mammograms earlier than would otherwise be recommended. She might also avail herself of other preventive or early-intervention strategies such as screening for ovarian cancer (a condition also linked to the BRCA1 gene), tamoxifen treatment to prevent breast cancer, and/or preventive surgery to remove the breasts before they become cancerous. Counseling may also be used to help identify carriers of certain defective genes—that is, people who carry a single copy of a defective gene and who therefore won't develop the disease themselves but may pass the gene on to offspring. A woman who finds that she is a carrier for Huntington's disease or breast cancer, for example, may use that information to influence her childbearing plans.

What do genetic counselors do?

Genetic counselors have several different ways of assessing an individual's genetic status. The first of these is through a family history. The counselor will first ask for information about the family tree to determine which relatives may have been affected by the condition in question as well as associated conditions. Questions may be asked about the age at which the condition developed in various relatives as well as the specific nature of the disease process (for example, whether cancer occurred in one breast or both). The counselor then analyzes this information—sometimes along with observations about visible traits or symptoms associated with the disease—to determine the patient's individual risk.

If the family history appears to put the patient at fairly high risk, the counselor may then discuss the possibility of DNA-based testing to identify genetic mutations associated with the disease. Genetic tests are available for several hundred conditions that run in families. These include inherited forms of breast and ovarian cancer, hemochromatosis (a disorder that causes the body to absorb too much iron), inherited colon and rectal cancers, Huntington's disease, and Alzheimer's disease. Depending on the test, a sample of saliva, blood, urine, stool, or other bodily substance may be required so that its DNA can be analyzed in a laboratory.

Who should have genetic counseling and testing?

People who have close family members with inherited adult-onset diseases may consider consulting a genetic counselor about their individual risk status—whether or not there is a known test available for the genes associated with this disease. In some cases, knowledge of a genetic predisposition for a particular disease can lead to individualized prevention and/or planning strategies. Eventually, geneticists hope that the results of genetic testing may also help prevent and even treat inherited diseases. In some cases this hope has already been realized. For example, infants identified as having the genes for phenylketonuria (PKU) can be given a special diet to prevent mental retardation and other neurological complications of this disorder. In many other cases, however, the ability to identify a specific genetic defect (such as sickle cell anemia) has not led to improved care.

When making a choice about the value of genetic testing for any individual, a genetic counselor will discuss the benefits and risks of these tests (see below), as well as various ethical, legal, and social issues. The decision made will reflect not only individual values but also views of family and friends. Other factors that can influence a decision to be tested include the economic repercussions (such as the effects that knowledge of a genetic predisposition might have on employability and insurance options), preexisting diseases, emotional factors, and lifestyle. The counselor will also go over the costs of available tests, since many genetic tests are expensive and are not necessarily covered by health insurance. In general, the more likely it is that knowledge of genetic status will affect prevention and treatment options, the more likely people are to choose to be tested.

What are the risks of genetic testing?

Whether or not an at-risk adult should actually have a genetic test is a highly controversial matter. This is true partly because the mere identification of a genetic predisposition to a disease does not necessarily yield useful information about when the disease will occur or how quickly or severely it will develop. Furthermore, knowledge of a genetic defect—or even the lack of a defect—can sometimes do more harm than good. For example, a woman who finds out that she carries genes for Huntington's disease, an ultimately fatal degenerative neurological disease for which there is no cure, will not be able to do anything to control the development of the disease, and at the same time may end up feeling more worried than ever, never knowing when the first symptoms will occur. She may also feel helpless or defective. In other people, belief that a disease is inevitable may be interpreted as a license to abrogate all responsibility for their health and well-being, even in areas that they actually can control.

Even a negative test can do serious damage that may outweigh the relief that comes from getting a clean bill of health. For example, some women who find out that they do not carry a breast cancer gene feel oppressive "survivor's guilt" when they learn that their sister or mother is a carrier. Family members who know that they carry a gene for a disease often develop a special bond with one another, and may, consciously or unconsciously, reject the non-carriers from this close inner circle.

Because genetic testing often gives murky results, it can leave people with even more uncertainty and fear than they had before they knew their status. For one thing, the presence of a genetic mutation does not necessarily mean that a person will develop the disease. Anywhere from 30 to 85 percent of women carrying the BRCA1 gene (a gene linked to a small percentage of breast cancer cases) will go on to develop breast cancer, and between 10 and 65 percent will develop ovarian cancer. There is no way for an individual woman to know if she will be one of the lucky ones, with or without the test. In some cases, too, there may be other, as yet unidentified genes that also play a role (pro or con) in determining the development of a disease. As a result, a woman who turns out not to have a particular defective gene may falsely assume that she is risk-free, when in reality she carries some other unidentified gene or risk factor for the disease. In addition, testing can sometimes reveal a genetic mutation of unknown significance, which again can lead to considerable fear and anxiety—perhaps more than existed before the testing took place.

The results of a genetic test can also bring about considerable stigmatization by other people, including potential employers and insurers. Whether or not a patient and/or her clinician is obligated to reveal the results of genetic tests to other family members, employers, and insurance companies remains the subject of considerable debate in both legal and ethical circles. While no federal law exists to prevent discrimination in employment and insurance coverage among private companies, several laws that prohibit discrimination in employment and health insurance (e.g., the Americans with Disabilities Act, the Health Insurance Portability and Accountability Act, and the Civil Rights Act) may offer some degree of protection. In addition, federal agencies are barred from using genetic information in hiring or promotion, and they are limited in their ability to obtain or release this information. Nonetheless, anyone considering genetic testing would be wise to learn as much about the test as possible—including who will have access to the results—and should discuss available state and local legal protections regarding the use of these results with a genetic counselor and, if possible, an attorney.

Related entries

Alzheimer's disease, breast cancer, cardiovasular disease, colon and rectal cancer, diabetes, preconception counseling, prenatal genetic counseling

Genital Warts

Genital warts are benign growths in the genital and anal area. A common form of sexually transmitted disease, they are caused by one of various forms of the human papilloma virus (HPV), other forms of which cause plantar warts of the foot and common warts of the skin. Also called venereal warts or condylomata acuminata, genital warts usually result from sexual contact with an infected partner, although they occasionally are spread by touching the genitals with wart-infested hands. In rare instances genital warts are spread from an infected mother to a newborn during delivery.

Although they are easily spread and hard to eradicate, genital warts are generally no more than an annoyance. Warts caused by certain types of the HPV, however, have been associated with cervical cancer. Treatment can be important for pregnant women because occasionally a large mass of warts on the vaginal walls can physically obstruct labor. In rare cases, untreated warts on the cervix, vagina, or anal area may necessitate a cesarean section so that they do not break open and bleed excessively during delivery.

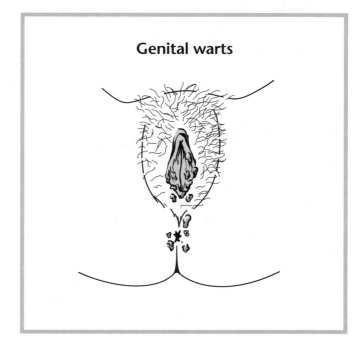

Genital warts

Who is likely to develop genital warts?

Genital warts can develop in any person whose genital area has been directly touched by another wart. Because these warts thrive in warm, moist environments, they are likely to proliferate in women who are pregnant or who have vaginal infections (see vaginitis) because at these times vaginal secretions tend to increase. Some investigators believe that warts are particularly likely to grow in people with compromised immune systems, including those who are infected with the human immunodeficiency virus (HIV), which causes AIDS.

What are the symptoms?

Genital warts in women can appear on the labia, inside the vagina, and on the cervix (opening to the uterus), as well as around the anal area. In men they generally appear on the head or shaft of the penis, and sometimes on the scrotum or around the anus. The warts start as pink, tan, or red swellings about the size of rice grains but often merge to resemble small cauliflowers. Some warts are so minute and painless that they are unnoticeable. Others are over 3 inches around and interfere with the ability to sit or to walk. Sometimes the warts itch or burn, and scratching them can cause irritation.

It can take between 1 and 6 months for warts to appear after infection.

How is the condition evaluated?

Some women (especially those with warts on the cervix) do not find out they have genital warts until they have an abnormal Pap test. Others may notice suspicious swellings on the vulva and consult a clinician. Since the naked eye can miss many warts, most clinicians use a magnifying glass or a colposcope (a special type of microscope used to examine the genital area) for a more thorough inspection. Often a vinegar-like (acetic acid) solution is applied to the affected area first to turn cells white and improve visibility. If warts are found, the clinician may do a biopsy (tissue sample) to make sure that there have been no cancerous changes in any surrounding cells. In some cases a blood test may be recommended as well to check for the presence of HIV, which seems to accelerate the growth and spread of the warts.

How are genital warts treated?

Because genital warts often recur and are so easily spread, eradicating them can be frustrating. Part of the treatment involves evaluating the woman's partner as well as discussing techniques to prevent the spread of the warts, since obviously it is pointless to remove warts in a woman who continues to have sexual contact with an infected partner.

For small warts, self-treatment with the prescription cream imiquimod (Aldara) is sometimes successful, although it can irritate surrounding skin. The cream is applied 3 times a week until the warts dissolve.

Larger or persistent warts can be dissolved with a topical agent such as podophyllin or trichloracetic acid applied directly. Because these medicines (especially podophyllin) can cause chemical burns if used incorrectly, women should not try to apply them at home. Podophyllin must be removed several hours after it is applied and usually needs to be reapplied several times at weekly intervals. It should not be used by women who are pregnant because it can cause birth defects. A topical cream, podofilox, which a woman can apply herself for 3 days a week up to 3 weeks, is also available by prescription and is effective.

If warts persist or return after this treatment, the clinician will make sure they are not cancerous by doing a biopsy, if necessary using a topical or local anesthetic. Once cancer has been ruled out, the clinician may try burning or freezing off the warts using electrocautery (see entry) or liquid nitrogen (see cryosurgery). These techniques are sometimes used instead of topical agents when warts are extensive or occur in particularly sensitive locations.

Some investigators have also had success removing a small number of warts by injecting them with alpha interferon several times a week for about 3 weeks. Though less likely to cause pain and scarring than other treatments, alpha interferon makes some women feel as though they have the flu and is not safe for use during pregnancy. Injection of Interferon B into the muscle of the arm or buttocks appears to be an effective and less painful treatment, but it is not yet available in the United States.

There is some psychological research to suggest that warts may respond to hypnosis in some individuals for whom medical treatments fail.

As a last resort for extensive or persistent infections, laser surgery may be used. Though quite effective in eradicating warts, laser surgery usually requires regional or general anesthesia, and many women experience incapacitating pain in the perineum (the skin between the vulva and the anus) after surgery, as well as persistent vulvar pain.

Because it is hard to tell if all warts have been removed, a woman should be rechecked by her clinician after about 6 months. Sometimes additional treatment may be necessary. To make sure no cancerous changes have occurred, a Pap test every 6 months thereafter for at least a few years is a good precaution.

How can genital warts be prevented?

Preventing the spread of genital warts involves the same safer sex practices required to prevent the spread of any sexually transmitted disease. Because abstinence from sexual activity while the warts are contagious is often impractical, condom use is important until all warts have been eradicated. Male condoms, however, do not provide total protection, since a man's scrotum can harbor the wart virus.

Related entries

Acquired immune deficiency syndrome, anesthesia, biopsy, birth control, cervical cancer, cesarean section, condoms, cryosurgery, electrocautery, laser surgery, Pap test, safer sex, sexually transmitted diseases, vaginitis, vulvar disorders, vulvar pain

Glaucoma

Glaucoma is a group of eye disorders, each of which involves an increase of fluid pressure within the eye. Together these disorders are among the leading causes of blindness in the United States, affecting approximately 2 million Americans. Much of the glaucoma-induced blindness is theoretically preventable with early detection. But there lies the catch—and the tragedy—of this disease, which often goes unnoticed until it is well advanced and severe vision loss is inevitable.

In the normal eye a fluid called the aqueous humor circulates between the lens and the cornea and nourishes structures within the eye (see illustration). Although this fluid is produced continuously, it is also drained out of the eye at an equal rate. The drainage takes place through a passageway between the iris and the cornea called the drainage angle, which in turn directs the fluid out of the eye through a tiny channel (Schlemm's canal). In the normal eye this endless cycling of production and drainage keeps the fluid pressure stable, but in people with glaucoma the drainage lags behind the amount of new fluid that is constantly being pumped into the eye. The result is an increase in pressure within the eye. If this pressure gets too high, it damages the optic nerve at the back of the eye, slowly deteriorating its fibers and destroying its ability to carry visual messages to the brain.

There are two basic forms of glaucoma: acute and chronic. In the acute form, which is considered a medical emergency, the iris of the eye blocks the drainage angle and thus prevents fluid from draining properly. This often occurs when the lens, which enlarges with age, pushes the iris forward and thus narrows the angle between the iris and the cornea, eventually closing the drainage channel between them. In the much more common chronic form of glaucoma, the drainage angle is not blocked—which explains why this form of glaucoma is sometimes called open-angle glaucoma. Pressure still builds up, however, presumably because other factors (perhaps poor absorption, for example) interfere with drainage.

Who is likely to develop glaucoma?

Although some forms of glaucoma can occur in infancy and childhood, the most common form (chronic open-angle) occurs more frequently as people age. This form of glaucoma af-

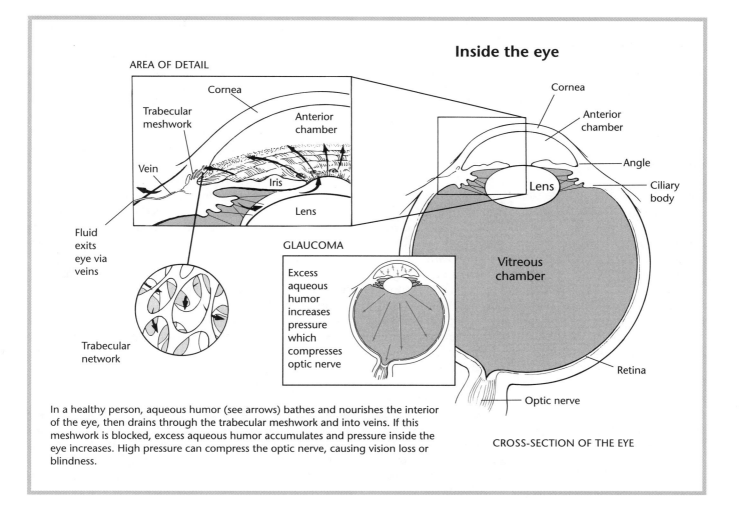

In a healthy person, aqueous humor (see arrows) bathes and nourishes the interior of the eye, then drains through the trabecular meshwork and into veins. If this meshwork is blocked, excess aqueous humor accumulates and pressure inside the eye increases. High pressure can compress the optic nerve, causing vision loss or blindness.

fects 1 to 2 percent of all Americans over the age of 40, 5 percent of those over the age of 65, and up to 14 percent of those over the age of 80. It is also particularly common in African Americans and in people with diabetes, as well as in people who have a family history of the disease.

Occasionally eye injuries, inflammation, or cataracts may provoke acute glaucoma, as may treatment with corticosteroid eyedrops or medications that dilate the pupil (which may result in closure of the Schlemm's canal by the iris). This is particularly true in vulnerable people, such as elderly individuals who are farsighted, as well as in people whose close relatives have had acute glaucoma.

What are the symptoms?

Many people pass through the early stages of chronic glaucoma without noticing anything amiss—which is the biggest handicap in treating this disease. Often the only symptom is the gradual loss of peripheral (side) vision, a phenomenon not usually observable without an eye examination until considerable irreversible damage has already occurred. Only at this relatively late point in the disease do most people notice that their field of vision is significantly narrowed. At this point, too, they may notice that their vision is blurry or that it is increasingly difficult for their eyes to adapt to dimly lit environments.

In contrast, the symptoms of acute glaucoma are almost always blatant. This is fortunate, since acute glaucoma requires immediate medical attention if blindness is to be prevented. Most of the time one eye will become extremely painful and red, often coupled with visual blurriness or the visualization of colored halos around lights. Occasionally vomiting may occur as well. In the preceding months some people have preliminary attacks of "subacute" glaucoma in which these same symptoms occur to a milder degree, particularly when light is dim.

How is the condition evaluated?

The best way to head off irreversible damage from glaucoma is for all adults over the age of 40 to be screened for this condition on a regular basis—approximately every 2 years. People at unusually high risk—such as those with diabetes or with a family history of glaucoma—should be evaluated starting at a younger age. Part of this glaucoma evaluation is a normal accompaniment of virtually any routine eye examination. It includes a painless measurement of the pressure within the eye, an inspection of the optic nerve with a handheld ophthalmoscope to look for signs of damage, and a simple (or possibly computerized) test of peripheral vision.

A clinician who is screening for glaucoma in particular measures the pressure in the eye by using one of several forms of tonometry. This is accomplished by anesthetizing the cornea with drops, placing an instrument called a Schiotz tonometer directly on top of the eye's surface, and then using the weight of the indentation it makes to estimate pressure. Ophthalmologists and most optometrists sometimes use an even more precise method called applanation tonometry, in which a pressure probe is applied to the front surface of the eye and the resistance to its force is measured. Another commonly used way to estimate fluid pressure involves using an air-puff tonometer, a device that measures eye pressure by puffing small bursts of air against the eyeball. Of these three techniques, applanation tonometry is the most accurate, although it is not generally done (or necessary) as a part of routine screening. A suspicious reading from a regular tonometer or an air-puff tonometer, however, warrants additional testing by applanation tonometry.

In addition, an eye specialist who suspects glaucoma will do a thorough eye examination, including an assessment of peripheral vision and an evaluation of the internal drainage system of the eye to determine whether or not the drainage angle is closed. The back of the eye is examined to check for damage to the optic nerve and to assess blood vessels near the retina and other areas in order to rule out additional disease. Once glaucoma has been diagnosed, an eye specialist will ask the patient to return for periodic assessment and treatment.

Anyone who suspects that she may have acute glaucoma should consult an ophthalmologist or local emergency room immediately to be evaluated and treated.

How is glaucoma treated?

There are a number of different treatments for chronic open-angle glaucoma. Which ones are tried depends partly on the nature and severity of the glaucoma itself as well as the patient's overall health and medication history. In its earliest stages (that is, before there is evidence of damage to the optic nerve and the pressure is only marginally elevated), treatment may involve nothing more than frequent eye examinations to monitor the pressure, optic nerve, and visual field, and to allow more aggressive treatment at the first sign of potentially damaging pressure. At that point an eye doctor will usually prescribe one of three classes of drugs: beta blockers, miotics, or epinephrine. More recently a fourth type of topical medication has been developed, a carbonic anhydrase inhibitor called Trusopt. All of these drugs work by reducing the production rate of aqueous humor, increasing the drainage rate, or both.

The most commonly prescribed of these drugs today, and those with the fewest side effects, are beta blockers such as timolol (Timoptic) eyedrops. These decrease pressure within the eye by slowing the production of aqueous humor. Beta blockers, even eyedrops, must be used with caution in people with certain heart diseases (such as congestive heart failure) or asthma, since they enter the bloodstream and may occasionally exacerbate the symptoms of these diseases.

People who cannot use beta blockers may be prescribed miotic drugs (such as pilocarpine), which work by increasing the rate of drainage. Because pilocarpine narrows pupil size, it sometimes results in blurry vision or difficulty seeing in dimly lit environments, especially among those who also have cataracts. This side effect is particularly common in younger patients.

Another alternative to beta blockers is epinephrine eye-drops. This drug appears both to decrease the formation of aqueous humor and to increase its rate of drainage. Epinephrine also dilates (widens) the pupil, which can sometimes blur vision. It occasionally causes side effects such as heart palpitations and nervousness, as well as allergic reactions, and should be used with care by people with certain types of heart disease. Patients who use epinephrine chronically may also have a reactive vascular congestion (red eye) when the effect of the medication wears off.

If none of these drugs works or can be used, carbonic anhydrase inhibitors (such as Trusopt) may be given as drops. These drugs also work by decreasing the production of aqueous humor.

All of the drugs used to treat glaucoma may lose their effectiveness over time, and all may produce a number of unpleasant side effects. If such problems arise, many ophthalmologists will recommend surgical treatments. The least invasive of these, a form of laser surgery called laser trabeculoplasty, involves vaporizing small amounts of eye tissue to improve the eye's drainage capacity. Laser trabeculoplasty is usually performed on an outpatient basis with only local topical anesthesia and is effective in relieving eye pressure in about 70 percent of cases. On the minus side, it may be only a temporary measure in staving off high pressure; eventually incisional surgery (successful in 90 to 95 percent of cases) may be necessary to create new openings for drainage.

When it comes to treating acute glaucoma, a type of surgery called iridotomy is the only permanent cure. This can now often be accomplished with lasers rather than a physical incision, and the entire operation can be done in an ophthalmologist's office. In some cases after an iridotomy, adhesions (scar tissue) may form and close the angle permanently; medication or even additional surgery may then become necessary.

How can glaucoma be prevented?
Although glaucoma itself cannot be prevented, the best way to avoid associated vision loss is to have regular eye examinations, particularly after age 40, and earlier if there are individual or family risk factors.

Related entries
Cataracts, contact lenses, diabetes, dry eye, eye care, laser surgery, macular degeneration, nearsightedness and farsightedness, retinal detachment

Goiters and Thyroid Nodules

A goiter is any enlargement of the thyroid gland (see thyroid disorders). Although toxic goiters may sometimes occur in conjunction with other thyroid disorders such as hyperthyroidism or hypothyroidism (see entries), simple (or "diffuse") goiters exist in people with normally functioning thyroids. People with diffuse goiters have uniformly and symmetrically enlarged thyroids and may have visible swelling at the bottom of the throat. Diffuse goiters are often no more than cosmetic problems, unless they obstruct the windpipe or esophagus, in which case swallowing may become uncomfortable.

When enlargement is limited to one area of the thyroid, the swelling is called a thyroid nodule or, if there are many nodules, a multinodular goiter. Most thyroid nodules are benign and have no effect on thyroid function, though about 5 percent turn out to be cancerous.

Who is likely to develop a diffuse goiter or thyroid nodule?
Before the introduction of iodized table salt, goiter was an endemic problem in the United States, but today iodine-deficiency goiter is prevalent only in some undeveloped regions of the world. Nonetheless, goiters that occur for unknown reasons (sporadic goiters) continue to be common. In the United States, sporadic goiter or single thyroid nodules are present in 5 to 7 percent of women and are at least 4 times more common in women than in men.

Multinodular goiters are even more prevalent and can be felt in 5 percent of women. Nodules that cannot be palpated may occur in many more women: when the thyroid gland has been examined in ultrasound studies, 20 percent of women have been found to have thyroid nodules, and autopsies of the thyroid gland found nodules in as many as 60 percent of women studied.

How are these conditions evaluated?
Any person with a thyroid nodule should be screened for thyroid cancer, though most of these nodules will turn out to be benign. A physician evaluating a nodule will first consider the patient's history and assess her thyroid function with various laboratory tests, including blood tests to measure levels of thyroid stimulating hormone (TSH). Since "hot" nodules (that is, those producing excessive amounts of thyroid hormone) are almost always benign, this test can eliminate the need for additional testing. Often a nodule can be quickly diagnosed using a fine-needle aspiration, done in the clinician's office under local anesthesia. In some cases the clinician may want to do a thyroid scan to see if the nodule is "hot." In a thyroid scan, done on an outpatient basis, the patient first swallows or is injected with radioactive iodine and then returns the next day. A special camera produces an image of the thyroid based on the amount of tracer that has collected at various sites. Since iodine is a key component of thyroid hormones, nodules with high levels of radioactivity will be assumed to be synthesizing large amounts of these hormones.

If the nodule is "cold" (that is, does not absorb any radiation), cancer remains a possibility, though still a small one, since most nodules turn out to be benign adenomas or cysts.

To exclude further the possibility of thyroid cancer, a fine-needle aspiration is needed.

How are goiters and thyroid nodules treated?

If a nodule turns out to be cancerous, the patient will be treated accordingly (see thyroid cancer). If a thyroid nodule is producing excessive amounts of thyroid hormone, the person will be treated for hyperthyroidism (see entry).

Noncancerous nodules and diffuse goiters not associated with impaired thyroid function may require no treatment at all unless they grow large enough to become uncomfortable, pose a cosmetic problem, or recur following treatment. Younger people with diffuse goiter may also want to consider treatment because their longer life expectancy alone increases the risk that mechanical problems will eventually develop.

The standard treatment for goiters is levothyroxine (a synthetic form of the thyroid hormone thyroxine), which usually shrinks goiters or inhibits further growth. Whether this drug can reduce the size of individual thyroid nodules remains controversial. Anyone taking levothyroxine should have blood levels of TSH monitored regularly to make sure that she does not develop subclinical hyperthyroidism, a condition that can result from overtreatment of goiter and, if undetected, can increase the risk of developing osteoporosis (a disease in which the bones gradually lose their store of calcium and other minerals and become less dense and more susceptible to fracture).

The goiter itself should also be monitored regularly to make sure that it is responsive to treatment. It usually takes at least 6 months for signs of regression to appear in a diffuse goiter, and several years may pass before there is obvious improvement in long-standing multinodular goiters.

Related entries

Hyperthyroidism, hypothyroidism, osteoporosis, thyroid cancer, thyroid disorders

Gonorrhea

Gonorrhea is a sexually transmitted disease (STD) caused by the bacterium *Neisseria gonorrhoeae*, also known as the gonococcus. Although only about 650,000 cases are reported each year in this country, the actual occurrence is probably closer to 1 to 2 million cases annually.

Because gonorrhea in women often produces no symptoms, it is more likely to go untreated in women than in men, causing serious consequences. Despite the fact that the progression of this disease can be readily halted with antibiotics, gonorrhea still accounts for 20 to 40 percent of all cases of pelvic inflammatory disease (PID), which can result in infertility and increase the risk of ectopic pregnancy. PID can also lead to chronic pelvic and abdominal pain as a result of adhesions (scarring). Furthermore, a single episode of PID seems to predispose women to recurrent bouts, probably because the infection somehow alters their defense mechanisms against invading microorganisms.

Gonorrhea ("the clap") is usually spread from one person to another through sexual contact—vaginal, anal, or oral. Because the gonococcus dies within seconds once it is outside the body, it is extremely unlikely to be transmitted in other ways. The bacterium thrives in a warm, moist environment and tends to develop in mucous membranes such as those found in the vagina, cervix, urethra, rectum, and throat. It can also spread to the mucous membranes of the eye if transmitted by a hand that has touched infected genitals. The result can be gonococcal conjunctivitis, an inflammation of the membranes lining the eyelids (the conjunctiva) which can produce blindness if it goes untreated (though this rarely occurs).

Occasionally the gonococcus spreads into the bloodstream, in which case the disease is described as a disseminated gonococcal infection. Depending on which parts of the body become infected, this can lead to arthritis, heart valve disorders, skin lesions, and meningitis (an infection of the lining of the brain and spinal cord). Women seem to be slightly more prone to disseminated infection than men.

Gonorrhea can be spread to newborns as they pass through an infected mother's birth canal. The conjunctivitis that can result was once a major cause of blindness, but today it is a rare occurrence owing to state laws requiring the routine instillation of antibiotic drops into the eyes of all babies at birth—whether or not the mother is known to be infected with gonorrhea.

Who is likely to develop gonorrhea?

Like most STDs, gonorrhea is primarily a disease of the young and the poor. Low-income city-dwelling women are at greatest risk for the disease, with more than half of those infected under the age of 25.

Other risk factors are a prior history of infection and having a recent sexual partner with urethral discharge. Anyone who has sexual contact—vaginal, oral, or anal—with an infected person can get gonorrhea, however, whether or not the infected partner shows any symptoms of the disease. Women are more likely than heterosexual men to acquire the disease from an infected partner. In addition, women who perform oral sex (fellatio) on an infected man are more likely to get gonorrhea of the throat than a man who performs oral sex (cunnilingus) on an infected woman.

Because infection is particularly likely in women who are still in their early reproductive years, women under the age of 25 who have had at least one sexual encounter should seriously consider appropriate screening tests even if they have no symptoms. And regardless of age, any woman with a sexual history that puts her at risk for STDs should also seek regular screening.

What are the symptoms?

Because about 80 percent of all women infected with gonorrhea have no symptoms, many begin to suspect a problem only when symptoms arise in a male partner. The most common symptoms of gonorrhea in men are a thick, milky discharge from the penis and a burning sensation during urination—the same symptoms associated with other forms of urethritis (inflammation of the urethra). As many as 1 in 5 men with gonorrhea may experience no symptoms, however.

Symptoms in women, when they occur at all, seem to develop within 10 days of infection (researchers still are not exactly sure about the timing). Usually the vagina and cervix are the first sites of infection, and this can result in a thick vaginal discharge, abnormal uterine bleeding, pelvic pain, or pain and swelling of the labia. If the infection becomes more severe, symptoms of pelvic inflammatory disease—such as pelvic pain, fever, vomiting, and menstrual irregularities—may also develop. In most women the bacteria also travel into the urethra. In women who have had a hysterectomy (surgical removal of the uterus), the urethra is almost always the primary site of infection. As a result, pus in the urine is a common symptom of gonorrhea, together with painful urination and the need to urinate frequently (both also signs of a urinary tract infection).

About 30 to 50 percent of women with gonorrheal infection have rectal infection as well, usually because of infected vaginal secretions and less often because of rectal intercourse. Most rectal infections have no symptoms, but occasionally they may result in constipation, painful straining at stool, and pain, bleeding, or discharge from the anus.

When the throat is infected, there are usually no symptoms whatsoever. Occasionally, however, there may be a mild to moderate sore throat, and lymph nodes in the neck may be enlarged and tender. These symptoms are easily confused with those of strep throat.

The 1 to 3 percent of infected people who develop a disseminated gonococcal infection may experience fever, chills, lack of energy, and lack of appetite. In women, disseminated infections often occur around the time of menstruation or during pregnancy. A disseminated infection can cause a form of arthritis (inflammation of the joints) and tendinitis (inflammation of the tendons), especially of the knees, elbows, ankles, and wrists. There is often a skin rash on the extremities, often near the joints of the hands and feet. It begins with between 5 and 30 red sores or pimples which later evolve into pustules with clearly defined centers.

Occasionally people with gonorrhea develop pain in the upper quarter of the abdominal region, together with fever, nausea, and other symptoms. Together these symptoms are called Fitz-Hugh-Curtis syndrome, or perihepatitis, and they signal an inflammation of the surface of the liver.

How is the condition evaluated?

No simple blood or urine test can detect the gonococcus—even if the microorganism has spread into the bloodstream. Accurate diagnosis can be done only by taking pus, mucus, or other potentially infected material from the body and examining it to see if it contains gonococci. The sample is usually taken from the cervix, although it may be taken from the throat, urethra, or rectum, depending on the woman's specific symptoms and sexual history. In the most rapid and inexpensive method of analyzing this material—Gram's stain—the sample is spread onto a slide, stained, and examined under a microscope. This method, however, which is reliable in men, misses as much as 40 to 60 percent of all gonorrhea in women.

A more accurate method of diagnosing gonorrhea in women requires growing (culturing) the sample in a nutrient jelly—which takes up to 2 days—so that the bacteria (if any) can multiply. This culture technique picks up about 90 percent of all infections. Newer and faster techniques using DNA amplification are very accurate and are now done instead of cultures.

If the culture or other test is negative, many clinicians will automatically assume that the problem is chlamydia. Because chlamydia is so common—and because it readily coexists with gonorrhea without necessarily producing any symptoms—it makes sense for anyone being screened for one of these diseases to be checked for the other as well.

A woman found to have gonorrhea should also be screened for syphilis, since having gonorrhea is one of the major risk factors for this even more serious STD. She should also consider testing for HIV (the virus that causes AIDS). Any sexual partners who have been exposed to the woman within the past 30 days should be evaluated for gonorrhea.

How is gonorrhea treated?

The once-standard practice of dosing everyone suspected of having gonorrhea (or anything else) with penicillin has now been abandoned. Penicillin-resistant gonococci constitute as many as a quarter of all strains in certain urban areas, and penicillin cannot treat chlamydia, which infects 35 to 50 percent of women who have gonorrhea. For these reasons, treatment is given according to guidelines issued periodically by the Centers for Disease Control (CDC), which reflect changing patterns of antibiotic resistance. Most cases of confirmed gonorrhea today are treated with forms of cephalosporin antibiotics (for example, Suprax) or fluoroquinolones (Cipro or Noroxin), together with antibiotics aimed at chlamydia—usually either doxycycline (a kind of tetracycline) or azithromycin. An advantage of using ceftriaxone (a cephalosporin given by injection) to treat gonorrhea is that it may be effective in eradicating any incipient syphilis as well.

If a woman has symptoms of gonorrhea but tests negative for the gonococcus, many clinicians will treat both the woman and her partner(s) for chlamydia first—which is now more common than gonorrhea and often accounts for urethritis and other symptoms also associated with gonorrhea.

During pregnancy the safest regimen is ceftriaxone to treat gonorrhea, and erythromycin or amoxicillin to treat any possible chlamydia. Tetracyclines and the fluoroquinolones are not used during pregnancy or breastfeeding, nor are the fluoroquinolones considered safe for use by anyone under the age of 18, since they can interfere with bone growth. Women allergic to cephalosporins are usually prescribed either spectinomycin or a fluoroquinolone antibiotic plus treatment for chlamydia.

Treatment needs to take place as soon as possible—whether or not any symptoms are present. A sore throat associated with pharyngeal infection, for example, will disappear on its own within about 12 weeks, but unless antibiotics are taken, the throat will become a reservoir of infection.

How can gonorrhea be prevented?

All sexually active women in their early reproductive years who are not in mutually monogamous relationships should, in addition to having regular pelvic examinations, be screened annually for gonorrhea. Any woman who knows or even suspects she may have gonorrhea should avoid having unprotected sexual relations until both she and her sexual partner or partners have been examined and, if necessary, treated for the disease. Following the safer sex practices recommended to help prevent the spread of all STDs can help prevent the spread of gonorrhea in particular (see safer sex).

Related entries

Adhesions, antibiotics, arthritis, chlamydia, condoms, ectopic pregnancy, pelvic examinations, pelvic inflammatory disease, safer sex, sexually transmitted diseases, syphilis, urinary tract infections

Gum Disease

Gum disease, also known as periodontal disease, is a process in which the tissues surrounding the teeth become damaged. Periodontal disease is the major cause of tooth loss in people over the age of 35, and almost everyone who lives past middle age develops at least a mild form of it. Still, most people today can expect to keep their teeth throughout their lives by getting regular dental care, watching their diet, and practicing good dental hygiene.

In its mildest form, known as gingivitis (inflammation of the gingiva, or gums; see illustration), healthy pinkish gums turn red and may bleed during brushing or flossing. Women with gingivitis may find that the condition worsens if they are taking oral contraceptives or if they become pregnant. Gingivitis is thought to be due to certain types of bacteria found in the saliva which cling to the teeth and gumline in a gelatinous substance called plaque. Plaque consists of bacterial colonies together with residues of sugar and carbohydrates from the diet. Over time it can calcify into a brittle, hard-to-remove substance called calculus (tartar).

A more severe form of periodontal disease is called periodontitis. Most dentists believe that periodontitis results from

progressively worsening gingivitis, although some recent data suggest that two separate processes may be involved. In periodontitis the gums separate from the tooth, both at and below the gumline, leaving deep pockets where bacteria and sometimes pus can accumulate. As the bacteria invade the tooth's root, they destroy the ligaments anchoring the tooth to the bone, gradually detaching the gums from the teeth. Eventually the infection may erode the bony socket holding the tooth in place. Evidence is also mounting that chronic gum disease may be linked to systemic ailments, including an increased risk of stroke and cardiovascular disease and, in women, increased odds of delivering a low birthweight infant.

Who is likely to develop gum disease?

Some dentists estimate that gingivitis affects as many as 4 out of every 5 people over 45. It is particularly likely to develop in people who do not practice good dental hygiene, who have badly aligned teeth (which can trap plaque), and who smoke. Gingivitis may also develop during times of hormonal change. For this reason it often begins at puberty and is common in women who are pregnant or who are using oral contraceptive pills. In postmenopausal women, estrogen deficiency appears to increase the risk of severe gum disease and tooth loss, although estrogen replacement therapy (see entry) may help alleviate this risk.

People with uncontrolled diabetes are also susceptible to gingivitis. Three types of drugs commonly cause gingival hyperplasia—overgrowth of the gums. They are phenytoin (Dilantin, an anticonvulsant drug used to treat epilepsy), calcium-channel blockers (used to treat high blood pressure and heart diseases), and cyclosporine (an immunosuppressive agent used to prevent rejection after organ transplants). Periodontitis may affect at least half of all people over 45.

What are the symptoms?

The most common symptom of gingivitis is swollen, tender gums that bleed easily. A little space (gingival pocket) may also develop between the gum and the crown of the tooth. Because gingivitis is generally painless, it often goes undetected in people who do not have regular dental examinations.

In its early stages periodontitis has symptoms similar to gingivitis. As the disease develops, the gingival pockets extend below the gumline, and there is more swelling and recession of the gums. Teeth may become particularly sensitive to hot or cold foods, and there may be an unpleasant taste in the mouth, as well as bad breath. In the later stages, teeth may shift position, loosen, or fall out.

How is the condition evaluated?

A dentist or periodontist (a specialist in periodontal disease) examines teeth and gums carefully, looking for the degree of inflammation, depth of pockets, and amount of plaque and calculus along the base of the teeth. Questions about general health may also be asked to learn if the gum prob-

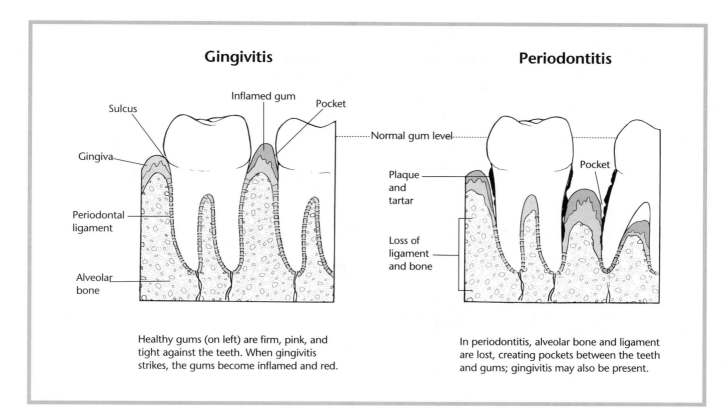

Gingivitis

Sulcus

Inflamed gum

Pocket

Gingiva

Periodontal
ligament

Alveolar
bone

Healthy gums (on left) are firm, pink, and
tight against the teeth. When gingivitis
strikes, the gums become inflamed and red.

Periodontitis

Normal gum level

Plaque
and
tartar

Pocket

Loss of
ligament
and bone

In periodontitis, alveolar bone and ligament
are lost, creating pockets between the teeth
and gums; gingivitis may also be present.

lems could be due to some systemic disease or drug use, and x-rays may be performed to assess the level of bone loss under the gums.

How is gum disease treated?

Gingivitis is usually treated with a combination of thorough cleaning (scaling) to remove plaque and calculus, followed by scrupulous home care. If there are any misaligned teeth or misshapen fillings, crowns, or bridges, these will also be repaired, since they can make it difficult to remove plaque. Brushing the teeth at least twice a day, and flossing at least once, is still the best way to keep plaque in check and keep gingivitis from progressing.

The first and most conservative steps in treating periodontitis are essentially the same as those for gingivitis. Usually a dentist or dental hygienist removes tartar with a deep scaling (which may need to be repeated every 2 or 3 months), to be followed by daily brushing and flossing. If pockets continue to enlarge and support structures continue to erode, the clinician may try combining traditional scraping and planing with short-term use of antibiotics such as metronidazole or doxycycline, which are effective against the anaerobic bacteria often associated with gum disease. These drugs are usually administered as pills or tablets, but if only a few teeth are involved, it may merely be necessary to apply antibiotic gels, chips, or films directly to the pockets between the teeth and gums.

If these nonsurgical approaches fail, surgery may be necessary. Various procedures can be done to clean out the infec-

tion, recontour the underlying bone, or trim and reshape the gums so that pockets become shallower. One cosmetic drawback to these procedures, especially if they involve teeth in the front of the mouth, is that they tend to expose some of the tooth's root. Also, however good the surgery, problems almost always return within a couple of years unless good dental hygiene is practiced at home.

How can gum disease be prevented?

The best way to avoid gum disease is to brush thoroughly at least twice a day, floss at least once a day, limit intake of sweets (especially those that leave a film on the teeth), avoid cigarette smoking (which increases the risk of periodontal disease), and have a dental examination once or twice a year. Women who are pregnant or who are using birth control pills should be especially vigilant and may need to schedule extra dental visits.

Tartar control toothpastes have not been proven to be particularly helpful, mainly because—although they do remove tartar from tooth surfaces—they do not get at the problem tartar below the gumline. There is some evidence that mouth rinses containing antimicrobial (bacteria-killing) substances such as chlorhexidine (Peridex, available only by prescription in the United States) may help remove plaque. Side effects, however—including tooth staining and tissue irritation—may outweigh benefits, especially since there is still no solid evidence that any mouthwash, including antimicrobial mouthwashes, can actually cure gingivitis. Nor are there any good data yet to show whether nonsteroidal antiinflammatory drugs (such as Motrin and Indocin) might be able to slow destruction of bone.

For people who are predisposed to heavy deposits of plaque and tartar, it may be necessary to use special irrigation devices, toothpicks, or gum stimulators. Frequent cleanings by a dentist or dental hygienist may also be desirable. Although most dental insurance policies cover basic dental services, including preventive services, many do not cover such frequent preventive care. Ultimately, however, the cost of a few extra cleanings is far less than the cost (and pain) of periodontitis.

Related entries

Antibiotics, antiinflammatory drugs, cosmetic dentistry, dentures/bridges/implants, diabetes, epilepsy, orthodontia

Hair Care

Americans of both sexes—though still largely women—spend millions of dollars each year on hair care products, and subject their hair to curling, blow drying, oiling, straightening, spiking, permanent waving, bleaching, dyeing, removing, and restoring. Most of these efforts are made to improve appearance, which plays a major role in self-esteem and psychological well-being.

The basics of hair growth

Hair is composed of dead cells that grow out of tiny pockets, or follicles, of actively dividing cells just under the skin (see illustration). These follicles are nourished by small blood vessels and fed by sebaceous (oil) glands, which give hair its shine.

Like the nails, hair is hardened by a protein called keratin, which is found in smaller quantities in living skin cells. Each strand of hair consists of three layers: the outer cuticle, the middle cortex, and the inner medulla. The thin, colorless cuticle serves basically to protect the thicker cortex, which contains melanin, the pigment that gives hair its color. Women with blond hair have less melanin in the cortex of their hair than do women with darker hair. The shape of the cortex in cross-section also determines the hair's curl: the cross-section of the cortex is oval in curly hair and round in straight hair. The innermost layer of the hair, the medulla, reflects light and gives hair its characteristic color tones. The color, curliness, sheen, and manageability of hair are controlled to a large extent by heredity. So is the time in life at which the hair begins to turn gray or white—a result of a depletion of the hue-giving melanin.

A few unlucky women have hair with odd grooves along the strands and cross-sections in the shapes of triangles, ellipses, and kidney beans rather than the normal circles and ovals. This makes their hair unmanageable no matter what they do. "Uncombable hair syndrome," as this condition is

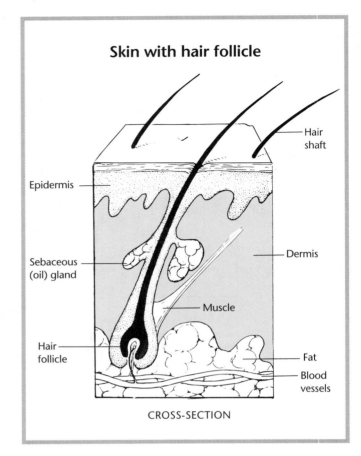

Skin with hair follicle

Hair shaft

Epidermis

Sebaceous (oil) gland

Dermis

Muscle

Hair follicle

Fat

Blood vessels

CROSS-SECTION

called by dermatologists, apparently can be present from birth and currently has no treatment.

Hair strands usually grow at the rate of about half an inch per month, and continue at this clip for 2 years or so. After this point the strand goes into a period of stasis, or rest, and then eventually falls out. Normally about 50 to 100 strands are lost per day. This usually does not pose a problem, since the 100,000 or so hairs on the average person's head fall out at staggered intervals.

Having generally good health and eating a nutritious diet seem to play a role in the health of hair, although there is no evidence that supplementing the diet with any specific nutrient—such as proteins or amino acids—makes a difference. Nutritional deficiencies, however—such as occur during crash diets or eating disorders such as anorexia nervosa—do seem to damage hair significantly.

Some of these effects attributed to nutritional deficiencies may actually be related to hormonal changes that occur in women who lose excessive amounts of body fat. In fact, hormonal changes in general seem to have considerable influence on hair throughout a woman's life cycle. For example, hormonal changes during puberty increase oil secretion by the sebaceous glands, leaving hair oilier and less manageable than usual. During pregnancy, another time of rapid hormonal changes, many women find that their hair becomes either more or less manageable. Some women also find that permanent waves do not "take" during pregnancy. And during the postpartum period, as well as during menopause, hormone withdrawal often increases hair loss.

Despite much-hyped claims to the contrary made by beauty salons, there is no scientifically sound evidence that "hair analysis" provides any useful information about the hair's nutritional imbalances—or anything else for that matter.

The basics of hair care

With all the time, effort, and money entailed, it would be nice to think that hair care products and treatments have some effect on the appearance and manageability of hair. Some purists argue that these investments cannot possibly affect the health of hair, since hair, after all, is dead. Although this is true in a literal sense, there is no question that products and treatments can change the appearance of hair, if only through temporary cosmetic alterations. There is also no question that these products and treatments can damage hair if they are overused. Fortunately, even damaged hair is eventually replaced with new, healthy hair, although this can take years.

Hair needs to be treated gently to prevent damage. This usually means minimizing excess exposure to wind, sun, and chlorine. It also means regular but gentle brushing to rein in stray hairs and eliminate tangles. The proverbial "hundred strokes a night" is too harsh a treatment for most hair and merely results in excessive hair loss. Certain hairstyles—such as tight pony tails, braids, buns, or cornrows—as well as teasing and back-combing, tend to split and damage hair, as does rolling the hair too tightly on curlers. Hair should be brushed from the scalp to the ends so that oil from the scalp can be distributed evenly over the strands. Split ends, which often appear at the tips of older hairs, are best eliminated with regular trims.

Daily shampooing with a gentle shampoo does not harm hair, but it is certainly not necessary for all types of hair—or for all types of lifestyle, physical activity, weather, or occupation. Hair that is clean, shiny, and manageable is being washed frequently enough.

To shampoo, the hair should first be wet with warm (not hot) water and then lathered outward from the scalp with a small amount of a gentle shampoo. Although protein shampoos cannot penetrate the hair shaft or render any permanent changes, they can coat the shaft temporarily and give the hair a fuller, thicker appearance. Massaging with fingertips rather than nails helps prevent dandruff, and, for women with oily hair, keeping massage to a minimum helps avoid stimulating oil production. The shampoo should be rinsed out thoroughly. One application of shampoo is generally sufficient, despite admonitions on the back of most shampoo bottles to "rinse and repeat" (undoubtedly in the interest of selling more shampoo). A cream rinse or conditioner can be applied after the hair is rinsed. By coating the hair, these products can minimize damage from brushing, combing, and drying and may also temporarily increase the sheen or bulk of the hair.

Because wet hair is particularly susceptible to stretching and subsequent damage, it should be towel dried and then gently untangled with fingers or a wide-toothed comb, not a hairbrush. If blow drying or hood drying is preferred to air drying, it should be done on low heat and the hair should be left slightly damp for minimum damage. Heated rollers and curling irons used frequently can cause split ends.

For women with dandruff—flakes of skin from the scalp that are obvious on the hair and clothing—there are over-the-counter dandruff shampoos which contain chemicals that suppress overproduction of skin cells. For maximum effect the hair should be shampooed daily and the shampoo left on about 3 to 5 minutes before being rinsed out thoroughly. The most effective nonprescription dandruff shampoos contain zinc pyrithione (such as Head and Shoulders, Zincon, and Danex). Others may contain salicylic acid and sulfur (Ionil, Sebulex, Vanseb) or coal tar (Pentrax, Sebutone, Zetar). If a dandruff problem persists, a clinician can prescribe stronger shampoos (containing 2.5 percent selenium sulfide), a steroid lotion, or an antiyeast shampoo, since one current theory is that dandruff is caused by an overgrowth of a particular type of yeast that lives on the oils of the sebaceous glands. Once dandruff is eliminated, it is a good idea to use a dandruff shampoo every so often to prevent recurrences.

Sprays, spritzes, mousses, and gels can temporarily change the appearance of the hair without causing permanent damage. Some gels and mousses may dry out the ends, however. Also, it is important to avoid inhaling hair sprays and to choose products in general which do not irritate underlying skin or clog pores of the scalp and which are environmentally safe. Hair spray should be avoided near acne-prone skin, especially on the forehead.

Both permanent waves and straightening procedures use chemicals to unlock certain molecular links in the strands and then other chemicals to relock them into different positions. These chemicals are generally thought to be safe, although they can damage hair if used excessively. It is best to have hair straightening and waving done by an expert, because of the danger of chemically burning the scalp or hair.

Related entries
Body image, cosmetic safety, hair dyes, hair loss, hair removal, hirsutism, ovarian cancer, skin care and cosmetics, skin disorders

Hair Dyes

Over half of all American women dye their hair. Some of them do it to cover gray, while others simply prefer to sport a shade other than the one nature intended. Hair can be bleached (lightened) or tinted (darkened) at home or in a salon relatively neatly and conveniently. Whereas hair dyeing once meant spending tedious hours in the bathroom coated with gloppy, acrid-smelling goos, today there are many fast-acting, pleasantly scented gels and shampoos available. New technology allows these products to produce a much more sophisticated, multihued effect so that it is harder than ever before to answer the question "Does she or doesn't she?"

Modern dyes also often include conditioners that coat and reinforce the hair shaft and enhance the hair's luster and sheen. As a result, many women find that they can achieve an equally satisfactory and much less expensive effect by dyeing their own hair at home, although it is probably a good idea for a novice to start out at a beauty salon, if only to make sure the color is right.

Overusing hair dyes, particularly permanent dyes containing ammonia and peroxide, can split, dry, and dull the hair. And some evidence, though controversial, suggests that certain types of hair dye may increase a woman's chances of developing particular forms of cancer, such as non-Hodgkin's lymphoma.

Types of hair dyes

Permanent dyes. To be permanent, a dye has to be able to penetrate the cuticle of the hair (the thin, clear outer layer of overlapping scales). This usually means that it must contain harsh chemicals such as ammonia and peroxide. Ammonia opens up the scales on the cuticle so that the peroxide and dye can enter the cortex. There the peroxide bleaches away the natural pigment, while the dye undergoes a chemical reaction that enlarges and entraps it in the cortex. The result is a color that will stay on the hair until newer hair grows out.

The problem is that new hair grows out relatively quickly. In fact, telltale roots often appear within a week or so of the treatment. So there is a great temptation to dye the hair frequently, and therein lies the danger: over time, the ammonia and peroxide used in permanent dyes take their toll on the hair. When the cuticle is disrupted too often, the scales stop overlapping completely, so that moisture can easily enter and swell the hair shaft. Initially this may make the hair look fuller, but soon the damaged hair shaft will break and split, and the hair will lose its luster. The hair roots underneath the scalp remain undamaged, however, and eventually new, healthier hair will grow in.

Some of these problems can be minimized by using products that have reduced levels of peroxide or contain conditioners to bolster the damaged cuticle. Other products, which brighten the hair without lightening it, contain no ammonia at all and only small amounts of peroxide. Whatever product is chosen, it is always a good idea to test it on a small, hidden area of the scalp first to make sure that it causes no irritation.

Semipermanent dyes. Another way to avoid ammonia and peroxide is to use semipermanent dyes. Although these dyes usually fade within about 6 weeks, they are much kinder to the hair. Semipermanent dyes essentially paint over the hair's natural color, and so they are often appealing to women who want to cover up gray hairs with something close to their natural color. Since there is generally no blatant change in color,

revealing roots are usually less of a problem than with permanent dyes. But semipermanent dyes are not an option for a raven-haired woman who wants to go blond, since they do not penetrate the cortex of the hair and bleach away the melanin.

Cellophane wraps. These are a form of semipermanent hair dye. Although they cannot completely mask gray, they enhance the hair's volume and natural highlights. In this procedure, which must be performed in a salon, the woman sits under the hood of a hair dryer for about half an hour while hair dyes, called cellophanes, are baked onto the cuticle of her hair. These dyes color the outside of the hair shaft without actually penetrating the cuticle. They usually last about 8 weeks.

Hair dye and cancer

There is some reason to believe that using hair dyes for several years may slightly increase a woman's risk of developing ovarian cancer, as well as certain cancers of the immune system. It also seems that the risk increases with the darkness and permanence of the dye, as well as the length of time over which it is used.

For many years, investigators have known that hair dyes—particularly the darker shades—contain certain chemicals, including aromatic amines, that are recognized carcinogens in animals. This in itself, however, did not necessarily implicate hair dyes in human cancers. Nor did the reports during the 1970s indicating that hairdressers were at increased risk of developing non-Hodgkin's lymphoma, multiple myeloma, and leukemia. Although these findings were enough to have cosmetology classified as an occupation that involved exposure to carcinogens, they did not prove that it was the hair dyes and not some other environmental or sociological factor that led to the increased risk.

More compelling, however, are recent studies indicating that women who dye their hair on a regular basis have an increased risk of developing non-Hodgkin's lymphoma, leukemia, or ovarian cancer. For example, one study of 573,369 women found that those who had used black hair dye for more than 20 years had a slightly increased risk of dying from non-Hodgkin's lymphoma and multiple myeloma. It is not clear from this study whether these women also had a higher risk of developing—as opposed to dying from—these cancers. Another recent study did show that the risk of developing leukemia was 50 percent higher in women who used hair dyes, and that the rate jumped to 150 percent in women who had used the dyes for 16 years or more. Still another study indicates that dyeing hair 1 to 4 times a year increases the risk of developing ovarian cancer by 70 percent, and dyeing hair 5 or more times a year increases the risk by 100 percent.

What these studies have not yet shown is precisely which compounds in the dyes may be causing the problems. In fact, these studies do not even necessarily implicate the hair dye in the increased cancer rates, since women who dye their hair may have other common factors in their lives which could contribute to developing cancer. Also, even if hair dyes do turn out to cause certain cancers, all of the figures from the studies need to be interpreted with caution. Having a greatly increased risk is not necessarily cause for panic, after all, if the original risk is extremely low. As it turns out, the 50 percent increase in leukemia risk means that 1.5 in 100 women who dye their hair can expect to develop leukemia, as opposed to 0.6 out of 100 women who do not dye their hair. Similarly, a 100 percent jump in the risk of ovarian cancer means that 3 out of 100 women who dye their hair for over 16 years can expect to develop ovarian cancer, as opposed to 1.5 women who do not dye their hair.

Even more encouraging is new information from the Nurses' Health Study, an investigation by researchers at the Harvard School of Public Health involving nearly 100,000 women. This study could find no connection between hair dyes and leukemia, lymphoma, or multiple myeloma. Although this study did not distinguish between women who used dark or light dyes—the assumption being that originally dark-haired women were more likely to use dark dyes—the researchers still expected to see some kind of increased cancer rate in this large group of women if, indeed, hair dyes in general led to an increased risk.

In short, women have to balance the low and uncertain risk against the benefits they receive from dyeing their hair. From this perspective, many women—as well as many investigators—still consider hair dyes to be relatively safe, at least until there is better evidence to the contrary.

Nonetheless, most clinicians advise pregnant women to avoid dyeing their hair, at least until after the first trimester. They also suggest that women who want to use a dark dye use a product containing henna or lead acetate—both of which are believed to be safe—rather than chemicals such as 4MMPD (4-methoxy-m-phenylenediamine) and 4MMPD-sulfate.

Related entries

Body image, cosmetic safety, hair care, hair loss, hair removal, hirsutism, ovarian cancer, skin care and cosmetics, skin disorders

Hair Loss

Hair loss from the scalp, or alopecia, can occur in women as well as men, although in women the loss is usually from the top of the scalp rather than from the sides or forehead (see illustration). Men losing their hair may rue the passage of their youth, but there are plenty of bald, virile actors and athletes to help bolster the male ego; balding women have no such positive role models. Because physical appearance is still a fundamental part of many women's self-esteem, it is no wonder that hair loss in women is often much more emotionally devastating than in men.

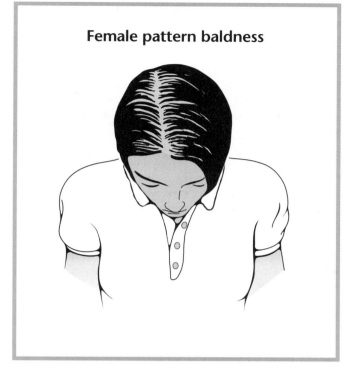

Female pattern baldness

What are the causes of hair loss in women?

Permanent hair loss in women is usually related to virilizing hormones called androgens which all women have circulating in their blood. For reasons still little understood, the hair follicles in some women may process these hormones abnormally so that levels become elevated in the scalp only, or the follicles may be oversensitive to even low levels of androgens. The tendency toward this kind of baldness seems to be inherited but not in any kind of obvious, direct fashion.

Women with excess body hair (hirsutism), acne, and menstrual abnormalities, in addition to scalp hair loss, often have relatively high levels of androgens throughout the body. This may be the result of various underlying conditions, including an underfunctioning thyroid gland or a problem with the adrenal glands or ovaries (see hypothyroidism, hyperandrogenism).

Temporary hair loss is also common in women. Several months or so after childbirth, many women notice that their hair is falling out, probably as a delayed reaction to abrupt hormonal shifts. Some women find that their hair starts falling out when they stop or start using birth control pills. Other prescription drugs are a common cause of reversible hair loss as well. Major emotional stress or severe illness can cause temporary hair loss, as can chemotherapy or radiation therapy used to treat cancer. Except with chemotherapy, hair loss generally does not begin until about 2 to 6 months after the precipitating event. In all of these cases, hair growth almost always resumes on its own.

In a rare condition called alopecia areata, hair loss occurs rapidly, often within 24 hours, leaving a smooth bald patch on the affected area—usually the scalp but occasionally other regions of the body. People with alopecia areata may also have fingernails with fine pitting or abnormal shapes. The course of alopecia areata varies from person to person, from complete reversal of symptoms to temporary remission to permanent hair loss. The cause is not known, but it may run in families, and some researchers suspect that it may be an autoimmune disorder influenced by hormone levels and stress.

How is hair loss treated?

Baldness has been notoriously difficult to reverse, although there has been some success with the drug minoxidil (Rogaine). This drug, applied topically, appears to stimulate some hair regrowth in both men and women. Drugs such as spironolactone (generally used to treat high blood pressure) or birth control pills that are high in estrogens may also be somewhat effective. In many cases, however, the only answer is to wear wigs or hairpieces or to consider hair transplantation.

The drug finasteride (Proscar, Propecia), more frequently used to treat hair loss and prostate problems (benign prostatic hyperplasia) in men, may promote hair growth on women's scalps as well, although it is not currently approved for treating hair loss in women. Side effects are generally mild but may include breast enlargement and increased sex drive. Any sexually active woman of reproductive age using finasteride should be sure to use one or more effective means of birth control.

Hair transplantation, which is usually performed under local anesthesia, involves removing small plugs of scalp containing only a few hairs from areas of healthy terminal (coarse) hair and using them to replace plugs of scalp from hairless patches. Getting the best results requires transplanting several hundred plugs over several sessions. It is wise to get a referral to a dermatologist rather than go to a hair replacement clinic. Insurance does not cover this cosmetic procedure.

There is no cure for alopecia areata, but spontaneous hair regrowth occurs in 90 percent of people with the disorder. Treatments that may be effective for women with mild cases include steroids, immune suppressors (cyclosporine), minoxidil, and ultraviolet light therapy.

Related entries

Autoimmune disorders, chemotherapy, estrogen, hirsutism, hyperandrogenism, hypothyroidism, radiation therapy, stress

Hair Removal

Although hair removal is usually not necessary to ensure health or hygiene, many women—and some men—wish to remove body hair that they consider excessive or unsightly. There are a variety of methods available, which vary considerably in cost, ease, speed, and degree of pain involved. With the exception of electrolysis, all of these methods are temporary. Some women find that bleaching fine hairs is an acceptable alternative to hair removal.

Shaving

Shaving is the quickest—and one of the least expensive—forms of hair removal, but it is also the one that results in the quickest regrowth of hair. Many women shave their underarms and legs, but it is also perfectly effective to shave facial hair. Contrary to popular belief, shaving does not result in the regrowth of coarser, thicker, or darker hair, although, if done improperly, it can roughen or irritate surrounding skin. Also, because razors cut the hair perpendicular to the skin, a rough tip is created (instead of the original tapered tip), and this may give hair a coarser or harsher feeling.

To shave without irritating the skin, the hair should first be softened with water, and coarse or thick hair should be lathered with soap or shaving gel. Then the hairs should be shaved with a sharp blade in the direction of growth. Electric shavers usually do not give as close a shave, although they are less likely to produce razor burn. Also, shaving creams cannot be used with electric razors.

Tweezing

Tweezing is another quick and inexpensive—if somewhat painful—method of hair removal. It is particularly useful for a few isolated hairs on places such as the eyebrows, chin, or upper lip, or around the breasts. To minimize the possibility of infection in the hair follicle, the surrounding skin should be washed before tweezing and dabbed with a little bit of alcohol. The hair should then be pulled out in the direction of growth. A clinician should be consulted before plucking hair from a mole, since irritation or folliculitis can result.

Tweezed hairs eventually regrow, but the new hairs are not any darker or thicker than the original ones. Also, because the hairs are plucked from underneath the skin, the results tend to be longer-lasting than with shaving.

Abrasives

Another way to remove a few scattered hairs involves rubbing the area with a pumice stone or other abrasive material. While an effective short-term way of removing fine hair, abrasives can also easily irritate the skin, and it can take a lot of rubbing to achieve a minor effect. Abrasives are generally too harsh to be used on the face, but some high-grade abrasives (Delete) are safe, especially above the lip.

Waxing

Waxing is essentially tweezing on a large scale. In this method, melted wax is applied to the hairy area and allowed to cool. Then it is quickly stripped off in the direction of hair growth, carrying the hairs along with it. Results are about as long-lasting as with tweezing, since the hairs are ripped out from under the skin. It is usually best to have a trained cosmetologist perform waxing, which can irritate the skin or cause an infection of the hair follicles if done by someone without experience. Though more expensive than shaving or tweezing, waxing is a relatively popular way to remove hair on the legs, upper lip, and chin.

Depilatories

Depilatories are chemical agents (usually thioglycolate) sold over the counter in scented cream, foam, or lotion form (Neet, Nair). They are used by many women to remove leg, underarm, or facial hair temporarily. These products all work by dissolving the protein in hair while leaving the root in place. After wetting the skin and allowing the depilatory to work for about 10 minutes, the woman can wipe away the dissolved hair.

Because these chemicals can severely irritate and even burn the skin, especially on the face, it is important to do a patch test on a small area of skin before any widespread application and to avoid using them on inflamed or broken skin.

Electrolysis

Electrolysis is considered the only permanent method of hair removal. It is also quite frequently time-consuming, tedious, and expensive. In this technique a trained electrologist inserts a very fine needle into the hair follicle and then delivers a current of electricity which destroys the hair root. This usually prevents regrowth, although destruction is often incomplete, necessitating a number of retreatments. Multiple treatments may be needed anyway, since only a limited number of hairs can be worked on at each session.

It is important to make sure that the electrologist has proper training and—to help prevent the spread of HIV (the virus that causes AIDS) and hepatitis—uses a fresh needle for each patient. Sometimes electrolysis can result in pitting or scarring of surrounding skin, as well as infections of the hair follicle, but otherwise the procedure is considered relatively safe.

Related entries

Acquired immune deficiency syndrome, cosmetic safety, hair care, hair loss, hirsutism, moles, skin care and cosmetics, skin disorders

Hay Fever and Perennial Allergic Rhinitis

Allergic rhinitis is a common condition affecting 10 to 20 percent of the population. Characterized by inflamed mucous membranes of the nasal passages, it can occur either seasonally (hay fever) or year-round (perennial allergic rhinitis). Working in certain industries (such as laboratories using lab-oratory animals) may trigger yet another kind of allergic rhinitis, called occupational rhinitis, in susceptible individuals.

All forms of allergic rhinitis occur after repeated exposure to common airborne substances (allergens) that trigger white blood cells to make immunoglobulin E (IGE) antibodies in allergic individuals. These antibodies bind to the surface of mast cells, another kind of white blood cell, in the mucous lining of the nasal passage. When these mast cell–antibody complexes are stimulated by an allergen, they release irritating substances (histamine, leukotrienes, and neuropeptides) that lead to the production of excess mucus, dilated blood vessels, itchiness, and sneezing. They may release other substances that inflame the mucous lining as well. Repeated exposure to the allergen can leave nasal passages chronically inflamed.

Who is likely to develop hay fever and perennial allergic rhinitis?

Symptoms of allergic rhinitis develop when susceptible individuals are repeatedly exposed to triggering allergens. People who are allergic to certain tree pollens, grasses, or weeds, for example, may develop symptoms on a seasonal basis; others, with allergies to cockroaches, animal dander, molds, or dust mites (microscopic insects that feed on human skin scales), may have symptoms on a year-round or nearly year-round basis. Susceptibility itself is largely a matter of genetics: people with a family history of allergies, as well as those with asthma (see entry), are particularly vulnerable.

The prevalence of allergic rhinitis, as well as asthma, appears to be increasing in industrialized nations, perhaps because exposure to indoor allergens appears to be rising. Increasing evidence implicates cockroaches as the source of many allergic attacks, especially in urban areas. People who are sensitive to molds are more likely to be exposed in basements, bathrooms, or other areas of high humidity, as well as in buildings contaminated with mold from water damage.

Most cases of allergic rhinitis begin before the age of 20 and persist into adulthood.

What are the symptoms?

The most common symptoms of allergic rhinitis are an itchy, runny nose and sneezing. Postnasal drip and nasal congestion are also common, as are itchy eyes and a red, itchy palate. Often symptoms occur only during a specific season of the year or after contact with animals or other known triggers.

How is the condition evaluated?

Before diagnosing allergic rhinitis, a clinician will do a thorough history and physical examination, including an inspection of the nasal passages, to rule out nonallergic forms of rhinitis (inflammation of the nose) as well as other structural abnormalities (such as nasal polyps or a deviated septum) or systemic inflammatory diseases. If allergies are suspected, the clinician will conduct a skin test in which suspected allergens are either scratched onto the surface of or injected just under the skin to see if they produce a local reaction (a rash). In some cases, particularly in hypersensitive patients, blood tests (called RAST testing) may be done instead of skin tests. In addition, CT scans and other imaging tests may be used to examine the nasal passages and sinuses more closely.

How is the condition treated?

A number of medications are available to treat the symptoms of allergic rhinitis, both over the counter and by prescription. Although many are effective, at least some of the time, choosing the right approach is a matter of trade-offs.

While nonprescription drugs can help clear a runny or stuffy nose at minimal cost, for example, they occasionally have disturbing side effects. Over-the-counter decongestants such as pseudoephedrine (Sudafed, Dimetapp) can provide relief but sometimes cause insomnia, palpitations, headache, and nervousness. They should be used with caution by anyone with high blood pressure or glaucoma, and avoided by women in the first trimester of pregnancy as well as those taking MAO inhibitors. Similarly, over-the-counter antihistamines such as chlorpheniramine (Actifed, Contac, Coricidin) or diphenhydramine (Benadryl) can relieve sneezing, runny nose, and congestion but sometimes lead to drowsiness, dizziness, blurred vision, dry mouth, and difficulty urinating.

If side effects are a problem, several other antihistamines, some available over the counter, some by prescription, work just about as well without causing as much drowsiness. These drugs—which include loratidine (Claritin), cetirizine (Zyrtec), and fexofenadine (Allegra)—are more expensive, however, and some people find that they lose their effectiveness after they have been taken for an extended period of time.

For many people with hay fever, nasal sprays containing corticosteroids can control symptoms, used alone or in combination with antihistamines. They prevent allergy attacks by blocking substances that inflame the nose. Cromolyn sodium sprays (such as Nasalcrom) are somewhat less effective than corticosteroids but also result in fewer side effects. These sprays may relieve mild symptoms within a few hours; relief for more severe symptoms may take a week or more. Any nasal spray can lead to excessive dryness in the nose.

Non-corticosteroid nasal sprays can provide relief as well. Decongestant sprays such as phenylephrine and oxymetazoline, found in products such as Afrin, Dristan, and Neo-Synephrine, should not be used for more than 4 to 5 days, however, or they may lead to "rebound" congestion. The prescription antihistamine nasal spray azelastine (Astelin) causes sedation just like over-the-counter antihistamines. Other nasal sprays such as ipratropium bromide (Atrovent) contain anticholinergic drugs that can reduce symptoms of runny nose but have no effect on itchiness, sneezing, or congestion. Atrovent contains peanut oil and should not be used by anyone allergic to peanuts, soybeans, or soya lecithin.

Women who want a nondrug alternative to nasal congestion may want to try an external nasal dilator (e.g., the Breathe Right nasal strip), an adhesive-backed plastic strip applied to the nose that holds the nostrils open to ease breathing. Before using one of these strips, makeup should be removed and the skin cleansed around the outside of the nose.

While these can be aesthetically problematic, a new transparent version is increasing the appeal of this approach.

If all else fails, and there is a known allergen causing symptoms, immunotherapy (allergy shots) should be considered. The idea here is to reduce individual sensitivity to a given allergen over a long period of time by injecting gradually increasing amounts of that allergen under the skin. Immunotherapy is helpful for some—especially those allergic to tree, grass, and weed pollen, as well as dust mites and animal dander. The cost is substantial, however, since it's usually necessary to make weekly visits to an allergist for 6 months to a year for shots, followed by biweekly to monthly visits for another 3 to 5 years.

Pregnant women should discuss all of these options with their clinicians, who can help develop a treatment plan based on severity of symptoms. Ideally all medications should be avoided during the first trimester of pregnancy. Traditionally the over-the-counter antihistamines such as chlorpheniramine and diphenhydramine have been suggested as the antihistamines of choice during pregnancy. Although loratidine (Claritin) and cetirizine (Zyrtec) are in the same class of drugs, their effects during pregnancy have not yet been as widely studied. If corticosteroid nasal sprays must be used during pregnancy, beclomethasone (Beclovent) is usually the one recommended. Pregnant women are generally advised against starting allergy shots until after delivery, but it's generally considered safe to continue a series of shots that was started before the pregnancy began.

How can allergic rhinitis be prevented?

Preventing hay fever or any other form of allergic rhinitis boils down to eliminating or reducing exposure to substances that trigger allergic attacks. While this is often not possible, taking steps to minimize exposure to a known allergen can often help reduce symptoms. The following tactics may help reduce exposure to specific substances.

Dust mites and animal dander. If hay fever or allergic rhinitis is due to dust mites and/or animal dander, someone other than the allergic person should do the household dusting and vacuuming when possible. An alternative is to invest in a double-filtered vacuum cleaner or a high-efficiency particulate arresting (HEPA) vacuum cleaner. HEPA air cleaners are often recommended to reduce airborne particles, but there is increasing debate about whether their use results in any noticeable improvements in symptoms. Many allergists also recommend ripping out carpeting, eliminating all stuffed and upholstered furniture, and removing books and dust-catching knickknacks, but not everyone can take such drastic—and not necessarily effective—measures. Covering the affected person's mattress and pillowcase with airtight rubber covers, wiping these down with water on a weekly basis, washing bedding frequently in very hot water, and keeping the bedroom in particular as dust-free as possible can be an effective alternative. Forced-air heating systems (which disperse dust even more than other heating systems) should be equipped with an effective air filter to trap offending particles.

Specific allergens found in dust can also be attacked directly. Agents lethal to dust mites can be applied to carpeting—although these agents, called acaricides, are probably unsafe for use in the home of a pregnant woman. Eradicating cockroaches can be challenging. Regular fumigation of the home by an exterminator can help, although irritating fumes from certain insecticides can aggravate underlying respiratory symptoms. People allergic to animal dander are best off if they forgo keeping furry pets altogether and avoid lengthy visits to homes of pet owners. If this is impossible, however, it can be very helpful to have someone who is not allergic wash the pet on a weekly basis.

Molds and pollens. The best tactic for avoiding many molds and pollens is to stay indoors—ideally in an air-conditioned environment—as much as possible during certain seasons, especially on days when pollen and mold counts are unusually high. These counts are often available in local newspapers, as well as on the Internet (e.g., *www.aaaai.org/nab/pollen.stm*). At all times of the year, shampoos and skin creams should be checked to make sure they do not contain extracts of cottonseed, flaxseed, or other natural substances that are sometimes allergenic. Investing in a dehumidifier can reduce levels of mold and dust mites in the home, as can adding a few drops of chlorine bleach to cut flower arrangements and changing the water daily. Cleaning humidifiers regularly and keeping indoor plants to a minimum can also help prevent the growth of molds and other allergens.

Related entries
Asthma, colds

Headaches

Headaches are an extremely common problem in women, particularly during the reproductive years. A full three-quarters of premenopausal women experience pain in the head or neck region, usually more than once a month. Headaches in women also seem to occur more frequently and to be more intense, more disabling, and longer-lasting than headaches in men. In 15 percent of women, headaches are severe enough to interfere with daily activities. While symptoms of headaches are similar in both sexes, headaches in women generally occur more frequently, are more intense, last longer, and are more disabling than those in men.

The reasons for this predominance in women remain unclear, though many experts believe that chronic and acute stress plays a major role in many cases. Headaches in women also seem to be related in some way to the menstrual cycle (so-called menstrual headaches). Many premenopausal women find their headaches are worse during menstruation and ovulation, whereas other women develop headaches just prior to their periods, with the symptoms disappearing at about the time menstruation begins (see premenstrual syndrome). Headaches that come and go according to the menstrual cycle are more likely to begin at menarche (the first menstrual period) and to abate during pregnancy. Using oral contraceptives aggravates menstrual headaches in some women.

Estrogen is among the most potent substances known to cause headache, and that may explain why premenopausal women often suffer relatively severe symptoms compared with postmenopausal women. It would also help explain why many women who are not taking estrogen replacement therapy find that their headaches subside after menopause—particularly menstrual headaches. Other women find that new headaches develop for the first time during the menopausal years, but again this could be traced to fluctuations or irregularities in hormone levels. And still other women who never had headaches start getting them after they have completed menopause.

Headaches are usually divided into three broad types: tension (muscle-contraction) headaches, migraines (vascular headaches), and combination headaches (muscle-contraction vascular headaches). Another rare headache condition (which affects mostly young men) is called a cluster headache. This type of headache involves episodes of burning, boring pain in the eye, temple, cheek, or jaw. Symptoms usually begin in the midst of deep sleep.

The different types of headaches are part of a continuum ranging from mild headaches that appear occasionally to severe headaches that occur almost continuously. Over time a woman with a mild syndrome can develop a much more severe condition, or with treatment can revert to milder symptoms.

It is important to know that some aches in the head are not attributable to muscle contraction, vascular changes, or a combination of the two. Toothaches, sinusitis (inflammation of the sinuses owing to an upper respiratory infection; see colds), allergies (see hay fever and perennial allergic rhinitis), temporomandibular joint syndrome (see entry), and especially caffeine withdrawal can cause the head to ache. More important, some head pain can signal a serious, potentially life-threatening condition. Although absolute guidelines are difficult to formulate, a woman should seek prompt medical attention if she has any of the following symptoms:

- sudden, severe headache accompanied by fever and a stiff neck that resists bending forward (this suggests meningitis)

- headache accompanied by difficulty with speech, paralysis, double vision, imbalance (this suggests an impending stroke)

- sudden, excruciating head pain that is unlike one's normal pattern of headaches (this too might indicate bleeding within the brain)

- a headache that inexorably worsens over days or weeks, especially in one part of the head (this suggests a possible blood clot or tumor)
- pain at the temple in people over 60 (this could be temporal arteritis, which can permanently affect eyesight if not treated promptly)

Tension headaches

On the mild end of the pain scale are episodic tension (muscle-contraction) headaches. These involve a band of pain that presses over the top of the head or back of the neck. This pain is usually mild to moderate, although in some people tension headaches can be just as severe and debilitating as migraines (see below). Episodic tension headaches often start in the late afternoon and last for several hours. The muscle contraction that causes tension headaches is thought to be a result of poor posture, eyestrain, stress, or psychological factors, any of which can lead to a tightening of neck or facial muscles. This type of headache is equally common in men and women.

Over time, tension headaches can start occurring daily or almost daily and last most of the day. This type of headache is called a chronic tension headache. Often a woman will wake with a headache or develop one soon after rising and find that the intensity builds as the day progresses. The progression from episodic to chronic headaches is frequently caused by treating the headache with painkillers (analgesics).

Chronic tension headaches that suddenly develop on their own in a person who has not been taking painkillers for episodic headaches are usually related to some physical injury such as a whiplash injury of the neck or a flulike illness.

Migraines

Migraines are two to three times more common in women than in men. They involve a whole complex of symptoms, including numbness, prickling, tingling, nausea, vomiting, intolerance to light or sound, depression, and irritability. Some neurologists believe that not all of these episodes, which they call migraine equivalents, necessarily include a headache. Because these episodes share certain related symptoms but have different and still unknown underlying causes, they are sometimes misdiagnosed as other conditions and are therefore treated ineffectively.

In general, however, a migraine headache involves moderate to severe throbbing in the head, with pain felt typically in the temple or behind the eye. A migraine usually begins on one side of the head and then gradually spreads and intensifies within several hours. The most frequent symptoms accompanying this headache are nausea, vomiting, and intolerance to light or sound.

Some women with "classic migraine" have a premonition or aura about an hour before a migraine begins. Sometimes the aura takes the form of a small blind spot (scotoma) surrounded by bright, flickering light or colorful and expanding zigzag lines. An aura might involve a feeling of numbness or pins and needles that starts in the fingers of one hand and gradually extends upward into the arm and eventually to the nose and mouth area. Some migraines are also preceded by mood changes, hallucinations, feelings of déjà vu, and thinking and language disorders. Auras last between 10 and 30 minutes.

Although these attacks can occur on a weekly or yearly basis, many migraines occur once or twice a month, perhaps as a result of changing hormone levels during menstruation or ovulation. Migraines generally begin in the first 3 decades of life, and in women most start around the time of puberty. Many women develop headaches—particularly migraines—during the first trimester of pregnancy but often find that the condition improves as the pregnancy progresses. If headaches occur in the last trimester of pregnancy, especially in conjunction with high blood pressure, swelling, and rapid weight gain, they may signal preeclampsia, which if not treated promptly can progress to eclampsia (see entry), a life-threatening condition.

Migraines are sometimes called vascular headaches because they seem to involve sudden changes in the blood vessels of the head (see illustration). Recent research suggests that migraine headaches may be related to disturbances in the function of serotonin, a neurotransmitter that acts as a vasoconstrictor (a chemical that contracts blood vessels). Inflammation is also an important mechanism.

Investigators at Harvard Medical School have found evidence that men who reported migraines had 80 percent more strokes than those who did not; and for strokes caused by blocked blood vessels, as opposed to bleeding vessels, the risk for men with migraine was twice that of nonsufferers. Since strokes kill about 144,000 people in the United States each year, 60 percent of whom are women, and migraines are also more common in women than in men, it is clear that studies need to be done to determine if female migraine sufferers are at greater risk for stroke than women who do not get these headaches.

It is not yet known whether migraine itself (in either men or women) is directly related to stroke, or whether the high rate of stroke has something to do with the drugs that are taken to relieve the headache. In any case, migraines seem to rank far below the other risk factors for stroke, which include high blood pressure, high blood cholesterol, obesity, diabetes, smoking, and a family history of stroke.

There is some evidence linking migraine headaches to certain foods. Among the commonly cited culprits are red wine, chocolate, aged cheese, milk, legumes, cured or smoked meat, coffee, tea, chicken livers, nitrates, and monosodium glutamate (MSG).

Combination headaches

If migraine headaches occur frequently, they may develop into muscle-contraction vascular headaches—the third type of headache particularly common in women. These head-

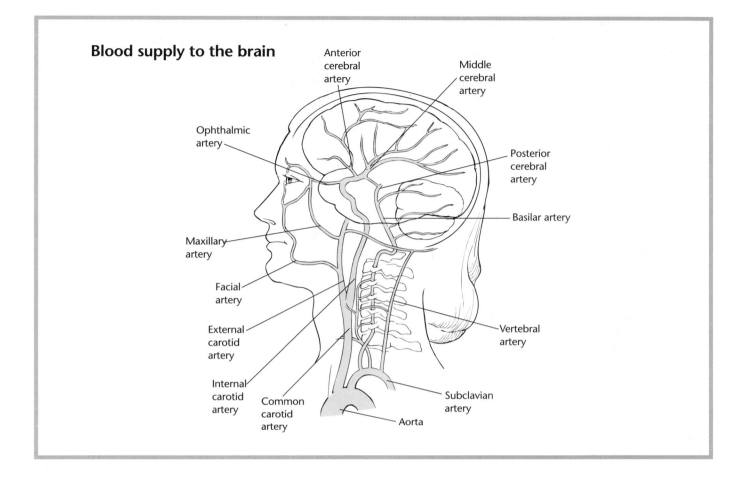

Blood supply to the brain

- Anterior cerebral artery
- Middle cerebral artery
- Ophthalmic artery
- Posterior cerebral artery
- Basilar artery
- Maxillary artery
- Facial artery
- External carotid artery
- Internal carotid artery
- Common carotid artery
- Aorta
- Vertebral artery
- Subclavian artery

aches involve all the symptoms of migraine headaches on top of all the symptoms of chronic tension headaches. Combination headaches can also happen the other way around: they can result from the worsening of a chronic tension headache which occurs daily, or almost daily, and builds up in intensity to migraine headaches. Sometimes combination headaches are therefore misdiagnosed as simple migraine headaches, which usually do not occur so frequently.

How are these conditions evaluated?

Women who have severe, frequent, or long-lasting headaches—as well as women who suddenly develop headaches or marked changes in headache patterns later in life—should see a clinician to determine the underlying cause of the pain. Usually the clinician will examine the head, neck, and nervous system and ask about the timing and nature of the headaches, as well as any emotional, social, or job-related factors that could play a role. Occasionally, other diagnostic tests such as a CT scan or MRI (magnetic resonance image) of the head or x-rays of the upper spine may be needed as well.

How are headaches treated?

After the physician has ruled out serious diseases that sometimes underlie head pain, the first aim of treatment for moderate to severe headaches is pain relief. For occasional headaches, aspirin, acetaminophen, ibuprofen, or combination preparations such as Excedrin Migraine can be used. Tension headaches and combination headaches, however, may actually be perpetuated by frequent use of painkillers that are commonly used to treat them—a phenomenon known as a "rebound headache." Rebound headaches can develop if any of the over-the-counter pain medications are used on a daily basis.

To prevent the worsening of headaches, these medications should therefore not be used more than 1 or 2 days per week. If a woman needs over-the-counter painkillers more frequently, she should consider taking a prescription medication instead.

Usually a doctor will first prescribe a stronger oral antiinflammatory medication or a combination pill with a vasoconstrictor and a muscle relaxant. Commonly prescribed pain pills include Midrin or a nonsteroidal antiinflammatory drug (NSAID) such as naproxen sodium (Naprosyn) or ibuprofen (Motrin). For tension headaches, prescription muscle relaxants such as carisoprodol (Soma) or metaxalone (Skelaxin) can be helpful. Stronger medications such as Fiorinal/Fioricet, Tylenol 3, or Percodan/Percocet should be avoided if possible because they contain potentially addictive substances.

Sometimes drugs such as Midrin or ibuprofen are ineffective because the stomach is not absorbing them efficiently (often moderate to severe headaches are accompanied by some degree of gastrointestinal dysfunction). Another drug called metoclopramide hydrochloride (Reglan), taken 15 minutes before the analgesic, can help. This approach works only if the headache starts during the day. For women who wake with headaches, rectal suppositories such as indomethacin (Indocin) or ergotamine (Cafergot) may be tried. indomethacin is a potent nonsteroidal antiinflammatory painkiller. Cafergot, an antimigraine drug, contains caffeine as well as ergotamine tartrate, a potent vasoconstrictor which also reduces inflammation. This drug commonly causes nausea and leg cramps and is not safe for use during pregnancy or breastfeeding.

By far the most effective medications for migraines are the so-called "triptans," which boost the effect of the neurotransmitter serotonin. They attack the migraine cycle by causing vasoconstriction and blocking inflammation. Among available triptans are almotriptan (Axert), naratriptan (Amerge), sumatriptan (Imitrex), and zolmitriptan (Zomig). All have similar effectiveness and side effects, including tingling in the fingers and tightness in the throat, tiredness, lightheadedness, and nausea.

If migraine headaches do not respond to these pills, a variety of non-oral medications can be tried. Sumatriptan is available as a nasal spray and an injected medication; the latter is packaged in autoinjector form for easy use. Another vasocontrictor, dihydroergotamine mesylate (DHE45), is also available as a nasal spray, and, for severe headaches, is available in injectable form together with an antiemetic drug such as compazine to prevent nausea. The triptans and DHE45 are dangerous in women who have uncontrolled high blood pressure or coronary artery disease.

Though all medications should be avoided if possible during pregnancy, probably the safest available drug is the rectal suppository promethazine hydrochloride (Phenergan). It is only somewhat effective in relieving headaches, but it can also relieve nausea and vomiting and, because it causes drowsiness, it helps promote sleep—which itself can facilitate recovery from the headache.

How can headaches be prevented?

Stopping a headache that has already begun is rarely enough. The ultimate goal is to prevent new headaches from starting—or at least to reduce their frequency and severity.

In the case of headaches that routinely begin 18 to 36 hours after her last cup of coffee, a woman might consider tapering off her use of caffeine. Caffeine withdrawal headaches are among the easiest to prevent. If head pain is the result of chronic sinus infections, allergies, or dental problems, getting treatment for these underlying conditions can diminish the severity of the headaches.

In the case of migraines, a woman might want to start by experimenting with her diet, avoiding for a couple of weeks all of the foods that are thought to provoke migraine. If the headaches subside, she may then restore these foods, one per

---

Common headache triggers

General

Stress/tension
Fatigue
Lack of sleep
Skipping meals

Food/drinks

Caffeine
Tyramine in aged cheese and red wine
Phenylethylamine in dark chocolate

Food additives

Sodium nitrate
Monosodium glutamate
Aspartame

Alcohol

Menstruation and ovulation

---

week, to see if she can identify those that exacerbate her headaches. If this dietary experiment works, she will know which foods to stay away from in the future.

Tension headaches can sometimes be relieved through muscle relaxation techniques, which are described in detail in numerous popular books, audio cassettes, and videos. Some women have also found that biofeedback, acupuncture, shiatsu (Japanese finger pressure massage; see alternative therapies), hot or cold showers, massage, yoga, or physical therapy may help relieve tension headaches. Because nutrition, sleep, and exercise patterns may play a role in headaches, it can be useful to keep a "headache diary" to see if the headaches are associated with any particular habits, foods, or situations. Fasting for a prolonged period of time or making radical changes in sleep habits can also produce headaches in some people, and therefore these behaviors should be avoided. Taking supplements of magnesium may also help prevent migraines, particularly those associated with the menstrual cycle.

Some women find that discontinuing oral contraceptives reduces the frequency of headaches. For women on estrogen replacement therapy, the estrogen should be reduced to the lowest effective dose.

If a woman is having more than 2 or 3 headaches per month, preventive medications are usually worth trying. The physician will generally prescribe one of a number of different medications that seem to help prevent headaches or at least reduce their frequency and severity. Among the most effective drugs to prevent migraines, as well as tension headaches in some cases, are beta blockers such as propranolol (Inderal), atenolol (Tenormin), nadolol (Corgard), metoprolol (Lopressor), and timolol (Blocadren), which are generally used to treat hypertension and abnormal heartbeat. Some beta blockers may cause fatigue, depression, or insomnia.

Tricyclic antidepressants such as amitriptyline (Elavil) are commonly used to prevent both migraines and chronic tension headaches. These drugs—which have the added advantage of helping to regulate sleep cycles—are sometimes used at the same time as beta blockers. Antidepressants may cause sedation, dry mouth, constipation, and weight gain (but usually only in higher doses than in those used to treat headaches). They should not be used by women with epilepsy, irregular heartbeat, or glaucoma. A drug that is less effective than the others but has the fewest potential side effects is verapamil (Calan, Isoptin), a calcium antagonist that is usually prescribed to relieve rapid heartbeat. Verapamil should not be taken by women with disorders of the conduction system in the heart. Constipation is the most common side effect.

Simple aspirin in low doses (1 coated tablet per day) is effective as a prophylactic agent in approximately 20 percent of cases. Side effects are minimal with this dose.

During pregnancy, beta blockers are safe for prevention. Often physical therapy or relaxation exercises can be used to help relieve tight neck and shoulder muscles. Headaches frequently improve by themselves after the first trimester. Any headache that occurs during the third trimester needs to be evaluated to rule out other pregnancy-related causes (such as preeclampsia).

Related entries
Alternative therapies, antidepressants, antiinflammatory drugs, eclampsia, estrogen replacement therapy, insomnia, preeclampsia, premenstrual syndrome, stress, stroke, temporal arteritis

Heart Disease

Heart disease, also called cardiovascular disease, includes a myriad of disorders involving the heart and its blood vessels. Many of these fall into the category of coronary heart disease, a term that itself encompasses a variety of conditions.

Most coronary heart disease is due to a process known as atherosclerosis, in which fat and cholesterol are deposited in the inner walls of arteries throughout the body. Over the years, scar tissue and other debris build up as more fat and cholesterol are deposited. If one or more of the arteries that supply the heart muscle with blood are seriously narrowed, a condition called coronary artery disease (CAD; see entry), and especially if a blood clot forms at a site of the narrowing

(see illustration), the heart cannot get enough oxygen from the bloodstream. The result is chest pain (angina pectoris; see entry)—and possibly a heart attack.

In addition to coronary artery disease and angina pectoris, coronary heart disease includes other disorders that are complications of atherosclerosis, including congestive heart failure and arrhythmias (see entries).

Other heart disorders
Women are likely to encounter several other problems of the heart that are not (or are not always) caused by atherosclerosis.

Hypertrophic cardiomyopathy. The left ventricle of the heart is the main pumping chamber. If it becomes excessively thick and stiff, it will not be able to "relax" and fill with blood (see congestive heart failure). Consequently, not enough blood will flow from the heart to the arteries. Many people with hypertrophic cardiomyopathy have no symptoms until the condition is quite advanced, and, too often, the condition is only diagnosed upon autopsy. Others experience difficulty breathing, fluttering heartbeat, lightheadedness, fainting during exercise, and perhaps chest pain. If detected early enough, this condition can be treated with drugs such as calcium-channel blockers or beta blockers.

Hypertrophic cardiomyopathy has many causes (including coronary artery disease and high blood pressure). There is also a genetic form, so women from families in which several members have died suddenly from a heart problem should consult a physician.

Aortic stenosis. Another cause of a thickened ventricle is aortic stenosis (see entry). In this condition the valve that separates the heart from the aorta—the main artery leaving the heart—narrows. As a result, the heart has to pump harder to keep the blood flowing through the valve, and the left ventricle eventually becomes enlarged from overexertion. Despite the heart's efforts to compensate, various vital organs—including the brain and the heart itself—become deprived of oxygen. When the heart is oxygen-starved, chest pain may result. When the brain is not getting enough oxygen, dizziness or fainting may result. Breathlessness is another common symptom—the body's reaction to its sense that not enough oxygen is reaching life-sustaining organs.

Aortic regurgitation. In this condition, the three leaflets that make up the aortic valve do not create a tight seal (see illustration). Consequently, blood leaks back through the valve into the left ventricle, making it have to pump harder to move adequate blood throughout the body.

Mitral valve prolapse. Many women have a condition in which the mitral valve—which connects the upper left to the lower left chamber of the heart—balloons out (prolapses). This condition usually causes no symptoms, but some blood may flow back (regurgitate) into the atrium whenever the

How the body's natural wound healing can cause a heart attack

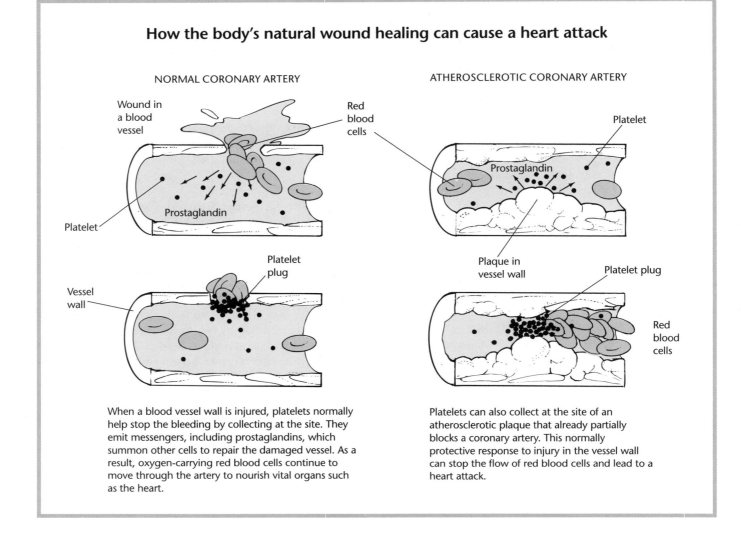

NORMAL CORONARY ARTERY

ATHEROSCLEROTIC CORONARY ARTERY

When a blood vessel wall is injured, platelets normally help stop the bleeding by collecting at the site. They emit messengers, including prostaglandins, which summon other cells to repair the damaged vessel. As a result, oxygen-carrying red blood cells continue to move through the artery to nourish vital organs such as the heart.

Platelets can also collect at the site of an atherosclerotic plaque that already partially blocks a coronary artery. This normally protective response to injury in the vessel wall can stop the flow of red blood cells and lead to a heart attack.

ventricle pumps it in the other direction. Mitral valve regurgitation seems to put people at increased risk for infective endocarditis, an infection and inflammation of the membrane that covers the interior of the heart. People with mitral valve prolapse (see entry) may also be at slightly increased risk for stroke.

Congestive heart failure. This disorder occurs when the heart fails to pump blood out efficiently, and as a result blood that would normally enter the heart backs up in the veins. This inefficient pumping of blood causes tissues throughout the body to be deprived of oxygen, and the backed-up blood in the veins causes fluid to collect in the lungs, lower legs, ankles, and liver.

Congestive heart failure (see entry) can result from a variety of underlying problems, including mechanical problems of the heart valves, damaged heart muscle from previous heart attacks, or long-standing high blood pressure. In women it is less likely to be associated with coronary artery disease than in men.

Arrhythmia. Abnormalities in heart rhythm can be an important complication of heart disease. Arrhythmia is often signaled when a person complains of a racing or pounding heart, but sometimes it is experienced as fatigue, faintness, or blackouts, or it may have no symptoms at all. Coronary artery disease is a major cause of arrhythmia leading to heart attacks, but other causes of arrhythmia include weakened heart muscles (heart failure); imbalances of blood electrolytes, especially potassium; high epinephrine levels (as may occur with excitement); the effects of certain drugs, such as amphetamines, cocaine, caffeine, and alcohol; and thyroid disorders.

There are several types of arrhythmia (see entry), some much more serious, even life-threatening, than others. The first step in evaluating a woman with palpitations is to determine which type is occurring.

Pericarditis. Chest pain similar to that of a heart attack or angina is sometimes due to a totally unrelated condition called pericarditis. This inflammation of the membranous sac surrounding the heart muscle is equally common in both sexes but is more common in younger people. Pericarditis is often due to a viral infection and frequently begins with a cold (upper respiratory tract infection). It can also result from the viruses that cause mumps, influenza, mononucleosis, chicken pox, rubella (German measles), and hepatitis B.

Viral pericarditis, while often dramatic and quite painful, is generally not a serious condition. It disappears on its own after 1 to 3 weeks, and pain can usually be relieved with aspirin or other mild analgesics. But because the symptoms of pericarditis are so similar to those of a heart attack (except that moving the chest rarely exacerbates heart attack pain), anyone who suspects she has pericarditis needs to see a physician immediately. The two conditions can be differentiated by means of blood tests, a physical examination, and an electrocardiogram.

Women and heart disease

There is a slow-dying myth that heart disease is a problem from which women are somehow exempt. This myth flies in the face of the reality that 2.5 million American women are hospitalized annually for cardiovascular disease. Approximately 500,000 American women die of heart problems each year, half of them because of coronary artery disease. In fact,

coronary artery disease is the most frequent cause of death among women in the United States. On top of that, at least 300,000 American women, most of whom are of childbearing age, have a congenital malformation of the cardiovascular system.

Despite these statistics, astoundingly little research has been conducted on the best ways to diagnose, treat, and prevent cardiovascular disease in women. Nor have there been extensive studies of the different psychological, social, or economic factors that may bear on the way heart disease affects women. Until quite recently most studies of heart disease involved only men. Women of childbearing age, for example, were excluded because researchers claimed that compounding variables such as menstrual cycle changes would only complicate results. And older women were excluded because they tended to have more coexisting illnesses than men of the same age. What these studies failed to address was that these very "confounding" factors might have some bearing on how cardiovascular disease manifests itself in women and on the methods that might work in preventing and treating it. Studies under way today are attempting to take the other variables into account.

Many of the risk factors for cardiovascular disease are thought to be similar in both sexes—obesity, cigarette smok-

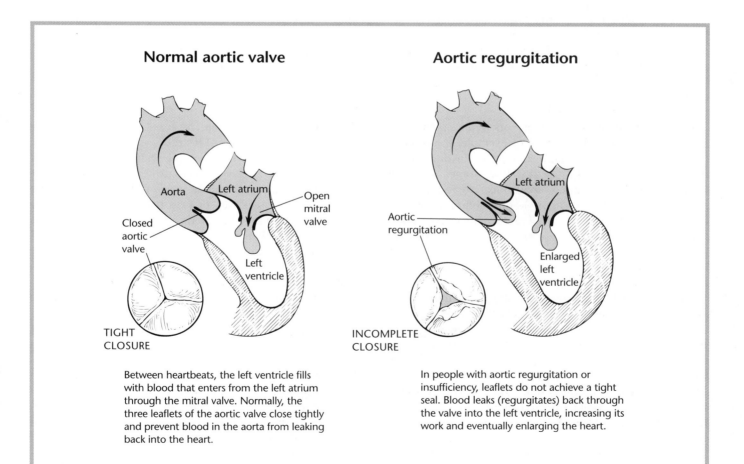

Normal aortic valve

Aorta
Left atrium
Open mitral valve
Closed aortic valve
Left ventricle

TIGHT CLOSURE

Between heartbeats, the left ventricle fills with blood that enters from the left atrium through the mitral valve. Normally, the three leaflets of the aortic valve close tightly and prevent blood in the aorta from leaking back into the heart.

Aortic regurgitation

Left atrium
Aortic regurgitation
Enlarged left ventricle

INCOMPLETE CLOSURE

In people with aortic regurgitation or insufficiency, leaflets do not achieve a tight seal. Blood leaks (regurgitates) back through the valve into the left ventricle, increasing its work and eventually enlarging the heart.

ing, hypertension, diabetes, a sedentary lifestyle, a family history of heart disease, and possibly stress, high blood cholesterol, and high blood fat levels. Other major differences between the sexes do exist when it comes to the heart. These differences are biological, medical, and social.

Biological differences between the sexes. The rate of coronary heart disease is low in women during the reproductive years, whether or not they are using oral contraceptives. Only 1 in 1,000 women aged 35 to 44 and 4 in 1,000 women aged 45 to 54 can expect to develop coronary heart disease. (These statistics are true for all women except diabetic women, who are at the highest risk of all groups.)

After menopause women's risk of cardiovascular disease rises by a factor of 2 or 3. Surgical removal of both ovaries (called oophorectomy) before natural menopause occurs can increase the risk of having a heart attack by a factor of 3. This is usually attributed to a decrease in estrogen production, which is thought to encourage atherosclerosis in the arteries that supply blood to both the heart and the brain.

Although cardiovascular disease tends to develop later in life in women than in men, it is more likely to be fatal once it does develop. Women with heart disease are twice as likely as men to die within 2 months of their first heart attack and are more likely to suffer a second heart attack.

The biological reasons for these differences have not been well studied, but it is known that both the heart and the coronary arteries in women are smaller and lighter than those of men, and this may have some effect on the atherosclerotic process or on the response to treatment. An added factor is that women with heart disease (because they are generally older than men when it develops) tend to have other systemic diseases at the same time.

Medications and operations that work well for men are not always as successful in women. For example, thrombolytic therapy, which involves administering clot-busting drugs to treat heart attacks, works just as well in women as in men at dissolving life-threatening blood clots. Women, however, more frequently develop serious bleeding complications after taking these drugs. In addition, because many women's heart attacks are more severe, because they have other health problems, and because they are older on average than men who have heart attacks, they are less likely to be good candidates for this therapy in the first place.

Surgical procedures to treat coronary heart disease—such as balloon angioplasty (which stretches the arteries with an inflatable balloon), coronary atherectomy (in which atherosclerotic plaques are removed from the arteries), and coronary bypass surgery (in which detours are built around blocked arteries)—are not offered to women as frequently as to men, partly because they simply do not work as well in women. Although long-term survival after these operations seems to be comparable in both sexes, women tend to experience more complications following surgery and are twice as likely as men to continue having symptoms of their disease 4 years after coronary angioplasty.

It is still not clear whether various medications, including aspirin, beta blockers, and calcium-channel blockers, have the same efficacy in both men and women, at least for all applications. Lipid (blood fat) lowering drugs (including Mevacor and Lopid) do appear to have favorable effects in women as well as men, however.

Medical differences between the sexes. Heart disease is not diagnosed until later stages in women, in part because both clinicians and women themselves are less apt to recognize symptoms for what they are. In most medical centers, women with symptoms of heart disease such as chest pain are considerably less likely than men with similar symptoms to receive tests such as a stress electrocardiogram (ECG), which determines how well the heart performs during exercise. When women are given stress tests, their hearts seem to respond differently to exercise than men's and give different readings. As a result, it is sometimes difficult to interpret abnormalities in a woman's ECG according to standards established in studies of men.

Women are also less likely to be referred for coronary angiography, which can show blockage of coronary arteries. They receive fewer invasive surgeries and cardiac medications than men with similar or less severe symptoms. In addition, women are referred less frequently to rehabilitation centers, enroll less frequently, and have poorer attendance than men, possibly because relatively few rehabilitation programs have been developed that pay special attention to the exercise abilities and psychosocial needs of older women.

Whether all of this means that women are receiving too little care, men are receiving too much, or both are getting appropriate amounts remains to be determined.

Social differences between the sexes. Another part of the answer to why the course of heart disease is different in men and women may lie in social factors. Older women (who tend to be the ones who develop cardiovascular disease) may be less likely than men of the same age to have a spouse who pushes them to seek care or who helps them with household duties once they have returned from the hospital. This may in part explain why women who are referred to cardiac rehabilitation programs tend to go much less frequently than men.

Women are more likely than men to suffer from anxiety and depression after they have had a heart attack or surgery for CAD. Some investigators have postulated that these psychological symptoms may be related to the fact that women who have had heart attacks tend to be relatively sicker than their male counterparts and less able to resume normal activities. Women seem to take longer than men to recover from heart attacks and lose more days of work because of heart symptoms in general. Women also return to paid employment after a heart attack less often than do men, although this may reflect the fact that many older women do not work outside the home.

Because depression and anxiety disorders are very common

in women, sometimes women experiencing chest pain and rapid heartbeat are incorrectly assumed not to have coexisting cardiovascular disease. In fact, depression and panic disorders can complicate heart disease further and increase the mortality risk. Women who are taking psychotropic drugs for the treatment of depression or anxiety should mention this fact to their clinician. Not only can many of these drugs have effects on the heart, but certain heart medications (such as beta blockers) can have psychiatric effects as well.

Women with cardiovascular disease also need to speak up about work and family responsibilities that may interfere with their treatment plans. If necessary they may discuss ways to juggle these tasks with a clinician, psychologist, or socialworker, so that outside responsibilities do not jeopardize their health and well-being.

Related entries

Angina pectoris, anxiety disorders, aortic stenosis, circulatory disorders, congestive heart failure, coronary artery disease, diabetes, estrogen replacement therapy, high blood pressure, mitral valve prolapse, panic disorder, stress, stroke

Heartburn

Heartburn is estimated to affect 1 in 10 American adults on a weekly basis and as many as 1 in 3 on a monthly basis. Known in medical jargon as gastroesophageal reflux disease (GERD), it occurs when acid contents of the stomach wash back up (reflux) into the esophagus (food tube). The source of the problem seems to be laxity in the muscle separating the esophagus from the stomach (the lower esophageal sphincter, or LES), which normally opens to allow food to pass into the stomach but otherwise remains tightly shut (see illustration).

Gastroesophageal reflux has long been seen as a nuisance, but it is now recognized as having potentially serious complications in some people. Of greatest concern is the development of Barrett's esophagus, a change in the lining of the esophagus that increases the risk of esophageal cancer.

Who is likely to develop heartburn?

Heartburn is particularly apt to occur in conditions that decrease pressure on the sphincter muscle—such as being pregnant or taking calcium-channel blockers or other smooth muscle relaxants—and in conditions in which pressure in the abdomen increases, such as obesity. It can also happen when a person has a hiatus hernia, a disorder in which part of the stomach protrudes into the chest area through an opening in the diaphragm, the muscle that separates the abdomen from the chest (see illustration).

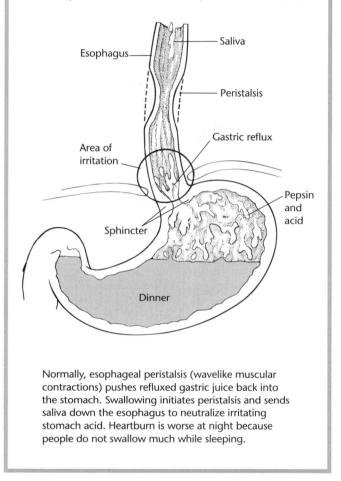

Gastric reflux

The lower esophageal sphincter normally relaxes only to allow swallowed food to enter the stomach or permit gas to escape. If it is looser than normal, heartburn can result.

Esophagus — Saliva
— Peristalsis
Gastric reflux
Area of irritation
Pepsin and acid
Sphincter
Dinner

Normally, esophageal peristalsis (wavelike muscular contractions) pushes refluxed gastric juice back into the stomach. Swallowing initiates peristalsis and sends saliva down the esophagus to neutralize irritating stomach acid. Heartburn is worse at night because people do not swallow much while sleeping.

What are the symptoms?

The pain of heartburn begins as a gnawing or burning sensation in the chest, which may radiate to the arms or jaw. Sometimes sour-tasting materials back up as far as the throat or even the mouth. Over time the irritating acid may lead to esophagitis, or inflammation of the esophagus, a condition that can make swallowing difficult and result in bleeding. Occasionally there may be hoarseness, coughing, or wheezing as well. Symptoms of heartburn generally occur soon after eating and when a person is lying down. Sitting up and having a drink is often enough to provide temporary relief.

How is the condition evaluated?

Because the chest pain characteristic of heartburn is sometimes indistinguishable from that of angina or a heart attack,

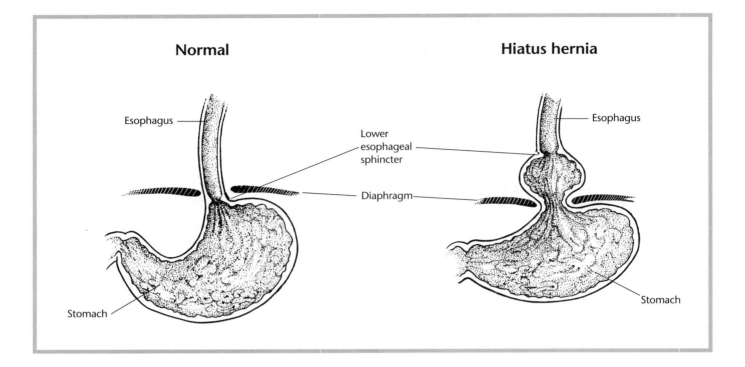

Normal

Esophagus

Lower
esophageal
sphincter

Diaphragm

Stomach

Hiatus hernia

Esophagus

Diaphragm

Stomach

it is important to rule out these more serious conditions—particularly in anyone who is already at risk for cardiovascular disease. If pain in the chest is relieved by sitting up or drinking fluids, if the symptoms occur only after eating or are accompanied by difficulty swallowing, if the pain is not aggravated by exertion, and if over-the-counter antacids provide relief, chances are good that the problem is heartburn. If there is any uncertainty, however, or if symptoms are worrisome, a clinician should be consulted.

Usually the clinician will be able to diagnose heartburn from a simple description of the symptoms, although occasionally more extensive tests—such as an endoscopic examination or barium x-ray of the esophagus—may be necessary. And because gastroesophageal reflux has been linked to precancerous changes in the esophagus, some experts have advocated routine testing with endoscopy for people who have long-standing heartburn. Others point out that because heartburn is so common, and esophageal cancer is so rare, the chance of precancerous changes or cancer being found in a given individual is extremely low. In addition, there are no scientific studies to show whether routine endoscopy can cut down on cancer incidence or deaths. For the time being, women with chronic reflux symptoms should discuss the pros and cons of endoscopy with their physician on an individual basis.

How is heartburn treated?

People with heartburn should try to avoid spicy or fatty foods, alcohol, coffee, citrus juice, and other substances that irritate the esophagus or relax the sphincter muscle. Medications that may aggravate reflux include birth control pills, antihistamines, calcium-channel blockers, nitrates, sedatives,

and some heart and asthma medications. Since lying down on an empty stomach makes reflux less likely, it is a good idea to avoid eating for 2 or 3 hours before going to bed. Some people find it even more helpful to elevate the head of the bed with 6- to 8-inch blocks or to purchase a special wedge that is placed under the shoulders and upper back while reclining (regular pillows, by contrast, tend to increase abdominal pressure and thus aggravate symptoms). It also helps to cut out cigarette smoking—which relaxes the esophageal sphincter muscle even more—and to lose weight if one is overweight. Women who find that their symptoms worsen when taking oral contraceptives should talk to a clinician about adjusting the dosage or changing to another method of birth control.

If heartburn persists, taking antacids such as Mylanta, Maalox, or Gelusil in either tablet or liquid form can provide quick relief. Sometimes stronger drugs, which reduce acid production in the stomach—such as H_2 beta blockers cimetidine (Tagamet), ranitidine (Zantac), famotidine (Pepcid), or proton pump inhibitors such as omeprazole (Prilosec)—may be prescribed as well. Cimetidine, ranitidine and famotidine are available in low doses without a prescription. Alternatively, metoclopramide (Reglan) may be taken to increase the speed with which food is emptied out of the stomach. In rare cases, a surgical procedure called fundoplication may be performed to prevent reflux of stomach acids into the esophagus. In some cases, it may be possible to use a newer, less invasive form of this procedure (laparoscopic Nissen fundoplication), which allows shorter hospital stays and faster recuperation times. The long-term efficacy of this approach, however, remains to be established.

Pregnant women should try lifestyle modifications, dietary

changes, and antacids before resorting to stronger medications. Antacids should be used with caution, however. Not only can they interfere with iron absorption, but also those containing sodium bicarbonate can lead to metabolic problems and fluid overload. Antacids containing magnesium should be avoided in the latter stages of pregnancy because they can slow down or stop labor and can even cause convulsions. Although there is no evidence that H_2 beta blockers or proton pump inhibitors pose a danger during pregnancy, because evidence remains limited, it is prudent to avoid using them unless reflux symptoms are intolerable.

Related entries

Angina pectoris, chest pain, coronary artery disease, obesity, peptic ulcer disease, smoking

Hemorrhoids

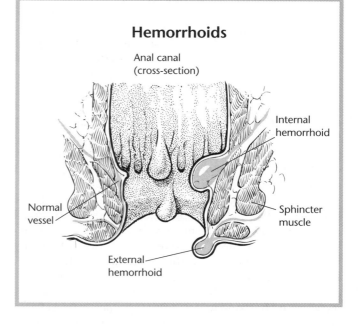

Hemorrhoids

Anal canal (cross-section)

Internal hemorrhoid

Normal vessel

Sphincter muscle

External hemorrhoid

Hemorrhoids are clusters of dilated or swollen veins located at the anal opening or just inside the anus (see illustration). Like other forms of varicose veins (see entry), hemorrhoids (also called piles) are caused by increased pressure which eventually destroys the valves in the veins. Blood pools in the veins, stretching the walls and making them more likely to rupture and bleed during a bowel movement. And because blood flow is slowed in a distended blood vessel, it is also more likely to clot, which increases both swelling and pain.

Who is likely to develop hemorrhoids?

Hemorrhoids are particularly common in people with constipation. Not only can painful hemorrhoids make it more difficult to pass stool, but also straining can itself cause or aggravate hemorrhoids. A vicious cycle can develop when a person overrides the urge to defecate because of hemorrhoids, since this can produce constipation, which can in turn cause even more severe hemorrhoids.

Hemorrhoids are very common in pregnant women, partly because of increased abdominal pressure and partly because constipation is a frequent problem in pregnancy. They may also tend to develop more often in people who are obese.

What are the symptoms?

The classic symptom of hemorrhoids is bright red blood passed during a bowel movement. Sometimes there may be itching or burning around the anus as well, although most hemorrhoids are painless unless blood clots have formed. External hemorrhoids can be seen as small purplish mounds protruding from the anus. Internal hemorrhoids cannot be seen from the outside but may be suspected if there is blood or mucus passed together with hard stools.

How is the condition evaluated?

Usually hemorrhoids are diagnosed on the basis of symptoms, although another relatively minor condition called an anal fissure can lead to rectal bleeding and pain. This deep crack in the mucous membrane of the anal canal can result from constipation, anal surgery, or anal intercourse. Because the treatment for anal fissures is almost identical to treatment for hemorrhoids, there is no particular danger in confusing one with the other.

Nonetheless, rectal bleeding can signal more serious conditions such as colon polyps (noncancerous growths; see bowel disorders) or colon cancer. To rule out these possibilities, a woman who thinks she has hemorrhoids should always be examined by a clinician. Most of the time all that will be necessary is a visual inspection of the anus, sometimes with the aid of a flexible lighted tube called a proctoscope or anoscope. This procedure is mildly uncomfortable, but it takes only a few minutes.

How are hemorrhoids treated?

There is no evidence that any of the heavily advertised ointments and creams sold to relieve hemorrhoids is effective. These products may produce allergic reactions or other side effects in some people. Pregnant women in particular should always consult their clinician before trying an over-the-counter hemorrhoid remedy. Often hemorrhoids that develop during pregnancy will disappear on their own after delivery. In addition, if hemorrhoids are mild, they may require no treatment at all other than taking basic steps to prevent them from worsening.

Some safe home remedies that often help include eating a high-fiber diet and drinking plenty of fluids (to increase stool bulk and decrease constipation), as well as soaking in warm baths. Using a bulk stool softener such as psyllium (Metamucil), methylcellulose (Citrucel), or calcium polycarbophil (Fiberall, Fibercon) is very effective for reducing hemorrhoid discomfort and preventing recurrence. Wiping the affected area with witch hazel, petroleum jelly, or certain herbal preparations (such as combinations of witch hazel leaves, bayberry, and goldenseal) can also be soothing, and many women advocate sitting on hard surfaces or in a "yoga" (tailor) position to take weight off the pelvis. Gently pushing protruding hemorrhoids back into the anus can bring relief. There is no evidence that taking vitamin B$_6$ in any amount will clear up hemorrhoids.

When hemorrhoids continue to burn or itch despite home remedies, or if blood loss seems excessive, a woman should consult her clinician. Sometimes pain and swelling can be relieved by opening the vein and removing a clot or by gently pushing a protruding hemorrhoid back up into the rectum. Internal hemorrhoids can sometimes be removed in a procedure called banding, which involves tying off the blood vessel with a rubber band until it falls off painlessly several days later. (There are so many veins in this area that losing a few makes no difference.) Alternatively, a chemical can be injected into the vein to seal off internal hemorrhoids and prevent further bleeding. This technique is called sclerotherapy (see entry).

External hemorrhoids are too sensitive to pain to make banding or sclerotherapy feasible, but with local anesthesia they can be burned out with an infrared device (a photocoagulator or a laser beam, which may be less painful though more expensive). If hemorrhoids persist or recur, they may need to be surgically cut, tied, or frozen out (hemorrhoidectomy). The more extensive this operation, the more effective it is, and the less chance that hemorrhoids will recur. More extensive operations can also result in an uncomfortable recovery period of a few weeks.

How can hemorrhoids be prevented?

Establishing regular bowel habits, preventing constipation through good nutrition and exercise, and practicing Kegel exercises can all help prevent hemorrhoids or keep them from becoming worse.

Related entries

Bowel disorders, colon and rectal cancer, Kegel exercises, laser surgery, nutrition, polyps, sclerotherapy, varicose veins

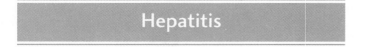

Hepatitis

Hepatitis means inflammation of the liver. It can result from a variety of causes, including viruses that specifically infect the liver, less specific viruses and other infectious microor-

ganisms, and exposure to alcohol, toxic chemicals, or certain medications. Most forms of hepatitis clear up by themselves within a few months, but a small minority of people with certain types of hepatitis go on to develop a chronic and sometimes fatal liver condition.

Types of hepatitis

The most common forms of viral hepatitis are hepatitis A (caused by the hepatitis A virus, or HAV); hepatitis B (caused by the hepatitis B virus, or HBV); hepatitis C (caused by the hepatitis C virus, or HCV, and also known as Type C hepatitis); and noninfectious hepatitis.

Hepatitis C was previously called non-A, non-B hepatitis. This rather vague name arose because, until quite recently, it could not be traced to any one identifiable virus. It is now known that most cases of this form of hepatitis in the United States are due to the hepatitis C virus, although non-A, non-B hepatitis can also be caused by at least one other, rather rare virus, which usually occurs epidemically in nondeveloped areas and sporadically in more developed areas. Unlike other viruses that cause hepatitis, infection with hepatitis C can lead to serious liver disease, often many years after infection. Hepatitis C currently accounts for most cases of liver transplantation in this country. Generally spread through food or water that has been contaminated with feces, this virus seems to be particularly lethal when acquired during pregnancy.

Type A. This is the most common and least serious form of hepatitis. It is usually acquired through contaminated food or water and is present in the stools, blood, and other body fluids of an infected person for 2 to 3 weeks before symptoms develop. This means that a person infected with HAV can infect other people for several weeks before realizing that she is infected.

Most healthy people who acquire HAV recover completely within a month or two. The odds are somewhat lower for elderly people or those with medical problems such as severe anemia, diabetes, or heart disease. Unlike other forms of hepatitis, Type A never becomes a chronic (persistent) condition, nor are there any "carriers"—symptom-free people who carry the virus for life with the potential to infect others. Once a person has had hepatitis A, she becomes immune to future infections.

Type B. Of much greater concern is hepatitis B, which accounts for 9 percent of all deaths worldwide. Hepatitis B is spread mainly through sexual intercourse. It is about a hundred times more contagious than the AIDS virus (HIV) and can be passed through any bodily fluid (including blood, sweat, tears, saliva, semen, and vaginal secretions), as well as through contaminated needles. Thus, HBV can be acquired through kissing or shared toothbrushes, razors, and tattooing, acupuncture, or body-piercing instruments as well as through more intimate contact. During pregnancy or, more frequently, childbirth, HBV can be passed from mother to child.

The great majority of people infected with HBV recover within a few months and after recovery have a lifelong immunity to hepatitis B. About 10 percent, however, become carriers of the virus, with the potential to infect others although they have no further illness themselves. About 3 to 5 percent of all people with hepatitis go on to develop chronic hepatitis and cirrhosis (hardening of the liver). Four out of 5 pregnant women with chronic HBV can expect to pass the infection on to their babies, generally during delivery. Most of these infants become chronic carriers and risk developing serious complications of hepatitis B later in life. Chronic hepatitis B currently accounts for approximately 6,000 deaths a year in the United States.

Type C. The third main category of viral hepatitis, hepatitis C, has only recently been recognized as an even more serious threat to health than hepatitis B. While most people infected with hepatitis B overcome the infection, about 85 percent of those who acquire hepatitis C will retain the virus indefinitely (chronic infection), 70 percent will go on to have lifelong liver disease (chronic hepatitis), 20 to 30 percent will develop cirrhosis after 10 to 20 years, and 5 percent will eventually die from liver cancer or cirrhosis. According to the Centers for Disease Control (CDC), an estimated 3.9 million Americans (1.8 percent) may be infected with HCV, many of them unknowingly.

Hepatitis C already accounts for about 10,000 deaths per year, and increasing evidence suggests that these numbers will grow substantially, possibly killing as many as 30,000 people annually by the year 2010. Because many young people acquire hepatitis C, many experts fear that in the years to come, large numbers of people in their productive midlife years will require liver transplants or develop life-threatening liver disease.

Noninfectious hepatitis. Noninfectious forms of hepatitis are caused by alcohol abuse, exposure to toxic chemicals, and many medications, ranging from painkillers to oral contraceptives, antihypertensive drugs, and steroids.

Who is likely to develop hepatitis?
In the United States hepatitis A occurs in people who eat meals prepared and served by infected food handlers, as well as in people who live or work in mental institutions, day care centers, and the like. It is particularly common among relatively young people.

Hepatitis B is most likely to be found in intravenous drug users who share contaminated needles or in people whose sexual partners have hepatitis B. In addition, health care workers or others who have frequent contact with potentially contaminated blood or needles are at high risk, as are people who work in or have been treated in hemodialysis units (for kidney failure) or homes for the mentally retarded or who have regular household contact with HBV carriers. The rate of chronic HBV infection tends to be higher than average in women of Asian, Alaskan Eskimo, or Pacific Island descent, as well as in women who were born in Haiti or sub-Saharan Africa, and in women who have a history of liver disease or multiple blood transfusions or who have been previously rejected as blood donors.

Type C hepatitis is most commonly acquired by sharing contaminated intravenous needles while using illegal drugs, or after an accidental "needle stick" in a health care setting. Less commonly, hepatitis C can be acquired via sexual contact with an infected partner. Before the hepatitis C virus was identified and blood supplies were screened more effectively (i.e., before July 1992), many people were infected with HCV after transfusions with tainted blood. Anyone who received blood clotting factors made before 1987 is also at risk. As with hepatitis B, infection with hepatitis C is unusually likely in hemodialysis patients, health care workers, persons with multiple sex partners, and infants born to infected women.

Noninfectious forms of hepatitis occasionally occur in people with diffuse bacterial infections (septicemia), as well as in people who have abused alcohol or who have been exposed to toxic chemicals such as carbon tetrachloride.

For reasons that are poorly understood, some people are also susceptible to developing a noninfectious form of hepatitis after they use certain medications, including phenylbutazone (a nonsteroidal antiinflammatory drug), 6-mercaptopurine (used in chemotherapy and to treat Crohn's disease), alpha methyldopa (Aldomet, used to treat hypertension), isoniazid (used to treat tuberculosis), halothane (an anesthetic), high doses of acetaminophen (Tylenol), anabolic steroids (to increase muscle mass), erythromycin (an antibiotic), or chlorpromazine (a tranquilizer).

Anyone with a history of hepatitis or other liver disorders (including jaundice) should always describe these to a clinician before taking oral contraceptives or any of these other medications. Women who have active hepatitis or a history of jaundice (yellowing of the eyes and skin) during pregnancy are usually advised against using birth control pills as a form of contraception.

What are the symptoms?
Whatever the specific cause, all forms of hepatitis can have an acute or active (short-lived) form which involves basically similar symptoms. Many of these resemble symptoms of the intestinal flu: nausea, vomiting, diarrhea, lack of appetite, headache, muscle aches, abdominal pain, and low-grade fever. Often jaundice develops. These symptoms can range from mild or imperceptible to severe and life-threatening.

Hepatitis B, hepatitis C, and, occasionally, medication-induced hepatitis may develop into a persistent form, either as chronic persistent hepatitis or chronic active hepatitis. The former is generally a milder version of acute hepatitis, which frequently has no symptoms and does not progress to more serious complications. It may eventually disappear on its own. Chronic active hepatitis, however, which generally follows hepatitis B or hepatitis C infection, can sometimes progress to cirrhosis, liver cancer, liver failure, or death.

Many people with hepatitis, including hepatitis C, can feel well for many years, or may simply feel fatigued, but may still be experiencing liver damage.

How is the condition evaluated?

Anyone with several symptoms suggesting hepatitis, particularly jaundice, should consult a clinician. Usually urine tests will be done to check for bilirubin, and blood tests will be done to check for certain enzymes called transaminases (aminotransferases) and other indications of liver dysfunction. Blood tests for hepatitis B surface antigen and hepatitis C antibody can also be measured. Often the clinician will feel the right side of the abdomen to check for tenderness or enlargement of the liver. The clinician may also ask for a sexual, occupational, and medical history (including past blood transfusions) and for information about any medications taken in the past few months or any history of drug or alcohol abuse.

If the diagnosis is still uncertain, or if symptoms continue for more than 6 months, a liver biopsy (tissue analysis) may be done to distinguish chronic persistent from chronic active hepatitis.

How is hepatitis treated?

Except in the case of hepatitis C, the symptoms of hepatitis disappear spontaneously within 2 to 3 months or, in some cases, after the discontinuation of the alcohol, toxic chemicals, or medications thought to be causing them. Anyone with hepatitis needs to have blood tests done by a clinician every 1 to 3 weeks until all laboratory results are normal. Patients with hepatitis do not need to restrict their physical activity so long as they do not become overtired. Nor is there any reason to isolate oneself from family members or to stay home from work. It is important for a person infected with hepatitis A to wash her hands thoroughly after going to the bathroom and to make sure other people have no contact with her feces or other body fluids. Dishes and other eating utensils should be heated to at least 120°F for 15 to 20 minutes (in a dishwasher, for example) before they are used by another person.

People with hepatitis should avoid drinking alcoholic beverages during the course of the disease and for at least a month after all laboratory tests have returned to normal. Alcohol (as well as other drugs) cannot be metabolized effectively by a damaged liver. Because the hormones estrogen and progesterone are also metabolized in the liver, premenopausal women with hepatitis should substitute some other form of birth control for oral contraceptives, and postmenopausal women with hepatitis will probably be taken off estrogen replacement therapy.

Because symptoms of nausea, vomiting, and anorexia often worsen as the day goes on, it helps to pack most of the day's calories into a big breakfast. Sometimes drugs such as Benadryl or Compazine may be prescribed to relieve nausea. A person unable to eat or drink adequately may require hospitalization and intravenous feeding for a few days to prevent malnutrition and dehydration.

Treatment with injections of interferon, usually in combination with an oral antiviral drug called ribavirin, may help patients with chronic hepatitis B and C infections, and, in some cases, may lead to the elimination of the hepatitis virus from the body. Side effects of these treatments can include debilitating muscle aches and fever, and because ribavirin can cause anemia, it may be inappropriate for people with heart, vascular, or kidney disease. When interferon is taken alone by patients with hepatitis C, relapse is common after the drug is discontinued. New antiviral and other drugs are currently under investigation, and a drug called lamivudine has recently been approved as an alternative to interferon injections in the treatment of hepatitis B. Liver transplantation may be an option when none of these medications works and symptoms are severe.

How can hepatitis be prevented?

The risk of acquiring hepatitis B and C can be reduced by abstaining from use of illegal drugs and from contact with contaminated tattooing or piercing instruments, by practicing safer sex (including the use of condoms), and by avoiding multiple sexual partners. Women who think they may have been exposed to hepatitis B should have an injection of immunoglobin (hepatitis B immune globulin), a kind of antibody produced by the white blood cells to fight infection, within 8 days. This can sometimes prevent infection, or at least the development of serious symptoms. It is still not known whether administering the standard immune serum globulin after a blood transfusion or high-risk behavior can help prevent hepatitis C. For the time being, a better means of prevention seems to be refraining from high-risk behavior (unsafe sex and the use of intravenous needles), as well as screening blood donors for the hepatitis C antigen and avoiding the use of commercial blood donors.

Women who are at high risk for acquiring hepatitis B—including those with an infected family member or who work in a high-risk profession—should consider immunization, as should women planning to visit regions where HBV is widespread, such as sub-Saharan Africa, Southeast Asia, the Pacific islands, and the Amazon region. The vaccine against hepatitis B, which has been widely used only in recent years, is made through recombinant genetic techniques. This should calm any fears about being infected with the AIDS virus during a hepatitis B vaccination.

For complete immunization three separate injections are necessary, the first two a month apart and the third 5 months later. Though somewhat inconvenient and expensive (running about $100 to $150), this vaccine provides immunity for 5 years or more. Side effects, if any, are almost always mild and transient. Before vaccination is undertaken, however, it makes sense to have blood tests for preexisting immunity.

Because many of the symptoms of hepatitis (such as nausea and vomiting) can be mistaken for symptoms of pregnancy, and because the risk of hepatitis in newborns is high, many clinicians now routinely test the blood of pregnant women for HBV early in pregnancy. If infection has developed during pregnancy, immunoglobin can be given to reduce the severity of symptoms. Because most newborns infected at birth go on to become chronic carriers or develop serious liver disease, arrangements should be made to vaccinate the newborn within 12 hours of birth and again at 1 and 6 months. A dose of immunoglobin is given to the newborn with the first injection of the vaccine.

It has recently become standard practice to immunize *all* newborns—whatever their risk—with hepatitis B vaccine within 1 week of birth, 1 month later, and again at 6 months of age. The American Academy of Pediatrics also recommends hepatitis B immunization for children about to enter kindergarten and for all 12-year-olds.

Hepatitis A can sometimes be prevented by injection with another immunoglobin (standard immune serum globulin) which contains antibodies against HAV. Protection against hepatitis A lasts for only a few weeks, however. If given just before a trip to an area of the world where hepatitis A is prevalent, immunoglobin often can prevent infection. If given within 2 weeks of known exposure to contaminated food or water or other source of infection, it can prevent serious symptoms from developing, if not infection itself.

There is still no immunization available to prevent infection with hepatitis C.

Related entries
Acquired immune deficiency syndrome, alcohol, antiinflammatory drugs, biopsy, birth control, condoms, estrogen replacement therapy, headaches, prenatal care, sexually transmitted diseases

Herpes

Genital herpes is a sexually transmitted disease (STD) that affects as many as 10 million Americans. Its main symptoms are recurrent outbreaks of painful sores in the genital region. The disease is caused by the herpes simplex virus, which takes two forms—herpes simplex virus 1 (HSV 1) and herpes simplex virus 2 (HSV 2). About 80 percent of herpes sores in the genital region (that is, genital herpes) are due to HSV 2. HSV 1, in contrast, accounts primarily for cold sores and fever blisters on the mouth or lips. But because either virus can be passed from genitals to mouth during oral sex (fellatio or cunnilingus), genital herpes is sometimes due to HSV 1, and cold sores and blisters on the mouth and lips can occasionally be caused by HSV 2. Sometimes a person with HSV 1 infection of the mouth can spread the virus to her own genitals with her hands.

Both HSV 1 and HSV 2 belong to the same family of viruses that includes the Epstein-Barr virus (the cause of mononucleosis) and the herpes zoster or varicella zoster virus (the cause of chickenpox in children and shingles in adults). All of these viruses have the ability to remain dormant in the body for long periods of time without making their presence known. Symptoms occur only when the virus is activated, which means an infected person can go weeks, months, or even years between recurrences.

The herpes simplex virus is no exception. After first entering the body—usually following close bodily contact with the mucous membranes of an infected person—it travels into the nerve endings, where it can remain dormant. Outbreaks may continue intermittently for years—particularly during illness or stress—but they are self-limited. Recurrences also tend to become less severe and more infrequent as time goes by.

For most people, herpes does not cause physical complications any more serious than occasional outbreaks of painful sores, and these can usually be satisfactorily controlled with comfort measures and drugs. But because there is still no cure, many people with herpes feel stigmatized by having an ineradicable STD. Some feel depressed because there is little they can do about it, while others feel angry at a former sexual partner for giving them a lifelong disease over which they have little control. Many people worry about how to tell potential sexual partners about their infection without jeopardizing an incipient relationship. Women also worry about whether having herpes will affect future pregnancies.

Who is likely to develop herpes?
Like all sexually transmitted diseases, herpes is most common in the young, the poor, and the urban. But it can develop in anyone who has skin contact with the genital region, lips, mouth, or cheeks of an infected person. Although the virus is more contagious when a person has obvious sores, occasionally it can also be spread through secretions, breaks in the skin, or mucous membranes even during the latent periods. A contaminated finger can transmit the virus to the eyes.

The herpes simplex virus can be passed to an infant as it travels through the birth canal of an infected mother. This is a relatively rare event in the United States, occurring in no more than 1 in 3,000 live births, and possibly in as few as 1 in 20,000. When it does occur, however, it can result in brain damage, blindness, or even death. Infants born to women who contract a new herpes infection just around the time of delivery are at greatest risk of infection: about 50 percent will contract the disease. Although there is some risk in infants born to mothers experiencing a recurrent outbreak at the time of delivery, the chances are much lower (about 5 percent), probably because the baby has acquired antibodies to the herpes simplex virus through the placenta.

What are the symptoms?
About 2 to 7 days after initial infection, many people develop flulike symptoms such as fever, chills, headache, malaise, and muscle aches. There may be pain or itching in the genital region, accompanied—or soon followed—by clusters of small red bumps on the labia, vagina, cervix, perineum, buttocks,

urethra, or bladder. Within a few days these bumps become painful, watery blisters that soon rupture into open, oozing sores. They then scab over and heal themselves within about 3 weeks. Some women develop tender or painful lymph nodes in the groin. These symptoms also disappear by themselves.

Not all women infected with the HSV 2 have symptoms of a primary outbreak. As many as 3 in 5 women infected with the virus are unaware of their infection. Sores on the cervix in particular often go unnoticed. Furthermore, some of the symptoms of the initial outbreak are easily interpreted as symptoms of other conditions. For example, the red bumps that first appear sometimes develop in a shallow linear groove that could easily be attributable to trauma or chafing. The oozing from blisters may be mistaken for abnormal vaginal discharge. And the painful urination that may occur when the urethra or bladder is involved may lead a woman to think she has a urinary tract infection.

After the initial outbreak, some people with herpes never have symptoms again. In others, the virus becomes reactivated periodically—especially during the first year after infection—and the sores may recur, usually in the same place as before. Recurrences are generally milder and shorter than the initial outbreak. In women they are particularly common around the time of menstruation. About half of all infected women have a "prodromal" period anywhere between 30 minutes to 2 days before sores appear. This usually involves stinging, itching, or pain around the area of eruption. People whose initial infection was asymptomatic may remain free of symptoms forever. Often, however, they experience a recurrence later in life without ever having had (or noticed) the primary outbreak.

How is the condition evaluated?

If sores are present, the clinician can often make the diagnosis by examining them, although scrapings from the sores will usually be cultured to confirm that the herpes simplex virus is the culprit. Positive results can be detected in 1 or 2 days but often can require several days. If the sores were healing by the time the culture was done, a false negative result can occur. Women with a new sore in the genital area can increase the accuracy of diagnosis by seeking medical attention immediately.

It is difficult to test for herpes if no symptoms are present, although blood tests that detect antibodies to the herpes virus can be tried. The problem is that the antibodies are present forever once infection has occurred, and most tests cannot differentiate between antibodies to HSV 1 and HSV 2. As a result, many people who already have HSV 1 infections (as manifested by occasional cold sores) will test positive for herpes even if they are not infected with HSV 2. A person recently infected with HSV 2 may show a jump in levels of antibodies several weeks after infection (since it takes awhile for the antibodies to develop), but unless blood was drawn during the initial attack there will be no basis for comparison.

After a person has been diagnosed with herpes, most clinicians will test for other STDs at the same time, since some—like chlamydia and gonorrhea—are often spread along with herpes but may produce no symptoms in women. Women with new herpes outbreaks or outbreaks that are resistant to therapy should consider HIV testing.

How is herpes treated?

Although there is still no cure for herpes, the antiviral drug acyclovir (Zovirax) is often successful in treating outbreaks and reducing the frequency of recurrences. During an attack, the oral form, taken every 4 hours 5 times a day, can alleviate the pain of sores as well as any systemic symptoms, and promotes healing. A topical cream is also available for treating painful sores, but it has no effect on systemic symptoms or speed of healing. The newer antiviral drugs valacyclovir (Valtrex) and famciclovir (Famvir) are just as effective as acyclovir and can be taken less frequently.

Women who have frequent or severe recurrences may be prescribed acyclovir to help suppress potential attacks. This "suppressive therapy" should be stopped periodically (about once a year) to see if the symptoms may be abating on their own; some people, however, will have a severe outbreak as soon as they stop taking the drug.

With or without medication, it is important to keep the sores as clean and dry as possible. Many people believe that reducing stress—or trying various relaxation techniques—can reduce the chances of an outbreak, but there are no solid data to back this up.

Treatment for herpes infection in pregnant women is the same as for non-pregnant women. Delivery by cesarean section may be advisable if there are active sores present when labor begins.

Various self-help measures can provide some degree of pain relief. These include taking aspirin or acetaminophen, soaking the sores in warm baths with baking soda, and drying them with a hair dryer. It is also a good idea to wear cotton underpants that "breathe" so that sores are exposed to the air as much as possible. If urination is painful, it may help to urinate while squirting warm water over the genitals or while sitting in a bath.

Many people with herpes find that talking to other people with the disease—especially in the setting of a support group—helps them feel less isolated and makes it easier to cope with the disease.

How can herpes be prevented?

Avoiding sexual contact with persons who have active herpes sores can greatly reduce the chances of acquiring the disease. It is especially important to avoid direct contact with the sores. And incorporating the basic strategies of safer sex—such as always using a condom unless one is in a mutually monogamous relationship with an uninfected person—can reduce the chances of acquiring herpes from an infected but symptom-free partner. Women who are already infected with the virus can help prevent its spread by avoiding sex when they have active lesions and by using condoms whenever they have sex with an uninfected partner. (Sexual partners who are in a monogamous relationship and who are both already infected with herpes do not need to take these precautions.)

The chance of transmitting herpes during sexual contact can also be reduced by half by taking valacyclovir (Valtrex) daily. The FDA recently approved use of Valtrex for reducing the risk of transmission.

Pregnant women who have active sores or prodromal symptoms in the weeks prior to the expected time of delivery (or when they unexpectedly go into early labor) should be sure to alert their clinician so that a cesarean section can be arranged if necessary.

Related entries
Cesarean section, chlamydia, condoms, gonorrhea, safer sex, sexually transmitted diseases, urinary tract infections

High Blood Pressure

Consistently high blood pressure—hypertension—is a common problem in this country and is considered a major cause of stroke and heart disease. At least 1 in 5 American adults is thought to have high blood pressure. Although the disease is more common in men than in women overall, the numbers balance out with age because women tend to live longer.

Hypertension is not a unitary condition with a single cause but seems to result from a combination of environmental influences in people who are genetically susceptible. There are two basic forms: primary and secondary. Primary hypertension (sometimes called essential hypertension), which accounts for the vast majority of cases, arises on its own without any underlying disease or disorder. In contrast, secondary (or organic) hypertension results from some preexisting condition.

Blood pressure is the amount of pressure exerted by the blood against the arterial walls. It is measured twice: during a contraction of the heart muscle (systolic blood pressure) and during the longer periods of rest between contractions (diastolic blood pressure). Thus, a blood pressure measurement always consists of two numbers, such as 120/80 (read as "120 over 80"). In this case, 120 stands for the systolic pressure, while 80 stands for the diastolic pressure. The systolic pressure is always higher than the diastolic pressure.

A clinician measures blood pressure by using a sphygmomanometer or similar device. The sphygmomanometer consists of a rubber cuff that wraps around the arm just above the crook of the elbow and is connected to a calibrated tube filled with mercury. By pumping the cuff with air so that it squeezes the arm and then listening for pulse sounds with a stethoscope, the clinician gets a numerical reading that corresponds to the height of a column of mercury supported by the blood pressure. Thus, a systolic reading of 120 means that the blood pressure during the contraction of the heart supported a column of mercury 120 millimeters high.

Blood pressure is affected by many factors, some of which are long-standing—such as the pumping power of the heart or the resistance (elasticity and smoothness) of the arteries. But many more transient factors can also account for blood pressure changes: time of day, medications, or current level of emotional stress (including the stress of having one's blood pressure measured!). Only a consistently high reading—measured in at least two different settings by competent clinicians with accurate equipment—is enough to justify a diagnosis of hypertension. The diagnosis of hypertension is not something to be made lightly, since it may result in a lifetime of medication.

The medical community has been steadily lowering its definition of just how high blood pressure has to be before it is considered "hypertension." That is partly because the health risks of high blood pressure increase on a continuum: a woman with a systolic blood pressure of 100 has a lower risk of cardiovascular disease than a woman with a pressure of 120. The U.S. government's Joint National Committee on the Detection, Evaluation, and Treatment of High Blood Pressure defines the following categories:

	Systolic	Diastolic
Optimal	<120	<80
Normal	<130	<85
High Normal	130–139	85–89
Hypertension	>140	>90

Women with blood pressure in the "high normal" range are more likely to develop hypertension later in life than women with "optimal" or "normal" blood pressure.

Whether the same blood pressure should be considered dangerous in people of different age, sex, or ethnicity remains the subject of debate. It is well known that various demographic factors have a major bearing on the consequences of hypertension. For example, serious complications are much more likely to develop in African Americans than in whites with the same degree of hypertension. Similarly, complications are much more likely to develop in men than in women with identical levels of hypertension.

Who is likely to develop high blood pressure?
In the population at large, men are more likely than women to develop hypertension, and African Americans are more likely to develop it than whites. African American women over the age of 40 are twice as likely to have hypertension as white women of the same age. There seems to be a higher than average rate of hypertension among Filipinos and lower than average rates in people of Chinese or Hispanic descent. Because the prevalence of hypertension tends to increase with age, however, these general statements can be misleading. Although blood pressure in young white women tends to be lower than blood pressure in young white men, for ex-

ample, white women aged 60 to 74 are just as likely as white men the same age to have hypertension. For African American women the statistics are grimmer: they are just as likely to have hypertension as African American men their age by the time they reach 45.

Excess sodium in the diet and inadequate potassium and calcium have all been linked to hypertension in certain susceptible people. There is evidence that taking birth control pills may be associated with hypertension in some women. Psychological and social factors—most notably stress—also seem to be involved, although the precise cause-and-effect relationship between stress and hypertension and the role that stress plays in the differentials between men and women need more extensive study. Women who drink 1 or 2 alcoholic beverages per day seem to be at lower risk for developing hypertension than those who do not drink at all; women who drink heavily are at much higher risk.

Women who are obese—that is, who weigh at least 20 percent more than their ideal weight (see weight tables)—develop hypertension 4 times more frequently than nonobese women of similar background. White women who are obese are 8 times more likely to develop high blood pressure, and 10 times more likely to have heart disease, than other women. Losing weight seems to be a good way to lower blood pressure.

The link between diabetes and high blood pressure is equally complicated. Not only are women with diabetes at increased risk for developing hypertension, but also hypertension can exacerbate the complications of diabetes. In addition, both hypertension and diabetes tend to occur together with high levels of blood fats and with obesity, both of which are risk factors for atherosclerosis and heart disease.

Other factors, such as smoking cigarettes, seem to increase the risk of complications once hypertension sets in. Serious complications of hypertension (such as kidney failure) are more likely to develop in African Americans than in people of other ethnic backgrounds. Whether this is because their hypertension is more severe or because there are differences in the arteries themselves is still unclear. Other factors such as differences in the sodium content of the diet, social stressors, lifestyle (especially exercise), and access to medical care may also help explain the disparate nature and rate of hypertension among people of different racial backgrounds.

Secondary hypertension tends to develop in women with various underlying conditions, including atherosclerosis and kidney disorders (see entries). In the case of kidney disease, it is not always easy to know if the hypertension is primary or secondary, since high blood pressure can be either the cause or the effect of kidney disease.

If blood pressure is already high before pregnancy, it often rises even more during pregnancy. If hypertension develops after the 20th week, it can be a sign of preeclampsia—a serious condition that requires close monitoring by a clinician. Women who had hypertension before they became pregnant are considered to be at high risk for complications, and their fetuses are at risk for low birth weight. With good prenatal care and tight control of blood pressure, however, women prone to hypertension during pregnancy can usually deliver healthy, normal babies.

What are the symptoms?

Primary hypertension is a disease without symptoms. The only sure way to know that the blood vessels and organs are at risk for being damaged is a consistently high blood pressure reading.

Hypertension constricts the arterioles—the smallest and thinnest of the arteries throughout the body. One result can be an enlarged heart, since the heart muscle expands as it works more vigorously to pump blood into these vessels. As the heart enlarges, it begins to pump less effectively. Damage to arteries from high blood pressure can cause bleeding into the brain (a stroke) and into the retina of the eye (which can lead to blindness).

Kidney disease, heart attacks, stroke, and congestive heart failure can also occur because hypertension sets the stage for atherosclerosis—the process whereby blood vessels become clogged with fatty deposits and scar tissue (see illustration). The lining of a normal artery permits blood to flow unimpeded. When this lining is damaged, as occurs after years of excessively high pressure on the artery walls, platelets gather at the site to heal the wound. Cholesterol accumulates in the flat muscle cells that line the artery, and these cells start to proliferate. The resulting combination of fat and scar tissue in the arterial wall—called plaque—clogs the artery, and platelets cause the blood flowing over the abnormal lining of the artery to clot. Eventually a clot may become large enough to block abruptly the flow of blood through the artery.

If the clogged or blocked artery supplies blood to the heart, the result is chest pain (angina) and perhaps a heart attack. If the blocked artery supplies blood to the brain, the result may be a stroke. If it supplies blood to the kidney, the result can be kidney failure.

How is the condition evaluated?

If a woman has elevated blood pressure on one or two occasions, the clinician will want to obtain several readings before making a diagnosis of hypertension. It is common for blood pressure to go up when a person is seen in a physician's office or emergency room with an acute illness or injury.

With the advent of easy-to-use home blood pressure monitoring machines, it is now possible to use readings taken outside the doctor's office to determine whether a person has hypertension (as well as to track the effectiveness of blood pressure medications). Home monitoring devices can vary in accuracy, however; the most accurate are those that measure blood pressure in the arm (above the elbow). It is a good idea to bring a home monitoring device to the clinician's office on occasion to compare it for accuracy against the clinician's measurement.

If hypertension is diagnosed, a clinician will do a thorough

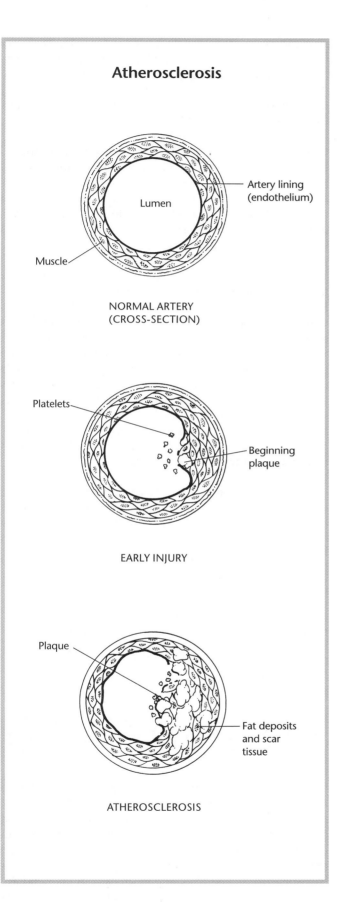

Atherosclerosis

Artery lining
(endothelium)

Lumen

Muscle

NORMAL ARTERY
(CROSS-SECTION)

Platelets

Beginning
plaque

EARLY INJURY

Plaque

Fat deposits
and scar
tissue

ATHEROSCLEROSIS

physical examination to determine the extent of damage to the arteries, if any. Part of this examination will include a detailed family history of hypertension, hormonal abnormalities, and kidney disease, as well as a search for risk factors for heart disease. Various blood and urine tests (including a complete blood count and urinalysis) will also be performed to check the levels of glucose, cholesterol, triglycerides, uric acid, calcium, blood urea nitrogen (BUN), and creatinine. Sometimes an electrocardiogram will be done to evaluate heart rhythm. An ultrasound image can also indirectly give information about the effect of hypertension on the heart muscle.

In some cases a clinician may order additional tests to see if the problem is secondary hypertension (which occurs only 5 to 10 percent of the time). Indications for additional testing include hypertension that came on rapidly without any family history of the disease, or unusually severe and difficult-to-treat hypertension.

How is high blood pressure treated?

People who have blood pressure in the high normal range (>130/85), as well as people with newly diagnosed hypertension, are now being advised to make lifestyle changes to lower blood pressure. This is because mild to moderate hypertension can often be controlled without resorting to medications. Weight reduction in an overweight woman is often enough to bring blood pressure down to normal. Women who are sodium-sensitive will find that their blood pressure responds to a low-sodium diet. People who eat a diet high in potassium, magnesium, and calcium tend to have lower blood pressure. One diet high in these elements, the DASH diet (Dietary Attempts to Stop Hypertension), has been shown to be especially effective in lowering blood pressure. The diet is high in grains, fruits, vegetables, and low-fat dairy products.

If one drinks alcohol, limiting oneself to 7 drinks per week, cutting out cigarettes altogether, and increasing exercise may be helpful, although certain forms of exercise (such as lifting heavy weights) may actually increase blood pressure temporarily. If a woman with high blood pressure is taking oral contraceptives, her clinician will suggest that she stop taking them and switch to another form of birth control. Finally, biofeedback, stress management, as well as regularly practiced meditation or self-hypnosis, and other relaxation techniques can be effective in some cases.

Women with known hypertension often find it helpful to purchase a blood pressure cuff to monitor their blood pressure at home. This allows more accurate assessment of average blood pressure than can be obtained with occasional readings done in the doctor's office.

If these lifestyle changes are unable to control hypertension, or if a woman is at high risk for complications, a clinician will prescribe one of several medications as well. Despite the prevalence (and, in the oldest age group, preponderance) of hypertension among women, most studies of hypertensive medications have involved only men. As a result, there is considerable controversy about whether drugs routinely prescribed for this condition are as effective in women as in men, and whether they have comparable side effects.

Until more studies are done, however, women with otherwise uncontrollable hypertension should continue to use the same drugs men take. Among the most effective and best tolerated are diuretics (water pills), beta blockers, calcium-channel blockers, ACE inhibitors, and angiotensin receptor blockers (see below). Although all these medications control high blood pressure extremely well, only diuretics and beta blockers have been proven to decrease the odds of hypertension-related death from a heart attack. Just which drug is appropriate can vary according to a woman's overall health status. Many other medications (such as hydralazine, aldomet, prazosin, and clonidine) can control high blood pressure, but they must be taken more frequently, and they produce more potential side effects than diuretics, beta blockers, calcium-channel blockers, and ACE inhibitors. But no matter which drugs are chosen, none is a cure for primary hypertension. It is vital for anyone with high blood pressure to keep taking medications for as long as they are prescribed—which often means for a lifetime. Because hypertension has no symptoms, many people stop taking their medications so long as they feel relatively healthy. Once the drugs are stopped, blood pressure rises again and eventually takes its toll on the arteries. And even when medications are taken faithfully, they are less effective in women who smoke, who are obese, and who do not get adequate exercise. Lifestyle changes in these areas can help lower blood pressure and decrease the risk of coronary artery disease.

If a woman needs more than 3 medications to control her blood pressure, she should consult a physician about testing for secondary causes of hypertension. Secondary hypertension is treated with some of the same drugs that are used for primary hypertension. If the underlying disease can be treated effectively, the associated hypertension will disappear as well.

Diuretics. These are the longest-studied and least expensive drugs for controlling high blood pressure and are among the most effective. Also known as water or fluid pills, they seem to work by increasing the output of salt and water by the kidneys, thereby decreasing the volume of blood. Side effects are relatively minimal, generally limited to an increased frequency of urination. Occasionally fatigue or lightheadedness occurs. Anyone using diuretics needs occasional laboratory tests to check for chemical imbalances, especially low potassium, and a lipid profile.

Beta blockers. Propranolol (Inderal), metoprolol (Lopressor), and atenolol (Tenormin) are excellent medications for controlling high blood pressure and for preventing coronary artery disease. They work by blocking the blood vessels' ability to contract. Most patients notice no side effects from using beta blockers, especially the "cardioselective" ones such as atenolol. Among the possible side effects are slow pulse, fatigue, dizziness, depression, diarrhea, cold or tingling fingers or toes, and dry mouth, eyes, or skin. Less often, people may develop insomnia, hallucinations, anxiety, confusion, depression, or breathing difficulties. Beta blockers should be used with caution by people with asthma.

Calcium-channel blockers. Verapamil (Calan, Isoptin), diltiazem (Cardizem, Tiazac), and nifedipine (Procardia, Adalat) reduce pressure in the arteries by preventing the entry of calcium into small blood vessels. Generally these drugs are well tolerated, but fatigue is an occasional side effect, and, less frequently, rapid heartbeat, dizziness, nausea, constipation, and swollen feet, ankles, or legs.

ACE inhibitors. Angiotensin concerting enzyme inhibitors, including captopril (Capoten), enalapril (Vasotec), and lisinopril (Zestril, Prinivil), work by interfering with the production of a protein that constricts blood vessels. ACE inhibitors seem to cause even fewer side effects than some of the other antihypertensive medications and are one of the first-line therapies for hypertension. Occasional side effects include dry cough and in rare cases allergic reactions. ACE inhibitors are often preferable for the many women with diabetes as well as hypertension, since they do not have adverse effects on carbohydrate metabolism and seem to help preserve kidney function. These medications cannot be used during pregnancy because they cause birth defects.

Angiotensin receptor blockers. These drugs are similar in action to ACE inhibitors but do not cause cough as a side effect. Because they are relatively new drugs, they are usually reserved for people who were treated successfully with an ACE inhibitor but developed cough or other side effects.

Related entries
Alternative therapies, birth control, blood tests, cholesterol, circulatory disorders, coronary artery disease, diabetes, diuretics, exercise, heart disease, kidney disorders, obesity, oral contraceptives, preeclampsia, smoking, stress, stroke, weight tables

Hirsutism

Hirsutism means excess hair growth. It is a common problem for women, partly because there are many unrealistic social norms about the amount and distribution of body hair, and partly because different ethnic groups vary considerably in normal amounts of body hair. Asian and Native American women have relatively little body hair of any type, for example, whereas women of Mediterranean extraction often have moderately heavy facial and body hair. It is normal for women to have a few dark hairs on the upper lip, on the breasts, and on the line from the navel to the pubic region (the linea alba), and many women have coarse pubic hairs on the inside of the thighs.

What are the symptoms?

In women, hirsutism involves an increase in the growth of coarse hairs in places where they would ordinarily occur only in males, such as the upper back, lip, chin, upper abdomen, chest, or chin. When hair growth increases all over the body, but particularly on the arms, legs, and scalp, the condition is called hypertrichosis.

Who is likely to develop these conditions?

Hirsutism in women is usually due to an excess of hormones called androgens. Many women with this condition may have other symptoms associated with hyperandrogenism, such as acne, obesity, and irregular menstrual periods. Women taking some medications may also develop hirsutism. Some oral contraceptives contain certain progestins that can have androgenic effects. One of these progestins, norgestrel, has a relatively potent effect, as does the drug danazol, which is sometimes prescribed for endometriosis.

Other medications, including glucocorticoids (antiinflammatory drugs), phenytoin (Dilantin, an anticonvulsant), minoxidil (an antihypertensive drug), and phenothiazines (tranquilizers), can produce hypertrichosis, as can conditions such as hypothyroidism, anorexia nervosa (an eating disorder), malnutrition, porphyria (a disease marked by elevated levels of a blood component called porphyrin), and a disease of the connective tissue called dermatomyositis (see polymyositis and dermatomyositis). Virilization may also be seen with adrenal or ovarian tumors.

How is abnormal hair growth treated?

Treatment for hirsutism and hypertrichosis depends on the cause. Once serious conditions such as a tumor of the adrenal glands or ovaries have been excluded, the condition is often treated cosmetically—with tweezing, bleaching, shaving, electrolysis, or laser therapy. Veniqa is a new topical cream which can inhibit hair growth. In other cases a medication may have to be changed. The oral contraceptive pill slows hair growth in approximately 60 to 100 percent of hyperandrogenic women and is considered the first line of therapy; formulations containing norgestrel or levonorgestrel should be avoided, however. Sometimes excess hair growth is helped by treatment with an antiandrogen, like such as spironolactone (Aldactone). This medication, which is a mild diuretic, has few side effects, but it must be used for at least 6 months before any improvement is evident. It can take up to 18 months for hairs to disappear, even if the excess androgen has been eliminated from the woman's system.

Another antiandrogen, finasteride (Proscar, Propecia), which is better known for treating hair loss and prostate problems (benign prostatic hyperplasia) in men, can also be used to treat hirsutism in women because it promotes the growth of hair on the scalp but blocks it on the body. It can be as effective as spironolactone for hirsutism. Side effects are generally mild but may include breast enlargement and increased sex drive (in contrast to *decreased* sex drive in male users). Because of the potential of antiandrogen drugs to cause male fetuses to develop with female genitalia, they should not be administered to sexually active woman of reproductive age unless they are taking birth control pills.

Related entries

Acne, anorexia nervosa and bulimia nervosa, antianxiety drugs, antiinflammatory drugs, birth control, body image, endometriosis, epilepsy, hair loss, hair removal, high blood pressure, hyperandrogenism, hypothyroidism, infrequent periods, menstrual cycle disorders, nutrition, obesity, oral contraceptives, polymyositis and dermatomyositis

Hormonal Contraception

The pill is the most popular method of birth control in the Western world today, and it is the best-known type of hormonal contraception (see oral contraceptives). In recent years, however, many other methods of delivering hormonal contraceptives have become available. These include injections, implants, rings, patches, and morning-after pills. Some of these methods involve the administration of a hormone similar to the progesterone made by the ovaries (synthetic progesterone, or progestins); others involve a combination of a progestin with estrogen.

The newer progestin-only and combination methods require no interruption of sexual activity for insertion, and, unlike the birth control pill, do not have to be remembered on a daily basis. The progestin-only methods can also be used by women who are breastfeeding or who are unable to use estrogen for other reasons. And while we cannot say with certainty until these methods have been used for a longer period of time, most experts suspect that the newer means of hormonal contraception probably have noncontraceptive benefits similar to those of the birth control pill. These include shorter, more regular menstrual periods; ability to resume fertility quickly once the method is stopped; reduced risk of ectopic (tubal) pregnancies; and reduced menstrual flow and cramping as well as a decrease in acne, excess body hair, iron-deficiency anemia, and premenstrual symptoms. Other possible benefits may well include a lowered risk of ovarian and uterine cancers, ovarian cysts, benign breast lumps, pelvic inflammatory disease, and osteoporosis.

All forms of hormonal contraception, including oral contraceptives (see entry), produce side effects that make them unacceptable to some women. These may include menstrual irregularities, headaches, acne, breast tenderness, weight changes, excess hair growth or hair loss, nausea, and depression. Yet these methods of birth control are extremely reliable and relatively safe, and for some women they represent the best trade-off when convenience, cost, and impact on future fertility are all taken into account. On the downside, none of these methods provide any protection against sexually transmitted diseases.

Hormone injections

Currently only one injectable form of hormonal contraception is available in the United States, the injectable progestin Depo-Provera (medroxyprogesterone acetate). The first and oldest form, it is considered to be a safe and effective method of contraception. Administered in a clinician's office 4 times a year, Depo-Provera may circumvent some of the side effects of the oral birth control pill because it contains no estrogen.

The synthetic hormone in Depo-Provera is chemically similar to progesterone, the hormone produced by the ovaries during the second half of the menstrual cycle. It works by preventing ovulation. Without the release of an egg from the ovary, fertilization and pregnancy cannot occur. Depo-Provera also thickens cervical mucus, which reduces transport of sperm, and induces changes in the uterine lining that make it more difficult for a fertilized egg to implant, should conception occur.

Depo-Provera is injected by a clinician into a woman's buttocks or upper arm. To be fully effective, this injection must be repeated every 3 months. It should also be given only during the first 5 days after the beginning of a normal menstrual period to make sure that the woman is not already pregnant. The exception is women who have just had a baby, who will still not have resumed normal menstrual patterns. New mothers who choose not to breastfeed can have an injection within 5 days of childbirth. Nursing mothers should ideally have an injection 6 weeks after the delivery. If more than 3 months have passed, however, the clinician will probably want to do a pregnancy test before giving the first injection.

When taken as scheduled—every 3 months—Depo-Provera is over 99 percent effective. That is, out of every 100 women using this method each year, fewer than 1 will become pregnant. It is also one of the easiest and most convenient methods of contraception available because a single injection protects a woman against pregnancy for months—during which time it is not necessary to think about contraception at all. Women using this method must return to a clinician's office 4 times a year, however.

At $30 to $75 a shot (4 times a year), the cost of a year's worth of Depo-Provera injections can be about the same as a year's worth of oral contraceptives, that is, roughly $200. But added to this is the cost of visiting a doctor's office or clinic for the injections, as well as the cost of pregnancy tests for women who are more than 2 weeks late for their shots. For some women these charges can bring the cost of a year of Depo-Provera to well over $500.

Many women who use Depo-Provera have some irregular vaginal bleeding and weight gain. About a third of women experience irregular bleeding for the first 3 months, although this bleeding decreases over time. In one large study, women who used Depo-Provera for 2 years gained an average of 8 pounds (about 4 pounds a year), women who used it for 4 years gained an average of 14 pounds (about 3.5 pounds a year), and women who used it for 6 years gained an average of 16.5 pounds (about 2.75 pounds a year). This weight gain, however, is not as common as that associated with birth control pills or hormonal implants (see below). Many women also eventually stop having monthly periods while using Depo-Provera, although this is usually no cause for concern. Some women may also experience depression.

Another area of concern is osteoporosis. This concern stems from one study which showed reduced bone density after 5 years of use. Other research indicates, however, that the only women who experience this side effect are those who smoke cigarettes, a risk factor for osteoporosis in and of itself. Current thinking is that most effects on bone density in adult users are reversible, although there is still some concern about long-term effects in adolescent users.

Depo-Provera should not be used by women with a history of liver disease, major depression, or vaginal bleeding of unexplained origin, nor should it be used by any woman who might already be pregnant. As with the birth control pill, it is important to have a physical examination before the first injection and to tell the doctor about any history of breast cancer, hypertension, diabetes, liver disease, asthma, migraine headaches, epilepsy, abnormal mammograms, benign breast lumps, kidney disease, menstrual irregularities, or depression. Women should also tell health care providers that they are using Depo-Provera for contraception, since the hormone it contains can affect blood tests and the efficacy of certain medications.

Unlike some other forms of hormonal contraception, Depo-Provera is generally considered safe for use during breastfeeding, though it is usually advisable to wait at least 6 weeks after childbirth to have the first injection. The hormone can be passed through the breast milk, but so far there do not appear to be any harmful effects on the infant.

The contraceptive effects of Depo-Provera are fully reversible once the hormone is eliminated from the body—no matter how long the contraceptive has been used. Most women who want to become pregnant can conceive within a year after the last injection of Depo-Provera, and over 90 percent will become pregnant within 18 months. Once a woman has received a shot, however, she has to wait at least several months before changing her mind about having a baby.

Some public health investigators and women's health advocates worry that Depo-Provera is too often given to poor, young, and uneducated women who are not provided with sufficient information about potential side effects.

The ring

A relative newcomer to the hormonal contraception front is Nuvaring, a soft, flexible transparent ring that is inserted into the vagina and steadily emits low levels of estrogen and progestins (ethinyl estradiol and etonogestrel, a breakdown product of desogestrel). The ring is 4 mm thick, 54 mm around, and contains two plastic cores surrounded by silicone tubing and separated by impermeable glass stoppers. It is 95 to 99 percent effective if used correctly.

Although it is necessary to visit a clinician for the initial prescription, a woman can insert the ring at home. The ring is then left in place for 3 weeks and removed for 1 week (during menstruation). Unlike barrier methods of contraception (see entry), the ring doesn't require a fitting or proper placement, nor is there any need to use spermicidal creams or jellies. It generally costs around $30 to $35 per month, plus the cost of the initial examination.

Like so many of the newer forms of hormonal contraception, the ring doesn't require daily motivation for use. Because it releases the hormones in a steady dose, too, it keeps blood levels of hormones relatively constant and leads to better-controlled menstrual cycles than does the birth control pill. Its effects can also be reversed fairly quickly should a woman wish to become pregnant.

On the downside, about 1 in 4 women using the ring can expect to experience some degree of spotting even after the ring-free week has passed. Some women also complain that the ring can be felt—or even fall out—during sexual intercourse. The side effects of the ring include a somewhat elevated risk of blood clots probably similar to those associated with the birth control pill, as well as headaches, vaginal discharge, and vaginitis in some women. Oil-based medicine to treat yeast infections cannot be used while the ring is in place, nor can barrier methods be used as back-up methods of contraception or to help prevent sexually transmitted diseases.

The patch

One of the newest means of hormonal contraception is Ortho Evra, an adhesive patch attached to the skin that releases a combination of hormones (norelgestromin and ethinyl estradiol) into the body through the skin. Ortho Evra is a square (20 cm per side) made up of three layers: an outer layer of polyester, a medicated adhesive middle layer, and a clear inner liner that is removed before the patch is applied to the buttocks, stomach, upper outer arm, or upper torso. It is sold in packets of 3 for a single menstrual cycle, with individual replacement patches sold separately.

Like most of the other newer forms of hormonal contraception, the patch is extremely effective if used correctly. Its effectiveness can be as high as 99 percent, although the rate is slightly lower in women who weigh more than 198 pounds. Other advantages include the fact that the patch needs to be applied only once a week, and, unlike some other hormonal methods, it only rarely causes spotting or other abnormal vaginal bleeding. Fertility is resumed quickly once patch use is stopped.

Risks are similar to those associated with birth control pills. Other adverse effects may include breast discomfort, nausea, menstrual cramps, headaches, and, occasionally, irritation around the site of application. Some women who wear contact lenses have also complained that Ortho Evra has led to blurry vision or has made it impossible to wear the lenses.

The price of the patch is comparable to that of many other forms of hormonal contraception: about $30 to $35 a month, plus the cost of the initial examination.

The morning-after pill

In many cases it is still possible to prevent conception from occurring even after sexual intercourse has taken place. The most effective methods include taking a high dose of estrogen alone or a high dose of estrogen combined with a progestin—in other words, taking oral contraceptives in higher than normal doses. Such agents probably prevent conception or implantation by interfering with ovulation, slowing the movement of the egg through the fallopian tube, or altering the uterine lining so that implantation is less likely.

One widely used method of morning-after contraception involves taking 2 birth control pills (such as Ovral) containing a synthetic estrogen (often ethinyl estradiol) combined with a progestin (often levonorgestrel) within 72 hours of unprotected intercourse, and then taking 2 more of these pills 12 hours later. Before using any form of morning-after contraception, a woman should be evaluated by a clinician. This can sometimes be done over the telephone if the woman and the clinician already know each other. Two prescription drugs are marketed specifically as a morning-after pill. "Plan B" contains levonorgestrel only, with one pill taken within 72 hours of intercourse and one 12 hours later. Because there is no estrogen in this pill, there are fewer estrogen-related side effects such as nausea or vomiting. "Preven kits" are also available by prescription and include four pills (a combination of levonorgestrel and ethinyl estradiol) that either delay or stop ovulation or prevent a fertilized embryo from implanting in the uterus. A urine pregnancy test is included. Morning-after pills cost about $15.

A newer method of morning-after contraception—which may also disrupt a pregnancy that has already begun—involves taking a single dose of the antiprogesterone mifepristone. More widely known as RU-486 (see nonsurgical abortion) or the "French abortion pill," mifepristone also shows promise as a daily contraceptive, since low daily doses can inhibit ovulation with an efficacy rate comparable to that of progestin-only oral contraceptives. And since RU-486 taken just after midcycle prevents the buildup of the uterine lining, it may even be effective as a once-a-month contraceptive if taken around the time of ovulation. Even so, there are practical problems preventing its widespread use as a contraceptive—most notably the problem of how to make it widely available without encouraging its unauthorized use as an abortion drug.

It is impossible to measure the efficacy of morning-after pills precisely, simply because no one knows for sure if conception would have occurred if the pills had never been taken in the first place. Still, by most estimates, taking these pills probably reduces the risk of pregnancy after unprotected intercourse by 90 to 95 percent.

Although it is easy enough to take the morning-after pill, women must consult a clinician within days of having unprotected intercourse if this method is to work. To be effective, a morning-after pill must be taken within 72 hours. In some states women can now obtain "emergency contraception" directly from a pharmacist. In others, it is available over the Internet through the Planned Parenthood Federation of America and at least one for-profit Web site. Under these programs, a woman reads a consent form and provides personal information, after which she gives her credit card number to pay a screening fee of between $40 and $74. After a doctor or nurse practitioner reviews the form, she is given dosage instructions and can phone her prescription in to a nearby pharmacy.

The morning-after pills used today are not associated with any serious side effects, although some women do experience unpleasant but brief bouts of nausea, vomiting, breast tenderness, and disturbed menstrual cycles. The effects of these drugs on a preexisting embryo are unknown. Women who have used morning-after pills should have normal fertility if they attempt to conceive later on.

Male hormonal contraception

Despite many years of research, the prospects for finding a safe, effective male contraceptive pill remain dim. One of the basic problems is that the mechanisms that lead to sperm production in a man are closely linked to the mechanisms for sex drive and potency. As a result, drugs that interfere with the development of sperm also interfere with a man's desire or ability to have sexual intercourse in the first place. Complicating matters further is the fundamental truth that it is ultimately the woman who gets pregnant. The motivation in most men to use contraception or risk its side effects is therefore not comparable to most women's. This means that even if and when an effective male contraceptive becomes available, most women would be able to rely on it only in close and trusting relationships.

One way researchers have tried to inhibit sperm production (spermatogenesis) is to give injections of the hormone testosterone. Large amounts of this androgenizing hormone inhibit the secretion of follicle stimulating hormone and luteinizing hormone from the pituitary gland, which in turn inhibits spermatogenesis. The many variations on this approach seem to block sperm production completely in some men but not in all.

An alternative approach involves taking testosterone together with drugs called gonadotropin releasing hormone (GnRH) agonists, which suppress the secretion of luteinizing hormone and follicle stimulating hormone. This approach seems to be more effective in bringing the sperm count down to zero. But because this method requires daily injections, it is impractical. On top of that, it often leads to unacceptable side effects, including blood clots, an enlarged prostate gland, and changes in blood lipoprotein levels.

Related entries

Abortion, acquired immune deficiency syndrome, birth control, condoms, diaphragms and cervical caps, douching, intrauterine devices, lubricants, menstrual cycle, natural birth control methods, nonsurgical abortion, oral contraceptives, pregnancy testing, safer sex, sexual response, sexually transmitted diseases, spermicides, tubal ligation, vacuum aspiration

Hyperandrogenism

In hyperandrogenism a woman has an excess of hormones called androgens. Although all women have relatively low levels of these hormones circulating in their blood, at higher levels these hormones (which include testosterone) produce traits associated with masculinization. As androgens increase above normal levels, certain symptoms may appear sequentially—first acne, hirsutism (excess hair growth), and irregular or absent menstrual periods, and at higher levels, male pattern balding, deepening of the voice, increased muscle mass, and, finally, enlargement of the clitoris.

Excess androgens can be produced by either the adrenal glands (two glands that sit above the kidneys) or the ovaries or both; levels so low that they may not even be measurable in a laboratory test can sometimes result in symptoms. By far the most common cause of hyperandrogenic symptoms is polycystic ovary syndrome (PCOS). In this noncancerous condition the ovaries contain rings of tiny follicles (cysts) around overgrown central tissue and may also be enlarged (see illustration).

About half the women with PCOS are obese. But whether or not they are in fact obese, hyperandrogenic women appear to have several metabolic abnormalities that are typically associated with obesity. For example, they are significantly more resistant than average to the effects of the hormone insulin, which means that they may have abnormally high blood sugar levels. It is not yet clear whether elevated levels of insulin cause the production of excess androgen or vice versa. Because of insulin resistance, women with PCOS are at substantial risk of developing Type 2 diabetes—about 7 times greater than women without PCOS (see diabetes).

Preliminary studies also indicate that hyperandrogenic women have higher total cholesterol levels and lower high-density lipoprotein levels than other women of similar weight. They may also have larger waist-to-hip ratios than women with normal androgen levels. All of these symptoms in the general population have been associated with an increased risk of atherosclerosis and heart disease, although it has not yet been shown that women with hyperandrogenism actually have a greater incidence or earlier onset of heart problems than other women.

Who is likely to develop hyperandrogenism?

Most women with hyperandrogenism have polycystic ovary syndrome. But hyperandrogenism may also occur if androgens are taken by female athletes to help build muscles or by transsexuals to promote a conversion to a male body type. Medications given for other purposes may sometimes have androgenic side effects as well. For example, oral contracep-

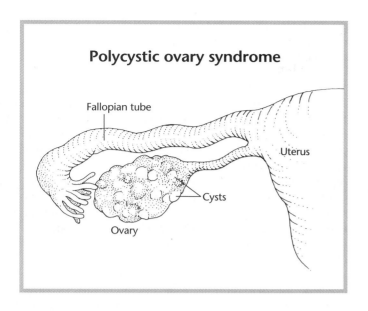

Polycystic ovary syndrome

Fallopian tube

Uterus

Cysts

Ovary

tives containing a progestin (synthetic progesterone) called norgestrel can produce androgenic effects, as can Danazol, a drug prescribed for endometriosis.

Certain genetic defects can alter the production of androgen, producing symptoms indistinguishable from those of PCOS. The most common of these defects is called congenital adrenal hyperplasia. Newborn females with this syndrome have ambiguous genitalia and certain sodium and potassium imbalances. In a milder form of the defect, symptoms such as menstrual irregularity appear at puberty.

Elevated levels of one type of androgen, as well as excess body hair, have been linked to high levels of prolactin, a hormone produced by the pituitary gland which stimulates breasts to produce milk. Prolactin inhibits the production of hormones that induce ovulation. One indication of high prolactin levels is galactorrhea, the production of breast milk in a woman who has not recently had a baby.

Usually the prolactin levels associated with hyperandrogenism are only mildly elevated and there is no sign of a pituitary tumor. In rare cases, however, the excess androgen may be coming from a tumor of the adrenal glands or the ovaries. If symptoms appear abruptly or rapidly, when they are especially severe in light of the woman's family history, and if they are not associated with puberty, a tumor is suspected.

How is the condition evaluated?

The most important step in evaluating hyperandrogenism is to determine its cause. Any woman with symptoms suggesting this condition needs to see her primary care physician, who will first take a detailed history. This will include a review of symptoms (including when they started and how they have changed over time), as well as a complete menstrual history (to be correlated with body weight) and a list of all medications that might have produced excess androgens as a side effect. A family history can also be very helpful in ruling out various causes or suggesting a possible genetic predisposition.

Next the physician will conduct a thorough physical examination, focusing on the symptoms that may be due to excess androgen. Blood tests will be performed, including a check of androgen and probably prolactin levels, as well as various other tests, depending on the results of the history and physical exam. Ultrasound may be used to identify any abnormalities of the ovaries.

If a serious condition such as a tumor or genetic defect is suspected, or if androgen levels are particularly high, the woman probably will be referred to an endocrinologist (a physician who specializes in glandular disorders) or other specialist for further evaluation.

How is hyperandrogenism treated?

If there do not seem to be any underlying diseases causing hyperandrogenism, the first line of therapy is the oral contraceptive pill containing a non-androgenic progestin. It may take at least 6 months for excess body hair to begin disappearing, so women with hirsutism should consider cosmetic approaches as well (such as tweezing, bleaching, shaving, or electrolysis). If contraceptive pills are ineffective, an antiandrogen therapy may be added.

Spironolactone (a diuretic drug) is the most potent antiandrogen currently available in the United States. Women taking it should increase their daily fluid intake and also have their potassium level checked within a few weeks of starting therapy. Although spironolactone can produce menstrual irregularity in women who previously had regular periods, in women with irregular periods it can help normalize the menstrual cycle.

Women of reproductive age who are taking antiandrogens should use an effective contraceptive because the drugs can cross the placenta and block the normal development of a male fetus. Often oral contraceptives are recommended in conjunction with antiandrogens because they regulate menstruation and further reduce androgen levels. Because of their low failure rate, they are also the preferred form of birth control for women with excess androgens. Women diagnosed as having excess levels of prolactin should avoid oral contraceptives because the estrogen in them tends to increase prolactin levels and could induce tumor growth. Women with irregular menstrual periods and few cosmetic symptoms (such as hirsutism and acne) may prefer cyclic progestin therapy (such as Provera) over daily oral contraceptives.

Another aspect of treatment involves monitoring for the health effects associated with hyperandrogenism. Women with irregular menstrual periods, for example, need to be treated (with birth control pills or cyclic progestins) to prevent endometrial hyperplasia, a thickening of the uterus which is sometimes a precancerous condition.

All women with PCOS should also be assessed for cardiovascular risk factors, including a family history of heart disease, high cholesterol in the blood, high blood pressure, and a history of smoking. Because many women with hyperandrogenism are resistant to insulin, a doctor may also want to perform a blood test to look for early diabetes in women who are obese or who have other cardiovascular risk factors. Any treatment that reduces insulin resistance in both lean and obese women with PCOS can have additional beneficial effects, including menstrual regularity, decreased hair growth, and (presumably) improved fertility. Weight loss has been shown to be effective in reducing insulin resistance. Several drugs, such as metformin, are also effective in decreasing insulin resistance and the symptoms of PCOS. Although there is still no concrete evidence that women with PCOS are more susceptible than other women to cardiovascular disease, a woman and her doctor may decide to treat these risk factors directly through weight loss or dietary changes. Obesity itself tends to intensify the hirsutism, menstrual irregularity, and insulin resistance typical of this condition.

If a woman with hyperandrogenism is infertile, she can be referred to a reproductive endocrinologist. Usually anovulation (the failure to release an ovum) is the cause of infertility in hyperandrogenic women. Clomiphene citrate (Clomid or Serophene), a fertility drug, triggers ovulation in about 80 percent of women with PCOS, and about 50 percent of these women will successfully become pregnant. This drug slightly increases the chance of conceiving twins. Insulin-sensitizing drugs such as metformin further improve the effectiveness of clomiphene in producing ovulation and are increasingly used for women with PCOS that proves resistant to clomiphene alone.

If an ovarian or adrenal tumor is identified, removing it usually results in a complete cure. Many small ovarian tumors can now be removed by laparoscopy (see entry), a procedure that involves making a small incision just below the navel. It requires a shorter recovery time than more traditional abdominal surgery. Congenital adrenal hyperplasia may be treated with glucocorticoid replacement therapy, antiandrogens, or oral contraceptives.

Elevated prolactin levels may improve with low-dose bromocriptine therapy. It is important to start with very low doses taken with food at bedtime to avoid the nausea and confusion that are frequent side effects. Usually the endocrinologist will increase the dose at weekly intervals until prolactin levels are in the normal range.

Related entries

Acne, amenorrhea, birth control, cholesterol, coronary artery disease, diabetes, dilatation and curettage, diuretics, endometrial hyperplasia, endometriosis, galactorrhea, hair loss, high blood pressure, hirsutism, hyperprolactinemia, infertility, infrequent periods, menstrual cycle disorders, obesity, osteoporosis, ovarian cancer

Hyperprolactinemia

Hyperprolactinemia is a condition in which the pituitary gland at the base of the brain secretes excess levels of the hor-

mone prolactin into the bloodstream. Prolactin plays a major role in stimulating the breasts to secrete milk and, indirectly, in inhibiting ovulation.

Who is likely to develop hyperprolactinemia?

Prolactin levels rise temporarily under many normal conditions, including pregnancy, breastfeeding, sexual intercourse, nipple stimulation, stress, and exercise. It is also normal for prolactin to increase when estrogen levels rise at various times in the menstrual cycle and after a meal. Persistently high levels of prolactin, however, may be due to a noncancerous tumor of the pituitary gland. The majority of these tumors (called prolactinomas) diagnosed in women are less than 10 mm in diameter, although occasionally a larger tumor may be present. Often, however, no tumor can be seen radiologically.

Another condition that can lead to hyperprolactinemia is a deficiency of thyroid hormone (a condition called hypothyroidism). Hyperprolactinemia may also result from excess growth of the pituitary gland and from a disorder of the adrenal glands called Cushing disease (a variant of Cushing syndrome; see entry). Various tumors and disorders of the hypothalamus (the part of the brain that regulates hormone release), kidney failure, and liver disease can also be responsible, as can ulcer medications, tricyclic antidepressants, and some tranquilizers, narcotics, and antihypertensive medications.

What are the symptoms?

Elevated prolactin levels can cause abnormalities in the menstrual cycle, ranging from irregular periods to absence of periods. Sometimes women with hyperprolactinemia have what is known as the amenorrhea-galactorrhea syndrome, a condition in which menstrual periods stop and milk can be expressed from the breasts of a woman who has not recently breastfed a baby. Sometimes excess levels of prolactin can lead to infertility. Many women with hyperprolactinemia have decreased levels of ovarian hormones, which in turn can cause abnormal menstrual cycles, vaginal dryness, and pain on intercourse, as well as fatigue and diminished sex drive. Women with both excess levels of prolactin and abnormal menstrual periods are also more prone to losing bone mass, a condition that can lead to osteoporosis.

Women with hyperprolactinemia may have signs of hyperandrogenism (excess levels of hormones called androgens) such as hirsutism (excess body hair). Large tumors on the pituitary may cause visual difficulties, headaches, and numerous other symptoms that result from the pressure of the tumor on the gland and surrounding brain structures.

How is the condition evaluated?

An evaluation involves taking a history (which should include information about any menstrual irregularities) and a blood test to measure prolactin levels. This test is most accurate if done after an overnight fast and in a nonstressed condition. Because prolactin levels fluctuate, a repeat test is usually done to confirm any abnormality that may appear the first time around. Even relatively modest elevations of prolactin may indicate a number of diagnoses, including hypothyroidism and pregnancy, both of which can be checked with a blood test.

If these possibilities, as well as chronic kidney disease, are eliminated, and if medications are not the cause, an MRI (magnetic resonance imaging) scan will be done to see if there is a visible tumor. An MRI will also be done if prolactin levels are extremely high. The painless procedure uses magnetic fields to produce images of internal structures. Because MRI is still expensive and not available in all medical centers, an alternative scanning procedure, a CT scan (computerized axial tomography), may be used instead.

How is hyperprolactinemia treated?

Women with regular menstrual cycles who have small tumors or no evidence of a tumor may just be watched carefully by the physician. Prolactin levels will be measured regularly, and MRI scans will be taken to make sure tumors have not developed or enlarged. Prolactin levels sometimes remain stable and may even return to normal, particularly in women who had no initial menstrual irregularities.

Women with higher levels of prolactin or whose periods are irregular or absent usually require drugs or surgery. And treatment is always necessary in the case of large tumors. Most commonly drug therapy is tried first, usually with bromocriptine, which lowers prolactin levels. Bromocriptine shrinks tumors, sometimes making surgical removal unnecessary, or at least making very large tumors easier to remove. It can also normalize menstrual cycles and stop the production of breast milk.

Starting the drug at very low doses and taking it with food at bedtime can help minimize common side effects, which include nausea, nasal congestion, headache, dizziness, and constipation. The dosage can then be increased at weekly intervals until prolactin is in the normal range. In rare cases, chronic use of bromocriptine can produce alcohol intolerance, involuntary movements, fatigue, depression, and anxiety. For women who develop side effects, a newer drug, cabergoline (Dostinex), is as effective as bromocriptine; it can be taken once or twice a week, and causes fewer side effects but is more expensive.

There is no evidence of any abnormalities in babies born to women who became pregnant after bromocriptine had normalized their menstrual cycle. Nor does bromocriptine therapy appear to damage the fetus or breastfeeding infant. Women with hyperprolactinemia, however, are generally advised to stop using bromocriptine if they find they are pregnant. Because the normal hormonal changes of pregnancy increase the size of the pituitary gland, pregnant women may experience visual difficulties, headaches, and excessive thirst and increased urination (a condition called diabetes insipidus, caused by a shortage of an antidiuretic hormone produced in the pituitary). Any pregnant woman with hyperprolactinemia should see a specialist on a monthly basis so that her symptoms can be monitored and treated if necessary.

Women whose tumors are unresponsive to bromocriptine or cabergoline may require surgery to remove the tumor. When performed by an experienced surgeon, this can often be accomplished without damaging the function of the pituitary gland, and there are rarely complications. Some evidence indicates, however, that hyperprolactinemia may recur after 4 to 5 years in up to half the people who have surgery, even though the tumor itself seems to be gone. Radiation therapy may be necessary following surgery, especially in women who are not considering bearing a child.

Surgery is usually not an option for large tumors, but bromocriptine can reduce prolactin levels, relieve symptoms, or shrink tumors to a size at which surgery may be more successful.

When hyperprolactinemia is caused by a lack of thyroid hormone, it can be treated with thyroid hormone supplements. Eliminating the responsible drug or underlying defect (when possible) will alleviate hyperprolactinemia arising from other causes.

Related entries

Amenorrhea, antianxiety drugs, antidepressants, birth control, blood tests, Cushing syndrome, high blood pressure, hirsutism, hyperandrogenism, hypoglycemia, hypothyroidism, infertility, kidney disorders, menstrual cycle disorders, osteoporosis, pain during sexual intercourse, sexual dysfunction, substance abuse, vaginal atrophy

Hyperthyroidism

Hyperthyroidism is a condition that results from an excess of thyroid hormone, which in turn increases the body's metabolic rate. It occurs 5 to 10 times more often in women than in men. Some studies estimate that 4 to 20 out of every 1,000 women have this disorder, although judging the exact prevalence is difficult, since mild forms may go unnoticed, and inadequate screening tests in past years may have missed many symptom-free cases. Most cases of hyperthyroidism can eventually be cured with drugs or surgery.

Produced by the thyroid gland at the base of the neck (see thyroid disorders), thyroid hormones are crucial for both growth and development. Without sufficient thyroid hormones (hypothyroidism), the whole body slows down, leading to tiredness, weight gain, constipation, and other symptoms. Too much thyroid hormone (hyperthyroidism), however, can cause increased appetite accompanied by weight loss, heat intolerance, insomnia, sweating, hand tremors, heart palpitations, goiter, shortness of breath, mood swings, muscle weakness, diarrhea, and hyperactivity or apathy.

The most common form of hyperthyroidism is Graves disease. It occurs when an abnormal antibody stimulates the thyroid to secrete excessive amounts of thyroid hormone. Other sources of too much thyroid hormone are toxic nodules. These involve one or more discrete lumps which develop in part of the thyroid gland and manufacture excessive amounts of thyroid hormone. Toxic nodules are almost never cancerous.

DeQuervain's thyroiditis and silent (or painless) thyroiditis (part of the spectrum of autoimmune thyroid disease) are two other forms of hyperthyroidism which occur when part of the thyroid gland becomes inflamed and destroyed, resulting in the release of large amounts of stored thyroid hormone. Occasionally exposure to excess iodine can also result in hyperthyroidism.

Who is likely to develop hyperthyroidism?

Graves disease can occur at any age, but it is most common in women in their 20s and 30s. Toxic nodules occur most often in women over age 60, and these older women are more likely to develop a form of hyperthyroidism called subclinical hyperthyroidism. Although often so mild that there are no apparent symptoms, subclinical hyperthyroidism can increase the risk of irregular heartbeat, reduce bone density, and exacerbate angina or congestive heart failure.

DeQuervain's thyroiditis often follows a viral respiratory illness, while silent or painless thyroiditis is relatively common in the postpartum period.

In rare instances women exposed to radiocontrast dye (used in various medical tests including hysterosalpingograms), kelp tablets, povidone-iodine douches, iodine-containing expectorants, and amiodarone (Cordarone, used to treat heart arrhythmias) may develop iodine-induced hyperthyroidism.

What are the symptoms?

The most common symptoms of Graves disease are increased appetite accompanied by weight loss, heat intolerance, insomnia, sweating, hand tremors, heart palpitations, enlarged thyroid gland (a goiter), shortness of breath, mood swings, muscle weakness, bowel disorders such as frequent bowel movements and diarrhea, hyperactivity (or apathy in elderly people), and, rarely, anorexia and vomiting. Bulging eyes, sometimes severe enough to impair vision, are characteristic of this disease.

In addition, women often have irregular menstrual periods and fertility problems, including frequent miscarriages. Sometimes there may be accompanying blood disorders or pernicious anemia. Osteoporosis (porous bones) may develop because thyroid hormone can directly reduce bone density. Osteoporosis (see entry) is a systemic and often debilitating skeletal disease in which the bones gradually lose their store of calcium and other minerals. As a result they become less dense and more susceptible to fracture from even slight trauma.

Symptoms of toxic nodules and iodine-induced hyperthyroidism are similar to those in Graves disease except that the eyes do not protrude. By contrast, deQuervain's and silent thyroiditis often involve a period of hyperthyroidism when the stored hormone is first released, followed by a period of hypothyroidism and, eventually, recovery. Sometimes there are very few if any symptoms.

How is the condition evaluated?

Thyroid function is most reliably evaluated by measuring the levels of thyroid stimulating hormone (TSH) in the blood serum. TSH is the hormone produced by the pituitary in the brain which controls thyroid hormone production via a very sensitive feedback loop between the brain and the thyroid gland. As the level of thyroid hormone is increased, the message gets back to the brain to decrease production of TSH. If an abnormally low TSH level is detected and thyroid hormone levels are higher than normal, hyperthyroidism is present. Appropriate treatment depends on determining the specific form of hyperthyroidism.

These can be differentiated with a radioiodine uptake test—a thyroid scan to measure the amount of iodine that collects in the thyroid gland over a 24-hour period. If hyperthyroidism results from the production of new thyroid hormone (as it does in Graves disease and toxic nodules), radioiodine uptake will be elevated. This happens because iodine is a vital component of thyroid hormone and is taken up in large amounts when the hormone is being produced. A thyroid scan can then distinguish Graves disease from toxic nodules.

Thyroid scans are done on an outpatient basis. The patient first swallows or has an injection of radioactive iodine and then returns the next day. A special camera produces an image of the thyroid, based on the amount of radioiodine that has collected at various sites. Since iodine is a key component of thyroid hormones, nodules with high levels of radioactivity will be assumed to be synthesizing large amounts of these hormones.

If a woman who is breastfeeding develops hyperthyroidism, she must interrupt nursing to have a thyroid scan. For mild cases, such as painless thyroiditis, the radioiodine uptake test can be deferred until after the baby is weaned. In the meantime, the ratio of thyroid hormone levels in the blood can often be used to determine if some other form of hyperthyroidism may underlie the symptoms.

How is hyperthyroidism treated?

Graves disease can be treated by taking drugs that suppress thyroid function and eventually lead to remission of symptoms, or by drinking concentrated solutions of radioiodine, which render the thyroid inactive. More rarely the thyroid gland may be surgically removed. If the thyroid has to be removed, or if, as a result of treatment, it becomes underactive after iodine therapy, the patient will have to take thyroid replacement hormones for the rest of her life.

Choice of treatment may vary according to an individual woman's reproductive plans and status. Radioiodine cannot be used during pregnancy, for example, because it can destroy thyroid tissue in the fetus. Pregnant women with Graves disease are usually treated with the antithyroid drug propylthiouracil (PTU), with careful monitoring of the fetus throughout pregnancy.

A woman with Graves disease who wishes to become pregnant in the near future is generally treated with radioiodine or surgery. Ideally, pregnancy should be avoided until Graves disease has been resolved. Antithyroid drugs take at least a year or two (and frequently much longer) before there is any chance of remission, and many doctors recommend waiting yet another year before attempting pregnancy. By contrast, pregnancy is believed to be safe 6 months after receiving radioiodine therapy. The waiting time is even shorter following a thyroidectomy, although this procedure is riskier than the other treatments, requires general anesthesia and a hospital admission, and leaves a scar on the neck.

Unlike Graves disease, toxic nodules and other forms of hyperthyroidism are much less likely to go into remission following treatment with antithyroid drugs. For this reason, radioiodine therapy or surgery is usually the better option, although antithyroid drugs may be taken before these treatments to modulate symptoms. In addition, antithyroid drugs are not effective in treating deQuervain's or painless thyroiditis because these forms of hyperthyroidism do not involve synthesis of new thyroid hormone. More effective for these conditions are beta blockers, drugs that are most commonly used to treat irregular heartbeat or hypertension. Beta blockers can relieve symptoms of hyperthyroidism while the thyroid recovers. Any pain can be relieved with aspirin or other nonsteroidal antiinflammatory drugs, or, if necessary, corticosteroids.

New mothers may choose to delay radioiodine or surgical therapy, since women who receive radioiodine should avoid close contact with children and pregnant women for about 5 days. Surgery would also require a short absence from the baby. Women who develop postpartum hyperthyroidism caused by thyroiditis may not require any treatment, since this condition often resolves on its own.

Related entries

Anemia, angina pectoris, bowel disorders, congestive heart failure, infertility, insomnia, menstrual cycle disorders, miscarriage, osteoporosis, platelet disorders, thyroid cancer, thyroid disorders

Hypoglycemia

Hypoglycemia is a much-abused term which in reality means nothing more than low blood sugar—that is, levels of glucose in the bloodstream that are too low to meet the body's energy needs. In recent years it has become common for people who feel faint or lethargic upon arising or after eating to think they are hypoglycemic, even though they often have perfectly normal blood sugar levels. Even when blood sugar levels do drop temporarily—as they sometimes do normally after excess alcohol or sugar consumption or prolonged fasting—this does not justify calling a person "hypoglycemic" as though it were some specific and chronic condition.

Bona fide hypoglycemia is relatively rare and is usually a sign of one of a number of different diseases and disorders. Hypoglycemia that occurs on an empty stomach is known as fasting hypoglycemia, and people with this condition often wake up feeling dizzy or lethargic. In contrast, people with hypoglycemia that occurs only after eating (postprandial hypoglycemia) may wake up feeling fine and have no symptoms until several hours after the first meal. People who have regular postprandial hypoglycemia for no obvious reasons are said to have idiopathic reactive hypoglycemia. The term idiopathic means that there are no apparent causes, while the term reactive means that the response follows a specific stimulus—in this case a meal.

Who is likely to develop hypoglycemia?

Occasionally people with early (and probably still unrecognized) Type 2 diabetes develop hypoglycemia after eating, as do some pregnant women.

Fasting hypoglycemia may develop following prolonged starvation (as occurs in anorexia nervosa; see entry). In addition, people with diabetes (see entry) who are on insulin can develop fasting hypoglycemia if they skip meals, exercise excessively without compensatory food intake, or take too much insulin (in which case the hypoglycemia may be called an insulin reaction). Some of the antidiabetic oral agents such as glyburide can also induce hypoglycemia.

What are the symptoms?

When blood sugar levels are low, the body tries to normalize levels by releasing epinephrine, a hormone that not only increases the heart rate and blood pressure but also speeds up metabolism so that more glucose is released from storage. High epinephrine levels can result in sudden symptoms similar to those of a panic or anxiety attack, including faintness, weakness, sweating, shakiness, hunger, anxiety, and, more rarely, irritability and heart palpitations. Many people have mild forms of these symptoms when they have gone too long without eating, even when measured blood sugar levels are normal.

Other symptoms may develop because the nervous system is being deprived of an essential energy source. These include headache, confusion, personality changes, muscle weakness, fatigue, and lack of coordination (which can make a person appear intoxicated). Vision may become dim, blurry, or double, and in more severe reactions seizures or unconsciousness may result.

How is the condition evaluated?

The symptoms of hypoglycemia are shared by a number of different disorders, including panic attacks, anxiety disorders, depression, and even alcoholic intoxication (which can also induce hypoglycemia). The only way to pinpoint the problem as hypoglycemia is to have a clinician run a test of blood sugar levels at a time when symptoms are occurring.

Usually multiple blood tests are needed, during a 6-hour fast (if fasting hypoglycemia is suspected) or following meals (if postmeal symptoms are the problem). In nondiabetic women, there is no absolute level of blood sugar that is "too low" if symptoms are not present. Thus the diagnosis of hypoglycemia is made only when symptoms correlate with low blood sugar levels.

The diagnosis of hypoglycemia is only the beginning. The clinician will next try to determine the underlying cause of the disorder. The evaluation will include a thorough physical examination as well as a consideration of the patient's dietary habits and the nature and timing of the symptoms.

How is hypoglycemia treated?

The only effective treatment for true hypoglycemia is to treat the underlying condition. People who have diagnosed themselves as having "hypoglycemia" or "low blood sugar" often embark on a special diet which they have heard helps relieve this condition. Even when blood sugar levels are normal, many people feel better when they eat frequent small high-protein meals, with an emphasis on complex carbohydrates (grains, fruits, and vegetables) rather than simple sugars (sweets). This diet appears to help people whose hypoglycemia is attributable to ulcer surgery as well.

Sudden hypoglycemia in a person with diabetes can be promptly relieved by eating or drinking anything high in sugar such as a candy bar or a glass of orange juice. If the person is already unconscious, however, the best response is to seek immediate medical attention so that glucagon or glucose can be injected directly. Trying to force foods or liquid down the throat of an unconscious person may result in choking.

Related entries

Alcohol, anorexia nervosa and bulimia nervosa, anxiety disorders, congestive heart failure, depression, diabetes, epilepsy, fatigue, headaches, kidney disorders, panic disorder

Hypothyroidism

Hypothyroidism is a condition in which a deficiency of thyroid hormones slows the body's metabolic rate. Produced by the thyroid gland at the base of the neck, thyroid hormones are crucial for both growth and development. Without sufficient thyroid hormones, the whole body slows down, leading to tiredness, weight gain, constipation, and other symptoms. People with hypothyroidism may also have high levels of cholesterol and triglycerides in their blood and are therefore at increased risk for atherosclerosis (clogging of the arteries) and heart attacks. Thyroid hormone deficiency is usually diagnosed long before serious consequences develop and is readily remediable with medication.

Iodine deficiency is the most common cause of hypothyroidism (and goiter) throughout the world. This rarely occurs in the United States today, however, because of the use of iodized table salt and other iodine-rich foods. Instead, almost all hypothyroidism in the United States is due either to Hashimoto's disease—an autoimmune disorder in which an abnormal antibody response destroys the thyroid gland—or to prior treatment for an excess of thyroid hormone. Hashimoto's disease is 3 to 5 times more common in women than in men.

Who is likely to develop hypothyroidism?

Hypothyroidism is particularly common in women over the age of 60, 6 to 7 percent of whom have this condition. Sometimes it may develop in people who are taking lithium to treat manic-depressive disorder, possibly because of some underlying autoimmune disease of the thyroid as well.

Women who have recently given birth to a baby are particularly susceptible to developing silent thyroiditis—inflammation of the thyroid which leads to a transient period of hypothyroidism sometimes following a period of overproduction of thyroid hormone. In addition, 2 to 4 percent of women do not produce enough thyroid for a period of time following childbirth, and they are sometimes misdiagnosed as having postpartum depression (see postpartum psychiatric disorders). Women who have had part of their thyroid gland removed because of cancer are at risk for hypothyroidism. Hypothyroidism can sometimes be acquired later in life after damage to the thyroid gland by radiation therapy.

What are the symptoms?

Symptoms of hypothyroidism often develop slowly and may not be noticeable for years. The most common of these—weight gain, fatigue, intolerance of cold temperatures, and muscle cramps—are shared by many people with normal thyroid function. Other symptoms may include constipation, lethargy, excessive menstrual bleeding, anemia, scant menstrual bleeding, brittle nails, dry skin and hair, goiter, slowed heart rate, and sleep apnea (see sleep disorders). Women may have difficulty becoming pregnant and often have a reduced sex drive.

If hypothyroidism persists for several years without treatment, it sometimes progresses to a state called myxedema (although this term can also be used interchangeably with hypothyroidism). Patients with myxedema typically have a puffy face, dry skin and hair, hair loss on the head and part of the eyebrows, and brittle nails; in teenagers, menarche may be delayed or absent. In severe hypothyroidism abnormal discharge of milk from the breasts may occur (a condition called galactorrhea), as well as accumulations of fluid around the heart and lungs, hearing loss, carpal tunnel syndrome (see entry), and swollen ankles, feet, and calves. Extreme hypothermia (low body temperature) and life-threatening coma (called myxedema coma) can be precipitated by exposure to cold, illness, trauma, infection, or sedatives.

How is the condition evaluated?

Hypothyroidism can easily be detected with a simple blood test that measures levels of TSH (thyroid stimulating hormone). To look for causes of the condition, a clinician will ask if the patient has a history of radioiodine therapy or surgery for hyperthyroidism or of exposure to external radiation, and will check to see if she may be using any medications that can cause hypothyroidism. A blood test for antithyroid antibodies can help determine if the hypothyroidism may be due to some autoimmune disorder such as Hashimoto's disease.

How is hypothyroidism treated?

Most clinicians treat hypothyroidism with a synthetic form of the thyroid hormone thyroxine, called levothyroxine (Synthroid, Levoxyl). Usually patients with more severe symptoms, elderly patients, and those with coexisting cardiopulmonary or other complicating illness (such as congestive heart failure or coronary artery disease) start with small doses which are increased gradually, while younger patients start with almost a full dose of medication. Symptoms generally disappear within a few months, but, except in cases of silent thyroiditis, treatment must be continued for life.

Any woman being treated for hypothyroidism should have blood serum levels of TSH checked regularly so that subclinical hyperthyroidism can be avoided. This results from overtreatment with thyroid preparations. Subclinical hyperthyroidism can lead to heart problems as well as reductions in bone density (see osteoporosis).

Related entries

Autoimmune disorders, blood tests, carpal tunnel syndrome, cholesterol, congestive heart failure, coronary artery disease, galactorrhea, hyperprolactinemia, hyperthyroidism, infertility, manic-depressive disorder, obesity, osteoporosis, postpartum psychiatric disorders, radiation therapy, sexual dysfunction, sleep disorders, thyroid disorders

Hysterectomy

Hysterectomy is the surgical removal of the uterus. When the uterus alone is removed, the operation is sometimes called a total (or simple) hysterectomy (see illustration). If the cervix (opening to the uterus) is left in place, it may be called a partial (or subtotal) hysterectomy. A radical hysterectomy—removal of the uterus and cervix, their supporting ligaments, the upper portion of the vagina, and the pelvic lymph nodes—may be used to treat some cancers.

With approximately 590,000 performed each year, hysterectomy is second only to cesarean section as the most frequently performed major operation in this country. Indeed,

it has been estimated that over a third of all American women have a hysterectomy by their 60th birthday. And the annual hospitalization costs for this operation are in excess of $5 billion per year.

The appropriateness of some hysterectomies has been the subject of debate for several decades. Feminists, consumer advocates, and medical economists alike—as well as some physicians—go so far as to claim that almost all hysterectomies are unnecessary, and their claims get considerable attention in the popular media. Although many of their figures are grossly exaggerated, there is growing consensus that a sizable minority of the hysterectomies done in this country are unjustified. Most convincing is a recent large-scale study which suggests that approximately 15 percent of all hysterectomies may be unnecessary.

Consistent with this study is the fact that rates of hysterectomy in industrialized nations vary markedly without any obvious differences in women's health. The rate in the United States, for example, is much higher than in Norway, Sweden, and England. Similarly, there is substantial variation from one region of this country to the next, with the highest rates in the South and Midwest. Furthermore, a woman's choice of practitioner influences her chances of being told she needs a hysterectomy: hysterectomies are less likely to be recommended by recently trained gynecologists (male or female) than by older ones (who tend to be male).

These differences in medical culture and tradition account for some of the variations in hysterectomy rates. Other factors include difficulties in diagnosis, limited information about the consequences of hysterectomy versus alternatives, and a discrepancy between the judgments of doctors and the preferences of patients—all factors that can make it difficult to determine whether a hysterectomy is truly necessary in any given case. As insurance companies become tighter with their financing and doctors agree on appropriate guidelines for hysterectomy, the number of unnecessary surgeries should drop.

Who is likely to have a hysterectomy?

A hysterectomy is often essential in women who have cancer of the uterus, ovaries, or cervix. Under some life-threatening circumstances, it may be the best means available to stop massive bleeding or curb infection after childbirth or abortion, but these instances are rare. More commonly, hysterectomy is one of several options available to treat a variety of less life-threatening conditions. The most frequent use of hysterectomy in this country (30 percent) is for treating uterine fibroids—benign growths in the uterus which sometimes cause pelvic pain and heavy or prolonged menstrual periods (menorrhagia). Heavy or otherwise abnormal vaginal bleeding that cannot be tied to any specific cause or controlled by other means accounts for 20 percent of hysterectomies, while another 20 percent are done to treat endometriosis and adenomyosis (see entries).

Among other conditions that occasionally necessitate hysterectomy are a dropped (prolapsed) uterus (sometimes with

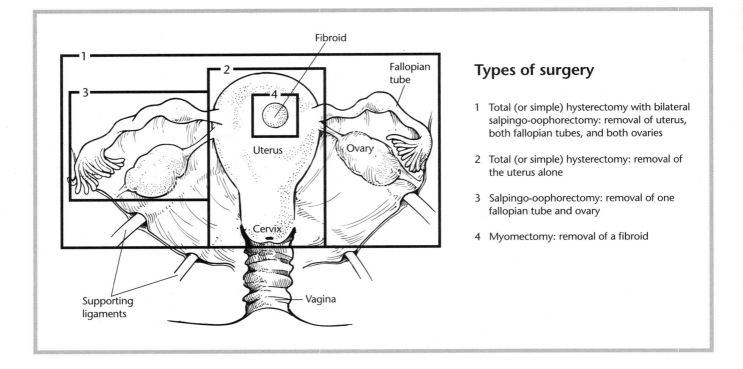

Types of surgery

1 Total (or simple) hysterectomy with bilateral salpingo-oophorectomy: removal of uterus, both fallopian tubes, and both ovaries

2 Total (or simple) hysterectomy: removal of the uterus alone

3 Salpingo-oophorectomy: removal of one fallopian tube and ovary

4 Myomectomy: removal of a fibroid

protrusion of the bladder or rectum into the vagina; see prolapsed uterus and cystocele/urethrocele/rectocele), pelvic inflammatory disease (PID), and pelvic adhesions (which may be related to some of these other conditions; see adhesions). Endometrial hyperplasia (overgrowth of the uterine lining) may also call for a hysterectomy, especially if the woman is nearing or past menopause, a time when this condition is most likely to become cancerous.

Very controversial are hysterectomies used to sterilize women or to treat conditions such as painful menstrual cramps, premenstrual syndrome, nonspecific pelvic pain, lesser degrees of uterine prolapse, and precancerous cell changes in the cervix—conditions that, in most cases, can be treated with less drastic measures. Some physicians also question whether hysterectomy is appropriate in women who have more than one condition, each of which alone would not justify surgery.

Another question women considering hysterectomy often face is whether one or both ovaries should be removed along with the uterus. Removal of the ovaries often makes good sense if the ovaries are themselves seriously diseased, or if there is a strong family history of ovarian cancer. Most doctors will also remove the ovaries in a woman nearing or past menopause, on the assumption that the ovaries produce little estrogen at this point and may eventually become cancerous if left in place.

The practice of removing the ovaries in a premenopausal woman strictly for the sake of cancer prevention is increasingly coming under fire, however. There is a growing consensus that the benefits (zero cancer risk) have to be weighed carefully against the adverse effects of hormone loss and the premature menopause that it produces. Some of these effects (such as hot flashes) can often be reversed by estrogen replacement therapy (ERT). But other possible effects—such as decreased sex drive—may be irreversible. Thus, more and more doctors now advise women under 45 with healthy ovaries and without extremely high risk for ovarian cancer to keep their ovaries, even if they need to have a hysterectomy.

How is the procedure performed?

The uterus can be removed either through an abdominal incision or through the vagina. The method used depends on the specific reason for the surgery, the number of adhesions (from scarring) a woman may have as a result of previous surgeries or infections, and the surgeon's individual preferences and experience.

Both operations require hospitalization and general or regional anesthesia. Abdominal surgery usually involves 3 to 5 days of hospitalization and 4 to 8 weeks or more to recover, whereas vaginal hysterectomy may call for only 1 to 2 days in the hospital and 2 to 4 weeks for full recuperation. Vaginal hysterectomy also is generally less painful, involves less bleeding and a reduced chance of complications, leaves less visible scarring, and is less likely to result in adhesions. Although visualizing the internal organs can be more difficult in vaginal hysterectomy, new laparoscopic techniques can help the surgeon overcome this obstacle. Abdominal surgery is often unavoidable if there are many adhesions from previous surgery or infection, or if the woman has large uterine fibroids.

Before any hysterectomy various blood and urine tests will

be done, and an enema is sometimes given to cleanse the colon. Often the pelvic area will be shaved as well. In an abdominal hysterectomy (see illustration), the surgeon makes an incision 4 to 6 inches long into the abdomen. This can be either a vertical (midline) incision extending up from the pubic bone toward the navel, or a transverse (bikini) incision across the pubic hairline from hipbone to hipbone. Although the transverse incision leaves a more discreet scar, some surgeons prefer the greater visibility afforded by a vertical incision.

Once the incision is made, the surgeon cuts and ties off the fallopian tubes, ligaments, and blood vessels of the uterus, and then lifts out the uterus through the incision. Some surgeons (with the patient's prior permission) also remove the appendix at the same time, since this takes only a few minutes and prevents any future possibility of appendicitis. Recently there has been some interest in preserving the cervix if possible, since it is believed that the cervix (and uterus itself) play a role in sexual response and orgasm. At present, however, there is not enough evidence about the benefits of this procedure to justify routinely leaving the cervix in place.

In a vaginal hysterectomy the woman is given regional or general anesthesia and lies in the position she assumes for a regular pelvic examination. The surgeon makes an incision near the top of the vagina at the cervix, through which the uterus is removed.

What happens after surgery?

In the case of an abdominal hysterectomy, there is often some discomfort in the incision area for the first few days after surgery. Most women are up and walking by the third day. Normal activities—including driving, exercising, and working—can be resumed gradually over the next month or two. Some women find they are easily fatigued for several months, and should adjust their schedules accordingly. Recovery is generally faster after a vaginal hysterectomy. Most doctors advise waiting 4 to 8 weeks before resuming sexual activity.

The psychological effects of hysterectomy can obviously vary greatly from one woman to another. It is clear that losing a uterus may have a very different impact on a 20-year-old woman with cancer than on a 45-year-old mother of three who is bothered by painful fibroids. Many women report feeling relieved to be rid of pain-provoking organs—not to mention the monthly menstrual period and risk of pregnancy in premenopausal women—but a small minority seem to rue the loss of fertility and see themselves as less feminine or complete.

At present only two consequences of hysterectomy can be stated definitively: menstruation ceases (because there is no uterine lining to be shed), and the woman can no longer bear children. Unless the ovaries have been removed, they continue to function until menopause, producing hormones

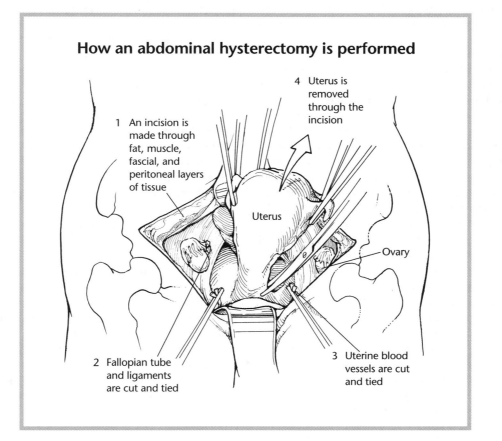

How an abdominal hysterectomy is performed

1 An incision is made through fat, muscle, fascial, and peritoneal layers of tissue

4 Uterus is removed through the incision

Uterus

Ovary

2 Fallopian tube and ligaments are cut and tied

3 Uterine blood vessels are cut and tied

that affect sexuality and releasing eggs on a monthly basis (these are absorbed by the body). Hysterectomy may be followed by a premature menopause—even (for reasons not fully understood) if the ovaries remain in place. Among the symptoms are hot flashes, sweating, vaginal dryness, painful sexual intercourse, and a loss of interest in sex or the ability to enjoy sexual relations (see sexual dysfunction).

Women who have both ovaries removed along with their uterus and do not take estrogen replacement therapy (ERT) are at increased risk for cardiovascular disease. Whether or not this risk increases if one or both ovaries are preserved is more controversial. While the large Nurses' Health Study indicated that women who kept at least one ovary were at no increased risk, smaller studies (including the Framingham Heart Study) have reported slight increases in risk after hysterectomy alone.

Although many women feel a sense of loss after hysterectomy—even if they did not wish to bear children in the future and are glad to be rid of the source of symptoms—the available studies indicate that hysterectomy rarely causes long-term mood disturbance or depression. For the small number of women who do become depressed or anxious after a hysterectomy, there is no solid evidence that these changes are due to the operation itself or to other aspects of the woman's life, to societal attitudes about women in general, or to lack of participation in the decision to have a hysterectomy in the first place. Women who have had psychological problems prior to the surgery are most likely to have adverse psychological reactions afterward. Not receiving enough support from family and friends can predispose a woman to these problems.

As better data about the outcomes of hysterectomy begin to trickle in, it is beginning to look as though hysterectomy is more likely to improve a woman's quality of life—at least for women who undergo the surgery to treat benign uterine conditions. In part this is because hysterectomy means the end to painful symptoms. In the Maine Women's Health Study, for example, 798 women (418 of whom had had a hysterectomy between 1989 and 1991) were surveyed. The study found that hysterectomies done to correct moderate or severe symptoms such as bleeding and pelvic pain left a majority of the women (71 percent) feeling better—mentally, physically, and sexually—than before the operation. Such happy outcomes were less likely for the women who had nonsurgical treatments (such as hormonal therapy or antiinflammatory drugs) for the same symptoms, a quarter of whom ended up opting for hysterectomy within a year of the study because their symptoms continued to plague them.

Only a small minority of the women in the Maine study reported symptoms such as reduced interest in sex, loss of enjoyment of sexual activity, hot flashes, weight gain, and depression. And many of these problems—particularly the depression and reduced interest in sex—were just as common in women who had not had a hysterectomy, who were also more likely still to be bothered by their original symptoms.

Possible alternatives to hysterectomy	
Condition	**Alternative**
Uterine fibroids	Hormonal therapy
	Myomectomy (surgical removal of the fibroids)
	Uterine artery embolization
Dysfunctional uterine bleeding	Nonsteroidal antiinflammatory drugs (NSAIDs)
	Hormonal therapy
	Endometrial ablation
Chronic pelvic pain and dysmenorrhea	Nonsteroidal antiinflammatory durgs (NSAIDs)
	Hormonal therapy
	Laparoscopic surgery
Endometriosis	Hormonal therapy
	Laparoscopic surgery
Genital prolapse	Pessary
	Surgical repair without hysterectomy

Many women worry that hysterectomy will change sexual response. This fear is not borne out by research, however. Older studies that focused on measuring sexual outcomes of hysterectomy reported improved sexual function in 50 percent of subjects, no change in 25 percent, and worsening in 25 percent. More recent studies have found that sexual functioning improves overall; fewer than 5 percent of women report developing pain with intercourse, low sex drive, or difficulty with orgasm after hysterectomy.

What are the risks and complications?

Hysterectomy, though a relatively safe operation, is major surgery. And like all major surgery it carries certain risks, including reactions to anesthesia, bleeding (possibly requiring transfusion), infection, blood clots, damage to other organs, abnormal scarring, and a chance of death (about 1 in 1,000). Abdominal hysterectomy generally carries a somewhat higher risk of complications than vaginal hysterectomy.

Some women find that they have a slight fever after surgery or problems emptying the bowel or bladder, but these are usually easily correctable. The surgeon should be notified

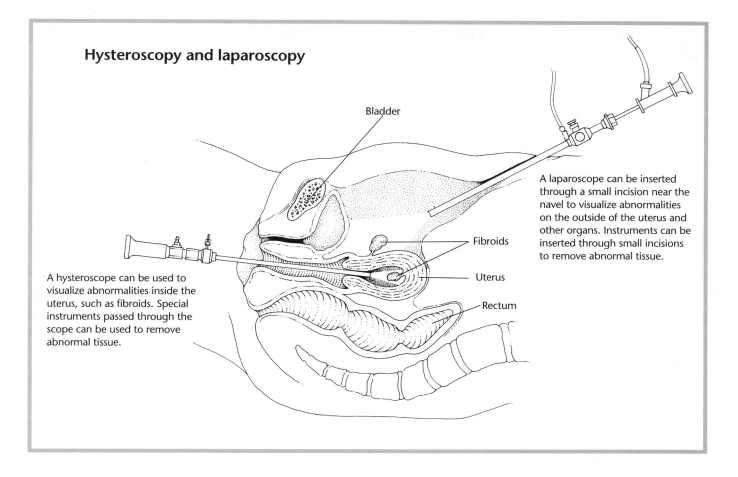

Hysteroscopy and laparoscopy

Bladder

A laparoscope can be inserted through a small incision near the navel to visualize abnormalities on the outside of the uterus and other organs. Instruments can be inserted through small incisions to remove abnormal tissue.

Fibroids

Uterus

Rectum

A hysteroscope can be used to visualize abnormalities inside the uterus, such as fibroids. Special instruments passed through the scope can be used to remove abnormal tissue.

promptly, however, if these problems persist for more than a few days, or if fever reaches 100°F or higher. Medical attention is also necessary if there is any unremitting pain, bright red or heavy vaginal bleeding, foul-smelling vaginal discharge, large blood clots, swelling or tenderness in the leg, breathing difficulties, cough, or chest pain.

How can unnecessary hysterectomy be avoided?

Until more questions are answered about hysterectomy and its outcome, the best way for a woman to avoid an unnecessary hysterectomy is to be a fully informed partner in the decision-making process. Among the chief issues a woman should discuss with her clinician are the severity of the symptoms, her desire to preserve reproductive organs (and childbearing potential), concern about future cancer risks, possible adverse effects of both the hysterectomy and its alternatives, the feasibility and costs of a hospital stay and recuperation time, attitudes of the woman's sexual partner, and any alternative treatments. Women should also ask if a vaginal hysterectomy is possible, and should find out if (and why) it is necessary to remove the ovaries as well as the uterus.

Premenopausal women in particular should learn whether a nonsurgical alternative might be available. Most hysterectomies in this country among women of reproductive age

are done to treat conditions that interfere with quality of life but are not life-threatening (such as uterine fibroids, endometrial hyperplasia, chronic pelvic pain, and endometriosis). Often some other therapy is available that would allow a woman to keep her reproductive organs intact until menopause, a time when most of these conditions abate on their own (see chart). For example, a woman with fibroids might consider hormonal therapy, or myomectomy (surgical removal of the fibroids alone) instead of a hysterectomy. In addition to discussing all options carefully with a clinician, women may also want to consider getting a second opinion before making any final decision.

Related entries

Antiinflammatory drugs, cervical cancer, coronary artery disease, cystocele/urethrocele/rectocele, depression, endometrial cancer, endometrial hyperplasia, endometriosis, estrogen replacement therapy, fatigue, laparoscopy, menopause, menorrhagia, menstrual cramps, menstrual cycle disorders, myomectomy, osteoporosis, ovarian cancer, ovary removal, pelvic inflammatory disease, pelvic pain, premenstrual syndrome, prolapsed uterus, sexual dysfunction, urinary tract infections, uterine fibroids, vaginal bleeding (abnormal)

Hysteroscopy

Hysteroscopy is a procedure in which the clinician inserts a telescopelike instrument called a hysteroscope through the vagina and cervix to view the inside of the uterus (see illustration).

Hysteroscopy can be performed to diagnose a condition such as abnormal vaginal bleeding, or for treatment. Diagnostic hysteroscopy, usually done on an outpatient basis using local anesthesia, can help a gynecologist locate uterine fibroids and polyps. It may also be used during an infertility evaluation.

In an operating room, hysteroscopy can be used, along with appropriate instruments, to remove fibroids, polyps, and IUDs that have become embedded in the uterine wall. Tubal ligations can also be performed by hysteroscopy; in this procedure an electrocautery probe is passed through the scope and used to coagulate the tubal openings.

How is the procedure performed?

When hysteroscopy is performed mainly to diagnose a condition (rather than for treatment), it can be done in the gynecologist's office. With the woman lying on her back and her feet in stirrups, a local anesthetic is injected around the cervix, causing mild discomfort. After a few minutes, when the anesthetic has taken effect, the gynecologist inserts a narrow lighted tube through the cervix into the uterus and carefully views the inner cavity of the uterus. The whole procedure takes about half an hour.

When hysteroscopic surgery is performed to treat a condition, such as to remove a fibroid tumor, it is usually done in a day surgery setting using general or regional anesthesia. Surgical instruments inserted through the hysteroscope are used to snip polyps or scoop out fibroids.

What are the risks and complications?

Diagnostic hysteroscopy is a relatively safe procedure which rarely results in complications. A woman often has light bleeding and occasional cramping for several days afterward. When prolonged bleeding—the main complication of hysteroscopy—occurs, it usually follows operative hysteroscopy, during which some abnormality is removed. Very rarely, a woman may develop an infection or a perforation (small puncture) of the uterus. Hysteroscopy performed in the operating room carries the additional risks associated with general or regional anesthesia (see entry).

Related entries

Adhesions, anesthesia, electrocautery, infertility, laparoscopy, polyps, tubal ligation, uterine fibroids

Immunizations

In contrast to the uncertainty associated with many screening tests, immunizations have proven to be very effective in preventing life-threatening diseases. They often are a low priority for clinicians, however, and many patients unjustifiably fear adverse reactions. The result is that many people, especially women of childbearing age, are not properly immunized.

How does immunization work?

Immunization is accomplished with vaccines, which work by training the immune system to attack and destroy specific viruses, bacteria, or toxins. They do this through the use of antigens—molecules that identify these disease-causing agents as "foreign." The antigens in vaccines may come from killed or weakened viruses, from bacterial molecules, or from inactivated toxins. They are harmless, but the immune system reacts to them as though they were the viruses, bacteria, or toxins themselves, and mounts an attack.

White blood cells called macrophages, T-cells, and B-cells all participate in the immune response (see illustration), and certain B-cells and T-cells will "remember" the antigen. If it shows up again in the future—this time attached to a real microbe or toxin—they will be prepared to get rid of it before it can do any damage.

What are the risks and complications?

Adverse reactions to vaccines are very rare. Sometimes they are the result of a previously unknown allergy to certain stabilizers or preservatives used in the production of the vaccine. Patients are often asked if they are allergic to eggs, since vaccines for measles, mumps, and influenza are prepared from viruses grown in eggs and therefore contain small quantities of egg protein; a person who is allergic to eggs should not be immunized for these diseases.

Women who are known to be pregnant will not be given vaccines made from live viruses, particularly rubella and measles, because they can potentially cause birth defects in the fetus. Other vaccines such as those for hepatitis, influenza, and tetanus are safe. All nonpregnant women of childbearing age should be vaccinated for rubella 3 months or more prior to attempting pregnancy. (Measles, mumps, and rubella immunizations are often combined in a vaccine abbreviated MMR.)

Contrary to popular belief, the following conditions are *not* good reasons to avoid an immunization: ‣ reaction to a previous vaccination that involved only local soreness, redness, swelling, or low-grade fever; ‣ mild upper respiratory or gastrointestinal symptoms with low-grade fever; ‣ current antibiotic treatment; ‣ current recuperation from an illness; ‣ a household member who is pregnant; ‣ recent exposure to an infectious disease; ‣ breastfeeding; ‣ personal or family history of general allergies; ‣ allergy to penicillin; ‣ family his-

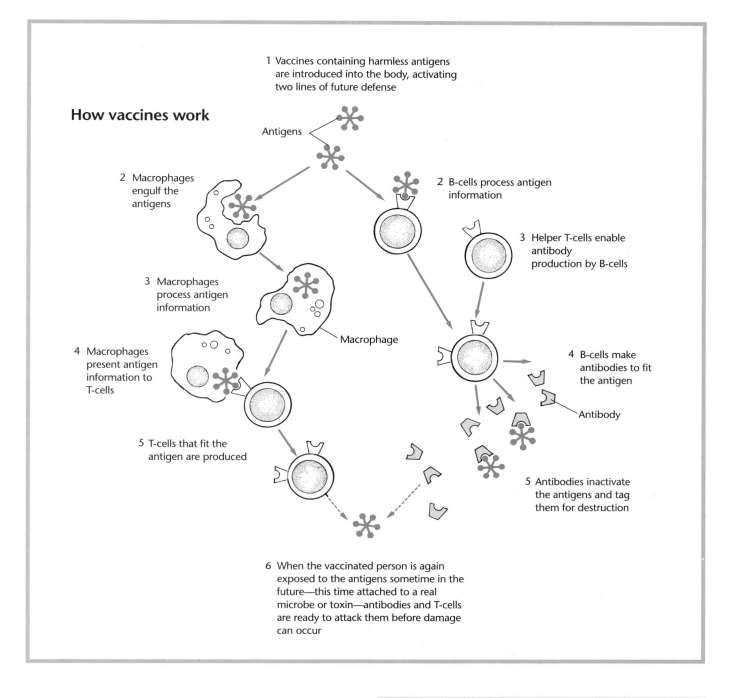

How vaccines work

1 Vaccines containing harmless antigens are introduced into the body, activating two lines of future defense

Antigens

2 Macrophages engulf the antigens

2 B-cells process antigen information

3 Macrophages process antigen information

3 Helper T-cells enable antibody production by B-cells

Macrophage

4 Macrophages present antigen information to T-cells

4 B-cells make antibodies to fit the antigen

Antibody

5 T-cells that fit the antigen are produced

5 Antibodies inactivate the antigens and tag them for destruction

6 When the vaccinated person is again exposed to the antigens sometime in the future—this time attached to a real microbe or toxin—antibodies and T-cells are ready to attack them before damage can occur

tory of an adverse event after vaccination, such as a heart attack.

Immunizations that all nonpregnant women should receive are listed in the chart on page 300.

Related entries
Colds, hepatitis, physical examinations, prenatal care, rubella, screening

Incontinence

The word incontinence can refer to the involuntary loss of urine or feces. In women urinary incontinence is extremely common, especially as they grow older. Not only can urine escape easily from the relatively short female urethra (see illustration), but also both childbirth and menopause can decrease the muscular support necessary to control the flow of urine. As a result, approximately 5 to 10 percent of all women have some kind of urinary incontinence, with numbers grad-

Immunizations recommended for women

Vaccine	Who should have it	Who should not have it	Possible reactions
Tetanus-diphtheria (primary series of 3 shots)	All adults who have not been previously immunized	People who had a neurologic reaction or hypersensitivity to a previous tetanus-diphtheria shot	Local pain, swelling
Tetanus-diphtheria booster	All previously immunized adults	People who had a neurologic reaction or hypersensitivity to a previous tetanus-diphtheria shot	Local pain, swelling which tend to be more severe if boosters are given less than 5 years apart
Rubella	Unimmunized women of childbearing age and health care workers	Pregnant women, people whose immunity is compromised, and people hypersensitive to neomycin	Joint pain in up to 40% of nonimmune adults
Measles (may be combined with mumps and rubella in the MMR)	All nonimmune people born after 1957; a second dose should be considered for young adults entering college, travelers to foreign countries, and health care workers	Pregnant women	Low-grade fever, rash, local pain, and swelling in people previously immunized
Hepatitis A	Women at increased risk of infection or complications of infection, including those planning travel to countries with relatively high rates of infection, people who work in high-risk occupations, food handlers, day care center staff, and those with chronic liver disease or who receive clotting factor concentrates	No data available on use during pregancy	Local soreness, headache, loss of appetite, tiredness
Hepatitis B	Intravenous drug abusers, heterosexual women with multiple sexual partners, recipients of certain blood products, health care workers frequently exposed to body fluids, and all children; safe during pregnancy	None	Local soreness

Influenza	People with chronic heart or lung disease, diabetes, asthma, allergy, or kidney disease, as well as residents of chronic care facilities, health care workers, people with a compromised immune system, and all adults over 50; appears safe during pregnancy	People who are allergic to eggs	Infrequent fevers, chills, and muscle aches lasting 1–2 weeks
Pneumococcal	Same as influenza vaccine, above, as well as those who have chronic liver disease, who are alcoholics, or who have had their spleen removed	No data available on use during pregnancy	Local soreness in about half of those immunized
Varicella (chicken pox)	Nonimmune adults, particularly those who live or work in settings where transmission of varicella is probable, including schools, day care institutions, and residential care and military facilities; non-pregnant women of childbearing age; adolescents and adults living in households with children; international travelers; and health care workers	Pregnant women	Allergic reaction rare

ually increasing after menopause. Incontinence is often one justification for admitting women into nursing homes, and as many as half of women in nursing homes have a significant degree of urinary incontinence. By their mid-80s this problem affects 7 out of 10 women living in nursing homes.

All of these estimates are probably too low because many women are hesitant to admit incontinence to their clinician or mistakenly regard it as an inevitable accompaniment of aging. Yet the growing number of television commercials for protective pads and adult diapers (such as Attends, Depends, and Tranquility) bear witness not only to the prevalence of the problem but also to the lifting of this old taboo.

Incontinence is not always a serious concern. Some women find that they can learn to live with the occasional leakage of urine that occurs when they cough or laugh. For many others, however, the inability to control voiding is an embarrassing, agonizing, time-consuming, and even expensive affliction (given the cost of supplies, laundry, and medical care). Severe incontinence, which occurs most often in elderly women, can lead to skin irritation and aggravate pres-

sure sores. The dependence on diapers and the scarcity of public toilets can keep otherwise relatively healthy women homebound, resulting in social isolation and loneliness.

Types of incontinence

Urinary function depends on complex neurologic processes which can be disrupted by diseases of the brain, spinal cord, or nervous system, as well as any abnormalities in the anatomy or muscular support of the urinary tract. Normally the bladder, a sac that lies between the pubic bone and the uterus, stretches to accommodate urine, which has been delivered through the ureters from the kidneys. A ringlike muscle called a sphincter keeps urine from escaping through the urethra, which is a thin tube about an inch and a half long attached to the bladder. When the bladder fills to a certain critical level, a muscle called the detrusor spontaneously contracts, the sphincter relaxes, and urine squeezes into the urethra and out of the body through the urethral opening.

Most people can override this reflex by sending a message from the brain to keep the detrusor from contracting and the

The urinary tract

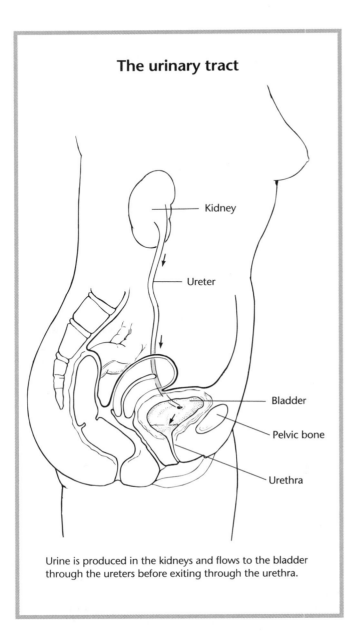

Kidney

Ureter

Bladder

Pelvic bone

Urethra

Urine is produced in the kidneys and flows to the bladder through the ureters before exiting through the urethra.

Urge incontinence. As women grow older, they may experience sudden and completely irresistible urges to void. Also called spastic bladder or uninhibited urinary bladder, this problem is thought to result from an overactive detrusor muscle combined with poor tone in the urethra due to aging and reduced levels of estrogen. When the bladder fills to a certain critical level, it goes into spasm, and involuntary voiding occurs almost immediately. Often older women have stress incontinence in combination with urge incontinence.

Overflow incontinence. With this type the bladder continues to fill with urine until it becomes overdistended, yet the woman cannot void or does not feel the urge to void. Eventually the bladder becomes so full that urine overflows, even if the detrusor never contracts. Overflow incontinence can occur when the detrusor is working inadequately, when there is a physical obstruction to urine flow, or when neurological problems interfere with sensations of bladder fullness. Because there is always residual urine sitting in the bladder, women with this form of incontinence are particularly susceptible to chronic bladder infections (cystitis; see urinary tract infections).

Functional incontinence. Incontinence that cannot be traced to any physical abnormality of the genitourinary system is called functional incontinence. Many elderly women receive drugs that can increase the need to urinate so much that it becomes difficult to control. Other women, especially older women, have physical disabilities such as arthritis which prevent them from getting to the bathroom quickly. This is especially a problem in public, where facilities for women are notoriously inadequate and lines may be long. As certain "potty parity" laws pending in several states mandating additional facilities for women are passed, many instances of functional incontinence will be alleviated. The notion that lines for women's rooms are excessively long because women spend so much time primping in front of the mirror turns out to be wrong when subjected to scientific scrutiny. The difference in the amount of time women take in the restroom, compared with men, is largely due to differences in anatomy and clothing, as well as to the fact that it is women more often than men who have to attend to the potty needs of young children.

Who is likely to develop urinary incontinence?

Stress incontinence can occur at any age, particularly in a woman who has borne children, because childbirth can weaken the pelvic floor muscles. But often symptoms worsen—or first appear—after menopause, when a deficiency of estrogen can lead to further weakening and thinning of these muscles and surrounding tissues, which in turn destabilizes the angle of the urethra. Women who have transient episodes of stress incontinence during or shortly after pregnancy may go on to have more severe stress incontinence in the years to come.

Stress incontinence can also be a symptom of other conditions that result when weakened pelvic floor muscles can no

sphincter from relaxing until voiding is socially acceptable. Incontinence occurs when some part of this system breaks down. The result is one of four basic types of incontinence: ▸ stress incontinence, ▸ urge incontinence, ▸ overflow incontinence, and ▸ functional incontinence, as well as certain inherited or acquired physical defects that can interfere with bladder control. Some women can have two or more forms of incontinence at the same time. This is particularly true as a woman grows older.

Stress incontinence. This is by far the most common type. It is due to a weakening in the pelvic floor muscles which support the bladder and other internal organs. This in turn alters the angle of the bladder and urethra so that the sphincter surrounding the urethra can no longer resist much abdominal pressure from above. As a result, urine leaks out after any kind of excess pressure or stress on the abdominal region.

longer support the internal organs. These conditions include cystocele, urethrocele, rectocele, and prolapsed uterus (see entries), all of which are more likely to occur in women who have given birth—particularly if they have had many children or have histories of difficult or long labors.

Urge incontinence often cannot be traced to a specific cause but may be due to bladder infections or anxiety. It may also occur in women with diabetes, multiple sclerosis, or other diseases that affect the nerves. It is a common symptom of interstitial cystitis (see entry), a poorly understood bladder disorder which occurs primarily in women. There is some evidence that urge incontinence may sometimes be linked to excess caffeine (from coffee, tea, cola, or chocolate), which, in addition to increasing the overall secretion of urine, has been linked to a hyperactivity of the detrusor muscle. Women who have a history of voiding and bladder difficulties, including childhood bedwetting, seem to be particularly likely to develop urge incontinence in their later years.

Overflow incontinence frequently occurs in women with nerve or sensory disorders that prevent them from controlling urination or from sensing when their bladder is full. Using muscle relaxants can also decrease bladder tone and can result in overflow incontinence. Similarly, the chronic use of drugs with anticholinergic effects, including antidepressants, may interfere with control of the bladder. Elderly women with very large cystoceles (fallen bladders) are also prone to develop overflow incontinence.

Functional incontinence is common in women with physical limitations which prevent them from getting to a bathroom before voiding occurs. It is particularly common in hospitals and nursing homes, as well as in women who are away from familiar settings and access to toilet facilities. It can also be a side effect of certain drugs, including some anticholinergics, antidepressants, and diuretics (used to treat high blood pressure).

Finally, there is some evidence that women of different ethnic groups are prone to different types of incontinence as well as different symptoms and risk factors. Most of our current knowledge about incontinence is based on studies of white women, but at least one recent study has suggested that black women have a much lower prevalence of pure stress incontinence (without other symptoms) than white women. It could be the case, however, that white women seek, or have access to, more medical care for this symptom than black women do, so that the differences may reflect socioeconomic rather than ethnic factors.

What are the symptoms?

The classic symptom of stress incontinence is the sudden loss of urine whenever an activity increases pressure or stress within the abdomen. Laughing, coughing, sneezing, exercising, or lifting heavy objects, as well as wearing a tight girdle or corset, can cause a small amount of urine to leak out. Over time the amount that leaks out may increase. Women with stress incontinence usually do not leak urine just from changing position or while sleeping.

Unlike stress incontinence, the symptoms of urge incontinence can fluctuate over weeks, months, or even years, sometimes in response to changes in a woman's life situation. Some women find that their symptoms vary from day to day. In general, however, women with urge incontinence frequently succumb to an overwhelming urge to urinate and also often need to urinate excessively at night—a problem known as nocturia. When women experience urge incontinence, they usually respond by voiding more frequently. This behavior, however, worsens the situation by "training" the bladder to hold smaller and smaller volumes of urine.

In contrast to stress incontinence, in urge incontinence there are usually at least several seconds separating the urge and the onset of leakage. In addition, because urge incontinence tends to occur when the bladder is moderately full, a large volume of urine may be lost, whether in the form of gushes, a steady stream, or prolonged dribbling. This problem can occur in any position, even in bed, and often a change in position can trigger leakage, as can walking, running, or listening to the sound of running water. Women with urge incontinence usually have trouble stopping the stream of urine during normal voiding.

In overflow incontinence the bladder is chronically overdistended. When it becomes full enough to surpass the resistance of the sphincter muscle, urine dribbles out of the urethra. Some women with overflow incontinence are unable to maintain a strong stream of urine.

How is the condition evaluated?

Any woman who has symptoms of urinary incontinence, painful urination, or excessive urination at night should see her clinician for evaluation (unless she is pregnant or has some other obvious and temporary explanation for the problem). Even women with disorders such as painful sexual intercourse or chronic pelvic pain should be checked for urinary tract problems, since often a dysfunction in the reproductive organs can have an effect on the bladder or urethra—and vice versa. Women past menopause should also have regular evaluations of the urinary system, since incontinence is such a common problem in older women.

A clinician evaluating incontinence will first want to make sure the problem is not due to any easily reversible cause—such as medication, urinary tract infection, or vaginal atrophy (see entry). The next step involves determining what type—or types—of incontinence is involved. This is particularly important because in some cases the treatment for one type of incontinence can actually exacerbate another type.

Although there are now many complicated (and expensive) tools available for evaluating problems of the urinary tract, these are usually not necessary in diagnosing incontinence. Often all that is required is a careful personal and family history and a pelvic examination, with emphasis on the organs of the urinary system.

Usually a preliminary examination will be performed when the bladder is full, first while the woman is lying down and then while she is standing. The clinician will look for any displacements of the genitourinary organs and will also note any thinning or smoothing of the vaginal tissues that may signal vaginal atrophy. Later, during the pelvic exam, the clinician may ask the woman to tense and release her pelvic muscles. She may also be asked to cough to see if any urine is lost. A urinalysis and culture will be done to rule out infection.

Many clinicians ask women with incontinence to complete a "voiding diary." For a set number of days the woman records her urinary output and episodes of incontinence and also notes fluid intake and medications, as well as any potentially relevant activities and events. From this record the clinician may discover, for example, that urge incontinence occurs only after the woman takes her morning dose of a diuretic medication. Then the problem can be easily remedied by splitting this dose into two smaller portions or stopping the pill altogether. Similarly, if the diary shows that the woman is drinking excessive fluids, she may be asked to limit fluid intake to 64 ounces daily.

If the type of incontinence is still unclear—or if there is a history of unsuccessful prior surgery, abnormal voiding, or underlying neurologic disease—the woman will probably be referred to a specialist (urologist or gynecologist) for more sophisticated tests of urine flow (urodynamic tests) before any decisions are made about further therapy. These include cystometry (the measurement of bladder function), a relatively painless office procedure done with equipment that records bladder pressure and detrusor activity. Occasionally cystoscopy—an outpatient procedure in which a urologist inserts a small viewing instrument through the urethra into the distended bladder to see if there is any inflammation—is necessary. Usually it can be done in the urologist's office with local anesthesia. When a more detailed examination or treatment is needed, it is done in a day surgery setting with regional or general anesthesia.

Sometimes a woman thought to have urge incontinence will be prescribed a trial course of antispasmodic drugs such as oxybutynin (Ditropan) or tolteridine (Detrol) and asked to report her symptoms after a few days. If the drug seems to relieve incontinence significantly, the clinician will probably continue to prescribe it in conjunction with some form of behavioral therapy to retrain the bladder. If successful, this trial can save a great deal of time and money.

How is urinary incontinence treated?

Although it is often difficult to eradicate incontinence completely, there are many ways to make symptoms more tolerable. Depending on the underlying cause of the problem, these methods may include exercises, hormonal therapy, behavior therapy, drugs, or surgery. They may also involve substituting a different medication or alleviating an underlying disorder or infection. If a woman has several types of incontinence, the one with predominant symptoms should receive the primary treatment.

Sometimes all that is necessary to reduce mild incontinence is doing Kegel exercises (see entry) to strengthen the muscles of the pelvic floor. In these exercises, a woman tightens her pelvic muscles 25 times in a row for 3 seconds, 3 times a day. Trying to stop or deflect the urine stream by squeezing these muscles can be done now and then to monitor progress. Women with weaker pelvic muscles may need to have biofeedback training (see alternative therapies) to regain control, or they may need supervised training with electrical stimulation before they can perform Kegel exercises at home. Wearing a tampon can also help prevent stress incontinence that occurs during exercise or other relatively infrequent but predictable activities.

Special pessaries—rubber devices inserted into the vagina—can also help control incontinence due to pelvic organ prolapse (the dropping of the bladder, uterus, or nearby organs). The effectiveness of these devices varies depending on the type and severity of incontinence, as well as the woman's individual anatomy.

Various forms of physical therapy can also help strengthen pelvic floor muscles. Women who find it difficult to perform Kegel exercises can sometimes use biofeedback techniques to learn how to contract pelvic muscles more effectively. Biofeedback is a technique in which a person learns to control actions that are normally involuntary. In this technique, which can be performed either in a clinician's office or at home, balloon pressure or electromyogram (EMG) probes are placed in the vagina to measure the strength of pelvic floor contractions as the patient does Kegel exercises. The patient can view the strength of these contractions on a screen, thus seeing just which movements are most effective. At the same time, the EMG probe provides electrical stimulation that helps strengthen muscles as well.

Another effective—and relatively affordable and convenient—biofeedback technique for stress incontinence involves using sets of 4 or 5 progressively heavier vaginal cones. A woman places a cone into the vagina and contracts the pelvic floor muscles enough to keep the cone in while walking. Once she learns to retain the smallest cone for 15 minutes twice a day, she moves on to the next, slightly heavier, cone. She continues this process until she is able to retain the heaviest cone. This technique can be performed at home.

A newer form of physical therapy that can help strengthen pelvic muscles is extracorporeal magnetic stimulation. In this approach, the patient sits in a chair, from which a focused magnetic field is generated. This field stimulates the pelvic muscles to contract by stimulating pelvic nerves. Preliminary evidence suggests that this approach can help approximately 60 percent of women with either stress or urge incontinence. Also effective for these types of incontinence is peripheral nerve stimulation, which involves a device called the sensory afferent nerve stimulator, or SANS. In this approach, nerves in the pelvis are stimulated with a needle on a weekly basis.

The drawback to all these advanced forms of physical therapy, however, is that treatment is often not covered by insurance.

Other treatments are necessary to relieve moderate or severe stress incontinence. If the incontinence is associated with vaginal atrophy, for example, topical vaginal estrogen creams can often provide significant relief by improving muscle tone. Estrogen replacement therapy may also help alleviate incontinence associated with low estrogen levels after menopause. Also helpful can be Estring, an oval-shaped ring that gradually releases estrogen into the vagina. Estring is inserted into the upper third of the vagina and replaced every 3 months. It should not be used by women who have breast cancer or any other cancer stimulated by estrogen, or by women who are pregnant, who have unexplained genital bleeding, or who develop allergic reactions.

Stress incontinence without symptoms of urge incontinence, vaginal atrophy, or weakened pelvic support may be relieved by taking pseudoephedrine (a nonprescription decongestant, such as Sudafed), usually in doses of 30 to 60 mg 3 times a day. This seems to work by increasing the muscle tone of the urethral sphincter. Some women cannot take pseudoephedrine, however, because it can cause heart palpitations and nervousness.

Another approach involves injections of collagen to treat stress incontinence, a procedure that can be performed under local anesthesia. Collagen is a protein that provides structural support and stability to connective tissues. In this procedure it is injected into tissue surrounding the urethra. This increases pressure by adding bulk, with the result that urine leakage is minimized. Effects wear off in 1 to 7 years, at which point it is necessary to have additional injections. Injection of a newer product, called Durasphere, which consists of graphite beads suspended in a gelatin matrix, is expected to last longer, perhaps permanently.

If stress incontinence seems to result from uterine prolapse or a rotated bladder neck, surgery may be considered. Surgery is also necessary to repair fistulas that (rarely) underlie incontinence. Many of the available techniques can be performed with relatively low risk, even on elderly women, and some of the newest procedures are minimally invasive and can be performed under local or spinal anesthesia. No form of surgery for incontinence is 100 percent effective, however, and sometimes the operation can actually cause new bladder problems. Also, women with mixed incontinence (both stress incontinence and urge incontinence, for example) should not expect a "successful" operation for stress incontinence to relieve their urge incontinence. For this reason, surgery usually works less well in elderly women, who tend to have more than one form of incontinence.

Even so, surgery is worth considering if stress incontinence seriously interferes with daily life and if it cannot be relieved with less invasive methods. Women should discuss the various procedures available with their clinician to determine which is most appropriate for their particular symptoms and life circumstances. Ideally, a urodynamic evaluation in a referral center should be performed before any surgical procedure is undertaken.

The most common surgery performed for stress incontinence involves repositioning the bladder and urethra (bladder neck suspension). This can be done through either the abdomen or the vagina, with general anesthesia. Since there is a high rate of recurrence, a bladder neck suspension may need to be repeated after several years. Some women also experience sexual dysfunction afterward because the angle or length of the vagina may change.

Urge incontinence is more effectively treated with non-surgical methods, including a form of behavioral therapy called timed voiding. Behavioral therapy is like adult toilet training in that it gradually transfers control of the bladder from involuntary (spinal reflex) to voluntary (cerebral) control. In timed voiding the woman is told to urinate at preset intervals—say every hour—throughout the day, whether or not she feels an urge. Gradually the intervals are increased until the woman can go an acceptable length of time without involuntary leakage. Timed voiding is an effective treatment for 4 out of 5 women with urge incontinence who have no other form of incontinence. Also, it has no systemic side effects.

Some women with urge incontinence find it helps to cut out all caffeine and acidic foods (including decaffeinated coffee), and to limit the intake of fluids in the evening. Paradoxically, however, drinking ample water can actually help relieve urge incontinence.

Various drugs, including propantheline (an anticholinergic) and oxybutynin (an antispasmodic), are often prescribed for urge incontinence, as is imipramine (Tofranil), an antidepressant which decreases bladder activity while increasing urethral sphincter tone. Some women find that even in low doses they cannot tolerate the common side effects of these drugs, which can include blurred vision, dry mouth, constipation, confusion, and dizziness on standing. Anticholinergics should also not be used by women with glaucoma, a condition involving increased fluid pressure within the eye. Newer, improved anticholinergic drugs for urge incontinence such as tolterodine (Detrol) and extended-release oxybutinin (Ditropan) may lead to fewer disturbing side effects, although even these drugs still lead to drowsiness, blurred vision, and impaired thinking and memory in elderly users. Because tolterodine doesn't readily cross the blood-brain barrier, however, it may be the best choice for elderly women.

Occasionally severe problems can be treated with surgery such as bladder augmentation or urinary diversion, although both approaches have serious drawbacks. After bladder augmentation, a woman has to catheterize herself for the rest of her life. And after urinary diversion surgery, she has to deal with a drainage bag that collects urine. A newer technique called chronic stimulation of S3, or InterStim, may be preferable if the problem is an overactive detrusor muscle. Performed in a clinician's office under local anesthesia, this approach involves placing an electrode into the lower part of the spine (containing nerves that stimulate the bladder) which is worn for a week or two. If incontinence abates, the problem may be amenable to a neurostimulator, which can be implanted into the spine under general anesthesia. This implant resembles a cardiac pacemaker and must have its battery changed every 6 to 10 years.

Overflow incontinence is usually treated by treating any underlying disorder. Alpha blockers—medications that relax the bladder outlet, such as prazosin (Minipress) and terazosin (Hytrin)—can also be tried.

Addressing functional incontinence is largely a societal problem, depending on improved access to public restroom facilities and better-staffed nursing homes. Adjusting doses of medication to a woman's individual schedule, providing bedside commodes, and replacing buttons and zippers with easier-to-open Velcro fasteners can also help.

Although a variety of treatment options are available for incontinence, for some women the use of adult diapers can provide an acceptable means of coping with symptoms. It is important, however, that a woman not hesitate because of embarrassment to discuss with her physician other ways of eradicating the problem of incontinence.

Related entries

Alternative therapies, antidepressants, arthritis, back pain, cystocele/urethrocele/rectocele, diabetes, diuretics, high blood pressure, interstitial cystitis, Kegel exercises, menopause, multiple sclerosis, pain during sexual intercourse, pelvic examinations, pelvic pain, prolapsed uterus, stroke, urinary tract infections, vaginal atrophy

Infertility

Infertility is defined medically as the inability to conceive a pregnancy after at least a year of regular sexual intercourse without contraception. An increasing problem in the United States, infertility is a major life crisis for many people, who have assumed from childhood that they would someday be able to have their own children. Today 10 to 20 percent of all married couples are infertile, and about a quarter of all women can expect to have at least one episode of infertility at some point during their childbearing years. According to surveys done in 1988 by the National Center for Health Statistics, 8.4 percent (4.9 million) of American women of childbearing age were infertile. Of these, 2.2 million never had children, and 2.7 million had at least one child but were unable to conceive additional children.

What causes infertility?

The increase in infertility in this country is largely attributed to an epidemic increase in sexually transmitted diseases and associated pelvic inflammatory disease (PID), coupled with a trend toward delayed childbearing. Evidence is overwhelming that fertility decreases with advancing age. A woman aged 35 to 44 is twice as likely to be infertile as a woman aged 30 to 34. Men also become less fertile as they grow older, though in a less dramatic fashion.

Various other factors can increase the likelihood of infertility. Cigarette smoking, for example, seems to alter fallopian tube function, which in turn seems to destroy eggs and impair the density, movement, and shape of sperm. Using illicit drugs—including marijuana, narcotics, and cocaine—not only can reduce sex drive and lead to sexual dysfunction but also may alter secretion of certain hormones vital to normal menstrual function and ovulation (the release of an egg from the ovary). In addition, women who exercise or diet excessively, to the point of reducing body fat below a certain critical point, often stop ovulating and become temporarily infertile. Finally, it is becoming increasingly clear that exposure to specific occupational and environmental toxins can affect fertility in both men and women (see occupational hazards).

About 40 percent of infertility occurs because of problems in the woman. These can include a failure to ovulate (anovulation), hormonal imbalances that leave the uterine lining unprepared for implantation of the embryo, physical abnormalities of the uterus, scar tissue (adhesions) within the fallopian tubes or on the ovaries or uterus (resulting from infections or a ruptured appendix), inadequate cervical mucus, production of antisperm antibodies, or habitual miscarriage (see miscarriage). Endometriosis, uterine fibroids, or uterine polyps in a woman can interfere with conception and implantation.

Male factors account for another 40 percent of infertility. These generally involve inadequate sperm production or function, which can occur for a variety of reasons, including hormonal deficiencies, anatomical defects, sexual dysfunction, and chromosomal abnormalities. In the remaining 20 percent of infertile couples, the reasons for infertility are never determined.

How is the condition evaluated?

Usually an infertility evaluation of both partners is done after a woman has been trying to conceive for at least a year without success. This is because only 15 percent of fertile couples can expect to conceive within the first month of trying, 63 percent within 6 months, and about 80 to 90 percent within a year. An infertility workup may be started after just 6 months or so for a woman who is over 35, has evidence of endometriosis, or is extremely anxious about her ability to become pregnant.

An initial examination, which can be performed by a primary care physician, generally begins with a history and physical examination (see illustrations). The clinician will check the woman for any obvious hormonal or reproductive tract disorders that may explain her infertility. These include irregular menstrual cycles without ovulation, an excess or deficiency of thyroid hormone, an excess of prolactin (a hormone involved in menstrual regulation), or an excess of androgens. Hirsutism and other symptoms of hyperandrogenism such as obesity, acne, and menstrual irregularities will be noted. A pelvic examination will be done to look for signs of endometriosis, uterine fibroids, cervicitis or other cervical abnormalities, cysts or other growths, and congenital abnormalities.

The clinician will ask the couple to give details about the

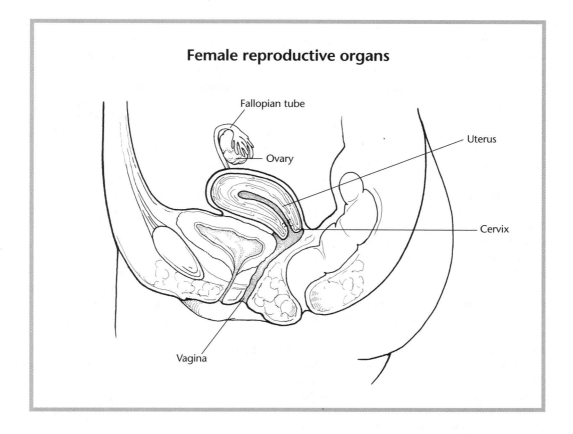

Female reproductive organs

Fallopian tube

Ovary

Uterus

Cervix

Vagina

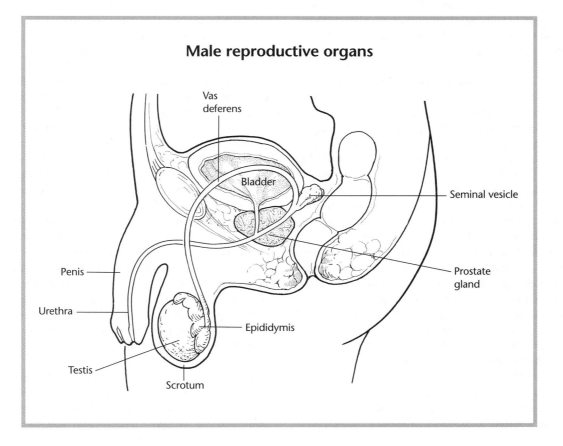

Male reproductive organs

Vas
deferens

Bladder

Seminal vesicle

Prostate
gland

Penis

Urethra

Epididymis

Testis

Scrotum

nature and duration of the infertility, and will review their medical, surgical, and family history and the menstrual, contraceptive, and obstetric history of the woman. The man will be asked if he has ever been responsible for a pregnancy, and the woman will be asked if she has ever been pregnant. Other questions will include any possible exposure to occupational toxins, as well as stress, eating disorders, exercise habits, and the use of alcohol, cigarettes, medications, and illegal drugs.

The clinician will also spend some time reviewing the normal menstrual cycle and basic steps required for pregnancy. The couple will be taught the optimal timing for intercourse based on the woman's typical cycle interval. Ovulation occurs about 14 days before the first day of the menstrual period, with the fertile period beginning from about 4 days before ovulation until two days after. The couple will be encouraged to have intercourse every other day during this period. For example, if a woman's typical cycle interval is 30 days, she most likely ovulates on cycle day 16, and optimal timing would include cycle days 12, 14, 16, and 18. Cycle day 1 is defined as the first day of menstrual bleeding heavy enough to require a pad or tampon.

After the initial evaluation the couple will be referred to a gynecologist—a physician who specializes in disorders of the female reproductive system and performs surgery when necessary—although sometimes a reproductive endocrinologist may handle the part of the evaluation that focuses on the hormonal system. The gynecologist or endocrinologist may decide to do more sophisticated tests and procedures to narrow the range of possible disorders. Because 10 to 30 percent of infertility cases have more than one cause, clinicians will eventually conduct most of the following tests even if a specific problem is detected early on.

Sperm analysis. A sperm analysis is done quite early in an infertility evaluation, partly because male factors so often account for infertility, and partly because finding a severe problem with the man's sperm may preclude—or at least delay—the more invasive tests that will need to be done on the woman. The man provides a sperm sample by masturbating into a sterile cup (or, if necessary for religious or psychological reasons, by ejaculating into a silicone condom during intercourse), and the volume, number, motion, and shape of sperm are assessed in a laboratory. If any abnormalities are found, a second analysis is done as confirmation.

If there is a problem with the sperm, the next step is to uncover its nature (too few sperm, no sperm at all, slow-moving sperm, misshapen sperm) and, when possible, its cause—which is usually low hormone levels, injuries, infections, or even a reversible drug reaction. Some of these causes—such as a large varicocele, an enlarged vein in the scrotum—are readily correctable with surgery. If testosterone levels are low, the man should be seen by an endocrinologist for further evaluation and therapy.

If a low sperm count cannot be corrected, another option is artificial insemination. In this technique concentrated samples of the man's semen are placed inside the woman's cervi-cal opening around the time of ovulation. Sometimes the semen is first processed to improve the chances of conception. Artificial insemination is usually an office procedure and is generally painless. ICSI (intracytoplasmic sperm injection) has improved the prognosis of fertility for men with very few sperm or low mobility. This technique involves directly injecting a single spermatozoon into the cytoplasm of a human oocyte (immature egg), usually obtained from follicles produced under hyperstimulation of the ovaries.

When the man produces extremely few or no viable sperm at all, artificial insemination with sperm from an anonymous donor is an option. In this case the semen is screened to make sure it does not contain dangerous viruses, including the virus that causes AIDS.

Basal body temperature charting. A failure to ovulate accounts for about 20 percent of the infertility problems in women. The least expensive way for a woman to find out if she is ovulating is to fill out a basal body temperature (BBT) chart. To do so, a woman takes her temperature each morning before getting out of bed, having intercourse, or going to the bathroom. She then records this temperature on a graph, with the vertical spaces indicating each degree of temperature and the horizontal spaces indicating each day of the menstrual cycle. The woman should also indicate days when bleeding occurs. Circles can be used to show the days when she and her partner have intercourse, and daily fluctuations in mucus can be noted at the bottom (see chart).

Most women measure their temperature with a special basal body temperature thermometer, available in pharmacies, although some find it easier to use a digital thermometer. Over the course of the menstrual cycle, the basal body temperature will jump to a markedly higher level once ovulation occurs—generally around day 14 to 16 of the cycle, with day 1 being the first day of menstruation. The catch is that temperature fluctuates somewhat from day to day, with the result that usually it is not possible to know if ovulation has occurred until several days afterward. Three consecutive days on which the temperature is at least 0.4 degrees above its previous level generally means that ovulation has occurred. Ovulation can be confirmed with an over-the-counter kit (such as OvuQuick, Q-Test, or Ovukit); these measure or detect luteinizing hormone (LH), which surges just before ovulation.

A clinician can confirm that ovulation has occurred by measuring progesterone levels in the blood. In a normal cycle peak progesterone secretion occurs around day 20, or about a week after ovulation, and stimulates the uterine lining (endometrium) to thicken. To time this test correctly, the clinician uses information from the woman's symptoms or from the basal body temperature chart.

Endometrial biopsy. If the BBT chart and progesterone test suggest a problem with ovulation, the next step is to have an endometrial biopsy. The presence of a thickened (secretory) endometrium as menstruation approaches is proof that ovu-

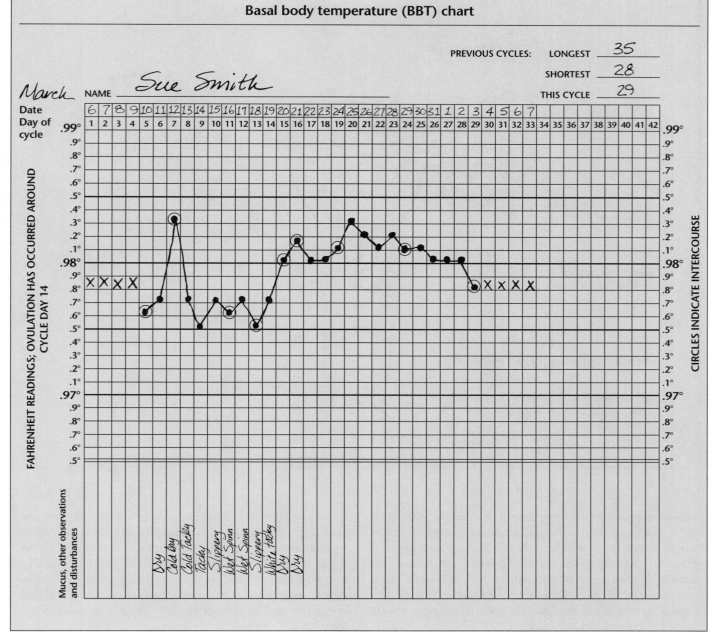

Basal body temperature (BBT) chart

March   NAME Sue Smith

PREVIOUS CYCLES: LONGEST 35   SHORTEST 28   THIS CYCLE 29

FAHRENHEIT READINGS; OVULATION HAS OCCURRED AROUND CYCLE DAY 14

CIRCLES INDICATE INTERCOURSE

Mucus, other observations and disturbances: Dry, Cold Dry, Cold Tacky, Tacky, Slippery, Wet Spinn, Wet Spinn, Slippery, White tacky, Dry, Dry

lation has occurred. The biopsy is performed toward the end of the menstrual cycle but before bleeding begins. Usually it can be done in a clinician's office without anesthesia. Cramping may occur for the short time required to remove the tissue. Even if a woman is already pregnant, the chance that the biopsy will disrupt the pregnancy is slim.

Sometimes an endometrial biopsy is performed to diagnose a luteal phase defect. In this condition ovulation occurs, but the endometrium does not thicken on time and is not ready to accept the fertilized ovum when it reaches the uterine cavity. In some cases this problem may be due to the premature failing of the ovaries, signaled by irregular men-

strual cycles and hot flashes. Occasionally a woman fails to ovulate because of excessive exercise or dieting. In these cases modifying exercise habits or putting on a little weight may be all that is necessary to solve the problem. Likewise, sometimes weight loss can restore ovulation in an extremely obese woman. But in most cases of failure to menstruate or ovulate, the hormonal imbalances that underlie anovulation must be corrected with medications.

Usually a drug called clomiphene citrate (Clomid), which is similar to estrogen, is used to stimulate the pituitary gland to secrete follicle stimulating hormone (FSH) and luteinizing hormone (LH), which in turn prompt the maturation and re-

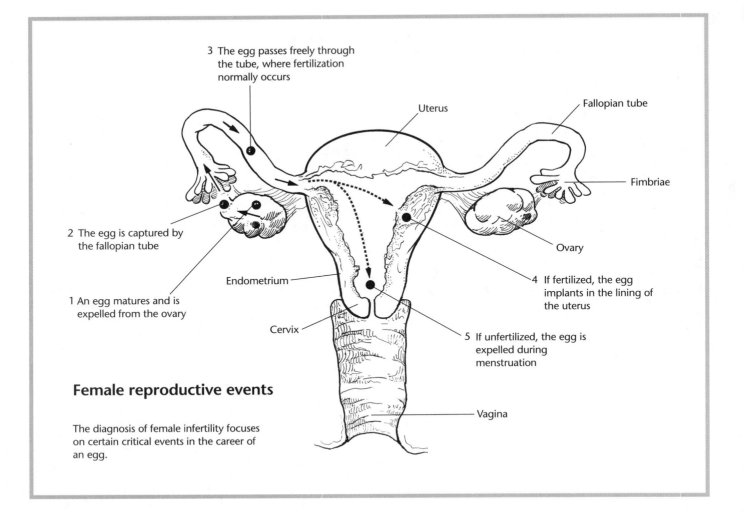

3 The egg passes freely through the tube, where fertilization normally occurs

Uterus

Fallopian tube

Fimbriae

2 The egg is captured by the fallopian tube

Ovary

Endometrium

4 If fertilized, the egg implants in the lining of the uterus

1 An egg matures and is expelled from the ovary

Cervix

5 If unfertilized, the egg is expelled during menstruation

Vagina

Female reproductive events

The diagnosis of female infertility focuses on certain critical events in the career of an egg.

lease of an egg from the ovary (see illustration). Clomiphene citrate comes in the form of pills that are usually taken for 5 days a month. Clomiphene citrate slightly increases the chances of having twins and may produce hot flashes and some lower abdominal pain. In women with polycystic ovary syndrome (PCOS) and insulin resistance, taking the insulin-sensitizing drug metformin in addition to clomiphene results in increased frequency of ovulation.

If pregnancy does not occur within 3 months of Clomid therapy—even though ovulation is documented with a BBT chart or a progesterone level check—the woman will probably be referred to an infertility specialist (if that has not happened already). An infertility specialist is a gynecologist or endocrinologist whose practice, and in some cases research, focuses exclusively on infertility. This physician will prescribe higher doses of Clomid, and if that is still unsuccessful, stronger drugs. Pergonal or Gonal-F may be tried. Pergonal, which is similar in form to both LH and human chorionic gonadotropin (a hormone produced during pregnancy by the developing placenta), is extracted from the urine of menopausal women and so is sometimes called human menopausal gonadotropin (hMG). Gonal-F is a highly puri-

fied form of follicle stimulating hormone (FSH), the hormone primarily responsible for stimulating the development of egg-containing follicles in the ovaries. It is produced by recombinant DNA technology. These drugs must be given by injection and require close monitoring by an infertility specialist, since they carry a 30 to 40 percent chance of multiple pregnancy and may result in serious side effects, including large ovarian cysts.

Hysterosalpingogram. This test can determine if the fallopian tubes are open and can reveal the shape of the uterine interior (in Greek *hystero* means "uterus" and *salpingo* means "tube"). It is a particularly important part of the infertility workup, because fertilization of the egg takes place in the fallopian tubes, and damaged tubes that interfere with passage of the egg or sperm account for about 30 percent of all infertility.

In this procedure, usually performed in the radiology department of a hospital, the gynecologist uses a catheter to pass a radiopaque contrast agent through the cervix. Using a special x-ray screen, he or she then watches the contrast agent flow up into the uterus and fallopian tubes. Any blockages or other abnormalities soon become apparent. Occasionally the contrast agent itself can solve the problem by removing or dissolving some minor blockages. Hysterosalpingograms are ideally performed early in the menstrual cycle, after the menstrual flow has stopped but before ovulation (and possible pregnancy) has occurred.

To minimize the abdominal cramping sometimes caused by a hysterosalpingogram, it may help to take a nonsteroidal antiinflammatory drug 30 minutes to 2 hours before the procedure. Women who have a past history of pelvic infections, ectopic pregnancies, tubal surgery, or a ruptured appendix are at increased risk for developing a pelvic infection after a hysterosalpingogram (3.5 percent risk versus a normal 1 percent risk). For that reason, they may be given antibiotics to prevent infections.

Depending on the results, the gynecologist or infertility specialist will advise the couple whether surgical correction of a blockage is possible or whether in vitro fertilization (which allows the egg to be fertilized outside the damaged tube) might be a better option. These decisions must take into account not only the relative risks and effectiveness of each therapy but also cost and emotional considerations.

Laparoscopy and hysteroscopy. A hysterosalpingogram cannot provide information about pelvic adhesions or other implants (such as those from endometriosis) which lie outside the fallopian tubes or other reproductive organs. These can only be identified by a laparoscopy, a surgical procedure that allows direct examination of the exterior of the reproductive organs, sometimes coupled with a hysteroscopy, another procedure in which a telescopelike instrument is inserted through the vagina and cervix to permit a view of the inside of the uterus. The hysteroscopy can often pick up defects in the uterus which were not clear from the hysterosalpingogram, although it is not known yet whether the added information actually improves a woman's chances of pregnancy.

These procedures take an hour or two to complete and are usually done as outpatient surgery under general anesthesia. They should be performed by an infertility specialist, who may be able to treat any problems uncovered during the surgery (fibroids, adhesions, blocked tubes), using methods such as laser vaporization, electrocautery, and excisional biopsy.

A surgeon who finds minimal or mild endometriosis implants will usually recommend taking clomiphene citrate to induce ovulation, combined with artificial insemination. In rare instances a uterine fibroid is found to be blocking the cervix and interfering with fertilization, in which case the growth can be removed at the time of the hysteroscopy. Although it is not always necessary to remove the growths in such cases, one major drawback to using drugs that induce ovulation is that these same drugs stimulate the growth of endometriosis implants and uterine fibroids. If the condition is severe, surgery will be necessary, sometimes followed by drug treatment to suppress the recurrence of growths. In all cases, if conception has not occurred after a mutually agreed upon period of time (usually 6 months to 2 years), in vitro fertilization will probably be recommended.

What additional methods of treatment are available?

After undergoing all of these tests, up to 20 percent of couples will still be told that they have "unexplained infertility." For these couples—as well as for those for whom drugs, surgery, and intrauterine insemination have failed—additional tests may be done by an infertility specialist. Among the problems looked for will be genital tract infections and immunological defects. The infertility specialist may also use ultrasound to look for relatively rare abnormalities related to ovulation. Detailed tests can be done to evaluate the binding of sperm and egg as well as the quality of the eggs.

Infertility specialists also have various techniques of "assisted reproduction" at their disposal. Other techniques—in vitro fertilization (IVF), gamete intrafallopian transfer (GIFT), and zygote intrafallopian transfer (ZIFT)—all involve the direct retrieval of eggs from the ovary. Intrauterine insemination (IUI) involves stimulation of the ovaries, followed by injection of sperm directly into the uterus via a catheter inserted through the cervix.

The woman is first given hormones (such as GnRH agonists, Pergonal, Clomid, or human chorionic gonadotropin) to stimulate the maturation of fertilizable eggs. Maturation is monitored with ultrasound and frequent measurements of hormone levels in the blood. If and when enough eggs mature, the surgeon, with ultrasonic guidance, inserts a long, thin needle into the vagina, through the vaginal wall, and into one of the ovaries. All recognizably mature eggs (there are usually many) are removed and placed into a glass dish. Most women are put under light sedation during this procedure (through an intravenous line), and sometimes local anesthesia is used as well.

In the process of in vitro fertilization, the eggs are then mixed with sperm (from either the woman's partner or a donor) in the hope that they will become fertilized and start to divide. If they do, they will be inserted directly into the uterus several days after retrieval. A pregnancy test can be done 12 to 14 days later.

IVF is a good option for women with blocked or damaged fallopian tubes, since fertilization takes place outside the body. For standard in vitro fertilization to work, however, a man needs to produce a fair number of healthy sperm. When the problem is an extremely low sperm count, a few in vitro fertilization centers in this country are able to inject a single healthy sperm directly into the egg and then insert the fertilized egg into the uterus.

If the woman's fallopian tubes are open, other techniques of assisted reproduction have a somewhat higher success rate. In GIFT, the eggs and sperm are placed into the fallopian tubes via laparoscopy before fertilization has occurred. Even more successful is ZIFT, in which fertilization of the eggs and their initial division into several cells is confirmed before they are placed into the tubes.

Although all of these procedures increase the chances of a multiple birth, most couples consider themselves lucky if even one of the eggs ends up developing. The success rates with assisted reproduction are as high as 80 percent, but only for those couples who make numerous costly and emotionally draining attempts—which most couples ultimately are unwilling to undergo. Each attempt takes at least 10 days, costs somewhere around $5,000 to $10,000, and brings with it slight risks of ovarian rupture, bleeding, infections, ectopic pregnancy, multiple pregnancy, and complications of anesthesia. Success rates vary from clinic to clinic and from surgeon to surgeon—not to mention from condition to condition, including the age of the woman.

Couples who have failed to achieve pregnancy through one of the lower-tech procedures such as Clomid and who are willing to try assisted reproduction techniques for a cycle or two have a greater chance of achieving pregnancy than with any other form of infertility therapy. In addition, the ability to freeze fertilized eggs indefinitely may increase the odds of ultimately achieving a pregnancy. Finally, these techniques provide new hope for fertile couples who carry lethal genetic traits—which, since the egg is fertilized outside the body, can sometimes be diagnosed before implantation.

No technique of assisted reproduction can help a woman who is not capable of ovulating (even with hormonal stimulation) or a man who is not able to produce at least a few viable sperm. These couples do have the option of using these techniques together with donor sperm or eggs, which of course will not carry the genes of at least one of the potential parents. It is even possible for a postmenopausal woman to bear a child by arranging for the donated egg from a younger woman to be fertilized by the older woman's partner and then implanted into her uterus, to be carried to term—although ethical, interpersonal, and legal issues associated with this procedure remain unresolved. Alternatively, a woman with a malformed or missing uterus can have her own eggs fertilized with her partner's sperm and then implanted in the uterus of a surrogate mother (this is called gestational surrogacy).

What are the alternatives to infertility treatment?

None of the new technologies for treating infertility comes without huge emotional and financial costs. Some of them have never been proved to be more effective than letting nature take its course, and insurance companies often do not cover them, even in their so-called comprehensive policies. The ones that do usually restrict the acceptable techniques or limit them to just a few approved laboratories.

Infertility itself is fraught with tremendous stress, anxiety, and feelings of isolation, in addition to the testing, treatment, and financial strain. Guilt feelings or accusations may arise between the infertile partners, and intrusive questions or pressures may come from well-intentioned friends, relatives, and co-workers. Infertile women often feel stigmatized for failing at what they perceive to be a fundamental part of womanhood and are overwhelmed by a sense of helplessness

and loss of control. Often sexual dysfunction develops in the relationship as a result, which does not help the infertility problem.

Given all of the technological, bureaucratic, and emotional obstacles, infertile couples might want to start by considering some less dramatic, and often equally fulfilling, options. One choice for couples who decide to eschew the newer technologies is doing nothing at all—since every month about 3 percent of all so-called infertile couples conceive on their own.

Another option, though one with its own costs and complications, is adoption. Since many agencies in the United States will not consider a couple over the age of 40 for the adoption of an infant, an infertile couple open to this option should start exploring it as early as possible. Agencies that specialize in international adoptions are sometimes more lenient about the age of the parents; it may be necessary, however, to travel to the country of the child's origin and to spend many uncertain weeks or even months there before the adoption can be finalized. Moreover, multiethnic families have their own special issues, in addition to the challenges that face all adoptive parents and children.

Still other couples forgo infertility treatments and adoption and instead come to accept their childlessness, often with the help of support groups. Self-help groups such as RESOLVE, a national organization for infertile couples, can help ease feelings of social isolation and secrecy and offer various practical alternatives. Sometimes they help childless couples recognize ways to channel their nurturing instincts into other pursuits such as teaching, coaching, or caring for disadvantaged children.

Couples who can afford to do so should consider couples counseling and perhaps, in addition, individual psychotherapy. (Many infertile couples whose relationship is threatened by infertility may feel that they cannot afford *not* to do so, whatever the cost.) Sometimes a priest, minister, or rabbi can serve in this role. Infertility can be the most trying experience of a person's life up to that point, and one of the most devastating blows to a relationship. Some individuals and couples sail through this experience with their self-esteem and sense of life's direction intact, but for many others the stresses associated with infertility are often too difficult to bear without the support and perspective that a caring, experienced counselor can offer.

How can infertility be prevented?

Infertility is usually unavoidable, and no one should be blamed for being or becoming infertile. Nevertheless, there are certain actions that can help reduce the risks of at least some forms of infertility.

The first is quite simply for women to consider having their babies in their 20s or early 30s, if they have that option. As much as many women would like to deny that fertility declines with age, the biological fact is that with every passing year over 30 a percentage of women will become infertile. Some develop conditions that can be corrected; but in a fraction of these women infertility cannot be overcome with the interventions currently available. For couples who rank having biological children high among their lifetime priorities, it may make sense to consider whether careers and other commitments can be juggled in some way so that childbearing can be attempted at an age when it has the best chance of success.

Taking steps to avoid contracting a sexually transmitted disease is extremely important to a woman's future fertility. These include using condoms during intercourse unless she is in a monogamous and infection-free relationship, keeping the number of her sexual partners low, and seeking immediate treatment if any suspicious symptoms develop. Because intrauterine devices carry a risk of uterine infections and thus possible infertility, clinicians will not generally recommend them for women who wish to have children at some time in the future. A woman who smokes can decrease her chances of infertility by quitting. If a woman has a substance abuse problem, getting help for it is a good idea whether or not a future pregnancy is in the picture.

Related entries

Adhesions, anorexia nervosa and bulimia nervosa, biopsy, ectopic pregnancy, electrocautery, endometriosis, hyperandrogenism, hyperprolactinemia, hysteroscopy, intrauterine devices, laparoscopy, laser surgery, menstrual cycle, menstrual cycle disorders, miscarriage, occupational hazards, pelvic inflammatory disease, sexual dysfunction, sexually transmitted diseases, stress, thyroid disorders, uterine fibroids

Infrequent Periods

Infrequent menstrual periods are generally defined as periods that occur more than 6 weeks apart. The condition is due to hormonal imbalances that lead to dysfunction of the hypothalamus, a part of the brain that regulates basic functions including eating, sleeping, and reproduction. Although infrequent periods often require no treatment, some women may have difficulty becoming pregnant.

Who is likely to have infrequent periods?

Infrequent periods (also called oligomenorrhea) are particularly common in the first few years after menarche (the first menstrual period) as well as in the years preceding menopause. Often in women of these ages, when menstruation does occur, it does not involve release of an egg from the ovary.

For reasons still not understood, some women menstruate as infrequently as every 2 months for all or most of their reproductive lives. So long as these periods are fairly regular, this type of oligomenorrhea does not usually require treatment. Infrequent periods that develop in women who have

had regular monthly periods are often due to stress, anxiety, excessive exercise, poor nutrition, chronic illness, or anorexia nervosa. All of these conditions can interfere with the function of the hypothalamus. In polycystic ovary syndrome, abnormally high levels of male-type hormones called androgens can also cause infrequent periods. (This condition is called hyperandrogenism; see entry.)

How is the condition evaluated?

A clinician will first do a physical and pelvic examination and take a history to find out if there are any underlying diseases or conditions that might explain the infrequent periods. Usually blood tests will be done to measure levels of hormones that play a role in the normal menstrual cycle.

How are infrequent periods treated?

Often menstrual periods become normalized when the underlying disease or condition is treated. Treatment for irregular bleeding that is not due to a systemic disease depends on the woman's age. If menstrual flow in an adolescent is not excessive, waiting a year or two is usually sufficient for the condition to resolve itself. If bleeding is heavy, it can be controlled with oral contraceptives. These are usually stopped after about 6 months to see if the cycles have normalized.

More mature women of reproductive age who ovulate infrequently, such as those with polycystic ovary syndrome, may take progesterone, such as medroxyprogesterone acetate (Provera), to regulate bleeding and prevent endometrial cancer, which has been associated with prolonged lack of periods. Usually the medication is taken for 10 to 12 days every 1 to 3 months, with menstruation (withdrawal bleeding) occurring just after the last day of medication. Alternatively, oral contraceptive pills may be prescribed to regularize menstruation. An added benefit of oral contraceptives is that certain kinds reduce androgen levels and therefore reduce hirsutism (growth of excess hair) in women with abnormally high levels of androgens.

Neither progesterone nor oral contraceptives induce ovulation, however. If pregnancy is desired, fertility counseling is usually necessary. Ovulation will probably have to be induced with either clomiphene citrate (Clomid) or human menopausal gonadotropins (Pergonal).

As menopause approaches, bleeding without ovulation may alternate with normal menstrual cycles for a couple of years as both become less frequent. This condition is common and requires no treatment. Before treatment is considered for a woman with infrequent periods who is approaching menopausal age, blood tests should be done to check for levels of follicle stimulating hormone (FSH) in the blood serum. This hormone is secreted by the pituitary and helps stimulate the development of ovarian follicles, one of which will eventually release a fertilizable egg. When the ovary stops responding to FSH, more FSH is produced by the pituitary, since there is no estrogen to shut off FSH production (see menstrual cycle). High FSH levels indicate that menopause has begun.

How can this condition be prevented?

Although infrequent periods are often unpreventable, some women may be able to normalize their menstrual cycle by maintaining a healthy body weight, exercising in moderation, and trying to reduce stress.

Related entries

Amenorrhea, anorexia nervosa and bulimia nervosa, anxiety disorders, blood tests, endometrial cancer, estrogen replacement therapy, hirsutism, hyperandrogenism, infertility, kidney disorders, menarche, menopause, menorrhagia, menstrual cycle, nutrition, obesity, stress

Insomnia

Insomnia, or the inability to get enough sleep, is an extremely common problem and can be a symptom of a host of physical and psychological disorders. Nevertheless, approximately a third of all people who think they have insomnia are actually getting enough sleep. Many people simply do not need the 8 hours of sleep that is often cited as ideal. Sleep needs among healthy people range from 4 to 10 hours, although the average adult gets between 7.5 and 8.5 hours of sleep per night. Also, as people age they sleep more lightly, with more frequent awakenings, and tend to need less sleep in general. This is partly so because certain medical problems—including certain kinds of heart disease and arthritis—can interfere with sleep, but also because sleep patterns change naturally over the course of one's life.

A good night's sleep consists of a series of sleep cycles, each representing a continuum of very light to very deep sleep and each lasting about 90 minutes. Throughout the night a sleeper goes back and forth from light to deep sleep a number of times. During the lightest phase, called non–rapid eye movement (or NREM) sleep, the sleeper is easily roused. It is in this stage that many people just beginning to doze may startle themselves awake, for example, after imagining a fall from some high place.

As a person passes through the NREM stages, sleep gradually deepens and at last reaches the deepest stage of the cycle, called rapid eye movement (REM) sleep. In this stage the eyes begin to move vigorously under the lids, perhaps because they are "looking" at the dreams that occur at this time. Sleep researchers believe that to wake up feeling fully rested, a person needs an average of 4 uninterrupted sleep cycles consisting of both NREM and REM sleep. People with insomnia may go through too few sleep cycles per night to feel rested, or they may be missing out on some crucial part of each cycle—particularly REM sleep.

Although the purpose of sleep is still not fully understood, most researchers today believe that at least one of its roles is to give the body and brain time to recharge after the stress and strain of waking activity. Even so, the occasional episodes of sleeplessness that afflict virtually everyone at one point or another are rarely of deep concern. It is usually easy to make up for the lost sleep by dozing a bit longer once life has returned to normal, and most people who experience transient insomnia can expect to function relatively normally during the day and should not expect any long-term health consequences. The same is true for people who experience "sleep fragmentation," a phenomenon well known to most mothers (and more than a few fathers), who have had to get up for several brief periods during the night to care for an infant or a sick child.

Losing sleep for more than a few days, however, is another matter. People with either short-term insomnia (which can last for several weeks) or chronic insomnia (which can last for months or years) can experience a variety of problems, including excessive daytime sleepiness, lack of coordination, mental and physical sluggishness, poor judgment, impaired concentration, sensory deprivation, and dangerous behavior such as dozing behind the wheel of a car. A lack of deep, dream-filled (REM) sleep may also interfere with a person's ability to learn and to process the information garnered during the day. Dozing during the day can also keep a person from noticing and registering events going on around her. There is even some evidence that sleep-deprived people may have weakened immune systems that leave them more susceptible to colds and other illnesses.

Who is likely to develop insomnia?

Among the many factors that can predispose a person to insomnia are emotional stress and anxiety, including the stress and anxiety that come from worrying about insomnia. Jet lag, conflicts at work, excitement or worry about a relationship or a new project—any of these can make sleeping difficult for a night or two. Traumatic life events such as the death of a loved one, the breakup of a relationship, the loss of a job, or the fear of having a serious illness can all induce short-term insomnia.

Chronic insomnia, by contrast, can result from underlying physical disorders (such as fibromyalgia) which make sleeping uncomfortable or from psychiatric problems, particularly depression. Although some depressed people sleep excessively, others find themselves waking in the wee hours of the morning. Shift workers who routinely alter sleeping and waking times, as well as people with sleep disorders such as "restless leg syndrome" or sleep apnea, may be prone to chronic insomnia as well (see sleep disorders).

Excessive caffeine consumption is another classic cause of insomnia. Although most people realize that drinking a couple of cups of caffeinated coffee after dinner may interfere with sleep, they often forget that there is caffeine in tea, cola, and chocolate, not to mention a number of over-the-counter drugs, including many allergy and arthritis medications, decongestants, cold remedies, and painkillers. Another medication that can prevent women from sleeping is appetite suppressants (see dieting). Finally, some people who take the older forms of beta blockers for high blood pressure, angina, and other heart problems are kept awake by the disturbing nightmares that are occasionally caused by these drugs.

Using over-the-counter sleep medications or alcohol to induce sleep may exacerbate insomnia. Alcohol induces sleep in the early part of the night, but it disrupts sleep later on. Over time, people develop a tolerance to both alcohol and over-the-counter sleep aids, so that increasingly large doses are needed to produce the same effect.

Bouts of sleeplessness are common during pregnancy. In the first trimester frequent trips to the bathroom in the middle of the night often interrupt sleep, and later in pregnancy vivid dreams, not to mention the difficulty of finding a comfortable position, can keep pregnant women from getting a good night's rest. Once the baby is born, new mothers are chronically robbed of sleep, not necessarily because of insomnia per se but because they simply do not have time to get enough rest. Besides having to spend the wee hours of the night feeding a hungry newborn, a mother of young children is often busy running a household, chauffeuring kids to activities, managing the entire family's schedule, and perhaps working a full-time or part-time job. A child who is sick or wakes with a bad dream—or a child who rises routinely at the crack of dawn—is often the source of a mother's sleep deprivation as well. Many new mothers sleep only 2 or 3 hours at a time and miss out on valuable REM sleep. A woman who suffers from postpartum depression is even more likely to have trouble sleeping.

Menopause is another time of life when insomnia becomes a problem for women. Here the source is usually hot flashes, which can be drenching and uncomfortable enough to rouse a woman from sleep several times during the night. Even in women unaware of nighttime hot flashes, a decrease in REM sleep related to falling estrogen levels can cause fatigue and occasionally can contribute to depression.

What are the symptoms?

A person who is not getting enough sleep will generally doze—or think about dozing—whenever she is bored or inactive. She will often need an alarm clock to get out of bed in the morning and use caffeine to get through the day. Another common symptom of sleep deprivation is irritability with family, friends, and co-workers.

How is the condition evaluated?

Anyone who feels excessively sleepy or fatigued during the day should suspect that she may have insomnia. Certain sleep disorders (particularly sleep apnea, which requires medical attention) can interfere with sleep while leaving the person unaware of the disruption. If the cause of the insomnia is elusive, or if the insomnia may be due to a serious sleep disorder, a visit to a physician is prudent. Often a thorough medical history is sufficient to identify the cause and guide the treatment.

When insomnia persists despite the best efforts of patient and clinician, referral to a sleep disorders center may be helpful. These centers, which can be found at many major medical centers, offer a multidisciplinary approach to evaluating and treating sleep disorders. Specialists in fields such as neurology, psychiatry, and pulmonary medicine review the patient's symptoms and consider her medical and psychiatric history. Sometimes the source of the problem can be identified only if the patient undergoes one or more overnight tests in which brain waves, breathing, and eye and muscle movements are measured during sleep. These evaluations can be quite costly, although many health insurance policies will cover them.

How is insomnia treated?

Short-term insomnia can sometimes be helped with over-the-counter sleep aids (such as Sominex, Nytol with DPH, Nervine, Sleep-Eze, or Unisom) or even a glass of wine. Most over-the-counter sleep aids rely on the action of antihistamines, such as diphenhydramine (in Benadryl). It may be cheaper to buy generic antihistamines than sleep aid products, although it is essential to choose an antihistamine that does not contain agents to counteract drowsiness.

When nonprescription medications are not effective for occasional insomnia, a physician will usually prescribe benzodiazepine tranquilizers such as lorazepam (Ativan). Like all tranquilizers, these drugs can be addictive if used over long periods of time, and because they suppress the dream stage of sleep, withdrawal can result in "rebound" nightmares. Nevertheless, for insomnia associated with anxiety, a short course of tranquilizers can sometimes be helpful.

Some physicians may prescribe low doses of antidepressant drugs such as amitriptyline (Elavil), trazodone, or doxepin instead. Although tolerance and rebound effects do not develop with these drugs, some people are bothered by side effects such as "drug mouth" or morning grogginess, even in low doses.

Newer drugs such as zolpidem (Ambien) can help with regularizing sleep cycles but should be used for only a month or two. There is renewed interest in a natural hormone, melatonin, produced by the pineal gland, which helps regulate sleep-wake cycles and other daily (circadian) body rhythms. Melatonin can be obtained over the counter in health food stores and can be taken at any time. It can be effective in preventing jet lag, and in helping people who are changing time zones get some sleep, but is clearly less effective for insomnia per se. There is good evidence that the herb valerian is effective and safe, although it's important to remember that the U.S. Food and Drug Administration does not strictly regulate herbs and dietary supplements and thus cannot guarantee the strength, purity, or safety of any given herb or supplement. People who are taking other prescription medications should also discuss possible interactions with their clinician before taking any over-the-counter herb or dietary supplement. Various nondrug strategies, used under the supervision of a sleep specialist or other clinician, may work better in the long run than sleeping pills. In chronotherapy, the hours of going to bed and waking up are gradually delayed until the biological clock is set to the desired time. Alternatively, various sleep restriction techniques can be used to extend gradually the time spent in bed. In these techniques the patient is first kept out of bed even when she is sleepy and forced to wake up before she is ready. Daytime naps are forbidden as well. Later she is allowed to wake up at her regular time but is forced to go to bed several hours later than usual until at last the time spent sleeping in bed has reached the desired level.

None of these techniques is effective if the insomnia is a symptom of some physical or psychological problem such as sleep apnea or depression. In such cases treatment for insomnia goes hand in hand with treating the underlying disorder. Estrogen replacement therapy is very effective in relieving the hot flashes that can cause insomnia during menopause.

How can insomnia be prevented?

A great deal of insomnia can be prevented or alleviated without professional help. Good "sleep hygiene" is generally the first line of attack against insomnia. This consists of following certain low-cost, self-help techniques that often help promote drowsiness and regular sleep cycles.

Stick to a regular sleep-wake schedule. Do not try to make up for lost sleep on weekends or holidays. This seems to help because every person has a built-in biological clock which regulates sleepy and wakeful periods (as well as times of peak metabolism). If the clock is "set" for 11 P.M. sleepiness, and a person tries to go to sleep at 9 P.M., problems are bound to arise. The most notorious example is shift workers, who must go to sleep in daylight hours for part of the week and nighttime hours for another part.

Avoid sporadic naps. Although taking a nap at the same time every day can be helpful (by decreasing the need for sleep at night), frequent catnaps and dozing just end up disrupting nighttime sleep. The optimal time for napping is about 12 hours after the midpoint of usual nighttime sleep.

Wind down slowly before going to bed. Avoid stressful activities such as sorting unpaid bills or picking a fight with one's spouse. Some people find it relaxing to stroll about the house, write a letter, read a book, or take a warm bath before attempting to sleep. Relaxation exercises can also be helpful, but vigorous exercise after dinner should be avoided. One relaxation exercise that helps many people is lying in bed and progressively tensing and then relaxing each muscle group, starting with the toes and working up to the shoulders and neck. Other people find it helpful to do abdominal breathing, which involves keeping the chest still and using the stomach muscles to take slow deep breaths.

Make the bedroom conducive to sleep. A comfortable bed, attractive linens, dark windowshades, adequate ventilation, temperature and humidity control during all seasons, air filters for people suffering from allergies or asthma, and eye coverings or earplugs if necessary can all make sleep come more easily.

Leave the bedroom if sleep is a problem. The last thing a sleep-deprived person wants to do is build up an association between the bedroom and sleeplessness. If relaxation exercises do not work, instead of tossing and turning in bed one might try going to some other room to read quietly or watch a dull television program. The goal is to provide a relaxing, comforting, and quiet environment.

Exercise regularly. Exercise during the day seems to make sleep come easier at night. Daytime or at least early evening exercise is best, since vigorous activity right before bed can keep a person up for hours.

Be careful about food and drink. Eating meals at the same time every day can help synchronize the body's biological clock. Some people find that drinking warm milk or having a high-carbohydrate snack just before bed helps them sleep. Some researchers maintain that this is because such foods are high in L-tryptophan, a naturally occurring amino acid that seems to promote drowsiness. (High levels of L-tryptophan are also found in turkey, which may help explain the "turkey narcolepsy" that many people experience after Thanksgiving dinner.) There is no scientific evidence thus far that the amount of L-tryptophan in food is enough to alleviate anything more than the most minor insomnia, however. Higher doses, in supplement form, often produce nausea and other side effects and should be avoided. Tryptophan as a supplement was removed from the U.S. market after a batch caused 1,500 cases of the chronic and debilitating eosinophilia-myalgia syndrome—including 40 deaths. One form of this amino acid, 5-hydroxytryptophan (5-HTP), is available in the United States, however, and is used to treat insomnia.

Related entries

Antianxiety drugs, antidepressants, anxiety disorders, breastfeeding, coffee, depression, dieting, estrogen replacement therapy, exercise, high blood pressure, menopause, postpartum issues, postpartum psychiatric disorders, sleep disorders, stress

Interstitial Cystitis

Interstitial cystitis is a chronic, noninfectious condition in which the tissue between the lining and the muscular wall of the bladder becomes damaged (see illustration). Although many women suffer from this condition (the exact numbers remain uncertain), it is still not widely recognized within the medical community and often is misdiagnosed.

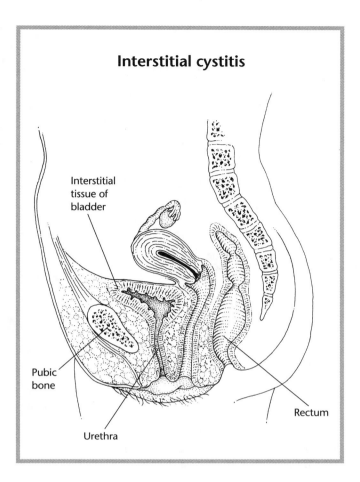

Interstitial cystitis

Interstitial tissue of bladder

Pubic bone

Urethra

Rectum

Who is likely to develop interstitial cystitis?

Interstitial cystitis seems to affect mainly middle-aged women and seems never to affect women under the age of 18. Its underlying cause remains unknown. Women with interstitial cystitis have a higher than average rate of allergic and autoimmune disorders, including medication and food allergies, hay fever, asthma, and rheumatoid arthritis.

What are the symptoms?

Many of the symptoms resemble those of a urinary tract infection: pain and pressure in the bladder and pelvis, a burning sensation on urination, and the need to urinate frequently—at least 8 times a day. Some women may need to urinate as often as once or twice an hour, and often several times throughout the night. Pain and discomfort increase as the bladder fills and are relieved as it empties, although sometimes there is a sensation of incomplete emptying. The symptoms can be chronic or recurrent, waxing and waning over months to years.

How is the condition evaluated?

Interstitial cystitis is often difficult to diagnose and can be mistaken for urinary tract infections, kidney disorders, sexually transmitted diseases, vaginitis, and endometriosis (see

entries). Any woman who suspects she may have this condition should first see a primary care physician for a physical examination. The clinician will probably obtain a urine test to determine if there is any bacterial infection. Once infection and anatomical defects have been ruled out, the physician will probably refer the patient to a urologist, who will perform a test called a cystoscopy. In this procedure the urologist inserts a small viewing instrument (a cystoscope) through the urethra (the thin tube that drains urine from the bladder to the outside of the body) into the distended bladder and looks for any signs of interstitial cystitis such as pinpoint areas of bleeding all over the bladder wall or Hunner's ulcer (a wedge-shaped erosion in the bladder wall). In order to diagnose interstitial cystitis, it is important that the bladder be distended with fluid during the examination, a procedure that is not routinely part of a cystoscopy. Some urologists may also want to do a biopsy of the bladder by removing tissue through the cystoscope and examining it for bladder cancer. Cystoscopy can usually be done with local anesthesia on an outpatient basis.

The urologist will also probably do another test called a cystometrogram. In this procedure, performed under local anesthesia, a tiny electronic sensor is threaded into the bladder through a catheter. As fluid is infused into the bladder, the sensor indicates contractions in the bladder wall by measuring changes in pressure. If contractions begin long before the bladder reaches normal capacity, interstitial cystitis is likely.

How is interstitial cystitis treated?

Drug therapy for interstitial cystitis includes amitriptyline, an antidepressant used in low doses, and hydroxyzine, an antihistamine, taken at bedtime. Pentosan pentosulfate (Elmiron) eases symptoms by making the lining of the bladder less permeable. Some women find that having a physician dilate the bladder with the antiinflammatory drug dimethyl sulfoxide (DMSO), instilled directly into the bladder, also seems to provide temporary relief. This treatment involves weekly visits to a clinician's office for 1 to 2 months. The FDA is testing several other promising drugs.

In the meantime, some women find that they can often prevent flare-ups by avoiding certain foods that stimulate the bladder. Among the common culprits are alcohol, caffeine, chocolate, carbonated beverages, fruits and fruit juices (especially citrus and cranberry), tomatoes, artificial sweeteners, and even brewer's yeast.

Another relatively easy source of relief involves trying to increase the time between urinations by a small increment each week to help retrain the nerves and muscles and increase bladder capacity. A urologist may also be able to relieve symptoms temporarily by filling the bladder with fluid—a procedure requiring anesthesia—in the hope of increasing bladder capacity. Only in the most severe cases are more drastic approaches attempted, such as laser treatment or surgery (usually to replace most of the bladder with a bag outside the body or with a pouch made out of part of the colon), and neither of these has been particularly successful in relieving symptoms so far.

Related entries

Antiinflammatory drugs, biopsy, incontinence, kidney disorders, sexually transmitted diseases, urinary tract infections, vaginitis

Intrauterine Devices

An intrauterine device is a small object inserted by a clinician into the uterus to prevent pregnancy. IUDs come in a variety of shapes and sizes, and some contain certain chemicals—such as copper or progesterone—to help increase their efficacy while permitting the size of the actual device to be reduced, and thus reducing the risk of complications.

The IUD is a very effective means of contraception, with an expected failure rate of about 1 to 2 percent and a typical failure rate of about 3 percent. After 7 years of use, only 1 woman in 100 using the progestin-impregnated IUD is expected to become pregnant.

Although the IUD was originally touted as an "ideal" form of birth control—no muss, no fuss, and highly effective—problems arose in the 1970s when a number of women developed serious complications, particularly pelvic inflammatory disease and sometimes fatal septic abortions (infected miscarriages) after using the IUD known as the Dalkon Shield. Even after the Dalkon Shield was banned from the U.S. market in 1974, liability and insurance concerns about IUDs in general led manufacturers to remove most of the devices from the market—although many of these products are still available in Canada and other countries.

There are now two kinds of IUDs available in the United States (see illustrations). The first of these, known as the Copper T 380A (ParaGard), which became available in 1988, is a white plastic device coated with copper. A more recently approved hormone-secreting device, Mirena, has been available in Europe for over a decade. Mirena releases minuscule amounts of the hormone levonorgestrel, a form of progesterone, providing contraception for up to 5 years. At the same time, it can dramatically reduce menstrual blood flow and may even shrink uterine fibroids.

Because the progestin-implanted IUD reduces menstrual blood loss, many clinicians consider it a plus for women who have heavy menstrual bleeding (and possibly even a reason to use this method regardless of contraceptive needs). About 75 percent of women using an IUD continue to ovulate and so do not suffer the side effects of changing estrogen levels sometimes associated with progestin-only oral contraceptives. Some investigators feel that this device may be particularly attractive to older women with menstrual irregulari-

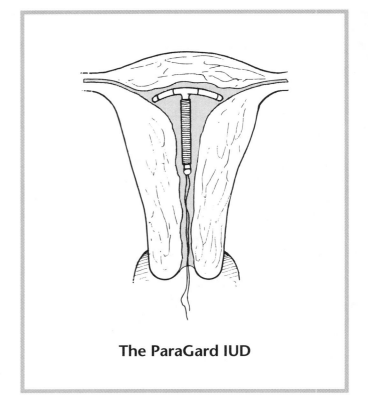

The ParaGard IUD

ties who do not plan to bear children in the future. No IUD offers protection against sexually transmitted disease.

Just how the intrauterine device prevents pregnancy continues to be a matter of controversy. Originally it was thought that the device worked by speeding the transport of the egg through the fallopian tube—thus reducing its chances for fertilization—or by producing a mild inflammation or chronic infection in the uterine lining that somehow prevented a fertilized egg from implanting. Today some investigators insist that neither of these theories is correct and suggest that IUDs work by interfering with the transport of both sperm and egg.

How is an IUD inserted?

Before obtaining an IUD, a woman needs to have a thorough physical examination. To make sure that she is a good candidate for this method of birth control, the clinician will do a Pap test, pelvic examination, and certain baseline tests to check for pregnancy and sexually transmitted diseases (STDs), and will ask about any history of pelvic inflammatory disease or STDs and number of sexual partners (all of which can have a bearing on the safety of the IUD).

If the results of the tests are satisfactory, the clinician will insert the IUD into the uterus through the vagina and cervix (opening to the uterus) using a strawlike instrument. Both the Mirena and Copper T 380A are made of plastic in the shape of a T which is flattened temporarily into a straight line during insertion and which springs back into shape inside the uterus. Both of these devices have a plastic string or strings which protrude through the cervical opening and can be felt in the upper part of the vagina. The string is used to remove the IUD, as well as to make sure that it stays properly positioned.

Some women feel uncomfortable cramping during insertion. After insertion many experience cramping and spotting for a few days.

The ideal time to have an IUD inserted is still a matter of controversy. On the one hand, some clinicians prefer to do the insertion during or toward the end of a woman's menstrual period, since the cervix is slightly open then and chances are slim that she is pregnant. On the other hand, clinicians who feel that the risk of infection is greater at this time prefer to insert the IUD around the time of ovulation (mid-cycle). Equally unclear is whether IUDs should be inserted immediately after an abortion or childbirth. Although some studies indicate that insertion at these times may increase the odds of expelling the device—or the chance of complications—others found no problems whatsoever. Until conclusive data are in, it probably makes sense to wait 6 to 8 weeks after an abortion or childbirth before having an IUD inserted.

Once inserted, the IUD is an extremely easy form of contraception to use. It does not interfere with sexual spontaneity, and there is no need to remember to take a pill or to keep a supply of spermicide on hand. The only regular effort required is to check the string about once a month (more frequently in the first month of use) to make sure that the device is still in place.

On the inconvenience side of the ledger, women who want to use an IUD usually need to visit a clinician's office at least twice before the device can be inserted (since it takes at least a couple of days for some of the test results to come back). In addition, it is usually necessary to have a checkup about 3 months after insertion and then return again every so often to have the device replaced. The Mirena device is effective for 5 years. The Copper T 380A can remain in place for much longer—up to 10 years of use.

The total cost of an IUD—including the cost of 2 initial office visits and the required screening tests—generally runs between about $320 and $400.

What are the risks and complications?

Many women find that they have some cramping and spotting for the first few days after an IUD is inserted. Although the Mirena actually diminishes menstrual flow, copper IUDs tend to induce heavier and longer-lasting menstrual bleeding, particularly during the early months of use. Continuing menstrual cramps and excessive menstrual bleeding—or associated anemia—lead a sizable minority of women to have their IUD removed during the first year of use.

Using an IUD appears to increase the risk of developing pelvic inflammatory disease, particularly in women who have not yet had children. For this reason many clinicians will not insert an IUD in a woman who has not yet completed her family. The risk is greatest during the first month after insertion, however, and can sometimes be circumvented altogether by taking antibiotics during this time. Women who have multiple sexual partners—or who have a partner who has multiple sexual partners—continue to be at increased risk for pelvic inflammatory disease when they use an IUD. Any woman who uses an IUD and experiences lower abdominal pain, pain during sexual intercourse, foul-smelling vaginal discharge, nausea, vomiting, and possibly fever and chills should contact a clinician promptly.

Expulsion of the IUD is another common problem, though less so with today's devices containing copper and progestin. Because expulsion is most likely to occur during the first few months of use, many women choose to use a barrier method of contraception in addition to the IUD for this period of time. Often the IUD is expelled during the menstrual period, though this may not even be noticed. That is why it is wise to check the string frequently: absence of the string indicates that the device may have shifted its position, in which case a clinician should be contacted.

In rare cases an IUD will perforate the uterine wall—a serious but sometimes unnoticeable problem that is most common during the early months of use. In rare instances the IUD can actually break through the uterine wall and travel to other parts of the body such as the abdomen, where it can become embedded and cause serious complications. This is another compelling reason to check the string on a regular basis—particularly because it is possible to have a perforated uterus without any symptoms—and to contact a clinician if there are any changes.

To locate a missing IUD, the clinician will use ultrasound or x-ray. If the device is still in the uterus, it can often be pulled back into place or removed without surgery. If the device is outside the uterus, abdominal surgery may be necessary to keep the IUD from perforating or otherwise damaging other organs or inducing scar tissue. Occasionally the lining of the uterus may grow around the IUD, embedding the device. Although this does not seem to impair the contraceptive effect of the device, it can lead to pain when the device is removed, sometimes to the point where a dilatation and curettage (D&C) or hysteroscopy is necessary for removal.

Women should not use an IUD if they are or may be pregnant or if they have active or recurrent pelvic inflammatory disease, any sexually transmitted disease, acute cervicitis or vaginitis, abnormal vaginal bleeding, or anomalies of the uterus (such as birth defects or uterine fibroids) which distort its shape. Nor is the IUD a good choice of contraception for women with multiple sexual partners or whose sexual partner has multiple sexual partners (see safer sex). In addition, women with a known or suspected allergy to copper should not use an IUD that contains copper.

Although an IUD does not directly reduce a woman's chances of becoming pregnant in the future, complications such as pelvic inflammatory disease and uterine perforation, though rare, can render a woman infertile or sterile. That is why IUDs are generally not considered a good choice of birth control for women who want to bear children in the future, though exceptions are sometimes made for women in monogamous relationships who cannot use other methods of contraception.

If a woman becomes pregnant while using an IUD, she has a 40 to 50 percent chance of having a miscarriage. Even if the IUD is removed during the pregnancy, the chances of a miscarriage remain as high as 25 percent. Having the IUD removed as soon as possible is a good idea whether or not the woman plans to continue the pregnancy, since leaving an IUD in place can lead to septic abortion. For women who do choose to continue the pregnancy, the presence of an IUD in the uterus can cause various complications in addition to miscarriage, including infection, stillbirth, premature delivery, and the delivery of a low birth weight infant.

Related entries

Abortion, birth control, condoms, diaphragms and cervical caps, ectopic pregnancy, hormonal contraception, hysterectomy, natural birth control methods, nonsurgical abortion, oral contraceptives, pregnancy testing, safer sex, sexually transmitted diseases, spermicides, tubal ligation, vacuum aspiration

Iron

Iron is one of 20 minerals that are essential micronutrients. Contained in hemoglobin, the component of red blood cells that carries oxygen to body tissues, iron is also stored for later use in the spleen, liver, and bone marrow. A deficiency of iron may lead not only to a sore tongue and hair loss but also to iron-deficiency anemia, the most common form of anemia.

Who is likely to develop iron deficiency?

Women who are pregnant are particularly vulnerable to iron deficiency because of the demands made on their iron stores by the fetus. Any situation that involves a large amount of blood loss—including surgery, gastrointestinal bleeding from an ulcer, colon polyp or tumor, unusually heavy menstrual periods, or the use of a copper intrauterine device (which often leads to heavy periods), for example—can also result in iron deficiency.

Because iron is commonly lost through menstruation, many premenopausal women require 18 mg of iron per day, compared with only 8 mg for men and postmenopausal women. Women who are pregnant, who are on a weight-loss diet, or who have recently lost a lot of blood may need to take iron supplement pills.

What are the best sources of iron?

Iron is found most abundantly in red meats, liver, rice, beans, potatoes, eggs, and dried fruits (see chart). Just because a food contains iron does not necessarily mean that the nutrient is

Good sources of iron in the diet		
Food	**Serving size**	**Mg of iron**
Calf liver	3.5 oz	14
Liverwurst	3 oz	9
Chicken livers	3.5 oz	8
Prune juice	½ cup	5
Ground beef (lean)	3.5 oz	4
Chickpeas	½ cup	3
Steak	3 oz	3
Raisins	½ cup	2
Molasses	1 tbsp	2
Prunes	4	2
Kidney beans	½ cup	2
Spinach	½ cup cooked	2
Chicken	¼ chicken	2
Turkey	4 oz	2

readily absorbed by the body, however. Iron is much less readily absorbed from vegetables and grains (including iron-fortified commercial food products) than from meat and fish. One way to increase the absorption of iron from food or a supplement is to drink citrus juice or take vitamin C at the same time. This is because vitamin C increases the absorption of iron.

Minerals compete for absorption in the gut, and so taking too much of any one of them often reduces absorption of another, equally vital one. Taking too much iron can interfere with the body's absorption of zinc. Also, minerals are most effective in the body when they are in balance with other minerals. Red blood cell formation requires both iron and copper working together, for example. For this reason, a balanced diet—which should contain a variety of minerals—is still usually the best way to ensure that the body gets enough iron.

Ferrous sulfate is the form of iron most frequently prescribed for women with iron deficiency. The usual dose is one tablet of 325 mg 2 or 3 times daily. Although taking iron supplements can cause constipation, reducing the daily dose of iron or changing to a different compound can help. One possibility is the drug Niferex—available over the counter under many different brand names—which combines iron with a low molecular weight polysaccharide to decrease the risk of nausea and constipation. To increase iron absorption, Niferex should be taken with vitamin C. Iron supplements usually need to be taken for several months to restore reserves in iron-deficient women.

Although iron supplements are available without a prescription, a woman should let her physician know how much she is taking. Taking iron can mask symptoms of other serious conditions such as blood loss caused by colon cancer. It is important to check with a clinician about the proper dose of iron supplementation and whether evaluation of underlying causes of the deficiency is necessary. Even though iron loss in women is commonly related to menstruation, it is important to make sure that one is not losing blood from the gastrointestinal tract.

Related entries

Anemia, colon and rectal cancer, constipation, dieting, fatigue, intrauterine devices, menorrhagia, nutrition, pregnancy, vitamins

Irritable Bowel Syndrome

Irritable bowel syndrome affects at least 15 percent of the U.S. population and is a fairly common cause of chronic abdominal and pelvic pain in women. The exact incidence in women is unknown because most people with symptoms probably never seek medical care, but it is estimated that in industrialized countries twice as many women as men report symptoms of IBS. In less developed countries most cases of IBS are reported in men, though this may be related to cultural biases in using the health care system rather than some inherent difference between the sexes.

The exact definition of IBS varies from one doctor to another, despite efforts to standardize diagnostic criteria. The condition is generally characterized by abdominal pain and changes in bowel habits. Although symptoms can be quite distressing and frustrating to treat, IBS does not predispose people to more serious disorders and has no known effect on life expectancy.

IBS is sometimes called spastic colon, nervous colon, irritable colon, or unstable colon, as well as mucous colitis or nervous colitis. The latter two terms are misleading because they can cause people to confuse IBS with ulcerative colitis, a more serious condition characterized by bloody diarrhea (see bowel disorders). In addition, the suffix "-itis" in colitis implies an inflammatory process, when in fact IBS has nothing to do with inflammation but instead is thought to be caused by exaggerated muscular contractions and function in the cells of the intestine.

Normally there are two different types of intestinal contractions: segmenting contractions, which keep waste products from moving down toward the rectum and anus, and propulsive contractions, which occur occasionally to force the contents forward. When segmenting contractions become excessive, constipation results. When propulsive contractions become excessive, diarrhea results. Exaggerated intestinal contractions can be stimulated by a number of factors, including eating disorders, emotional stress, anxiety, depression, certain medications, and conditions such as hyperthyroidism. Some women who have been diagnosed as having IBS find that their symptoms increase during menstruation or in the days just before menstruation.

Who is likely to develop irritable bowel syndrome?

IBS most often develops during adolescence or early adulthood. It is quite rare for the symptoms to begin after the age of 50. The prevalence of past sexual abuse seems to be higher in women with irritable bowel syndrome than among the general population, suggesting that a history of abuse may be a risk factor for IBS.

What are the symptoms?

The characteristic symptoms of IBS are crampy abdominal pain and some combination of constipation and diarrhea. Bowel movements may contain mucus and are frequently loose and watery or else resemble pellets, small balls, or ribbons. People with IBS commonly feel bloated and pass excessive gas, and many complain of indigestion and heartburn. Constipation is sometimes accompanied by nausea. If only some of these symptoms occur, many doctors prefer to diagnose the condition as functional bowel syndrome, although other doctors use this term interchangeably with irritable bowel syndrome.

Some people with IBS may actually be able to feel contractions in the intestine. It is also common to have an urgent or frequent need to urinate during the day or to wake at night in order to urinate. Many people with IBS have bouts of anxiety and depression, but whether these are causes, results, or symptoms of the condition remains unclear.

Typically symptoms of IBS occur after a meal and are temporarily relieved by a bowel movement. Specific foods such as milk, fried foods, peanuts, or caffeine sometimes produce symptoms in susceptible people. Although a few people have symptoms every day, most people with IBS go through days, weeks, or even months without experiencing any abnormal bowel function or pain.

In rare instances people with IBS may have significant weight loss (owing to depression) or bleeding in the gastrointestinal tract (owing to anal fissures or hemorrhoids which result from straining to move the bowels). More frequently, however, these symptoms signal more serious conditions and warrant a thorough medical examination.

How is the condition evaluated?

In examining a patient with chronic pelvic or abdominal pain and altered bowel habits, a doctor will make a diagnosis based on the nature of the symptoms reported. There is no test for diagnosing IBS, but the clinician will consider the possibility of other conditions associated with similar symptoms. These conditions include lactose intolerance (being unable to digest milk and milk products), duodenal ulcer (see peptic ulcer disease), allergies, various bacterial infections, and parasitic infections (including giardiasis and amoebiasis), as well as menstrual cramps, thyroid disorders, diverticular disease, uterine fibroids, colon cancer, ovarian cancer, and acquired immune deficiency syndrome (see entries).

A woman's description of her symptoms is one of the most helpful pieces of information a clinician uses in diagnosing IBS. A physical examination, including a rectal examination, will be performed, and blood will be tested for signs of infection, chronic inflammation, and anemia. An ultrasound may be done to make sure there are no visible abnormalities of the reproductive organs. Sometimes sigmoidoscopy, colonoscopy, or a barium enema may be used to exclude other inflammatory processes. In sigmoidoscopy the lower part of the colon is examined with a bendable lighted tube called a flexible proctosigmoidoscope. No sedation or anesthesia is needed; the procedure causes, at most, mild discomfort and takes only about 15 minutes. In colonoscopy the upper part of the colon is examined as well, and the patient receives light intravenous sedation during the procedure, which takes between 30 minutes and an hour. A barium enema outlines the structure of the gastrointestinal tract so that it can be examined by x-ray. In preparation for these procedures, enemas or laxatives are used to clean out the colon.

Any patient who is having problems with bloating should be checked for lactose intolerance, a disorder whose symptoms are similar to those of IBS. People with lactose intolerance have a deficiency of an enzyme called lactase, which normally digests lactose, the principal sugar found in cow's milk. Drinking milk or eating dairy products may lead to abdominal bloating and sometimes pain within minutes to hours. To test for lactase deficiency, a doctor will often prescribe a completely lactose-free diet for a week or two to see if symptoms disappear or decrease.

How is IBS treated?

Because IBS may have a number of different causes, there is no one treatment that works for every patient. For some the mere assurance that the symptoms are not caused by a more serious disorder can relieve stress and alleviate symptoms. For most people with IBS, however, certain dietary changes and sometimes medications are necessary.

Dietary changes generally involve decreasing fat and increasing fiber (roughage) intake. By increasing water retention in the intestine, fiber makes stools bulkier and can alleviate both constipation and diarrhea. High-fiber foods include fresh fruits and vegetables, whole grains (particularly wheat bran), nuts, prunes, raisins, figs, and dates. There are two sources of fiber that are also available in various over-the-counter preparations—insoluble fiber (the type found in bran) and soluble fiber (psyllium, methylcellulose, pectin, or calcium polycarbophil). The latter are "bulk formers" and are sometimes referred to as "natural laxatives." For many people with IBS, these supplemental fiber products are a more reliable source of fiber and are better tolerated than dietary sources. Even when diarrhea (not constipation) is the main symptom, fiber supplements are an essential part of treatment for most people with IBS. Stronger laxatives are needed for the rare intractable bout of constipation, but regular use leads to dependence and can eventually make constipation much worse.

Many people find that certain forms of fiber produce bloating and gas, and some experimentation may be necessary before a satisfactory diet or supplemental source of fiber is found. If bloating is a problem, it often helps to eliminate foods likely to cause gas. These include apricots, bananas, beans, brussels sprouts, carrots, celery, onions, peanuts, pretzels, prunes, raisins, and wheat germ. Flatulence that results from eating beans and peas may be reduced by using Beano, an over-the-counter preparation of the enzyme alpha-galactosidase. It works by partially metabolizing insoluble sugars found in beans and peas and so decreasing the amount of sugar available for fermentation in the colon—a process that otherwise produces gas. Medications containing simethecone (such as Riopan Plus and Mylanta II) can also help alleviate gas, as can agents that help speed the transit of food through the stomach, such as metoclopramide (Reglan, which is available by prescription only).

People who are lactose-intolerant should avoid foods and medications containing lactose to decrease or eliminate flatulence. Some people who cannot drink milk find that they can eat cheese and yogurt, which are lower in lactose. Adding a product called Lactaid (a form of lactase) to yogurt and certain milk products can prevent symptoms by breaking lactose down into simpler sugars.

If dietary changes have no effect on symptoms, drugs called anticholinergics (such as Bentyl or Donnatal) that alleviate muscle spasms are sometimes prescribed to relieve pain on a temporary basis, even though they still have not been proven to be beneficial in treating IBS. Low doses of antidepressants can be helpful for easing the abdominal pain of IBS, just as they can reduce pain from a variety of other chronic conditions. Tricyclic antidepressants such as amitriptyline, nortriptyline, or desipramine are used in low doses at bedtime. The class of antidepressants known as SSRIs (selective serotonin reuptake inhibitors) may also reduce discomfort from IBS, since these drugs regulate serotonin, a neurotransmitter that plays an important role in sensation and muscle activity in the gut. Drugs for IBS that specifically target serotonin, such as alosetron (Lotronex) have been fraught with complications but sometimes may be tried under close observation by a clinician. For chronic diarrhea or frequent stools, antidiarrheal drugs such as loperamide (Imodium) or diphenoxylate (Lomotil) taken on an occasional basis may be helpful as well. For women with IBS associated predominantly with constipation, the serotonin-active drug tegaserod (Zelnorm) has recently been approved by the FDA.

Stress management, biofeedback, and relaxation training (see alternative therapies), antidepressant or antianxiety medications, or professional counseling seem to help some people with irritable bowel syndrome.

Related entries

Alternative therapies, anorexia nervosa and bulimia nervosa, anxiety disorders, bowel disorders, colon and rectal cancer, constipation, depression, diverticular disease, hemorrhoids, laxatives, stress, thyroid disorders

Kegel Exercises

Kegel exercises are pelvic floor exercises to strengthen the muscles that surround part of the vagina, rectum, and urethra. These pelvic floor muscles often become weakened during pregnancy and childbirth, as well as after menopause. Although Kegel exercises cannot repair major anatomical defects, they can be a simple and inexpensive way to prepare for childbirth and improve muscle tone after delivery. They can also relieve symptoms from various problems that result from weakened pelvic floor muscles, including urinary stress incontinence, prolapsed uterus, cystoceles, urethroceles, and rectoceles. As an added bonus, many women find that sexual response improves when these muscles are strengthened.

How are Kegel exercises performed?

There are a variety of Kegel exercises, but all involve the alternating contraction (tightening) and release of the pelvic floor muscles. These muscles are the same ones used to stop the flow of urine when sitting with the legs spread apart. One simple Kegel exercise is to contract the muscles as far as possible, hold tightly for 3 seconds, and then release. Another exercise, often used in childbirth education classes, involves thinking of the muscle as a sort of elevator. The woman starts at ground level (completely relaxed) and then tightens her muscles slightly to reach the first floor, holding for several seconds. She then moves up floor by floor, pausing at each one, until she reaches the fifth floor with her muscles fully contracted. Then she gradually releases the muscles floor by floor in the same way. Each Kegel exercise should be done several times a day, for a total of 50 to 100 repetitions daily. Some women find that doing 2 sets of 25 repetitions each is convenient, and takes only a few minutes a day.

Because they can be done inconspicuously, Kegels can be fit into even the busiest routine. In fact, many women get in the habit of doing them whenever they talk on the phone, sit at a red light, or lie awake in bed, or even while having sexual intercourse (often to their partner's delight). A doctor, nurse, midwife, or childbirth education instructor can give more specific directions about appropriate exercises for a woman's individual condition or problem, as well as the number of times per day to repeat them. Biofeedback training (see alternative therapies) or supervised training with electrical stimulation may be necessary for women with weak pelvic muscles before they can properly perform Kegel exercises at home.

Related entries

Cystocele/urethrocele/rectocele, incontinence, pregnancy, prolapsed uterus, sexual response

Keloid Scarring

Keloids are elevated, fleshy, ridged scars that occur when the skin produces excess scar tissue beyond the bounds of the original skin injury. Unlike other large "hypertrophic" scars, keloids take on a size and shape of their own rather than conforming to the dimensions of the original wound. In susceptible people they can develop after any kind of skin trauma, including surgery, injury, or even a vaccination. They have also been known to occur for no apparent reason, especially on the face, neck, or chest.

Some women develop unsightly keloid scars on their face after cosmetic surgery or on the abdomen after a cesarean section. Although they pose no particular medical risks, such scars can cause considerable unhappiness, particularly when they develop on the face or other exposed areas of skin. Any woman who is undergoing surgery should discuss the possibility of keloid scarring with her surgeon, and any woman who knows from past experience that she is susceptible to keloids should be very cautious about undergoing elective procedures, such as cosmetic surgery.

Who is likely to develop keloid scars?

Certain ethnic groups—particularly those with dark skin—are especially susceptible to keloid scarring. Some researchers even insist that whites never develop true keloid scars, theorizing that these scars may reflect an aberration in the way the body metabolizes a hormone vital to skin coloration (melanocyte stimulating hormone). This theory is consistent with the fact that keloids virtually never occur on the soles and palms—which are usually light colored even in dark-skinned people. It is also consistent with the observation that keloids tend to be more common during puberty and pregnancy, times when melanocyte stimulating hormone levels are particularly high.

There is also some evidence that keloid scarring may be initiated by an abnormal immune response, in which case no group would necessarily be exempt. Whatever the explanation ultimately turns out to be, the fact remains that keloids are at least 15 times more common in people of dark-skinned ethnic groups than in whites.

Many women do not know that they are susceptible to keloids until a large scar has already formed, such as after a cesarean section. Women who may have developed unusually large scars from immunizations, chicken pox, or other small wounds should be wary about the possibility of keloid scarring following surgical incisions.

How is the condition evaluated?

Keloids actually have a number of characteristics that distinguish them from other forms of hypertrophic scarring. There are differences, for example, in the placement of collagen, a fibrous protein which normally serves as the support structure for skin but which also makes up scar tissue. When ex-

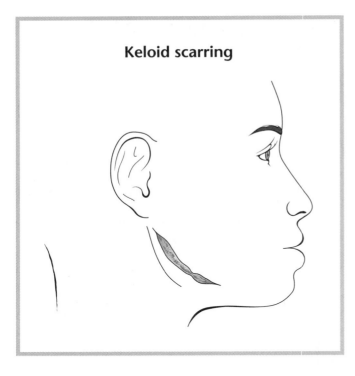

Keloid scarring

amined under an electron microscope, standard hypertrophic scars show bundles of collagen that run parallel to the skin surface. In contrast, in keloids the collagen is contained in randomly organized sheets with no clear orientation to the skin's surface.

There are also certain biochemical and immunologic differences between keloids and other enlarged scars. Such features, however, are not always apparent to the naked eye, and so most keloids are labeled as such simply because of their appearance. Since treatment is essentially the same for both keloids and other enlarged scars, this rarely poses a problem.

How are keloid scars treated?
Occasionally a keloid scar will recede on its own. The frustrating paradox of trying to treat the many that do not is that new keloids often result from the very process of removal. Trying to excise keloids surgically is particularly counterproductive, since the process necessarily involves making a new wound—which in about 50 percent of cases results in yet another keloid.

Over the years various surgical techniques have evolved to circumvent this problem, such as the use of skin grafts to help close the new wound with less tension. Together with injections of corticosteroids such as triamcinolone, tretinoin (Retin-A), or other drugs, these techniques are often successful. On the down side, many of these drugs have occasional side effects of their own, including skin discoloration and spider veins (telangiectasias; see varicose veins).

To help circumvent these kinds of effects, investigators have tried to remove keloids with laser surgery, using supplementary medications only if there are signs of recurrence. Currently there is no established and effective treatment for this condition.

How can keloids be prevented?
Most keloid scarring cannot be prevented. If a woman who knows that she is susceptible is having surgery, however, the same steps that are normally used to remove keloid scars can be taken during the operation, including special wound closure procedures and injection of antiinflammatory drugs.

Related entries
Antiinflammatory drugs, cesarean section, cosmetic surgery, laser surgery, pregnancy, varicose veins, wrinkles

Kidney Disorders

The kidneys are a pair of bean-shaped organs about the size of a fist that lie on either side of the spine at the back of the abdominal cavity. By serving as filters for excess fluids, salts, and acids, they produce urine and play a crucial role in removing waste material from the blood and maintaining the body's balance of fluids.

Blood enters the kidneys through blood vessels called the renal arteries and then passes through a series of about a million interconnected filter systems called nephrons. Each of these functional units contains a coil of blood vessels called a glomerulus and some winding tubules (see illustration). The glomerulus filters out blood cells, proteins, sugars, and large particles from the blood and returns them to the bloodstream through the renal vein. Whatever is left passes into the tubules, which filter out salts and acids required by the body. The waste products—including urea, uric acid, creatinine, and any excess water or salts—remain in the tubules as urine and are passed through the ureters for storage in the bladder.

When this complex waste removal system is injured, infected, or malfunctioning for some other reason, the consequences can be severe for just about every other part of the body. Although many of these consequences are the same in men and women, certain kidney problems can have particular effects on hormonal, reproductive, and sexual functioning in women. Conversely, pregnancy and other conditions unique to women can predispose them to developing certain kidney disorders.

Kidney infections
Acute urinary tract infection (UTI) occurs when bacteria colonize in the vaginal area and then travel up to the bladder. If they go beyond the bladder, up through the ureters, and colonize in the kidney, the infection is called pyelonephritis. Although any UTI can be uncomfortable, pyelonephritis can also be quite dangerous if left untreated. Signs and symptoms of this condition include fever, chills, flank pain, nausea, vomiting, burning during urination, and the need to urinate frequently. A person with a UTI will usually notice the burning sensation and the frequent urination, but will not have

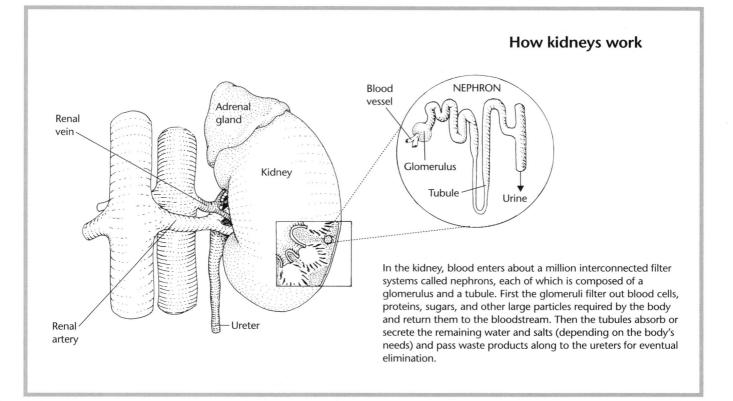

How kidneys work

In the kidney, blood enters about a million interconnected filter systems called nephrons, each of which is composed of a glomerulus and a tubule. First the glomeruli filter out blood cells, proteins, sugars, and other large particles required by the body and return them to the bloodstream. Then the tubules absorb or secrete the remaining water and salts (depending on the body's needs) and pass waste products along to the ureters for eventual elimination.

the systemic symptoms that characterize a kidney infection: nausea, vomiting, and fever.

Any woman who suspects she has a urinary tract infection should be checked by a clinician. This first involves having a urine sample analyzed (by urinalysis in the lab or dipstick in the office) for the presence of white cells and, if positive, having a urine culture done to determine the exact type of bacteria involved. Bacteria in the urine indicate a urinary tract infection. If flank pain, fever, or chills are also present, then the clinician may suspect that the infection has spread to the kidneys. Blood cultures may be done, and treatment may be more prolonged than for a UTI—perhaps calling for hospitalization and the use of intravenous medication.

If a woman has more than 6 urinary tract infections a year, her clinician may want to do an ultrasound to rule out the presence of kidney stones or some other obstruction of the urinary system, and to assess kidney size. The clinician may also want to do a special kind of kidney x-ray called an intravenous pyelogram to look for any underlying congenital defects or kidney stones. In this procedure a dye injected into the bloodstream collects in the kidneys, where it provides a detailed picture during an x-ray. UTIs are usually treated with antibiotics for 1 day, 3 days, or 7 days, depending on the individual situation and other medical problems.

Untreated recurrent pyelonephritis can progress to chronic kidney failure (see below), but it can usually be treated effectively with antibiotics. In general, if a woman is under 55, is relatively healthy, is not pregnant or diabetic, has no past history of kidney infection, and has a temperature under 101°F,

normal blood pressure, and no chills, most clinicians will treat her with oral antibiotics which she can take at home. But if the woman is over 55, has known or suspected urinary tract damage, has severe symptoms, has other medical conditions such as diabetes, or is pregnant, she may be hospitalized and treated with intravenous antibiotics and fluids and monitored closely for potential complications.

Acute pyelonephritis is the most common infectious complication of pregnancy, occurring in 1 to 2 percent of all pregnancies. This is why good prenatal care calls for screening urinalysis for all pregnant women during routine checkups and, if these are positive, urine cultures. Treatment of UTIs and even of asymptomatic bacteria in urine has been shown to prevent pyelonephritis during pregnancy. Pregnant women with kidney infections have a high risk of complications such as acute respiratory distress syndrome and septic shock (difficulty with cardiovascular functioning). Consequently, any pregnant woman who develops pyelonephritis will be hospitalized for management and observation and treated with intravenous antibiotics as well as intravenous fluids to avoid dehydration (which may cause premature uterine contractions).

Acute kidney failure

Kidney failure occurs when kidney filtration either stops or slows down. In acute kidney failure (also called acute renal failure, or ARF), the loss of function occurs suddenly. Urination becomes difficult or impossible, waste products appear in the bloodstream, and the body's fluid balance is disturbed.

In the most serious of cases, symptoms such as swelling of tissues (edema), listlessness, nausea, diarrhea, rapid breathing, bleeding from the gastrointestinal tract, convulsions, and coma may develop. Although acute kidney failure is potentially life-threatening, it is often fully reversible after a few weeks or months of proper treatment.

Acute kidney failure can result from a myriad of causes. Usually these are divided into three types, based on their cause.

Prerenal causes include all those that originate above the kidney and genitourinary system. Often these problems occur because of a reduced fluid content in the blood (hypotension) or a reduced output of blood by the heart, which means that the kidneys receive too little blood for effective filtration. Common prerenal causes of acute kidney failure include infections, traumatic injury, shock, severe bleeding after surgery, congestive heart failure and other heart disease, and drug poisoning.

Renal causes of kidney failure result from damage in the kidney itself. These include bacterial infection as well as inflammation of the glomeruli (glomerulonephritis) or the spaces between the glomeruli and the tubules (interstitial nephritis). Kidneys can also be damaged by diabetes, scleroderma, lupus, hypertension, and sickle cell anemia, as well as infiltration by cancerous cells and contact with certain heavy metals.

Postrenal causes of kidney failure involve some obstruction that prevents urine from flowing out of the kidneys. This problem is most common in men and results when enlargement of the prostate gland blocks the ureters that empty both kidneys. In women, however, it is possible for blockage to result from large cervical or ovarian cancers, fibroids, surgical accidents (during a hysterectomy, for example), or endometriosis. These obstructions can be detected and evaluated with ultrasound in many cases and repaired surgically.

Certain conditions related to reproduction also predispose women to acute kidney failure. Most cases of pregnancy-related acute kidney failure occur in the third trimester. Before abortion was legalized, acute kidney failure commonly occurred during the first trimester and early second trimester as a result of infections acquired during illegal abortions; these were a major cause of death in women having abortions.

Today acute kidney failure develops in about 1 out of every 10,000 pregnant women. It is usually due to complications of pregnancy such as placenta previa (a placenta that blocks the cervix), rupture of the uterus, preeclampsia, and eclampsia. Severe nausea and vomiting during pregnancy can lead to a significant loss of salt, potassium, and water, thus disrupting fluid balance in the body and occasionally, if left untreated, producing acute kidney failure (see morning sickness). This is a particular problem if the vomiting continues into the third trimester of pregnancy.

If the placenta detaches from the uterine wall prematurely (a rare cause of acute renal failure), cortical necrosis of the kidney may develop. This condition almost always causes death, especially among older mothers. Carrying a dead fetus in the uterus for a prolonged period of time (called a missed abortion) can also increase the odds of developing cortical necrosis.

Sometimes a retroverted (tipped) uterus (see entry) becomes trapped in the pelvis as a pregnancy progresses and blocks the neck of the bladder. A clinician may be able to correct this problem by exerting pressure through the vagina onto the back of the uterus. Otherwise repair can be accomplished surgically.

Other problems before and after pregnancy can also lead to acute kidney failure. These include hemorrhage after delivery, sometimes from retained placental fragments, lacerations of the cervix or vagina, or uterine inversion and rupture. Ovarian hyperstimulation syndrome, which sometimes develops during treatment for infertility with drugs that induce ovulation (the release of an egg from an ovary), can cause acute kidney failure. This syndrome usually clears up after treatment with intravenous fluids and bed rest.

Whatever the cause, acute kidney failure requires prompt treatment or it can result in death, usually from infection or gastrointestinal bleeding. The specific treatment depends on the nature and severity of the underlying illness, which in turn influences the chances of recovery. All women with acute kidney failure must be hospitalized for careful monitoring and nutritional therapy, and in severe cases may require dialysis treatments to remove excess wastes until normal kidney function returns. Recovery rates are particularly high in pregnant women with acute kidney failure, probably because most of the women affected are in good health in the first place. But fetuses carried by women with acute kidney failure resulting from bleeding problems, preeclampsia, or eclampsia have a greatly reduced chance of survival.

Chronic kidney failure

Chronic kidney failure is the progressive deterioration of kidney function over a number of years. It is most commonly caused by chronic inflammation of the glomeruli, which leads to protein and blood in the urine, secondary hypertension, and gradual kidney failure. Among the diseases that can damage the glomeruli are diabetes, lupus, AIDS, amyloidosis (a rare progressive blood disorder which involves deposits of a protein called amyloid in various organs), and myeloma (a form of cancer that can interfere with blood cell production).

Other kidney disorders that can lead to chronic kidney failure are chronic kidney infections, interstitial nephritis (see above), vesicoureteral reflux (a condition in which urine flows backward from the bladder into the kidneys), and polycystic kidney disease (an inherited condition involving clusters of cysts on the kidneys; see illustration). Chronic kidney failure in women is also often directly due to diseases such as diabetes, lupus, scleroderma, hypertension, amyloidosis, or, rarely, the chronic use of nonsteroidal antiinflammatory drugs.

Chronic kidney failure is incurable and, unless it is controlled, can progress to end-stage renal disease. In this condition, which usually appears a decade or two after the onset

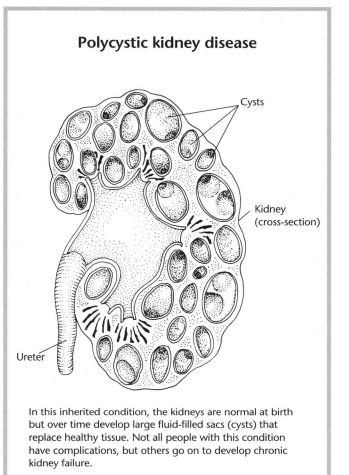

Polycystic kidney disease

Cysts

Kidney
(cross-section)

Ureter

In this inherited condition, the kidneys are normal at birth but over time develop large fluid-filled sacs (cysts) that replace healthy tissue. Not all people with this condition have complications, but others go on to develop chronic kidney failure.

of abnormal kidney functioning (although sometimes much sooner), the kidneys function at less than 5 to 10 percent of normal capacity, and severe complications may result. Once kidney function has declined to this level, chronic dialysis treatment or a kidney transplant is essential.

Milder forms of chronic kidney failure may involve few if any symptoms. As urea and other waste products accumulate in the blood, however, a condition known as uremia develops. Symptoms of uremia include nausea, vomiting, headache, abdominal pain, diarrhea, an unpleasant taste in the mouth, weight loss, fatigue, weakness, dizziness, blurred vision, muscle twitches or cramps, decreased mental acuity, convulsions, and coma. The skin can take on a yellowish-brownish tinge, and hypertension, gastrointestinal bleeding, and itching may develop. Congestive heart failure, pericarditis (inflammation of the sac encasing the heart muscle), anemia, and osteoporosis may occur as well. There is also some evidence that women with kidney failure may be predisposed to developing some forms of thyroid disease.

In a premenopausal woman with chronic kidney failure, menstrual cycle disorders (see entry) are common, particularly failure to menstruate, infrequent periods, or too fre-

quent periods. Symptoms of uremia begin at about the same time as these menstrual problems. In fact, the appearance of menstrual cycle disorders frequently marks the worsening of chronic kidney disease.

These menstrual abnormalities often stem from failure to ovulate. This, in turn, seems linked—at least in some cases—to elevated levels of the hormone prolactin (hyperprolactinemia), which seem to increase as kidney function declines. When prolactin levels are high, estrogen levels fall and ovulation is inhibited. Although moderately increased prolactin levels are common in women with chronic kidney failure, extremely high levels are quite rare and indicate the need for a CT scan or MRI to rule out a prolactin-secreting pituitary tumor.

Pregnancy is a problem for women with chronic kidney failure, although improved prenatal care in recent years has improved the outlook considerably—especially for women with mild disease. Today close to 9 out of 10 women with mildly to moderately impaired kidney function can expect to have a successful pregnancy. The prognosis remains grim for more severe kidney disease, as well as for women with persisting high blood pressure. Chances of miscarriage, stillbirth, neonatal death, prematurity (often induced by the clinician to protect either mother or baby), placenta abruptio, and fetal growth retardation are all greatly increased for these women.

Previously impaired kidney function often deteriorates even further during pregnancy in women with glomerulonephritis, as well as in women with moderate to severe kidney failure. Hypertension may worsen as well, and the kidneys continue to deteriorate even after the pregnancy is over. Researchers still are not sure whether the problems are due to pregnancy itself or to the associated hypertension.

Deterioration of kidney function can persist whether or not the pregnancy is terminated. When a woman with kidney failure becomes pregnant, often a clinician will suggest terminating the pregnancy because of risks to both the mother and the fetus. This decision—ultimately made by the mother—hinges on the assessment of a pregnancy's long-term impact on her health and survival. The dilemma, of course, is that this assessment must be made on the basis of incomplete knowledge, since there is still no consensus about the risk of complications during pregnancy in women with moderate to severe forms of kidney failure. What is known is that pregnancy appears to pose no significant risks for women with mild disease.

Chronic kidney failure is usually treated by controlling the many symptoms as they develop, including hypertension, osteomalacia (softening of the bones), osteoporosis, and congestive heart failure. In women with end-stage renal disease there is no evidence that exercise or, in postmenopausal women, estrogen replacement therapy can retard bone loss from osteoporosis. Calcium supplementation may be helpful. ERT is still important, however, in reducing the risk of heart disease.

Women with chronic kidney infection who also have menstrual irregularities should see a gynecologist for a possible biopsy of the uterine lining, since chronic failure to ovulate and low levels of estrogen increase the odds of developing endometrial (uterine) cancer and endometrial hyperplasia. Treatment usually involves taking progesterone supplements or combination (estrogen plus progesterone) oral contraceptives. If a woman with chronic kidney failure has other health problems, however, the gynecologist may want to do an endometrial ablation (destruction of the uterine lining) using either electrocautery or laser surgery. This usually requires only local anesthesia and takes under an hour to accomplish. If irregular or profuse bleeding continues after the ablation, a hysterectomy (removal of the uterus) may become necessary.

The severe anemia that often results from kidney failure—and almost always occurs in end-stage renal disease—used to be treated with transfusions, but more recently blood transfusions have been replaced with human erythropoietin (EPO). Produced through recombinant DNA techniques, it is usually administered intravenously during dialysis treatments. Though quite costly, it is often covered by Medicare (which pays for people of any age with end-stage renal disease). Not only does EPO (a substance necessary for production of red blood cells) reverse anemia, but also many people find that it improves their overall sense of well-being. In addition, it may help regularize the menstrual cycle in many premenopausal women.

It is important for women with severe kidney disease to make sure that they are receiving routine health maintenance examinations, including pelvic examinations, Pap tests, and mammography. Too often there is a tendency on the part of both the woman and her clinician to focus only on the kidney disorder. As a result, other problems may be overlooked. Because women who routinely use kidney dialysis machines may be at increased risk for developing certain cancers, and because women who have had a kidney transplant have an increased risk of developing leukemia and lymphoma, routine health screening is a critical part of treatment.

Dialysis and women

Kidney dialysis is an artificial means of removing waste products from the blood when the kidneys can no longer do so effectively. Most people who use dialysis have end-stage renal disease and, because of poor overall health from conditions such as diabetes, are at risk for complications. These people often receive kidney transplants sooner rather than later, depending on other medical problems and the availability of a donor kidney. Dialysis is also used for the temporary treatment of acute kidney failure or for patients who are waiting for a donor kidney to become available. Although dialysis cannot remove all waste products from the blood or completely eliminate the symptoms of uremia, it does allow people to survive who would otherwise die without functioning kidneys.

There are several different forms of dialysis in use today.

Hemodialysis, for example, removes waste products directly by pumping the blood through a filtering machine and then returning the cleansed blood to the body. In peritoneal dialysis the filtering of fluid is done within the peritoneal wall (the covering of the abdominal cavity) with the aid of a dialysis solution that is frequently infused into and drained from the cavity.

Until recently dialysis almost always involved spending 9 to 48 hours per week at an outpatient dialysis center—a disruption that takes its toll on both work and family life. Today some people can perform dialysis on their own (or with the help of a willing partner or visiting nurse). Although many women simply do not have the support to allow home dialysis, those who are able to do it find that it makes maintaining their independence much easier.

Both men and women with severe kidney failure who need dialysis treatments have unusually low libido (sexual desire), frequency of intercourse, and overall sexual satisfaction. The reason may seem obvious, in the sense that anyone in ill health who has to spend a good part of the week hooked up to a dialysis machine is likely to lose interest in sex. It is hardly surprising that people on dialysis also have unusually high rates of depression, an emotional disorder that often leads to low libido. Some doctors feel that people on dialysis, especially those with decreased sexual function, should be evaluated by a psychiatric support team (psychiatrist, psychologist, or social worker) as a routine part of their health care.

The fact that women's sexual problems seem to correlate with prolactin levels suggests that there may also be a biochemical component to their sexual dysfunction. The higher the prolactin levels, the greater the sexual dysfunction. Some investigators have hypothesized that the estrogen deficiency associated with high prolactin levels may in turn cause thinning and drying of vaginal tissue, which makes sexual intercourse uncomfortable or painful. This discomfort may explain a good part of the decrease in the frequency of, and satisfaction from, sexual relations.

One drug that lowers prolactin levels—bromocriptine—apparently improves sexual function in men who have high levels of prolactin. Its effects on sexual dysfunction in women with hyperprolactinemia who are on dialysis have not yet been studied. Similarly, while erythropoietin has been reported to improve libido and sexual performance in men (even though it has no effect on hormone levels), its effects on women still need to be investigated.

Menstrual irregularities are almost universal in premenopausal women undergoing chronic hemodialysis. But researchers still are not sure how much of this is due to dialysis and how much to kidney failure in and of itself. Also, it is still unclear whether menstrual periods become more or less frequent after dialysis is started or whether or not the type of dialysis has an impact on the severity of the problems.

Because of the combination of menstrual irregularities—particularly lack of ovulation—and low libido, it is rare for women on dialysis to conceive. Undoubtedly the high levels of circulating waste products also play a role, perhaps by creating an environment toxic to implantation or to embryonic development. Chances of conception are somewhat higher for relatively young dialysis patients who do not have hypertension or who are taking drugs to regularize their menstrual periods.

In the rare event that conception does occur, the outcome is usually bleak. The risks of miscarriage, prematurity, placenta abruptio, ruptured uterine membranes, fetal distress, fetal growth retardation, stillbirth, and excessive amniotic fluid accumulation are all very high. The mother's hypertension may become worse during pregnancy, and preeclampsia is common, often necessitating delivery before the fetus is sufficiently mature. (If the pregnancy does go to term, a cesarean section is almost always necessary because of dangers to either mother or child.) For all of these reasons, therapeutic abortions are performed in half of pregnancies that occur in women on dialysis.

For some women, however, the desire to bear a child may override these risks. All in all, the prognosis depends on the nature and severity of the woman's kidney failure, her general health in other respects, and the expertise of her obstetrician, neonatologist (a physician who specializes in newborn care), and nephrologist (a physician who specializes in kidney disorders). Also, when the conception occurs before dialysis treatments have to be started, the chance of having a successful pregnancy increases somewhat. This may be because, once the pregnancy is established, removing waste products from the blood improves the fetal environment and decreases the incidence of excess amniotic fluid accumulation. Near the end of the pregnancy the woman may need to have longer or more frequent dialysis treatments to compensate for the increased production of waste products by the fetus.

Kidney transplantation

When a person with end-stage kidney disease is relatively young (under age 60) and healthy, kidney transplantation is preferable to dialysis, which is inconvenient and associated with various complications (including infections, heart and lung problems, high blood sugar levels, seizures, hernias, and peritonitis). For premenopausal women who want to bear children, kidney transplantation is the only treatment that can restore normal reproductive capacity.

Kidney transplants are among the more frequently performed transplant operations in this country, but finding a compatible donor kidney (matched for blood type and antibodies) usually takes quite a while. If a kidney is incompatible, the body will reject it. Usually the best donors are siblings or other relatives, although donation by a family member may be complicated by emotional or other factors. If a compatible kidney from a family member is not available for whatever reason, there are tissue-typing centers that can locate kidneys from organ donors. Even with a compatible kidney, moreover, a person must still take immunosuppressant drugs (such as cyclosporine) for the rest of her life to pre-

vent rejection of what remains a "foreign" body. The downside of immunosuppressant drugs is that they increase the risk of infections by suppressing the immune system.

Women, especially those in minority groups, are less likely than men to have kidney transplants. When they do have them, their chances of retaining the new kidney and returning to normal functioning are excellent. Quite often libido and the ability to have orgasms return to the same level as before the kidney failure, and menstrual periods become regular again. Because ovulation usually occurs as well, conception becomes much more likely. The growing fetus generally tolerates immunosuppressive drugs quite well, and so most women who have had a kidney transplant can expect to have successful pregnancies if they wish to have children.

Many women seem to grow excess body hair after a kidney transplant, for reasons that are not understood but are partially related to immunosuppressive therapy. Though no cause for medical concern, excess hair can pose an obvious cosmetic problem, but one that is readily remediable with tweezing, bleaching, shaving, or electrolysis.

Related entries

Abortion, antiinflammatory drugs, congestive heart failure, depression, diabetes, eclampsia, edema, endometrial cancer, endometrial hyperplasia, endometriosis, estrogen replacement therapy, heart disease, high blood pressure, hirsutism, hyperprolactinemia, hysterectomy, infertility, laser surgery, lupus, menstrual cycle disorders, osteoporosis, pregnancy, sexual dysfunction, urinary tract infections, vaginal atrophy

Knee Pain

Knee pain is a problem that is particularly common among women—partly because their joint structure differs from that of men, and partly because women are more apt to be engaged in activities such as picking up (and picking up after) small children.

Anterior knee pain

Anterior knee pain (chondromalacia patella)—that is, pain at the front of the knee—is probably the most common cause of knee disability in people under 40, with many more women affected than men. It occurs when excessive tension in supporting ligaments causes the kneecap to deviate to the side of the thigh bone (see illustration). Pain is usually felt just behind the kneecap and usually intensifies during kneeling, squatting, or walking downstairs. Over time excessive tension can break down the cartilage (fibrous connective tissue) in the joint.

To evaluate pain at the front of the knee, a doctor will physically examine the kneecap and may take x-rays to look

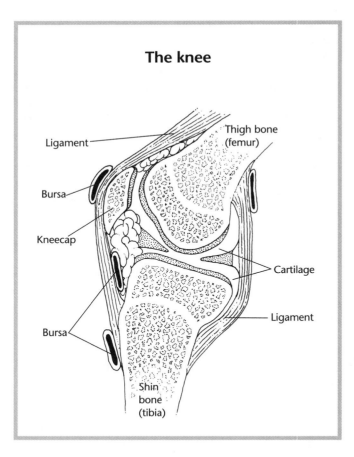

The knee

Ligament

Bursa

Kneecap

Bursa

Thigh bone
(femur)

Cartilage

Ligament

Shin
bone
(tibia)

for signs of arthritis, although symptoms often do not correlate well with the radiologic findings. In 4 out of 5 cases anterior knee pain can be treated successfully with simple measures, usually by eliminating or modifying activities that produce symptoms and by doing progressive resistance exercises (under the supervision of a physical therapist or other specialist in sports medicine) to strengthen the muscles around the knee so that they counterbalance any tight ligaments.

When pain flares up, ice packs, painkillers such as Tylenol, and nonsteroidal antiinflammatory drugs can provide temporary relief. When symptoms have subsided, a maintenance program of muscle strengthening should be continued indefinitely. Sometimes knee pads, a heavy elastic brace (which is commercially available) to stabilize the kneecap, or an orthotic device in the shoe to correct a tendency of the foot to turn inward can also help prevent future problems. Wearing flat-heeled shoes rather than high heels can minimize misalignment of the knee joint. A combination of these measures usually allows about two-thirds of people with anterior knee pain to return to unrestricted activity, including sports activities, within a year.

If problems persist, surgery may be necessary to relieve tension in the ligaments. Surgery to relieve anterior knee pain has a high rate of success, especially in people who have noticeable deviation of the kneecap.

Osteoarthritis of the knee

Osteoarthritis of the knee is a leading cause of knee pain and disability in people over 50. It is often due to mechanical wear and tear and is aggravated by obesity, occupations that involve repeated trauma to the knee, and previous knee injuries. Osteoarthritis of the knee is detectable by x-ray in over a quarter of women aged 65 to 69 and over half of women over 80. But only about 8 percent of women aged 65 to 69 and 15 percent of women over 80 have symptoms of knee pain attributable to osteoarthritis. Symptoms can include a dull aching pain deep within the knee which increases with activity and, in advanced cases, may occur at night.

Osteoarthritis of the knee is evaluated with a physical examination of the knee joint and nearby muscles. X-rays may also be taken to see if there is any bone thickening, narrowing of the joint space, bone spurs (osteophytes), or cysts under the cartilage, all of which are characteristic of osteoarthritis. Treatment involves modifying the activities that produce pain, using a cane (which relieves weight on the affected joint), and taking pain medications such as acetaminophen (Tylenol). Since this is a disease of joint destruction rather than inflammation, antiinflammatory drugs such as aspirin and NSAIDs are often no more effective than acetaminophen. Occasionally injections of corticosteroids (antiinflammatory agents derived from adrenal hormones) can bring dramatic relief for chronic joint pain (see antiinflammatory drugs).

If these measures fail, a type of surgery called total knee arthroplasty (joint replacement) can be very effective—with a success rate approaching 80 percent in appropriate patients. In this procedure a steel ball on a stem and a polyethylene cup are glued with an acrylic cement onto the bones (see arthroplasty). Although the rate of complications is only about 1 to 2 percent, women tend to undergo this surgery when the disease is relatively advanced, thus potentially increasing risks. Other drawbacks include the fact that artificial joints often loosen over time and may need to be repaired or replaced, though seldom within 12 years. In younger patients other procedures such as osteotomy (the surgical removal of part of a bone to reduce deformities that can promote cartilage damage) are sometimes tried first.

Pes anserine bursitis

Before treating osteoarthritis of the knee, it is also important to diagnose and treat any associated conditions that may be more amenable to therapy. One of these, seen more often in women than in men, is called pes anserine bursitis. Bursitis means inflammation of the bursa, a fluid-filled sac found in joints which limits friction between the bone and the muscles and tendons. In pes anserine bursitis the inflammation occurs in the bursa cushioning the spot where the hamstring tendons on the back of the thigh insert into the shin bone (tibia) at the side of the knee. It can occur after athletic activities or in chronic osteoarthritis and produces pain and tenderness just below the knee joint which gets worse when the knee is bent. Pes anserine bursitis can be diagnosed in a phys-

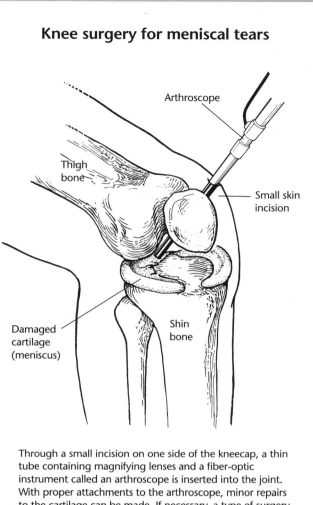

Knee surgery for meniscal tears

Arthroscope

Thigh bone

Small skin incision

Damaged cartilage (meniscus)

Shin bone

Through a small incision on one side of the kneecap, a thin tube containing magnifying lenses and a fiber-optic instrument called an arthroscope is inserted into the joint. With proper attachments to the arthroscope, minor repairs to the cartilage can be made. If necessary, a type of surgery called arthroscopic partial meniscectomy can remove a torn flap of meniscus.

an outpatient procedure called arthroscopy (see illustration). With the patient under local or general anesthesia, the surgeon makes a small incision on one side of the kneecap through which a small tube containing magnifying lenses and a fiber-optic instrument called an arthroscope is inserted. This allows the interior of the knee to be visualized and, with proper attachments, also allows minor repairs to be made at the same time. Although complete healing takes only a few days, arthroscopy is an invasive procedure. For this reason some doctors prefer to diagnose torn menisci using arthrography, a special kind of x-ray procedure in which a dye is injected into the joint, or, more commonly, magnetic resonance imaging (MRI), which produces a computerized picture based on magnetic fields within the knee.

Nonsurgical therapy (such as decreased activity and antiinflammatory drugs) is effective for many patients with meniscal tears and even works in about a quarter of patients with severe tears. If symptoms have not improved after several months, however, a type of surgery called arthroscopic partial meniscectomy can remove the torn flap of meniscus, under the guidance of an arthroscope. Most people do well with the procedure and are happy with the results. In some more difficult cases, such as those with osteoarthritis, the success rate may be lower.

Aftereffects of the surgery can include swelling and pain (which is managed with medications), and the procedure is generally followed by months of vigorous rehabilitation exercises. If surgery is not an option, maintaining strength in supporting muscles can help minimize impact on the knee joint and associated pain—as it can in any painful knee condition.

Related entries

Antiinflammatory drugs, arthritis, arthroplasty, exercise, musculoskeletal disorders, obesity, osteoarthritis, sports injuries

ical examination and relieved by injecting a corticosteroid mixed with lidocaine or xylocaine (local anesthetics) into the affected area.

Torn cartilage

Another knee problem common in women over 50 with osteoarthritis is torn cartilage (meniscal tears) from degeneration rather than from injury (which more often occurs in young men). The menisci are wedges of crescent-shaped cartilage that cushion the thigh and lower leg bones and stabilize them against rotational forces. They can degenerate in older people and tear easily, producing swelling and pain. Sometimes people with meniscal tears will feel that their knee is "giving way" or feel it "locking" into a fixed position. Often there is a painful click when the knee is bent or the leg is rotated.

The most precise way to diagnose a meniscal tear is with

Laparoscopy

Laparoscopy is a procedure that allows a doctor to observe directly a woman's uterus, fallopian tubes, and ovaries (see illustration page 297). Also sometimes called a "belly-button operation" or "bandaid surgery," it is often used to diagnose or detect ovarian cysts, adhesions (scar tissue), pelvic or abdominal pain, endometriosis, ectopic pregnancy, or blocked fallopian tubes, and therefore is an important tool in an infertility evaluation. Laparoscopy can be used to help locate and remove an IUD (intrauterine device) which has perforated the uterus, as well as to sterilize a woman through tubal ligation. It is also used during some vaginal hysterectomies.

Although many of these procedures can be done through a laparotomy (a regular abdominal incision; see entry), laparoscopy generally involves less pain, risk, and scarring. Performing the procedure requires special skill and training on the part of the surgeon, however.

How is the procedure performed?

Laparoscopies are usually done in a hospital day surgery unit. After anesthesia (usually general) has taken effect, the surgeon makes an incision half an inch to an inch long just below the navel. Carbon dioxide or nitrous oxide gas is then pumped into the abdominal cavity through a long, thin needle. This gas, which lifts the intestines and exposes the underlying pelvic organs, may cause a feeling of discomfort or bloating in women relying on regional anesthesia. Next the surgeon inserts a sharp metal instrument called a trocar into the abdominal cavity through the incision. The trocar is contained inside a cannula (tube), which remains inserted in the incision as the trocar is removed. The surgeon then inserts the laparoscope—a long, lighted optical instrument that works much like a periscope—through this cannula, as well as any other necessary surgical instruments or materials. Once the procedure is over, gas is removed from the abdominal cavity. The surgeon sutures the incision with a stitch or two and covers it with a small bandage.

What happens after surgery?

If there are no complications, the woman can usually leave the hospital within 4 to 8 hours of a laparoscopy and resume normal activities (including sexual intercourse) after about a day. She may feel some pain under her ribs or in her shoulder for a few days to a week if any gas remains in the abdomen. A few women have some vaginal bleeding following a laparoscopy.

What are the risks and complications?

Although laparoscopy is a relatively safe procedure, in rare instances it can result in complications. These may include inflammation of the lining of the abdominal cavity, abscess formation, or organ damage from surgical instruments, as well as the usual risks associated with general anesthesia. Risks are reduced if the laparoscopy is done by a gynecologist experienced with this procedure.

Related entries

Adhesions, anesthesia, ectopic pregnancy, endometriosis, hysterectomy, infertility, intrauterine devices, laparotomy, menstrual cycle disorders, ovarian cysts, pelvic pain, tubal ligation

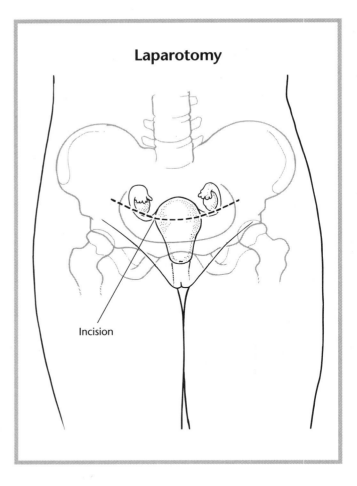

Laparotomy

Incision

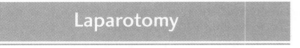

Laparotomy

A laparotomy is abdominal surgery whose purpose is to explore, diagnose, or treat a range of conditions in women. Appendicitis, ovarian cancer, ectopic pregnancy, pelvic inflammatory disease, and pelvic adhesions (scar tissue) are frequently diagnosed with a laparotomy. The procedure is also used to treat endometriosis, remove uterine fibroids, free adhesions from pelvic organs, remove ovaries (oophorectomy), reverse a tubal ligation, or remove an appendix (appendectomy). Because a laparotomy is major surgery, less risky procedures such as laparoscopy are often considered first for many of these conditions.

How is the procedure performed?

Laparotomies must be done in the hospital using general anesthesia. They require an incision 4 to 5 inches long in the lower abdomen just above the pubic region (see illustration).

A minilaparotomy is a related procedure, usually used for tubal ligations (see entry), which involves a much smaller incision, local anesthesia, a shorter recovery time, and fewer risks of complications.

What happens after surgery?

After surgery is complete, the woman must stay in the hospital for a few days and then rest at home for about 2 weeks more. Complete recovery usually takes about 6 weeks.

What are the risks and complications?

Like all major surgery, laparotomy carries certain risks, including reactions to anesthesia, bleeding (possibly requiring transfusion), infection, blood clots, damage to other organs (including perforation of the lower portion of the small intestine), abnormal scarring (see keloid scarring), and, in rare cases, death.

Related entries

Adhesions, anesthesia, ectopic pregnancy, endometriosis, keloid scarring, laparoscopy, ovarian cancer, ovary removal, pelvic inflammatory disease, tubal ligation, uterine fibroids

Laser Surgery

Lasers are devices that use a gas (such as carbon dioxide, krypton, or argon), solid (such as ruby or alexandrite crystal), or liquid (such as a dye) to concentrate light waves into tiny but powerful beams. Laser surgery was first used in the 1960s to treat eye diseases, since the transparent eye tissues were ideal for accurately focusing the early laser instruments. Continually refined since then, lasers now enjoy widespread use in many medical fields. The last decade has witnessed an explosion in the medical use of and public interest in lasers.

No field has benefited more from lasers than that of skin care and cosmetic surgery. Today lasers are the treatment of choice for many dermatologic conditions including varicose veins, birthmarks, liver spots, and precancerous growths. The pulsed dye laser was specifically developed to treat vascular conditions such as port wine stains and hemangiomas but is also used to treat scars and small blood vessels on the face or legs. Lasers are used to induce permanent hair removal and to remove tattoos. Probably the most dramatic of all the cosmetic developments has been skin resurfacing with the carbon dioxide or erbium:YAG laser, which can remodel or resurface facial wrinkles and acne scars.

Surgical lasers are also being used increasingly as an alternative to electrocautery, cryosurgery, and cone biopsy in certain gynecological procedures—such as stopping abnormal uterine bleeding; performing tubal ligations; removing genital warts and precancerous cells; and treating endometriosis, ectopic pregnancies, and adhesions from pelvic inflammatory disease (PID). Lasers are also commonly used in treating many different eye disorders, including glaucoma and retinal degeneration and detachment, and the carbon dioxide laser is used (though rarely) to perform eyelid surgery (blepharoplasty). In addition, lasers such as the argon laser are used to stop bleeding from abnormal blood vessels of the retina in people with diabetes, and excimer lasers are widely used in corneal refractive surgery.

How is the procedure performed?

Lasers work as "bloodless scalpels" to vaporize or cut tissue as well as seal off blood vessels without requiring an incision. They also can target an area without damaging surrounding tissue. As a result, laser surgery generally involves less pain, bleeding, healing time, and risk of infection or other complications than other forms of surgery.

For treating skin and eye conditions and certain gynecological problems (such as precancerous cells in the cervix), the procedure is done on an outpatient basis. Many people compare the feeling of a laser treatment to the snap of a rubber band on the skin. Most conditions are treated without anesthesia, although aggressive procedures such as laser resurfacing of the skin require anesthesia. After laser surgery, the treated area should be washed gently twice a day, followed by the application of a healing ointment.

What are the risks and complications?

Like any surgery, laser surgery can sometimes be associated with excessive bleeding, although blood loss tends to be less than with other forms of surgery. The likelihood of other complications, such as infection or difficulty healing, varies according to the nature and location of the surgery. The lasers used to treat vascular conditions, pigmented lesions, and excessive hair are extremely safe. Side effects such as increased or decreased pigmentation are rare. In contrast, because laser resurfacing removes superficial layers of the skin, leaving a denuded surface, risks are somewhat greater. While healing is usually rapid, patients should allow some downtime. Risks of laser resurfacing include scarring, infection, and changes in skin pigmentation.

Choosing an experienced and well-trained laser surgeon can help minimize these risks. And because lasers pose a significant risk of damage to the eyes, it is essential for both patient and surgeon to have appropriate eye protection during any laser procedure.

Related entries

Adhesions, biopsy, cervical cancer, cryosurgery, diabetes, ectopic pregnancy, electrocautery, endometriosis, eye care, genital warts, keloid scarring, macular degeneration, pelvic inflammatory disease, retinal detachment, skin disorders, tubal ligation, vaginal bleeding (abnormal), varicose veins

Laxatives

Laxatives are agents that help the bowel empty itself by increasing the bulk and water content of feces. In some circumstances they have a useful medical function, but because they are available without a prescription, they are easy to obtain and to overuse (or abuse).

When are laxatives necessary?

Occasional use of the so-called natural laxatives (bulk stool softeners)—such as psyllium (Metamucil, Konsyle, Effersyllium), methylcellulose (Citrucel), calcium polycarbophil (Fiberall, Fibercon), and pectin (Kaolin-Pectin, Donnagel)—can help relieve mild constipation. These agents work by absorbing water in the colon. Sometimes stronger laxatives are necessary in the short term, such as when narcotic painkillers, which cause constipation, must be taken for several days.

Using certain herbal tonics—in tea, powder, or extract form—for no more than a month or two may also be tried. Among the most commonly recommended by herbalists (and generally considered nontoxic if used as directed) are dandelion (which has only a slight effect), yellow dock, and cascara bark. Chinese rhubarb, the most potent of the bunch, should only be used in small amounts and never for longer than 2 weeks at a time. Burdock is often recommended as another herbal laxative, but to date there is no solid evidence that it has any effect. With any herbal remedy, it is important to remember that inspection procedures are not as stringent as with conventional medicines; as a result, there is always a possibility that the label may misrepresent the potency or that the product is contaminated.

What are the risks and complications?

Many people use laxatives frequently because of an erroneous notion that a daily bowel movement is a necessary part of good health. Used over long periods of time, however, laxatives can have an effect that is opposite to the one intended: they can increase constipation by weakening intestinal muscles so that they do not function efficiently. This is true even of mineral oil (Haley's M-O) and nonabsorbable sugars (lactulose, sorbitol, and glycerin), as well as stronger agents such as milk of magnesia, magnesium citrate, castor oil, Dulcolax, senna, phenolphthalein, and cascara, which work by irritating the lining of the intestine or by stimulating intestinal contractions.

Another reason for overuse of laxatives, especially common in women, is a fear of gaining weight. Actually, laxatives are not an efficient way to shed pounds, since even when they are taken in huge quantities, they eliminate only a small fraction of ingested calories. Overuse of laxatives not only can result in diarrhea or constipation, but also can deprive the body of necessary vitamins and other nutrients and may result in sodium (salt), potassium, and water depletion.

People with eating disorders and people who abuse narcotics are particularly vulnerable to laxative abuse, sometimes to the point of endangering their health and life. Although laxatives do not produce a physical "high" in the same sense as drugs such as heroin or cocaine, abusing them can lead to psychological dependence. Young women with anorexia or bulimia often convince friends and families that they are suffering from constipation when in fact they are hoarding laxatives in the attempt to lose additional weight.

Many women with anorexia also genuinely suffer from constipation—as does anyone who does not get enough bulk in the diet. When these women start to eat, they frequently feel uncomfortable abdominal pressure and bloating, which leads them to rely excessively on laxatives.

Frequent use of over-the-counter laxatives may explain why anemia is often so difficult to treat in women with bulimia, even after their eating habits have improved. Compounds such as Ex-Lax and Correctol, which rely on the drug phenolphthalein for effect, can suppress bone marrow and destroy some early forms of red blood cells. Conscious of all these dangers, the parents of some young women with anorexia and bulimia have petitioned the U.S. Food and Drug Administration to legislate more stringent regulations for over-the-counter laxatives (as well as diet pills).

Anyone dependent on laxatives requires medical supervision because serious symptoms can occur when they are cut out abruptly.

Related entries

Anemia, anorexia nervosa and bulimia nervosa, bowel disorders, constipation, hemorrhoids, irritable bowel syndrome, substance abuse

Lipectomy and Liposuction

Diet and exercise are generally the best ways to reduce overall body fat and improve muscle tone; but localized deposits of fat or excess, stretched-out skin may be resistant to these measures. The areas of fat, though not generally considered hazardous to health, may pose cosmetic concerns. Plastic surgical techniques called liposuction (aspiration of fat) and lipectomy (surgical removal of fat) are available to deal with these problems.

To many women the idea of liposuction (also called lipolysis) sounds too good to be true: it promises to deliver firm buttocks, flat tummy, and taut underarms without diet and exercise. On top of that, liposuction actually decreases the number of fat cells in the body; dieting and exercise merely leave shrunken fat cells lying in wait for future engorgement.

As with most things that sound too good to be true, it turns out that liposuction has serious limitations. For one thing, it is simply not an option for many women—specifically, women over 50, women who are not in adequate health, and women without the means to pay for an operation that is rarely covered by medical insurance. Even women who are good candidates for liposuction should realize that this dream does not come without costs.

Liposuction works best where there are areas of localized fat deposits and good overlying skin tone. Once the fat is surgically sucked out of the area, the skin reshapes itself through its own elasticity. If the skin has been stretched out, however, or if skin tone is lax, the skin will not shape itself to conform to the changed contour. In these cases some type of skin removal or "tuck" must be considered.

Removing excess skin can be combined with lipectomy—the surgical excision of larger amounts of fat—if more extensive changes in contour are desired. Skin and fat removal on the abdomen can also be combined with deeper procedures to tighten the abdominal muscles after pregnancy, a procedure called an abdominoplasty. In each of these procedures, the structures of skin, fat, and underlying muscle must

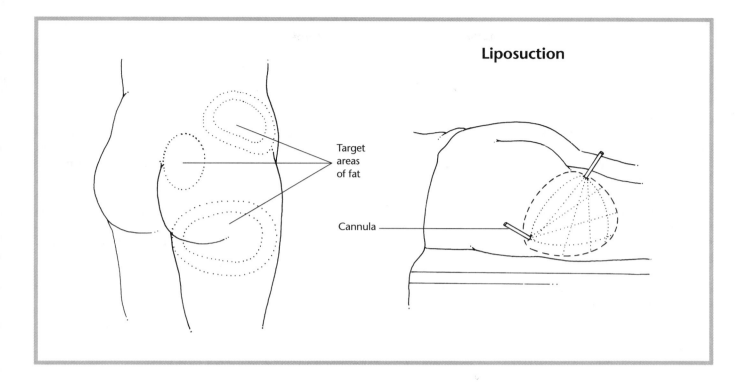

Liposuction

Target
areas
of fat

Cannula

be evaluated so that the most appropriate surgery can be planned.

This kind of body contouring surgery is in almost every case a purely cosmetic procedure. Occasionally the removal of excessively stretched skin can be justified for medical reasons, for example, after extreme weight loss. But contouring surgery should not be thought of as an alternative to diet for weight control. The surgery is designed to work on local areas of excess fat or skin that persist despite exercise, diet, and muscle toning. It is usually recommended that a woman try to reach a stable, healthy weight before undertaking this kind of surgery, since subsequent weight gain or weight loss may distort the result achieved by the operation. And unlike weight loss that follows diet and exercise, lipectomy and liposuction offer no proven health benefits, such as a reduced risk of diabetes, high blood pressure, heart disease, or stroke.

How are lipectomy and liposuction performed?

Liposuction may be performed by itself or in combination with the more extensive surgical removal of skin and fat. Liposuction is used to remove fat from many different areas of the body, including the isolated pockets of fat in the abdominal region, hips, thighs, or upper arms, as well as fat deposits on the chin, breasts, ankles, or inner knee. It can also be used to siphon off some excess fat cells before a more extensive surgical removal of fat and skin is performed. Whatever the specific goal, liposuction is usually performed in a hospital setting on an outpatient basis, although some surgeons prefer that the patient be hospitalized for observation the night after the procedure.

Before the procedure begins, some form of anesthesia will be administered. For small areas of fat, a local anesthetic is injected into the designated area along with a vasoconstrictor (usually epinephrine) to limit blood loss. This is supplemented with intravenous sedation. For treating larger areas of fat, general anesthesia may be necessary.

Once the anesthesia has taken effect, the surgeon makes a small incision, preferably in an inconspicuous location near the fat deposit. Then an instrument called a cannula (a blunt, hollow tube with perforations at the end) is inserted through the skin at the outer edge of the fat deposit (see illustration). This cannula tunnels through the loose connective tissue that separates muscle from skin. Then some dislodged fat cells, along with some liquified fat and blood, are suctioned out through it. The cannula is reinserted again and again at various angles to the first insertion point in an approximately radial pattern until enough fat has been removed to achieve the desired result. The incisions are stapled or sutured shut, and a pressure dressing much like a panty girdle is placed over the wound to help prevent excessive scarring and bruising.

After the fat has been sucked out, a honeycomb of connective tissue that resembles a sponge is left behind. Tissue fluid and blood from small blood vessels fill the spaces in the honeycomb where the fat cells have been removed, leaving the area swollen and black and blue. As healing progresses, the swelling gradually recedes and the discoloration goes away. The honeycomb, no longer filled with fat deposits, flattens out and the skin conforms to the new, flatter shape.

Lipectomy involves more extensive surgery. Longer incisions are required to remove the fat and then take up the excess skin and tighten it—just like taking in the seams in an article of clothing that is too large. The surgeon tries to place these incisions in natural folds or inconspicuous areas of the skin, but it is difficult to hide the scars completely. Once the incision is made, the surgeon frees up the skin and fat in the region so that the desired amount can be removed. Liposuction is employed at times to help with the contouring. After the tissues are freed up, they are draped over the body so that the excess can be identified. The excess skin is then removed, and the rest of the tissues are sewn together.

One of the most common uses of skin and fat removal is to reshape the abdomen, especially after pregnancy or abdominal surgery. Pregnancies can cause stretched muscles, stretched skin, and stretchmarks. Even with exercise, the muscle tone of the abdominal wall might not be restored, and excess skin may never return to its pre-pregnancy shape. Abdominal operations can leave unsightly scars that the woman finds disfiguring. Lipectomy and liposuction can help with many of these problems.

Abdominal recontouring (a "tummy tuck") requires a long, curved incision at and above the pubic line. This allows all the loose skin and fat of the abdomen to be freed up and tightened. It also exposes the muscle layer so that the surgeon can tighten the muscles with stitches or sew them closer together. This type of surgery usually requires that the belly button be detached from the skin around it and then reattached after the abdominal skin and fat have been pulled more tightly together. Although stretchmarks cannot be erased with this operation, they can sometimes be cut away with the excess skin; and even if they remain, they may appear less conspicuous once the defatted skin becomes tauter.

Similar techniques of making incisions, freeing up the skin and fat in a region, tightening it up, and removing the excess can be applied to many areas of the body besides the abdomen. Women concerned about saggy fat in the upper arms or upper thighs can have these areas "tucked" and "lifted" in this way. Even though the result is tighter skin tone and better shape, however, the scars are often quite visible. A woman considering this kind of surgery should be aware that she will be trading shape for lasting scars.

What happens after the surgery?

Although liposuction is usually done on an outpatient basis, lipectomy and other, more involved forms of body contouring may require a night or two in the hospital. Patients are encouraged to get up and walk soon after surgery to help restore circulation. The surgeon will usually employ some type of dressing or support garment to keep swelling and bruising to a minimum after surgery. Nonetheless, it is normal to be quite black and blue, especially after liposuction. The areas where the surgery took place will be tender immediately afterward and can stay that way for several weeks. The liposuction patient may not want to apply pressure to the area for a while, because it will feel bruised and sore: a desk worker, for example, may not be able to work right away if she finds sitting uncomfortable. Some kind of support garment is useful for weeks to months after surgery to help resolve swelling.

Exercise and strenuous activity must be avoided for several weeks after surgery. Each surgeon will have a list of restrictions, based on the specific type of procedure. The more surgery that is done, the more restrictions the woman will face. By 3 or 4 weeks after surgery, though, most women will have returned to their usual activities.

What are the risks and complications?

As with any major surgery, lipectomy can be complicated by excessive bleeding or infection, as well as problems with anesthesia. Furthermore, the surgery will necessarily leave scars. Women who tend to scar excessively may find the risks of surgery unacceptable (see keloid scarring).

After surgery of this magnitude, swelling in the tissues is also inevitable. As the swelling recedes, it is replaced by scar tissue which contracts as it heals, causing a sensation of tightness. The area will eventually stretch out. But especially after liposuction, there may be ridges, dimples, or lumpy areas after the swelling settles down and scar tissue sets in. The more thorough the fat removal, the more likely it is that these surface irregularities will show up.

Fluid may collect under the skin after the surgery, especially if large areas of skin and fat have been recontoured. Drainage tubes may be placed to remove this fluid, less commonly with liposuction and more commonly with skin and fat excision. Even after the drainage tubes are removed, fluid may continue to collect and will need to be drained in the surgeon's office.

Elevating the skin and fat to redrape it damages the small sensory nerves that enter the area. This damage results in changes in sensation, usually temporary but possibly permanent. It can take over a year for sensation to return to normal. The procedure also detaches some of the small blood vessels that feed the skin and fat. This can lead to circulation problems in the skin, especially in women with certain risk factors. Nicotine, for example, causes small blood vessels to go into spasm. Smokers, therefore, are at much greater risk than nonsmokers for circulation problems in the skin. Women with diabetes run similar risks. If a circulation problem develops, the tissues may not heal promptly, scarring may be severe, or some of the skin may form large scabs and even die. These complications may require further surgery to correct. Many surgeons insist that their patients avoid any nicotine exposure for several weeks before surgery to minimize the chances of these sorts of healing problems.

Any woman considering body contouring surgery must recognize that these procedures are major ones that are not without medical risk. Patients immobilized after any type of surgery, for example, are at risk for blood clots forming in the legs and, though rare, traveling to the lungs. Good candidates for lipectomy must be in excellent health. Women with diabetes, kidney disorders, or heart disease, for example, are not good candidates. It is imperative to have a thorough physical examination and consultation with a physician beforehand so that any potential risk factors can be identified.

Liposuction, while involving less surgery than lipectomy, entails particular risks of its own. One problem is that the small size of the incision makes it hard for the surgeon to see under the skin to determine how much blood and fluid have been lost. If too many fat cells are removed, the accompanying blood loss can cause life-threatening shock—although this complication is increasingly rare as surgeons become more experienced with the procedure. Another risk, though small, is the formation of a fat embolism—a fragment of fat which can be lethal if it migrates to some vital organ. Furthermore, the need for unusual positioning in the operating room to allow access to the buttocks or the thighs may introduce problems for the anesthesia team. Although these risks are not common ones, they indicate that these procedures should not be taken lightly. A woman should make sure that her surgeon is well trained and experienced in these operations and that her anesthesia team is competent and credentialed.

Related entries

Anesthesia, body image, cosmetic surgery, dieting, exercise, keloid scarring, obesity, skin disorders, smoking, weight tables

Liver Spots

Liver spots (also known as age spots) are harmless flat patches of increased pigmentation that frequently appear on the face and hands of people as they age. Despite the name, liver spots have nothing to do with the liver (although they were once believed to) but seem to result from cumulative ultraviolet light exposure.

Who is likely to develop liver spots?

They most often develop in light-skinned people over the age of 55, but they are not uncommon in people over the age of 40.

What are the symptoms?

Liver spots most often appear on the forehead or on the back of the hands. Usually light brown, reddish brown, or black in color, they can be as small as a freckle or spread to several inches in diameter.

How is the condition evaluated?

Liver spots are generally harmless and require no professional evaluation. If a growth on the skin suddenly feels sore, changes color, or thickens, however, a dermatologist or other clinician should be consulted to make sure that it is not skin cancer.

How are liver spots treated?

Liver spots generally require no medical treatment, but if they are bothersome for cosmetic reasons it is possible to lighten them with skin bleaching products that inhibit pig-

mentation or with special cosmetic creams containing alpha hydroxy acids or retinoids. They can also be frozen off with liquid nitrogen (see cryosurgery).

How can liver spots be prevented?

It may be possible to prevent some new liver spots by applying a sunscreen (sun protection factor 15) to areas routinely exposed to the sun, such as the hands and lower arms.

Related entries

Cryosurgery, melanoma, skin care and cosmetics, skin disorders

Lubricants

Lubricants are substances that reduce friction. Many of these can be used to decrease dryness in the vagina so that sexual intercourse is comfortable. Normally, mucus secreted during sexual arousal serves as lubrication during intercourse, but for many reasons this natural lubricant may be inadequate. These include the hormonal changes of menopause or breast-feeding, certain sexual dysfunctions, or simply a lack of sufficient foreplay prior to penetration. Other common causes of vaginal dryness are birth control pills, hysterectomy, menstruation, pregnancy, vaginal infections, douching, strenuous exercise, and emotional stress.

Inadequate lubrication is easily remedied with various unscented, nonstaining, and water-soluble lubricants. These include K-Y Jelly, Lubifax, Probe, Lubrin, Surgilube, and Astroglide. These are available at pharmacies and many supermarkets without prescription. Also sold over the counter—though much more expensive—are moisturizing gel tampons which provide continuous vaginal moisture if they are inserted into the vagina 3 times a week. These slightly acidic lubricants, which closely match the body's pH, also help inhibit the growth of some organisms that cause vaginitis.

Women using birth control can use lubricated condoms or spermicidal jellies, creams, or foams as lubricants with a diaphragm. Women who rely on condoms or diaphragms for birth control, however, should never use oil-based lubricants (such as butter or vegetable oil) or petroleum jelly (Vaseline), which rapidly deteriorate rubber. These products can also stick to vaginal walls, where they may promote bacterial growth.

Related entries

Birth control, douching, menopause, pain during sexual intercourse, sexual dysfunction, stress, vaginal atrophy, vaginitis

Lumpectomy

A lumpectomy is a surgical procedure increasingly used to treat breast cancer, usually in combination with radiation therapy. It is also used to remove benign breast lumps, such as fibroadenomas—noncancerous tumors composed of connective tissue and other cells which have multiplied faster than normal (see breast lumps, benign).

How is the procedure performed?

Unlike more extensive types of mastectomies, a lumpectomy for cancer involves the removal of only the cancerous lump itself, along with a small amount of surrounding normal breast tissue, so that the breast often appears essentially unchanged except for a small scar (see mastectomy). If slightly more surrounding tissue is removed (with some more disfigurement), a lumpectomy is sometimes called a partial mastectomy, wide excision, wedge resection, or segmental resection. Frequently lymph nodes in the underarm region need to be removed during a lumpectomy for cancer, to help the surgeon estimate the chance that the cancer has spread. Lumpectomy can be performed with local anesthesia in an ambulatory surgery unit; partial mastectomy is performed in a hospital under general anesthesia.

Why is the procedure performed?

For most cancers lumpectomy, when combined with radiation therapy, appears to be just as effective in saving lives as having the entire breast removed. Nonetheless, lumpectomy is not the right choice for every woman with breast cancer. It is not appropriate for women who have more than one primary cancer in the breast or whose workup prior to surgery (with x-rays, blood tests, bone scans, or mammography) shows strong signs that the cancer may recur.

Lumpectomy also offers no particular advantage for women who have only a small amount of breast tissue or whose cancer is very large or centrally located, for in these cases there will be little cosmetic difference between removing just the cancer and removing the entire breast. Studies are now under way, however, to see if shrinking very large tumors with chemotherapy may make it possible to remove them later with lumpectomy followed by radiation. The initial results of these studies are favorable.

A large number of women choose mastectomy even though they might otherwise seem to be good candidates for a lumpectomy. Some simply feel safer ridding their body entirely of the cancerous breast, while others fear the effects of radiation treatment, which is almost always necessary after a lumpectomy. For elderly women or those living in remote areas, radiation therapy may simply be an impractical option.

There have been some studies showing that the region of the country in which a woman lives affects the likelihood that her physician will recommend lumpectomy as opposed to mastectomy. Women living in the South seem to have much higher rates of mastectomy than those living in the Northeast. Some cancer surgeons may encourage women to have mastectomies because they have difficulty changing the way they have done things in the past, or because they truly believe that women will feel safer, and be safer, if they have the entire cancerous breast removed.

A woman who must decide between a mastectomy and a lumpectomy should never feel that she has to make her decision on the spot. Breast cancer is not an emergency. It makes eminent sense to take 2 or 3 weeks after a diagnosis to consider the options, talk to other women with breast cancer, and get a second opinion from another breast surgeon.

What happens after surgery?

After the lumpectomy 5 daily trips to the hospital for 6 weeks are required for radiation treatments, which last a few minutes each. Although the side effects of lumpectomy itself are minimal, the side effects of radiation include swelling and redness of the breast, fatigue, muscle pain, and sensitivity to sunlight. These effects usually end when therapy is completed, but in some cases they may last for several months or much longer after treatment.

Frequent physical examinations and mammograms are necessary after a lumpectomy and radiation therapy to make sure that no cancer recurs in the breast tissue. The first follow-up mammogram is usually done 6 months after the completion of radiation therapy, and follow-up physicals generally take place every 3 months for the first year after radiation, every 4 months in the second year, and every 6 months thereafter.

Related entries

Biopsy, breast cancer, breast lumps (benign), breast reconstruction, chemotherapy, mammography, mastectomy, radiation therapy

Lung Cancer

Lung cancer is the most lethal cancer that occurs in women. Cigarette smoking is the leading cause of lung cancer, but even among women who do not smoke, lung cancer is nonetheless the third leading cause of cancer-related death, after breast and colon cancer. Unless detected in its earliest stages, lung cancer is often fatal, although survival rates have been slowly improving in recent years.

Many researchers believe that this improvement would be greater if more research dollars were poured into studying lung cancer. One explanation for this apparent oversight (besides possible conflicts of interest between federal officials and the tobacco industry) may be the public perception that lung cancer is a self-inflicted disease. This perception is unfortunate, not only because people who choose a self-destructive lifestyle still deserve sympathy and care, but also because—in a surprisingly large number of cases—lung cancer turns out to have little to do with lifestyle choice.

There are many types of lung cancer, the most common of which—squamous cell carcinoma (see illustration) and oat cell carcinoma—are associated with heavy cigarette smoking. But the number of cases of "nonsmoker's" cancer—a type of cancer called adenocarcinoma—has been steadily increasing at an astounding rate as well. This increase is particularly dramatic among women. Adenocarcinomas accounted for only 12 percent of all lung cancers in 1965, whereas today they account for 40 percent. A subtype of adenocarcinoma—bronchoalveolar cancer—is also becoming increasingly common in this country, and it too does not seem to be associated with cigarette smoking.

Some of this apparent increase in nonsmoking-associated lung cancers may be an artifact of better technology: as the means of differentiating types of lung cancer in the laboratory have improved, physicians may be identifying these adenocarcinomas more accurately than in the past, even though they may have been relatively common all along. But many scientists believe that, in addition to this improvement in identification, there has been a true increase in the incidence of adenocarcinomas, most probably attributable to environmental pollutants. Recognizing lung cancer for the epidemic that it is—an epidemic that afflicts many "innocent" people—and providing federal research dollars to investigate it is vital to controlling this devastating disease.

Who is likely to develop lung cancer?

Many investigators suspect that lung cancer of any type develops over the years owing to a series of insults to the lungs—whether from toxic gases (as in the case of cigarette smoke), other environmental carcinogens (such as radon or asbestos), or long-term lung disease (such as scleroderma). Most investigators suspect that these factors work together, so that a cigarette smoker who is also exposed to carcinogens would be at particularly high risk. Unavoidable genetic factors also play a role in making some people more susceptible to external carcinogens than others. Bronchoalveolar cancer seems to be particularly common in people with a history of preexisting lung damage.

Nevertheless, it is well established that the most common forms of lung cancer are most likely to develop in cigarette smokers. Fifteen percent of smokers will eventually develop it, and the rate among women smokers appears to be rising. Between 1960 and 1986 lung cancer increased more than 4 times among women smokers, surpassing breast cancer as the leading cause of cancer death in this group. In 1991 cigarette smoking contributed to 79 percent of all lung cancer deaths in women.

There is preliminary evidence that women run about twice the risk of developing lung cancer from smoking compared with men. A recent study sponsored by Britain's Institute of Cancer Research and Norway's National Institute of Occupational Health has suggested a possible reason why: cigarette

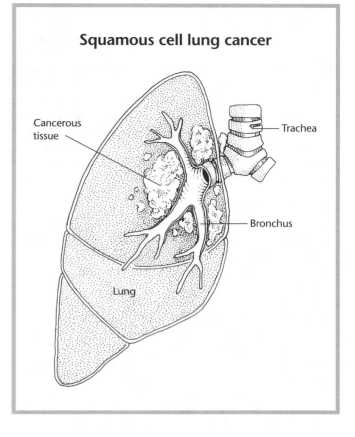

Squamous cell lung cancer

Cancerous tissue

Trachea

Bronchus

Lung

smoke apparently does relatively more damage to the DNA in women's lung cells.

What are the symptoms?

The most common symptoms of lung cancer are a persistent cough ("smoker's cough"), weight loss, breathing difficulties, and chest pain. Often the cough brings up pus or blood-streaked sputum. As the disease progresses and spreads (metastasizes) to other organs, hoarseness, fever, fatigue, weakness, dizziness, headache, and lack of appetite may also develop, depending on the type, extent, and location of the cancer. In its early stages, however, lung cancer rarely causes symptoms at all, and by the time it is diagnosed, it commonly has spread.

How is the condition evaluated?

Many people who smoke think that by having periodic chest x-rays they can identify lung cancer while it is curable. Most clinicians no longer feel that routine chest x-rays to screen healthy people for lung cancer—or even to screen ex-smokers and asymptomatic smokers on a routine basis—reduce the overall number of deaths from lung cancer. Well-designed studies of screening with chest x-rays and sputum tests in heavy smokers (all men) have shown that such testing does not alter the high mortality rate of lung cancer, even though it picks up more asymptomatic cases.

It is certainly worthwhile, however, for smokers who have

symptoms suggestive of the disease to undergo testing, and recent thinking is that CT scans may be a better test than chest x-rays. If a clinician suspects lung cancer, one of several imaging studies (initially a chest x-ray, sometimes followed by a CT scan) will be done to look for a tumor, and a sputum sample may be examined for the presence of malignant cells. The clinician may also use a tube called a bronchoscope to view the air passages and to obtain a sample of any suspicious tissue by biopsy (and laboratory analysis). These tests and possibly a PET (position emission tomography) scan or surgical check of the chest (mediastinoscopy) can help the clinician determine whether a tumor can be removed surgically.

How is lung cancer treated?

The 5-year survival rate with most types of lung cancer is low compared with other cancers that afflict women, although these rates can be as high as 80 percent in the few people who have their cancer diagnosed while their tumor is still operable. As with most forms of cancer, treatment for lung cancer depends on the type of tumor, as well as its stage of development and the patient's overall health.

If the cancer is diagnosed at an early stage, surgical removal offers the best chance of survival. There is some recent evidence that radiation to help shrink tumors before surgery may improve the outcome even further in some patients.

Quality of breathing after surgical removal of a lung cancer is affected by how much functional lung tissue remains, but most patients can resume normal activities within a month or two. Helpful advice is offered on *www.lungcancer.org* or *www.cancerguide.org*. It is advisable to see a clinician for frequent follow-up examinations to make sure that the cancer has not spread or recurred.

Surgery is usually not possible in the case of rapidly spreading small cell carcinoma, which is notoriously difficult to cure. Chemotherapy, sometimes combined with radiation therapy, can often be dramatically effective in shrinking the tumor, however, and this may result in a temporary remission. It cannot offer a cure, however, if disease is extensive.

How can lung cancer be prevented?

For the time being, the only obvious—though rarely easy—way to reduce the risks of developing at least some forms of lung cancer is to stop cigarette smoking. Although there is some debate about just how long it takes for the risks of lung cancer in an ex-smoker to fall to the level of those who have never smoked—estimates range from 5 to 20 years—the risks do fall, no matter how long or how much a person has smoked in the past. Two smoking-free years halves the risk of heart attack, and ten smoke-free years halves the risk of lung cancer.

Even without cigarette smoking, prevention will remain a problem until the causes of the "nonsmoker's" cancers are better understood. Current efforts to find chemical markers in the blood or urine that may one day be used to identify malignant cells early in the course of the disease offer some hope. If these efforts bear fruit, earlier detection—and there-

fore better chances of cure—may someday be a simple and relatively inexpensive approach to reducing deaths from lung cancer.

Research is under way to find less invasive ways to stop lung cancers early on and to arrest the carcinogenic (cancer-causing) properties of smoke. Indeed, some investigators believe that it may one day be possible to use drugs (such as synthetic vitamin A analogs called retinoids) or certain chemicals isolated from dark green vegetables to nip lung cancers in the bud. These studies have been very disappointing to date, however. If this is indeed a solution, it is by no means simple: a major study in Finland recently showed that taking antioxidant vitamins (vitamin E and beta carotene) actually increased the risk of lung cancer in male smokers over the age of 49. Further studies are necessary to clarify these results.

Related entries
Biopsy, breathing disorders, chemotherapy, chest pain, occupational hazards, radiation therapy, smoking

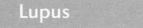

Lupus

When the term lupus is used by itself, it usually refers to systemic lupus erythematosus, or SLE. This is a chronic autoimmune disease of unknown origin which afflicts 8 to 10 times as many women as men around the world. Classed with diseases of arthritis and autoimmunity, lupus involves inflammation in many parts of the body, including the joints, blood vessels, heart, lungs, brain, and kidneys and appears to stem from an immune system disorder in which the body produces antibodies that injure its tissues. The word *lupus* is Latin for "wolf," and refers to a rash or mask over the nose and cheeks (in the shape of a butterfly) which frequently appears in people with this disease.

Who is likely to develop lupus?

Lupus most frequently develops in women between the ages of 20 and 40. This prevalence in women of reproductive age, as well as the increased incidence of lupus in older women using hormone replacement therapy, suggests that female hormones may play a role in this disease. Lupus shows a slight tendency to run in families. It is found worldwide but is more common among certain groups than others. In the United States the disease occurs about twice as frequently in Native American women as in white women, and nearly 3 times as frequently in African American women. Serious complications also tend to appear more frequently in African American women with lupus. This may be because genetic factors predisposing people to lupus vary from one ethnic group to another, or it may reflect social factors such as access to health care and education, or it may represent a combination of the two.

Women using certain drugs can sometimes develop the symptoms of lupus. These include hydralazine (for hypertension) in high doses, certain tranquilizers, procainamide (used to regulate heart rhythm), and isoniazid (to treat tuberculosis). The role of oral contraceptives in inducing lupus remains controversial.

What are the symptoms?

Symptoms of SLE tend to appear episodically, with flare-ups alternating with periods of remission. In addition to the butterfly mask on the face (which often worsens after exposure to sun or ultraviolet light), symptoms can include painful, swollen joints, particularly in the fingers and wrists; rashes, fevers, and pigmentation changes after exposure to sunlight; mouth and vaginal sores; hair loss; inflammation of the membranes around the heart and lungs which can result in chest pain and coughing; fatigue; disturbances of the central nervous system, including migraine headaches and seizures; abdominal pain due to inflammation of the abdominal cavity; and Raynaud's phenomenon, a condition in which fingers become white and blue after exposure to cold. Some women have problems with attention and memory.

Kidney disorders are the most common serious illness resulting from lupus; 50 to 70 percent of patients with severe disease show evidence of renal involvement on biopsy of the kidneys. Many people with lupus have abnormal levels of white cells, red cells, or even platelets and may have symptoms associated with these conditions (see anemia and platelet disorders). Overall 90 percent of people with lupus can expect to be alive 5 years after diagnosis, and 80 percent after 10 years. About 20 to 30 percent of patients have mild disease with no life-threatening complications. Perhaps 4 percent of people with lupus eventually recover completely.

Symptoms of drug-induced lupus include low-grade fever, aching joints and muscles, chest pain, and skin rashes. These usually disappear when the drug is stopped, though laboratory evidence of antibodies associated with the disease may persist for months.

Occasionally symptoms of lupus appear for the first time during pregnancy. Some studies of pregnant women with lupus show that pregnancy can cause mild flare-ups of symptoms, while others refute this finding. Women with lupus who have not been treated with cytotoxic drugs (Cytoxan) or who do not have kidney disease usually do not have difficulty conceiving. Women with lupus are more likely than other women, however, to develop preeclampsia (see entry), to have both early and late miscarriages (particularly if they also have the autophospholipid antibody syndrome; see entry), and to deliver prematurely. Occasionally the fetus can develop neonatal lupus, one manifestation of which is congenital heart block, a form of abnormal heartbeat in which electrical conduction is slowed or interrupted.

Depression can occur in SLE for a number of reasons. The disease itself can cause depression and, in rare cases, psychosis. The strain of coping with a long-term illness and the discomfort of the symptoms may trigger depression. Disability related to complications is another contributing factor. Changes in physical appearance—for example, hair loss and pigmentation changes (both increased and decreased pigment)—may seriously impair self-esteem for some women. Finally, depression is an occasional side effect of the corticosteroids often used to treat SLE.

Another form of lupus, also more common in women, is discoid lupus erythematosus (DLE). DLE can exist as an independent condition or as one symptom of SLE. In DLE round, red scaling patches appear on the skin, usually on the cheeks, bridge of the nose, scalp, or ears, and sometimes on the upper trunk and extremities. In many cases these appear after exposure to the sun, and in some instances they scar. About 10 percent eventually develop more internal and systemic inflammatory symptoms, sometimes resulting in full-scale SLE.

How is the condition evaluated?

In evaluating a woman with some of the symptoms of lupus, a doctor will first want to exclude conditions with similar symptoms such as rheumatoid arthritis, polymyositis and dermatomyositis, and other diseases of the connective tissue (see autoimmune disorders). This requires testing the blood for the presence of specific proteins as well as a careful consideration of more subtle symptoms that characterize each of these conditions. Almost always a test for proteins called antinuclear antibodies (ANA) will be done, since these proteins are found in the blood of nearly 95 percent of people with systemic lupus (these are rarely present in DLE). A complete blood count may detect unusually low numbers of red or white blood cells, or platelets. Blood and urine may be tested for a substance called creatinine, which appears in high levels if kidney function has been disturbed. If there is evidence of damage, tissue may be taken from the kidney (through a biopsy) for laboratory analysis. Blood tests for antiphospholipid antibodies may also be done, because 20 to 50 percent of patients with SLE will have these antibodies, and they have been associated with complications in pregnancy as well as other risks from abnormal clotting, such as strokes and heart attacks. If there is any chest pain, a cardiac ultrasound or chest x-ray may be done to see if any fluid has collected around the heart or lungs.

How is lupus treated?

Many patients with lupus, even if asymptomatic, are treated with antimalarials (Plaquenil), since there is some evidence that this therapy may prevent long-term complications of their disease. When mild symptoms occur, patients are usually treated with aspirin and other antiinflammatory drugs as well as corticosteroids. Corticosteroids and other stronger immunosuppressive medications are unavoidable in treating kidney and central nervous system complications of lupus, but they require careful monitoring by a physician, since long-term use can cause multiple side effects such as glucose intolerance, hypertension, acne, cataracts, stretchmarks, and osteoporosis. Mood swings and insomnia may develop with these drugs, and, at higher doses, depression. In rare cases, other forms of mental illness can occur. Patients need to be monitored for opportunistic infections—infections that do not ordinarily affect healthy people.

Regular exercise, especially when coupled with sufficient rest, may be beneficial in combating the fatigue of this disorder. Patients should avoid direct sun exposure and other forms of ultraviolet light as much as possible, and use topical sunscreens when they must be exposed to sunlight. Rashes can be treated with topical corticosteroid creams or ointments.

Reconstructive surgery, although rarely necessary, can reduce any joint deformities that may have appeared (see arthroplasty). Other complications of SLE (such as coronary artery disease) are treated as appropriate for the specific condition. Treating kidney disorders as early as possible may minimize permanent damage. This usually involves taking combinations of cyclophosphamide (an anticancer drug), corticosteroids, and immunosuppressive agents such as azathioprine (which is also used in transplant patients). The antimalarial Plaquenil (hydroxychloroquine) lessens skin problems, arthritis, and other manifestations of the disease.

Any woman with SLE who is pregnant needs to be monitored closely. She and her clinician should weigh the pros and cons of continued medication therapy during pregnancy. Very early in her pregnancy she should have her blood tested for certain antibodies associated with neonatal lupus (a rare condition).

To prevent scarring, DLE must be treated promptly by applying a topical corticosteroid ointment or cream to the lesions. Hydroxychloroquine or another medication, dapsone, can also be helpful. Exposure to sunlight and ultraviolet light should be minimized. Taking corticosteroids can sometimes restore hair growth.

Related entries

Anemia, antiinflammatory drugs, arthritis, arthroplasty, autoimmune disorders, coronary artery disease, depression, estrogen replacement therapy, hair loss, headaches, high blood pressure, insomnia, kidney disorders, miscarriage, musculoskeletal disorders, oral contraceptives, osteoporosis, platelet disorders, polymyositis and dermatomyositis, preeclampsia, Raynaud's phenomenon, rheumatoid arthritis, skin disorders, stroke

Lyme Disease

Lyme disease is a multistage, multisystem infection caused by small bacteria called spirochetes *(Borrelia burgdorferi)* that are transmitted by *Ixodes* ticks. This species of tick, also called the deer tick, is much smaller than the type of tick usually found on dogs—it is only about size of a poppy seed—and thrives on wildlife such as the white-tailed deer that live in grassy, woody, brushy, or marshy regions. These ticks can also survive on domestic animals, including dogs, cats, and horses.

Lyme disease was first identified in Old Lyme, Connecticut, in 1975 (though it may have been recognized earlier in Europe). Over 103,000 cases were reported to the Centers for Disease Control (CDC) between 1982 and 1997 alone, with about 16,000 new cases reported each year. Long-term consequences and optimal treatment are still being explored, but we already know that this disease is usually amenable to antibiotic therapy if treated early. Without effective treatment, however, Lyme disease can lead to serious and possibly recurring disorders of the joints, nerves, and heart.

Who is likely to develop it?

While people of all ages can be infected with Lyme disease, the highest reported rates occur in people under 15 and between 30 and 59 years of age. Cases have been reported in 48 states, as well as the District of Columbia, but the disease is most often contracted in the northeastern, north central, and Pacific coastal regions of the United States—areas in which the *B. burgdorferi* spirochete is endemic. Lyme disease has also been reported in Europe, Japan, China, and Russia. Residents and visitors to endemic areas are at risk. The spirochete can be transmitted year-round, but most cases are contracted between April and July.

What are the symptoms?

A bull's-eye or circular red ring or rash, which develops around the tick bite after about 3 to 10 days, often signals Lyme disease, although many women never develop a rash. This ring can grow to 5 inches or more in diameter. Other early symptoms (stage 1 of the disease) may include flulike symptoms such as mild fever, headache, fatigue, listlessness, muscle and joint pains, and swollen glands.

Over the next 3 to 4 weeks, the rash gradually fades, with or without treatment. During this time (stage 2 of infection), malaise, skin lesions, and stiff neck may develop, together with continuing fatigue, headaches, and pain in the joints and muscles. Without early antibiotic treatment, the body begins to develop antibodies to the spirochete. In rare cases, dizziness, fainting, irregular heartbeat, and breathing difficulties may develop, possibly signaling heart problems such as arrhythmias, myocarditis, pericarditis, and, rarely, congestive heart failure.

In later stages, which can occur weeks or months after the tick bite, a small proportion of patients may develop Bell's palsy (partial or total paralysis of one side of the face) or other forms of facial paralysis and inflammation of the lining of the spinal cord or brain (meningitis; see entry) or of the peripheral nerves. Eye inflammation (keratitis) may also develop at this stage, and possibly memory impairment, excessive sleepiness, irritability, or other behavior changes. Some people also experience intermittent arthritis of the knee, with episodes often lasting weeks, months, or longer.

How is the condition evaluated?

Because the symptoms of Lyme disease involve so many different organ systems, this disease is easily confused with other conditions. Often the afflicted patient and the clinician must work together to review symptoms and experiences over many months before even considering the possibility of Lyme disease. Having the characteristic bull's-eye rash or remembering being bitten by a suspicious tick (especially in a high-risk locale) can make diagnosis easier, but more often than not a patient comes in with joint pains, heart irregularities, or vague behavioral symptoms weeks or months after the initial infection. Frequently the patient has no particular memory of a tick bite, either, especially if she has not been in an area in which Lyme disease is endemic.

Tests for specific antibodies to the Lyme disease spirochete can sometimes be helpful, but many tests are still unreliable and inaccurate (for example, a person infected with the spirochete that causes syphilis will have a positive result in these tests). As more and more clinicians use the next generation of tests, accuracy should improve considerably.

How is Lyme disease treated?

Treatment for Lyme disease varies according to the stage of the disease at which it is diagnosed. Antibiotic treatment begun within about a month of the tick bite is usually effective, but the symptoms can be more difficult to eradicate if treated at later stages. Oral antibiotics (usually amoxicillin or doxycycline) are usually prescribed for about 10 to 30 days. There is some evidence that a one-time dose of doxycycline may be effective early after exposure. If these are ineffective, intravenous antibiotics (usually ceftriaxone or penicillin G) for 2 or 3 weeks may be required.

Arthritic symptoms are often treated with nonsteroidial antiinflammatory drugs (NSAIDs) or, if necessary, steroids injected directly into the affected joint.

How can Lyme disease be prevented?

Using tick repellants such as permethrin or DEET, wearing protective clothing, and promptly removing attached ticks are the best ways to prevent Lyme disease, together with community efforts to control the ticks. Anyone hiking or camping in woody, grassy, or marshy areas—particularly where Lyme disease is prevalent—should wear a hat, long-sleeved shirt, and long pants tucked into socks. Getting in the habit of brushing off clothing before going inside and checking the entire body for ticks after hiking or visiting high-risk areas can also reduce the risk of infection, as can removing suspicious ticks promptly. Wearing light-colored clothing and using a flashlight can make the tiny deer ticks easier to spot. Pets should also be inspected regularly for ticks and should wear tick collars. Vaccinations, while not 100 percent effective, are also worth considering for pets that live in or will visit a high-risk area.

To remove a tick, wear gloves if possible and grasp the tick with a fine-point tweezers, pulling gently but firmly until the tick releases its grip on the skin. Squeezing the tick too tightly—or using matches, Vaseline, or alcohol—can be counterproductive because infected material may be released through the skin before the tick is removed. Hands should be washed thoroughly with soapy warm water afterwards and the bite area cleaned with rubbing alcohol or other antiseptic.

A bite is no reason for alarm: the tick may not turn out to be a deer tick, and even if it is one, it may not have carried the spirochete or transmitted it during the bite. For these reasons, preventive antibiotics are rarely administered unless signs or symptoms of Lyme disease develop. To be safe, however, it's a good idea to save the tick in a jar filled with alcohol and label the jar with information about when and where the bite was acquired and where it occurred on the body. If there is no sign of a bite, the tick should be drowned in a sealed jar of alcohol and disposed of carefully.

If the tick appears to be a deer tick, a visit to a clinician is probably in order. The clinician may give preventive antibiotics if he or she considers the patient to be at high risk for developing Lyme disease. To determine risk, the clinician will ask about the size of the tick, whether or not it was attached to the skin, and how long it was attached. Only ticks that were engorged (globular and somewhat enlarged, the signs of just having finished a blood meal) at the time of removal warrant preventive treatment with antibiotics—except in the case of a pregnant woman, who will probably be given amoxicillin. This is not because the risk of getting Lyme disease is any greater during pregnancy, but only because preventive treatment may alleviate anxiety about the health of both mother and fetus. In other cases the clinician will simply instruct the patient to call if there is any change in health, particularly any redness at the site of the tick bite other than the transient redness that sometimes develops over the first 24 to 48 hours as an allergic reaction to tick saliva.

In late 1998 the Food and Drug Administration (FDA) licensed a new vaccine against Lyme disease for use in persons 15 to 70 years of age. This vaccine is ineffective in about half of people vaccinated, however, and it is as yet unclear how long the effects last, whether booster shots are required, or what the long-term effects might be. Requiring 3 different injections administered over the course of a year, the vaccine must be timed to correspond to the beginning of the transmission season (which usually starts in April). It can produce side effects resembling a flulike illness and provides no protection against other tick-borne illnesses. Even so, the vaccine may be worth considering for anyone who will have frequent and prolonged exposure to ticks in areas where Lyme disease is endemic. The series of shots costs about $200 and is covered by some insurance policies.

Related entries

Antibiotics, arrhythmias, arthritis

CIRCULATORY SYSTEM

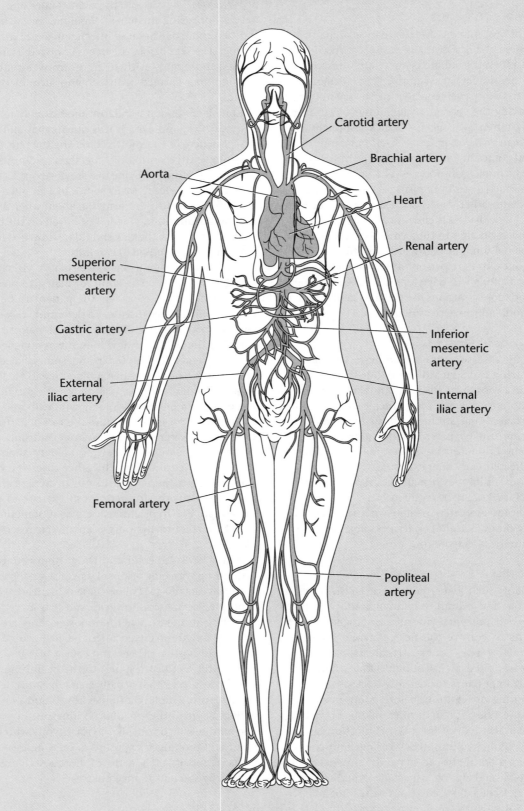

Carotid artery

Brachial artery

Aorta

Heart

Renal artery

Superior
mesenteric
artery

Gastric artery

Inferior
mesenteric
artery

External
iliac artery

Internal
iliac artery

Femoral artery

Popliteal
artery

DIGESTIVE SYSTEM

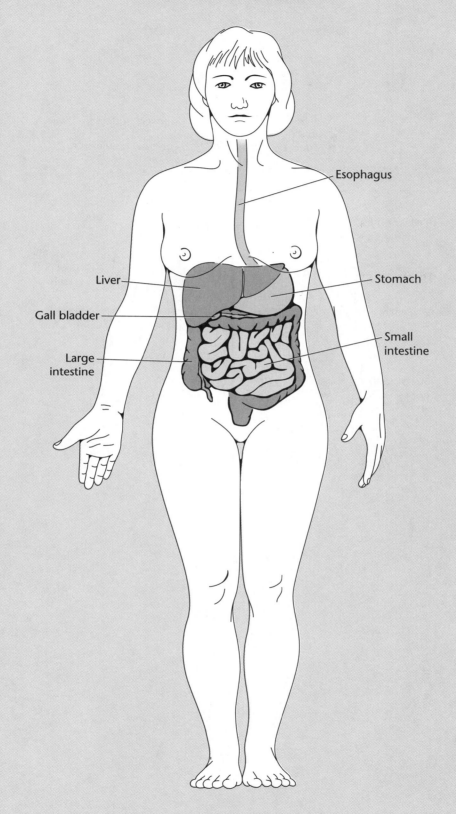

Esophagus

Liver

Stomach

Gall bladder

Small
intestine

Large
intestine

LYMPHATIC SYSTEM

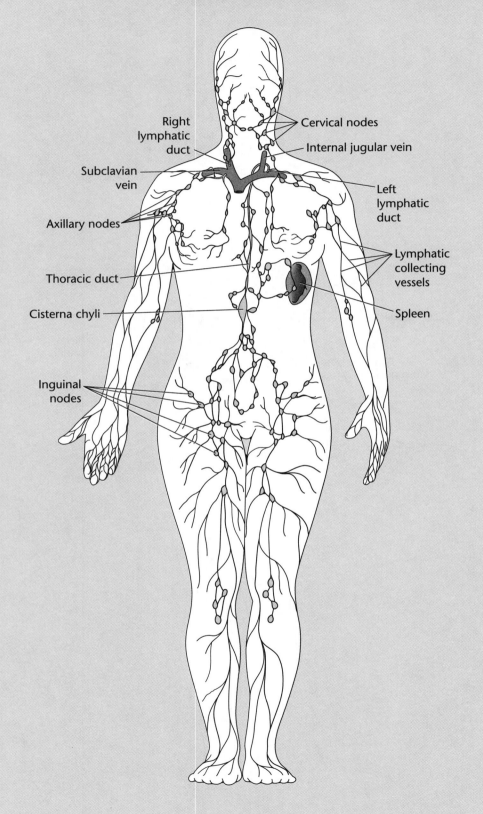

Right lymphatic duct

Cervical nodes

Internal jugular vein

Subclavian vein

Left lymphatic duct

Axillary nodes

Lymphatic collecting vessels

Thoracic duct

Cisterna chyli

Spleen

Inguinal nodes

MUSCULAR SYSTEM

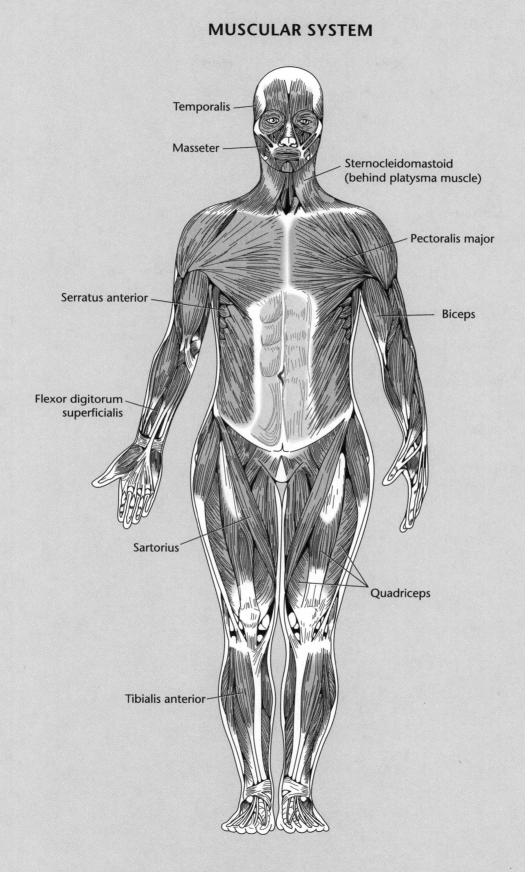

Temporalis

Masseter

Sternocleidomastoid
(behind platysma muscle)

Pectoralis major

Serratus anterior

Biceps

Flexor digitorum
superficialis

Sartorius

Quadriceps

Tibialis anterior

NERVOUS SYSTEM

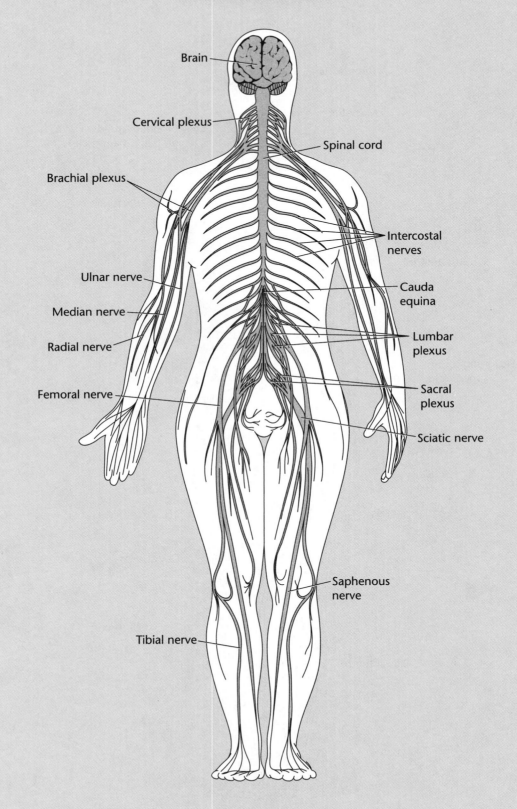

Brain

Cervical plexus

Spinal cord

Brachial plexus

Intercostal nerves

Ulnar nerve

Cauda equina

Median nerve

Lumbar plexus

Radial nerve

Femoral nerve

Sacral plexus

Sciatic nerve

Saphenous nerve

Tibial nerve

SKELETAL SYSTEM

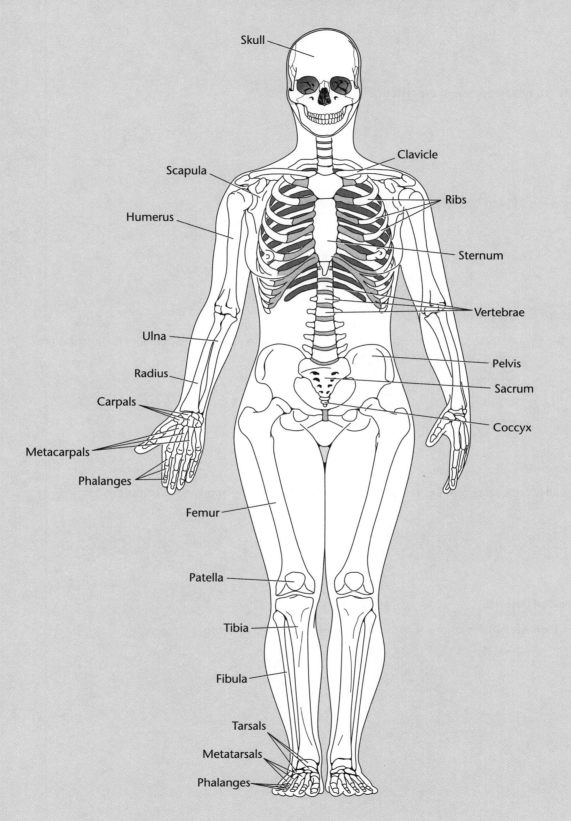

Skull

Clavicle

Scapula

Humerus

Ribs

Sternum

Ulna

Vertebrae

Radius

Pelvis

Carpals

Sacrum

Metacarpals

Coccyx

Phalanges

Femur

Patella

Tibia

Fibula

Tarsals

Metatarsals

Phalanges

RECORDING YOUR MEDICAL HISTORY

Who to notify in case of emergency

Location of your health care power of attorney

Health insurance information

Include your health insurance provider's name and phone number for approval of hospitalization, emergency room care, and surgical procedures.

Allergies

List all allergic reactions, like rashes and hives, to such things as food and medications.

Medical illnesses

List such ailments as angina, heart disease, and high blood pressure.

Surgical procedures

Note operations such as gallbladder and bypass surgery. Include dates and other details such as medical anesthesia and their side effects.

Hospitalization or emergency room visits for other reasons

List such ailments as broken bones, concussions, serious burns, sprains, and lacerations.

Medications

List all of your current prescriptions and over-the-counter medications, as well as prior medications you've tried, along with their side effects. Consider writing these down on a note card and carrying them with you in your wallet in case of an emergency.

Preventive health/health maintenance

Include dates of and any idiosyncratic reactions to immunizations and vaccinations.

Test results

List dates and results of mammograms; Pap smears; PSA tests and prostate exams; sigmoidoscopies; bone density tests; and periodic lipid panels. Also keep copies of any other significant diagnostic test results and X-rays.

Family history

Include family history, from your maternal and paternal grandparents to parents and siblings. List illnesses treated both medically and surgically, concentrating on those diseases that are often hereditary, for example, hypertension, coronary artery disease, diabetes, and breast and colon cancer.

Mental illnesses

Note here any mental illnesses, such as depressive and panic disorders.

FOOD PYRAMIDS

Food pyramid created by the U.S. Department of Agriculture

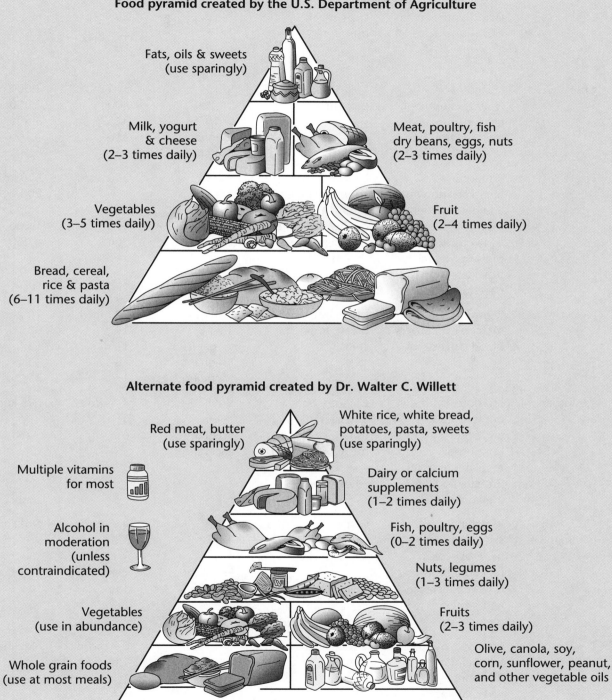

Fats, oils & sweets
(use sparingly)

Milk, yogurt
& cheese
(2–3 times daily)

Meat, poultry, fish
dry beans, eggs, nuts
(2–3 times daily)

Vegetables
(3–5 times daily)

Fruit
(2–4 times daily)

Bread, cereal,
rice & pasta
(6–11 times daily)

Alternate food pyramid created by Dr. Walter C. Willett

Red meat, butter
(use sparingly)

White rice, white bread,
potatoes, pasta, sweets
(use sparingly)

Multiple vitamins
for most

Dairy or calcium
supplements
(1–2 times daily)

Alcohol in
moderation
(unless
contraindicated)

Fish, poultry, eggs
(0–2 times daily)

Nuts, legumes
(1–3 times daily)

Vegetables
(use in abundance)

Fruits
(2–3 times daily)

Olive, canola, soy,
corn, sunflower, peanut,
and other vegetable oils

Whole grain foods
(use at most meals)

VITAMINS

Nutrient	What it Does	Selected sources	Age or group	RDA	Upper limit (no adverse effects)
Biotin	Helps synthesize fat and amino acids	Liver, meat, fruit	9–13 14–18 > 19 Lactating	20 μg/d* 25 30 35	Not known
Choline	Promotes healthy fetal development, cell function, and metabolizing fat	Milk, liver, eggs, peanuts	9–13 14–18 > 19 Pregnant Lactating	375 mg/d* 400 425 450 550	2,000 mg/d 3,000 3,500 3,500 3,500
Folate	Promotes red blood cell growth and development; may help prevent certain cancers; prevents neural tube defects in developing fetus	Enriched cereal, dark leafy green vegetables, whole grains; women of childbearing age should take a folate-only supplement	9–13 14–18 > 19 Pregnant Lactating	300 μg/d 400 400 600 500	600 μg/d 800 1,000 1,000 1,000
Niacin	Regulates metabolism; lowers blood cholesterol	Meat, fish, poultry, bread, fortified cereals	9–13 14–18 > 19 Pregnant Lactating	12 mg/d 14 14 18 17	20 mg/d 30 35 35 35
Pantothenic acid	Promotes synthesis of progesterone and other hormones; regulates energy, protein, and fat metabolism	Chicken, beef, potatoes, oats, tomatoes, organ meats, yeast, egg yolk, broccoli, whole grains	9–13 > 14 Pregnant Lactating	4 mg/d* 5 6 7	Not known
Riboflavin (vitamin B$_2$)	Maintains healthy skin, vision, nervous system function; promotes disease resistance and protein metabolism	Organ meats, milk, whole grains and fortified cereals	9–13 14–18 > 19 Pregnant Lactating	0.9 mg/d 1.0 1.1 1.4 1.6	Not known
Thiamin (vitamin B$_1$)	Promotes good heart and nerve function, carbohydrate metabolism	Whole grains, fortified cereals, pasta	9–13 14–18 > 19 Pregnant or lactating	0.9 mg/d 1.0 1.1 1.4	Not known

Vitamin A	Promotes good eyesight, bone growth, and epithelial tissue function; antioxidant; may help prevent heart disease and some cancers	Liver, whole milk, butter, fish, sweet potatoes, carrots, pumpkin, dried apricots	9–13 14–18 > 19 Pregnant Lactating Vegans may need more	600 μg/d 700 700 770 1,300	1,700 μg/d 2,800 3,000 3,000 3,000
Vitamin B$_6$	Promotes normal cell function and metabolism of amino and fatty acids	Fortified cereal, organ meats, soy-based products	9–13 14–18 19–50 > 50 Pregnant Lactating	1.0 mg/d 1.2 1.3 1.5 1.9 2.0	60 mg/d 80 100 100 100 100
Vitamin B$_{12}$ (cobalamin)	Promotes healthy red blood cells and DNA	Fortified cereal, meat, fish, poultry	9–13 >14 Pregnant Lactating Vegetarians may need more	1.8 μg/d 2.4 2.6 2.8	Not known
Vitamin C	Promotes collagen formation, circulatory function, and wound healing; serves as antioxidant	Citrus fruits and juice, tomatoes and their juice, potatoes, cruciferous vegetables, strawberries, cabbage, spinach	9–13 14–18 > 19 Pregnant Lactating Smokers need an additional 35 mg/d	45 mg/d 65 75 85 120	1,200 mg/d 1,800 2,000 2,000 2,000
Vitamin D	Builds bones, muscles, and nerves; aids in the absorption of calcium and phosphorus	Fortified cereal, fatty fish, fish liver oil, dairy products	9–50 59–70 > 70	5 μg/d* 10 15	50 μg/d 50 50
Vitamin E	Protects cells from oxidation damage	Vegetable oils, wheat germ, whole grains, nuts, fruits, vegetables, meat	9–13 14–18 > 19 Lactating	11 mg/d 15 15 19	600 mg/d 800 1,000 1,000
Vitamin K	Promotes normal blood clotting and bone formation	Vegetables, plant oils, margarine	9–13 14–18 > 19	60 μg/d 75 90	Not known

* Indicates adequate intake (AI), rather than recommended daily allowance

Source: National Academies Press and the Office of Dietary Supplements, National Institutes of Health

ELEMENTS

Nutrient	What it does	Selected sources	Age or group	RDA	Upper limit (no adverse effects)
Calcium	Promotes blood clotting, muscle and nerve function, normal bones and teeth	Dairy foods, corn tortillas, tofu, green leafy vegetables	9–18 19–50 >50	1,300 mg/d* 1,000 1,200	2,500 mg/d 2,500 2,500
Chromium	Helps maintain normal blood glucose levels	Some cereals, meats, poultry, fish	9–13 14–18 19–50 >50 Pregnant Lactating	21 µg/d* 24 25 20 30 45	Not known
Copper	Promotes enzyme regulation of iron metabolism	Organ meats, seafood, nuts, wheat bran, whole grains, cocoa	9–13 14–18 >19 Pregnant Lactating	700 µg/d 890 900 1,000 1,300	5,000 µg/d 8,000 10,000 10,000 10,000
Iodine	Promotes healthy thyroid function; prevents goiter	Iodized salt, seafood	9–13 14–18 >19 Pregnant Lactating	120 µg/d 150 150 220 290	600 µg/d 900 1,100 1,100 1,100
Iron	Necessary for hemoglobin and hormone function; prevents anemia	Fruits, vegetables, fortified cereal and bread, meat, poultry, molasses	9–13 14–18 19–50 >50 Pregnant Lactating Vegetarians may need more	8 mg/d 15 18 8 27 9	40 mg/d 45 45 45 45 45
Magnesium	Necessary for enzyme function	Green leafy vegetables, whole grains, nuts, meat, milk	9–13 14–18 yrs 19–30 yrs >30 Pregnant	240 mg/d 360 310 320 350	350 mg/d 350 350 350 350
Manganese	Promotes bone formation; aids enzyme function	Nuts, legumes, tea, whole grains	9–13 14–18 >19 Pregnant Lactating	1.6 mg/d* 1.6 1.8 2.0 2.6	6 mg/d 9 11 11 11

Molybdenum	Promotes enzyme function	Legumes, whole grains, nuts	9–13	34 μg/d	1,100 μg/d
			14–18	43	1,700
			>19	45	2,000
			Pregnant or lactating	50	2,000
Phosphorus	Promotes normal growth and development; aids in processing foods and maintaining blood sugar levels	Dairy products, peas, meat, eggs, some whole grains	9–13	1,250 mg/d	4,000 mg/d
			14–18	1,250	4,000
			>19	700	4,000
			Pregnant	700	3,500
			Lactating	700	4,000
			Athletes may exceed upper limit without adverse effects		
Selenium	Antioxidant; regulates thyroid function and helps body metabolize vitamin C	Organ meats, seafood, some vegetables grown in selenium-rich soil	9–13	40 μg/d	280 μg/d
			>14	55	400
			Pregnant	60	400
			Lactating	70	400
Zinc	Promotes regular gene expression, bone metabolism, normal vision, and regulation of blood sugar level	Fortified cereals, red meat, some seafood	9–13	8 mg/d	23 mg/d
			14–18	9	34
			>19	8	40
			Pregnant	11	40
			Lactating	12	40
			Vegetarians may need more		

* Indicates adequate intake (AI), rather than recommended daily allowance

Source: National Academies Press and the Office of Dietary Supplements, National Institutes of Health

Lymphedema

Lymphedema occurs when lymphatic fluid pools in the layer of fat just under the skin and in other interstitial tissues, resulting in swelling and inflammation. Most often, lymphedema involves the arms and/or legs. It occurs most commonly in the arms of women who have had a radical mastectomy and/or radiation therapy for breast cancer, and it can appear weeks or even years after the surgery, serving as a painful reminder. While most forms of lymphedema cannot be eliminated, in many cases special care and exercises can keep symptoms under control.

Lymph is a nearly colorless fluid that contains lymphocytes, a kind of white blood cell essential to the body's ability to fight infection. It circulates through a network of lymphatic vessels that runs throughout the body, much like the circulatory system. Normally, the lymphatic vessels drain excess lymph from the skin and superficial tissues, filtering out impurities through lymph nodes before channeling it into the blood system. If lymph nodes are missing, damaged, or malfunctioning, however, or if the lymph vessels are blocked, lymph starts collecting under the skin, leading to lymphedema. As these collections of fluid build up, oxygen becomes less available to the tissues, and this in turn interferes with wound healing. In addition, infections may develop because protein-rich lymph is an excellent medium for bacterial growth.

By far the most common form of lymphedema, secondary (or acquired) lymphedema, develops when an infection or medical or surgical procedure leads to the damage or removal of some of the lymph nodes. Much rarer is primary lymphedema, a form of the condition that occurs when lymph nodes are missing or defective.

Who is likely to develop lymphedema?

Primary lymphedema is rare. It can sometimes be traced to inherited abnormalities and may occur together with certain malformations of the blood vessels (including port wine stains). Symptoms can develop at any time in life and may involve any of the limbs, as well as other parts of the body.

Secondary lymphedema, by far the more common form of the condition, most frequently results from surgical procedures that involve cutting or removing the lymph nodes—particularly radical mastectomy, but also pelvic and abdominal surgery as well as procedures to remove melanomas (a form of skin cancer). As many as one-quarter of all women who have had a mastectomy involving removal of the lymph nodes in the underarm develop arm lymphedema.

Secondary lymphedema can also develop if the lymphatic vessels are blocked as the result of infections or scarring from radiation therapy. That is why over half of all women who have both lymph node surgery and radiation therapy for breast cancer can expect to develop lymphedema.

What are the symptoms?

Lymphedema is characterized by swelling in the arms or legs—and sometimes other parts of the body—accompanied by a feeling of heaviness or fullness. The first sign of a problem may be shoes, rings, watches, or bracelets that start feeling tight, since the swelling usually starts at the outer end of the limb and progresses upward over time.

Feelings of tightness, dull achiness, and reduced flexibility and mobility of the affected limb may also occur. In the early stages of the disease, gently pressing the affected area will produce small but temporary indentations ("pitting"). The arm or leg may be normal or almost normal upon waking in the morning and swell only as the day goes on. As the condition worsens, however, tissue becomes spongy, skin begins to harden, and limbs increase in girth. In the most severe stage, swelling becomes extreme, skin and underlying tissue feel hard and unyielding to pressure, and using the affected arm or leg may be difficult if not impossible.

Symptoms that are due to a temporary injury may resolve within a week, but in many cases last indefinitely. Symptoms can also develop weeks or even years after lymph node surgery. Injury to the arm, overuse (even by gardening or playing an instrument), or infection can aggravate symptoms.

Over time, persistent lymphedema may result in inflamed skin and infection (lymphangitis). Symptoms of lymphangitis include pain in the affected area, red blotches on the skin, discoloration, hot and swollen skin, increased feelings of heaviness in the limb, and, often, high fever and chills.

How is the condition evaluated?

A woman who has had a mastectomy or pelvic or abdominal surgery and who develops swelling or pain in a limb should consult a clinician about the possibility of lymphedema. The clinician will take a detailed medical history and perform a physical examination to distinguish lymphedema from circulatory disorders (see entry) and determine the cause of the swelling. Part of the exam will involve applying gentle pressure to the affected limb to check for pitting, as well as measuring the circumference of the limb to gauge progression of the swelling. Various tests (such as lymphoscintigraphy or lymphangiography) may be done to distinguish patterns of lymph flow that can help differentiate primary and secondary forms of lymphedema, and, in some cases, additional tests may be performed to rule out the possibility that a tumor is obstructing lymphatic vessels.

How is lymphedema treated?

While there is still no cure for lymphedema, simple self-help measures, with guidance from a clinician, can often provide substantial relief. Elevating the affected limb and doing special exercises are the best ways to minimize swelling. Keeping the skin clean and dry and occasionally applying lubricating lotions can also help prevent associated skin lesions, tightness, and toughening. Elastic stockings, compression sleeves, or special bandages can often help as well. Use of such aids at times when more swelling is likely, such as during air travel, may prevent worsening of lymphedema. Diet can make a difference, too. Sticking to a low-salt, protein-rich diet helps some women, and losing weight may also help relieve pressure on the legs and feet.

If self-help fails to provide relief, it may be necessary to visit a hospital or clinic several times a week for treatment with pneumatic compression devices. These devices, which are worn for several hours at a stretch, several days a week, alternately inflate and deflate around the affected limb. Another possibility is a form of massage therapy called manual lymph drainage, usually administered by a specially trained massage therapist on a daily basis for about a month. After each session, the therapist wraps the affected limb in compression bandages. Cancer patients should consult a knowledgeable clinician before undergoing this therapy, however, because of (so-far unsubstantiated) concern that certain types of massage therapy may help promote the spread of metastatic cancer.

A clinician should be contacted immediately if a limb affected with lymphedema becomes red, hot, or painful, or if it develops open sores. These are all indications of a possible infection and may require treatment with antibiotics. All other lymphedema treatments should be stopped until a clinician has diagnosed and treated the infection.

Surgical procedures to relieve lymphedema have so far yielded disappointing results, although researchers hope that someday microsurgical techniques may be able to repair damaged lymphatic vessels.

How can lymphedema be prevented?

Women who have had mastectomies or any other lymph node surgeries can reduce the chance of developing problems by avoiding overuse of the affected limbs, meticulously treating cuts, scrapes, and bug bites with antibacterial ointment, and reporting any signs of infection immediately to a clinician. If possible, too, affected limbs should not be used for blood pressure measurements, blood draws, or injections. Special exercises tailored to the patient by a physical therapist can often help as well. Arm and hand exercises can help reduce the risk of arm lymphedema after mastectomy, for example, while foot and leg exercises can reduce the risk of lymphedema after pelvic surgery. In addition, keeping weight under control can also make lymphedema less likely to develop and minimize swelling and pain if it does.

Prior to breast cancer surgery, it is often advisable to discuss the possibility of lymphedema with the surgeon as one of the many factors that help determine the most desirable type of surgery.

Related entries

Antibiotics, breast cancer, circulatory problems, edema, mastectomy, melanoma, radiation therapy, Turner syndrome

Macular Degeneration

Macular degeneration is an eye disease in which the central part of the retina gradually deteriorates. It is the major cause of blindness among elderly people living in Western countries and the leading cause of legal blindness in the United States. (The definition of legal blindness varies from state to state but often means that the better eye has a vision of 20/200 or worse, even with glasses.)

The retina lies at the back of the eye and processes light in a way somewhat similar to the way film processes the light that enters a camera. Unlike photographic film, however, each of the light-detecting cells (rods and cones) in the retina processes the rays that are focused on it separately and sends its own independent signals about brightness and color to the brain (via the optic nerve). This independent processing system means that if one portion of the retina is destroyed, the portion of the visual field normally processed by that portion will be lost.

In macular degeneration the lost portion is the highly detailed, central part of the visual field. This loss occurs because the light detectors in the center of the retina (macula)—which are responsible for processing light from the center of the visual field—degenerate. As a result, central vision fades, making tasks such as reading and driving difficult if not impossible. So long as there is no other eye damage, peripheral (side) vision is retained, allowing many people with macular degeneration to see well enough to carry out the tasks of daily life independently.

In approximately 90 percent of people with macular degeneration, the problem can be attributed to the atrophy (thinning out) of the macula alone. This form of macular degeneration is sometimes called "dry" macular degeneration. About 10 percent of the time new, abnormal blood vessels growing between the retina and its supporting tissue leak, resulting in scar tissue that interferes with normal vision. This less common form of macular degeneration, also known as "wet" macular degeneration, is sometimes amenable to treatment with laser surgery if detected early enough. Some of the age-related changes may be accelerated by exposure to ultraviolet rays in sunlight.

Who is likely to develop macular degeneration?

Although little is known about the cause, it often seems to be the result of aging and affects as many as 1 in 5 people over the age of 75. It also is more common in women than in men. Other populations at higher than average risk are whites, cigarette smokers, and people with a family history of the disease.

What are the symptoms?

Macular degeneration is ultimately marked by the loss of central vision. In the beginning, however, symptoms are more likely to appear as lines or irregular patches of dimness run-

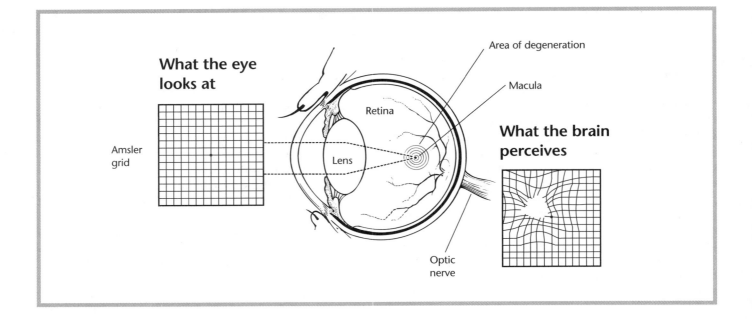

What the eye looks at

Amsler grid

Retina

Lens

Area of degeneration

Macula

What the brain perceives

Optic nerve

ning across the visual field. As the condition progresses, fine print in the center of a page may appear blurred or a blind spot may develop, straight lines may appear somewhat curvy, colors may fade, objects may look larger or smaller than they should, and it may be increasingly difficult to see street signs and other distant objects.

How is the condition evaluated?

Because changes that suggest macular degeneration can also be symptoms of a number of other eye conditions, anyone who develops them needs to be evaluated by an ophthalmologist (eye specialist). This is accomplished easily enough in anyone receiving regular eye examinations—which are generally advisable at least every 2 years in all people over the age of 40 and probably once a year after 50. Because some forms of macular degeneration are treatable if detected soon enough, early detection is vital.

To test for macular degeneration, an eye doctor will examine the eyes to check for the presence of drusen, tiny yellow deposits in the retina that may mean the eye is at risk for developing more severe macular degeneration. He or she may also ask the patient to look at a checkerboard-like pattern called an Amsler grid while covering one eye and staring at a black dot in the grid's center. People with macular degeneration may not be able to see some of the lines or may perceive the straight lines as wavy.

An eye doctor may also evaluate the blood vessel pattern in the eye by using a test called fluorescent angiography. The vessels of the eye are highlighted with a special contrast agent (which is first injected into a vein of the arm) and then photographed so that the doctor can look for abnormalities.

How is macular degeneration treated?

Little can be done to stop or reverse most cases of macular degeneration. When the underlying problem is macular atrophy—rather than leaking blood vessels—the only workable approach usually involves certain lifestyle changes to make life with limited vision more liveable. These changes include reading with special high-magnification lenses, finding large-type reading material, and increasing the level of brightness in rooms whenever possible. Some ophthalmologists also suggest monitoring vision at home by checking patterns daily on an Amsler grid card (see illustration) and reporting any changes in perception.

When degeneration is due to new and abnormal blood vessels, laser surgery (photocoagulation) can sometimes slow deterioration—or stop it entirely—by sealing off leaking vessels with a laser beam. This technique is effective, however, only if attempted early in the course of the disease, since it cannot reverse damage that has already occurred.

There is no convincing evidence so far that macular degeneration can be treated successfully with vitamin and mineral supplements. One study has suggested that adding zinc supplements to the diet may be helpful, but these findings must still be borne out in clinical trials.

How can macular degeneration be prevented?

There is no guaranteed way to prevent this condition, although regular eye examinations to allow early detection may prevent some forms of the disease from progressing. To some extent wearing sunglasses that absorb ultraviolet light may help reduce the risk of damage to both the macula and other parts of the eye.

Eating plenty of foods rich in the natural pigments called

carotenoids probably cannot hurt either, and may well have benefits beyond preventing macular degeneration. A recent study of 800 people by researchers at the Massachusetts Eye and Ear Infirmary found that those whose diets contained the highest levels of carotenoid-rich foods had a risk of developing macular degeneration 43 percent lower than for those whose diets contained the lowest levels. Even more protective than the much-touted carotenoid beta carotene were the carotenoids lutein and zeaxanthin, which are found in dark green leafy vegetables such as spinach and collard greens. More research must be done to find out if it was indeed the carotenoids or some other characteristic shared by the study subjects that helped ward off macular degeneration.

Related entries

Cataracts, contact lenses, dry eye, eye care, glaucoma, laser surgery, nearsightedness and farsightedness, retinal detachment, smoking

Magnetic Resonance Imaging

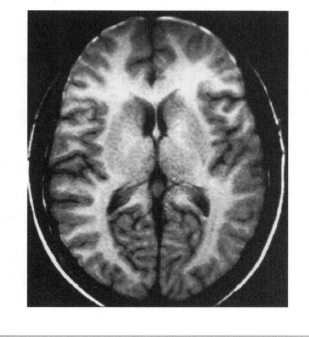

**Magnetic resonance image
of the brain**

Magnetic resonance imaging is a noninvasive procedure, available since the early 1980s, that provides pictures of the body's interior (see illustration). One great advantage of MRIs—in contrast to other imaging techniques such as x-rays and CT scans—is that they frequently involve no potentially damaging radiation or contrast dyes. They also often yield different information than conventional x-rays, particularly of soft tissue. These advantages have allowed MRIs to supplant x-rays in evaluating multiple sclerosis, spinal disk disease, stroke, brain tumors, and many disorders of the musculoskeletal system. MRI is also useful for evaluating certain breast disorders.

How is the procedure performed?

A patient having an MRI lies inside a large tunnel-like machine which produces a strong magnetic field. When radio waves are directed through the body in this field, the nuclei (centers) of the hydrogen atoms in various internal structures react in a characteristic way—depending on the type of tissue and its water content. By summing the reactions of these atoms to radio waves sent from many different angles around the body, a computer then produces images that appear as sections or slices of the body. These slices may be obtained in a variety of image planes.

As far as the patient is concerned, this whole process—which generally takes no more than 30 to 45 minutes—is completely painless, although some people find it a bit difficult to lie still or feel somewhat claustrophobic inside the tunnel. Some examinations require the intravenous injection of an MR contrast agent. Sedatives are sometimes given to re-duce anxiety. And newer, open design MR scanners are less likely to cause claustrophobic reactions, although the magnetic field is not as strong. Even so, this "open magnet" design may suffice for many conditions in lieu of a conventional MR scanner.

What are the risks and complications?

There are no known health risks associated with magnetic resonance imaging. MR contrast agents, however, are not recommended during pregnancy

Related entries

Antianxiety drugs, back pain, computerized axial tomography scans, mammography, multiple sclerosis, stroke, ultrasound

Mammography

A mammogram is a special kind of breast x-ray that can detect malignant (cancerous) tumors and other breast abnormalities (see illustration). It is used both to evaluate the breasts of women with symptoms (such as a lump or pain in

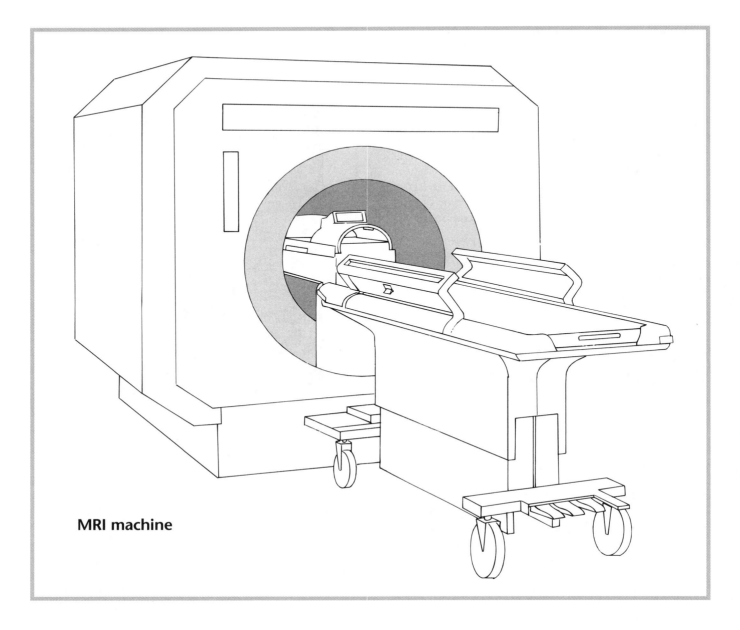

MRI machine

the breast) and to screen for breast cancer in women who have no symptoms. Mammography can detect tumors so small that they cannot yet be easily felt, a point at which they are highly treatable. For certain groups of women it has been shown to reduce—moderately—the risk of dying from breast cancer.

Mammography is most effective when used in conjunction with regular breast exams done by clinicians and with breast self-examination (BSE) done by women at home. Even if a mammogram is negative, a doctor may decide to follow a woman with a breast lump closely for a month or two, or to perform a biopsy of the mass, depending on the woman's age and other risk factors for breast cancer. In most cases a discrete breast lump that is clearly different from adjacent breast tissue will require biopsy.

How is the procedure performed?

In the procedure itself the breast is compressed between two flat plates (see illustration). Most women experience only minor discomfort, although some find the compression fairly painful. Premenopausal women may want to have the mammography done in the week following completion of a menstrual period, since breasts tend to be least tender (and lumpy) at this time. A radiologist or radiologic technician will then x-ray each breast twice, once from above and once from the side. To avoid unnecessary radiation exposure to other organs, women are given a lead apron to wear during the procedure.

If any suspicious areas appear, some radiologists will also use ultrasound to help distinguish benign (noncancerous) breast lumps such as cysts and fibroadenomas from malignant tumors. This technique produces an image of the breast using sound waves rather than radiation. Computer-aided detection devices (ImageChecker) can also be used to double-check suspicious areas and identify subtle signs of breast cancer, particularly clusters of bright white specks called microcalcifications and dense regions of radiating lines that indicate masses, some of which may be cancerous.

Women having a mammogram should avoid using deodorants, lotions, or powders on the day of the procedure because these can block the image. It is also a good idea to find out whom to call if results are not received within 3 weeks. No news is not always good news, and a call to the mammography center is a perfectly appropriate reminder after this length of time.

If results from the mammogram are unclear, a newly approved device called the T-Scan 2000 may be used to evaluate suspicious areas. This handheld device is placed on the breast and connected to a computer, which displays images of the areas in question. Bright spots on the computer image suggest possible malignant tumors. While its ultimate worth remains to be seen, the T-Scan 2000 has the potential to save women from having biopsies on breast lesions that turn out to be noncancerous, as well as help identify women who need an early biopsy.

Who should have a mammogram?

There is currently considerable controversy about the appropriate age at which to begin regular screening for breast cancer with mammography. Mammography has been shown to reduce deaths from breast cancer by 30 percent in women between 50 and 70 years of age. This means that there will be 1 less death per year for every 15,000 women screened.

For women under 50, by contrast, screening mammography has not clearly shown a reduction in deaths from breast cancer. Younger women have a much lower incidence of breast cancer, and their breasts are often too dense to x-ray accurately. They have a much greater chance of getting a false-positive result—a mammogram falsely suggesting breast cancer—and may end up undergoing unnecessary and costly tests, as well as months of needless anxiety even after finding out they're perfectly healthy. Some studies of younger women have also found a higher rate of death from breast

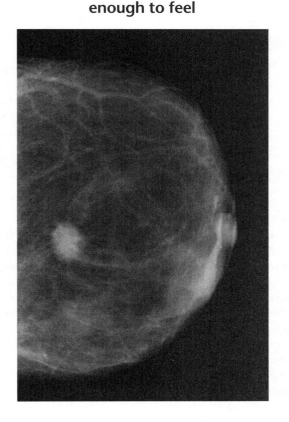

A breast tumor large enough to feel

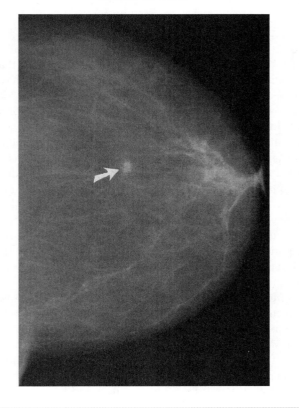

A breast tumor too small to feel

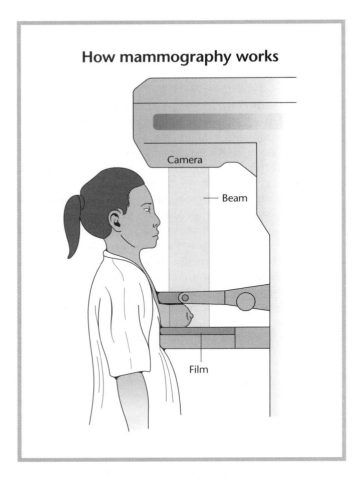

How mammography works

Camera

Beam

Film

cancer in those who had screening mammography than in those who were not screened. But this does not mean that the mammography *caused* the cancer. This link may have arisen because false-negative tests led women and their doctors to overlook breast abnormalities that they would ordinarily biopsy, or because the generally small tumors detected by mammography were less likely to be treated with chemotherapy, or simply because the younger women being screened already had some risk factor or suspicious finding that led their physicians to order a mammogram in the first place.

As for women over 70, to date there has not been a study of the effects of screening on cancer deaths. But because the risk of acquiring breast cancer increases with advancing age, the decision not to screen should be determined on an individual basis.

Computer models also call into question the cost-effectiveness of mammography. For older women the cost-effectiveness ratio was found to be $21,400 per year of life saved. For women in their 40s it was $150,000 per year of life saved.

For an individual woman, however, these population-based studies are of little relevance; the only question is how best to protect herself from breast cancer and how to catch it at its earliest possible stage. That is why most organizations still recommend regular screening for breast cancer

with mammography and clinical breast examination, so long as women recognize their limitations and drawbacks. These considerations can be summarized by the following guidelines:

- Most clinicians recommend that all women over 40 have a mammogram at least every 1 to 2 years, and all recommend annual mammograms for women 50 and older. Even though some studies excluded women over 70, active and healthy elderly women should consider screening every 2 years as well.

- Women of all ages who are at average risk for breast cancer should have a clinical breast examination at the time of their periodic health examination. For high-risk women with a family history of premenopausal breast cancer, most authorities recommend beginning yearly mammograms and clinical breast examinations at age 35. Some authorities also say that women with a positive genetic test for BRCA1 or 2 should have annual mammograms beginning at age 25.

- Women at high risk should also consider genetic testing to see if they might benefit from preventive drug or surgical therapy. Although breast self-examination should not be regarded as a foolproof screening procedure, most clinicians encourage women to familiarize themselves with normal breast texture so that they can seek medical attention if unusual changes develop.

- A doctor may also want to do a mammogram when a woman has a suspicious lump, discharge, or thickening of the skin.

- No woman should let cost keep her from having a mammogram. Many states now require health insurance companies to cover mammograms, at least for women over 50, and Medicare covers annual mammograms for women eligible for Medicare. Women without health insurance can find out about low-cost mammography programs through the American Cancer Society (see resources).

What are the risks and complications?

Mammography is not infallible. Sometimes it will produce a false-positive result. This means that it identifies as a possible cancer calcium deposits and masses in the breast that turn out to be benign. But a mammogram can also produce false-negative results: that is, it fails to pick up a cancer, thus falsely reassuring women and their doctors by leading them to believe that no potentially cancerous cells exist. A false-negative mammogram despite the presence of a lump that a woman or her physician can feel is a primary cause of delayed diagnosis of breast cancer, especially in younger women. Noncancerous lumps are very common in younger women, and mammography is less sensitive in them because of the dense texture of their breast tissue.

Mammography involves exposure to radiation, which may

itself slightly increase the risk of breast cancer. Potential hazards owing to radiation exposure from a modern mammogram are considered negligible for women over 40. Risk is greatest for women in their teens and 20s. Risks can be minimized by choosing a mammography facility certified by the Food and Drug Administration (FDA) as employing properly trained workers and modern equipment. Although density and size of the breast will determine the amount of radiation (measured in rads) received, total absorption per mammogram should not exceed a maximum of 1 rad.

Are there alternatives to mammography?

In the past, thermography—another method of visualizing the interior of the breast—was used to screen for breast cancer. It works on the principle that certain breast cancers and abnormalities are hotter than normal breast tissue. The different heat patterns in each breast were mapped out in a photographic image (thermogram) produced by a heat-detecting device.

Although "hot spots" on a thermogram may indicate cancer, they may also indicate other nonmalignant breast disease in which there is increased blood distribution. For this reason thermography yields many false-positive results. It has been abandoned by many centers in recent years and should never be relied on as a sole means of screening for breast cancer.

Another alternative to mammography, the breast ultrasound, may eventually become a true alternative to the mammogram. By using pulses of high-frequency sound waves to detect breast abnormalities, ultrasound can distinguish a generally benign fluid-filled cyst from a potentially cancerous solid lump. The handheld ultrasound device can also access the underarm breast tissue, which is often missed in a mammogram, and can help locate masses that may be missed in a normal mammogram in women with dense breast tissue. Because the accuracy of the breast ultrasound varies greatly with the skill of the technician performing it, and because it doesn't always detect microscopic calcium deposits that often signal breast cancer, it is still not recommended as a routine screening tool for all women. As easier-to-use technology evolves, however, this situation may change.

Related entries

Biopsy, breast cancer, breast lumps (benign), breast pain, breast self-examination, ultrasound

Manic-Depressive Disorder

Manic-depressive disorder is a form of mood disorder that involves cycles of mania and depression. During the manic episodes the person is euphoric or irritable and as a result may be prone to wild, reckless, or belligerent behavior. During the depressive episodes the same person becomes overwhelmed by feelings of sadness and hopelessness. A person with this disorder (also called manic depression, manic-depressive illness, or bipolar disorder) can swing from mania to depression at long or short intervals or can experience symptoms of both at the same time. Between manic and depressive episodes the same person may function normally, sometimes for months or years.

In recent years a certain cachet has become attached to this illness as people have been made aware that celebrated writers (such as Virginia Woolf, Sylvia Plath, and William Styron), famous movie stars (such as Patty Duke Astin), and brilliant politicians (such as Winston Churchill) suffered from this disease. It has come to be associated with creativity, and some patients with the diagnosis fear the loss of their creative "edge" if they treat the disease. Untreated, however, this devastating disorder, which affects almost 2 million Americans, can lead to divorce, job loss, bankruptcy, alcohol and substance abuse, even suicide.

Manic depression is a chronic illness that can be controlled only with long-term medication. People who experience one episode almost always have additional ones, and without treatment these usually occur more frequently over time. Symptoms may worsen during and immediately following pregnancy (see postpartum psychiatric disorders).

Who is likely to develop manic-depressive disorder?

This disorder typically begins in adolescence or early adulthood and continues throughout the rest of the person's life. It occurs in both men and women with about equal frequency. Recent data suggest that there may be at least one form of the disorder that can start in childhood, with manic phases characterized by extreme irritability, moodiness, and violent, out-of-control behavioral storms.

Although we are only beginning to understand why some people develop this disorder, new imaging technologies have already suggested that it involves alterations in the function of certain parts of the brain. Some studies implicate impaired regulation of neurotransmitters, the chemical messengers that help nerve cells to communicate, while others implicate certain hormones, such as those that regulate the way the body handles stress.

Some of these malfunctions may be shaped by a person's experiences, which can produce actual physical changes in the central nervous system and affect the brain's capacity to regulate moods. There also seems to be a genetic component. Manic-depressive disorder tends to run in families, and there is increasing evidence linking it to a specific inherited genetic defect.

What are the symptoms?

During an episode of mania a person may feel immune to the laws of human biology and society. As a result, she may initiate grandiose projects, abuse drugs (particularly cocaine, alcohol, and sleeping pills), embark on spending sprees, engage in risky sexual encounters, provoke fights with employers, and generally exercise poor judgment. Other symptoms of mania include feelings of euphoria or elation, excessive energy or activity, extreme irritability, distractibility, restlessness, racing thoughts, rapid speech, and a reduced need for sleep. A person having a manic episode may also deny that anything is wrong. Sometimes mania is preceded by a period of hypomania, a mild form of mania characterized by high energy levels, excessive moodiness, and impulsive behavior.

Symptoms of clinical depression (which is more intense and longer-lasting than everyday feelings of sadness) include persistent feelings of numbness, helplessness, hopelessness, worthlessness, sadness, and guilt. People who are clinically depressed often lose interest in previously pleasurable activities, including sex, and may consider life so meaningless that suicide seems the only solution.

Other symptoms of depression include changes in appetite; weight gain or loss; decreased energy; difficulty thinking, concentrating, remembering, or making decisions; headaches; fatigue; sleep disorders, including insomnia; chronic pain; and somatization disorders (in which a person experiences physical symptoms that do not seem to stem from any physical disease; see psychosomatic disorders).

How is the condition evaluated?

People with manic-depressive disorder may suffer needlessly because their illness often goes unrecognized for years or even decades. One reason for this lack of recognition is that periods of mania (or hypomania) may feel good, making it all too easy for the person to deny that anything is wrong. Because many of the symptoms are so broad, too, manic-depressive disorder is readily misinterpreted as some problem other than mental illness, for example, as poor work or school performance or as alcohol or substance abuse.

A person who suspects that she or some family member may have manic-depressive disorder should mention this possibility to a clinician and arrange for an evaluation by a qualified physician, generally a psychiatrist.

How is manic depression treated?

Even the most severe forms of manic-depressive disorder can now be alleviated under the care of a psychiatrist or other experienced physician. Often a person in the throes of mania may need to be committed to a mental hospital for her own protection as well as for treatment. Because manic-depressive disorder is a chronic condition, it requires long-term treatment and supervision even when symptoms seem to be under control.

The most common and generally most effective treatment today is lithium carbonate or lithium citrate (which goes under brand names such as Eskalith and Lithonate). These are salts of the naturally occurring mineral lithium and are administered by mouth in capsule, tablet, or syrup form. Because lithium can take 1 to 3 weeks for full effect, sometimes tranquilizers, such as haloperidol or chlorpromazine, may be given to someone in the midst of a severe manic episode.

These tranquilizers are gradually withdrawn as the lithium begins to act.

Lithium can prevent the recurrence of both manic and depressive episodes, as well as control mania once it has begun. It often must be taken indefinitely and is as vital to the continuing health of a person with manic-depressive illness as insulin is to many people with diabetes.

Some women stop taking their lithium when they find it stops the glow they feel during periods of hypomania, or simply when they feel they no longer need it. Like medicine for hypertension, however, lithium must be taken even when there are no symptoms. This does not mean that lithium must, in every case, be taken for a lifetime; but the decision to discontinue it should be made with a clinician, who will closely monitor the patient for any recurrences.

An oddity of lithium is that the levels necessary for effectiveness are close to the levels that are toxic. Toxic levels of lithium in the blood can cause confusion, stupor, vomiting, extreme thirst, severe diarrhea, weight loss, muscle twitching, slurred speech, dizziness, blurred vision, and pulse irregularities. People using lithium therefore need to have the lithium levels in their blood checked regularly. They also need to notify their doctor of any significant changes in weight or diet, since these can modify lithium levels.

There is also evidence that, at least in some women, lithium levels may rise and fall at various times of the menstrual cycle. More studies need to be done, however, before any general conclusions can be drawn. A woman using lithium who notices that her symptoms are worsening at different times of the month should certainly consult her clinician to see if dosages need to be altered, and if she is taking birth control pills she should mention that fact.

Long-term lithium therapy can worsen certain skin conditions, especially acne and psoriasis, and may produce swelling. It may also cause the thyroid gland to enlarge in people who have hypothyroidism (see entry). This problem can be overcome by taking supplementary thyroid medications.

Although some studies have shown that taking lithium during the first 3 months of pregnancy can slightly increase the risk of having a baby with malformed heart and blood vessels, more research needs to be done before the effects of lithium in pregnancy are known with certainty. In the meantime, women who become pregnant while taking lithium should carefully discuss with their physician the risks and benefits of continuing the drug.

If lithium is discontinued early in the pregnancy, it will often be restarted during the final weeks of pregnancy to help prevent postpartum depression and mania. Again, a woman using lithium should discuss with her physician the advisability of breastfeeding.

Lithium is excreted by the kidneys and may accumulate to dangerous levels if the kidneys cannot eliminate enough of it. The less sodium (salt) there is in the body, the less lithium is excreted and the more it accumulates. For this reason, people with severely impaired kidney function cannot use lithium. Also, anyone with heart disease, problems with excessive sweating, or a diet that involves significantly altered salt intake needs to have her lithium levels monitored particularly closely.

For all of these people—as well as for the 1 person in 10 with manic-depressive disorder who is not helped at all by lithium—alternative medications are available. Usually these involve an anticonvulsant drug such as carbamazepine (Tegretol) or valproate (Depakote), which was recently approved by the Federal Food and Drug Administration for this use. Women who are pregnant or trying to become pregnant should consult their clinician about alternative treatment, as these drugs are not considered safe for use in pregnancy.

Specific symptoms may also be treated separately. If severe depression is a problem, for example, antidepressants may be prescribed, usually in combination with mood stabilizers to prevent mania (see entry on antidepressants). These drugs can take up to 6 weeks to work, however, and many may lead to bothersome side effects. Mania, delusions, and hallucinations are sometimes treated with antipsychotic drugs, which can also be used in lower doses to reduce anxiety and insomnia. In other cases, antianxiety drugs (see entry) such as benzodiazepines may be prescribed to reduce anxiety, panic attacks, and/or insomnia.

Many people with manic-depressive disorder find that psychotherapy helps them to recognize manic or depressive episodes early on, as well as to understand the feelings they have about living with this chronic condition. Others find that they are helped by support groups consisting of people with similar experiences. The National Alliance for the Mentally Ill, the National Depressive and Manic Depressive Association, and the National Mental Health Association all sponsor support groups for people with manic-depressive disorder, as well as support groups for their family and friends.

Related entries

Alcohol, anxiety disorders, depression, insomnia, postpartum psychiatric disorders, psychosomatic disorders, psychotherapy, seasonal affective disorder, sleep disorders, stress, substance abuse

Mastectomy

Mastectomy is the surgical removal of the breast. It is most often done as a treatment for breast cancer, although occasionally it is used to remove a very large noncancerous growth. In addition, some women at high risk for breast cancer choose to have prophylactic mastectomies to prevent the possibility of developing breast cancer later in life.

Types of mastectomy

The types of mastectomies performed today are differentiated according to how much breast tissue, along with surrounding muscle and lymph nodes, is removed. Which of the current procedures a woman and her surgeon will choose depends on a number of factors, including the size and cell type of cancer, the extent of spread, the woman's age and general health, the size of her breasts, and—increasingly—her personal preferences. It appears that, for most women, the chances of surviving breast cancer are about the same no matter which type of surgery is done. Thus, making a decision is primarily a matter of considering each procedure's degree of disfigurement, side effects, and associated treatments (such as follow-up radiation), along with the peace of mind that may come from removing as much of the cancerous breast as possible. Before making the decision, a woman should carefully review the pros and cons of each operation and get the opinion of at least two breast cancer surgeons.

To understand the choices available today, a bit of history is in order. Until the mid-1970s, the classic treatment for breast cancer in this country was a procedure called the radical mastectomy. In this operation (also called the Halsted procedure, after its originator) the surgeon removed the cancerous breast and overlying skin, the underlying muscle of the chest wall, and all lymph nodes and surrounding fat from the adjacent armpit. To do so it was necessary to make an incision that extended from the armpit to the midline of the chest, and the result was a prominent scar. Radical mastectomies left women disfigured, disabled (because muscles were removed), and susceptible to infections (because all of the lymph nodes were removed).

These complications turned out to be a high price to pay for little if any benefit. The entire procedure was premised on the now outdated notion that cancer (like its namesake, the crab) spreads in an orderly fashion from the breast to the lymph nodes and then out to more distant sites in the body. From this perspective it made sense to think that cutting out the lump, breast, lymph nodes, and adjacent muscles early enough in the disease process could rid the body of cancer once and for all. Eventually investigators learned that even the smallest cancers can metastasize (spread) to more distant sites through the bloodstream without first entering nearby lymph nodes. This explains why radical mastectomies did not cure most women with breast cancer.

Among the first of the alternatives to radical mastectomy was the modified radical mastectomy (see illustration). In this procedure the entire breast, most of the underarm (axillary) lymph nodes, and a small pectoral muscle in the chest are removed, but the chest wall retains its shape and the arm preserves normal mobility and strength. By 1979 the modified radical mastectomy had virtually replaced the Halsted. It is no longer commonly performed today, however, since in most cases total mastectomy—removing just the breast (see illustration)—produces equivalent results. (The surgeon will probably also remove a few underarm lymph nodes for biopsy, to help determine the need for subsequent therapy; the more cancer found in the lymph nodes, the greater the chance that it has spread elsewhere in the body.)

Scarring is less extensive with a total mastectomy than

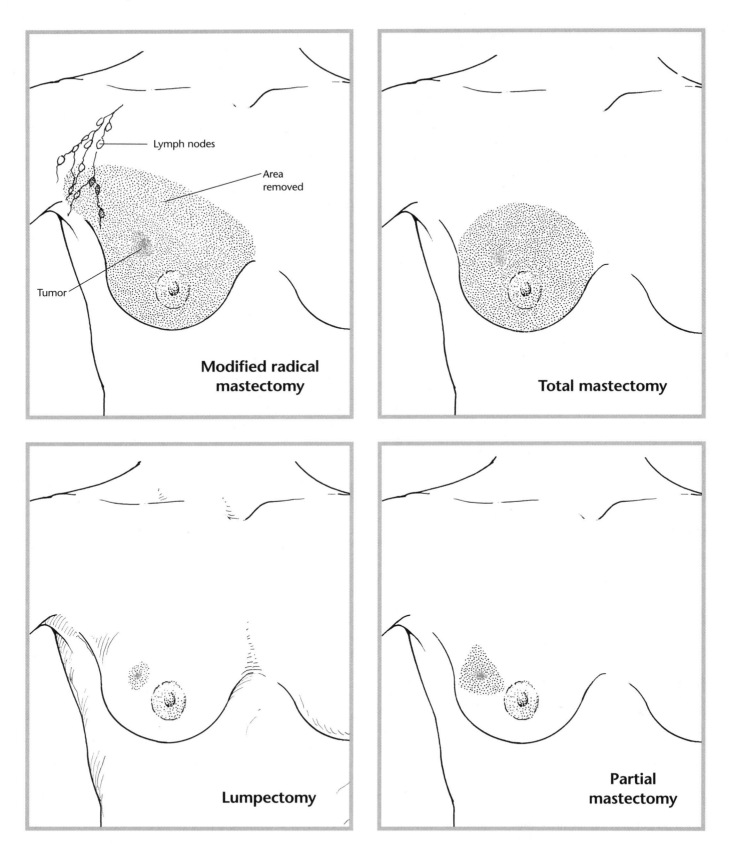

Lymph nodes

Area removed

Tumor

Modified radical mastectomy

Total mastectomy

Lumpectomy

Partial mastectomy

with a modified radical mastectomy, and because almost all of the lymph nodes and all of the chest muscles are left intact, the chances of swelling, infections, and other problems are greatly reduced. Total mastectomies are still performed frequently today, and they are the treatment of choice in certain situations.

By 1990 a consensus report issued by the National Institutes of Health stated that a new procedure called lumpectomy—removal of just the lump itself and some of the surrounding tissue, rather than the entire breast (see illustration)—followed by radiation is preferable to total mastectomy for stage 1 and 2 breast cancers because the survival rate is equivalent to that for total mastectomy, and most of the breast is spared. (Stage 1 breast cancer is defined as a cancer that consists of a lump less than or equal to about three-quarters of an inch in diameter that has not yet spread to lymph nodes or other parts of the body. If the tumor is slightly larger, or if the lymph nodes are enlarged but there is still no concrete sign of spread, the cancer is said to be at stage 2.) Lumpectomy has become an increasingly popular choice among women with breast cancer because it leaves the breast looking almost completely normal, except for a small scar and possibly a slight change in the contour of the breast. The only other long-term complication of the surgery itself is some possible numbness at the site of the incision. Of all the surgical options available, lumpectomy is the least disfiguring.

When the lump and a larger segment of the breast (but not the entire breast) is removed, the procedure is called a partial mastectomy (see illustration). The overlying skin at the incision site and part of the lining of the underlying muscle is removed as well, along with a few adjacent lymph nodes for analysis. Although the shape of the remaining breast is noticeably altered after a partial mastectomy, it can be reconstructed at some later time. (Partial mastectomy is also called segmental mastectomy, quadrantectomy, or wide excision.)

Both lumpectomy and partial mastectomy must be followed by radiation therapy to give a survival rate comparable to that for total mastectomy. The uncomfortable side effects associated with radiation therapy are swelling and redness of the breast (which in some cases can last for months after treatment is over), fatigue, muscle pain, and sun sensitivity. Getting to and from the treatment facility for radiation 5 days a week for approximately 6 weeks can be inconvenient as well. But for many women these side effects and disruptions pale beside the physical and psychological effects of losing an entire breast to a mastectomy.

When do women choose mastectomy over lumpectomy?

Some women with early-stage cancers prefer mastectomy over lumpectomy because they want to rid their bodies of the cancerous breast or because they fear undergoing radiation treatments. Other women, particularly elderly women or women who live far from a radiation treatment facility,

may want to get the whole thing over with as quickly as possible and may therefore choose total mastectomy.

Total mastectomy may be the only option for a woman who has more than one cancerous lump in a breast or a very large cancer (stage 3). In women with small breasts, lumpectomy or partial mastectomy may not preserve much of the breast anyway, even in the case of stage 2 cancers. If it ever becomes practical to shrink tumors with chemotherapy before surgery—as some investigators are already attempting to do—lumpectomy may one day become more feasible in some of these cases, but for now mastectomy is usually recommended.

In the case of ductal carcinoma in situ—that is, a mass of cancerous cells that has not yet invaded breast tissue but remains in the mammary duct (see breast cancer)—the traditional cure was total mastectomy. Some women still choose it, preferring the peace of mind that may come from totally eliminating the risk of invasive cancer (at least in one breast). It now appears that if these tumors are relatively small, lumpectomy plus radiation is as effective as mastectomy in curing this disease. Many women choose not to treat the condition at all, however, until there is evidence that the cells have invaded the surrounding breast tissue, which may never happen.

Removing *both* breasts entirely was the classic treatment for lobular carcinoma in situ—abnormal cell growth in the breast lobes (see breast cancer). This condition, despite the name, is probably better thought of as a risk factor for cancer than as cancer itself. Today, women with LCIS are usually followed carefully with regular mammograms, and surgery is recommended only if there are signs of spread. But some women may feel that preserving the breasts is simply not worth the cost of living with the risk of developing invasive cancer, and so they may choose mastectomy. This is particularly true for women with a strong family history of breast cancer or who have dense breast tissue, since the denser the tissue, the less accurate a screening mammogram tends to be.

Occasionally a procedure called a subcutaneous mastectomy is done in a woman at high risk for breast cancer. Many breast cancer surgeons caution against this operation—which involves removing tissue under the skin while leaving the overlying skin, nipple, and areola intact—because it leaves open the possibility that cancer may still develop in the remaining breast tissue.

What happens during and after surgery?

Modified radical, total, and partial mastectomies are performed in a hospital under general anesthesia. The length of the operation varies from 1 to 2 hours, depending on the amount of tissue being removed. Lumpectomy can be performed with local anesthesia in an ambulatory surgery unit.

After a mastectomy a woman remains hospitalized for a few days, with less time required for the less extensive operations. Drainage tubes are left in place for several days, dressings on the wound are changed regularly, and stitches are gradually removed beginning about the fifth day. Often women have a combination of numbness and oversensitivity in the area of the operation, which may last for months, coupled with some pain and swelling in the adjacent arm, which may or may not disappear entirely with time.

It takes about 2 weeks for the initial wound to heal. Fatigue and tightness in the chest may be present for several weeks, and it usually takes a month before the patient can begin to resume normal activity.

A woman should have a thorough physical examination—including a liver function test, complete blood count, and mammogram of the other breast—approximately every 3 months after the surgery. In addition, she should immediately tell her clinician about any new swelling in the arm or changes near the scar or in the remaining breast. Whenever there is a reasonable risk after surgery that a cancer has or will spread, chemotherapy, hormonal therapy, or radiation therapy will be recommended to destroy the errant cells.

Women who have had a mastectomy must decide whether they want to live with a missing breast. To some women doing so is a symbol of freedom and self-esteem, a message to themselves and the world that their self-worth does not depend on having a breast. To others it is yet another constant reminder of the cancer. For women who feel uncomfortable—or who are bothered by the back strain or awkward posture or balance which occasionally results from having only one breast—options include using a prosthesis (artificial breast) or having breast reconstruction (see entry).

Most hospitals provide women who have had mastectomies with a lightweight artificial breast form that fits into a brassiere without irritating the tender scar tissue; later a better-fitting prosthesis can be custom-made. A variety of prostheses are available which mimic the weight, shape, and feel of real breasts. Some of these fit into a bra cup or are held on with ribbons or Velcro; alternatively, the prosthesis can be permanently installed in a special brassiere.

Women considering using a prosthesis can get in touch with the American Cancer Society's Reach to Recovery Program, which is staffed by volunteers who themselves have used prostheses. The volunteers are excellent sources of information about prostheses and related problems and will accompany a woman to her fitting. Information about this program is usually provided by the hospital staff or by the woman's clinician. The YWCA also sponsors a program called ENCORE, which provides help in finding a prosthesis and appropriate clothing, as well as support from other women who have had breast cancer. In addition, starting 3 weeks after surgery, ENCORE provides group exercise programs for mastectomy patients who want to strengthen their affected arm.

More and more women are considering breast reconstruction as a permanent alternative to a prosthesis. Many find that prostheses are awkward or uncomfortable, and of course even the best prosthesis will leave a woman (and her sexual partner) to face her scar whenever she removes her bra. The decision to have breast reconstruction (see entry) can be made at any time—even decades after the original mastectomy.

The psychological aftermath. For most women breasts are more than mere body parts; they are symbols of attractiveness, sexuality, fertility, and/or nurturing capacity. As a result, the loss of a breast carries with it the potential for considerable emotional pain in realms far removed from the fears of death, and debility that are often associated with cancer and other serious illnesses.

Fortunately, women today are often better prepared psychologically for mastectomies than they once were. Not so long ago women frequently went under anesthesia to have a potentially cancer biopsied and woke up to find themselves missing a breast. In recent years the recognition that breast cancer is not an emergency has fostered a trend toward separating the biopsy from the mastectomy. This leaves the woman a few weeks to ponder the pros and cons of various procedures and also to prepare herself emotionally for the loss of a breast.

Most hospitals also now provide some form of counseling in the days immediately following the operation to help a woman deal with her sense of loss. But this does not prevent many women—who often are simultaneously facing the fear of dying and the long course of radiation or chemotherapy—from coming out of a mastectomy feeling disfigured. Many develop symptoms of anxiety or depression, including feelings of helplessness, uncertainty, low self-esteem, and lack of emotional expression. Others worry about interpersonal relationships and fear that they will be unattractive sexually.

It is now clear that having a mastectomy in and of itself does not interfere with the ability to desire or enjoy sex. Nevertheless, in one study as many as 30 to 40 percent of women who had a modified radical mastectomy reported significant sexual dysfunction—even a year or two later.

Interestingly, women who had a lumpectomy reported similar difficulties with sexual desire and arousal, although they retained more of their original body image and felt more comfortable with nudity and discussions of sexuality. Overall, there was little long-term difference in the general psychological and sexual recovery of women who had total mastectomies compared with those who had lumpectomies. The major difference—as one would expect—was that women who had mastectomies had more problems with their body image. This drawback has been greatly alleviated for some women by making reconstructive surgery available immediately after mastectomy.

Whatever the form of mastectomy, a woman whose cancer recurs or who is crippled by the side effects of surgery or drug therapy is going to have less interest in, and ability to engage in, sexual activity. Still, a mastectomy is unlikely to damage or destroy a relationship that was basically solid before the operation. There will almost certainly be some stresses and strains, relating to both the cancer and the loss of a breast; and (as in numerous other situations) many women find it frustrating and isolating to have a partner who tells them to "put the surgery behind you" when they would like to talk about their concerns and memories.

Considerable support can be found in joining a self-help group that consists of other women who have gone through a similar experience. Emotional reactions can be shared, as well as practical advice about living and dealing with breast cancer. Women with more serious symptoms of depression and anxiety should also seek the help of a professional psychotherapist, who can provide cognitive therapy and, if necessary, prescribe psychotherapeutic drugs.

Related entries

Biopsy, body image, breast cancer, breast reconstruction, chemotherapy, depression, lumpectomy, mammography, psychotherapy, radiation therapy, sexual dysfunction

Mastitis

Mastitis is a breast infection that sometimes occurs in women who are nursing a baby or who have recently stopped nursing. It is caused by bacteria, usually *Staphylococcus aureus*, which enter the breast from the baby's mouth or surrounding skin through cracks in the nipple.

What are the symptoms?

Women with mastitis have a red, painful swelling or lump in the affected breast, and sometimes a fever, which can be quite high. Chills and an achy, flulike feeling are common. If mastitis is not treated, an abscess (collection of pus) can develop under the skin.

Sometimes the lymph glands in the breasts or near the armpit swell during mastitis, and these can be confused with breast cancer. Still, if a woman with mastitis has a small lump that does not go away, she should be checked for the remote possibility of a malignancy.

How is mastitis treated?

Treatment involves taking antibiotics to kill the bacteria, as well as analgesics to relieve the pain and fever. Hot showers, compresses, or towels can also relieve the pain. Although women with mastitis were once advised to nurse only on the opposite breast, it is now clear that frequent nursing on the affected breast, though quite painful at first, can help relieve mastitis by draining the milk that promotes bacterial growth. Neither the bacteria (which generally came from the baby) nor the antibiotic that will be prescribed to a nursing mother should harm the baby. An abscess usually requires drainage, either with aspiration or an incision.

How can mastitis be prevented?

Some lactation experts believe that breast infections can result from a plugged milk duct that is not treated. Skipped feedings and engorgement are causes as well. Women who have signs of a plugged duct—which include a small, red, and painful breast lump—may try offering the sore breast first so that it can be better emptied, breastfeeding more often and for a longer time, changing position with every feeding to exert pressure on different ducts, and expressing milk from the affected breast if the baby has not nursed long enough. Keeping clothing from pressing on the ducts, soaking the breast in warm water prior to nursing, washing the breasts gently after nursing, and getting more rest—though often difficult for the nursing mother—also help. Sudden weaning should be avoided if possible since it may predispose a woman to plugged milk ducts.

Related entries

Antibiotics, antiinflammatory drugs, breast lumps (benign), breast pain, breastfeeding

Melanoma

Melanoma—also called malignant melanoma—is the least common but most lethal form of skin cancer. Involving skin cells that produce pigment (melanin), a melanoma is usually painless but readily burrows into the skin and, if untreated, can rapidly spread (metastasize) to distant organs via either the blood or lymphatic systems.

Melanoma can arise out of normal skin or from a preexisting mole that has suddenly changed size or color, developed irregular borders, or begun to itch, bleed, swell, or hurt (see moles). Occasionally melanomas appear in the eye or in some parts of the central nervous system as well. About 5 percent of all vulvar cancers are melanomas. In women melanomas are more likely to appear on the legs than on the torso.

The earlier a melanoma is detected and treated, the greater the chance of long-term survival. Altogether about 60 to 80 percent of people with melanoma can expect to be alive 5 years after diagnosis, but the chances are as low as 30 percent if the cancer has already spread by the time it is detected. Although melanomas are about as common in women as in men, women seem less likely to die from them, perhaps because they are more likely to seek early medical attention.

In the past few decades there has been a marked increase in the number of melanomas throughout the world. This is usually attributed to the popularity of suntanning. Even one severe sunburn in early childhood can increase the chances of developing a melanoma much later in life. And despite the claims of many commercial tanning parlors, there is no such thing as a safe form of ultraviolet light. It is true that the lion's share of sun damage can be attributed to "burning" rays from the sun—the short-wave UVB light—which make up only about 10 percent of the energy that reaches the earth on a bright, sunny day. This is because the UVB rays are about

1,000 times more powerful than long-wave UVA light. Nevertheless, even UVA rays in large and concentrated amounts (such as those used by tanning parlors) can cause skin damage.

Types of melanoma

There are four different kinds of malignant melanomas.

Superficial spreading melanoma. By far the most common, this accounts for about 70 percent of all melanomas. It often appears on the arms, legs, or torso as a small spot with an irregular border. It may contain red, pink, white, or blue dots or tiny blue-black nodules, and sometimes there are small indentations on the surface.

Nodular melanoma. The next most common kind, this melanoma can appear as a rapidly enlarging pearly, gray, black, or colorless bump anywhere on the body. Sometimes nodular melanomas ulcerate and look like little sores that never completely heal.

Acrolentiginous (acral lentiginous) melanoma. This third kind of melanoma usually consists of a dark patch on the mucous membranes or on the soles, palms, or tips of fingers or toes. It is more common in dark-skinned people.

Lentigo-maligna melanoma. This final kind of melanoma develops on the face in elderly people as a large (1 to 2 inch) flat, tan or brown spot speckled with darker brown or black pigmentation. Sometimes a lentigo-maligna melanoma begins as a benign spot which can exist for several years before becoming cancerous.

Who is likely to develop melanoma?

The fairer the skin, the greater the susceptibility to melanoma—and all forms of skin cancer, for that matter. That is why melanoma is most common in blue-eyed blondes or redheads with fair skin and almost nonexistent in African Americans or others with very dark skin. People who are already susceptible to melanoma increase their risk even further by spending long periods of time in the sun without using an adequate sunscreen.

Some experts argue that exposure to x-ray radiation and various chemical pollutants or other environmental toxins may increase the odds of developing melanoma, although this point is controversial. Susceptibility to melanoma can be inherited: certain families have a preponderance of a type of mole called a dysplastic or atypical nevus, which sometimes turns into melanoma; this condition is called atypical nevi syndrome.

Different forms of melanoma are more likely to occur at different ages. Whereas superficial spreading melanomas may occur at any age, nodular melanomas are most likely to appear in people between the ages of 20 and 60. Lentigo-maligna is more prevalent in the elderly.

Melanomas seem to be more common in pregnant than in nonpregnant women. There is no evidence, however, that pregnancy increases the chance that a preexisting mole will transform itself into a melanoma.

What are the symptoms?

There are often no symptoms associated with melanoma other than the characteristic appearance of the growth itself. A preexisting mole that develops irregular borders, becomes asymmetrical, changes color, enlarges, or begins to bleed, itch, swell, or hurt may be a sign of melanoma and warrants a prompt visit to a dermatologist. The same is true of a black spot that suddenly appears on the white of the eye.

How is the condition evaluated?

A clinician who suspects melanoma from the appearance of a growth on the skin will do a biopsy to confirm the diagnosis. This involves cutting out the suspicious growth, as well as a margin of normal adjacent skin, and then examining the cells under a microscope for signs of malignancy. If there is a chance that the cancer has spread to other parts of the body, a complete physical examination, a chest x-ray, a CT scan, and liver function tests may be necessary.

How is melanoma treated?

If melanoma is diagnosed with the original surgical biopsy, the surgeon will go back and remove more of the surrounding skin. The size of the excision depends on the depth of the original tumor. Occasionally, however, nearby lymph nodes may have to be removed as well, particularly if there is any chance that the cancer has spread, and it may also be necessary to graft skin from elsewhere on the body to replace the removed skin. Intensive radiation therapy is sometimes used as well, but it tends to be much less effective than surgery.

If the melanoma is relatively thick or has spread to other parts of the body, the clinician may refer the patient to a cancer specialist (oncologist). In advanced cases chemotherapy (treatment with drugs that slow the growth of malignant cells) or immunotherapy (treatment with drugs that activate antibodies to fight the cancerous tissue) may be warranted.

Whatever the treatment, anyone who has had a melanoma should see a clinician on a regular basis so that any recurrence of the cancer (or development of a second cancer) can be detected early. All first-degree relatives (children, parents, and siblings) should also be examined by a dermatologist because of their increased risk for malignant melanoma.

How can melanoma be prevented?

The best way to prevent melanomas from developing is to avoid excessive exposure to the sun or to any ultraviolet light intense enough to cause tanning or burns. Ultraviolet radiation is generally most intense between the hours of 10 A.M. and 2 P.M. Direct exposure to sunlight is necessary to promote the synthesis of vitamin D by the skin, which helps prevent osteoporosis by promoting the absorption of calcium. But only a few minutes per week of exposure without sunscreen are needed for adequate vitamin D production. Vita-

Self-examination for melanoma and other skin cancers

Women should regularly inspect their skin for suspicious pigmentation or changes in the shape, size, or color of moles. Most melanomas in women appear on the arms, legs and torso.

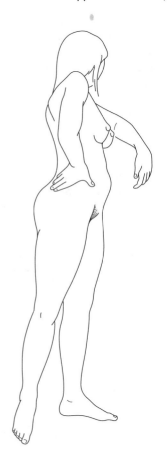

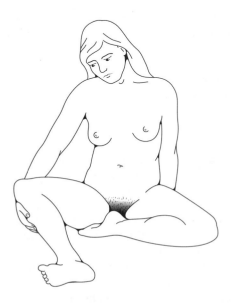

Moles on the back, buttocks, and scalp should not be neglected, even though they are hard to see. A black spot that suddenly appears on the white of the eye may signal melanoma and should be called to the attention of one's clinician.

Even in people with dark skin, mottled or light areas on the feet and hands should be examined by a physician. Moles on the vulva and around the nails are more likely than others to become cancerous and should be monitored regularly.

min D can also be obtained by eating fortified foods or by taking multivitamin supplements.

When in the sun, the best protection is a sunblock with a sun protection factor (SPF) of 15 to 30. The SPF indicates the multiple by which the sunblock extends the safe period of exposure—which will vary from person to person. In a person who could normally stay out for 15 minutes (0.25 hours) without burning, for example, using a sunblock with an SPF of 15 would extend the safe exposure time to 3.75 hours (15 × 0.25 hours). It is usually necessary to reapply even the most effective sunblock after swimming or excessive sweating.

A recent study in mice suggests that sunscreens may provide a false sense of security. Although sunscreen in this study seemed to protect the animals from sunburn, it did not reduce the incidence of melanoma. This study cannot necessarily be extrapolated to humans, of course, and it is certainly no excuse to forgo sunscreen. Still, the safest bet at this point is to keep sun exposure within reasonable limits and to wear protective clothing, a sun hat, and sunglasses, as well as sunscreen whenever one is out in the sun. Even on cloudy days, or in the winter in most parts of the United States, ultraviolet light can still cause overexposure in people not using sunscreen.

Because melanomas can become quite advanced without producing any symptoms, women should make a habit of regularly inspecting their skin for suspicious areas of pigmentation or sudden changes in preexisting moles (see illustration). Anyone with atypical nevi (moles with irregular borders and a mottled appearance) should be particularly vigilant about doing these self-examinations at frequent intervals. People with partners should exchange examinations on a regular basis, since moles on one's own back and buttocks are difficult to see. Even in people with dark skin, mottled or light areas on the hands and feet may signal melanoma and should be examined by a dermatologist or other clinician.

Related entries

Biopsy, chemotherapy, moles, radiation therapy, skin care and cosmetics, skin disorders, vulvar cancer

Menarche

Menarche is a young woman's first menstrual period. In most women it normally occurs anytime between the ages of 10 and 16.5, generally several years after the first signs of puberty appear. Just what triggers menarche is still unknown, but there is little doubt that nutrition and overall health play a role in addition to genetics. Improved health care and diet are usually used to explain the drop in the average age of menarche in middle-class American girls, which has fallen from about 15.5 a century ago to about 12.5 today. Improved

nutrition may also explain why the proportion of body fat to lean tissue increases at an earlier age in today's young women. This relationship between fat and lean, termed critical weight, is an essential factor in determining just when menarche will occur, possibly because of the role fat plays in the manufacture of certain hormones.

If levels of fat fall below 15 to 22 percent of total body weight, as they often do before the growth spurt that precedes menarche, menstruation may not begin. The concept of critical weight also helps explain why some female athletes, ballet dancers, models, and actresses, as well as women with eating disorders such as anorexia nervosa, often stop menstruating or have light, irregular periods until they return to normal weight.

In the first year following menarche, menstrual periods may be sparse and irregular, and 75 percent of menstrual cycles are anovulatory—that is, no egg is released by an ovary. This is usually attributed to the immaturity of the intricate feedback system between the hypothalamus, pituitary gland, and ovary. Within 5 years of menarche, however, only 1 woman in 5 still has anovulatory cycles.

By the time menarche takes place, most young women have nearly completed their growth spurt and are within an inch or two of their adult height. In girls who show signs of sexual development before the age of 8 or so (a condition known as precocious puberty), drugs such as gonadotropin releasing hormone (GnRH) analogs may be given to delay menarche and prevent the premature halting of growth that would otherwise occur. Since these girls generally have the emotional maturity expected for their age, it is particularly important that the basic facts of menstruation are explained to them at an age-appropriate level before menarche occurs.

Related entries

Amenorrhea, anorexia nervosa and bulimia nervosa, menstrual cycle, menstrual cycle disorders, nutrition

Menopause

Menopause—popularly known as "the change of life," or simply "the change"—means the permanent cessation of the monthly menstrual period. The term is generally used to include a much larger set of events, however, both before and after the end of menstruation. All of these events—physical, emotional, and social—are related to a woman's changing hormone levels at mid-life, which end the phase of life when childbearing is possible.

Once a taboo subject relegated to silent fears or, at best, private whispers between the closest of friends, menopause was for many years falsely associated with erratic mood swings, overwhelming depression, and the loss of sexual desire and pleasure. Only recently have these negative stereotypes begun to crumble, owing largely to the widespread attention now paid to menopause by popular books and magazines, television talk shows and specials, and government agencies. As a result, menopause is increasingly being seen as a natural part of life, with both positive and negative aspects. Many women now readily discuss their observations and decisions about how to handle menopause with one another as well as with their clinicians.

One of the reasons why menopause has recently become a leading women's health issue has to do with changing demographics. Whereas a woman's average life expectancy at the turn of the twentieth century was only 50 years, today women can expect to live on average to about 78. Given that the typical woman undergoes menopause around age 51, this means that women still have a third or more of their life remaining after menopause begins. There are now some 40 million American women in or past menopause, and another 20 million women will reach it within the next decade as the baby boomers age.

Menopause is also being taken more seriously because of a better understanding of the impact it can have on a woman's health, as well as a renewed respect for quality of life issues. Concerns about menopause were once dismissed as either vain or emotional, unworthy of serious medical attention. New evidence that physical changes after menopause (as well as those in all the stages of life preceding it) significantly increase a woman's risk of developing debilitating, life-threatening, and costly diseases, particularly heart disease and bone fractures from osteoporosis, has put menopause in a whole new light.

What are the "symptoms" of approaching menopause?

Although on average a woman can expect to go through menopause at the age of 51, the normal range of ages at which menopause may occur extends from 42 to 58. If a woman younger than 40 undergoes menopause naturally, she is said to be experiencing premature menopause. Women who undergo premature menopause should be carefully evaluated by a clinician to make sure that there is no disease underlying the changes. No known factor can predict whether an individual woman will undergo an early or a late menopause, with the exception of cigarette smoking: women who smoke undergo menopause an average of 2 years earlier than nonsmokers. Whatever her age, a woman who has both her ovaries removed will experience "surgical" menopause.

For 5 to 10 years before menstrual periods actually cease, the body begins to undergo various neuroendocrine and ovarian changes leading up to menopause. This period is called the perimenopausal transition. During the initial stage of the perimenopausal period, estrogen levels may fluctuate wildly, with more dramatic highs and lows than in a normal cycle. Some endocrinologists speculate that this fluctuation may underlie the emotional lability that some women experience during the transition. During this early phase monthly bleeding continues more or less regularly. The next phase of

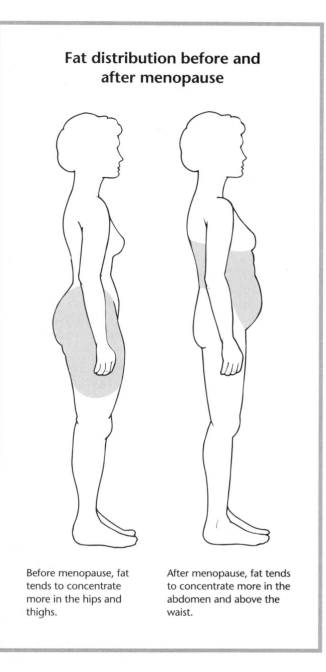

Fat distribution before and after menopause

Before menopause, fat tends to concentrate more in the hips and thighs.

After menopause, fat tends to concentrate more in the abdomen and above the waist.

the transition is marked by changes in the menstrual cycle: shorter periods, irregular periods, shorter cycle length, heavy menstrual flow, or a combination of all of these, differing from cycle to cycle. (Bleeding that occurs more frequently than every 21 days, lasts more than 8 days, or occurs between periods is considered abnormal bleeding, however, and should be evaluated by a clinician.) Because many perimenopausal women are still ovulating (releasing an egg from the ovary) despite irregular periods, contraception is necessary until menses have stopped for at least a year.

In all women there is a gradual decline in the production of estrogen hormones by the ovaries. This decline accelerates as menopause approaches and periods become more erratic.

As a result, changes occur in the many bodily tissues that are responsive to estrogen, including the vagina, vulva, uterus, bladder, urethra, breasts, bones, heart, blood vessels, brain, skin, hair, and mucous membranes. Even after menopause small amounts of estrogen continue to be produced by the adrenal glands, as well as by fatty tissue, which converts some of the androgens (virilizing hormones) produced by the adrenals into estrogen. There is some speculation that the release of estrogen by fatty tissue may help explain why heavier women seem to have relatively fewer menopausal symptoms. (Heavier women, however, are at higher risk for menorrhagia during the perimenopausal transition and are also at increased risk for endometrial cancer.)

Perhaps the most common of the symptoms associated with estrogen loss—affecting approximately 75 percent of women having a natural menopause and 90 percent of those having a surgical menopause—are hot flashes. Technically, a hot flash is the subjective feeling of warmth that a woman feels before there is any measurable change in her temperature. This is followed by the hot flush, a physiologically measurable change marked by visible redness and sometimes sweating in the chest, neck, and face.

Hot flashes are more common at night than in the daytime. These night sweats are often severe enough to interfere with sleep, and they seem to account for a good deal of insomnia among menopausal women. It is likely that many of the negative attributes once chalked up to menopause itself—mood swings, irritability, depression, fatigue—can be traced to the sleep disturbances caused by night sweats. Most people, male or female, who are awakened every time they are about to enter deep sleep will develop signs of emotional or mental instability. Hot flashes and flushes tend to subside with time and disappear after about 1 to 5 years, although in some women they last indefinitely.

The reduction in estrogen levels often leads to vaginal atrophy—the drying and thinning of the tissues of the vagina and urethra. Many of the sexual problems once thought to be inevitable and irreversible aspects of menopause may simply be due to this phenomenon, which can produce vaginal inflammation, inadequate lubrication, and pain with sexual activity. Vaginal atrophy is also associated with urinary symptoms that mimic urinary tract infections, including urinary frequency, painful urination, and stress incontinence (the involuntary loss of urine after laughing, sneezing, coughing, or vigorous exercise). At the same time, decreased estrogen levels predispose some women to true urinary tract infections (which can be prevented by estrogen replacement). A loss of muscle tone in the pelvic muscles—also related to declining estrogen levels—can exacerbate problems with incontinence and also increase the risk that the uterus, bladder, urethra, or rectum may protrude into the vagina (see prolapsed uterus, cystocele/urethrocele/rectocele).

Some women may notice increased growth of facial hair around menopause and a thinning of hair on the scalp. Sometimes women prone to adult acne find that it gets worse. These symptoms are attributed to the relative increase in the effects of testosterone, a virilizing hormone that is produced by the ovaries both before and after menopause.

There is no evidence that menopause itself predisposes women to depression. Women in their 20s and 30s are much more likely to develop a major depression than are older women. Nonetheless, the many life crises that can occur around the time of menopause may precipitate depression—including divorce, illness or death of parents, job loss, or children leaving home—as well as the very fact of aging in a society that values youth in women. At mid-life a woman's focus may shift from the time lived to the time left to be lived. The prospect of mortality, sometimes underscored by the development of new medical problems, may contribute to mild melancholy in some women. Women who have a prolonged perimenopause with many symptoms also appear more prone to transitory depression.

How is menopause "treated"?

The great variation in the way women experience the "symptoms" of menopause cannot be overstressed. Nevertheless, these developments cause significant problems for only 5 to 15 percent of women. From this perspective, being menopausal may require taking no action at all, other than perhaps enjoying the freedom from menstrual periods or the need to use contraceptives. Medical attention should be sought, however, if vaginal bleeding occurs more frequently than every 21 days or if there is heavy bleeding or bleeding that lasts more than 8 days. Sometimes an endometrial biopsy and a pelvic ultrasound may be necessary to rule out endometrial cancer, uterine fibroids, polyps, or other conditions that may account for these symptoms. A woman should also seek medical attention if hot flashes, insomnia, or other symptoms are severe enough to interfere with normal activities.

There is no question that estrogen is the most effective treatment for hot flashes. Estrogen in pill or patch form is generally given with progestin, a synthetic form of progesterone, to offset the risk of estrogen-induced endometrial cancer. The lowest dose of estrogen that provides relief of symptoms should be prescribed. The use of estrogen should be periodically reassessed by a woman and her clinician, with the goal of tapering and discontinuing estrogen within 5 years if possible. The Women's Health Initiative and other studies have consistently shown that the increased risk of breast cancer associated with estrogen replacement therapy does not start to accrue until after 4 to 5 years of use.

For women whose main menopausal symptoms are vaginal dryness, recurrent urinary infections, or pain with intercourse, estrogen therapy administered vaginally is very effective. There are various forms of vaginal estrogen treatment, including a cream, vaginal tablets, and an estrogen-impregnated vaginal ring. These forms of estrogen produce few if any systemic effects and do not require concomitant treatment with a progestin.

Some women cannot take estrogen replacement therapy (ERT; see entry), including those who have a personal history of breast or uterine cancer, active liver disease, or active thrombophlebitis (see circulatory disorders). For these women, as well as for those who are wary of hormone therapy in general or who dislike the concept of treating menopause with hormones as though it were a kind of deficiency disease, there are alternatives. Symptoms related to vaginal atrophy can be ameliorated with vaginal lubricants such as Replens, Kegel exercises, and frequent intercourse. To minimize hot flushes, many women try to avoid factors that might precipitate them—such as stress, hot weather, warm rooms, hot drinks, alcohol, caffeine, and spicy foods. Some studies have shown that paced deep breathing, acupuncture, biofeedback, and other relaxation techniques are helpful.

When estrogen is not appropriate for a woman with hot flashes, her clinician may prescribe low doses of certain antidepressants, such as venlafaxine (Effexor) or paroxetine (Paxil), or drugs that relax blood vessels, such as clonidine (Catapres). Both types of drugs have been shown to relieve hot flashes. Natural estrogens—such as those found in soy-based foods—may also be helpful, although high levels may be necessary to produce any noticeable effects. Herbal supplements such as black cohosh (Remifemin) are widely used for menopausal symptoms in Europe and show some evidence of being effective. These products, however, likely have a mild estrogen-like effect in the body, and their long-term safety has not been proven.

Many women are concerned about their risk of developing osteoporosis after menopause. The bone loss characteristic of this condition begins to outpace bone formation by the time a woman reaches her late 30s or early 40s, and as menopause begins, the loss accelerates for several years, eventually leveling off to about 1 percent annually. The consequent decline in bone density predisposes women to fractures, particularly of the hip and spine. About one-quarter of women in the United States already have lower than normal bone mass at the time of menopause, as measured by a bone density test. These women are more likely to develop osteoporosis with increasing age.

The best approach for menopausal women at risk of osteoporosis depends on a number of factors that must be weighed by a woman and her clinician. Drugs used to treat osteoporosis, such as bisphosphonates (Fosamax, Actonel) and raloxifene (Evista) are also FDA-approved for the prevention of osteoporosis. Estrogen replacement therapy is also effective for reducing bone loss after menopause. All these medications have side effects, however, and to date there are no studies proving that preventive treatment at menopause prevents fractures later in life. For this reason, many women may prefer simply to monitor their bone health with periodic bone density tests, holding off on any drug therapy unless bone density declines significantly.

Whatever decision is made about estrogen replacement therapy, menopause is an excellent time to reassess exercise, nutrition, and health care patterns with an eye to preventing chronic disease. For women who smoke cigarettes, quitting is the most powerful step they can take to reduce the risk of

future heart disease. For all women, having more frequent screenings of blood cholesterol, moderating alcohol intake, and eating a low-fat diet rich in fruits, vegetables, and whole grains makes good sense. Eating soybeans or other foods such as chickpeas and lentils containing phytoestrogens or isoflavones (estrogen-like compounds found in certain plants) may be prudent as well. Women living in parts of the world where the diet is high in these compounds seem to have milder menopausal symptoms, and several studies are under way to determine the role these substances may play in relieving menopausal symptoms and preventing heart disease.

To help prevent osteoporosis, the diet should also include 1,000 to 1,500 milligrams of calcium per day, as well as 400 to 800 international units of vitamin D. A regular program of weight-bearing exercise not only helps prevent osteoporosis but also contributes to maintaining an appropriate body weight.

Related entries
Alternative therapies, circulatory disorders, coronary artery disease, cystocele/urethrocele/rectocele, depression, estrogen replacement therapy, exercise, fatigue, hair loss, heart disease, incontinence, insomnia, Kegel exercises, lubricants, menstrual cycle disorders, nutrition, osteoporosis, ovary removal, pain during sexual intercourse, prolapsed uterus, smoking, urinary tract infections, vaginal atrophy, vaginal bleeding (abnormal)

Menorrhagia

Menorrhagia means having excessively heavy or prolonged menstrual periods. Soaking a sanitary napkin or tampon every hour or so, as well as menstruating for longer than 7 days, are both considered forms of menorrhagia. For some women heavy or prolonged periods may be little more than an inconvenience which at worst may cause anemia because of excessive blood loss. For others excessive menstrual bleeding may make it impossible to meet their usual responsibilities for several days each month.

Who is likely to develop menorrhagia?
Menorrhagia (also called hypermenorrhea) may result from a hormonal imbalance, most commonly in adolescents in the years following menarche and in women nearing menopause. Menstrual periods tend be irregular at these times of life and do not always involve the release of an egg from the ovary. In other cases hormonal cycles are normal, but a problem in the blood vessels of the uterus results in a failure to control bleeding. Uterine fibroids are another common cause of excessive bleeding, sometimes heavy enough to soak a sanitary napkin or tampon every hour, with passage of clots.

Occasionally menorrhagia, especially in a woman nearing

menopause, can result from more serious conditions, such as endometrial cancer. A late but very heavy period in a possibly pregnant woman who has not had heavy periods previously could signal a miscarriage or ectopic pregnancy. All of these require medical attention.

Other conditions that can underlie menorrhagia include cervical or endometrial polyps, hypothyroidism, pelvic inflammatory disease, and adenomyosis. Women with kidney failure who are on dialysis may have heavy or prolonged menstrual periods as well. In addition, intrauterine devices (IUDs) occasionally cause menorrhagia. They should in that case be removed and replaced with some other form of birth control.

In rare instances, menorrhagia may be due to a bleeding disorder. These are usually detected at menarche when a young woman first starts to menstruate. The bleeding disorders underlying menorrhagia tend to be platelet disorders, the most common of which is von Willebrand's disease. In this condition there is a defect of a clotting factor or factors in the blood necessary to cause platelets to aggregate at the site of blood vessel injury. As a result, women with von Willebrand's disease may experience not only menorrhagia but also nosebleeds, easy bruising, and blood in the stool. Administering factor VIII, a blood clotting factor that is defective in this condition, usually alleviates the symptoms.

How is the condition evaluated?

Most clinicians will evaluate the possible causes of menorrhagia by doing a pelvic examination, including a Pap test, as well as various blood tests to check for underlying disorders. Women of reproductive age who have been heterosexually active should also have a pregnancy test. An ultrasound is often performed to discover any uterine fibroids. An endometrial biopsy, dilatation and curettage (D&C) procedure, or hysteroscopy may also be done to further evaluate abnormalities of the uterus. For conditions such as polyps, these procedures can be therapeutic as well.

How is menorrhagia treated?

Treating the medical disorder or physical cause (such as an IUD) underlying menorrhagia is often the key to alleviating it. Menorrhagia that does not appear to be due to an underlying disorder is often correctable with progesterone supplements, either alone or in combination with estrogen. Often these supplements are given in the form of oral contraceptive pills.

Nonsteroidal antiinflammatory drugs such as ibuprofen and naproxen can reduce bleeding and any accompanying menstrual cramps.

Any woman who has had several bouts of menorrhagia should be checked regularly for anemia. Treatment involves taking daily iron supplements. Occasionally a blood transfusion may be necessary as well.

If menorrhagia persists after several months of medication, a hysteroscopy or D&C may be done to further explore causes and possibly treat them as well. The clinician may also try gonadotropin releasing hormone agonists, which produce a false and temporary state of menopause. At present these are not used for more than 6 months because of complications resulting from low estrogen levels (particularly bone loss).

If these fail, endometrial ablation may be performed in women who no longer want to bear children but wish to avoid hysterectomy. Under the guidance of a hysteroscope, this procedure uses lasers or electrocautery to destroy the endometrium, or lining of the uterus. Although it is 80 to 90 percent effective at reducing or abolishing excessive bleeding, the bleeding can recur. This procedure usually renders a woman sterile, although it is not considered a reliable form of birth control. In addition, the long-term risks of the procedure remain unknown. Newer techniques, such as the thermal balloon, have similar effectiveness and can be peformed in the doctor's office.

Women with severe anemia or particularly bothersome bleeding may want to consider a hysterectomy if they have no desire to bear children in the future. As today's insurance companies and HMOs become more cost-conscious, however, this is becoming a less available option for some women.

Any woman with menorrhagia who suspects she may be pregnant and may be having a miscarriage should contact a doctor immediately. She will need to be checked to see if all the contents of the uterus have been expelled. Any remaining gestational products will be removed through a D&C or vacuum aspiration procedure.

Medical treatment is usually not necessary for a woman who knows she is not pregnant and who has a single heavy period. Getting as much rest as possible often reduces bleeding, but she should seek medical attention if heavy bleeding persists for more than 24 hours.

Related entries

Anemia, antiinflammatory drugs, biopsy, birth control, cervical cancer, dilatation and curettage, ectopic pregnancy, electrocautery, endometrial cancer, hypothyroidism, hysterectomy, hysteroscopy, iron, kidney disorders, laser surgery, lupus, menopause, miscarriage, oral contraceptives, pelvic inflammatory disease, platelet disorders, polyps, thyroid disorders, uterine fibroids, vaginal bleeding (abnormal)

Menstrual Cramps

The medical term for painful periods or menstrual cramps is dysmenorrhea. Most women probably experience primary dysmenorrhea—painful menstruation not attributable to some underlying physical abnormality—at some point in their lives. Once attributed to psychosomatic factors, dysmenorrhea is now believed to be caused by an excess of prostaglandins, a group of naturally occurring fatty acids that cause uterine contractions and stimulate the intestines. These are produced by the tissue lining the uterus which is sloughed off during menstruation.

If the pain is caused by some physical abnormality of the reproductive organs such as endometriosis, adenomyosis, pelvic inflammatory disease (PID), an ovarian cyst, or uterine fibroids (see entries under these terms), or by an intrauterine device (IUD), it is called secondary dysmenorrhea.

Who is likely to develop menstrual cramps?

Primary dysmenorrhea usually begins within a year or two of menarche (the first menstrual period). Although some women continue to suffer from dysmenorrhea until reaching menopause, most find that symptoms gradually subside by their mid-20s or after their first pregnancy. Why some women are prone to particularly severe symptoms remains unknown.

What are the symptoms?

Dysmenorrhea involves crampy, spasmodic pain in the lower abdomen which sometimes spreads to the hips, lower back, or thighs. Other common symptoms include nausea and frequent diarrhea or constipation, or both at different times within the same menstrual period. In severe cases vomiting and fainting may occur. A few women have symptoms so severe that they cannot carry on their normal daily routine.

Secondary dysmenorrhea is likely if the pain also occurs between menstrual periods or lasts longer than the first few days of the period, or if standard treatment for primary dysmenorrhea fails to control the pain.

How is the condition evaluated?

Menstrual cramps must be distinguished from other causes of recurring pelvic pain such as endometriosis, uterine fibroids, irritable bowel syndrome, diverticular disease, and psychological conditions. Usually a pelvic examination, as well as applicable blood tests, will help eliminate most of these causes. Occasionally an ultrasound examination of the pelvic area or a surgical procedure such as a laparoscopy may be necessary as well.

How are menstrual cramps treated?

Treatment involves decreasing prostaglandin production by reducing the buildup of the uterine lining. Usually this is accomplished with antiprostaglandin medications or oral contraceptives. Aspirin is a mild antiprostaglandin that works essentially as a painkiller and relieves mild cramping; the painkiller acetaminophen (Tylenol) seems equally effective for these purposes even though it is not an antiprostaglandin.

For more incapacitating symptoms, stronger antiprostaglandins called nonsteroidal antiinflammatory drugs (such as ibuprofen and naproxen) which were originally developed to treat arthritis can be used to treat dysmenorrhea. These drugs are available over the counter (under names such as Motrin IB, Nuprin, and Advil), as well as in stronger prescription forms. They generally should not be used by women who have a history of ulcers or aspirin allergies; some women with asthma also find that these NSAIDs aggravate their condition.

Various self-help measures may also alleviate menstrual cramps. Many women find that uterine spasms are relieved by placing a heating pad over the abdomen or taking warm showers; others find that massage can eliminate backache. Deep breathing and muscle-relaxing exercises may also provide relief, as well as elevating the knees while lying down or tucking the knees up to the chest in a fetal position. Some women also find that mild to moderate exercise may augment the effects of medication, as does orgasm.

Treating secondary dysmenorrhea involves treating the underlying disorder.

Related entries

Adenomyosis, alternative therapies, antiinflammatory drugs, birth control, endometriosis, menarche, menopause, menorrhagia, menstrual cycle, ovarian cysts, pelvic inflammatory disease, pelvic pain, uterine fibroids, vaginal bleeding (abnormal)

Menstrual Cycle

The menstrual cycle involves the periodic release of a fertile egg or ovum from the ovary, the preparation of the uterine lining for pregnancy, and, if fertilization does not occur, the shedding of the lining as a bloody vaginal discharge—menstruation. This cycle occurs in premenopausal women and is controlled by finely tuned feedback between hormones of the pituitary gland, hypothalamus, and ovaries.

Phases of the menstrual cycle

In healthy women of reproductive age the menstrual cycle consists of three phases: the follicular, ovulatory, and luteal. If a woman does not become pregnant during a given cycle, these phases are followed by menstruation (a "period"), and the cycle begins anew.

Follicular phase. In the follicular (also called preovulatory or proliferative) phase, a portion of the brain called the hypothalamus secretes gonadotropin releasing hormone (GnRH), which in turn stimulates the pituitary gland at the base of the brain (see illustration, step 1) to secrete follicle stimulating hormone (FSH) and luteinizing hormone (LH). FSH stimulates the growth of a small group of follicles in the ovary (see step 2), only one of which (the Graafian follicle) will eventually produce a mature egg. After about a week the Graafian follicle has increased approximately a hundredfold in diameter (to about three-quarters of an inch in size), while the

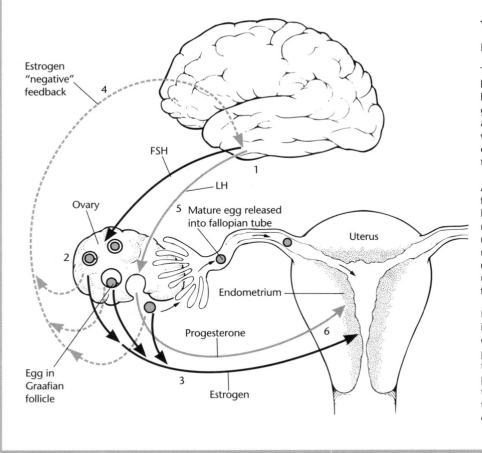

The normal menstrual cycle

The pituitary gland at the base of the brain secretes follicle stimulating hormone (1), which stimulates growth of follicles in the ovary (2). It also secretes luteinizing hormone, which stimulates the production of estrogen by the ovary (3). Estrogen thickens the lining of the uterus.

As estrogen levels rise, FSH secretion falls and LH secretion surges (4). High levels of LH cause the release of a mature egg from the Graafian follicle (5). The now-empty follicle produces more estrogen as well as progesterone (6), which build up the lining of the uterus in preparation for receiving a fertilized egg.

If fertilization does not occur, increased levels of progesterone and estrogen eventually inhibit the production of LH and FSH, which in turn causes estrogen and progesterone levels to fall. When these hormones become too scarce to maintain the thickened endometrium, menstruation occurs.

other follicles have shrunk and been reabsorbed back into the body.

Ovulatory phase. Meanwhile, LH stimulates the ovaries and part of the Graafian follicle to secrete estrogen (see step 3), a hormone that thickens the endometrium in preparation for the implantation of a fertilized egg. Estrogen also has a "negative feedback" effect on FSH secretion (see step 4), so that as estrogen levels rise, FSH secretion falls.

High levels of ovarian estrogen change the pattern of GnRH pulses to a high-amplitude, high-frequency pattern which triggers an "LH surge" in the pituitary. The large amounts of LH act directly on the ovary to cause the rupture of the Graafian follicle and the release of the mature egg into the fallopian tube (see step 5), where it is available for fertilization. This process is called ovulation.

Normally only one ovary releases an egg each month. Some women feel a pain or cramp in the lower abdomen or back around the time of ovulation, sometimes painful enough to be confused with appendicitis or ectopic pregnancy. This is called mittelschmerz ("middle pain") and may be accompanied by slight vaginal bleeding.

The quality of a woman's cervical mucus (secreted by glands in the cervix) normally changes throughout the men-

strual cycle because of variations in hormone levels. Following menstruation there may be a few days of dryness, followed by a gradual change from tacky, sticky mucus to creamy, milky, and, eventually, watery mucus. Around the time of ovulation, the cervical mucus becomes thinner, clearer, and increasingly abundant, sometimes resembling egg white; and just before ovulation it can be stretched between two fingers into strands an inch or more long—a phenomenon called spinnbarkeit. Mucus in this state is most hospitable to sperm, which can readily swim through it into the uterus and on to the fallopian tubes, where an egg is available for fertilization.

Luteal phase. After ovulation the quality of the mucus changes abruptly, becoming tacky, creamy, or sparse, depending on the individual woman, until menstrual flow begins. Body temperature rises slightly after ovulation.

The empty Graafian follicle becomes the corpus luteum, a yellow-colored structure that synthesizes more estrogen as well as progesterone (see step 6). Progesterone is a hormone that stimulates the endometrium to build up glands, blood vessels, and supporting tissue which give it a spongy appearance. This is the beginning of the luteal (or secretory) phase. The thickened endometrium begins to produce various substances, including prostaglandin, which has been shown to cause symptoms associated with ovulatory cycles such as uterine cramps, mood swings, and back pain.

If the egg is fertilized by a sperm, the corpus luteum will be maintained for about 6 to 8 weeks by a hormone called human chorionic gonadotropin (hCG) produced by the placenta. If fertilization does not occur, increased levels of progesterone and estrogen eventually inhibit (through negative feedback) the production of LH and FSH. The corpus luteum is reabsorbed into the body, leaving a whitish scar near the ovary's surface, and stops producing estrogen and progesterone.

Without enough estrogen and progesterone, the thickened endometrium, or uterine lining, is shed through menstruation. The lowered hormone levels also stimulate the hypothalamus to produce more GnRH, which stimulates the pituitary to produce FSH and LH, and the cycle begins again.

Menstruation

The average menstrual cycle is 28 days long from the first day of one menstrual period to the first day of the next, with normal menstrual cycles lasting anywhere between 21 and 38 days. Menstrual flow normally lasts from 3 to 7 days. Most women lose only about 3 to 4 ounces or 4 to 6 tablespoonfuls of menstrual fluid (which is actually composed of cervical mucus, vaginal secretions, and endometrial tissue in addition to blood) each month. This fluid is usually reddish-brown and odorless until it is contaminated by bacteria.

Most women today use commercially produced sanitary napkins, tampons, or menstrual sponges (natural, noncellulose sponges which can be rinsed out and reused) to absorb the menstrual fluids. Some women prefer using a cervical cap (see birth control) or rubber menstrual cup, a soft plastic device which is worn near the vaginal opening and can be washed and reused many times. Deodorized products are usually unnecessary (and potentially irritating). To reduce the risk of toxic shock syndrome (TSS; see entry) and possibly vaginal irritation, women should try to use tampons with as low an absorbency as is effective. In addition, most doctors advise women with a history of toxic shock to alternate tampons or sponges with napkins and to replace tampons or sponges after about 4 hours.

Recently an "urban legend" has been circulating on the Internet claiming that some commercial tampons contain potentially cancer-causing substances including asbestos and dioxins. Women are urged to buy only unbleached, all-cotton feminine hygiene products, which are claimed to be much safer. Much of this legend is nothing but "scarelore." No tampon product on the market contains asbestos—period. And while some brands may contain dioxins (produced through the chlorine bleaching of wood pulp), quantities are minute and are deemed safe by the Food and Drug Administration. Women concerned about dioxin exposure should also bear in mind that dioxins are everywhere, and given the extremely low levels of dioxins in tampons, changing brands of feminine hygiene products will make essentially no dif-

ference in overall exposure. As for switching to unbleached, all-cotton products, it should be noted that conventionally grown cotton is rich in pesticides, which are also potentially cancer-causing. Perhaps the most prudent approach to this whole issue is simply to follow the advice given to reduce TSS risk—that is, use the lowest-absorbency tampon that does the job and switch to pads overnight and on days of lighter flow.

Healthy women do not usually need to change their daily activities or exercise habits during menstruation, unless they are incapacitated by severe menstrual cramps. Sexual intercourse during menstruation appears to be harmless. Some women use a diaphragm, lubricated with spermicidal jelly or a vaginal lubricant (if another form of contraception is used), to catch menstrual flow temporarily during intercourse.

Changes over a lifetime

The menstrual cycle begins at menarche (the first menstrual period), which normally occurs between the ages of 10 and 17, and stops at menopause, which generally occurs in the late 40s or early 50s. The process that leads up to the mature menstrual cycle, however, begins before birth (see illustration). Primordial egg cells can be identified in a female embryo that is only 1 week old, and by 20 weeks of gestation there are 6 to 7 million egg cells surrounded by primordial follicles, tiny sacs that will eventually contain the eggs in the ovaries. From this point on these primitive egg cells are steadily absorbed by the body until, by birth, there are only 1 million of them. By the time of menarche about 400,000 remain, only 300 to 500 of which will develop into mature eggs during a woman's reproductive life.

Shortly before a girl reaches puberty, her pituitary gland begins to secrete more FSH and LH. Menstruation begins when LH is produced in a rhythmic pattern and in sufficient quantities.

The menstrual pattern changes again in the later reproductive years. Often women over the age of 35 notice that their cycles have shortened. Whereas the average length of the menstrual cycle in women in their early 20s is 32 days, many women over the age of 35 have cycles of 28 days or less. This occurs because the aging corpus luteum does not produce enough progesterone, resulting in a shortened luteal phase. Eventually, the poorer quality and diminished number of follicles lead to a decline in the production of estrogen, until ultimately there is not enough estrogen to produce the LH surge and ovulation. Women at the perimenopausal stage of the reproductive life cycle, like adolescents, usually go through a phase of irregular (and anovulatory) bleeding before menses stop altogether. In both adolescents and perimenopausal women, this type of bleeding without ovulation is called dysfunctional uterine bleeding.

It is important to realize that minor fluctuations in the menstrual cycle are normal at every age. It is rare for a woman to go through her reproductive years without experiencing variations in her usual menstrual pattern, given the complexities of the hormonal interactions that occur every month. A variety of external events—travel, stress, acute ill-

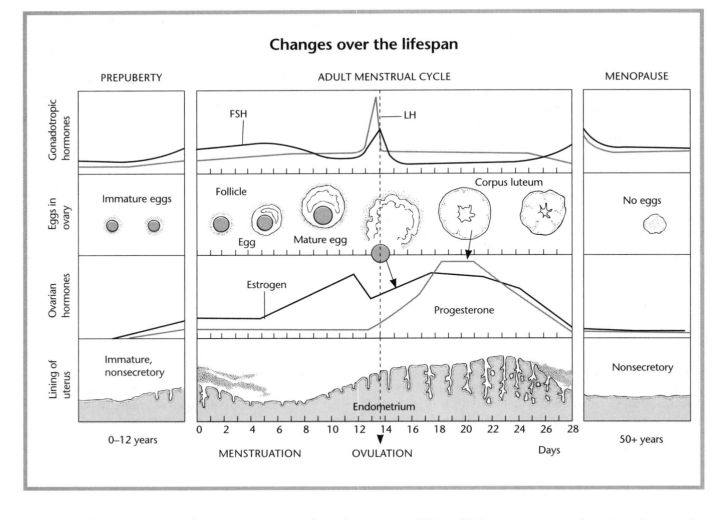

Changes over the lifespan

PREPUBERTY — ADULT MENSTRUAL CYCLE — MENOPAUSE

Gonadotropic hormones: FSH, LH

Eggs in ovary: Immature eggs | Follicle, Egg, Mature egg | Corpus luteum | No eggs

Ovarian hormones: Estrogen, Progesterone

Lining of uterus: Immature, nonsecretory | Endometrium | Nonsecretory

0–12 years   0 2 4 6 8 10 12 14 16 18 20 22 24 26 28   50+ years

MENSTRUATION   OVULATION   Days

---

ness—can affect one's periods. Sometimes even a single deviation from normal, such as a missed period in a sexually active woman, should be checked out with a physician. In other cases—for example, when a period is heavier or lasts longer than usual—a woman may be advised to wait and see if the problem corrects itself in future cycles.

Related entries

Amenorrhea, infrequent periods, menarche, menopause, menorrhagia, menstrual cramps, menstrual cycle disorders, premenstrual syndrome, toxic shock syndrome, vaginal bleeding (abnormal)

Menstrual Cycle Disorders

Most disorders of the menstrual cycle occur because of a malfunction in some part of the endocrine system (see illustration). Menstrual cycle disorders take the form of periods that are absent, scanty, infrequent, irregular, too frequent, heavy,

or painful. In addition, many women have irregular episodes of spotting, staining, or light bleeding between menstrual periods, a phenomenon known as breakthrough bleeding.

Absent periods

The absence of menstruation in a nonpregnant premenopausal woman is called amenorrhea (see entry). Primary amenorrhea is the term used if menstruation has not begun by the age of 18. Secondary amenorrhea is the term used if previously normal menstrual periods stop for more than 6 months in a woman who is not pregnant or breastfeeding and is not nearing menopause.

In most cases amenorrhea is not a cause for concern, but if it persists for more than several months it should be treated, for over time the lack of ovulation can affect fertility and increase bone turnover, thus raising the risk of osteoporosis (a disease that causes the bones to become porous and weak and to be highly susceptible to fracture; see osteoporosis).

Primary amenorrhea is most often due to delayed puberty, a condition in which maturation is slower than average because of genetic or environmental factors such as poor nutrition. Sometimes, however, the first menstrual period (menarche) is delayed when a girl is undergoing excessive stress or

The endocrine system in women

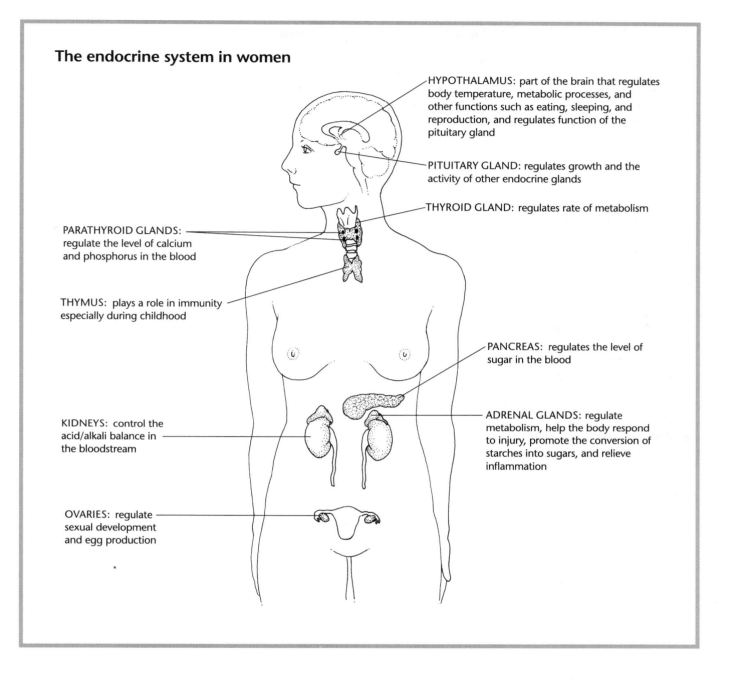

HYPOTHALAMUS: part of the brain that regulates body temperature, metabolic processes, and other functions such as eating, sleeping, and reproduction, and regulates function of the pituitary gland

PITUITARY GLAND: regulates growth and the activity of other endocrine glands

THYROID GLAND: regulates rate of metabolism

PARATHYROID GLANDS: regulate the level of calcium and phosphorus in the blood

THYMUS: plays a role in immunity especially during childhood

PANCREAS: regulates the level of sugar in the blood

KIDNEYS: control the acid/alkali balance in the bloodstream

ADRENAL GLANDS: regulate metabolism, help the body respond to injury, promote the conversion of starches into sugars, and relieve inflammation

OVARIES: regulate sexual development and egg production

intense athletic training, or when she is anorexic (see anorexia nervosa and bulimia nervosa). More rarely, primary amenorrhea may result from some anatomical obstruction such as an imperforate hymen, which blocks the flow of blood out of the vagina.

Even more infrequently, primary amenorrhea may result from genetic disorders such as Turner syndrome and testicular feminization syndrome (see entries), pituitary gland disorders and tumors, thyroid or adrenal disorders, diabetes, and obesity.

Periods that start and then stop for many months are common for the first few years after menarche, as well as in the years preceding menopause. This type of secondary amenor-rhea, which is perfectly normal in adolescents, is the result of the imperfectly coordinated function of the hypothalamus, a part of the brain that regulates basic functions including eating, sleeping, and reproduction. In perimenopausal women, irregularity is related to decreasing production of estrogen by the ovary.

Some female athletes, ballet dancers, models, and actresses, as well as women with eating disorders, develop irregular periods or stop menstruating altogether when their ratio of body fat to overall weight drops too low. Another relatively common cause of amenorrhea during the childbearing years is polycystic ovary syndrome, a condition marked by multiple ovarian cysts and excessive production of male-type hormones called androgens (see hyperandrogenism). If untreated, amenorrhea and hyperandrogenism may lead to chronic stimulation of the uterine lining by estrogen, which in turn has been associated with an increased risk of endometrial hyperplasia and endometrial cancer (see entries). About 1 woman in 5 with amenorrhea has elevated prolactin levels. Prolactin is a hormone that stimulates the breasts to secrete milk and, indirectly, inhibits ovulation (see hyperprolactinemia).

Scanty periods

Short or scanty menstrual periods (hypomenorrhea) are particularly common in women using oral contraceptive pills. This is because the relatively low estrogen content of most birth control pills produces an unusually thin endometrium, leaving relatively little uterine lining to be shed during menstruation. Though it is technically an abnormality, most women welcome this "side effect" and rarely find it reason for complaint.

It is important to distinguish this kind of hypomenorrhea from that due to systemic disorders. Among the disorders that may account for short or scanty periods are hyperthyroidism (overproduction of thyroid hormone; see entry), kidney failure (see kidney disorders), or certain kinds of endometrial inflammation (endometritis) in women with pelvic inflammatory disease (see entry). Once these underlying conditions are corrected, menstrual flow usually returns to normal levels.

Infrequent periods

Infrequent menstruation (a condition called oligomenorrhea) is generally defined as menstrual periods that occur 6 weeks or more apart. Infrequent periods (see entry) are often due to hormonal imbalances that lead to dysfunction of the hypothalamus. Although this condition usually requires no treatment, it may cause some women to have difficulty becoming pregnant.

Infrequent periods are particularly common in the first few years after menarche (the first menstrual period) as well as in the years preceding menopause. Often in women of these ages, when menstruation does occur, it does not involve release of an egg from the ovary. For reasons still not understood, some women menstruate as infrequently as every 2 months for all or most of their reproductive life. So long as these periods are fairly regular, this type of oligomenorrhea does not usually require treatment.

Infrequent periods that develop in women who have previously had more frequent periods can often be due to chronic illness or to stress, anxiety, excessive exercise, poor nutrition, or anorexia nervosa. All of these conditions can interfere with the function of the hypothalamus. In polycystic ovary disease, abnormally high levels of androgens can also cause infrequent periods (see hyperandrogenism). Treating secondary oligomenorrhea involves treating the underlying condition.

Irregular periods

Instead of having cycles of some predictable length (whether average, more frequent than average, or less frequent than average), women with irregular menstrual periods have cycles of inconsistent length. These cycles usually involve some combination of short, long, and normal intervals between periods.

Irregular periods are most common at both ends of the reproductive cycle—in the first 5 years following menarche (the first menstrual period) and in perimenopausal women (women nearing menopause). In both of these instances the most frequent cause is a hormonal imbalance which upsets the intricate feedback mechanism normally responsible for ovulation (the release of an egg from the ovary) and the production of progesterone (see menstrual cycle).

Occasionally irregular periods in women of any age may be related to stress, anxiety, crash dieting, eating disorders, or a variety of serious systemic diseases including liver, kidney, and thyroid disease or a disorder of blood clotting (see platelet disorders).

In the case of adolescents, menstrual cycles usually stabilize themselves over time. Some women continue to have irregular periods throughout their childbearing years (or at least into their mid-20s), but this generally presents no particular problem—other than difficulty predicting fertility.

Irregular periods that develop in older women also often resolve themselves in the form of menopause (cessation of menstruation). Women taking estrogen replacement therapy—although technically beyond the age of menstrual cycle disorders—may experience irregular bleeding when treatment first begins. Taking daily estrogen together with a low dose of progesterone can produce irregular, unpredictable bleeding for 3 to 6 months.

Too-frequent periods

Some women have menstrual periods that occur more frequently than every 21 days, a problem known as polymenorrhea. Frequent periods are most common in adolescents and in women in their late 30s and 40s (perimenopausal women) because of hormonal adjustments and imbalances that occur when the reproductive system is in transition. Any woman who thinks she has polymenorrhea, however, should consider the possibility that what seem to be frequent menstrual periods may actually be breakthrough bleeding (bleeding between menstrual periods) resulting from nonmenstrual causes such as uterine fibroids, cervical polyps, or cancers of the reproductive system. Too-frequent periods are particularly likely in older women, as well as in women using oral contraceptives.

Over time, polymenorrhea and other menstrual cycle disorders in adolescents often resolve spontaneously. Because frequent periods can result in anemia, using natural progesterone suppositories or taking oral contraceptives containing both estrogen and progesterone to help lengthen the cycle may be recommended.

In older women approaching menopause, time is also often the answer to polymenorrhea. Frequent periods may begin to alternate with infrequent periods, resulting in a phase of irregular periods before menstruation ceases altogether. If necessary, various hormonal and surgical therapies can be used to reduce debilitating or uncontrolled bleeding.

Occasionally systemic illnesses such as a deficiency of thyroid hormone (hypothyroidism) or excess levels of prolactin (hyperprolactinemia) can increase the frequency of menstruation. In these cases cycle length usually increases once the underlying condition is corrected.

Heavy or prolonged periods

Having excessively heavy or prolonged menstrual periods is called menorrhagia (see entry; also called hypermenorrhagia). Soaking a sanitary napkin or tampon every hour or so, as well as menstruating for longer than 7 days, are both considered forms of menorrhagia.

Like most menstrual cycle disorders, heavy or prolonged periods are usually due to a temporary hormonal imbalance most common in adolescents in the years following menarche and in women nearing menopause. Heavy bleeding is generally little more than an inconvenience that at worst may cause anemia because of excessive blood loss.

Occasionally, however, heavy periods can result from a more serious condition. If bleeding is heavy enough to soak a sanitary napkin or tampon every hour and clots are passed, a medical evaluation is appropriate to rule out fibroids or endometrial cancer. A late but very heavy period in a possibly pregnant woman who has not previously had heavy periods could signal a miscarriage or ectopic pregnancy (see entries). All of these conditions require medical attention; an ectopic pregnancy in particular can quickly become life-threatening.

Other conditions that can underlie menorrhagia include cervical or endometrial polyps, hypothyroidism, lupus, pelvic inflammatory disease, and adenomyosis (see entries). Women with kidney failure who are on dialysis may have heavy or prolonged menstrual periods as well. In addition, intrauterine devices (IUDs) occasionally cause menorrhagia and should be removed and replaced with some other form of birth control.

Painful periods

Dysmenorrhea (painful periods) involves crampy, spasmodic pain in the lower abdomen which sometimes spreads to the hips, lower back, or thighs. Other common symptoms include nausea and frequent diarrhea or constipation, or both at different times within the same menstrual period (see menstrual cramps).

Most women probably experience primary dysmenorrhea—painful menstruation not attributable to some underlying physical abnormality—at some point in their lives. Once blamed on psychosomatic factors, dysmenorrhea is now believed to be caused by an excess of prostaglandins, a group of naturally occurring fatty acids which cause uterine contractions and stimulate the intestines. These are produced by the tissue lining of the uterus, which is sloughed off during menstruation.

Primary dysmenorrhea usually begins within a year or two of menarche. Although some women continue to suffer from dysmenorrhea until reaching menopause, most find that symptoms gradually subside by their mid-20s or after their first pregnancy. Why some women are prone to particularly severe symptoms remains unknown.

If the menstrual cramps are caused by some physical abnormality of the reproductive organs such as endometriosis, adenomyosis, pelvic inflammatory disease (PID), an ovarian cyst, or uterine fibroids (see entries), or by using an intrauterine device (IUD), the condition is called secondary dysmenorrhea. Treating secondary dysmenorrhea calls for treating the underlying disorder.

Breakthrough bleeding

Breakthrough bleeding (or metrorrhagia) means bleeding between menstrual periods. In some women it occurs as a normal and harmless part of ovulation. Women with mittelschmerz (acute mid-cycle abdominal pain around the time of ovulation) frequently have some concurrent spotting. Using an IUD or oral contraceptives may lead to breakthrough bleeding as well. If these problems persist beyond the first three cycles of oral contraceptive use, a woman should have her prescription changed to a pill containing higher dosages of progesterone or estrogen.

Intermittent spotting or bleeding between periods can stem from any of a number of reproductive system disorders, including vaginal tears, vaginal atrophy, cervical polyps, cervicitis, endometriosis, endometrial hyperplasia, adenomyosis, uterine fibroids, ectopic pregnancy, incomplete miscarriage, pelvic inflammatory disease, or cancer of the vagina, fallopian tubes, ovaries, cervix, or endometrium. Some women may mistake the bleeding resulting from these conditions for menstrual bleeding and erroneously conclude that they are having unusually frequent periods.

Related entries

Amenorrhea, infertility, infrequent periods, menarche, menopause, menorrhagia, menstrual cramps, menstrual cycle, vaginal bleeding (abnormal)

Midwifery

A midwife is a person specially trained to assist with childbirth. Two kinds of midwives—most of them women—practice in the United States today: certified nurse-midwives and lay (independent) midwives. They vary widely in their training and experience. Most midwives approach childbirth as a natural, nonpathological process; for some there is a disinclination to rush the natural timing of labor or to resort to medical intervention (including anesthesia, episiotomies, cesarean sections, fetal monitors, forceps, and prenatal testing). Others feel comfortable using many modern techniques for controlling labor (such as the drug pitocin). Midwives are not licensed to do forceps deliveries, but some do perform vacuum deliveries. In countries where most deliveries are by midwives, the frequency of cesarean section and the cost of care are lower, while the health of mothers and infants is not compromised.

Midwives try to stay with a woman during the entire course of childbirth and also teach her about early care of the infant. Midwives were early advocates of natural childbirth, freestanding birth centers, birthing rooms in hospitals (where a woman can undergo both labor and deliver without being moved to another room), birthing chairs (which allow a woman to give birth in what many believe is a more natural and efficient position), and rooming-in (which allows mother and baby to stay together immediately after delivery).

The dominant form of childbirth assistance for centuries, midwifery gradually declined in this country beginning in the early nineteenth century, as women of the upper social strata began turning to physicians to deliver their babies (although at first many found the idea of males attending childbirth morally repugnant). The decline in midwifery, and the eons-old tradition of female lay healers in general, was part of a larger social trend toward the professionalization of health care and the domestication of women's work.

Real momentum in the revival of midwifery came in the late 1960s, when women associated with the counterculture movement fought against high-tech hospital procedures for what they regarded as a healthy, natural process. Some began to practice as lay midwives. By 1971 the American College of Obstetricians and Gynecologists (ACOG) officially recognized certified nurse-midwives, sanctioning them to take responsibility for uncomplicated births so long as they had some formal tie to a medical doctor. Many insurance policies also began to cover care by a midwife, which tends to be much less costly than that by an obstetrician.

Conflict still existed, however, between lay midwives and some obstetricians, who argued that home births were unconscionably risky; and often hospital privileges (and sometimes medical licenses) of doctors who offered backup services to lay midwives were revoked. Lay midwifery continued to grow, however, and today the practice is licensed by 10 states and is ambiguously legal in 30 others as well as in the District of Columbia.

Lay midwives

Lay midwives are the modern counterparts of the granny midwives of rural America. Most assist in home births or, occasionally, hospital births (but only when accompanying a physician). Some also provide prenatal care, nutritional advice, emotional support, and postpartum care.

Lay midwifery is still illegal—or actively discouraged by medical professionals—in some localities and may not be covered by insurance policies. Also, because there are no uniform standards or regulations for practice in most states, determining a lay midwife's competence can be difficult. Some have learned their trade through apprenticeship to older, more experienced midwives, while others have attended schools that teach midwifery. Some practice in conjunction with physicians and readily transport women to hospitals if there is an emergency; others invariably see births through on their own, letting nature take its (sometimes fatal) course. Some of these problems may subside if the Midwives Alliance of North America (MANA) gets its way and develops national certification guidelines for lay midwives.

Certified nurse-midwives

Many women see nurse-midwives as offering the best of both worlds. Not only do they generally subscribe to the same philosophy as other midwives, spend large amounts of time with the laboring woman, and cost less than many doctors, but also they undergo standardized training and are always associated with a physician should complications arise. Required to have a registered nursing degree and a certificate of midwifery from the American College of Nurse-Midwives (obtained after a year's training in obstetrics and gynecology), nurse-midwives sometimes also take a master's degree after doing a year of internship.

Nurse-midwives attend childbirths in hospitals and clinics or (more rarely) in the mother's home. In uncomplicated pregnancies the nurse-midwife may perform all the prenatal care from the very first visit and continue to help the mother after delivery with postpartum care. Some also teach childbirth education classes or continue to see women after delivery for routine checkups.

Despite the number of women who would like to follow this route for their labor and delivery, nurse-midwives are in scarce supply. There are currently only about 4,000 certified nurse-midwives in this country, and fewer than 30 training programs.

Who is not a good candidate for a midwife-assisted birth?

Women with preexisting conditions such as heart disease, diabetes, kidney disorders, hypertension, severe anemia, or substance abuse are not good candidates for a midwife-assisted birth. Women who develop complications during pregnancy—such as gestational diabetes, preeclampsia, placenta previa (a placenta that obstructs or encroaches on the cervical opening), placenta abruptio (a placenta that prematurely detaches from the uterine wall), Rh incompatibility (see Rh disease), multiple pregnancy, or a fetus in breech position (feet or buttocks first)—are also at high risk and therefore not good candidates. Although some midwives can handle some of these complications some of the time, a good nurse-midwife will recognize her limitations and seek medical assistance when necessary. In fact, most midwives have relationships with local obstetricians and call upon them when emergency situations arise.

Finally, a woman over the age of 35, especially one having her first child, should carefully discuss the risks with an obstetrician before choosing midwifery, although most women over 35 are good candidates.

Related entries

Cesarean section, childbirth, preeclampsia, pregnancy over age 35, prenatal care

Miscarriage

Miscarriage is the spontaneous loss of a pregnancy during the first 20 weeks of gestation, counted from the first day of the last period. A threatened miscarriage is defined as vaginal bleeding or light spotting during the first 20 weeks of gestation, which may result in either miscarriage (spontaneous abortion) or the continuation of the pregnancy.

Who is likely to have a miscarriage?

Perhaps as many as 70 percent of conceptions are miscarried, often before a woman even misses her period or realizes that she is pregnant. In addition, 15 to 20 percent of recognized pregnancies end in miscarriage. Even after an embryo implants in the uterine lining, as many as 1 in 3 pregnancies may miscarry. After one miscarriage a woman who has never given birth still has about a 3 in 4 chance of eventually having a normal pregnancy; even after 4 consecutive miscarriages her chances of a successful pregnancy remain 3 out of 5. As a woman gets older, her chances of miscarrying increase.

Most of the time the reasons for miscarriages remain unclear, although in over half of the miscarriages that occur in the first 8 weeks of pregnancy, there are serious genetic defects that would have made it difficult or impossible for the fetus to survive. In about 17 percent of miscarriages there is some hormonal imbalance in the mother which seems to interfere with the production of progesterone or some other hormone necessary for successful implantation and subsequent growth and development of the fertilized egg. Perhaps 10 percent of miscarriages seem related to a structural problem of the uterus or cervix. Women whose mothers used diethylstilbestrol (DES) while pregnant may be predisposed to these defects. In rare and still little-understood cases, some women seem to produce antibodies or other factors toxic to the developing embryo or fetus.

Chronic illnesses—such as diabetes, maternal infection, or exposure to environmental toxins such as heavy metals, drugs, and radiation—can also play a role in miscarriages. There is no evidence at this point that exposure to video display terminals or microwave ovens causes miscarriage, nor does moderate exercise or sexual activity.

What are the symptoms?

The first symptom of a miscarriage is usually bleeding from the vagina, sometimes preceded by a brownish discharge. Flow can be light or heavy. A woman with a threatened miscarriage may feel mild cramping, but her cervix remains closed. These symptoms can continue for several days.

On the one hand, it is important to note that bleeding and spotting in early pregnancy can be signs of ectopic pregnancy, a dangerous and sometimes life-threatening condition which requires immediate medical attention. On the other hand, some women have slight vaginal bleeding after the fertilized egg implants in the uterus—about 7 to 10 days after conception, or at about the time they are expecting their period—and this can be mistaken for a threatened miscarriage. Indeed, some women bleed at the time of their monthly periods throughout pregnancy. A pelvic exam, ultrasound exam, and a blood pregnancy test can help differentiate some of these conditions.

In an inevitable spontaneous abortion nothing can be done to preserve the pregnancy because the embryo or fetus is no longer viable. Bleeding and cramping increase, and the cervix begins to dilate. If the abortion is allowed to follow its natural course, the fetus will be expelled in the form of solid material that passes through the vagina. In cases where the obstetrician can determine that the fetus is not viable (through ultrasound, which can show an abnormal gestational sac and lack of a fetal heartbeat in a pregnancy of 8 weeks or more), the pregnancy may be terminated with vacuum aspiration (see entry).

Inevitable spontaneous abortions can be either "complete" or "incomplete." In a complete abortion all the products of conception are expelled, and bleeding gradually decreases on its own. In an incomplete abortion, however, heavy bleeding and pain can continue for several days since only some of the products of conception have been expelled. In a missed abortion the fetus dies but remains in the uterus for up to several months without being expelled and without the woman experiencing symptoms of a miscarriage.

If a woman loses 3 or more pregnancies before 20 weeks' gestation, she is said to have experienced recurrent (habitual) abortion.

How is the condition evaluated?

If a woman thinks she has had or is having a miscarriage, her clinician will first listen for a fetal heartbeat and conduct a pelvic exam. The presence of a fetal heartbeat and a pelvic exam that reveals a uterus that is still enlarged—and the absence of passed tissue or severe pain—usually signal only a threatened miscarriage. If a heartbeat cannot be detected (sometimes ultrasound will be used in this diagnosis), or if the pelvic exam reveals fetal tissue or the placenta coming through the dilated cervix, the miscarriage is inevitable. If the uterus has shrunk since the last examination and the woman has had prolonged spotting without other symptoms, the practitioner may suspect a missed abortion, which can be confirmed through ultrasonography.

Since women who have experienced missed abortions may have no heavy bleeding or other symptoms, the fetal death may go undetected for weeks. A lack of uterine growth from one examination to the next or the absence of detectable fetal heartbeat after about 8 to 10 weeks' gestation will suggest a missed abortion.

How is miscarriage treated?

A woman experiencing bleeding or severe pain or cramping during pregnancy should report these symptoms to her health care practitioner immediately. In the case of an inevitable, incomplete, or missed abortion, the fetus and placenta may be removed from the uterus by means of a dilatation and curettage (D&C; see entry), either in the hospital or in the doctor's office. In the case of heavy bleeding, severe pain, or uterine infection, D&C is standard procedure.

If miscarriage occurs at home, it is a good idea to collect any tissue that is passed and put it in a clean container. Although psychologically difficult, this procedure will allow a laboratory evaluation of fetal tissue that may help determine why the miscarriage happened. Even if the miscarriage appears to be complete, the woman should contact her clinician immediately.

If a woman has 3 or more consecutive miscarriages, her clinician will probably want to start an infertility workup, even though it is still likely that the miscarriages were chance phenomena. The clinician will ask the woman about her previous pregnancies and any chronic illnesses, uterine surgery, sexually transmitted diseases, DES exposure, drug exposure, radiation, and possible environmental pollutants. The clinician may also want to check for infections, hormone irregularities, sperm-fighting antibodies, and abnormalities of the uterus and fallopian tubes, and will evaluate the chromosomes of both parents (see infertility, genetic counseling). As many as 80 percent of women who have 3 or more miscarriages eventually sustain a pregnancy and deliver a healthy child.

How can miscarriage be prevented?

Inevitable miscarriages cannot be prevented. Women experiencing a threatened miscarriage are usually advised to rest in bed for a day and sometimes to avoid sexual intercourse for a few weeks after bleeding stops. Some obstetricians feel, however, that a healthy woman with a threatened miscarriage, especially early in the pregnancy, should continue her normal activities rather than protect a vulnerable pregnancy that may have an unhappy outcome further down the road, when the consequences would be more severe. In women with diabetes, getting symptoms under control before conception occurs can greatly decrease the risk of miscarriage.

What happens after a miscarriage?

After a miscarriage spotting may continue for several weeks. Medical care should be sought if fever develops, flow increases, or discharge has a strange or unpleasant odor. To give the cervix time to close and thus decrease the risk of infection, sexual intercourse should be avoided for 2 to 3 weeks after the miscarriage. It is safe to start trying to conceive again after about 8 weeks (2 normal periods).

Any miscarriage can be emotionally painful for the mother, as well as for other relatives who were looking forward to the baby. The fact that the symptoms of pregnancy such as tender breasts and enlarged stomach can persist for weeks following a miscarriage may make the grieving process difficult. For women (and, though usually to a lesser degree, their partners) who are grieving after a lost pregnancy, the process is often accompanied by a number of other emotions. A miscarriage can represent a major blow to a woman's self-esteem and leave her with a strong sense of defectiveness and guilt, however unwarranted. Many women also feel anger toward other women whom they perceive as having easy or "normal" pregnancies. If a fetal anomaly was detected after the miscarriage, the initial shock and denial may soon be replaced by anxiety as the couple grapples with confusing statistics about the probability of a recurring problem in a subsequent pregnancy.

Not surprisingly, many couples who have undergone pregnancy-related loss suffer from significant sexual dysfunction as well, particularly as they come to realize the tragic implications of what was formerly a hope-filled and loving act. The end result is often marital distress, which can be aggravated by the frustration that many women feel when they cannot talk out their emotions and memories with their partner.

Some women find that a clinician's attempt to identify possible causes of the miscarriage can be helpful. Genetic or preconception counseling are often effective in assuaging grief, guilt, and fears about future pregnancies. Some women come to accept their situation after participating in support groups consisting of others who have undergone similar experiences or, when this is not possible, simply talking to friends who are willing to listen. In other cases psychotherapy can be invaluable.

Related entries

Diethylstilbestrol (DES), dilatation and curettage, ectopic pregnancy, genetic counseling, infertility, pregnancy over age 35, vacuum aspiration, vaginal bleeding during pregnancy

Mitral Valve Prolapse

The mitral valve connects the upper chamber to the lower chamber on the left side of the heart. In about 1 out of 20 Americans, most frequently women, one or both leaflets of this valve balloon out, or prolapse (see illustration). This condition is called mitral valve prolapse (MVP).

Often discovered by a clinician during a routine stethoscope examination, mitral valve prolapse is usually no cause

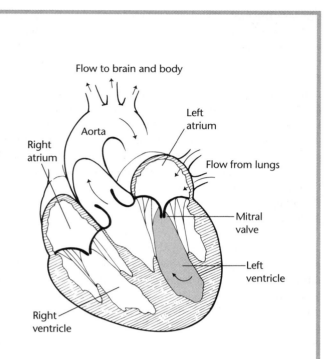

Flow to brain and body

Left atrium

Aorta

Right atrium

Flow from lungs

Mitral valve

Left ventricle

Right ventricle

Normal mitral valve

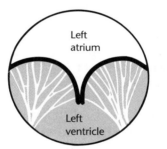

Left atrium

Left ventricle

Normally, the mitral valve closes tightly, and blood that has been pumped into the left ventricle does not reenter the left atrium.

Prolapsed mitral valve

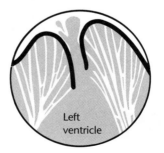

Left ventricle

When the mitral valve does not make a tight seal, blood may reenter the left atrium—a condition called mitral valve regurgitation.

for concern and in fact can be regarded as a variation of normal. On occasion, however, some blood may flow back into the upper chamber, or atrium, whenever the lower chamber, or ventricle, pumps blood in the other direction. This is called mitral regurgitation, and it seems to put people with mitral valve prolapse at increased risk for infective endocarditis, an infection of the membrane that covers the interior of the heart. People with mitral valve prolapse are also at slightly higher risk for stroke. An association between mitral valve prolapse and panic disorder, though once suspected, has never been confirmed.

Who is likely to develop MVP?

In some cases this seems to be a genetically determined condition which manifests itself predominantly in women. It is particularly common in those who have certain disorders of the thoracic skeleton, including scoliosis (curvature of the spine) and a sunken breastbone, or disorders of the connective tissue.

What are the symptoms?

Most of the time mitral valve prolapse produces no symptoms whatsoever. Sometimes, however, people with this condition experience chest pain, rapid heartbeat (palpitations), fatigue, anxiety, lightheadedness, or breathing difficulties. Occasionally women with mitral valve prolapse will develop symptoms because of hormonal changes that occur during menstruation or blood volume changes that occur during pregnancy.

Occasionally mitral valve prolapse progresses to mitral regurgitation (also called mitral valve insufficiency or mitral valve incompetence), in which a significant amount of blood flows backward into the left atrium. This condition can have other causes in addition to mitral valve prolapse (including infection, prior heart attack, or age-related wear and tear). In severe cases, shortness of breath, fatigue and leg swelling may develop, and, if untreated, ultimately life-threatening arrhythmias and/or congestive heart failure (see entries).

How is the condition evaluated?

A characteristic click-murmur sound heard through a stethoscope often signals mitral valve prolapse to a clinician. The clicks occur because of the prolapse itself, and if blood flows back into the atrium, a murmur can be detected shortly thereafter. To confirm the diagnosis a test called an echocardiogram may be done in a hospital's cardiac ultrasound department. This noninvasive and painless procedure transforms reflected sound waves into a continuous screen image of the heart tissues.

How is mitral valve prolapse treated?

Most people with mitral valve prolapse require no treatment. In some individuals, however, a clinician may recommend taking antibiotics before dental work or surgery to reduce the risk of developing endocarditis from a bacterial infection.

If chest pain caused by palpitations is troublesome, these

symptoms are usually treated with beta blockers (such as atenolol or propanolol), a class of medication that blocks certain actions of the sympathetic nervous system. These drugs should be used with caution by people with asthma as they can worsen symptoms. Some patients with mitral regurgitation need mitral valve surgery to repair or replace the defective valve.

Related entries

Angina pectoris, antibiotics, anxiety disorders, aortic stenosis, arrhythmia, asthma, chest pain, heart disease, menstrual cycle, musculoskeletal disorders, panic disorder, scoliosis, stroke

Molar Pregnancy

A molar pregnancy occurs when tissue around a fertilized egg which would normally develop into the placenta develops instead into an abnormal grapelike cluster of cells. Without this source of nutrients, the fetus degenerates, but the tissue (or hydatidiform mole) continues to grow—often yielding a positive pregnancy test and leaving the woman (and her clinician) with the impression that she is indeed pregnant. As a result, women who have a molar pregnancy often experience the same emotions and sense of loss as do women who have a miscarriage.

On top of that, they also have to contend with the possibility that any abnormal tissue left in place has the potential to become cancerous. About 80 percent of these moles are benign (noncancerous), but about 15 percent if left in place will become invasive, burrowing into the uterine wall and leading to serious bleeding and predisposing to infection as tissue is eroded. Another 5 percent will develop into fast-growing cancers called choriocarcinomas.

Molar pregnancies occur in approximately 1 out of every 2,000 pregnancies in the United States, although in some parts of Asia the incidence is as high as 1 in 200.

What are the symptoms?

Women with a molar pregnancy have a positive pregnancy test and often believe they are having a normal pregnancy for 3 or 4 months. The uterus often grows unusually quickly, however, and generally by the end of the first or beginning of the second trimester (if not earlier), there is some kind of vaginal bleeding. This can range from light spotting to outright hemorrhaging. Sometimes the cluster of tissue itself is discharged at the same time. Severe nausea, vomiting, and high blood pressure are often signs of a problem, as is the absence of fetal movement as the pregnancy progresses.

How is the condition evaluated?

A clinician may not suspect a molar pregnancy until the 12th week of pregnancy or later, when the absence of fetal heart-beat—or the presence of vaginal bleeding, plus severe nausea and vomiting—signals a problem. The first order of business will be to make sure the symptoms are not due to an ectopic (tubal) pregnancy—a potentially life-threatening situation. To do this, blood will be drawn and tested for levels of human chorionic gonadotropin (hCG), a hormone normally produced by the placenta (or the mole). Abnormally high levels of this hormone in combination with vaginal bleeding usually indicate a molar pregnancy, especially if there is no discernible heartbeat or fetal movement and if the uterus is larger than expected for that particular gestational age. An ultrasound examination will also usually be done to confirm this diagnosis by making sure that there is no amniotic sac with a fetus in it.

How are molar pregnancies treated?

Because molar pregnancies can sometimes become malignant, it is imperative that the abnormal growth is fully expelled from the uterus. If this does not happen spontaneously—which it often does, around the fourth month of pregnancy—a suction (vacuum aspiration) or dilatation and curettage (D&C) procedure is usually performed to remove it as soon as the condition is discovered. If hCG levels rise, some form of chemotherapy (usually methotrexate) is given after the procedure to kill any potentially cancerous cells that may lurk in the uterus. Levels of hCG will be checked regularly to make sure they return to normal. If they do not within about 8 weeks, the mole may have become cancerous.

Women are advised to use a highly effective form of contraception (such as oral contraceptives) and wait a full year after hCG levels have returned to normal before attempting another pregnancy. Otherwise it might be difficult to tell whether high hCG levels are due to the new pregnancy or to a cancer.

If the mole has become invasive or a choriocarcinoma has developed, it is often completely curable, usually with chemotherapy alone—in which case future childbearing is still possible. Occasionally, however, it may be necessary to remove the uterus (see hysterectomy).

Related entries

Chemotherapy, childbirth, dilatation and curettage, ectopic pregnancy, hysterectomy, miscarriage, oral contraceptives, pregnancy testing, ultrasound, vacuum aspiration, vaginal bleeding during pregnancy

Moles

Moles (nevi) are spots of various sizes on the upper layers of the skin. They can appear on any part of the body and are generally brown, blue, or black, although in light-skinned people they are sometimes pinkish. Some moles also contain hairs or rough yellow bumps. While moles may be present

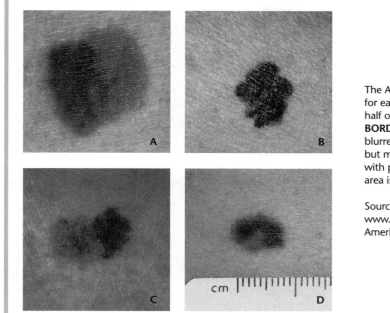

The American Cancer Society suggests using the ABCD rule for early detection of melanoma. **A** is for **ASYMMETRY:** One-half of a mole or birthmark does not match the other. **B** is for **BORDER:** The edges are irregular, ragged, notched, or blurred. **C** is for **COLOR:** The color is not the same all over, but may have differing shades of brown or black, sometimes with patches of red, white, or blue. **D** is for **DIAMETER:** The area is larger than inch or is growing larger.

Source: American Cancer Society's website www.cancer.org. Reprinted by permission of the American Cancer Society.

from birth, they also frequently appear or disappear spontaneously later in life. Moles that have been present since childhood often darken at puberty. Generally moles pose no health hazard whatsoever, but they should be watched carefully because certain changes may signal a potentially fatal form of skin cancer called melanoma.

One type of mole (called an atypical or a dysplastic nevus) is more likely than others to become cancerous. Unlike other moles, atypical nevi generally have irregular borders and a mottled appearance (see illustration). Some atypical nevi also have a raised center that sits on a colored base. Moles that are irregularly shaped and moles that are located around the nails or the vulva may have an increased likelihood of becoming cancerous.

Who is likely to develop moles?

Moles are extremely common, particularly in whites, and they tend to increase in number until middle age, after which they gradually fade or slough off. White adults have between 20 and 30 moles, on average. Atypical nevi tend to run in families and often develop in great numbers between the ages of 5 and 8.

What are the symptoms?

There are rarely any symptoms associated with moles. If a mole starts to itch, bleed, or change shape, size, or color, however, it should be evaluated by a dermatologist.

How are moles evaluated?

If a dermatologist or other clinician suspects melanoma, the mole will be biopsied—that is, cut out along with some surrounding skin and examined under a microscope. People with atypical nevi, as well as their close family members,

should have their skin examined regularly by a clinician, as should women with moles located near the vulva.

How are moles treated?

Moles generally require no treatment, but they can be removed surgically for cosmetic reasons. Potentially cancerous moles are also removed as part of the evaluation for malignancy.

Related entries

Melanoma, skin care and cosmetics, skin disorders

Mononucleosis

Mononucleosis is an infectious disease caused by the Epstein-Barr virus, a kind of herpes virus. Not highly contagious, it is acquired only by direct contact with the saliva of an infected person—generally through sneezing, coughing, or kissing (hence the nickname "the kissing disease"). It usually takes several weeks from the time of infection for the symptoms to develop. The virus remains present in the saliva for at least 6 months after recovery.

For a brief time investigators thought that chronic fatigue syndrome (see entry) might be a form of chronic mononucleosis because high levels of antibodies to the Epstein-Barr virus were frequently present in the blood of people with this often debilitating and hard-to-diagnose condition. It turned out, however, that people with chronic fatigue syndrome had high levels of antibodies to a number of different viruses in their bloodstream, not to mention that most Americans, whether or not they have chronic fatigue syndrome, have antibodies to the Epstein-Barr virus. This is because as many as 4 out of 5 children are infected with the Epstein-Barr virus between the ages of 4 and 15. They may or may not notice the symptoms, which generally include only a short-lived fever and mild tiredness.

Those who manage to escape Epstein-Barr infection during childhood usually contract it in adolescence or young adulthood. Over half of all college students have antibodies to the Epstein-Barr virus, and each year 12 to 13 percent of the remaining students acquire them—usually after experiencing the symptoms of full-blown mononucleosis, which is a much more prolonged and exhausting illness in adolescence and young adulthood than in childhood. Even so, mononucleosis is not usually a serious disease and clears up on its own after several weeks of bed rest or relative inactivity.

Who is likely to develop mono?

Mononucleosis (also known as mono and infectious mononucleosis) is most common in adolescents and young adults of either sex but can occur at any age.

What are the symptoms?

Mononucleosis almost always involves several weeks of low-grade fever, fatigue, weakness, sore throat, and swollen glands. There can be a large number of other symptoms, including a red rash, sore muscles and joints, nausea, nasal congestion, enlargement of the spleen, headache, abdominal pain, bleeding gums, lack of appetite, rapid or irregular heartbeat, and sensitivity to light.

After the initial symptoms subside, it may take several months before the body fully regains its normal energy levels, and sometimes relapses occur. Occasionally, a mild form of hepatitis (inflammation of the liver) may occur, too, resulting in jaundice (a yellowing of the skin). More severe complications are rare but may include certain neurological problems, infection of the heart, breathing difficulties, and, most seriously, rupture of the spleen.

How is the condition evaluated?

The vast number of symptoms associated with mononucleosis sometimes make it difficult to diagnose. When symptoms last at least a week, most people suspect that they have something more serious than a cold, and they seek medical attention. A clinician can use various blood tests to see if the Epstein-Barr virus is present in the bloodstream or to count the number of unusual lymphocytes (white blood cells), which tend to be quite numerous during an active infection.

How is mono treated?

There is no specific treatment available to eradicate the Epstein-Barr virus. Bed rest alone is usually sufficient to clear up the symptoms after 2 to 3 weeks—although it may take 2 to 3 months before normal energy levels return. Often a clinician will recommend gargling with saltwater or using throat sprays such as Chloraseptic to relieve a sore throat. Both sore throat and fever can be alleviated by drinking plenty of fluids, as well as by taking over-the-counter pain relievers. If there is nasal congestion, a decongestant such as pseudoephedrine hydrochloride (Sudafed), which does not cause drowsiness, can help.

After the initial symptoms have disappeared, it is still a good idea to avoid strenuous activity, and contact sports in particular, for several weeks. This is especially true if there is any evidence of an enlarged spleen because of the possibility of rupture. A ruptured spleen is life-threatening and requires emergency surgery. A physician should be contacted immediately if there is any sudden, sharp pain in the upper left side of the abdomen.

How can mono be prevented?

Unlike many other infectious diseases, mononucleosis is relatively difficult to spread from person to person. This is an advantage for someone with the disease—who should feel free to mingle with other people. About the only way to prevent the spread of the disease is to avoid direct contact with the saliva of those people with an active infection—that is, avoid kissing them.

Related entries

Abdominal pain, chronic fatigue syndrome, colds, fatigue, headache

---

Morning Sickness

Morning sickness is a term commonly used to describe the nausea or vomiting that occurs in at least a third of all pregnant women. Despite the name, the symptoms can occur at any time of day, either constantly or intermittently.

The cause of morning sickness is not well understood, but the increased level of certain hormones early in pregnancy probably plays a large role. Estrogen is thought to produce nausea and regurgitation of stomach acids in some women, but these symptoms may be aggravated by other factors such as hunger, fatigue, prenatal vitamins (especially those containing iron), odors, and diet, as well as psychosocial factors.

Who is likely to develop morning sickness?

Any pregnant woman can develop morning sickness, although many never do. Usually morning sickness is more pronounced during the early weeks of the pregnancy and disappears after the third or fourth month. Occasionally it lasts until delivery.

What are the symptoms?

Some pregnant women vomit every morning upon rising, while others find that symptoms appear daily in the late afternoon, and still others simply feel queasy constantly from morning till night. Many pregnant women are very sensitive to odors, which can trigger bouts of nausea. In a small percentage of pregnant women the nausea and vomiting become so severe that malnutrition, dehydration, and possibly even weight loss result. Often the balance of fluids and electrolytes in the body becomes disturbed as well. This condition is called hyperemesis gravidarum.

Women who are having their first baby or who have a relatively high body weight are at increased risk for developing this severe form of morning sickness, as are relatively affluent white women. Because this problem also develops frequently in women who are young, unmarried, and dependent, some investigators think that, at least in some instances, there may be a psychological component.

How is morning sickness treated?

For many pregnant women morning sickness is a minor annoyance that is relieved with the thought that it is part of the normal process of pregnancy. Sometimes the discomfort can be reduced by modifying eating patterns.

Women with morning sickness used to be prescribed various medications, but this has become less common in routine cases because of the concern about birth defects. In cases of hyperemesis gravidarum, however, intravenous fluids and medications to prevent vomiting are administered, and hospitalization is sometimes required. Among the medications frequently prescribed are Compazine, Tigan, Phenergan, and Reglan, all of which can be given orally, intravenously, or as rectal suppositories and are considered safe for use during pregnancy.

Sometimes it is possible to avoid hospitalization by switching to a diet of clear liquids and bland food rich in carbohydrates. Consulting a social worker or psychologist to discuss feelings about the pregnancy and explore any psychological component of the illness may help; hypnosis, too, has relieved symptoms in some cases. Even in the more severe cases of morning sickness the outcome of pregnancy is generally good.

How can morning sickness be prevented?

Many of the recommended changes in diet are based on women's collective experience rather than any hard scientific data. For this reason what may work for one woman may make matters worse for another, so personal experimentation is the best approach. Among the many practices that have helped relieve and prevent morning sickness in some women are:

- Spreading meals out throughout the day, and eating 5 to 6 light meals rather than 3 big ones, to keep the stomach from becoming completely empty
- Eating a light, sweet bedtime snack
- Munching on dry toast, saltine crackers, salted pretzels, a banana or peeled apple, or a peeled cooked potato

- Keeping saltine crackers or other foods at the bedside and eating them upon awakening
- Eating anything that seems appealing—potato chips, lemonade, watermelon cubes—since any calories kept down, even from junk food, are better than no calories
- Eating a high-carbohydrate diet which contains plenty of vitamin B_6 (found in foods such as leafy vegetables, whole grain breads, and pasta)
- Eating a high-protein diet (though many pregnant women cannot bear even smelling meat or other high-protein foods during the early part of their pregnancy)
- Avoiding citrus juice, coffee, and tea
- Avoiding greasy foods
- Drinking herbal teas, apricot nectar, ginger ale, or other non-diet carbonated beverages
- Drinking very hot or very cold beverages
- Rising slowly from bed and sitting quietly for a few minutes before rushing into the day
- Trying alternative therapies such as hypnosis and acupressure
- Taking capsules of powdered ginger root (available in health food stores), particularly if the ginger is contained in a gelatin capsule to prevent irritation of the esophagus
- Before getting out of bed, sampling some dry popcorn, crackers, or dry toast kept at the bedside

One study has confirmed the effectiveness of wristbands once used exclusively for motion sickness and seasickness. Worn around the wrist(s) at a point about 3 finger widths from the joint (a traditional acupuncture point), these bands are available at many pharmacies and marine supply stores and are sold under various brand names (including Sea Bands).

Related entries

Estrogen, nutrition, postpartum issues, postpartum psychiatric disorders, pregnancy, prenatal care, psychotherapy

Multiple Sclerosis

Multiple sclerosis is an often crippling disease of the central nervous system that afflicts an estimated 150,000 to 500,000 Americans. In MS, an extremely unpredictable disease, the fatty protective coating (myelin) that surrounds nerves in the brain and spinal cord is lost in numerous areas. This process, which is called demyelination, appears to be an autoimmune

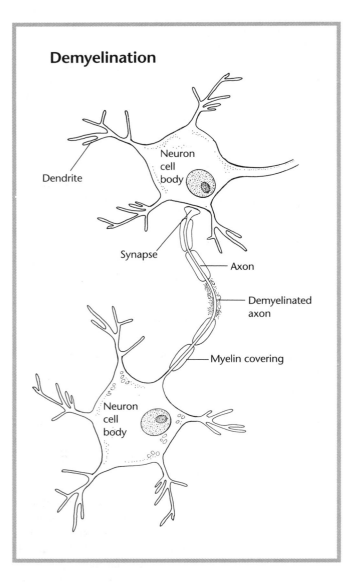

Demyelination

Dendrite

Neuron cell body

Synapse

Axon

Demyelinated axon

Myelin covering

Neuron cell body

process—that is, a process resulting from the body's directing antibodies and white blood cells against itself. The myelin is replaced by hardened (sclerotic) plaques and scar tissue (see illustration). Myelin normally facilitates the speedy and efficient transmission of messages between the brain and the body; once it is lost, these signals are slowed or even blocked completely.

Depending on just where the demyelination has occurred, the result can be loss of coordination, problems with balance, vision disturbances, bowel or bladder incontinence, or a wide variety of other symptoms. These usually occur in episodes (attacks) of 2 to 6 weeks in duration and then may disappear (remit) for months or even years. It is possible that these periods of remission occur at times when the myelin repairs itself. Much of the time, however, symptoms recur and become progressively more severe.

Most people with MS can expect to live an average of 35 years beyond the initial diagnosis. Although there is no cure, many continue to lead active and often quite mobile lives, especially during periods of remission. Slightly over 10 percent

of people with MS have only 1 or 2 attacks and never go on to have further problems. This form of MS is called benign sensory MS.

The vast majority of people with MS have a form of the disease called relapsing-remitting MS, which involves recurrent attacks and remissions, with attacks occurring every 1 to 3 years. These attacks usually last a few weeks or months and gradually subside. In some people, the attacks become more severe and disabling over time. Most of these people eventually (after 7 to 10 years, on average) go on to develop secondary progressive MS, a phase of the disease that involves continuous deteriorioration and sudden relapses.

About 10 percent have primary progressive MS, in which there are no real attacks but rather constant symptoms that progressively worsen over the years. Fewer than 5 percent of patients have a virulent form of MS called progressive relapsing MS, which, in rare cases, can be fatal within weeks.

The cause of MS remains a mystery. One school of thought is that it is an autoimmune disease, in which the body's immune system destroys its own myelin and myelin-making cells. People with MS do seem to have abnormally high concentrations of immune cells in their central nervous system. Other researchers contend that these immune dysfunctions may be traceable to some slow-acting virus which was acquired early in life and which decades later begins to damage either the immune system generally or the myelin directly.

Women are almost twice as likely as men to develop MS. The disease seems to have no relation to the menstrual cycle nor any effect on fertility. Women with MS can become pregnant and deliver healthy babies. But while the illness has no known effect on pregnancy, pregnancy's effects on the course of the disease are still poorly understood. For some women symptoms temporarily improve during pregnancy (possibly because the immune system is suppressed), but for others just the opposite occurs. In addition, the stress of pregnancy and child rearing can exacerbate symptoms for some women. For these reasons a woman with MS who is thinking about becoming pregnant should carefully consider her current health status, her ability to care for children should her condition worsen, and her individual response to stress.

Who is likely to develop MS?

Multiple sclerosis is usually diagnosed in people between the ages of 20 and 40. Neurological deficits in women often begin in their early 20s, while in men symptoms tend to appear about 5 years later. The disease is twice as prevalent in whites as in other ethnic groups and seems to occur more often in people of relatively high socioeconomic status. People living in northern (that is, colder) climates of the northern hemisphere—including the northern half of the United States—also seem unusually prone to the disease, with a predominance in the Western industrialized nations. MS rarely occurs in tropical and subtropical regions. In the southern hemisphere, the prevalence increases in groups of people living farther south of the equator. Geography seems to be most significant before the age of 15, however. People who move to southern climates of the northern hemisphere after that age are just as likely to get MS as people who still live in northern climates. The same is true for people who move north after a childhood in the South.

MS is not inherited or contagious, but there does seem to be a predisposition toward it in certain families. This may be because of some inherited factor that increases the likelihood of immune system malfunction—perhaps after exposure to a virus. Much more research must be done before these speculations can be confirmed. People of European, particularly Scandinavian, descent seem particularly prone to MS, and having a close relative with the disease increases the odds of developing it by a factor of 10.

What are the symptoms?

Most people with MS have symptoms in the form of attacks that come and go. The nature of the symptoms themselves depends on which part of the central nervous system has been demyelinated. Among the most common symptoms are loss of coordination, unsteady gait, dim or blurry vision, eye pain, tremors, involuntary movements, incontinence, fatigue, tingling, muscle weakness, numbness or paralysis in the arms or legs, and slurred speech. Stress and heat (even from taking a hot bath or spending too much time in the sun) often make symptoms worse.

Some degree of sexual disturbance or dysfunction is common in people with multiple sclerosis. Part of this may be due to pain, discomfort, and fatigue, as well as changes in body image that often accompany a chronic disease. There may be considerable anxiety about losing control of bowel or bladder function during sex as well. In many women damage to the nervous system may physically alter sexual response, making arousal more difficult or interfering with clitoral swelling and vaginal lubrication. Loss of muscle control and problems with balance can also be problematic.

Some of these problems can be overcome through communication with an understanding partner who is willing to try more satisfying or comfortable sexual techniques and positions. If incontinence is a concern, it may help to empty the bladder and bowels just before sex. Water-based vaginal lubricants can help relieve problems of vaginal dryness. In some cases couples may need or choose to express affection and receive sexual gratification through means other than sexual intercourse.

Virtually any method of birth control can be used effectively, although intrauterine devices (IUDs) are usually advised against in women with limited pelvic sensation because they may be unable to sense the pain of a pelvic infection. Women with poor hand coordination may also have trouble checking the IUD string for slippage each month. Poor coordination can also impede the use of a diaphragm, as can weak pelvic muscles. The many women with MS who are susceptible to urinary tract infections may find that use of a diaphragm increases the frequency of these infections.

How is the condition evaluated?

Multiple sclerosis can often be difficult to diagnose because the wide-ranging symptoms are shared by so many other dis-orders—including stroke, brain tumors, neuritis (inflammation of a nerve), syphilis, and chronic fatigue syndrome. If symptoms such as altered reflexes or sensation begin between the ages of 20 and 50, however, and tend to recur and remit, a clinician will almost certainly suspect MS and refer the patient to a neurologist.

The advent of magnetic resonance imaging (MRI) has made it easier to confirm the diagnosis of MS, since this technique can show the number and location of sclerotic lesions in the brain and spinal cord. Sometimes a computer analysis of the nervous system's electrical response to stimuli (an evoked potential test) may be used in the evaluation, as well as a lumbar puncture (spinal tap) to analyze the immune status of the spinal fluid.

How is multiple sclerosis treated?

There is no cure for MS, but many symptoms—including spasticity, bladder problems, depression, pain, fatigue, sexual dysfunction, and some forms of weakness—can often be relieved with a combination of medication, physical therapy, and psychological support.

Whenever possible, treating MS in its early stages (before it becomes progressive) is the most effective approach, although people with benign sensory MS usually benefit from counseling and careful observation alone. If attacks are becoming fairly frequent or intense, relatively new injectable medications—either of two beta-interferons (Avonex or Betaseron) or glatiramer acetate (Copaxone)—that help regulate the immune system can be used to prevent relapses and limit disability. These drugs are currently prescribed to people with active relapsing-remitting MS. Patients can inject themselves with these drugs, which can reduce flare-ups, at least over the short term. The beta-interferons, however, can produce intolerable side effects such as flulike symptoms in some people and may even lead to the development of antibodies that counteract their effects. In addition, neither the beta-interferons nor glatiramer should be used during pregnancy or breastfeeding. Occasionally high doses of immunoglobulin administered intravenously may be used as an alternative treatment, on the theory that these antibodies might stimulate the growth of new myelin. Whether or not this therapy is safe during pregnancy or breastfeeding remains unknown.

Symptoms such as unsteady gait, weakness, and vision loss are most commonly treated with high doses of corticosteroids, administered intravenously during the course of the attack. These drugs can be used in pregnancy. Muscle spasms can be treated with the muscle relaxants such as tizanidine hydrochloride (Zanaflex) or baclofen (Lioresal). Physical and rehabilitation therapy can play an important role in controlling symptoms of MS, as can avoiding excessive fatigue and high temperatures. Eating a balanced diet and getting adequate rest may be helpful in preventing minor infections and relapses. Regular exercise is important, too, although people with MS have to be careful to incorporate an appropriate recovery period into their routine. This may mean resting for as many as 3 to 4 days after each workout. Many people find that swimming, other water exercises, or even walking in water is particularly beneficial, so long as water temperature does not exceed 70 to 80°F. Regular massage can also improve muscle tone and boost circulation as well as provide relief from pain and stiffness.

Progressive forms of MS require different forms of treatment. Usually the drug of choice is an agent that suppresses the immune system such as cyclophosphamide, mitoxantrone, methotrexate, and azathiopine, sometimes while continuing beta-interferon treatments. These chemotherapeutic drugs, however, often used to treat cancer, are highly toxic, can be used for only a short time, and have limited benefits. Many can also cause particular problems for women. Cyclophosphamide, for example, can lead to premature menopause, and methotrexate cannot be used at any dosage during pregnancy.

Meanwhile, research in the pursuit of safer, more easily administered, and better-tolerated treatment options continues at a fast clip. One promising but still experimental therapy is plasma exchange, or lymphocytaphoresis, a technique in which white blood cells are mechanically removed from the blood; total radiation therapy of the lymph system; and treatment with octacosanol, which may help repair and strengthen myelin. Less-studied possibilities include acupuncture or acupressure treatments to reduce fatigue and relax stiff muscles; various forms of bodywork to preserve coordination; music therapy to relieve pain; drugs that stimulate the production of vitamin D-3, which appears to regulate the immune system; and even low-fat and other special diets to relieve symptoms in general.

Related entries
Antiinflammatory drugs, autoimmune disorders, birth control, body image, chronic fatigue syndrome, exercise, fatigue, incontinence, lubricants, preconception counseling, sexual dysfunction, sexual response, stress, stroke, urinary tract infections

Musculoskeletal Disorders

The musculoskeletal system includes the muscles and bones as well as the joints that connect one bone to another and the tendons that connect muscles to bones. This system, which protects internal organs and allows the body to move, can break down as a result of infection, inflammation, disease, injuries, or simple wear and tear.

One out of every 7 visits to primary care physicians is for musculoskeletal symptoms. Most of these are due to disorders of the connective tissues. Connective tissue disorders that are more common in women than in men include lupus, fibromyalgia, scleroderma, polymyositis and dermatomyositis, and rheumatoid arthritis (see autoimmune disorders for descriptions).

Women are also particularly likely to develop musculoskeletal disorders in distinct regions of the body such as the hands, wrists, elbows, lower back, jaw, and knees. Elderly women are particularly prone to osteoporosis, which can lead to broken bones. Many of these disorders are briefly described below.

Carpal tunnel syndrome. This painful but treatable condition of the hands and wrists results from the compression of the median nerve, which runs through a narrow passageway in the wrists to carry messages between the brain and the thumb, index finger, middle finger, and inner half of the ring finger. Occurring in about 1 out of every 1,000 people, carpal tunnel syndrome (see entry) is particularly common in women aged 50 to 70. It is also common in people who perform forceful, repetitive hand movements, particularly those that involve bending the wrist. These include typists, grocery store checkout clerks, factory workers, carpenters, upholsterers, meat packers, violinists, and waitresses, as well as people who knit, crochet, hook rugs, paint, do woodwork, or garden frequently. Conditions sometimes associated with carpal tunnel syndrome include rheumatoid arthritis, thyroid disease, diabetes, and pregnancy.

DeQuervain's tenosynovitis. Tenosynovitis (see tendinitis and tenosynovitis) is an inflammation of the protective membrane surrounding each tendon. In deQuervain's tenosynovitis, which occurs 9 times more often in women than in men, tendons in the thumb become inflamed and the sheaths surrounding them narrow. People with deQuervain's cannot flex their thumb fully, or else require external force to straighten it once it is flexed. DeQuervain's tenosynovitis occurs most frequently after activities involving repeated forceful extensions, pinches, or twists of the thumb, such as prolonged use of a screwdriver, typing, or lifting a baby or child by the armpits.

Osteoarthritis. The painful joints of osteoarthritis (see entry) are due primarily to gradual loss of cartilage rather than to inflammation. Cartilage (the connective tissue that lines joints and protects the ends of bones from rubbing against one another) can break down because of physical injury, mechanical stress, or some underlying metabolic abnormality. Women are particularly likely to experience degenerative changes in the joint at the base of the thumb as well as the knuckles (50 percent of women over 50 have some degree of osteoarthritis of the hands). Osteoarthritis also tends to occur in joints exposed to weight-bearing and stress, especially the knees, hips, spine, and big toe. Obesity can predispose people to osteoarthritis. About 30 percent of women aged 65 to 75 have noticeable symptoms of osteoarthritis of the knees.

Knee pain. Anterior knee pain involves pain in the joint connecting the kneecap and the thighbone. It is probably the most common cause of knee disability in people under 40, with many more women affected than men. It occurs when excessive tension in supporting ligaments causes the knee-cap to deviate to the side of the thighbone. Pain is usually felt just behind the kneecap and intensifies during kneeling, squatting, or walking downstairs. Over time excessive tension can break down the cartilage in the joint.

Knee pain (see entry) can also occur because of osteoarthritis and bursitis (see below).

Tennis elbow. Usually having nothing to do with playing tennis, this condition is probably caused by numerous small tears in the tendons that attach the lower arm muscles to the elbow. It often occurs after activities or exercises that involve repetitive rotating motion of the forearm. These can include various activities such as tennis, bowling, and badminton, as well as painting or using tools such as a screwdriver or wrench. The characteristic symptom of tennis elbow is recurrent pain on the outer, upper part of the forearm which may radiate down to the wrist. Usually moving the elbow or wrist worsens the pain. Symptoms generally develop gradually (see tendinitis and tenosynovitis).

Bursitis. Bursitis means inflammation of the bursa, a fluid-filled sac found in many joints that limits friction between the bone and the muscles and tendons. Because women are more apt than men to be engaged in activities such as lifting and carrying small children, they are at risk particularly for bursitis in the shoulders and knees (see knee pain). These conditions can also develop after athletic activities or in chronic osteoarthritis.

Temporomandibular joint syndrome. TMJ is a common disorder of the joint that connects either side of the jawbone (mandible) to the skull. Symptoms include sinus or jaw pain and tenderness, limited jaw movement, dull and diffuse earache, ringing in the ears, dizziness, headaches, and a clicking or popping sound while chewing. Pain may also affect the eyes, teeth, head, neck, shoulders, and back, and often worsens during or after eating or yawning. Between 70 and 90 percent of people experiencing symptoms of temporomandibular joint syndrome (see entry) are women between the ages of 24 and 40. The syndrome develops in 1 of 5 people with rheumatoid arthritis and is also common in people who have suffered from whiplash, trauma to the face, or emotional stress that leads them to grind their teeth (bruxism) or clench their jaw, particularly during sleep.

Osteoporosis. Osteoporosis (which literally means porous bones) is a systemic disease in which the bones gradually lose their store of calcium and other minerals and become less dense and more susceptible to fracture from even slight trauma. It occurs in both sexes and all ethnic groups but is particularly prevalent in women after menopause. As many as one-quarter of white women past menopause have some degree of osteoporosis, and 90 percent of all women past the age of 75 are affected. An activity as nonstrenuous as vigorous coughing is enough to fracture a rib in a woman with se-

vere osteoporosis. The result may be sharp pain that becomes worse with every inhalation of air or with bending or twisting the torso. Nearly a third of all women who live to age 90 can expect to have a hip fracture related to osteoporosis (see entry), and of these as many as 1 in 5 will die from complications within several months, usually from pneumonia or a blood clot in the lungs caused by prolonged bed rest.

Scoliosis. Scoliosis (the sideways curvature of the spine; see entry) is particularly common in women; approximately two-thirds of scoliosis patients are adolescent women. In most cases the cause is not well understood, although there is good evidence that genes are involved to some extent. The problem usually goes unnoticed—or does not develop—until a girl is between 10 and 16 years old.

Costochondritis. Inflammation of the junctions between the ribs and the cartilage is 3 times more common in women than in men. It can develop after excessive coughing, unaccustomed exercise, lifting heavy objects, or bruising nearby muscles. It takes the form of a dull, gnawing tenderness in the chest that lasts for hours or days, but occasionally it can be sharp and fleeting. Pressing on the front of the rib cage usually exacerbates this type of chest pain (see entry), as do bending, twisting, and other exercises that involve moving the ribs.

Related entries

Arthritis, autoimmune disorders, back pain, carpal tunnel syndrome, chest pain, fibromyalgia, knee pain, lupus, osteoarthritis, osteoporosis, polymyositis and dermatomyositis, Raynaud's phenomenon, rheumatoid arthritis, scleroderma, scoliosis, sports injuries, Sjögren syndrome, temporomandibular joint syndrome, tendinitis and tenosynovitis

Myasthenia Gravis

Myasthenia gravis is a rare autoimmune disorder characterized by episodes of muscular weakness. Because myasthenia gravis usually involves the voluntary muscles of the face, throat, chest, and limbs, it can cause considerable distress and complicate everyday activity. It becomes life-threatening when the muscles that control breathing are affected—as happens in about 1 of 10 people with the disease.

The most common form of myasthenia gravis is thought to occur when—for reasons that remain obscure—the body's immune system attacks receptor cells for acetylcholine, a neurotransmitter that induces muscles to contract. Most people with the disease also have abnormalities of the thymus gland, a small organ in the throat that produces T-cells, a form of white blood cells (lymphocytes) that play an important role in immunity.

Women with myasthenia gravis can become pregnant and deliver healthy babies, although special monitoring is advisable during the pregnancy. Some women even find that their symptoms disappear spontaneously during pregnancy. In 15 percent of cases, however, antibodies may be transferred through the placenta and result in a form of generalized muscle weakness in the newborn called neonatal myasthenia. Although symptoms of this disorder soon clear up as the abnormal antibody levels drop, special medical care may be needed for several weeks.

Who is likely to develop myasthenia gravis?
Estimated to afflict 1 in every 10,000 Americans, it can occur in anyone, but it most commonly afflicts women of reproductive age.

What are the symptoms?
Symptoms of myasthenia gravis usually occur following exercise or exertion and improve with rest. The most common symptoms are drooping eyelids and double vision. Many people with myasthenia gravis also go through periods when it is difficult to speak, chew, or even swallow, and they may have periodic weakness in the arms or legs. If the respiratory muscles are affected, breathing may become difficult as well—a situation that obviously calls for immediate medical attention.

How is the condition evaluated?
Because myasthenia gravis is a relatively rare disease and shares symptoms with other, less serious conditions, it sometimes goes undiagnosed for long periods of time. Usually, however, a clinician will suspect it in a young woman who complains of episodes of muscular weakness that improve after rest. To confirm the diagnosis, a drug called edrophonium may be administered. If myasthenia gravis is indeed the problem, symptoms will suddenly—but temporarily—improve. If there is any uncertainty, however, various neurologic and electrophysiologic tests may also be done to measure the function of the nerves and muscles, and blood may be drawn and checked to see if it contains the antibodies usually associated with the disease.

How is myasthenia gravis treated?
Approximately one-quarter of all cases resolve on their own. In those remaining, there are a number of different treatment options. Having surgery to remove the thymus gland (thymectomy) or taking certain corticosteroid or immunosuppressive medications (such as prednisone) can alter the course of the disease by slowing the body's immune response.

Symptoms of the disease can sometimes be relieved, too, with certain anticholinesterase drugs (such as pyridostigmine or neostigmine). Symptomatic relief can also be obtained through a procedure called plasmapheresis, in which blood is pumped from the patient's body and cleansed of the plasma which contains damaging antibodies.

Planning activities to take advantage of energy peaks and scheduling daily rest periods can help minimize the impact of this disease on one's everyday life. Taking medication about 30 minutes before meals can reduce chewing and swallowing difficulties. Double vision can be relieved by wearing an eye patch. Since stress can worsen the condition, patients and their families need to work out routines of cooperation that reduce day-to-day stress levels.

Related entry
Autoimmune disorders

Myomectomy

Myomectomy is a means of removing uterine fibroids surgically while leaving the uterus itself intact. An alternative to hysterectomy, myomectomy can be an effective way to alleviate some of the menstrual symptoms associated with fibroids if drug therapy has been unsuccessful. It is particularly appealing to women who want to retain childbearing capacity or to preserve the uterus for other reasons.

How is the procedure performed?
Usually large fibroids, which are difficult to extract through the vagina, are removed through an abdominal incision called a laparotomy (see entry). This procedure, which must be done in a hospital and involves general anesthesia, can take anywhere from 1 to 5 hours—in contrast with the hour or two that is typical of a hysterectomy. Depending on the size and location of the fibroids, however, it may be possible to have a less invasive type of myomectomy. Smaller fibroids, for example, are sometimes amenable to a hysteroscopic myomectomy, a procedure in which fibroids are removed through the vagina with a thin, telescope-like instrument called a hysteroscope (see hysteroscopy) which is inserted through the vagina into the uterus. No abdominal incision is necessary, blood loss is reduced, and hospitalization is much shorter.

Alternatively, a procedure called a laparoscopic myomectomy may be performed, in which the fibroids are removed with the aid of a laparoscope (see laparoscopy). This procedure is done under general anesthesia or, sometimes, regional anesthesia and requires a tiny incision (much smaller than the 4- to 5-inch incision required for a standard myomectomy) just under the navel.

What happens after surgery?
It can take as many as 4 to 6 weeks to recover from a standard myomectomy and return to normal activities. In contrast, women who have a laparoscopic or hysteroscopic myomec-

tomy can often go home from the hospital as soon as the surgery is over or the next day, and they generally recover completely in as few as 1 to 3 weeks.

What are the risks and complications?

The risks of a myomectomy performed by a skilled surgeon are similar to those of a hysterectomy and include a small chance of bleeding, infection, perforation of the uterus, and adverse reactions to anesthesia (including risk of death). In one-quarter of women fibroids may reappear after the myomectomy, sometimes leaving little choice but to do a hysterectomy after all. There is also a small possibility that adhesions (internal scarring) will develop after the surgery, possibly interfering with future fertility. For women who do become pregnant after a myomectomy, a cesarean section may be needed, depending on the specific nature of the myomectomy and the obstetrician's preferences.

Related entries

Adhesions, anesthesia, cesarean section, hysterectomy, hysteroscopy, infertility, laparoscopy, laparotomy, uterine fibroids

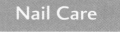

Nail Care

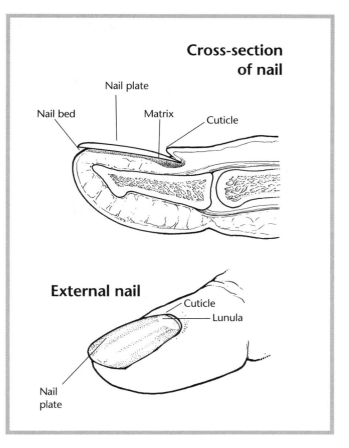

American women spend something on the order of $3 billion a year on nail care products and services. This is an astoundingly high figure, especially considering that there is virtually nothing that can be purchased to make nails grow faster or stronger. In fact, most dermatologists contend that the best way to ensure healthy nails is to clean and trim them regularly, protect them from injury and irritating detergents and chemicals, and eat a nutritious diet.

The basics of nail care

Healthy nails are pale pink, smooth, and shiny, and the surfaces are slightly rounded. They are made of dead skin cells that are hardened by a fibrous protein called keratin which grows out of living cells in the matrix below the cuticle (the whitish flap of skin at the base of the nails). Keratin is the same protein found in the hair.

Because nails are made of dead cells, no "growth formula" or "nail builder" is going to make the least bit of difference, other than coating the nail and possibly protecting it from daily trauma. Not only are most nail care products useless, but also many nail strengtheners can actually discolor or break nails, and cuticle removers can corrode the layer of keratin that naturally protects the nail.

Contrary to folklore, eating gelatin or taking calcium supplements does not have any effect on nail strength. Nails do seem to grow faster in hot weather, however, presumably because all metabolic processes speed up in the heat. Men's nails generally grow faster than women's, although hormonal changes during pregnancy and just before menstruation seem to spur nail growth in women. Nails of both men and women tend to grow more slowly and get thicker—as well as drier and more brittle—with age. They also grow more slowly during a serious illness.

Minor but frequent trauma to the nails—as experienced by typists, pianists, and nail biters—also seems to stimulate nail growth. Whether regular trimming has a similar effect is unclear, but in any case it seems to be essential for healthy nails. People who prefer their fingernails short will need to trim them about every week with nail clippers or manicure scissors. Women who choose to have long nails find that regular filing is necessary to prevent splits, which tend to attract dirt and therefore encourage infection.

Sometimes it is easier to clip nails after a bath or shower, especially if the nails tend to be thick or brittle. Despite the pronouncement of manicurists, cuticles should not be trimmed, since this may promote infection by opening up a route for the entry of microorganisms. Hangnails should be neatly clipped, not ripped off with the fingers, since this usually results in bleeding and possibly infection. Some dermatologists recommend softening the fingertips with hand lotion or hand cream to help prevent hangnails and cracked cuticles.

Toenails, which grow much more slowly than fingernails, need to be trimmed only about once a month. They should be clipped straight across and not too short. This helps prevent ingrown toenails, which form when the edge of the nail tip—which grows faster than the center—curls under and grows into the soft nail bed underneath. Wearing low-heeled, wide-toed shoes that fit properly also helps prevent ingrown toenails, since these can keep toes from being pinched or from sliding into the front of the shoe.

Wearing rubber gloves lined with cotton while doing housework may help prevent a variety of problems associated with excess exposure to water and detergents, including brittle and discolored nails as well as nail infection. Nondisposable gloves should be turned inside out to dry after each use to prevent the growth of bacteria and other microorganisms. Women prone to splitting nails should try to keep their hands out of water as much as possible and apply lotions both before and after washing hands. The best lotions contain alpha-hydroxy acids. At the same time, the cuticles should be pushed gently back from the nails with a soft cloth. This will help keep them from being torn.

Some women with long nails find it helpful to wear gloves during cold weather and for doing chores such as gardening, which can traumatize the nails. Some women even wear thin cotton or silk gloves or darkroom gloves (from camera stores) when putting away groceries and sorting laundry. Other women train themselves to use the pads of their fingertips instead of their nails and to learn various nail-saving tricks, such as dialing phone numbers with a pencil instead of a fingertip.

Manicures, pedicures, polishes, and press-ons

Many women find that manicures and pedicures improve the appearance of their nails and help prevent hangnails. Some women also feel that having a manicure motivates them to break a bad nail-biting habit. Aside from these benefits, however, elaborate manicures and pedicures, whether done at home or in an elegant salon, do not contribute to the strength or growth of nails.

Women who polish their nails should try to avoid extending the coat to the base of the nail—where it may cover up living tissue. A manicure will last longer if several thin coats of polish are applied rather than a single heavy layer. A few women are allergic to the formaldehyde that is often used as a hardening agent in nail polish. Signs of an allergy include a rash around the cuticles or separation of the nails from underlying tissue. These reactions can be avoided by using formaldehyde-free products and by making sure the polish never touches living tissue. Nail polish with nylon fibers may help protect fragile nails.

Most dermatologists also recommend limiting the use of nail polish remover to once a week, since it contains chemicals that tend to dry and weaken the nails. One way to cut down on use is to touch up chips or cracks with fresh polish or to repaint a new layer rather than redoing an entire nail after every mishap.

Women who bite their nails or have trouble growing them out sometimes elect to use artificial nails. These are available in relatively inexpensive "press-on" forms that can be applied at home, as well as in the form of costly salon treatments. A manicurist may apply acrylic tips, which are fake plastic nail ends stuck on with instant glue, filed, and then coated with an acrylic paste. Nail wraps are also available to extend nails that have grown out a bit on their own with a layer of fiberglass, linen, or silk. Whatever form of artificial nail is used, the natural nail continues to grow underneath it and eventually pushes it away from the growth zone at the nail base. The manicurist then has to fill in this space with acrylic paste every 2 weeks or so.

Not only can this whole business be quite costly—with the first application running around $50 and each "fill" costing close to $20—but also the gaps left at the nail base often trap moisture and provide a breeding ground for fungal infections. These infections can be severe enough to lead to the loss of the nail. The solvents and glues used in the acrylic powders encourage infection and also provoke allergic reactions in some women. Even the glue used to apply plastic press-on nails can pose problems.

Women who enjoy having manicures and pedicures may be able to minimize some of these risks by using a licensed manicurist—or, in states without adequate standards, looking for a manicurist with documented training, sufficient experience, and recent refresher courses. More important is making sure the manicurist sterilizes her tools in a heat-pressurized sterilizer. Nail polish remover and alcohol are not adequate to prevent fungal infections or warts.

Spots, splits, infections, and other problems

White flecks under the nail. For years many so-called experts have attributed these common little white dots under the nail to some kind of vitamin or mineral deficiency or even to some serious systemic disease. At present, however, there is no evidence confirming these theories. It seems much more likely that they are due to minor injury (such as excessive pressure exerted on the cuticle during a manicure). They may even be nothing more than pockets of air. Eventually these spots disappear on their own, although this sometimes takes years.

Discolorations and injuries. A black spot under a nail—often the thumbnail—is usually blood that has accumulated after the finger has been crushed or hit with a heavy object. In more serious injuries the entire nail may be lost. Sometimes nails also become discolored after exposure to harsh chemicals or as a reaction to certain medications.

Discolorations almost always disappear by themselves. (A permanent dark discoloration of a nail should be evaluated by a dermatologist for the possibility of melanoma.) Given that fingernails grow only about an eighth of an inch per month and toenails only about a twenty-fourth of an inch, however, it is no surprise that signs of injury take several months to grow out. It takes approximately 6 months for a new fingernail to grow in from start to finish.

Peeling and splitting. Brittle nails that peel or split easily most often signal inadequate nutrition or overexposure to strong detergents or chemicals. These conditions can be exacerbated by the overuse of nail-hardening products, which are often first applied after a peeling or splitting problem has begun. Dishwashing is a common culprit, not just because of the detergents but also because of the frequent immersion of hands in water, which temporarily swells nail tips. Repeated cycles of swelling and then shrinking back to normal eventually take their toll on the nail's durability. If nail breaking is associated with hair loss, weight gain, constipation, and bloating, a clinician should be consulted to rule out thyroid disease.

Ingrown toenails. Ingrown toenails are often an extremely painful condition, most common in the big toe. They occur when the edge of the nail tip grows under into the nail bed. This happens most commonly in women who wear tight, ill-fitting shoes or high heels, but it is also common in older people, whose nails often curve excessively.

An ingrown toenail can sometimes be treated at home by cutting off the excess nail and then elevating the affected edge by stuffing tiny pieces of sterile cotton between the nail and the underlying skin. This cotton should be changed every day, and comfortable, low-heeled shoes should be worn until all signs of inflammation have disappeared. If there is severe pain or a discharge of pus, the nail bed is probably infected and a clinician should be consulted as soon as possible. Usually ingrown toenails can be corrected with a simple surgical procedure.

Fungal and other infections. Any kind of cut, hangnail, or separation of the nail from the nail bed can open an easy entryway for microorganisms, leading to infection of the nail bed (called paronychia). Even frequent immersion of the hands in water can lay the groundwork for paronychia. Infections that develop slowly are usually due to yeast or fungi, particularly the kinds that cause athlete's foot and thrush. These infections, which often affect several nails at a time and can be quite persistent, can damage nail roots and result in discolored and deformed nails. If the nails themselves are infected, they may thicken and turn whitish and powdery.

In addition to keeping the nails as clean and dry as possible, one can treat fungal infections with oral antifungal medications. Topical medications applied directly to the nail are rarely effective. Itraconazole (Sporanox) is a newer oral drug that appears to be more effective than older ones (such as griseofulvin or ketoconazole). Oral drugs usually need to be taken for several months until the nail has grown out completely. Over-the-counter topical preparations are usually not strong enough to treat these infections, and oral preparations can be costly. Given the possibility of side effects—such as abnormal liver function, headache, rashes, insomnia, and confusion—some people simply opt to live with fungal infections, which are harmless if unsightly. Oral antifungal drugs are considered unsafe for use during pregnancy. A clinician should be consulted before use during breastfeeding.

Bacterial infections of the nails usually develop more quickly and tend to be more painful than fungal infections. Often there is redness, swelling, and severe pain at the side of the nail or near the cuticle, and pus may ooze out when the nail is pressed. If the skin along the side of the nail is infected, a blister of pus (a whitlow) may develop. Antibiotics may clear up these infections if used early enough, but sometimes it is necessary to have the blister lanced by a clinician to drain the pus.

Nail problems as signs of disease

Nails that are discolored, ridged, split, thickened, or misshapen may reflect improper hygiene and diet—or may simply be variants of normal nails. Occasionally, however, they can also serve as important clues to serious disease elsewhere in the body.

Pale nails, for example, may be an early sign of anemia. If the anemia is severe enough, the nails eventually become brittle, and their surfaces may become flat or concave like a spoon. They often also develop longitudinal ridges. Bluish nails (cyanosis), by contrast, can signal exposure to a toxic chemical such as excess copper or silver. If accompanied by shortness of breath and coughing, they can also indicate some degree of heart failure or a chronic lung disorder. Opaque, whitish nails may be a sign of liver disease, particularly chronic hepatitis or cirrhosis, while a whitish color at the base of the nail may signal chronic kidney disease. If the whitish half-moon (lunula; see illustration) that is normally present at the base of the nail (and most visible on the thumb) becomes faded, there may be a problem with the pituitary gland.

Nails that develop horizontal lines and ridges may reflect exposure to some toxic chemical or poison, or a recent serious illness or surgery. Nails may split or become deformed when arthritis inflames the finger joints. Brittle nails that separate easily from the nail bed sometimes suggest an underactive thyroid gland. But if the nails are concave in addition to being brittle and loose, the problem may turn out to be an overactive thyroid gland.

If the only problem is a separation of the trimmed end of the nail from the underlying skin (sometimes accompanied by little round pits), the problem may be psoriasis, a condition in which silvery white scales cover parts of the skin, or a fungal infection. If bacteria enter this space, the nail may appear black or greenish. In any case a dermatologist or other physician should usually be consulted, since the trimmed end of the nail may separate from the underlying skin in a variety of other conditions as well, including a vitamin deficiency or clogging of the arteries with plaque.

Clubbed fingernails, which are extremely rounded like the back of a spoon and, when viewed from the side, run into the skin in a straight line, may occur in many different diseases. These include congenital heart disease, lung cancer, long-standing infections, abscesses, chronic heart and lung disorders, and tuberculosis.

A woman who notices a painless "splinter" under her nail should consult a clinician right away, since this may actually be a small hemorrhage characteristic of bacterial endocarditis. This infection of the membrane that covers the interior of the heart is particularly likely in women with mitral valve prolapse (a "ballooning out" of one of the valves of the heart), heart murmurs, or other defects of the heart valves. Splinter-like hemorrhages under the nails can also be due to trichinosis, an infection that can result from eating raw or undercooked pork, as well as from a variety of autoimmune and connective tissue disorders.

Finally, chewed and bitten nails can be a sign of excessive emotional stress—particularly when nails are gnawed to the point of bleeding—though nail biting is sometimes nothing more than a disfiguring habit.

Related entries

Anemia, antibiotics, body image, cosmetic safety, foot care, hair loss, headaches, heart disease, hyperthyroidism, hypothyroidism, insomnia, kidney disorders, lupus, mitral valve prolapse, polymyositis and dermatomyositis, skin care and cosmetics, stress, thyroid disorders

Natural Birth Control Methods

The three natural—as opposed to "artificial"—birth control methods practiced most frequently are withdrawal, periodic abstinence, and fertility observation. Both withdrawal and periodic abstinence depend primarily on good timing and self-control. Sometimes they are assisted by fertility observation, in which a woman monitors her basal body temperature and cervical mucus changes in order to determine when she is and is not fertile.

The only health risk associated with natural birth control techniques (aside from the fact that they offer no protection from sexually transmitted diseases, including AIDS) is pregnancy if the method fails.

Withdrawal

Also known as coitus interruptus, this is a widely used method of contraception in which the man removes his penis from the woman's vagina and vaginal lips before ejaculation occurs. One major drawback to the method is that many men secrete a small number of sperm long before they actually ejaculate, and even one sperm can ascend the female reproductive tract and fertilize an egg.

Using withdrawal as a means of contraception requires that the man remember to pull his penis away from the vaginal area before ejaculation begins. No further intercourse or other penis-vagina contact can occur after the first ejaculation, since some sperm inevitably remain on the penis. The efficacy of withdrawal is comparable to that of barrier methods of contraception: the lowest expected failure rate is 4 percent if used perfectly, although a more typical failure rate is 19 percent.

The reality is that women who rely on the withdrawal method often end up pregnant, perhaps because it is a difficult method to comply with perfectly. Many couples find that withdrawal greatly interferes with sexual enjoyment. Not only does the man have to remember to withdraw in time, but also many men find withdrawal itself frustrating, and many women, who may not have reached orgasm before withdrawal has to occur, find the process unsatisfying. In addition, some women worry so much about premature ejaculation that they cannot relax, and this may further interfere with orgasm.

Still, couples who use this method for long periods of time often find ways to incorporate it into a satisfying sex life. Also, using withdrawal as a means of contraception involves no prior planning or effort. Some couples choose to combine withdrawal with fertility observation, so that during infertile times of the month ejaculation can occur inside the vagina.

Periodic abstinence

This term includes a number of subtly different practices including those known as natural birth control, fertility observation, and the rhythm method. All require no artificial devices to prevent conception but instead rely on timing acts of sexual intercourse so that they do not occur during the most fertile part of the menstrual cycle.

Natural birth control, or the rhythm method, is often used by members of the Roman Catholic Church (since this is the only means of contraception officially sanctioned by that religion). Fertility observation, in the form of basal body temperature charting and cervical mucus monitoring, is sometimes used by women who have philosophical objections to artificial devices or who are unwilling or physically unable to take on the risks associated with other forms of birth control. Some of these women consider abortion to be an alternative should their natural methods fail.

In any kind of periodic abstinence, couples refrain from sexual intercourse or direct penis-vagina contact (although they may engage in other forms of sexual activity) during the days of the menstrual cycle when the woman is believed to be fertile—that is, the times when there is an egg available for fertilization. After ovulation an egg is thought to be fertilizable for only about 12 to 24 hours, but since sperm can survive in the woman's reproductive system for up to 72 hours or more, having intercourse on any of about 3 to 4 days each cycle could theoretically lead to conception.

The obvious problem here is determining those exact days. To be relatively safe, most advocates of periodic abstinence suggest regarding the woman as fertile for about a third of the menstrual cycle, generally from a few days after menstruation ends until at least 3 days after ovulation has occurred (usually about 10 or 11 days before menstruation begins).

The drawback is that ovulation does not always follow a calendar-based schedule, even in women with the most "regular" of menstrual cycles. It is even possible for ovulation to occur during a menstrual period. For this reason, most women and couples who use this form of contraception rely on fertility observation (see below) to help estimate the likelihood that ovulation has occurred or is about to occur.

In general, birth control that relies strictly on refraining from intercourse on the days a woman thinks she is fertile is not very effective. The rhythm method in particular—which relies primarily on the calendar—is notorious for the number of children who can credit their existence to it. With the addition of fertility observation, the failure rate may be much lower, in some studies somewhere in the range of only 2 to 3 percent.

While convenient in the sense that it does not involve buying and using any paraphernalia or visiting a doctor or clinic, periodic abstinence can take a toll on a couple's sex life. Many women find that their desire for vaginal intercourse and orgasm peaks around the time of ovulation and declines considerably thereafter, which can leave them quite frustrated with this method (or quite careless). Other couples, however, have found ways to express their love and sexuality on the fertile days without engaging in vaginal intercourse.

Still other couples eventually take another course, which is to observe fertility and then use barrier methods of contraception on the days when a woman believes she is fertile. During the rest of the month no method of birth control is necessary. This combination method avoids the inconvenience of birth control devices on infertile days, and it avoids sexual frustration on days when the woman might become pregnant.

Fertility observation

A woman who practices fertility observation simply monitors signs within her own body that tell her when she is most likely to be fertile. The two most commonly used methods are basal body temperature (BBT) charting (see infertility) and cervical mucus monitoring.

Women monitor their fertility for a number of reasons. Some practice withdrawal or abstinence from vaginal intercourse during fertile days; others rely on barrier methods of birth control such as condoms, a diaphragm, or a cervical cap on days when they are likely to become pregnant. Because they know that on other days they are infertile, many women find that their sexual behavior can be more spontaneous and unencumbered with worry about pregnancy and bother with artificial devices.

Some women use fertility monitoring to increase the efficacy of other types of birth control. For example, a woman who generally relies on a diaphragm might want to have her partner use a condom as well on days when cervical mucus changes indicate that she may be fertile.

Basal body temperature charting. In this method a woman takes her temperature each morning before getting out of bed and charts it on a monthly graph (see infertility). Temperature will vary slightly from day to day, but at the time of ovulation, or just before, there will be a marked rise (at least 0.4°F) in the average temperature from one day to the next. This means that it is possible—in retrospect—to know that the fertile period is over once there have been at least 3 consecutive days of the higher average temperature (unless, of course, the woman has had a fever). On the day menstruation begins (or just before), temperature will return to the lower level. If the temperature remains high for more than 16 or 17 days, the woman is almost certainly pregnant.

Cervical mucus monitoring. Another way to estimate fertility (and not just in retrospect) is to examine the mucus which is normally secreted from the cervix. Cervical secretions—which can be felt on the outer vaginal lips or perhaps as discharge on the underpants or toilet paper—change during the course of the menstrual cycle, depending on the hormonal milieu, and, with a little practice, can be used to determine just where a woman is in her cycle.

In general, women tend to have very little or no discharge for a few days following menstruation, but soon after that a sticky discharge appears (this is considered to be the first fertile day). From day to day this discharge changes, first becoming thick and creamy, then thin and milky, and finally becoming translucent and stretchy (and thus hospitable to sperm transport). Within 2 days of ovulation (either before or after), there is a "mucus peak" when the mucus, which at this point resembles egg white, is thinnest, clearest, and most abundant. At this time some women can even stretch a long length of the mucus between thumb and forefinger (a phenomenon known as spinnbarkeit). Immediately after ovulation the mucus undergoes a marked change, sometimes becoming tacky or gummy and sometimes disappearing altogether. Women should consider themselves fertile until the fourth day after the mucus peak.

Although checking cervical mucus can be a good guide, it is not infallible—especially if a couple is having intercourse regularly, since semen left in the vagina can be mistaken for mucus or alter its characteristics. Thus, a woman who is gauging her fertility using cervical mucus should try to limit intercourse to every other day at most. She should also remember that a yeast infection or other vaginal infection (vaginitis) can alter the nature of cervical mucus, as can menstrual fluid, spermicidal cream or jelly, or medications inserted into the vagina.

Ovulation detection kits. Kits for estimating fertility are sold over the counter in many pharmacies. Again, the knowledge obtained from them can be helpful only in the latter half of the cycle, since sexual intercourse up to 3 days *be-*

fore ovulation occurs can still result in conception. In Germany, women can now use a handheld computer to determine when they are most at risk for conception; this device flashes red if risk is high, green if chances of fertility are slim.

Related entries

Abortion, birth control, condoms, diaphragms and cervical caps, douching, hormonal contraception, intrauterine devices, lubricants, nonsurgical abortion, oral contraceptives, pregnancy testing, safer sex, sexual response, sexually transmitted diseases, spermicides, tubal ligation, vacuum aspiration

Nearsightedness and Farsightedness

Probably the most common eye problems are refraction errors, which include nearsightedness (myopia) and farsightedness (hyperopia). In nearsightedness, objects at a distance are blurred; in farsightedness, nearby objects are blurred. These errors of vision occur when structures in the eye refract (bend) light in a way that is incoordinate with the length of the eye. The result is that images do not converge precisely on the retina, the light-sensitive membrane in the back of the eye which transforms light into electrical messages and sends them to the brain via the optic nerve (see illustration).

Who is likely to become nearsighted or farsighted?

Nearsightedness, which affects about 20 percent of the population and tends to run in families, is often noticed in childhood and may worsen during adolescence and after the age of 40. Farsightedness in people under 40 also tends to be the result of a congenital defect in the eye; after 40, farsightedness is caused (or exacerbated) by a loss of elasticity in the lens. This condition is called presbyopia, and it develops in everyone to some degree, whether the person previously was nearsighted, farsighted, or neither.

What causes refraction errors?

In normal vision, as light travels through the transparent cornea on the eye's outer surface it is bent and directed via the anterior chamber, which is filled with a fluid called aqueous humor (see illustration). From there the light travels through the pupil, a circular opening in the iris, or colored portion of the eye, which helps regulate the amount of light that ultimately reaches the retina. When light levels are low, the pupil dilates (widens) to allow more light to enter the eye; conversely, when levels are high, the pupil constricts (narrows) to protect the retina from excessive brightness. Various drugs can also affect pupil size.

After passing through the pupil, the light rays enter a capsule of transparent protein tissue called the lens. When vi-

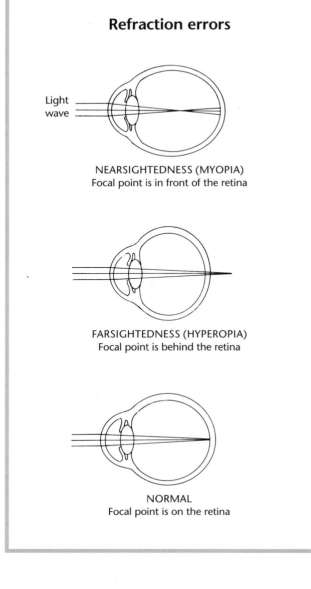

Refraction errors

Light wave

NEARSIGHTEDNESS (MYOPIA)
Focal point is in front of the retina

FARSIGHTEDNESS (HYPEROPIA)
Focal point is behind the retina

NORMAL
Focal point is on the retina

sion is normal, the lens, with the help of surrounding muscles (ciliary muscles), can change its shape to accommodate light from close or distant objects. By thinning to just the right degree, it bends rays from distant objects to converge precisely on the retina. Similarly, by thickening appropriately, it bends rays from nearby objects to a greater degree so that they, too, converge on the retina.

As the elasticity of the lens diminishes with age, its ability to accommodate light from different distances decreases. This results in presbyopia, in which images from nearby objects—such as the words on a page—become blurred.

After passing through the lens, the light is further refracted and enters the vitreous humor—a gel-like liquid—and then at last converges to form an image on the retina. In a person with normal vision, the rays converge precisely on the retina. In a nearsighted person the light from objects at anything but close range converges in front of the retina, blurring their

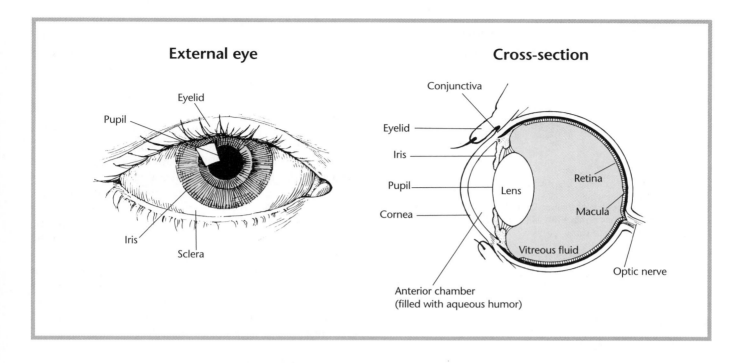

External eye

Pupil
Eyelid
Iris
Sclera

Cross-section

Conjunctiva
Eyelid
Iris
Pupil
Cornea
Lens
Retina
Macula
Vitreous fluid
Optic nerve
Anterior chamber
(filled with aqueous humor)

appearance. In a farsighted person just the opposite occurs: light from anything but distant objects is focused just behind the retina, making it difficult to see up close. Another kind of refractive disorder called astigmatism results when light is misdirected by an irregularly shaped cornea.

How are these conditions evaluated?

Although optometrists—who are not physicians but who have completed a specialized degree program—are prohibited in some states from diagnosing and treating eye diseases, young, healthy women should feel safe in consulting an optometrist for a routine eye examination and the prescription of contact lenses (see entry) or eyeglasses. An ophthalmologist—a medical doctor who has been specially trained in diagnosing and treating diseases of the eye—should be consulted, however, if there is any possibility of a disorder more serious than nearsightedness or farsightedness (see eye care). The medical evaluation and procedures conducted by ophthalmologists are generally more extensive and precise than the diagnostic tests conducted by optometrists.

How are these conditions treated?

Nearsightedness, farsightedness, and astigmatism can usually be corrected with eyeglasses or contact lenses. Problems caused by presbyopia may be treated with reading glasses, or with bifocal lenses if distance glasses are necessary. Many nearsighted people may correct their presbyopia simply by removing their glasses to read.

Most of the time contact lenses must be fitted by an optometrist or ophthalmologist. Opticians do not do any measuring or prescribing but rather grind and fit the lenses and sometimes make a replacement lens or polish an existing one. Optical shops that are part of national chain stores sell a large variety of frames and fit them with lenses prescribed by ophthalmologists and private optometrists, and some of these chains employ optometrists who examine eyes on the premises.

In some cases, a form of surgery known as radial keratotomy can permanently improve vision. Radial keratotomy (also called RK) is a microsurgical procedure used to correct nearsightedness. It may also be used to correct some forms of astigmatism. Considered risky and experimental until quite recently, this procedure may provide for many people a reasonable alternative to glasses and contact lenses.

In radial keratotomy, as in all refractive surgery, the cornea is altered and, along with it, the path of light heading for the retina. An ophthalmologist makes a series of delicate spoke-like incisions into the cornea of each eye (see illustration); these cuts, which go through only part of the thickness of the cornea, flatten its center, thereby reducing the refractive power of the cornea. This operation—which is rarely covered by insurance policies and which costs approximately $1,500 per eye—is done on an outpatient basis under local topical anesthesia. It takes between 15 and 30 minutes to perform. When both eyes require correction (which is usually the case), each eye is done on a separate day. The patient must wear an eyepatch or sunglasses for several days or longer after the procedure, until recovery is complete.

When performed by an experienced ophthalmologist, in 9 out of 10 patients whose conditions are suitable for the procedure radial keratotomy results in at least 20/40 vision (which is considered adequate for driving a car without glasses), and 6 out of 10 can expect to have 20/20 vision. Even so, a sizable minority of people who have radial keratotomy still may need to wear glasses, and a significant number may have trouble with glare permanently. In some cases

Surgery for refraction errors

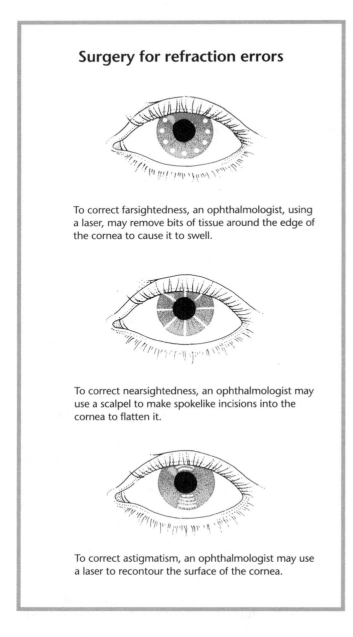

To correct farsightedness, an ophthalmologist, using a laser, may remove bits of tissue around the edge of the cornea to cause it to swell.

To correct nearsightedness, an ophthalmologist may use a scalpel to make spokelike incisions into the cornea to flatten it.

To correct astigmatism, an ophthalmologist may use a laser to recontour the surface of the cornea.

glasses may become their only option, since the altered cornea may be more difficult to fit with contact lenses. Finally, there is no guarantee that vision will not deteriorate further with age. Other forms of refractive surgery to correct nearsightedness as well as other problems such as farsightedness and astigmatism are currently under investigation. Astigmatism, for example, may be correctable with an operation called transverse keratotomy, which is similar to radial keratotomy except that the incisions are patterned differently (see illustration). Transverse keratotomy is often done in conjunction with radial keratotomy.

Another technique, called thermokeratoplasty, is being investigated as a possible way to correct farsightedness. In this form of laser surgery, the ophthalmologist uses an excimer laser to remove bits of tissue around the edge of the cornea (see illustration). As a result, the cornea swells slightly and so refocuses light onto the retina instead of behind it. A similar procedure, photorefractive keratectomy, has recently become available as an alternative to radial keratotomy for the correction of nearsightedness. Here the excimer laser is used in lieu of a scalpel to recontour the refracting surface of the cornea.

Finally, in extreme cases of nearsightedness or farsightedness, when glasses and contact lenses are inadequate, other possibilities, some of them still experimental, include extracting the lens and using an artificial lens, or replacing or rebuilding the cornea with synthetic or donated corneal tissue. In 1999 the U.S. Food and Drug Administration approved a technique in which tiny transparent plastic C-shaped rings called Intacs are implanted in the edge of the cornea. For mildly nearsighted people these implants can be an appealing alternative to laser surgery because they do not require the removal of any eye tissue and can be removed if they cause problems. Installation can be quite painful, however, and just as costly as laser surgery, with few if any health insurance policies covering the procedure.

What are the risks and complications of radial keratotomy?

Not all people respond equally well to radial keratotomy, since the same incision can flatten one cornea more than another. Excessive flattening is particularly likely to occur in older people, as well as in people with high pressure within the eye (such as people with glaucoma). Too many cuts can also overcorrect the nearsightedness, so that the patient becomes farsighted instead. A small minority of patients end up with worse vision than they had before the operation.

Blurred vision can occur owing to scarring of the cornea. A much rarer but even more serious complication involves infection of the cornea, which may ultimately rupture. In about 1 in 1,000 patients radial keratotomy results in a permanent loss of vision.

Related entries

Cataracts, contact lenses, dry eye, eye care, glaucoma, laser surgery, macular degeneration, retinal detachment

Nonsurgical Abortion

Nonsurgical abortion is a means of terminating a pregnancy within the first two months by using medications instead of surgical tools. This method, which is becoming increasingly available in the United States, appeals to women who find out they are pregnant soon after conception and do not have access to, or want to avoid, surgical abortion.

Unlike surgical abortion—which is usually performed safely at about week 8 or 9 of a pregnancy (about 4 to 5 weeks after a missed menstrual period)—nonsurgical abortions can be accomplished days after a woman discovers she is pregnant. Because the medications can be administered in a doctor's office and require no visits to an abortion clinic, they can be obtained relatively discreetly, and the process is often completed in a woman's own home. The idea that nonsurgical abortion involves no invasive instruments is also appealing to many women. Nonsurgical abortion is particularly appealing to younger women who find themselves pregnant, since many pediatricians and family practitioners who are not certified to perform surgical abortions on adolescents may well be able to prescribe medications to terminate a pregnancy.

Major conflict between prochoice and prolife groups has limited and delayed the availability of nonsurgical abortion in the United States until quite recently. The idea of a relatively easy, surgery-free abortion raises red flags for abortion foes. Many fear that nonsurgical abortions may make abortion too easy, thus cheapening the value of human life. Other opponents of nonsurgical abortions worry that they are simply not as safe and effective as they are often reported to be. Increasing evidence suggests, however, that these fears are unwarranted. Nonsurgical abortions appear to be generally safe and effective and do not seem to encourage women to have abortions they otherwise would not have. It also is now clear that nonsurgical abortions are by no means pain-free, and they can be even more emotionally grueling (and expensive) than quick surgical procedures. Just as with surgical abortions, too, some states require minors to have the permission of a parent or guardian before having a nonsurgical abortion.

What is RU-486?

RU-486, popularly known as the abortion pill or the French abortion pill, is a prescription medication (mifepristone) that blocks the effects of progesterone, a hormone necessary for fertilized eggs to implant and develop in the uterus. After a decade of struggles and setbacks in both the political and business arenas, RU-486 has now been approved for commercial use in the United States. It is also available in many other countries including China, France, England, Sweden, and Germany.

With RU-486 abortion can be safely accomplished before the 6th or 8th week of pregnancy. (Safe, early abortion may also now be possible with so-called manual vacuum aspiration, a surgical form of abortion; see entry on vacuum aspiration.) RU-486 can work as a "morning-after" contraceptive pill as well as an abortion pill (see hormonal contraception), and it appears to have other medical uses such as alleviating symptoms of endometriosis, uterine fibroids, and Cushing syndrome.

How does RU-486 work?

RU-486 essentially induces a miscarriage by either blocking the implantation of a fertilized egg (if it is taken during the luteal phase of the menstrual cycle) or interfering with the embryo's development soon after implantation (if it is taken a week or so after a period has been skipped). To be effective, the drug must be taken before the 9th week after the start of the last menstrual period. This limited window of time virtually guarantees that RU-486 will never replace surgical abortions, because 49 days into a pregnancy many women still do not know they are pregnant—and even fewer have had the time to decide on a termination or arrange for one.

A woman who wants to terminate a pregnancy with RU-486 first needs to visit a clinician to have her pregnancy confirmed and to exclude the possibility of an ectopic (tubal) pregnancy. She is then given the RU-486 pill and told to return 2 days later, at which time she is given other pills containing prostaglandin (usually the prostaglandin analog misoprostol), a hormone-like substance that initiates uterine contractions and helps soften and dilate the cervix (the opening to the uterus). Alternatively, a woman may be sent home with the prostaglandin, to be inserted vaginally 2 to 3 days later. The embryo or fetus is usually expelled within 4 hours after this second dose. If the actual abortion does not occur at the hospital or clinic, the woman must return later to make sure it has been completed successfully.

The logistics involved in using RU-486 can make it impractical for many women. In a country the size of the United States, women may be essentially prohibited from having nonsurgical abortions because it is too difficult, awkward, or expensive to arrange for transportation numerous times to a clinic or doctor's office that provides the drug, particularly one that is out of state. This is especially true for women living in rural or remote areas or for teenagers whose parents do not know about the pregnancy or who, in states requiring parental consent, won't approve the abortion. In addition, many office practices cannot accommodate women who are completing the 4-hour bleeding period after taking the prostaglandin. Multiple visits to a doctor bring the price tag of nonsurgical abortions up into—or above—the range of surgical abortions. The availability of a time-released form of prostaglandin would help reduce the number of trips to a doctor or clinic and make it possible to see a doctor only twice: before the prescription to rule out an ectopic pregnancy and again after taking the drugs to make sure the abortion is complete.

What are the side effects and risks of RU-486?

More than 150,000 European women have used RU-486 without any known long-term side effects. Approximately 20 major studies have also shown the drug to be generally safe and reliable, offering advantages over surgery such as a decreased risk of damage to the cervix and uterus. Still, RU-486 has a somewhat higher failure rate than surgical abortion. Approximately 2 in 100 women who use this drug will still need to have the abortion completed surgically. The failure rate is highest—perhaps as high as 14 percent—if the drug is used after the 7th week of pregnancy.

Many French doctors no longer recommend RU-486 for women who smoke because of fears about heart problems associated with prostaglandin, and any woman who has heart problems or high blood pressure needs special monitoring when using these drugs.

Prolonged and sometimes heavy bleeding and cramping can occur during the abortion, as well as occasional nausea and diarrhea. Despite the fears of those who oppose abortion, for some women nonsurgical abortions are actually more stressful and disturbing than surgical ones because the entire procedure takes several days. Women who choose this form of abortion are left alone to face the bleeding and a long waiting period during which they may agonize over their decision. As distressing as surgery may be, it is over and done with quickly and is in somebody else's hands. That is why even in France, where RU-486 has been available since 1988, women must undergo counseling and a one-week "period of reflection" before a doctor can prescribe the drug. Teenage girls must have the consent of a parent or government official. In Great Britain there is a 24-hour waiting period, and use of the drug is restricted to women living within a certain distance from a clinic, in case there are any side effects. Also, before RU-486 can be prescribed, two physicians must certify that the abortion is necessary for medical and emotional reasons.

What are other nonsurgical alternatives?

A growing number of physicians are using a combination of two drugs available by prescription in the United States to induce abortion before 9 weeks' gestation. The drugs are methotrexate, which has been used for years to terminate ectopic pregnancies (as well as to treat cancer, arthritis, and psoriasis), and misoprostol, an antiulcer medication that is used with RU-486. Methotrexate, which is given by injection, destabilizes the uterine lining, while misoprostol causes uterine contractions that expel the fetus. Misoprostol can also induce abortions on its own but is more effective when combined with methotrexate or RU-486.

The combination of methotrexate and misoprostol, which costs only about $10, is successful 90 to 95 percent of the time. Although two-thirds of women using this method abort the very first day, the rest may experience cramping and bleeding for an average of 28 more days until the abortion is complete. For another 5 to 10 percent of women, the combination of methotrexate and misoprostol leads to serious side effects or fails to work completely, in which case surgical abortion is necessary after the long waiting period.

The National Abortion Federation in Washington, D.C., an organization representing 350 abortion providers (see references), can refer hotline callers to clinics that offer nonsurgical abortions and other early surgical procedures.

Related entries

Abortion, birth control, Cushing syndrome, ectopic pregnancy, endometriosis, hormonal contraception, miscarriage, oral contraceptives, uterine fibroids, vacuum aspiration

Nutrition

For thousands of years people have recognized that the foods they eat affect their health and well-being. From graham crackers to castor oil to oat bran, various foods have been touted by healers, grandmothers, religious zealots, and nutritionists as the keys to good health, long life, and freedom from future ailments.

Women are particularly susceptible to nutritional claims because they are often responsible for shopping and cooking and because many are concerned with dieting and weight loss. Women are also prone to a number of diseases that may stem from, or be exacerbated by, diet, such as anemia, osteoporosis, diabetes, high blood pressure, diverticular disease, coronary artery disease, gallstones, and breast and colon cancers. Moreover, nutrient deficiencies become particularly common during certain stages of a woman's life—especially puberty, pregnancy, breastfeeding, and menopause.

There is no doubt that the foods we eat have something to do with the way our bodies work. Certain basic nutrients are absolutely necessary for human health—as scurvied sailors who went for months without eating citrus fruit used to learn the hard way. The body cannot produce some protein building blocks, vitamins, minerals, and fats on its own and must obtain these from the diet. Any healthy diet will include a certain amount of protein, carbohydrates, and fat. Many people in the United States do not get enough of these basic requirements and suffer from deficiency diseases—including some people who live in poverty, some who abuse alcohol, and others who deprive themselves of nutrients in the name of fashion or religious or philosophical beliefs.

In addition to being essential to life, some nutrients can have subtle druglike effects on bodily processes. The fact that spices have been used in Western cultures since the Middle Ages as both foods and drugs attests to this dual property of food (although the amount of spices required to produce a druglike effect is usually much larger than the amount commonly used in foods). These observations have led people to conclude that eliminating certain foods from the diet—as well as adding others—may have some beneficial effect on health.

There is a vast difference, however, between claiming that foods affect the body in general (for good or ill) and claiming that any specific food or diet has a direct influence. Nevertheless, the evidence accumulated in recent years has been impressive in suggesting links between the presence or absence of certain types of foods in the diet and a person's susceptibility to various diseases. For example, the amount and kinds of fat in the diet can affect blood levels of cholesterol, which in turn are associated with the risk of coronary artery disease. Extremely low fat intake over a lifetime is associated with a higher than normal risk of hemorrhagic stroke, whereas a diet high in fat seems to raise the risk of cardiovascular disease, as well as certain types of breast and colon cancers.

Diets high in fruits and vegetables may lower the risk of colon cancer, as well as cancers of the mouth, larynx, pancreas, and cervix. There is conflicting evidence about the role that whole grain (high-fiber) products play in reducing the risk of colon cancer, but it is known that high-fiber diets reduce constipation and the risk of diverticular disease. And one large prospective study found that breast cancer incidence was about 25 percent higher in women who included relatively few vegetables in their diet.

The temptation—especially for someone already at risk for one of these diseases—is to change dietary habits as soon as one of these results is announced. The extravagance with which nutritional claims are touted in the popular press, however, is not always proportional to the scientific evidence backing them up. Few nutritional studies to date can be considered conclusive; most of them merely provide intriguing clues about the complex relationships between different foods and human health. Most studies can only establish correlations rather than prove cause and effect, and do not account for a number of variables that undoubtedly play a role in human health and disease. Furthermore, since many nutrients interact with other nutrients in the diet, consuming large quantities of one type may cut down absorption of another—or may be ineffective without adequate intake of yet a third.

The fact that nutritional science is still in its infancy helps explain why nutrition has been so long neglected in medical schools and is often overlooked by physicians as a possible means of preventing and treating disease. It also helps explain the conflicting claims that so frequently appear in the popular press. One day oat bran is good, the next day it is a hoax; one day caffeine leads to breast cancer, the next day it is harmless. The result of so much hype, on the one hand, has been a growing skepticism among some members of the American public, who have come to believe that nutritional "breakthroughs" are not worth the newsprint required to announce them. On the other hand, because of media attention to nutrition, some people eagerly await the latest and presumably more accurate proclamation, assuming that there are easy, universal answers to the question, What should I eat?

For all the homage paid to scientific data, it is important to acknowledge that—consciously or not—most people choose foods more for reasons of cultural and national tradition, religious beliefs, economic considerations, and individual psychological experiences than for reasons of health. Susceptibility to a food fad occasionally arises from a genuine desire to be a healthier eater, but perhaps more often it reflects a person's philosophical beliefs or feelings of helplessness, insecurity, or anger.

What do nutritional experts currently recommend?

Nutritional needs vary according to a person's age, sex, and reproductive status, and they also vary from individual to individual within those groups, depending on a person's unique genetic makeup and life situation. The amount of vitamins needed by an adolescent girl often differs from that required by a woman in her 30s, or a woman who is pregnant or breastfeeding (see vitamins). In an attempt to help people plan balanced diets that reflect current understanding of nutrition, in 1992 the U.S. Department of Agriculture replaced the traditional "four food groups" with the "Food Pyramid," a guide to daily food choices. Although it is based primarily on well-documented studies, it represents a certain amount of educated guessing, and it is not without its critics. Many of them contend that the Food Pyramid was shaped as much by the interests of the U.S. meat and dairy industries as by objective nutritional knowledge. A food pyramid put out by the government of a Mediterranean country, for example, would probably look quite different, perhaps increasing the recommended amount of olive oil and lowering the amount of milk and meat. Even so, most nutritionists laud the Food Pyramid's overall goal of increasing U.S. consumption of grains, fruits, and vegetables. An alternative Food Pyramid was created by Dr. Walter C. Willett of the Harvard School of Public Health (see page 353).

Because of the heavy toll taken by heart disease in the United States, and the many studies linking blood cholesterol levels with coronary artery disease, the National Cholesterol Education Panel (NCEP) of the National Institutes of Health recommends that Americans reduce their fat intake (from meats, dairy products, and all types of oils) to 30 percent or less of total calories, reduce saturated fats (primarily from meats and from some oils such as coconut oil) to less than 10 percent of total calories, and reduce cholesterol in the diet (from eggs, shrimp, and some other seafoods) to less than 300 mg daily. The American Heart Association, noting that polyunsaturated fats can lower levels of HDL (the "good" cholesterol; see entry), advises limiting polyunsaturated fats to 10 percent of caloric intake as well. Monounsaturated fats such as olive oil and canola oil should make up the remaining 10 percent of daily caloric intake from fats and oils, since in some studies they seem to lower coronary risk by lowering LDL and increasing HDL cholesterol.

Useful as all of these recommendations may be, they are still open to interpretation when it comes to planning individual meals. Should fat be reduced to 30 percent—or 20 percent—of the diet? Should red meat be avoided altogether? Will eating more vegetables mean excess exposure to toxic pesticides? Will drinking more milk and eating more dairy products (to prevent osteoporosis) raise one's fat consumption (and perhaps increase the risk of coronary artery disease)? Is refined sugar harmful? What about salt? It is important to remember that there are no hard and fast answers to these questions.

Admonitions to cut back on calories, for example, or eliminate salt, or lower saturated fat intake do not necessarily apply to each individual woman. The recommended 2,100 calories a day can be perfectly fine for one woman, but it may lead another to gain unwanted pounds, while leaving a physically active woman constantly hungry. Although cutting down on salt does help lower blood pressure in some women, it has no effect on many others. And though some women's cholesterol levels do drop when they cut down on dietary cholesterol and saturated fats, many others compensate for this deprivation by producing more cholesterol in the liver. Dietary goals are blanket statements intended either to cover the widest segment of the population possible or to establish guidelines to protect the people most in need. These goals are not necessarily applicable to any one individual.

What makes sense, then, is for the individual woman to be aware of these general nutritional guidelines and then determine to the best of her ability if they seem to make sense for her, given her family and medical history and her personal lifestyle. In general, there is little evidence that gorging on or abstaining from any one particular food or group of foods is enough to overcome the many other factors that predict human health and longevity—factors including genetics, family history, and one's living and working environment, as well as exercise and other behaviors related to lifestyle.

Nutrition over the life span

Despite these caveats, some diets are, in general, clearly more healthful than others. The challenge is making everyday decisions in the face of conflicting information. This can be accomplished to some extent by aiming to eat a balanced, varied diet and modifying it according to individual needs. A healthful diet is low in fat, moderate in protein, and high in complex carbohydrates. It includes relatively large amounts of vegetables, fruits, and whole grains and sparing use of fats, oils, and sugar.

Adolescents. Between the ages of 10 and 15 many girls and young women do not consume a diet that meets their basic nutritional needs. Just before and during puberty, calorie requirements rise, and weight gain is common before menarche begins. In fact, unless a girl reaches a critical weight (and ratio of body fat to muscle), she will not begin to menstruate. These problems often persist into later adolescence, when young women continue to need higher levels of certain vitamins and minerals than most adult women. The average adolescent girl requires at least 2,200 calories per day, and more if she is involved in sports or is physically active. Calcium intake is particularly important in adolescent and young adult women to ensure attainment of peak bone mass by age 30, a time when bone mass begins to decline.

Often concerned about weight gain for the first time, teenage girls may subject themselves to low-calorie diets or fasts. The result can be not only nutritional deficiencies but also the emergence of various eating disorders and menstrual irregularities. Restrictive eating practices, if continued into young adulthood, can affect a woman's fertility.

Pregnant women. Not many years ago pregnant women were subjected to severe weight gain limits which required stringent dietary restrictions. The idea was that these restrictions not only would help a woman keep her figure but also would help prevent high blood pressure and preeclampsia during pregnancy. Today, however, most doctors feel that these weight restrictions seriously compromised the nutritional needs of both the mother and the growing fetus. It is now generally recommended that pregnant women gain between 22 and 27 pounds—somewhat less if they were overweight before they became pregnant, and somewhat more if they were underweight. Most of this weight gain comes not from excess fatty tissue but rather from the cumulative weight of the fetus, amniotic fluid, placenta, enlarged uterus and breasts, and increased blood supply and fluid volume.

For most women, eating only about 300 extra calories a day is enough to produce the desirable weight gain. Pregnant teenagers need slightly more calories and protein than pregnant adults, as well as additional calcium and phosphorus every day—400 mg more per day than a pregnant adult—because their bones are still growing. Other women who may need extra nutrients or special diets during pregnancy are those who have had 3 or more pregnancies within 2 years (including induced abortions and miscarriages), who smoke cigarettes or abuse alcohol or other drugs, who have certain chronic diseases, or who follow a vegetarian diet. Vegetarian diets can be problematic in pregnancy because they are often too low in protein, calcium, iron, zinc, and vitamins, particularly vitamins B_6 and B_{12}. Still, a varied vegetarian diet can meet the needs of both mother and fetus, so long as it is rich in fruits, vegetables (including leafy greens), whole grain products, nuts, seeds, and legumes, as well as dairy products and eggs.

Vegans—that is, vegetarians who choose not to eat animal products of any sort, including dairy products and eggs—can pose more of a challenge; meeting the needs of pregnancy will require eating ample quantities of cooked dried beans, peanut butter, nuts, and/or soy-based foods. Calcium requirements can be met in a vegan diet by eating tofu processed with calcium sulfate and by eating ample green leafy vegetables and products such as tahini, fortified soymilk, and fortified orange juice. Iron needs can be met by eating plenty of citrus fruits and juices, tomatoes, broccoli, raisins, watermelon, spinach, black-eyed peas, blackstrap molasses, chickpeas, and/or pinto beans. Eating cereals and other foods fortified with vitamin B_{12} is also a good idea for vegans because animal foods are the only source of this essential vitamin.

Adequate weight gain in pregnancy is usually a good sign that nutritional needs are being met. Rather than eating more (or "eating for two"), the idea is to try to select foods carefully and avoid gorging on empty calories. Fresh fruits, vegetables, and whole grains are preferable to cookies, candy, and other sugary treats. This is not all that different from advice given to nonpregnant women, of course, but many women are more apt to follow the advice when they are responsible for their baby's health as well as their own.

In general, the following daily diet should ensure a pregnant woman adequate nutrients:

- 2 or more servings of fruit or juice (rich in vitamin C)
- 2 servings of vegetables
- 4 servings of whole grain products
- 3 to 4 servings of dairy products or other calcium-rich foods (spinach, kale, sardines, or broccoli)
- 6 ounces of protein (meat, poultry, fish, eggs, cheese, lentils, nuts, beans, or brewer's yeast)

A sensible diet can generally provide adequate levels of all vitamins and minerals needed during pregnancy with the exception of iron, folic acid (folate), and possibly calcium. Just to be on the safe side, most doctors also recommend that pregnant women take a daily prenatal vitamin supplement during both pregnancy and the months when she is trying to conceive. There is now convincing evidence that supplementing folic acid in particular may reduce the incidence of neural tube defects in the fetus by as much as 60 to 72 percent. Currently the required daily allowance (RDA) for folate in a pregnant woman is 0.4 mg, an amount contained by most prenatal vitamins. Many doctors now feel that all women trying to become pregnant should consume at least 0.4 mg of folic acid per day beginning 1 to 3 months before conception and continuing through at least the 6th week of the pregnancy. Supplementation is particularly important for women with a multiple pregnancy, as well as women with certain blood disorders or who are taking antiseizure medications, since the need for folate increases in all of these situations.

Because an estimated 50 percent of pregnancies are unplanned, and because most women do not obtain even the minimum recommended amounts of folate in their diets, the Food and Drug Administration is now considering a proposal to supplement the country's flour supply with folate. Critics fear that universal supplementation may be dangerous because excessive intake of folate can mask a vitamin B_{12} deficiency, which if untreated can cause pernicious anemia and serious neurological damage. In one study to detect the prevalence of pernicious anemia, about 1 in 5 people with the disease were found to be black females, a quarter of whom were under age 40. Unless under the supervision of a physician, women should take no more than 400 micrograms of folate per day, regardless of their reproductive status.

Pregnant women were once admonished to avoid salt in the interest of preventing preeclampsia. It is now believed, however, that this practice may actually have contributed to the development of this serious disorder. The only women who should restrict use of salt during pregnancy are those with certain preexisting conditions such as salt-sensitive hypertension or congestive heart failure.

It is probably wise for pregnant women to avoid using products containing artificial sweeteners during pregnancy, as the effects on the fetus are unknown.

Postpartum and breastfeeding women. For many women, getting back to their pre-pregnancy weight and shape is a major goal after the delivery of a baby. Most women lose about 18 to 20 pounds within 10 days of the birth. After that, the rate of loss slows down, but many women find that they can return to their original weight within a few months merely by eating a well-balanced diet appropriate for their size, bone structure, and energy expenditure. Appropriate postpartum exercises can help restore abdominal and other muscle tone. Generally, it is not wise to try to lose more than about half a pound a week, and many sensible women adhere to the dictum, "Nine months to put it on, nine months to take it off."

Breastfeeding women may have to wait longer than a few months to get back into pre-pregnancy clothes. Some nursing mothers seem to shed the excess weight they gained during pregnancy effortlessly, but others find that weight loss is virtually impossible until the baby is weaned. In any case, this is definitely an undesirable time to embark on a stringent weight loss plan. Not only is breastfeeding physically demanding, but also the sleep deprivation and emotional stress of new motherhood can make dieting even more debilitating.

Moreover, to ensure an adequate milk supply, the lactating woman needs extra fluids, calories, calcium, and protein each day. In fact, she needs about 500 more calories per day than before pregnancy. Good food choices include high-protein foods as well as dairy products or calcium-rich foods. It is generally a good idea to continue taking prenatal vitamins until the baby is weaned. Drinking plenty of liquids helps ensure an adequate milk supply. One easy way to accomplish this is to have a glass of water or milk every time the baby is nursing. Beer was once considered the nursing mother's best friend, but most doctors now feel that alcoholic beverages are inappropriate for breastfeeding women, since the alcohol passes into the breast milk and can affect the baby.

Some women find that nursing babies are bothered by certain foods such as broccoli, cauliflower, cabbage, brussels sprouts, onions, garlic, and chocolate—either because the babies dislike the flavor of the breast milk or because they seem to develop diarrhea, colic, or other symptoms of indigestion after the mother eats these foods. Virtually everything the mother eats can enter the breast milk and alter its taste and nutrient content, so a little experimentation may be in order.

Postmenopausal women. After young adulthood, women's caloric needs gradually decline so that by menopause most women need only about two-thirds of the calories they needed at the age of 20. This can sometimes make it difficult for diet alone to meet a woman's needs for certain vitamins and minerals—particularly calcium, vitamin D, and the B vitamins—which stay the same or even increase as the years go by. Thus, selective vitamin and mineral supplementation may sometimes be necessary. Various dietary surveys have shown that women in their 40s and 50s consume far too little milk, fruit, and vegetables and consequently have deficiencies in both calcium and vitamin C.

After menopause, decreased estrogen levels in the body seem to make women more susceptible to osteoporosis and cardiovascular disorders, so many nutritionists suggest that postmenopausal women increase their calcium and vitamin D while restricting intake of fats, cholesterol, and possibly salt. Foods containing excess phosphorus (in the form of phosphates) should also be minimized, since excess phosphorus can increase bone loss by competing with calcium for absorption. Foods that may have proportionately more phosphorus than calcium include many soft drinks, meats, and processed cheeses.

Women with hypertension, heart disease, diabetes, or other chronic diseases should consult their clinician about more specific dietary modifications. Because many medications can interfere with the body's absorption of nutrients, a clinician should also be consulted about any necessary supplementation.

Elderly women. Nutrition is an even greater concern for elderly women, who are more likely to live alone than are elderly men, and are therefore less likely to shop for, prepare, and eat adequate meals. Having a chronic disease such as Alzheimer's, arthritis, or osteoporosis can make healthful cooking and eating habits particularly difficult to maintain. Even the able-bodied elderly who are living alone often find it a bother to prepare themselves balanced and nutritious meals and instead subsist on ready-to-eat snacks.

Many elderly women experience appetite loss, either because of depression or because of tooth and gum problems, poorly fitting dentures, medications, a sedentary lifestyle, or diminished (or altered) sense of taste. Many others take drugs that interfere with food absorption or live on a fixed income that precludes their buying fresh fruits and vegetables and protein-rich foods. For all of these reasons a large number of elderly women subsist without meeting their basic nutritional requirements. Nutritionists speculate that a sizable proportion of the depression, memory loss, and debility in elderly women can be attributed to nutritional deficiencies alone. It is therefore probably wise for all elderly women to take vitamin and mineral supplements to ensure that their basic needs are met. Eating a diet rich in high-fiber foods such as fruits, vegetables, and grains can help diminish constipation and diverticular disease, both of which are common in elderly women. If health permits, joining an exercise class or taking on some other form of regular exercise (such as swimming, dancing, or walking) can help build up an appetite.

Some nutritionists recently suggested revising the standard food pyramid to better meet the needs of adults over the age of 70. At the base of the revised pyramid is increased fluid consumption—eight 8-ounce glasses per day. This is because older people are less likely to perceive themselves as thirsty

and have to remind themselves consciously to drink more to stay hydrated. Water is essential to keep blood pressure at a safe level, prevent blood clots, avoid constipation, and promote healthy kidney function.

The revised pyramid also suggests that people over the age of 70 eat six or more servings of fiber-rich grain-based foods per day, with cereals in this group fortified with B vitamins such as B_{12} and folic acid, as well as two or more servings of fruit and three or more servings of vegetables, three servings of low-fat dairy foods, and two or more servings of fish, dried beans, or lean cuts of meat and poultry. As with the standard food pyramid, the revised pyramid suggests limiting intake of nutritionally empty high-fat and highly sweetened foods, and suggests using liquid oils in lieu of solid fats whenever possible.

Meals on Wheels, a federally funded program, is administered at the local level through 670 committees called Area Agencies on Aging located throughout the United States. Any person who is 60 or older, or has a spouse who is 60 or older, is eligible to receive home-delivered meals, although specific qualifications vary from state to state. In some states financial need and level of frailty factor heavily into eligibility. Meals administered through this program are limited to Monday through Friday delivery, although in some states independent organizations operated through churches, hospitals, or benevolent associations sponsor weekend delivery as well.

Elderly women who would like assistance with meals should contact their local Area Agency on Aging, or call information for the Meals on Wheels program nearest their home. Women who cannot find their local Meals on Wheels program should call the National Meals on Wheels headquarters in Washington, D.C.

Related entries

Anemia, anorexia nervosa and bulimia nervosa, artificial sweeteners, bowel disorders, breast cancer, breastfeeding, coffee, colon and rectal cancer, coronary artery disease, diabetes, dieting, diverticular disease, exercise, gallstones, heart disease, high blood pressure, menarche, menopause, miscarriage, obesity, osteoporosis, pesticides and organic foods, preeclampsia, pregnancy, smoking, stroke, substance abuse, vitamins, weight tables

Obesity

Obesity means having an excess of total body fat. In the past a woman was considered obese if she weighed at least 20 percent more than her ideal weight. It is quite possible, however, for a person to exceed the ideal weight for her height and still not have excess body fat if the weight of her bones and muscles is unusually high. In general, however, people who are

Risk of health problems associated with obesity

BMI Index	Risk for heart disease, hypertension, diabetes, some cancers, and early death
Under 19 (underweight)	Some risk
19 to 26 (normal)	Very low risk
26 to 27 (marginally overweight)	Some risk
27 to 32 (overweight)	Moderate risk
32 to 45 (severe overweight)	High risk
Over 45 (morbid obesity)	Very high risk

significantly overweight also tend to be obese, which explains why the two terms are frequently used interchangeably.

In the United States 27 percent of women and 24 percent of men between the ages of 20 and 74 weigh more than they should, according to standard height-weight charts (see weight tables p. 625). But as many as 40 percent of all American women claim to be "dieting" or actively engaged in some kind of weight control program. Study after study seems to confirm that the vast majority of them will fail in their efforts (necessary or not) to lose weight over the long haul.

Who is likely to be obese?

Obesity occurs when a person takes in more energy (in the form of food) than she uses up (by burning calories during physical activity); the excess energy gets stored as fat. But why some people are more prone to such an imbalance remains unclear. Overeating certainly has something to do with obesity, but some people seem to be able to eat everything in sight and stay at their ideal weight; others gain weight on very low calorie regimens.

Genetics certainly plays a role: if one parent is obese, each child has a 40 percent chance of also being obese, and if both parents are obese, the risk to each child rises to 80 percent. Overweight children and adolescents are more likely than others to become obese adults. Both genetic and cultural factors are thought to explain the higher prevalence of obesity in African American and Hispanic women, who do not seem to be as obsessed with thinness as white women are. For example, in one survey 64 percent of black teenage girls said it was better to be a little overweight than a little underweight; by contrast, the majority of white teenage girls in the survey claimed that they would "rather be dead than fat."

Both men and women are more likely to become overweight as they age. In men the peak incidence of obesity occurs between the ages of 45 and 54, whereas in women the peak incidence is between 65 and 74, when they are generally at their most sedentary and least inclined or able to undertake regular physical exercise.

How is the condition evaluated?

In recent years sophisticated measures of body fat have begun to be used in conjunction with weight to determine if a woman is obese. One of these measures is called the body mass index (BMI), which indicates how much of the weight comes from muscle or bone versus fat. It is calculated by multiplying weight in pounds by 700 and then dividing the product by the square of height in inches. That means that a woman who weighs 125 pounds and stands 5'5" (65 inches) tall would have a BMI of $(125 \times 700)/(65 \times 65)$ or about 21. A BMI higher than 25 is considered to be reason for concern. Therefore, a 5'5" woman weighing 170 pounds would have a BMI of $(170 \times 700)/(65 \times 65)$ or about 28 and would be labeled obese by this measure.

Another useful measure of obesity is waist-to-hip ratio, calculated by measuring the smallest area around the waist (with the stomach relaxed) and then dividing this number by the measurement of the widest area around the hips. A waist-to-hip ratio greater than 0.8 in women aged 40 to 59 has been associated with an elevated risk of diabetes, high blood pressure, and gallbladder disease (see illustration).

To determine both the causes and the effects of a patient's obesity, the physician will ask questions about the presence of any medical conditions, as well as the history of dieting and physical activity. Often some routine biochemical and metabolic tests will be performed to check for physiological problems, and overall physical fitness will be evaluated.

In addition to diabetes and high blood pressure, both of which are linked to an increased risk of coronary artery disease, obesity is also associated with osteoarthritis of the spine, endometrial cancer (because fat produces estrogen, an excess of which can stimulate abnormal cellular growth in the uterine lining), irregular menstruation, excess body hair, and, during pregnancy, increased risk of preeclampsia (toxemia).

How is obesity treated?

Diet and exercise. Dieting (see entry) is a constant national pastime among women, in part because most dieters eventu-

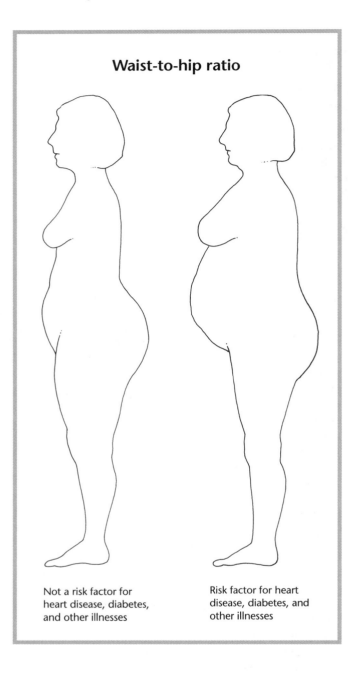

Waist-to-hip ratio

Not a risk factor for heart disease, diabetes, and other illnesses

Risk factor for heart disease, diabetes, and other illnesses

ber of pounds; for another, merely stabilizing a yo-yo pattern of repeated weight loss and gain or halting further weight gain can be considered a success. Setting as a goal an ideal weight that is inappropriate for a woman's particular body, or setting a weight loss target so high that achieving and maintaining it are too difficult, are the main reasons why most weight loss programs fail.

Anyone considering a weight loss plan must understand that obesity is a chronic condition. Therefore, maintaining lost weight is just as important as—and often more difficult than—losing it in the first place. Almost always, weight will be regained unless a woman changes her patterns of eating and exercise (see entry).

Medications. Occasionally long-term drug therapy may be appropriate in treating obesity in patients who cannot follow a reasonable diet or those with a lifelong history of weight loss and regain. Anti-obesity drugs available today include the appetite suppressants phentermine (Apidex-P, Fastin, Ionamin) and subitramine (Meridia), as well as orlistat (Xenical), a drug that works by blocking the body's absorption of dietary fat.

Surgery. As a last resort surgery may be considered, particularly if a woman has 100 pounds or more to lose. The two most commonly performed procedures aim at making it impossible to eat large amounts of food by shortening the amount of time it takes for food to get from the stomach to the small intestine. In the older and riskier of these two procedures, gastric bypass, most of the stomach is closed and reconnected to the small intestine. The second procedure, gastroplasty, is somewhat less effective but has fewer complications. Here the surgeon makes a small vertical passageway from the stomach to the small intestine by closing off the upper third of the stomach with sutures or staples.

With either procedure the patient can expect to lose approximately half her excess weight within the first year, although loss slows in the second year, and some weight may be regained after that. Few patients ever lose all their excess weight through surgery alone. Side effects and complications can include nausea, vomiting, and, over the long term, nutrient deficiencies (especially of vitamin B_{12}, folic acid, and iron).

Women who have had weight loss surgery are advised to postpone pregnancy until their weight has stabilized for a year or two. Once a woman becomes pregnant, she will need to be monitored carefully to make sure that she gains weight and that nutrition is adequate for the developing fetus.

Related entries

Antidepressants, artificial sweeteners, cholesterol, coronary artery disease, diabetes, dieting, endometrial cancer, exercise, gallstones, high blood pressure, hirsutism, lipectomy and liposuction, nutrition, osteoarthritis, preeclampsia, stroke, weight tables

ally regain the weight they lost and have to go on another diet. Many even end up weighing more than they did originally. But this should not discourage people who truly need to lose weight from trying. In fact, many people who were obese lose weight by focusing on realistic weight goals and healthy behaviors. The goal should be to improve or alleviate the symptoms and risks of obesity rather than striving for some ideal weight.

The specific weight loss plan needs to be determined on an individual basis, depending on a woman's history, concerns, and goals. One reason why so many attempts to treat obesity fail is that people assume that all obesity has the same cause and therefore can be treated in the same way. For one woman, successful treatment may involve losing a set num-

Obsessive-Compulsive Disorder

Obsessive-compulsive disorder (OCD) is an anxiety disorder characterized by persistent and repetitive thoughts or actions. Although these thoughts (obsessions) and actions (compulsions) appear senseless or destructive—even to the person with OCD—they are extremely difficult to resist. People with this disorder, which is somewhat more prevalent in women than in men, find themselves absorbed by various mental images or rituals—for example, checking again and again to make sure that the iron has been turned off or repeatedly washing their hands.

To some extent ritualistic behavior and routine thoughts are a part of every person's life; civilization might not exist—or at least not be very efficient—without them. Many perfectly normal people feel a need to recheck the door lock before retiring each night, while others worry for hours that they may have nicked another car in a parking lot. The diagnosis of OCD is made only if these repetitive thoughts or actions occupy so much time that they interfere with normal functioning or cause significant distress.

Just what causes OCD remains largely a mystery. Some psychiatrists attribute the disorder to early childhood experiences related to issues of control and authority. Others hypothesize that people with OCD may have some genetic predisposition that makes them oversensitive to change.

Who is likely to develop OCD?

As many as 50 percent of people with OCD show symptoms by the time they are 15. It is not uncommon for people with depression or anxiety to have symptoms of OCD as well. Recent research suggests that there are overlaps between eating disorders and obsessional symptoms. OCD is also hypothesized to be partly genetic, with increased rates of OCD in family members of people with the disorder.

Recently some evidence has also suggested that OCD in children may sometimes be a post-infectious autoimmune disorder. A subgroup of child patients with OCD are characterized by a sudden (acute) onset of symptoms (often including tics) following infections with group A B-hemolytic streptococci. This group of patients is identified by the acronym PANDAS (pediatric autoimmune neuropsychiatric disorders associated with streptococcal infections). Researchers still do not understand whether or not OCD in adults is related to this sudden childhood-onset form of the disorder.

What are the symptoms?

The main symptoms of OCD are recurrent ideas or behaviors that are unwanted and that may appear to be pointless. People with OCD usually have a good sense of reality and readily admit that their obsessions and compulsions are irrational, absurd, or superstitious. They are unable to stop themselves from yielding to these impulses, however, and become so completely absorbed in the obsession or compulsion that they think of nothing else until they have finished. If they are forcibly interrupted from completing their thought or behavior, they usually experience considerable anxiety.

OCD seems to worsen during pregnancy in some women. In others, pregnancy triggers symptoms of OCD that never existed before. After delivery some women seem to develop OCD as a form of postpartum psychiatric disorder (see entry). These women often have unwanted and intrusive thoughts of harming their baby. Perhaps as a result of these impulses, women with OCD tend to have trouble bonding with their infants and try to avoid situations, such as bathing the infant, in which they might try to enact their fantasies. Sometimes obsessive-compulsive symptoms accompany other psychiatric changes such as depression which may appear in the weeks or months after the birth of a baby.

How is OCD evaluated?

Clinicians experienced in diagnosing and treating mental disorders can usually identify OCD in a woman showing signs of obsession and compulsion. Certain obsessions, however, are difficult to distinguish from phobias (irrational fears), and in fact there may be overlaps between these two types of anxiety disorders. In addition, some people with OCD or obsessional characteristics also have other mental or emotional disorders, including depression or, rarely, an early stage of schizophrenia.

How is obsessive-compulsive disorder treated?

Many people with OCD respond well to antidepressants or other drug therapy, often in combination with cognitive or other forms of behavioral psychotherapy. Cognitive-behavioral therapy is also very helpful, using an exposure/response prevention technique in which the person is exposed to experiences of which she is fearful (e.g., touching something dirty) and is prevented from performing her habitual compulsive rituals (e.g., handwashing) following those experiences. With a therapist's support, this approach teaches people to tolerate their anxiety and to accept that their compulsive rituals are unnecessary.

In women with postpartum OCD or OCD that has been exacerbated by pregnancy, the antidepressants Prozac (fluoxetine), Zoloft (sertraline), and Paxil (paroxetine) seem to be safe and particularly effective, especially if combined with psychotherapy. In women who also have symptoms of depression, tricyclic antidepressants such as amitriptyline (Elavil) or desipramine (Norpramin) may also help. Since very little is understood about OCD in these women, however, the final word about effective treatment must await results of the various studies currently under way.

Related entries

Antianxiety drugs, antidepressants, anxiety disorders, depression, personality disorders, phobias, postpartum psychiatric disorders, pregnancy, psychotherapy, schizophrenia

Occupational Hazards

From the Lowell, Massachusetts, mills of the 1840s to the New York garment district of the early 1900s to the chicken processing plants of the South and the fields and orchards of California in the 1990s, occupational health hazards have always been a problem for women. Historically women have been employed primarily in service and clerical jobs and as semiskilled workers in manufacturing and nonconstruction industries. These occupations do not present as many catastrophic risks as the male-dominated heavy manufacturing and mining industries, but they have been no less threatening to long-term health and safety. For example, the U.S. Department of Labor's Bureau of Labor Statistics in 1989 identified the poultry processing industry as second only to shipbuilding and repair in the number of serious illnesses and injuries per 100 workers.

As women continue to enter the workforce and assume jobs that were traditionally performed by men, workplace safety and health is becoming even more of a women's issue. Women make up over half of the country's civilian workforce and already predominate in many of the industries most susceptible to work-related injuries. These include eating and drinking establishments, retail grocery stores, hospitals, nursing and personal care facilities, department stores, and hotels and motels.

Types of occupational hazards

Respiratory system. Diseases of the nasal passages, airways, and lungs are among the nation's 10 leading causes of work-related sickness and a major cause of occupational illness in women (see chart). As the numbers of potentially toxic chemicals continue to grow in the workplace as well as the general environment, the incidence of these diseases will undoubtedly increase as well.

Respiratory illness results from inhaling organic and inorganic dust, irritants, vapors, gases, and fumes, as well as from working in inadequately ventilated buildings. The specific nature and extent of the illness depends on just which toxic chemical was involved and how much of the toxin penetrated the respiratory tract. Room ventilation, temperature, humidity, the worker's rate of exercise and breathing, and any protective gear that may have been worn are all factors.

Some respiratory illnesses develop quite soon after exposure to a toxin. These include occupational asthma (symptoms are shortness of breath, cough, and wheezing); rhinitis (inflammation of the mucous membranes of the nose); industrial bronchitis (cough and sputum); and various disorders that arise from inhaling metal fumes. In pulmonary beryllium disease, for example, inhaling the lightweight metal beryllium can eventually lead to scarring of lung tissue and reduced breathing capacity. Early case reports of pulmonary beryllium disease came from a group of women exposed dur-

---

Some occupations that can be hazardous to the lungs and airways

Cleaning
Farming
Clerical work
Textile manufacturing
Laboratory work
Welding
Construction
Electronics
Tool, die, ceramics manufacturing
Detergent manufacturing
Baking
Paint, polyurethane, and plastics manufacturing
Shellfish processing
Service jobs

---

ing the course of working in the fluorescent lightbulb manufacturing industry.

Other respiratory diseases such as asbestosis, silicosis, and coal workers' pneumoconiosis (black lung disease) may take a decade or longer to develop after exposure. They result from inhaling inorganic dusts from asbestos fibers, silica (crystalline quartz), and coal, respectively, and have occurred historically in men as a result of exposure in the construction and shipbuilding industries and in mining and quarry work. Women have been exposed to asbestos primarily in textile and other end-product manufacture and as a result of household and residential contact. Symptoms of asbestosis can include chest pain, shortness of breath, and, occasionally, coughing.

Because women tend to hold most clerical and service jobs, they are at particular risk for developing "sick building syndrome," which has been reported among workers in buildings with inadequate ventilation. People with sick building syndrome generally suffer from rhinitis, laryngitis, coughing, and wheezing. These symptoms have been attributed to volatile vapors from chemicals such as formaldehyde in carpeting, draperies, and upholstered furniture; fiberglass dust from ceiling tiles and insulation material; low relative humidity; diesel fumes from outside traffic; and environmental tobacco smoke.

Musculoskeletal system. Injuries to the muscles and bones, as well as the structures connecting and supporting them, rate as the leading cause of disability in the United States for individuals of working age. At least half of the workforce in this country will be affected by musculoskeletal injuries at some point in their working life. Most of these injuries involve the back, upper spine, arms, hands, or fingers.

These injuries generally result from exceeding one's physical capabilities and limitations. This often happens in jobs that involve heavy lifting, repetitive motion (such as word processing), vibration, poor posture, and excessive bending, twisting, reaching, pushing, and pulling. The risk attached to each of these activities is modified according to the worker's age, sex, strength, physical fitness, fatigue, trauma, emotional stress, and certain preexisting conditions such as osteoarthritis and other degenerative disorders. Because many workstations, tools, and kinds of protective gear were designed for the average male stature and physical capacity, women may be particularly prone to on-the-job musculoskeletal injuries.

Physical capacities vary widely among individual men and women, however. The average woman tolerates lower maximum weights and forces than the average man, but these criteria often have nothing to do with actual job demands or a particular person's risk of injury, and have the potential to lead to discrimination. Any job applicant, whether man or woman, should therefore be evaluated on an individual basis for fitness to a particular task. Excluding applicants from jobs on the basis of sex is not the best means of protecting workers.

The best way to reduce the risk of musculoskeletal injuries in the workplace is to use mechanical aids and to redesign workstations and tools with the goal of reducing worker stress. Examples include the use of conveyor belts, hoists, lift tables, proper work surface heights, and contoured handgrips on tools.

Careful design of computer workstations is especially important to the many women who spend much of the day word processing and entering data into computers. Repeated forceful motions of the fingers, especially with the wrist flexed or extended, can produce carpal tunnel syndrome (see entry)—which involves tingling, numbness, and pain in the fingers—and tendinitis (see tendinitis and tenosynovitis). Headaches and backaches from muscle tension and strain can also result from poor design of computer workstations. Women who work at computers should make a habit of taking periodic breaks to avoid musculoskeletal strain, as well as eye strain.

Those who work for long hours at desks, whether the work involves computers or not, may want to try some exercises to reduce the muscle strain that comes from hours of sitting (see illustration). Taking a brisk walk during lunch breaks or to and from work can also help. Some larger companies offer exercise programs to their employees or health club memberships at reduced rates. In addition to relieving tension and preventing musculoskeletal disorders, activities such as these can help women maintain an appropriate weight, retain bone mass, and develop aerobic fitness.

Reproductive system. Disorders of the reproductive system rank among the nation's 10 leading categories of work-related injuries and illnesses. These disorders include any injury to the reproductive system itself or to a developing fetus or child whose health may be affected through the working parent. For women, these occupational hazards may lead to altered menstrual function, decreased sex drive, reduced fertility, miscarriage, pregnancy complications (such as babies born prematurely, underweight, or with abnormal body structures or functions), breast milk contamination, and childhood cancer in offspring.

Many chemical, physical, and biological agents have been suggested as possible reproductive hazards. Currently, most of the 60,000 chemicals in commercial use have not been thoroughly evaluated for reproductive or developmental toxicity.

The effects of certain physical hazards such as occupational exposure to noise are equally unclear. Excess noise has led to a reduction in the number of pregnancies and increased embryo and fetal death in some animal studies, but these results are not necessarily applicable to humans. As for the hazards during pregnancy of performing physically strenuous work, there seems to be no particular risk involved for healthy women who are receiving adequate nutrition and prenatal care. Growing evidence suggests, however, that repetitive heavy lifting in the last 3 months of pregnancy can cause uterine contractions.

Evidence is stronger regarding the effects of other physical hazards, particularly ionizing radiation, which is widely used in medicine, industry, government, and nuclear fuel operations. Depending on the dose, exposure to ionizing radiation during pregnancy can result in birth defects, mental retardation, childhood leukemia, and other childhood cancers in offspring.

The increasingly pervasive computer has caused widespread concern about the reproductive impact of video display terminals (VDTs), which emit minimal amounts of ionizing radiation as well as very low frequency (VLF) and extremely low frequency (ELF) radiation. Large-scale research in recent years, including a well-designed study by the National Institute of Occupational Safety and Health (NIOSH), has not found any solid link between VDT use and miscarriage.

Exposure to infectious disease is a particularly common occupational hazard among health care providers, housekeepers, laundry workers, laboratory technicians, day care providers, teachers, sanitation workers, and people who come in contact with animals or animal products. Acquiring the rubella virus, cytomegalovirus, hepatitis B virus, human immunodeficiency virus (HIV), human parvovirus B19 (Fifths disease), and chickenpox virus during pregnancy can result in fetal infections, miscarriage, and developmental defects.

Psychological hazards. A 1994 survey by the U.S. Department of Labor Women's Bureau reported that 60 percent of working women identified stress as the most important work-related health problem. Most of this stress comes from working in subordinate jobs with little control over work or work environment, coupled with the work-family conflicts, financial and economic strain, and sexual discrimination and ha-

Desk exercises

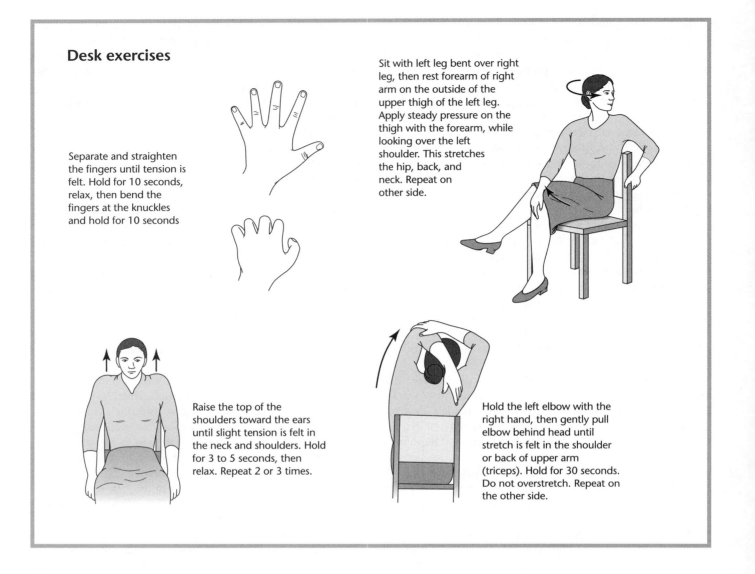

Separate and straighten the fingers until tension is felt. Hold for 10 seconds, relax, then bend the fingers at the knuckles and hold for 10 seconds

Sit with left leg bent over right leg, then rest forearm of right arm on the outside of the upper thigh of the left leg. Apply steady pressure on the thigh with the forearm, while looking over the left shoulder. This stretches the hip, back, and neck. Repeat on other side.

Raise the top of the shoulders toward the ears until slight tension is felt in the neck and shoulders. Hold for 3 to 5 seconds, then relax. Repeat 2 or 3 times.

Hold the left elbow with the right hand, then gently pull elbow behind head until stretch is felt in the shoulder or back of upper arm (triceps). Hold for 30 seconds. Do not overstretch. Repeat on the other side.

rassment on the job faced by many working women. Over 80 percent of working married women report having primary responsibility for household chores, and over 60 percent of them say they have primary responsibility for paying family bills. Working mothers generally also have primary responsibility for child and elder care on top of their jobs, and single mothers must often bear the entire responsibility themselves. Salary and promotion barriers add to the psychological strain: in 1997 women earned only 79 percent as much as men with equivalent training and responsibilities.

The health effects of all these stressors can be both physical and psychological and may include reactions such as anxiety and depression, gastrointestinal and sleep disorders, and increased job absenteeism. These symptoms can be difficult to recognize as stress- or workplace-related and even more difficult to treat. Once recognized, however, stress management strategies in the workplace—often together with individual psychotherapy—may be helpful. Unless the source of the stress can be identified and alleviated, however, these strategies will be limited in their effectiveness. Ultimately, job-related stress may require more opportunities for working women to participate in decision making, increased opportunities for job promotion and career advancement, flexible schedules that allow time for child and elder care, job redesign, and enforcement of policies against sex discrimination and sexual harassment.

How are occupational hazards evaluated and treated?

Even in the doctor's office, work is often overlooked as a potential source of medical problems in women. Not all primary caregivers will think that a fit of coughing and wheezing may be the first sign of occupational asthma, for example. Women who think they may have a job-related illness or disability should make a point of describing their work situation to their health care provider. Since some disabilities can take years to develop, a former job may be relevant as well.

In addition to a description of the symptoms, a clinician evaluating a possible job-related disorder will want to know about the tasks the patient performs at work; the types and amounts of chemicals, dust, fumes, gas, or radiation to which she has been exposed; the type of ventilation in the building and any protective gear worn; and complaints among other workers about similar symptoms.

Treatment of job-related diseases depends on the nature and severity of the particular disease.

How can job-related diseases be prevented?

Various cultural, biological, and economic factors complicate a woman's ability to protect her health and safety in the workplace. People in low-paying occupations with little job security—usually women and minorities—are obviously more hesitant to complain about unsafe working conditions or to enforce their right to know about potentially toxic exposures. Expressing concern about a job's effect on one's fertility or the health of an unborn child can threaten job security and create opportunities for subtle sex discrimination. The fact that women are often not members of trade unions probably increases their reluctance to speak up. Women struggling to balance home and work responsibilities or manage as single parents may simply not have time to pursue or even to investigate their rights as workers.

There are two basic categories of protections for workers in the United States: ▸ government regulations established to prevent hazards from occurring and, when these fail, ▸ compensation for injured workers.

Regulatory protections. The most fundamental regulatory protections are set by the Occupational Safety and Health Administration (OSHA). This federal body was established in 1970 to ensure "safe and healthful" working conditions for all American workers. Workers are encouraged to report dangerous conditions to OSHA, and OSHA is empowered to inspect workplaces for violations and to fine employers if violations occur. In cases where states have been allowed to take over OSHA's functions, their regulations must be at least as strict as those of the federal government.

In 1987 OSHA established the Hazard Communication Standards (HCS) to help provide better information to employers and employees about chemical hazards in the workplace. These standards require employers to label each container of hazardous chemicals with the identity and toxicity of the chemical. Employers must also provide information and training about hazardous chemicals to employees whenever they are assigned to a new work area or whenever a new chemical is introduced. In addition, under HCS, employees have a "right to know" what chemicals are being used in their workplace. This information exists in the form of Material Safety Data Sheets (MSDS) which give both generic and brand names, chemical composition, reported acute and chronic health effects, and steps to be taken if overexposure should occur. But because MSDSs are required only for chemicals, and because employers may resist providing them, employees may need to obtain additional information from other sources.

Any three employees can request a formal Health Hazard Evaluation from NIOSH (National Institute for Occupational Safety and Health), a part of the federal Centers for Disease Control (CDC) which conducts research on occupational disease. NIOSH also has educational resource centers around the country which can provide workers with literature and access to information about current research.

Well intentioned as government protections may be, they often remain more effective in theory than in practice. Government agencies simply do not have the means to investigate and survey any but the most flagrant violations. And many people who are the victims of violations remain unaware of their rights as workers, so the offenses often go unreported.

Finally, some of the regulations do not address the specific health concerns of women, particularly when it comes to reproductive risks. To date, only four agents have been regulated even in part to prevent reproductive damage. These are lead, radiation, dibromochlorpropane, and ethylene oxide. Although NIOSH has issued recommended exposure limits (RELs) for these agents, these are merely guidelines for estimating safe exposure limits and are not legally enforceable.

Any woman considering having children should try to reduce or eliminate reproductive hazards posed by her work situation before conception, since many harmful effects can occur even before a woman knows she is pregnant. In addition, the potential father's exposure to chemicals in the workplace can also have reproductive effects, depending on the frequency, timing, duration, and intensity of exposure.

The most effective protection is to eliminate the hazard (by substituting a safer chemical, for example). When this is not possible, exposure can often be reduced through engineering controls—such as making sure that the ventilation system is well maintained or that the toxic areas are well enclosed. As a last resort, using personal protective equipment such as respirators or masks may be tried, but this is only a short-term solution.

If protection is impracticable, a woman may want to ask her doctor to help her request a temporary job transfer or leave. By law, employers must treat requests by pregnant women for job transfers and leaves no differently from requests by other workers. The catch, of course, is that other requests may not be honored either. A woman may therefore hesitate to ask for leave or transfer if she knows this could adversely affect her income, seniority, health insurance, disability payments, or job security. If the law is violated, being able to bring an employer to court is often little consolation. Sometimes, however, it is the only solution.

In trying to protect themselves from occupational hazards, women often are tripped up by the fine line between protection and prohibition. The same laws set up to shield women from dangerous working situations sometimes end up keeping them from working at all. For this reason, women should be aware of antidiscrimination legislation that has been enacted over the past several decades. These acts are premised on the belief that, despite differences between men's and women's body stature, muscle strength, and childbearing capacity, differential treatment of women in the workplace is rarely justified. Title VII of the Civil Rights Act of 1964 explicitly prohibits sex-based discrimination with respect to hiring, discharge, compensation, terms, privileges, and other conditions of employment.

In 1978 the Civil Rights Act was further amended by the Pregnancy Discrimination Act. This act prohibits sex-based discrimination on the basis of pregnancy, childbirth, or related medical conditions, except in those circumstances in which sex is a bona fide occupational qualification (BFOQ), that is, when the employee's gender is reasonably important to the normal operation of a particular business or enterprise. To qualify as a BFOQ, a job qualification must relate to the essence or the central mission of the business. It would be legitimate, for example, for an employer to refuse to hire women as models for men's clothing. If "male" attributes are not fundamental to a job, however, women applicants with the necessary job-related skills must be judged by the same standards as male applicants.

Another victory for women in the workplace has come with the abolition of fetal protection policies (FPPs). These policies were used throughout the 1980s to exclude women of childbearing age from certain jobs on the grounds that these could have adverse reproductive effects. For example, in 1982 Johnson Controls, a lead battery manufacturer, instituted an FPP that excluded women of all ages—except those with medical documentation of sterility—from jobs that involved potential lead exposure.

Although ostensibly instituted to "protect" women from the reproductive effects of lead exposure (see illustration), FPPs in reality excluded women from certain male-dominated jobs. They also overlooked the adverse health outcomes for pregnant women and their offspring resulting from lost income and health insurance benefits. Furthermore, FPPs violated privacy rights by forcing women (but not men) to reveal their reproductive status to employers and co-workers. Because of FPPs some women even underwent surgery to become "officially" sterile. That women in other industries with equivalent reproductive hazards were not excluded from working (the workplace was cleaned up instead)—and that there was no concern for the reproductive health of men working in these ostensibly dangerous jobs—is testament to the sincerity of the "concern for health" supposedly underlying the FPPs.

This conclusion was supported by the landmark 1991 decision by the U.S. Supreme Court *International Union, UAW v. Johnson Controls Inc.*, which declared FPPs to be a form of sex discrimination. The court further held that sex was not a BFOQ in the battery business because sex and childbearing capacity did not relate to the central mission of battery manufacturing. Protecting the welfare of future children, noted the Court, is the burden of parents, not the employers of those parents.

The message was clear: If there are real concerns about hazards in the workplace, the solution is cleaning them up for all workers rather than excluding certain workers from dangerous sites.

Workers' compensation and other legal remedies. Because government does not always provide adequate protections, employees also have the option of resorting to the legal system for compensation. In theory, the threat of having to pay compensation is supposed to motivate employers to provide safe and healthful workplaces. But for certain workplace hazards, many of them particular to women, the compensation system is inadequate.

Workers' compensation is a no-fault system that was instituted in this country in the 1920s based on systems in Great Britain and Germany. It represents a compromise between labor and industry: employees give up their rights to sue employers, and employers accept all claims of work-related injuries and diseases. An employee is therefore automatically entitled to certain benefits after incurring a work-related injury, regardless of fault. These benefits include "reasonable" compensation for medical expenses and wage compensation if the disability prevents the job from being performed. Employers have been willing to grant this privilege because it saved them from facing unpredictable juries that might be likely to exact punitive as well as compensatory damages.

A major drawback to the workers' compensation system is that it does not adequately compensate for occupational diseases that take a long time to develop or that lack obvious symptoms or effects on the ability to work. To receive compensation, an employee has to prove the existence and extent of disability and then show that this disability arose out of conditions in the workplace. Usually the extent of a disability is determined by how much it reduces earning capacity. This can be a problem in the case of many work-related injuries common to women—such as those that cause infertility, decreased sexual desire, or miscarriage—which do not necessarily diminish employment opportunities or the ability to work. Some states, however, have specific provisions in their workers' compensation laws for effects such as "loss of reproductive function/organs."

If injury or disease results from the action of a third party (not the employer), employees may sue this third party under the toxic torts system. Workers exposed to asbestos on the job, for example, have successfully sued the manufacturers of products containing these substances for not putting warning labels on them. Under workers' compensation laws, however, these same workers could not have sued their employers for using these asbestos-containing products as part of the manufacturing process. Employees suing under tort law, as opposed to workers' provisions, are heard in a court of law (with a jury) and do not have to demonstrate impairment or disability.

Related entries

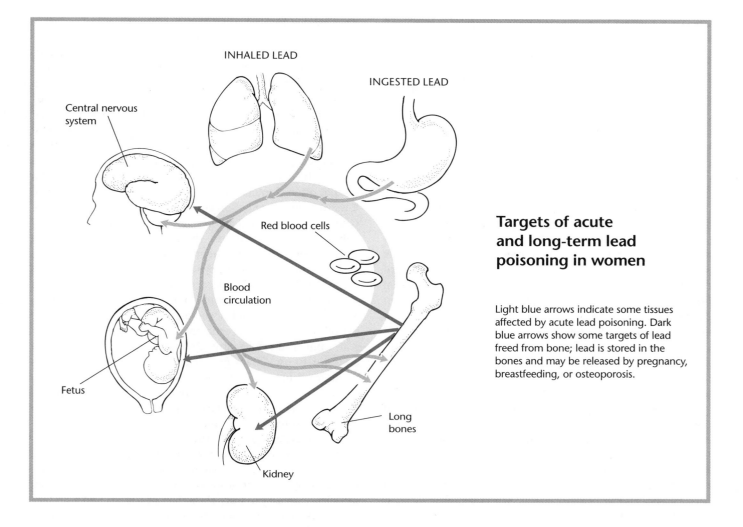

INHALED LEAD

INGESTED LEAD

Central nervous system

Red blood cells

Blood circulation

Fetus

Kidney

Long bones

Targets of acute and long-term lead poisoning in women

Light blue arrows indicate some tissues affected by acute lead poisoning. Dark blue arrows show some targets of lead freed from bone; lead is stored in the bones and may be released by pregnancy, breastfeeding, or osteoporosis.

dysfunction, sexual harassment, stress, tendinitis and tenosynovitis

Oral Contraceptives

Throughout most of the Western world, the birth control pill is today the most popular method of contraception. Ever since its introduction in the late 1950s, "the pill" has been recognized as a revolutionary force. It was first feared as an invitation to sexual promiscuity, but it was later hailed for giving women control over their bodies. Doubts arose in the 1970s, when new data revealed some serious side effects—especially blood clots, which could promote heart attacks, strokes, or circulatory disorders. Some feminists charged that the pill was in essence a massive experiment conducted on the women of the world.

Today, however, it appears that most of the dangers associated with oral contraceptives were due to the high doses of estrogen contained in earlier versions, and that most compli-

cations were limited to women over the age of 35 who also smoked cigarettes. Now newer and safer formulations of the pill which contain much less estrogen are available, and it is widely agreed that, for most women, oral contraceptives are a highly effective and safe method of birth control.

Although women over the age of 35 were formerly cautioned against using the pill (particularly if they smoked), it now appears that oral contraceptives are perfectly safe and possibly even beneficial for most nonsmoking women through their 40s. The long-term effects of taking these pills for 30 years or so remain unclear, however, largely because to this point there simply have not been enough women who have taken them for that long.

Oral contraceptives may help protect women against a number of health problems in addition to unwanted pregnancies. Not only does the pill seem to reduce the chances of developing both ovarian and uterine cancers, but also it may protect women against benign breast tumors. It seems to provide a significant degree of protection against pelvic inflammatory disease (PID)—which causes serious pelvic and abdominal pain as well as infertility—and may help increase bone density when taken by women nearing menopause. Finally, in many women regular use of the pill reduces menstrual cramps and heavy menstrual bleeding (menorrhagia), which in turn may help prevent iron-deficiency anemia. Some forms of oral contraceptives can also help clear up acne.

How do oral contraceptives work?

Most oral contraceptives prescribed today are called combination pills because they include two kinds of hormones: a synthetic estrogen and a synthetic progesterone (that is, a progestin). Normally, in the course of the menstrual cycle (see entry), fluctuating levels of these hormones are involved in a complex feedback loop which results in the release of an egg from the ovary (ovulation) and the growth of the uterine lining in preparation for the implantation of a fertilized egg. When a woman takes combination pills, a steady hormonal state throughout the month blocks this feedback mechanism: steady levels of estrogen prevent ovulation, while steady levels of progestin induce changes in the cervical mucus (which inhibit sperm transport) and in the endometrial lining (which inhibit its receptivity to implantation). Even the relatively small amounts of hormone contained in modern combination pills (generally 35 micrograms or less of ethinyl estradiol) are enough to effect these changes. A similar inhibition occurs during pregnancy, when much higher levels of estrogen released by the corpus luteum and placenta also serve to inhibit the cyclical release of hormones.

Most combination pills prescribed today contain a fixed dose of both synthetic estrogens and progestins. Among the most commonly prescribed of these "monophasic pills" are Loestrin, Lo/Ovral, Brevicon, Modicon, Ovcon-35, Norinyl 1 + 35, Ortho-Novum 1/35, Demulen 35, and Nordette. Also available are biphasic pills (Ortho-Novum 10/11) and triphasic pills (Ortho-Novum 7-7-7, Tri-Norinyl, Tri-Levlen, or Triphasil), which alter the relative proportion of hormones available throughout the course of the month to mimic more closely the hormonal changes of the menstrual cycle. These offer little if any advantage over the monophasic pills but may result in fewer side effects in some women. Recently pills with new forms of progestin (desogestrel and norgestimate) have become available. The progestins in these pills (sold under the brand names Desogen, Orthocept, and Orthocyclen) have less effect on blood pressure and are less likely to cause side effects such as breakthrough bleeding.

A new "extended cycle" birth-control pill, Seasonale, reduces the frequency of menstrual periods to four times a year. Containing the same combination of low-dose estrogen and progestin found in many other oral contraceptives, Seasonale is taken for 12 straight weeks, followed by a week of placebo pills, which results in menstruation. Breakthrough bleeding occurs about twice as often with Seasonale use as with other oral contraceptives, particularly in the first year. Women who view menstruation as an affirmation of health or a confirmation that they are not pregnant may prefer more traditional oral contraceptives.

Combination pills are generally taken for 21 days out of every menstrual cycle and then discontinued for 7 days, during which time menstrual period–like bleeding usually begins. Often the pills are started on day 1 of the menstrual cycle (that is, on the day when bleeding starts). Some monthly packets consist of pills that can be taken every day throughout the cycle: 21 days' worth of hormone-containing pills and 7 days' worth of differently colored sugar or iron pills. This type of packet is especially convenient for women who do not want to worry about remembering which days they are supposed to be taking a pill. Oral contraceptives work best if taken at about the same time every day. They can be taken with food if nausea is a problem. During the first month of use, a backup form of contraception should be used.

Once the body has adjusted to the new hormonal regimen, the pill often results in very regular menstrual cycles and allows women to predict precisely the first day of their period. Often, too, menstrual periods are lighter, shorter, and less painful. Problems with breakthrough bleeding (that is, bleeding between periods) frequently resolve themselves after the first few months. If not, switching to another formulation (with a different proportion of estrogen to progesterone) is usually the answer. Although some women do not menstruate while taking the pill, a woman who misses more than one period should have a pregnancy test to be sure.

If a pill is missed, many clinicians suggest that the safest course is to use a backup means of birth control (such as a condom) throughout the rest of the menstrual cycle, especially if the pill is skipped early in the cycle or if breakthrough bleeding occurs. Other clinicians argue that in most cases it is probably safe to make up for a missed pill by taking the previous day's pill with the current one.

Another form of oral contraceptive, sometimes called the minipill, contains only a small dose of synthetic progesterone (usually norethindrone or levonorgestrel). The minipill inhibits ovulation in only about half of the women who take it. It prevents pregnancy primarily by making the cervical mucus inhospitable to sperm and, to some extent, by slowing the transport of the egg through the fallopian tube. Though somewhat less effective than the combined oral contraceptive, the minipill is sometimes used by women who cannot take estrogens or in whom fertility is somewhat diminished (such as women nearing menopause). Progestin-only pills are taken every day of the menstrual cycle, even during menstruation, and preferably at the same time each day. As with the combined pill, it is wise to use a backup form of contraception during the first month of use.

The combined oral contraceptive pill is a highly effective form of birth control, with less than 1 pregnancy for every 100 women who take it in the course of a year. Oral contraceptives containing only progestins are somewhat less effective, with about 3 pregnancies resulting each year for every 100 users.

The oral contraceptive is relatively easy to use—provided the woman remembers to take a pill every single day. It is also an easy form of contraception to stop should a woman decide she wants to become pregnant or switch to another method. On the negative side, women using oral contraceptives must first see a physician in order to obtain a prescription and then return several months later for a checkup. Yearly checkups with a Pap test are also generally advisable.

In addition, if side effects are a problem, it may be necessary to return to the doctor's office or clinic several times until the right formulation is found.

A year's supply of birth control pills generally costs about $200 to $240. Added to this are the costs of physician or clinic visits for initial and follow-up examinations.

What are the risks and complications?

Among the many commonly cited side effects of the combination birth control pill are breast tenderness, swelling and bloating, weight gain, nausea, skin problems (especially eczema, rashes, and chloasma—large brown patches on the face), excessive hair growth or hair loss, depression, alterations in appetite and sexual response, vaginitis, and menstrual changes. Women with migraines—particularly women whose symptoms peak during menstruation—sometimes find that their headaches increase in either frequency or severity while they are using oral contraceptives. Others, however, find that their headaches become less severe. Although many women using the pill (especially versions containing relatively high levels of progesterone) develop acne, others find that oral contraceptives help clear up preexisting pimples. Many of these side effects disappear after the first few months or can be eliminated by switching to a different prescription. There is also some evidence that taking supplements of vitamin B_6 may help ameliorate the depression that sometimes occurs in women who take the pill.

Various studies have linked the pill with a somewhat increased risk of developing high blood pressure, gallbladder disease, and benign liver tumors. These risks have to be kept in perspective, however. For example, only about 5 percent of women who previously had normal blood pressure will develop hypertension after 3 months of pill use. And newer formulations of the pill (particularly desogestrel and norgestimate) have even less effect on blood pressure. The chances of developing the other disorders, though real, are similarly small.

In some studies oral contraceptives have been linked to certain forms of cervical cancer. Researchers have thought that this had less to do with any dangers inherent in the pill than with the fact that barrier methods of contraception (such as condoms and diaphragms) may have a protective effect against these cancers—or possibly with the fact that women who use oral contraceptives may have a higher level of sexual activity (which has also been linked to cervical cancer). Studies that take account of these factors nevertheless still show an increased risk.

Some of the progestins contained in combination pills may alter the body's ability to process glucose, at least temporarily. This alteration can present a problem for women with diabetes mellitus, who may need to increase their insulin dosage while using this form of contraception. Nevertheless, many doctors believe that this is a sacrifice worth making in return for a reliable method of birth control in women for whom pregnancy can often be problematic.

Earlier pills containing high estrogen levels were linked with an increased risk of cardiovascular disease, probably because of changes in triglyceride (blood fat) levels, though most studies of the link between triglycerides and heart disease have been done in men only. There is no evidence, however, that the lower-estrogen pills used today increase this risk, even though the progesterone they contain still has a minor effect on blood lipid levels. In fact, the estrogen may counteract the progesterone and actually protect against heart disease by preventing the buildup of atherosclerotic plaque. In women who smoke cigarettes, however, oral contraceptives seem to increase the risk of developing blood clots, which can result in heart attacks, strokes, and other circulatory disorders (see entry). Combined oral contraceptives are usually not recommended for women over the age of 35 who smoke cigarettes (and probably are not the best method for any heavy smokers).

Nor are they generally recommended for women with a history of hyperlipidemia, heart disease, lupus, stroke, circulatory or clotting disorders (such as thrombophlebitis), breast or uterine cancer, severe liver disease, or abnormal vaginal bleeding of unknown cause. Women who have migraine headaches, high blood pressure, diabetes, a history of depression, or sickle cell anemia should also consider other forms of contraception, though sometimes the pill can be used even when these conditions are present. Contrary to earlier belief, having uterine fibroids or bad varicose veins does not increase any health risks associated with oral contraceptives. To prevent premature suppression of bone growth, oral contraceptives are best postponed until a teenager has been menstruating for at least 6 months. Nor are oral contraceptives appropriate for women who are or may be pregnant. Combination pills are not usually prescribed for women who are breastfeeding.

Women with hypertension may want to consider the progesterone-only minipill, which has no known effect on blood pressure. The minipill also has minimal, if any, effects on glucose tolerance, and so may be a better choice for women with diabetes. It is also sometimes a reasonable alternative for women with migraine headaches. The minipill frequently results in menstrual disturbances, however, especially irregular bleeding, and may produce some of the same side effects as the combined pill—particularly appetite and weight changes, edema, depression, breast changes, acne, and hirsutism. It is also associated with an increased risk of ectopic pregnancy in the few women who do become pregnant while using it, probably because of the slowed transport of the egg through the fallopian tube. Little is known about long-term risks. In some countries, doctors do not consider the minipill safe for women who are breastfeeding, though it is widely prescribed as a contraceptive method for lactating mothers in both the United States and the United Kingdom.

Women considering oral contraceptives should first have a thorough physical examination which includes a pelvic examination, breast examination, Pap test, blood pressure measurements, and various blood and urine tests. They should tell their clinician about any personal or family history of blood clots, heart disease, stroke, breast cancer, or diabetes.

Women just starting to use the pill should have a checkup

within 3 months so that blood pressure changes and other possible side effects can be monitored. After that, a yearly physical examination is usually sufficient. It is important for a woman to tell her clinician that she is on the pill before any other tests or medical procedures are performed, since the pill can alter so many body functions. Because of the increase in risk of blood clots following major surgery, women taking the pill should stop before having elective major surgery. And all women should bear in mind that taking certain other medications—such as barbiturates, some epilepsy and arthritis drugs, and the antibiotics tetracycline and penicillins—can reduce the pill's efficacy as a contraceptive.

If a woman using oral contraceptives wants to become pregnant (or switch to another method of birth control), she should not stop taking the pills until after finishing a monthly packet. Sometimes ovulation does not resume for a few cycles, and periods may be absent or irregular during this time. Occasionally a phenomenon known as postpill amenorrhea occurs, in which menstrual periods fail to recur on their own (see amenorrhea). Most women who stop taking the pill, however, are fully fertile again within 3 months—about the time most clinicians recommend waiting before trying to become pregnant after going off the pill.

Related entries

Abortion, amenorrhea, birth control, circulatory disorders, condoms, diabetes, diaphragms and cervical caps, ectopic pregnancy, high blood pressure, hormonal contraception, intrauterine devices, menstrual cycle, natural birth control methods, nonsurgical abortion, pregnancy testing, safer sex, sexually transmitted diseases, smoking, spermicides, tubal ligation, vacuum aspiration

Orthodontia

Many women who missed out on braces as children or teenagers look in the mirror and rue what they think of as a lost opportunity. Contrary to earlier belief, however, it is still possible to fix crooked teeth, overbites, underbites, or even a protruding chin after the mouth has stopped growing. The biological process involved in tooth movement is the same in both adults and children, which means that so long as underlying gums and supporting bones are healthy, adjustments can be made well into adult life. They just take a little longer and may require some form of supplemental surgery because facial bones are no longer growing.

Crooked or crowded teeth can lead to a number of health problems. An imperfect bite (malocclusion) and crooked teeth, for example, increase susceptibility to temporomandibular joint syndrome (see entry) and its associated headaches, while a bad bite often leads to chewing difficulties and associated eating problems, unnecessary wear on tooth surfaces, and damage to underlying bone and gum tissue (see gum disease). Crowded teeth are more susceptible to decay, gum disease, and eventual loss because they are unusually difficult to keep clean. And protruding teeth are more susceptible to chipping and breaking. The prospect of extensive and expensive dental care and possibly even future dietary deficiencies may help make the considerable effort and expense of adult braces (a large portion of which usually has to be paid out-of-pocket) somewhat easier to bear.

What problems can be corrected?

Among the many problems that can be corrected through adult orthodontia (braces and/or surgery) are overbite, underbite, open bite (which occurs when back teeth contact each other but the front or side teeth do not), misaligned teeth, crowded or too-widely spaced teeth, extra or missing teeth, and a variety of jawbone discrepancies such as protruding or receding chin, excessive gum tissue above the upper front teeth, elongated face, and separated lips. A woman who thinks she may be a candidate for orthodontia should discuss her particular situation with an orthodontist (a dentist trained to correct bad bite and crooked teeth) or oral surgeon (a dentist trained to correct abnormalities of the face and jaw surgically).

How are these conditions evaluated?

If braces are a possibility, the orthodontist will probably want to see the potential patient once or twice before initiating treatment to review her medical and dental history. In these early visits the orthodontist will examine the mouth to check for overlapped, twisted, or improperly angled teeth and to see if there is enough room in the jaw for all the teeth or if there are abnormally large spaces between them. The size, position, and relationship of jaw and teeth will be determined, and the bite will be examined to see if the teeth of the upper jaw slightly overlap those in the lower one and if the points of the molars fit into the grooves of the opposing molars (considered an ideal bite). A plaster mold will usually be made of the teeth, and various x-rays and photographs will be taken to allow a closer inspection of both teeth and bite.

How are these conditions treated?

In the first visits possible treatment plans will be discussed, as well as expected results and estimated cost. If cost is an issue—which it often is—it is well worth asking the orthodontist if it might be possible to arrange a finance plan involving an initial down payment and monthly installments. Many orthodontists are quite willing to make such arrangements if asked. If the patient has dental insurance, it is worth checking the fine print, since some plans include orthodontic benefits which can at least help offset the cost of treatment.

Braces. Braces are bands or brackets on the teeth that are held together with a thin wire. As the wires are adjusted to greater tensions over a period of months or years, the teeth are gradually moved. Sometimes rubber bands (elastics) are also used to attach the upper and lower teeth, thus creating additional tension on either jaw. Special head or neck gear worn outside the mouth—usually only at night or for a certain number of hours per day—can also be used to create more tension. The resulting changes are often permanent because as the teeth move, the bone in front of them dissolves (resorbs) while the bone behind them accumulates, thus changing the structure of the mouth.

Today's braces are much less noticeable than the "tinsel teeth" that many adults may remember from their childhood. Instead of using ringlike metal bands to encircle the teeth, for example, orthodontists may now attach small brackets to the front surface of each tooth, leaving a large portion of natural tooth exposed. It is even possible to request clear or tooth-colored brackets in lieu of the more standard silver color. The nickel-titanium wires that are threaded through the brackets to pull the teeth into position are also much less conspicuous than ever before, as well as faster-acting and more comfortable. And although teenagers often rave over colored elastics, women interested in more discreet orthodontia can now opt for low-visibility white elastics.

Some orthodontic problems can even be corrected with "invisible" (lingual) braces which attach to the back surface of the teeth and thus cannot be seen from the front. These braces are harder to fit and adjust, however, and therefore tend to be much more expensive than regular braces. They are also more apt to irritate the tongue and interfere with speech.

Just how long braces must be worn depends on the extent of the problem, the overall health of the teeth, gums, and supporting bone, and the patient's age. It is quite common for treatment in adults to last for 2 years or so.

Wearing braces does not require any major lifestyle changes, but it is somewhat inconvenient at times. It is still possible to smile, sing, kiss, or even play a wind instrument (though serious musicians may have some difficulties), but some adults do take a while to stop feeling self-conscious about their new smile—even though they are usually much more secure about their decision than adolescents in the same situation.

Periodic discomfort is still part of the experience of wearing braces, especially for a day or two after each time the wires are tightened. The pain can be alleviated with Tylenol. Tenderness in the mouth and gums can make chewing difficult, however, and people who wear braces have to put certain foods on hold until the braces come off. Sticky treats such as bubble gum and caramels should be avoided, and other foods can be eaten comfortably only with some modification (such as scraping the kernels of corn off the cob).

People with braces must practice scrupulous oral hygiene, especially regular brushing and (if possible) flossing to help prevent food and plaque (a combination of old food and bacteria) from accumulating between the braces and the teeth. Besides predisposing teeth to decay, these accumulations can leave whitish deposits on the teeth once the braces are removed.

Surgery. In younger people, whose facial bones are still growing, braces are usually enough to correct most orthodontic problems. In adults, however, similar results are often impossible with braces alone, and so surgery (performed by an oral surgeon) may be necessary, usually after an initial period of bracing so that the teeth will fit together properly after the operation. Braces are usually left in place during the surgery to help stabilize the teeth and jawbone and are worn for some time after surgery to help finalize tooth alignment.

A protruding or elongated jaw can be corrected by removing part of the bone and resetting the remaining bone into the desired position. Other techniques can be used to lengthen a too-short jaw. These surgeries usually require a few days of hospitalization and are performed under general anesthesia. After the surgery it is difficult to speak or chew for a few days, especially if the jaws must be wired together (to promote faster healing). Though minimal, the risks of all these surgeries are infection, blood loss, reactions to anesthesia, and abnormal scarring.

What happens after the treatment?

Once the braces come off, the tissue surrounding the teeth still needs to be stabilized—a process that usually takes months or years but can sometimes go on indefinitely. Often the teeth are fitted with retainers (special plastic and wire devices designed to hold the teeth in place). At first these may need to be worn almost all the time, but eventually the wearing period may be reduced to just several hours a day or to nighttime alone.

Related entries

Body image, cosmetic dentistry, cosmetic surgery, dentures/bridges/implants, gum disease, keloid scarring, temporomandibular joint syndrome

Osteoarthritis

Osteoarthritis is the most common form of arthritis. Despite the suffix "-itis," which implies an inflammatory process, the painful joints characteristic of osteoarthritis are due primarily to gradual loss of cartilage rather than inflammation.

Cartilage is a form of connective tissue that lines joints and protects the ends of bones from rubbing against one another. It can break down because of physical injury, mechanical stress, or some underlying metabolic abnormality. As a result, bones begin to grate against one another, producing pain and further degeneration. Over time the bones may thicken and additional bone may grow along the sides, producing lumps (bone spurs or osteophytes). Fluid-filled cysts may also develop, and the surrounding area may become inflamed. Osteoarthritis (also called degenerative joint disease or wear-and-tear arthritis) tends to occur in joints most

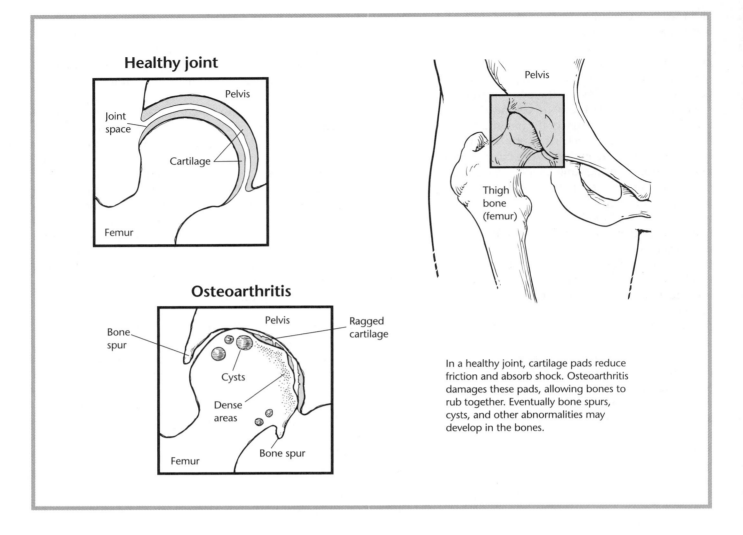

Healthy joint

Pelvis

Joint space

Cartilage

Femur

Osteoarthritis

Bone spur

Pelvis

Ragged cartilage

Cysts

Dense areas

Femur

Bone spur

Pelvis

Thigh bone (femur)

In a healthy joint, cartilage pads reduce friction and absorb shock. Osteoarthritis damages these pads, allowing bones to rub together. Eventually bone spurs, cysts, and other abnormalities may develop in the bones.

exposed to weight-bearing and stress, especially the spine, knees, hips, thumb, and big toe (see illustration).

Since cartilage does not normally deteriorate with age, this process should not be seen as an inevitable accompaniment to aging. Unlike bone, though, cartilage cannot repair or regenerate itself. As a result, any damage to cartilage is irreversible.

Who is likely to develop osteoarthritis?

Most cases of osteoarthritis occur after middle age, but the condition can develop in younger people who have sustained athletic or work-related joint injuries. Anyone who has previously injured cartilage is also at risk for developing osteoarthritis later in life. This may occur in conditions such as congenital dislocation of the hip, dislocation of the thighbone out of the hip, tissue death resulting from deficient blood supply, or a fracture within a joint. Obesity can predispose people to osteoarthritis because increased weight puts further stress on the joints, particularly the knees. Osteoarthritis that occurs after middle age is more common in women than in men.

What are the symptoms?

The pain of osteoarthritis tends to occur in joints subject to weight-bearing and stress. Women are particularly likely to experience degenerative changes in the base of the thumb, in the knuckles, and in the joint connecting the knee and thighbone (see knee pain). Unlike many other arthritic conditions (such as rheumatoid arthritis), pain usually occurs only when joints are moved. Women with osteoarthritis of the knee, for example, tend to feel pain only when they walk. In contrast, rest or inactivity is usually followed by joint stiffness. Only in the most advanced stages of the disease is there any joint pain during sleep.

Without treatment, pain and stiffness increase gradually over seasons or years without remission or significant improvement. An exception may be the symptoms of osteoarthritis of the hip, which can develop rapidly, perhaps because early symptoms (such as difficulty in putting on shoes) may go unnoticed.

Women are particularly likely to develop erosive osteoarthritis of the hands; in this condition lumps develop on the end or middle joints of the fingers (called Heberden's and

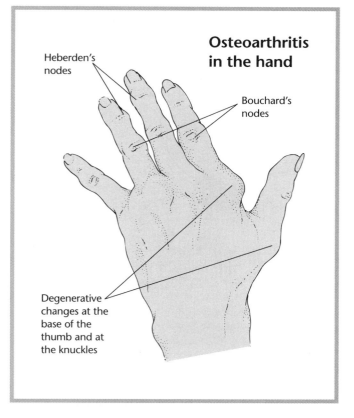

Osteoarthritis in the hand

Heberden's nodes

Bouchard's nodes

Degenerative changes at the base of the thumb and at the knuckles

Bouchard's nodes, respectively; see illustration). The pain and stiffness that may occur during the year or two of bone growth tend to subside over time, as the larger bone spurs stabilize the joint against motion and associated pain.

How is the condition evaluated?

A physician distinguishes osteoarthritis from other conditions by considering a number of different factors that together signal this disorder. Among the most important is the history of symptoms. For example, the doctor will want to know if symptoms appear after movement in mechanically stressed joints and if they have gradually and progressively increased over time. The doctor will suspect osteoarthritis even more if there have been no signs of inflammation and if symptoms have failed to respond to antiinflammatory drugs such as aspirin. A physical examination will be done to see if there are any Heberden's or Bouchard's nodes and whether a high-pitched grating noise called crepitus (which occurs when cartilage has deteriorated) can be heard when the joint is moved.

Finally, x-rays may be taken to find out if there is any evidence of osteoarthritis such as osteophytes or joint-space narrowing owing to cartilage loss. Other techniques used to visualize joints are magnetic resonance imaging (MRI) and arthroscopy. The latter allows the interior of a joint to be visualized through a small tube containing magnifying lenses and fiber-optic equipment (see knee pain); sometimes damaged cartilage can be removed during the same operation.

Even if osteoarthritis is suspected, a doctor may also want to do additional tests, including blood tests, to see if any other disorders are present that can be more readily treated. Disorders that can coexist with osteoarthritis include bursitis, a condition that involves inflammation of the fluid-filled sac (bursa) that limits friction in joints (see knee pain), as well as rheumatoid arthritis, gout (a condition in which crystals of uric acid accumulate in the joints), pseudogout (in which crystals of calcium salts accumulate in the joint), and polymyalgia rheumatica (see entry).

The base of the thumb is another area which is very prone to the development of osteoarthritis and must be distinguished from tenosynovitis (see tendinitis and tenosynovitis), while generalized stiffness must be distinguished from the stiffness that can result from Parkinson's disease (a progressive degenerative disease of the nerves) or hypothyroidism (see entry).

How is osteoarthritis treated?

Antiinflammatory drugs (see entry), including aspirin, are not effective in relieving, reversing, or preventing osteoarthritis, although they can be effective as pain relievers. This is probably because osteoarthritis rarely involves inflammation. An exception may be osteoarthritis of the hip, which for reasons not understood is often relieved with nonsteroidal antiinflammatory agents, particularly indomethacin. In general, it is probably best to substitute drugs such as acetaminophen (Tylenol) in moderation for pain relief, especially if complications such as stomach upset or bleeding arise after use of antiinflammatory agents. High doses (over 8 double-strength tablets per day) has been associated with kidney damage in some studies.

A commonly prescribed therapy that probably hurts more than it helps is immobilizing the affected joints with external braces or splints. Any brace that is rigid enough to stabilize the joint will also dangerously compress the soft tissue, and soft elastic braces do not provide enough stability and can cut off blood supply. Although splinting an affected joint or using a cervical collar around the neck can relieve pain, such treatments also eventually restrict the joint's mobility. This is because unused muscles tend to atrophy and because osteophytes may form and create a stabilizing effect. In certain joints that do not require much movement, such as in the thumb, this immobility is beneficial, but in most other joints specific muscle strengthening exercises done under the supervision of a physical therapist are a much better way to relieve pain and reduce stiffness.

Swimming and other water exercises may help, and some people find that merely improving posture can relieve pain associated with osteoarthritis of the spine. This disorder develops when disks wear out (owing to mechanical wear and tear or simple aging), with the result that the spaces between vertebrae narrow and are often filled in with bony spurs.

Advances in orthopedic surgery have made surgical reconstruction of the joints an effective alternative. Techniques are still evolving to help people with severely compromised

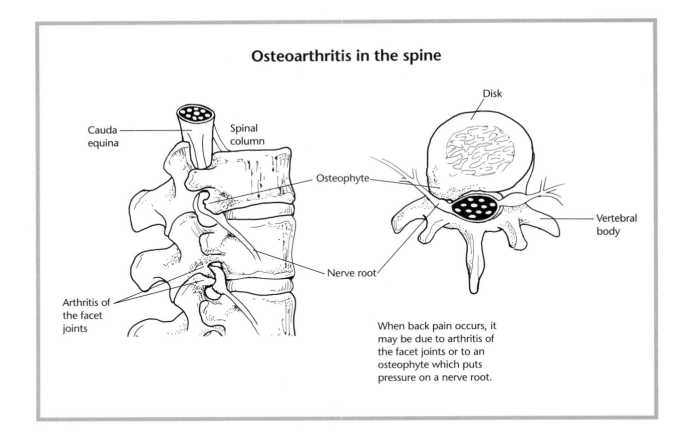

Osteoarthritis in the spine

Cauda equina

Spinal column

Arthritis of the facet joints

Osteophyte

Nerve root

Disk

Vertebral body

When back pain occurs, it may be due to arthritis of the facet joints or to an osteophyte which puts pressure on a nerve root.

joints, but today's procedures have been highly successful in relieving pain, restoring meaningful function, and dramatically improving the quality of life for people with osteoarthritis.

The definitive treatment for a destroyed hip or knee joint is a total joint replacement (arthroplasty; see entry) with an artificial device. This treatment should be considered by any patient whose pain is severe enough to interfere with sleep. The major drawback to arthroplasty is a risk of infection that increases with each operation; the artificial devices currently available also tend to need repair or replacement, though seldom within 12 years.

Occasionally an orthopedic surgeon may try less radical surgical procedures such as fusing (and thus immobilizing) osteoarthritic joints. This is usually done in joints of the hand, big toe, and thumb. Also, in relatively young (under 50) and physically active people with certain forms of knee deformities, such as bowlegs or knock-knees, which normally predispose cartilage to degeneration, a procedure called tibial osteotomy may be done to correct the deformity by removing a wedge of bone from the upper side of the shin bone. The major disadvantage of this procedure is that it must be followed by several months on crutches. In addition, it is most successful in people with only mild forms of osteoarthritis.

Most exercises require active effort on the part of the patient, although in early phases of therapy, heating pads, hot whirlpool baths, and massage may make it easier for a therapist to manipulate the joint passively.

Usually weight reduction has little effect on symptoms because it does not have sufficient impact to overcome the natural degeneration of cartilage once the process has begun. Nevertheless, many doctors still recommend weight loss to obese people with osteoarthritis because it can greatly decrease risks should surgery be required, and weight loss probably helps to defer or delay development of symptoms in other joints.

Related entries

Antiinflammatory drugs, arthritis, arthroplasty, back pain, hypothyroidism, knee pain, polymyalgia rheumatica, rheumatoid arthritis, tendinitis and tenosynovitis

Osteoporosis

Osteoporosis is a systemic and often debilitating skeletal disease in which the bones gradually become less dense and more susceptible to fracture from even slight trauma (see illustration). In the United States approximately 1.5 million fractures are caused by osteoporosis each year, and the an-

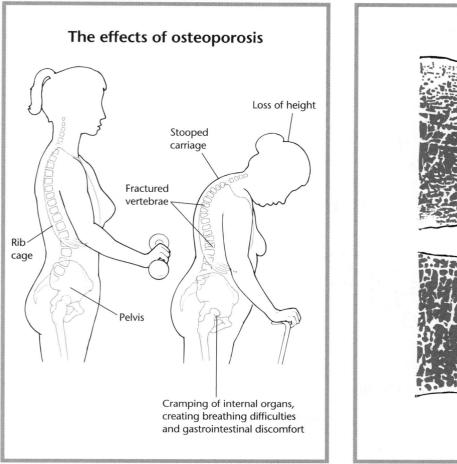

The effects of osteoporosis

Loss of height

Stooped carriage

Fractured vertebrae

Rib cage

Pelvis

Cramping of internal organs, creating breathing difficulties and gastrointestinal discomfort

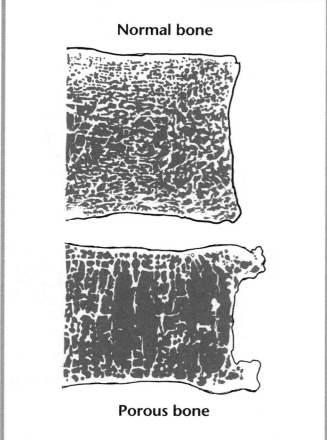

Normal bone

Porous bone

nual cost of caring for them is $10 billion. Fractures of the spine alone affect an estimated 500,000 people annually, the vast majority of whom are postmenopausal women. An estimated 10 million Americans have osteoporosis (8 million women and 2 million men), and 18 million more have low bone mass placing them at increased risk for osteoporosis and fractures.

As many as one-quarter of all white women past menopause have some degree of osteoporosis (which literally means porous bones; see illustration), and 89 percent of all women past the age of 75 are affected. Forty percent of all women in the United States will experience at least one fracture by the time they reach the age of 70.

Throughout the life span bone density is determined by a complicated mechanism regulated by hormones and growth factors. This mechanism balances the relative rate of bone formation and resorption (breakdown). Whenever the rate of formation exceeds the rate of resorption, bone density increases; whenever resorption exceeds formation, density decreases. The amount of available calcium in the body plays a major role in determining which of these processes will dominate. When there is not enough calcium in the bloodstream

to serve vital parts of the body such as the heart, nerves, and muscles, cells called osteoclasts will release the calcium from the bones, leaving tiny gaps in its place and a lower bone density (see illustration).

In childhood and adolescence bone formation exceeds resorption, and so bones increase in mass. Even though the bones stop growing lengthwise during adolescence, bone density and strength continue to increase. By their late 20s most people have reached their peak bone mass for a type of bone tissue called trabecular bone. Found in the interior part of bones, trabecular bone forms a series of uniformly distributed plates that are lost and converted to rod-like structures as the bone is resorbed. The other type of bone tissue—called the cortical bone—reaches its peak mass several years later. Cortical bone is densely packed and forms the exterior of bones as well as the shafts of the long bones.

Once peak bone mass is reached, usually several years of equilibrium follow in which bone formation and resorption are about equal. By the late 30s or early 40s, however, resorption starts to accelerate, and there is a cumulative loss of bone. As menopause approaches, women begin to lose bone mass at the rate of 3 to 5 percent per year, a process that con-

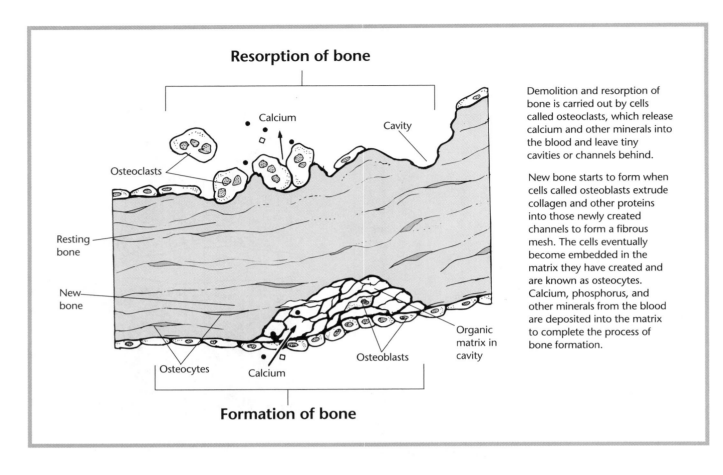

Resorption of bone

Calcium

Cavity

Osteoclasts

Resting bone

New bone

Osteocytes

Calcium

Osteoblasts

Organic matrix in cavity

Formation of bone

Demolition and resorption of bone is carried out by cells called osteoclasts, which release calcium and other minerals into the blood and leave tiny cavities or channels behind.

New bone starts to form when cells called osteoblasts extrude collagen and other proteins into those newly created channels to form a fibrous mesh. The cells eventually become embedded in the matrix they have created and are known as osteocytes. Calcium, phosphorus, and other minerals from the blood are deposited into the matrix to complete the process of bone formation.

tinues for several years until it eventually levels off at about 1 percent a year around the age of 50.

Bone loss in women is a result of several factors. Women usually start out with less bone mass and mineral reserve than men in the first place. The diet of many women contains insufficient calcium and other essential minerals, and loss of estrogen at menopause interferes with the body's ability to absorb calcium from the diet and incorporate it into bone. In addition, women are less likely than men to do weight-bearing exercise (performed against the force of gravity), which helps increase bone mass.

Who is likely to develop osteoporosis?

Afflicting more than 25 million Americans, osteoporosis occurs in all ethnic groups and both sexes, but women are 4 times more likely than men to develop the disease.

Risk factors for developing osteoporosis include: ▸ age; ▸ a family history of osteoporosis; ▸ being white or of Asian descent; ▸ having low bone mass; ▸ experiencing prolonged estrogen deficiency; ▸ a lifetime of low calcium intake; ▸ inactivity; ▸ smoking; ▸ excessive alcohol intake; ▸ excessive caffeine intake; ▸ and being chronically thin or of small bone frame.

A person's peak bone mass seems to be linked to the likelihood that osteoporosis will develop. The fact that African American women generally have a bone mass 10 to 15 percent greater than women of other ethnic groups may help ex-

plain why they are relatively less susceptible to developing osteoporosis.

Genetics probably plays a bigger role in this disease than was once suspected, and women whose mothers or other close female relatives have osteoporosis have a higher than average risk of developing the condition. As yet inconclusive evidence suggests that some women may carry a specific gene that predisposes them to osteoporosis. This gene seems to interfere with the body's use of vitamin D, which is required for calcium absorption.

Nutrition, exercise, and lifestyle are also linked to the amount of bone mass a person develops. These may also play a role in preventing bone loss later in life and reducing susceptibility to fractures. Cigarette smoking, alcohol abuse, and a diet deficient in calcium all seem to contribute to bone loss. Besides being associated with dietary deficiencies, alcohol abuse tends to make people more susceptible to falls and accidents. High levels of caffeine (over 3 cups of coffee per day) seem to deplete the body's stores of calcium, and thus may promote bone loss. But by consuming a single glass of milk a day—or otherwise upping calcium intake—a woman who drinks coffee in moderation can easily counteract this effect.

A sedentary lifestyle and a lack of regular weight-bearing exercise also decrease bone density. Older people, who are generally less agile than they were in their youth, tend to fall more often and thus create more opportunities for fractures.

People who do not get out into the sun often are at risk, since the skin needs to absorb ultraviolet light to synthesize vitamin D—which is generally not sufficiently available in non-fortified foods. As a result, virtually all people who live in the continental United States do not get enough natural vitamin D for at least 3 or 4 months a year. Older people are even less likely to go outdoors when the weather is inclement, and this puts them at greater risk of vitamin D deficiency. (These effects can be offset by eating foods fortified with vitamin D or by taking a vitamin supplement.)

All of these factors increase a person's odds of developing primary osteoporosis—that is, osteoporosis resulting from aging. Certain medical conditions and medications can also lead to the development of what is known as secondary osteoporosis at any time in life. These include hyperthyroidism, Cushing syndrome, diabetes, and some kidney disorders, as well as the excess use of certain drugs such as thyroid hormone (used to treat hypothyroidism), corticosteroids (used to treat asthma, arthritis, and other inflammatory conditions), and Dilantin (used to treat seizures).

Younger women who have had a low level of estrogen or a prolonged lack of periods (amenorrhea), or who have their ovaries removed are at increased risk for osteoporosis. Chronically low estrogen levels, especially during adolescence, when bones are normally growing, can decrease bone density at a dangerously high rate. Anorexia nervosa or excessive exercise—both of which lower the levels of body fat (which converts other hormones into estrogen)—are the main risk factors for weakened, porous bones in young women, and for developing osteoporosis later in life.

Women who are obese are actually less likely than average to develop osteoporosis, primarily because weight-bearing increases the mass of bones. Women over 50 who lose a significant amount of weight seem to increase their risk. None of this should be taken as an argument in favor of obesity, however, given all the other health risks (such as heart disease and diabetes) with which it is associated.

What are the symptoms?

The most common—and often the first—evidence of osteoporosis is a broken bone. Some women also experience aching in their lower extremities. The vertebrae, hip, and wrists are particularly susceptible to osteoporosis and fracture because they contain a relatively high proportion of trabecular bone tissue, which is lost earlier and more extensively than cortical bone tissue.

Sometimes all it takes for a person with osteoporosis to fracture one of these bones is stepping off a curb or coming to an abrupt halt. Osteoporotic vertebrae may collapse merely from the everyday pressure associated with walking, standing, or strenuous coughing. These are known as fragility (also compression) fractures. A series of fragility fractures can eventually lead to loss of height, as well as the dowager's hump which gives so many elderly women a stooped or humpbacked appearance. Although they often go unnoticed, fragility fractures sometimes cause severe pain. Normal activ-

ities can usually be resumed after a couple of weeks, though some women continue to have a chronic dull ache in the neck or back. Also, a severely curved spine can crowd internal organs, making breathing uncomfortable.

Hip fractures are about half as common as spinal fractures (approaching 500,000 per year in the United States), and they can be particularly devastating. Nearly a third of women who live to age 90 can expect to have a hip fracture related to osteoporosis. Women who fracture a hip often require long-term care or hospitalization, and a large proportion will die within a few months of the fracture from complications of surgery or from complications resulting from lengthy immobilization, such as pneumonia or blood clots in the pulmonary arteries (pulmonary emboli).

How is the condition evaluated?

Two groups of women generally should consult a clinician about the possibility of osteoporosis. The first group consists of women, often in their middle years, who have risk factors for osteoporosis and want to know the status of their bones. The second group consists of women who already have experienced symptoms of osteoporosis (such as a loss of height or a fracture from a mild fall). In addition, any woman in her mid-40s or younger who has either amenorrhea (absence of menstrual periods) or oligomenorrhea (infrequent periods) for any significant time should discuss the possibility of a bone density test with her clinician.

There are tests widely available at hospitals and freestanding imaging centers which can measure bone density in both these groups of women, as well as in the many women who are discovered to have osteoporosis after a routine chest or spine x-ray. These tests can be used to predict a woman's risk of developing fractures later in life, since it is now clear that the greater the degree of osteopenia (bone loss), the greater the risk of fracture.

There is no point in doing these tests, however, if the results will have no bearing on treatment or prevention plans. Often it is enough for a clinician to give advice—particularly to women in the first group (those with risk factors but no fractures)—about getting adequate calcium, vitamin D, and exercise, or, most important, the appropriateness of estrogen replacement therapy.

Nonetheless, assessments of bone density can be very useful in helping a clinician follow the progress of a woman who already has osteoporosis. Also, in a woman undergoing menopause, this assessment can tip off the clinician about the chances of bone fracture, and therefore influence the physician's decision about recommending estrogen early on, as well as the woman's decision about taking it. Young women with low levels of estrogen resulting from excessive exercise or anorexia nervosa might benefit from a bone density assessment if the results were to persuade them to modify their diet and exercise habits or to take estrogen supplements.

The National Osteoporosis Foundation in collaboration with many subspecialty societies has published clinical guidelines suggesting that bone density measurements be obtained for any woman in the following categories: ‣ all postmenopausal women under age 65 who have one or more additional risk factors for osteoporosis besides menopause (i.e., weight less than 127 lbs., personal or family history of fracture, and current cigarette smoking); ‣ all women aged 65 and older regardless of additional risk factors; ‣ postmenopausal women with fractures; ‣ women considering therapy for osteoporosis for whom bone density measurements would facilitate the decision; ‣ women who have been on hormone replacement therapy for prolonged periods.

In addition, the 1998 Bone Mass Measurement Act (BMMA) permits Medicare to reimburse the cost of bone density tests for individuals who: ‣ are estrogen-deficient and are considered by their clinicians to be at risk for osteoporosis; ‣ have abnormalities of the spinal column; ‣ take chronic glucocorticoid therapy; ‣ are being monitored to assess FDA-approved osteoporosis drug therapy.

The fastest, safest, and most precise of these tests is dual energy x-ray absorptiometry (DEXA), which measures the total bone content of the hips, spine, forearm, or entire body. Taking only a few minutes, DEXA has largely replaced dual photon absorptiometry, a technique that measures the total calcium and mineral content of the hip and spine but delivers relatively more radiation.

Single photon absorptiometry is more adept at measuring the amount of cortical bone in particular. A relatively simple procedure, it is used to assess bone density in the wrist or heel, locations where cortical bone is more predominant but may be lost if osteoporosis is fairly extensive. It usually takes no more than a few minutes to perform.

A CT (computerized tomography) scan is the best technique for assessing loss of bone mass (especially in the lower spine) because it measures the mineral content of the trabecular bone, which is lost most rapidly after menopause. CT scans deliver more radiation than the other available techniques, however, and are generally more expensive and take more time.

If osteoporosis is suspected, it will also be necessary to rule out other possible causes for the loss of bone mass or for low back pain. These may include degenerative arthritis, disk disease, and osteomalacia, a group of disorders that involve a loss of calcium and other minerals from the bones (see back pain). The clinician will also want to make sure that osteoporosis is due to aging alone and not to some other medical condition that requires specific treatment. Besides conducting a detailed history and physical examination, the clinician may run various blood and urine tests, including a complete blood count and a measure of thyroid stimulating hormone (TSH). He or she may also check for vitamin D deficiency, particularly in elderly women who live in northern climates.

How is osteoporosis treated?

Treatments for osteoporosis generally involve taking measures to prevent further degeneration and potentially increasing bone density or, in the case of secondary osteoporosis, treating whatever underlying condition is causing the bone loss. Until the introduction of drugs called bisphosphonates, there was no known way to reverse osteoporosis or to restore the skeleton to its original strength. The bisphosphonates, however, may actually increase bone density.

Backache, muscle spasms, and other discomforts associated with the fractures that result from osteoporosis can be relieved with painkillers or, when appropriate, heat, massage, and orthopedic supports. Emergency surgery may sometimes be required to set fractures, and when the hip joint becomes severely damaged, it may be replaced with an artificial joint (see arthroplasty).

Physical therapy is often used after a fracture to help restore mobility to the joint. To minimize the risk of falls and fractures, women with osteoporosis should accident-proof their homes—securing loose rugs, removing floor clutter, avoiding extension cords, installing tub and stairway railings, and arranging to have ice and snow removed from sidewalks and driveways. They should also talk to their clinicians about changing any medications that may cause dizziness or impair coordination.

Estrogen replacement therapy (ERT). Estrogen has a beneficial effect on bone by improving calcium absorption and reducing the amount of calcium excreted in the urine. Preventive effects are most dramatic when the therapy is started as close to the onset of menopause as possible, before the bulk of trabecular bone has eroded. The Women's Health Initiative showed that postmenopausal women taking standard doses of estrogen with progestin had about one-third fewer hip fractures than those taking no estrogen.

For all its benefits, ERT has risks and side effects that make it inappropriate for some women (see estrogen replacement therapy). A postmenopausal woman who is considering ERT should discuss relative risks and benefits with her clinician. Doctors try to prescribe as low a dose as is effective. The minimum amount needed to prevent bone loss (and relieve hot flashes at the same time) was thought to be 0.625 mg of conjugated estrogen (Premarin), available in pill form, although several recent studies have shown that 0.3 mg of conjugated estrogens *with* calcium is effective in maintaining bone mass as well. Estrogen patches also provide protection against osteoporosis.

Selective estrogen receptor modulators (SERMs). This group of compounds bind and interact with estrogen receptors, sometimes enhancing the effects of estrogen and sometimes counteracting it, depending on which tissue is involved. SERMs include tamoxifen, the synthetic antiestrogen that is used to treat breast cancer and that has been shown to reduce trabecular bone loss. Several years ago the Food and Drug Administration (FDA) approved another SERM, raloxifene (Evista), for the prevention and, more recently, treatment of osteoporosis. The Multiple Outcomes of Raloxifene (MORE) trial showed that raloxifene modestly increased trabecular bone mass and reduced new vertebral fractures by 40 to 50 percent. And in postmenopausal women with osteoporosis, raloxifene also decreased the risk of invasive breast cancer by 76 percent during 3 years of treatment. Raloxifene also lowers LDL ("bad" cholesterol) levels, although its effect on heart disease remains unclear.

Raloxifene is usually taken in a dose of 60 mg per day by mouth for both the prevention and treatment of osteoporosis. Unlike estrogen replacement, it does not relieve menopausal symptoms and may even cause hot flashes. Like estrogen, however, raloxifene increases the risk of blood clots by a factor of 2 or 3.

Bisphosphonates. Among the most promising (but costly) new drugs are the bisphosphonates. These agents act to reverse the progression of osteoporosis by inhibiting bone resorption and actually building up bone density in some patients. They can also help prevent fractures. Etidronate (Didronel), a drug approved by the FDA to treat Paget disease and other conditions characterized by increased bone turnover, has been used by physicians for several years to treat osteoporosis. It has been shown to increase the density of vertebrae and reduce the risk of spinal fractures when taken orally for 2 weeks every 3 months for a period up to 2 years. In late 1995 a newer bisphosphonate, alendronate (Fosamax), was approved by the FDA for treatment of osteoporosis in postmenopausal women. It has subsequently been approved for osteoporosis prevention in postmenopausal women, fracture prevention, treating glucocorticoid-induced osteoporosis, and treating osteoporosis in men. Studies have shown that alendronate increases bone density and reduces vertebral, hip, and wrist fractures significantly. Another study showed that alendronate prevents bone loss in early menopausal women as well. Side effects, mostly gastrointestinal upset, appear to be uncommon but may include irritation of the esophagus (esophagitis), abdominal or musculoskeletal pain, nausea, and heartburn.

More recently the FDA approved another bisphosphonate, risedronate (Actonel), for preventing and treating osteoporosis in postmenopausal woman, as well as glucocorticoid-induced osteoporosis. Both alendronate and risedronate are now available in a convenient once-a-week dosage.

While bisphosphonates can be quite effective in increasing bone mass and preventing fractures, using them properly can be somewhat inconvenient. Because these drugs are poorly absorbed, they have to be taken on an empty stomach to maximize absorption. Ideally these drugs should be taken with 6 to 8 ounces of water first thing in the morning, and patients should remain upright and eat or drink nothing for at least 30 more minutes. To prevent gastrointestinal side effects (including esophagitis), too, it is necessary to avoid lying down for at least 30 minutes after taking these pills. Women with GERD (gastroesophageal reflux disease; see entry on heartburn) may not tolerate bisphosphonates, although they may have an easier time with once-a-week preparations.

Calcitonin. There is evidence that this hormone inhibits the function of the osteoclasts, the cells that help break down bone tissue. As a bonus for women with painful vertebral fractures, calcitonin may also function as a pain reliever. This hormone appears to be relatively safe, and the side effects (most often facial flushing, nausea, and dizziness) almost always fade in a short period of time.

The major drawback of calcitonin is its high cost. Several years ago a nasal spray form of calcitonin (Miacalcin) was approved for the treatment of postmenopausal osteoporosis. To prevent the development of hyperparathyroidism (a condition that leads to kidney stones, fatigue, indigestion, and increased thirst and urination), women using calcitonin also need to supplement their diet with 1,000 mg of calcium and a multivitamin each day. This usually does not create a problem, since anyone undergoing treatment for osteoporosis should already be taking steps to ensure adequate intake of calcium and vitamin D (and exercise)—although by themselves these are usually not enough to overcome established osteoporosis.

Parathyroid hormone. The first of a new class of drugs called bone formation agents—marketed as Forteo (teriparatide)—appears to double the normal rate of bone formation. This drug is a 34-amino acid portion of the human parathyroid hormone, a bone-building hormone normally secreted by four tiny glands at the base of the neck. A recent large clinical trial reported in the *New England Journal of Medicine* by researchers at Massachusetts General Hospital showed that postmenopausal women with osteoporosis who took 40 micrograms of Forteo per day for 18 months lowered their risk of spinal fractures by two-thirds and lowered the risk of fractures elsewhere in the body by over one-half. Bone density in the spine, hip, and total body also increased significantly.

Forteo is often used with another drug that stops bone loss at the same time. It cannot be prescribed for more than 2 years, however, partly because knowledge about long-term effects is still limited and partly because its efficacy seems to dwindle over time. In some animal trials, teriparatide was found to cause a form of bone cancer (osteosarcoma) in rats, which led to a temporary suspension of clinical research. Researchers subsequently concluded that there was no reason to suspect—and no evidence of—a similarly elevated risk in people taking this medication.

Forteo, administered by injection, was approved by the Food and Drug Administration (FDA) in 2000 for use by postmenopausal women with osteoporosis who are at high risk for fracture. This treatment should not be used by children or adolescents, or by pregnant or nursing women. It is also unsafe for use in people with Paget's disease of the bone, unexplained elevated levels of alkaline phosphatase in their blood (which can signal Paget's disease), or high levels of calcium in the blood; who have had prior allergic reactions to it or its components; or who may have trouble giving themselves injections (or finding someone to help them do so). Women who have bone diseases should also discuss them with their clinician before taking parathyroid hormone.

Other drugs. Among the various other approaches being evaluated for the treatment of osteoporosis—and still considered "experimental"—are combinations of estrogen or raloxifene with bisphosphonates. These "combination regimens" may increase bone density more than either agent alone. Anabolic steroids, growth hormone and growth factors, vitamin D analogs (such as calcitriol, which is safest when calcium intake is relatively low), thiazide diuretics ("water pills" that reduce the amount of calcium excreted by the kidneys), and other substances to stimulate bone formation are currently subjects of research.

Increasing evidence suggests that statin drugs—used primarily to control blood cholesterol levels—may also restore strength to bones weakened by osteoporosis. Another promising substance, fluoride, has so far yielded disappointing results. Researchers have known for many years about fluoride's ability to increase trabecular bone density (probably by redistributing calcium into other types of bone), but they have never been able to credit it with actually decreasing the risk of bone fracture. In fact, studies so far show that, if anything, fluoride therapy increases stress fractures and may increase nonvertebral fractures. They also fail to confirm earlier findings that taking fluoride in conjunction with calcium reduces spinal fractures.

How is osteoporosis prevented?

The best way to reduce the risk of developing osteoporosis is to maximize bone mass in the years before osteoporosis has a chance to develop. Ideally, steps to build bones should be taken during the years of greatest bone growth and development (particularly adolescence), but it is never too late (or too early) to make a difference. Before menopause these steps essentially involve eating a balanced diet rich in calcium and vitamin D and participating regularly in weight-bearing exercise.

Calcium. Premenopausal adult women need at least 1,000 mg of calcium (see entry) per day. Requirements for adolescents and pregnant and breastfeeding women are 1,200 mg per day. Postmenopausal women not taking estrogen replacement therapy require 1,200 to 1,500 mg per day, while those who are taking ERT can continue at 1,000 mg per day. Most American women, however, do not get even the recommended dietary allowance of calcium (800 to 1,000 mg per day) established by the National Research Council. As women get older, calcium intake is likely to drop even more, partly because of a decrease in dietary intake of calcium and partly because of a decreased ability to absorb the calcium that is ingested. The typical postmenopausal American woman gets only about 400 to 500 mg per day.

Most clinicians advise taking calcium supplements in the form of calcium carbonate (which is contained in antacid tablets such as Tums) because it is less expensive and better tolerated than other forms and is more readily absorbed.

Taking calcium carbonate with food—particularly milk—improves absorption considerably in most women.

Vitamin D. Women in the reproductive years need to have at least 200 IU (international units) of vitamin D per day (assuming they are getting 1,000 mg per day of calcium); pregnant and postmenopausal women should be receiving 400 to 800 IU per day, especially during the winter months, when they may not be getting much sunlight exposure. Older women need additional vitamin D, partly because the aging intestine becomes less able to absorb vitamin D and also because as women grow older they are more likely to be poorly nourished or to be chronically ill or housebound.

Many foods are now fortified with vitamin D—enough so that most people who are eating a diet rich in calcium are probably also getting enough vitamin D. Just drinking two glasses of vitamin D–fortified milk a day, for example, provides a full 400 IU of vitamin D. If fortified foods are not being taken, however, an ordinary multivitamin pill can usually fill any woman's need for vitamin D, since most contain 400 IU of the vitamin. No one should take more than 800 IU of vitamin D per day because higher doses can increase calcium in the blood or urine to toxic levels.

Weight-bearing exercise. Exercises performed against the force of gravity put stress on the long bones and increase their mass; they also improve overall agility and balance and generally impart a sense of well-being. Brisk walking is one of the best weight-bearing exercises around, and many women find it relatively easy to incorporate a few long walks into their weekly schedule. Among the many other weight-bearing exercises are hiking, jogging, stair climbing, chair exercises, dancing, jumping rope, weight training, and tennis. Swimming and bicycling, while good aerobic exercises, do not put as much stress on the bones, although swimming can sometimes ease the pain of a vertebral fracture.

No one knows for sure just how long and how often exercise needs to be done to stave off bone degeneration, but starting slowly and working up to about an hour at least 3 times a week is a reasonable goal. All exercise programs and goals should be tailored to an individual's needs and abilities. Also, a woman with established osteoporosis should discuss with her clinician whether any weight-bearing exercises might be inappropriate for her, especially because some—such as jumping or jogging—can damage bones through repeated pounding. It might also help to consult a physical therapist (or any of the abundant literature about osteoporosis) to find gentle abdominal and back-strengthening exercises that do not require too much bending or sudden rotational movements. These can improve posture and also make it easier to perform weight-bearing exercises.

Fall prevention. Preventing falls is a matter of addressing the many different factors that contribute to falls, including poor vision, frailty, medication (especially medications for lowering blood pressure and relieving psychological problems), and balance disturbance. Some women may find that wearing padded hip protectors can dissipate the impact of a fall and help prevent hip fractures. In addition, simply rearranging objects in the home can also prevent many unnecessary spills. Simple steps include keeping rooms free of clutter, avoiding slippery floors, watching for thresholds, wearing supportive shoes, tacking down rugs, maintaining good lighting, installing "grab bars" in bathrooms, and using only cordless telephones. Older women with osteoporosis, particularly those who live alone, might also consider investing in a personal alarm activator that allows them to call for help should a fall occur and/or making arrangements to have someone check on them regularly.

Other lifestyle adjustments. Stopping smoking can help preserve bone and prevent osteoporosis, and cutting back on alcohol and caffeine may help women who are already at high risk. Although there is no evidence implicating relatively small amounts of caffeine (one or two cups of coffee a day) in osteoporosis, women who are already deficient in calcium should be aware that high caffeine intake seems to promote calcium loss. Maintaining a suitable body weight is also a good idea, given the association of osteoporosis with thinness and with rapid weight loss.

Related entries
Alcohol, amenorrhea, anorexia nervosa and bulimia nervosa, arthroplasty, back pain, breast cancer, coffee, coronary artery disease, diabetes, diuretics, endometrial cancer, estrogen, estrogen replacement therapy, exercise, high blood pressure, kidney disorders, menopause, nutrition, obesity, ovary removal, smoking

Otoplasty

Otoplasty literally means any kind of plastic or cosmetic surgery performed on the ear. Most commonly it is used to pin back protruding ears. Because "Dumbo" ears are often the source of deep embarrassment and can result in teasing from schoolyard peers as well as cruel remarks from thoughtless adults, this form of otoplasty is frequently done in childhood or early adolescence.

Some adult women may opt for otoplasty later in life, however, especially if they avoided childhood suffering by covering their ears with long hair and now want a more permanent transformation. Adults may also undergo otoplasty to repair damage suffered in an accident or from a disease, to reconstruct a missing ear, or to correct folded or "lop" ears.

How is the procedure performed?
If the goal is to pin back protruding ears, otoplasty is a relatively minor operation that can usually be done on an outpatient basis. Ears generally protrude either because the central portion of the ear (the concha) is too large or deep or because the upper fold (the auricle) is malformed. These defects can be corrected by making a cut between the back of the ear and the head (where scars will be hidden) and then stitching the ear back into a more desirable position. Many surgeons remove an elliptical piece of tissue from behind the ear.

An additional measure—which is usually necessary if ears stand out at right angles to the head—involves cutting the cartilage in the ear itself and then reshaping the ear into a new position. The ears are then bandaged with a pressure dressing (such as a turban) to hold the ears tightly against the head. This is left in place for about a week unless there is excess bleeding or pain.

What happens after surgery?
Pain usually subsides within several days, but the ears may feel somewhat numb for a few months. If the surgeon has fractured and reshaped the cartilage, a headband can be worn over the ears once the bandage is removed to hold the ears in place until the fracture is completely healed. This usually takes between 4 and 6 weeks.

What are the risks and complications?
Occasionally even the most minor otoplasty can result in complications. There is always the possibility of excessive bleeding and infection, for example, and some people may have adverse reactions to anesthesia. In addition, when the cartilage is cut, it does not always reunite with adjacent cartilage, in which case additional minor surgery may be necessary so that the cartilage can be stitched together again. The most common "complication" is assymetrical ears.

There is the rare but real possibility that otoplasty will result in ear distortions. The possibility of complications and undesirable cosmetic results is greater with the kinds of otoplasty done to reconstruct missing ears or parts of ears, especially when these procedures require the use of skin or cartilage grafts from other areas of the body.

Related entries
Anesthesia, body image, cosmetic surgery, keloid scarring

Ovarian Cancer

Cancer of the ovary is the second most common malignancy of the female reproductive tract (after endometrial cancer) and accounts for more deaths than the other gynecological malignancies combined. One out of every 70 women can expect to develop ovarian cancer at some point in her life.

It is generally thought that the cancer begins in the ovaries (see illustration), and if not treated promptly spreads to the pelvic organs, the membrane lining the abdominal cavity (peritoneum), nearby lymph nodes, and liver. The overall

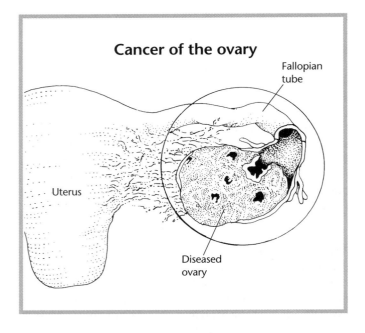

Cancer of the ovary

Fallopian tube

Uterus

Diseased ovary

outlook for most women with ovarian cancer is not much better today than it was half a century ago. This is largely because ovarian cancer is usually silent until after the disease has already spread (metastasized) to other parts of the body and because there is currently no proven screening method for detecting it at an early stage. So long as the cancer is confined to the ovaries, the chances of survival 5 years after treatment are over 90 percent, but once the cancer has spread to the vagina and other pelvic structures, the chances fall to 50 percent. Only about 20 percent of women whose cancer has spread outside the pelvis or into the lymph nodes can expect to be alive 5 years after treatment.

Who is likely to develop ovarian cancer?

Although ovarian cancer can develop at any time, the risk tends to increase with age. Whereas only 2 in 10,000 women between the ages of 30 and 50 in the United States are expected to develop this disease, the rate increases to 4 out of 10,000 after age 50. Ovarian cancer occurs more frequently in industrialized and developed nations and is more common in white than in African American women.

It appears more frequently in women whose female relatives have had the disease, but risks vary considerably depending on the kind of family pattern involved. A woman whose sister or mother had this cancer has a modestly increased chance of developing ovarian cancer compared with women in the general population. Women with the rare familial ovarian cancer syndromes, however, may have as much as a 50 percent risk of developing it at some point in their lives. Women with these rare syndromes often have several family members across two or more generations who have had ovarian, breast, endometrial, or colorectal (colon and rectal) cancers. They also tend to develop ovarian cancer at an earlier age than the average of 59 years. Breast cancer

survivors under the age of 50 also appear to be at increased risk of developing ovarian cancer.

Fewer than 5 percent of women diagnosed with ovarian cancer have any relatives with the disease, however. There is still very little conclusive evidence about what other factors might help predict risk in the many other women affected. Women who have borne at least one child or who have used oral contraceptives seem to have a considerably lower risk (by about 50 percent) of developing ovarian cancer, but there is still very little understanding of how these protective factors may interact with risk factors such as genetic predisposition.

What are the symptoms?

Occasionally ovarian cancer may be discovered when a woman develops persistent pelvic pain. More commonly, there may be no symptoms at all until the disease has spread beyond the ovaries. Then persistent indigestion, loss of appetite, a feeling of fullness in the abdomen, or merely a vague pain or pressure in the abdominal area may be noticed. In later stages of the disease, a woman may experience nausea, vomiting, constipation, or increasing abdominal size.

Because symptoms of ovarian cancer are often vague or absent during the early stages of the disease, many women are not diagnosed as having this cancer until the disease is at an advanced stage. That is why 80 percent of women diagnosed with ovarian cancer already have advanced disease.

How is the condition evaluated?

A clinician may first suspect ovarian cancer in a woman with various intestinal and pelvic complaints that persist after many appropriate remedies have been tried. The clinician who suspects ovarian cancer must first exclude gastrointestinal disease and other noncancerous conditions such as ovarian cysts or endometriosis. A careful physical examination will be performed, with particular care taken to locate a mass in the abdominal or pelvic region and to look for other signs of the cancer.

If a mass is suspected, an ultrasound examination can help the clinician estimate the likelihood of any growth's being malignant (cancerous). Depending on how high that likelihood is, the approach may be either to repeat the ultrasound in a month or two to see whether the mass has grown or to proceed to direct examination of the ovary. This is accomplished through either a laparoscopy or a laparotomy. Before these tests, a preoperative evaluation will include blood and urine testing, an electrocardiogram, a chest x-ray, and a CT scan of the abdomen and pelvis.

A simple blood test called the CA125 test is often performed in women suspected of having ovarian cancer. This test can detect levels in the blood of a protein shed into the bloodstream by most ovarian cancers. The test is most useful in postmenopausal women, in whom an elevated CA125 level rarely occurs unless there is indeed some kind of malignancy. In women who are still menstruating, however, a number of noncancerous conditions—such as uterine fibroids and endometriosis—can cause the CA125 level to rise.

How is ovarian cancer treated?

The first step in treatment is to determine the extent of the tumor at the time of surgery. A laparotomy, usually through a midline incision made from just above the pubic region, allows the surgeon to examine internal organs for signs of cancer and for fluid accumulation. A cell sample from the fluid can be taken and sent to a laboratory to determine if there are any cancerous changes.

If the cancer is limited to the ovary and there is no fluid accumulation, the surgeon will usually remove the ovaries, uterus, fallopian tubes, supporting ligaments, and possibly pelvic and aortic lymph nodes. Sometimes the appendix is removed at the same time. Cell samples will also be taken from nearby areas within the abdomen to make sure there are no other cancerous cells. Usually no further therapy is necessary.

If the cancer is extensive, sometimes portions of the gastrointestinal or urinary tract need to be removed. The more cancerous tissue removed, the greater the chances of long-term survival.

If the woman wants to preserve her childbearing abilities and only one ovary seems to be involved, it is sometimes possible to remove only the affected ovary and its associated fallopian tube. If the cancer is confined to that one ovary, and if cell characteristics are favorable, no further treatment is necessary.

What happens after surgery?

Following surgery, almost all women with more extensive disease will receive chemotherapy or, less commonly, radiation therapy. The drugs most often used in chemotherapy are a combination of carboplatin and paclitaxel (taxol). These drugs can often be given on an outpatient basis.

Because chemotherapy often works for only a limited period of time, however, more surgery may be required after a year or so to see if a different combination of drugs should be tried. At this point participating in a clinical trial at a tertiary center should be considered. These clinical trials include new chemotherapy combinations, as well as newer treatment techniques such as genetic therapy, monoclonal antibody therapy, and vaccine trials.

How can ovarian cancer be prevented?

Although there is no completely effective screening, having an annual pelvic examination is still a good idea. There is great interest in developing a better method to detect it at the earliest stage and thereby reduce the chance of death from this disease. The most promising of the methods under investigation are the tumor marker CA125; an assay that detects elevated blood levels of lysophosphatidic acid (LPA), a lipid found in high quantities in the blood of ovarian cancer patients; and transvaginal ultrasonography (in which a probe is inserted into the vagina to allow a better view of the ovaries).

Neither of these techniques, however, has been proven to be an effective screening test for the general population.

Because the risk of developing ovarian cancer is so great for women with the rare familial ovarian cancer syndromes, many doctors recommend that they have their ovaries removed (oophorectomy). The surgery is usually done after completion of childbearing or by the age of 35, since familial ovarian syndromes tend to occur at a relatively early age. Women who have the more common type of family history (ovarian cancer in just one or two relatives) should talk with their physician about the best way to be monitored. For example, they may want to discuss the possibility of frequent pelvic examinations, transvaginal ultrasonography, or possibly periodic blood tests to check CA125 levels. Women using oral contraceptives have an almost 50 percent decrease in risk of ovarian cancer over their lifetime. Those at high risk should consider this method of contraception as a preventive measure.

Related entries

Chemotherapy, constipation, endometrial cancer, endometriosis, infertility, laparoscopy, laparotomy, menopause, ovarian cysts, ovary removal, radiation therapy, uterine fibroids

Ovarian Cysts

A cyst is an abnormal tissue sac filled with fluid or a semifluid gel. Cysts can develop on one or both ovaries in women of any age, and they can grow to astounding proportions—sometimes reaching the size of an orange or larger. Although many ovarian cysts are harmless, they occasionally cause severe pelvic pain, particularly if they become very large or if they twist or rupture (the bigger the cyst, the greater the chance of rupture). And in older women in particular, it is vital that an ovarian cyst be distinguished from ovarian cancer.

In women of reproductive age, ovarian cysts often result from events that take place during the normal menstrual cycle; thus, they are called functional cysts. In the course of a normal cycle, a single cystlike follicle in the ovary (the Graafian follicle; see illustration) matures and ruptures to release an egg into the fallopian tube. What remains of the follicle is a yellow structure called the corpus luteum, which—unless pregnancy occurs—soon disintegrates on its own. Occasionally, however, the Graafian follicle does not rupture but instead continues to grow. This results in a type of functional cyst known as a follicle cyst. Another type of functional cyst called a corpus luteum cyst can develop if the corpus luteum keeps growing after the egg is released. Functional cysts of both types usually disappear on their own in the course of one or two menstrual cycles.

Occasionally a woman develops many tiny follicle cysts on the ovaries. This is called polycystic ovary syndrome, and it

Ovarian cysts

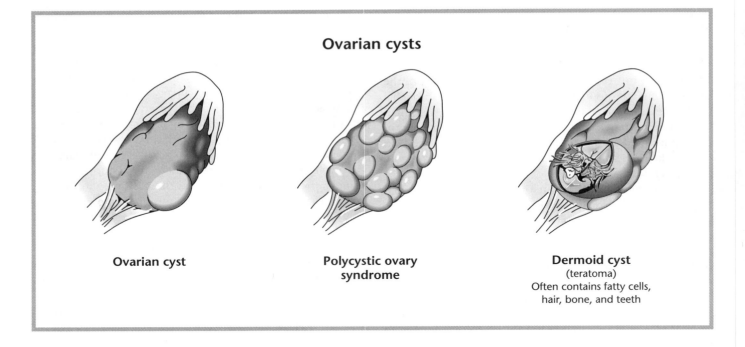

Ovarian cyst

Polycystic ovary syndrome

Dermoid cyst
(teratoma)
Often contains fatty cells,
hair, bone, and teeth

is generally associated with hormonal abnormalities and a number of other symptoms (see hyperandrogenism).

The ovaries are prone to a variety of other cysts and abnormal growths, many of which are noncancerous. Common in young women, for example, are dermoid cysts (teratomas). Often containing fatty cells, hair, bone, and even teeth, these are believed to result not from a pregnancy but from the woman's own cells, which for unknown reasons are stimulated to grow and become differentiated into these organs. Also fairly common are ovarian cystadenomas, benign tumors which contain fluid-filled cysts as well as some tissue. In rare cases, cystadenomas appear to become cancerous, although just how often this occurs remains unclear. Among the most common solid (noncystlike) growths on the ovaries are endometriomas, which are composed of tissue from the uterine lining—as can occur in endometriosis.

In a postmenopausal woman an ovarian growth is more likely to be due to ovarian cancer than to a benign cyst. The increasing use of ultrasound has made it clear, however, that postmenopausal women can also develop noncancerous cysts much more frequently than was previously believed. Cysts in postmenopausal women are sometimes called postmenopausal enlarged ovary.

Who is likely to develop ovarian cysts?

Functional ovarian cysts can—by definition—occur only in premenopausal women. Other than that, there are no known risk factors for them. Using oral contraceptives is known to be a *reverse* risk factor, in that women who are using birth control pills almost never develop functional ovarian cysts.

Other benign ovarian cysts and tumors are common in all age groups. Cystadenomas are more common in women with a family history of ovarian cancer.

What are the symptoms?

Ovarian cysts often produce no symptoms and are discovered only during the course of a routine pelvic examination. Occasionally, however, there may be pelvic or abdominal pain, especially if a cyst is pressing on nearby organs or is growing rapidly, or if it has ruptured or twisted. Some women may also experience pain during sexual intercourse. If the cyst has ruptured, there may be nausea, vomiting, or pain in the shoulder. Delayed, irregular, or painful periods may be yet another symptom of ovarian cysts. Symptoms generally reflect the size of the cyst or growth rather than its specific tissue type.

How is the condition evaluated?

The symptoms of ovarian cysts can suggest many other conditions—including ovarian cancer, pelvic inflammatory disease (PID), and ectopic pregnancy. The likelihood of having these and other conditions depends on a number of factors, including the woman's age, reproductive history, risk factors for ovarian cancer, and specific symptoms. In addition to doing a thorough physical examination—including a palpation of the uterus and pelvic region—a clinician evaluating a potential ovarian cyst will ask questions about all of these issues. Any woman with pelvic pain will be asked about risk factors for pelvic inflammatory disease, including previous sexually transmitted diseases and multiple sexual partners. And premenopausal women will be asked for the dates of their last and previous menstrual periods and for their contraceptive history.

An ultrasound (either transabdominal or transvaginal) may be done of the pelvic region as well. This can be extremely useful in determining the exact location of the abnormality and in differentiating ovarian cysts from ectopic pregnancies. And since malignant growths often have a characteristic appearance, the ultrasound can help the clinician assess the likelihood that a growth is cancerous.

Other parts of the evaluation depend on the woman's age. If there is even a remote possibility of pregnancy in a premenopausal woman, a pregnancy test will be done. If a premenopausal woman has pain on one side of the pelvic area and abnormal vaginal bleeding, the problem could be ectopic pregnancy or a corpus luteum cyst. To differentiate between these two conditions, a clinician may take a blood sample so that levels of the pregnancy hormone human chorionic gonadotropin (hCG) can be measured. This blood test may be done even if an earlier pregnancy test of the urine was negative, since urine tests are not always accurate in diagnosing an ectopic pregnancy. If there is no hCG in the blood, ectopic pregnancy can be ruled out.

Once the possibility of pregnancy has been eliminated, most premenopausal women with ovarian cysts are told to wait a month or two—unless the cyst is large or there is pelvic pain. After this waiting period the physical examination and ultrasound are repeated. If an ultrasound examination shows suspicious or equivocal results, or if the symptoms have not resolved themselves after one or two menstrual cycles, a number of other blood tests may be done as well.

One of the most useful, the CA125 radioimmunoassay, measures the amount of a specific antigen (a protein capable of inducing an immune response) which is shed into the bloodstream by certain·malignant cells and in other abnormal conditions. If levels of this antigen are low in a premenopausal woman, the clinician can be reasonably sure that an ovarian growth is due to a functional ovarian cyst rather than the outgrowth of endometrial tissue (an endometrioma). CA125 levels may be measured even before an ultrasound is done in a postmenopausal woman. This is because the chances of ovarian cancer are much greater after menopause, and levels of CA125 are elevated in about 80 percent of all ovarian cancers.

If a cyst is larger than about 6 to 8 cm in diameter, surgical exploration—and possibly removal—of the cyst by a gynecologist is usually necessary. Using a procedure called a laparoscopy, the gynecologist can inspect the cyst directly and remove tissue for study to determine its exact nature (see biopsy).

How are ovarian cysts treated?

An ovarian cyst in a premenopausal woman often requires no immediate treatment unless the cyst is unusually large or unless there is severe pelvic pain. If the cyst remains after one or two menstrual cycles, the clinician may prescribe birth control pills to see if these help suppress the cyst.

Persistent functional cysts can be left in place or removed surgically. Among the factors to be considered are the size and nature of the cyst and extent of the symptoms, as well as the woman's age and future childbearing plans. If the cyst ruptures or twists, or if pain is severe for other reasons, it can be removed surgically in a procedure called a cystectomy.

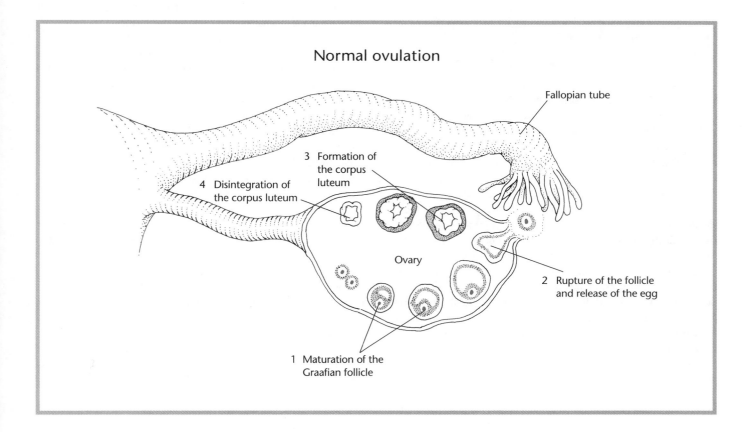

Normal ovulation

Fallopian tube

3 Formation of the corpus luteum

4 Disintegration of the corpus luteum

Ovary

2 Rupture of the follicle and release of the egg

1 Maturation of the Graafian follicle

This can usually be accomplished in conjunction with a laparoscopy.

In postmenopausal women, the usual practice has been to remove a cyst surgically because of the higher likelihood of ovarian cancer in this age group. As ultrasound techniques have become more refined, however, some doctors feel comfortable leaving a very small, clear-cut cyst in place in a postmenopausal woman, provided that the CA125 test results are normal. In this situation, it is important for the woman to be monitored periodically to detect any change in the cyst.

Because some ovarian cystadenomas appear to become cancerous, they are usually removed surgically when diagnosed during laparoscopy. But a premenopausal woman who still wishes to bear children should discuss her pregnancy plans with her gynecologist. Although it is often possible to preserve an ovary while removing a cyst, very large ovarian cysts may require the removal of the ovary (unilateral oophorectomy). So as long as the other ovary is functional, however, childbearing is still possible.

Although dermoid cysts are considered harmless, they are generally removed surgically.

Related entries
Ectopic pregnancy, endometriosis, hyperandrogenism, laparoscopy, menstrual cycle, oral contraceptives, ovarian cancer, ovary removal, pain during sexual intercourse, pelvic inflammatory disease, sexually transmitted diseases

Ovary Removal

The removal of one or both ovaries is called an oophorectomy or ovariectomy. If the fallopian tubes are removed as well, the procedure is called a salpingo-oophorectomy (salpingo means fallopian tube). When both ovaries are removed, in a procedure called bilateral oophorectomy, it is generally to treat ovarian cancer, other gynecological cancers that may have spread to the ovaries, or infections of the ovaries caused by pelvic inflammatory disease (PID). Occasionally removal of one or both ovaries may also be done to treat endometriosis as well. In rare instances bilateral oophorectomy (with hysterectomy) has been found helpful in alleviating severe forms of premenstrual syndrome, but an extensive evaluation and trials of less drastic treatments should be made before this radical step is considered. Both ovaries are sometimes removed to reduce the risk of ovarian cancer in women whose family history puts them at very high risk for the disease.

The removal of only one ovary—a procedure called a unilateral oophorectomy—is usually done when there is an ovarian cyst (noncancerous growth) so large that it cannot be removed without removing the ovary as well. Occasionally unilateral oophorectomy may be done for a cancer or infection that has not spread to the other ovary.

Before the 1970s it was common for surgeons to remove both ovaries routinely in premenopausal women over the age of 45 whenever a hysterectomy (removal of the uterus) was done for a noncancerous condition. The reasoning for this procedure was that the ovaries were going to stop functioning in a few years anyway, and the risks of developing ovarian cancer or requiring a second operation for a noncancerous ovarian condition were so high that removing the ovaries while the abdomen was already open was a reasonable means of prevention. Adding credibility to this argument is the virulence of ovarian cancer (which spreads rapidly), and the fact that, in most cases, it goes undetected until it is well advanced.

In the past few decades, however, most surgeons have concluded that the risks of removing the ovaries probably outweigh these benefits. Not only do women undergo premature menopause with this procedure, but also their risk for osteoporosis and cardiovascular disease starts to increase once the ovaries are removed. In addition, there are some data suggesting that the ovaries continue to produce androgens (virilizing hormones) even after menopause, and that loss of them can reduce a woman's sex drive. Finally, ovarian cancer is still a relatively uncommon disease. Epidemiologic data show that the future risk of ovarian cancer faced by any given woman is quite small—about 1 percent for a woman of 50.

For all of these reasons, most surgeons today offer premenopausal women the option of preserving the ovaries if they are undergoing a hysterectomy for a noncancerous condition. A woman with a family history of ovarian cancer, however, may want to discuss preventive ovary removal with her clinician, since her risk of developing cancer is higher (up to 5 percent for a woman of 50). Women who have a single copy of a BRCA1 or BRCA2 gene with mutations associated with ovarian cancer have an estimated lifetime risk of 16 to 60 percent for developing the disease at some point. In rare families that appear to carry a gene for ovarian and other cancers, preventive ovary removal is often recommended after childbearing is completed or at age 35.

How is the procedure performed?
Oophorectomy is major surgery and involves 2 to 5 days of hospitalization and 3 to 6 weeks to recover. Before the surgery various blood and urine tests will be done, and an enema may be given to cleanse the colon.

The actual procedure is performed much like an abdominal hysterectomy. The surgeon makes an incision 4 to 6 inches long into the abdomen. This can either be a vertical (midline) incision extending up from the pubic bone toward the navel, or a transverse (bikini) incision across the pubic hairline (see laparotomy). Although the transverse incision leaves a less visible scar, some surgeons prefer the greater visibility afforded by a vertical incision.

In some cases the ovaries can be removed through a laparoscope (see laparoscopy); this procedure avoids an abdominal incision and markedly shortens the recovery period.

What happens after surgery?

There is often some discomfort in the incision area for the first few days after the operation. Most women are up and walking immediately. Normal activities—including driving, exercising, and working—can be resumed gradually over the next month or two.

Prior to menopause the ovaries are the body's major source of the hormone estrogen. If only one ovary is removed, or even if just a part of an ovary remains, the woman will continue to have monthly menstrual cycles and will still be fertile. If both ovaries are removed in a premenopausal woman, the sudden loss of estrogen will produce premature menopause—often with abrupt and severe symptoms, including hot flashes, vaginal dryness, painful intercourse, and loss of sex drive. (This condition is sometimes called surgical menopause.) Often estrogen replacement therapy (ERT) is prescribed to help relieve these symptoms.

Androgen replacement therapy is at least partially effective in restoring sexual response in women who have had both of their ovaries removed. When testosterone (one of the androgens) is administered orally or through injection in a dosage sufficient to restore libido, however, masculinizing effects may occur, such as lowered voice, acne, and excess hair growth. A way of administering androgens with greatly reduced side effects is through a small slow-release pellet inserted under the skin in the hip region. This simple office procedure, which must be repeated every 6 months, is readily available to British women, but American women may have difficulty finding a physician familiar with it.

What are the risks and complications?

As with almost all other forms of major surgery, ovary removal involves certain initial risks, including the risks of infection, hemorrhaging, and adverse reactions to anesthesia. Most abdominal surgery results in at least a small degree of internal scar tissue formation as well, and some susceptible women develop an unsightly scar at the incision (see keloid scarring).

Recent research indicates that much of the misery associated with the loss of ovaries (and uterus) in a premenopausal woman is due to the physical discomforts of the surgery itself. In the past this discomfort was frequently attributed to psychological rather than physical causes (supposedly having to do with feelings of lost femininity and reproductive capacity). But a number of newer studies indicate that many women feel relief after oophorectomy or hysterectomy, especially if the procedure is done to alleviate a painful or life-threatening condition.

In short, reactions to these surgeries depend on many factors, including the woman's age, the nature of the condition that prompted the surgery, her reproductive history, her level of social support, her role in the workplace, and her previous history of psychiatric disorders and depression. Women who

have a history of multiple gynecological surgeries or chronic pelvic pain seem particularly predisposed to developing adverse psychological reactions after oophorectomy.

Related entries

Adhesions, anesthesia, depression, ectopic pregnancy, endometriosis, estrogen replacement therapy, hysterectomy, keloid scarring, menopause, menstrual cycle, osteoporosis, ovarian cancer, ovarian cysts, pain during sexual intercourse, pelvic inflammatory disease, psychotherapy, salpingectomy, sexual dysfunction

Pain Management

The universal sensations and emotions commonly known as "pain" result from a complicated series of complex biochemical mechanisms. While related to the release of chemicals in the nervous system, the experience of pain is as much a subjective and emotional process as a physical response. As everyone knows, the same injury or illness can plague one person considerably more than another, depending on individual emotional factors. Women and men appear to experience pain differently as well, and to react differently to pain relief. It is therefore no surprise that the effective management of pain, particularly the chronic pain that afflicts millions of Americans each year, often requires more than one approach, involving a combination of both conventional and nonconventional methods.

What is chronic pain?

Chronic pain is usually defined as pain that does not subside in the expected time of healing after an injury. This usually means pain—constant or intermittent—lasting at least as long as 3 to 6 months and sometimes years or even decades. Among common causes of chronic pain are arthritis, cancer, muscle strain, nerve damage related to diabetes or other conditions, osteoporosis, herniated disks in the back, endometriosis, fibromyalgia, and regional myofascial pain (a condition similar to fibromyalgia but involving a localized area and trigger points that produce involuntary twitches when pressed). Other common causes of chronic pain include headaches, interstitial cystitis, irritable bowel syndrome, dental problems, peripheral neuropathy (tingling or numbness in the hands and feet), and shingles. Long-lasting pain that can't be traced to any specific physical injury or disease also falls into the "chronic pain" category.

Pain that persists month after month not only is distressing physically but also often wreaks havoc on work, personal relationships, and just about every other aspect of life. Sometimes this condition is called chronic pain syndrome. Women who have a history of psychological trauma or domestic abuse (see entry) can experience chronic pain syndrome, often involving pelvic pain. Debilitating pain is often accompanied by anger, irritability, mood swings, alienation, demoralization, and, frequently, dependence on narcotic painkillers and/or alcohol. Symptoms of depression such as insomnia, lack of appetite, and loss of interest in sex are also common. Opportunities for exercise shrink, often resulting in weight gain and weakness. Medical bills mount just at a time when income may decline or dry up altogether. These social, financial, and emotional problems, together with side effects from pain medications, often exacerbate the physical discomfort, leading to a vicious cycle of pain and suffering.

How can chronic pain be managed?

Treating chronic pain begins with having the source of the pain properly diagnosed. Usually this means seeing a primary care clinician, preferably one who takes pain complaints seriously and deals with the problem aggressively.

In many cases, making the pain more tolerable is a more realistic goal than making it disappear altogether. Doing so generally involves mixing and matching various approaches, with a little trial and error to be expected along the way. Whatever the cause of the pain, successful control of chronic pain often requires some combination of painkilling medications, physical therapy, behavioral changes, and relaxation exercises.

A primary care clinician may refer a patient with chronic pain to a "pain clinic" for this kind of care. These clinics can put together a coordinated pain management plan that involves input from a team of health care providers, including physicians, nurses, psychologists, physical or occupational therapists, and nontraditional therapists (e.g., acupuncturists or massage therapists).

Medications. Both acute and chronic pain can be controlled to some extent with medications. Among the most effective are the nonsteroidal antiinflammatory drugs, or NSAIDs, that relieve pain by blocking the synthesis of pain-causing chemicals called prostaglandins. The most recently approved NSAIDs are the COX-2 inhibitors. These drugs appear to block pain while avoiding some of the gastrointestinal and bleeding problems associated with older medications.

Other pain-relieving drug treatments sometimes used to relieve chronic pain include acetaminophen (Tylenol); tramadol (Ultram), a synthetic version of codeine; and long-term opioid therapy. In some cases these medications are taken around the clock, with supplements if pain worsens. Side effects, the most common of which is constipation, can usually be controlled, though people taking opiates for chronic pain are at risk for addiction.

Certain types of pain, particularly pain related to nerve damage, may be more responsive to antidepressant medications (see entry). Of these, the tricyclic antidepressants (such as amitriptylene or Elavil) seem to be the most effective in blocking pain, and possibly the new serotonin-specific reuptake inhibitor (SSRI) venlafaxine (Effexor) as well. Some anticonvulsant drugs—including phenytoin (Dilantin), carbamazepine (Tegretol), valproic acid (Depakote), clonazepam (Klonopin), and gabapentin (Neurontin)—also seem to relieve pain related to nerve damage or dysfunction.

Physical therapy. To supplement painkilling medications, various physical approaches can help relieve pain, depending on its nature and location. Aching muscles and joints often respond to either heating pads or ice packs, the latter of which can also soothe itching. Massage, vibration therapy, and monitored exercise programs can often help relieve both bone and muscle pain.

Nerve stimulation therapies. Chronic pain including postoperative pain, low back pain, nerve pain, headache, rib pain, arthritis, phantom limb pain, and cancer pain often respond to transcutaneous electrical nerve stimulation (TENS). In this technique electrode pads are applied to the skin and stimulated with electric current that stops the conduction of pain messages to the brain. Acupuncture, a technique that involves placing fine needles at distinct points along energy "meridians" on the body surface, has also been shown in controlled and randomized trials to help control back pain, menstrual pain (dysmenorrhea), and dental pain, as well as the nausea and vomiting often associated with cancer chemotherapy. This may be because acupuncture appears to stimulate the body's natural painkillers (endorphins) as well as other neurotransmitters such as serotonin and norepinephrine.

Psychological support. Because the mind has some power over the perception of pain, an integrated approach to pain management often involves both behavioral and cognitive therapies (see entry on psychotherapy). Cognitive therapies focus on thoughts and perceptions that shape interpretations of bodily sensations. They may include relaxation techniques, guided imagery, meditation, support groups, and hypnosis (see entry on alternative therapies). Biofeedback, a technique through which a person learns to control bodily processes that are normally involuntary, can also be used to control pain.

Other approaches. Pain specialists may recommend more specialized approaches if pain is unremitting. Many of these approaches (e.g., cryoanalgesia, radiofrequency lesioning, spinal cord stimulation) involve cooling or electrically stimulating key nerves to block the conduction of pain sensations either temporarily or permanently. Other approaches, such as implantable drug delivery systems, are particularly helpful in treating pain traceable to physical injury and involving multiple areas on the body.

Related entries

Alternative therapies, antidepressants, antiinflammatory drugs, back pain, diabetes, endometriosis, fibromyalgia, gum disease, headaches, interstitial cystitis, irritable bowel syndrome, knee pain, osteoporosis, pain with sexual intercourse, psychosomatic disorders, psychotherapy, shingles

Pain during Sexual Intercourse

When a woman frequently experiences vaginal pain before, during, or after sexual intercourse, the condition is called dyspareunia. Approximately 1 in 5 women may suffer from this disorder at any given time, and many more experience it at some point in their lives. Dyspareunia results when there is not enough lubrication in the vaginal walls to relieve friction between the penis and vagina. It may also occur when penetration puts pressure on abnormal tissue deep within the pelvis (as with endometriosis).

Vaginismus, by contrast, is a relatively rare form of sexual pain disorder in which muscles in the outer third of the vagina (pubococcygeus muscles) involuntarily contract to prevent penetration, making sexual intercourse difficult, painful, or impossible. Many unconsummated marriages of long duration can be attributed to vaginismus in the woman. Partners of women with vaginismus can develop impotence as well.

Who is likely to develop dyspareunia or vaginismus?

Dyspareunia can occur in any woman who has intercourse without adequate stimulation, as well as in women with disorders of desire or excitement (see sexual dysfunction), or who are anxious about their sexual performance. Dyspareunia can initiate a vicious cycle in which fear and anticipation of pain interfere with arousal and the natural lubrication that it would otherwise produce. At certain points in a woman's life, too, vaginal lubrication is reduced because of hormonal changes. These include menopause (see vaginal atrophy), breastfeeding, and during or just following menstruation.

Pain may also develop after an episiotomy—a cut made by the clinician during delivery to prevent the perineum from tearing—as well as during radiation therapy for cancers of the reproductive organs. Some women may develop pain because of local irritation or infection which is further aggravated by sexual intercourse. Common causes of irritation are yeast infections; urinary tract infections; sexually transmitted diseases such as trichomonas, herpes, or genital warts; as well as allergic reactions to spermicides, vaginal deodorants, or the latex in condoms or diaphragms.

When the pain is felt deep inside the vagina, there may be an underlying disorder of the pelvic organs. These disorders include endometriosis, pelvic inflammatory disease (PID), adhesions, ovarian cancer, ovarian cysts, or tears in the ligaments that support the uterus. Occasionally deep vaginal pain may occur when the penis hits the cervix (the opening to the uterus) during thrusting. This can often be alleviated by changing positions.

Vaginismus, by contrast, seems to be a way for the body to avoid sexual contact. It is particularly common in women who experienced sexual trauma such as rape.

How are the conditions evaluated?

Women with dyspareunia should have both a physical and a pelvic examination, including a sexual history. If no obvious cause of the pain can be found, the clinician may order tests to see if there are any underlying disorders of the pelvis that might account for the problem. These may include various blood tests, a Pap test, a colposcopy, a pelvic ultrasound, and a laparoscopy.

Sometimes a practitioner will diagnose vaginismus when it is difficult to insert a finger or speculum into the vagina during a pelvic examination.

How are dyspareunia and vaginismus treated?

Any underlying gynecological problem will be treated first, often alleviating dyspareunia at the same time. Insufficient lubrication can be relieved by using a water-soluble vaginal lubricant (such as K-Y Jelly, Lubrin, Astroglide, or Replens), a lubricated condom, or a spermicidal cream, foam, or jelly. Also sold over the counter—though much more expensive—are moisturizing gel tampons which provide continuous vaginal moisture when inserted into the vagina 3 times a week. These slightly acidic lubricants, which closely match the body's pH, also help inhibit the growth of some organisms that cause vaginitis. Estrogen replacement therapy is another option for women past menopause. A woman who chooses not to take systemic estrogen can use estrogen cream periodically to relieve symptoms of painful intercourse.

For women with dyspareunia, treating the symptom is often all that is required. Women with vaginismus can be helped further with behavioral modification techniques. Usually a doctor will recommend a series of desensitization exercises, to be practiced at home, in which the vaginal muscles are gradually trained to accept penetration. First the woman is encouraged to insert a finger into the vagina, then several. Vaginal dilators of graduated sizes are usually the next step in training the vaginal muscles to relax. Doing Kegel exercises while the dilators are in place can help the woman develop a sense of control over her own muscles. Eventually she will be encouraged to attempt intercourse in a female-superior position, using her partner's erect penis, coated with extra vaginal lubricant, as a dilator. In some cases psychotherapy or hypnosis may also be helpful.

Related entries

Estrogen replacement therapy, Kegel exercises, laparoscopy, lubricants, psychosomatic disorders, psychotherapy, sexual abuse and incest, sexual dysfunction, sexual response, sexually transmitted diseases, vaginal atrophy, vaginitis, vulvar disorders

Panic Disorder

Panic disorder comprises a constellation of symptoms that begin with panic attacks and eventually develop into phobias that center on situations in which panic symptoms were previously experienced.

Panic attacks are brief, unexplained, and unexpected episodes of intense fear accompanied by heart palpitations, shortness of breath, dizziness, and other physical symptoms. These attacks are not just episodes of everyday anxiety or nervousness but overwhelming physiological reactions identical to the fight-or-flight response—the body's way of reacting to a physical threat. In the case of panic attacks, however, the threat exists only in the mind of the individual.

After a person has experienced one of these attacks, she may develop irrational fears—called phobias—about having another attack and will avoid situations or places associated with the initial attack. A woman who panicked while behind the wheel of a car may believe that she will die if she tries driving again; a woman who experienced a panic attack while out shopping may refuse to leave her house alone. The combination of this "fear of fear" and of recurring panic attacks is called panic disorder.

Panic disorder can be so devastating that people with it often truly believe they are going to die, lose their mind, or undergo insufferable embarrassment. The fear can be incapacitating enough to keep a woman from running errands, commuting to work, or maintaining normal relationships. The fear can also foster extreme dependence on family members or close friends. About 1 person in 3 with panic disorder goes on to develop agoraphobia, the fear of public places. People with agoraphobia may be unable to be in a crowd, ride public transportation, visit a shopping mall, or even leave their own home for fear of having a panic attack outside the familiar safety zone.

Panic disorder is often accompanied by other psychological and physical conditions as well. These may include depression, obsessive-compulsive disorder, alcohol abuse, substance abuse, suicidal tendencies, and irritable bowel syndrome. Sleep disturbances are common, either because the person wakes up in the middle of a terrifying attack or because daytime anxiety makes it difficult to sleep. How these symptoms relate to panic disorder—whether each might be caused by some common underlying disorder, for example, or whether some might themselves cause or be caused by the panic disorder itself—is still not understood.

Who is likely to develop panic disorder?
More than 3 million people in the United States have had a panic attack at some point in their lives. Women are twice as likely as men to have them. Full-blown panic disorder usually develops in young adults, but even children can have panic attacks and begin to avoid situations which are associated with panic. Often the initial attacks are brought on by some

kind of extraordinary external stress, including loss of a job, a death in the family, a serious illness or surgery, a divorce, or childbirth. Panic attacks can also arise from excessive caffeine consumption or from using cocaine or other stimulant drugs or medications. Some evidence even suggests that exposure to volatile organic compounds, such as those found in oil-based house paints and cleaning solvents, may cause panic attacks in some individuals.

Women who suffer from panic disorder before or during pregnancy may find that attacks become more frequent or severe after the baby is born. The attacks characteristically worsen within the first 2 or 3 weeks after delivery, often escalating to several panic attacks a day. Postpartum depression may also develop at the same time.

People with panic disorder show evidence of certain biochemical peculiarities that may make them particularly susceptible to panic attacks. Some investigators have associated panic disorder with increased activity of the hippocampus and locus ceruleus, portions of the limbic system in the brain that monitor external and internal stimuli and control the brain's responses to them. There may also be abnormalities in parts of the brain that, in people without the disorder, normally react with anxiety-reducing substances. In people with this disorder the portion of the nervous system that regulates heart rate and body temperature (the adrenergic system) also seems to be overactive. It is not clear whether this overactivity causes the symptoms of panic disorder or is merely another of the symptoms.

There is little doubt that emotions, thoughts, and interpersonal stress (such as marital conflict) play a role in panic disorder. A genetic component may be involved as well, since panic disorder seems to run in families. Several studies are under way to elucidate the importance of each of these factors.

What are the symptoms?
The hallmark symptom of panic disorder is recurrent panic attacks. A panic attack can involve a host of terrifying and distressing symptoms. These include a sense of doom, a sense of unreality, fear of dying or going crazy, fear of humiliation or losing control, racing or pounding heartbeat, chest pains, dizziness, shortness of breath, tingling or numb hands and feet, flushes, tremors, sweating, and chills. These symptoms can last from several seconds to several minutes, although the attack may seem longer to the person experiencing it. Between attacks, a person with panic disorder has a "fear of fear" that is often intense enough to interfere with daily functioning.

How is the condition evaluated?
Often people with panic disorder fear that they have a serious physical disability—that something is wrong with their heart, lungs, nerves, or gastrointestinal system, for example. They may go from doctor to doctor, undergoing many uncomfortable and expensive tests, looking for an acceptable diagnosis. If patients focus on their physical symptoms and

deny their feelings of anxiety, their clinicians may fail to recognize panic disorder as such. A person with panic disorder may be diagnosed as suffering from somatization disorder, a psychiatric condition in which physical complaints cannot be traced to any specific physical defect (see psychosomatic disorders).

Nevertheless, before panic disorder can be diagnosed, it is important to rule out other possible causes of the symptoms. These can include thyroid disorders, epilepsy, or heart disease. Even asthmatic symptoms and the allergic reactions associated with asthma may be confused with panic attacks.

How is panic disorder treated?

If panic disorder is successfully diagnosed, it can almost always be cured, either with psychotherapy, medications, or a combination of the two. Just which of these should be used depends on the preferences and reactions of the individual patient. There are several studies under way (supported by the National Institute of Mental Health) to determine the most effective therapy. For now a combination of medication and cognitive-behavioral therapy seems to offer many people the best chance of rapid and effective relief with a low rate of relapse.

Cognitive-behavioral psychotherapy is particularly effective in treating panic disorder. The cognitive part of the therapy involves learning to recognize thoughts and emotions that may underlie the panic attacks. This approach assumes that people with panic disorder have distorted thought processes that provoke a vicious cycle of fear. By learning to identify some of the thoughts and emotions that trigger the cycle—such as a fear of having a heart attack—it may be possible to modify and eventually control the responses to them. The behavioral portion of therapy usually involves systematic training in relaxation techniques, including breathing exercises, and in desensitization (repeated exposures to the situation that provokes the panic attacks, but with adequate social support) to help the patient learn to master her body's responses to anxiety. Cognitive-behavioral therapy is often successful after about 8 to 12 weeks.

Some people with panic disorder find it useful to join self-help or support groups composed of other people with the disorder. These groups are also the least expensive form of therapy available. In addition, psychodynamic therapy—which seeks to help the patient uncover early life experiences and deep-seated fears that might be the source of the anxiety—can help relieve some of the stress associated with panic attacks, though this type of therapy usually cannot stop the attacks from occurring.

Certain antidepressants and antianxiety drugs (tranquilizers) can prevent panic attacks or at least reduce their frequency and severity. Tricyclic antidepressants such as imipramine (Tofranil) were the first medications shown to be effective against panic disorder. Today, high-potency benzodiazepines such as clonazepam (Klonopin) and alprazolam (Xanax) are used more frequently. These antianxiety drugs work quickly and have few side effects. People who use benzodiazepines, however, run the risk of developing drug dependency, although clonazepam has a relatively low addictive potential. The risk is highest among people who have already had problems with alcohol or drug dependency. A newer antianxiety drug, buspirone (BuSpar), seems to work well at controlling panic attacks and has fewer side effects in some people than do the benzodiazepines.

As with tricyclic antidepressants, the high-potency benzodiazepines are usually started at low dosages which are gradually raised and then continued for 6 months to a year. After they are stopped, withdrawal symptoms such as weakness and malaise may occur.

Another kind of antidepressant, monoamine oxidase inhibitors (MAOIs), is also sometimes used to treat panic disorder. Because MAOIs can cause a dangerous increase in blood pressure when used with certain foods and drugs, they must be used with particular caution. The most commonly prescribed MAOI for panic disorder is phenelzine (Nardil).

Increasingly, the class of antidepressants known as selective serotonin reuptake inhibitors (SSRIs)—fluoxetine (Prozac), sertraline (Zoloft), paroxetine (Paxil), citalopram (Celexa), and fluvoxamine (Luvox)—and the related antidepressant venlafaxine (Effexor) are being used to treat panic disorder as well. To minimize side effects, all of these antidepressants are started at low dosages and are gradually increased until an effective dose is found; it can take several weeks before there is any noticeable effect. Antidepressant therapy must be continued for 6 months to a year to prevent panic attacks from recurring.

Because panic disorder is a chronic, relapsing illness, panic attacks sometimes recur even after treatment. Skills learned in treating the initial episodes can often make it easier to cope with setbacks. Sometimes people who have recovered from panic disorder continue to have occasional panic attacks for years to come, but these attacks no longer incapacitate them or dominate their lives.

Related entries

Alcohol, antianxiety drugs, antidepressants, anxiety disorders, depression, irritable bowel syndrome, mitral valve prolapse, obsessive-compulsive disorder, phobias, postpartum psychiatric disorders, psychosomatic disorders, psychotherapy, sleep disorders, stress, substance abuse, thyroid disorders

Pap Test

The "Pap" test—named for its 1943 originator, G. N. Papanicolaou—is an office procedure that helps identify abnormal cells from the cervix and other parts of the female reproductive tract. Because precancerous changes of the cervix usually take years to develop into cervical cancer, regular Pap tests can reveal cancer in its early stages when it is most easily cured. This test can also detect about 50 percent of endometrial (uterine) cancers and a much smaller percentage of other female reproductive tumors. Widespread screening programs based on this procedure have decreased the incidence of invasive cervical cancer and the number of deaths from this and other reproductive tract diseases.

Occasionally the Pap test will incidentally show signs of other conditions—for example, trichomonas vaginitis.

How is the procedure performed?

The Pap test is usually performed during a routine pelvic examination or in a woman with symptoms suggestive of cervical cancer. While the vaginal walls are held open with a speculum (see illustration), the clinician inserts a cotton swab or fine brush and a small spatula into the vagina and scrapes cells from the outside of the cervix and just inside the cervical canal. The scraping feels slightly uncomfortable to some women. The cells are then "fixed" to a slide and sent to a laboratory for microscopic analysis. A newer procedure called "Thin-Prep" involves placing the cells into a jar of special solution; they are transferred to a slide only after reaching the lab. While more expensive than the standard Pap test, this procedure gives more accurate results because it lowers the chance that blood, mucus, and preservatives will obscure the results.

The laboratory classifies cells according to one of several systems, the newest (and most consistent) of which is called the Bethesda system. According to the Bethesda system, a Pap test is graded into one of the following levels according to the nature of cell changes and how much of the cervix is affected: normal (no evidence of malignant cells), atypical cells of undetermined significance (ASCUS), low-grade squamous intraepithelial lesion, high-grade intraepithelial lesion, and invasive cancer (which would also be described according to its specific stage; see cervical cancer). The new classification includes any changes in cervical cells which are associated with the human papilloma virus, a sexually transmitted microorganism that has been linked to cervical cancer. It also determines if changes associated with the virus are linked to any precancerous changes.

An abnormal Pap test does not necessarily mean that the woman has cancer. Atypical cells (ASCUS, pronounced "ask-us") are usually due to infection of the cervix (cervicitis) or vagina (vaginitis) or to precancerous cell changes (dysplasia) that sometimes spontaneously revert to normal. If a Pap test does indicate atypical cells, however, the practitioner will probably recommend repeating the test in a few months. If there is any evidence of infection, the infection will be treated first. If atypical cells are still present on the repeat test, the next step is to examine the cervix and vagina with a special type of microscope called a colposcope. Colposcopy (see entry) usually causes minimal discomfort and can be done in the gynecologist's office. If there is a visible abnormality on the cervix, a small piece of tissue will be removed from the cervix and examined under a microscope for cancerous

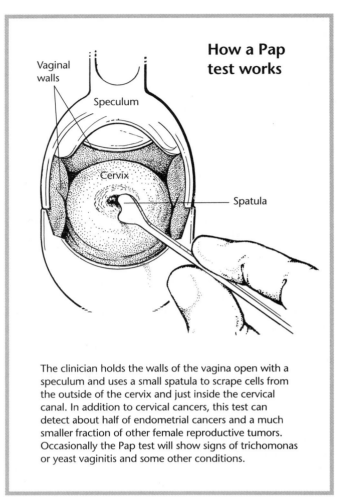

How a Pap test works

The clinician holds the walls of the vagina open with a speculum and uses a small spatula to scrape cells from the outside of the cervix and just inside the cervical canal. In addition to cervical cancers, this test can detect about half of endometrial cancers and a much smaller fraction of other female reproductive tumors. Occasionally the Pap test will show signs of trichomonas or yeast vaginitis and some other conditions.

changes (see biopsy). It is important to remember, however, that most women who have mild dysplasia never go on to develop more serious problems. The decision to undergo a colposcopy needs to be made by the individual woman and her clinician.

Women whose Pap test shows low-grade or high-grade squamous intraepithelial lesions, or women with HIV whose test shows atypical cells, are referred directly for colposcopy.

Are Pap tests accurate?

Accuracy of Pap test results has been a source of considerable and well-publicized concern in recent years. Manual reading of the slides led to a certain amount of inevitable fatigue and human error, no matter how well trained or well intentioned the technicians. Inevitably, some early-stage cancers were overlooked, and some women who ultimately turned out to be healthy were subjected to needless alarm and expensive follow-up care.

Newer automated screening devices for Pap smears are helping not only to speed up the process of interpretation but also to minimize these kind of errors. Using a high-speed microscope and image interpretation software, these machines can quickly and thoroughly analyze slides made from Pap smears. These machines can only identify "normal" slides, however, they can't be used to make positive diagnoses (i.e., definitively diagnose cancer). A pathologist must still manually review any slides that might contain abnormalities.

Who should have a Pap test, and how often?

Annual Pap tests are recommended starting at age 18 or at the onset of sexual activity, whichever occurs earlier. After 3 or more consecutive negative tests, many doctors recommend a regular exam about every 2 years. Women at high risk for conditions that could lead to cervical cancer (including first intercourse before age 17, more than 5 sex partners, or history of human papilloma virus infection) should have a Pap test annually. Also, any woman whose mother took diethylstilbestrol (DES) while pregnant should have a Pap test done at least once a year.

Because there is an increased risk of developing cervical cancer with increasing age, women over 65 who have never or rarely had a previous Pap test should ask their physician to perform one. Women who have had frequent negative Pap tests before age 65 benefit less from routine screening after 65.

Cone biopsy, laser surgery, and cryosurgery can produce temporary cell changes that can give false-positive Pap tests or make the test difficult to interpret accurately. Women who have undergone these procedures should wait 3 or 4 months before having a Pap test.

Related entries

Biopsy, cervical cancer, cryosurgery, diethylstilbestrol (DES), laser surgery, pelvic examinations, sexually transmitted diseases, vaginitis

Patients' Rights

The patients' rights movement grew out of concerns in the 1960s that medicine was becoming increasingly specialized, technical, and depersonalized. Together with a desire to foster an active role for the patient in the healing process, these concerns led to the 1973 publication of a patients' bill of rights by the American Hospital Association. After that date all accredited hospitals were required to accept this bill of rights.

In the years that followed, various hospitals and women's organizations issued their own versions of these rights, and many health care facilities routinely offer a written document describing them to all patients. More and more, hospitals are providing patient advocates (also called patient representatives) as intermediaries who can help patients ensure that their rights are enforced. Some institutions even em-

ploy medical ethicists to explore deeper implications of these rights.

It is customary for hospitals to include a list of patient responsibilities along with the list of rights. Typical patient responsibilities include being considerate of staff and other patients, as well as recognizing the effects of lifestyle and personal behavior on health.

What rights do patients have?

Here is a brief description of the issues covered in virtually all versions of the patients' bill of rights.

Quality care for all patients. Regardless of race, creed, color, sex, age, disabilities, or financial status, every patient is entitled to receive the highest-quality services available at the facility. Although this may sometimes mean going to a less crowded facility in a non-life-threatening situation, it does ensure prompt and equal access to the best care available. Patients have a right to expect that the hospital will make a reasonable response to requests for care, including evaluation, services, and, when necessary, referral to a more appropriate facility.

Informed consent. Patients have a right to know what will happen to them before it happens and to refuse any offered service or treatment. For nonemergency hospital admissions, this means having the right to know all the rules and regulations of the hospital. In the case of nonemergency tests and treatments, it means having the right to know exactly what the procedure involves, how much pain and disability may occur and for how long, what the risks are, and what the alternatives are (and the risks of the alternatives).

Before any procedure a patient is given a consent form to sign, which should include a written explanation of these matters. Patients—together with the physician—have the right to modify any part of the consent form that does not pertain to their particular situation.

Access to information. Patients have a right to know the name of the doctor responsible for their care and to receive information about their diagnosis, treatment plan, anticipated outcome, and expected length of hospitalization. This information should be given in terms that a patient can reasonably be expected to understand. Patients also have the right to obtain information about the relationship of the hospital to other health care and educational institutions and about any professional relationships that may exist between specific individuals involved in their treatment.

In the case of minors or others deemed incapable of understanding this information, the information should be made available to a parent, guardian, or other person acting on the patient's behalf.

Transfer to another institution. If the hospital cannot provide all the services necessary for care, it must make arrangements for the patient to be transferred to another facility. The patient has the right to know the reasons for the transfer as well as any alternatives. Before the transfer takes place, the new facility must accept the patient for transfer.

Declining treatment. Patients have the right to refuse treatment (although some state laws do not grant this right to psychiatric patients who are potentially dangerous to themselves or others). They also have the right to prepare advance directives (such as a living will or durable power of attorney), with assistance if needed, and to be assured that their wishes will be honored.

Leaving against medical advice. In almost all cases a patient has the right to leave the hospital even if her physician or other hospital staff advise against doing so. The exceptions are those patients who have infectious diseases or who might otherwise be dangerous to society. A patient who chooses to leave the hospital against medical advice will have to sign a form absolving the doctor and hospital from responsibility for any harm that may occur to the patient or others if the patient's condition worsens.

Privacy and dignity. Every patient has the right to be treated with dignity and respect and to have consideration given to personal privacy and individual beliefs.

Confidentiality. All patient records are confidential and cannot be shared with any person or agency who is not authorized by the patient or the law.

The right to see records. Many states now give patients the legal right to inspect their hospital records.

Participation in research and teaching. Many university-affiliated hospitals provide training programs for new health care professionals and conduct clinical trials to test new drug therapies. All patients in these facilities have the right to refuse to participate in these activities. This means that patients have the right to know if their doctor plans to use experimental drugs or procedures in their care, as well as the right to refuse to participate in these experiments. They also have the right to know the purpose of the research, its possible benefits to the individual patient and to humanity in general, and available alternatives. A patient who does not want medical students or other trainees to be present during any consultation or procedure can refuse to allow their attendance and should not have to fear repercussions in terms of the quality of care she will be given.

Continuity of care. After discharge from the hospital, the patient has the right to be informed about the clinician who will be taking responsibility for her continuing care. She also has the right to know appointment times and physician availability in advance.

Payment. Patients have the right to an itemized bill that describes all the hospital charges related to their care. They also have the right to question any portion of the bill they do not understand and to request information and help in receiving any financial benefits to which they may be entitled.

Pelvic Examinations

A pelvic examination is a physical evaluation of a woman's reproductive organs—vulva, vagina, cervix, uterus, ovaries, and fallopian tubes. Often done by itself as a routine checkup, a pelvic examination is sometimes done in conjunction with a complete physical examination or as part of regular prenatal care. It may also be done when a woman consults a clinician about a specific problem involving the reproductive organs.

Clinicians can use pelvic examinations to help determine if a woman is pregnant; if she is having a miscarriage; if her uterus or ovaries are enlarged, her cervix inflamed, her pelvic muscles slack; or if she has any vaginal infections (vaginitis), cystoceles, urethroceles, rectoceles, vaginal atrophy, genital warts, vulvar disease, abnormal growths, or suspicious tenderness in the ovaries. Unless the hymen is intact (which it sometimes is not, even in women who have never had sexual intercourse), the clinician will not be able to determine from a pelvic examination whether or not the woman has ever had sexual intercourse. An intact hymen, however, indicates that she is a virgin.

Many clinicians recommend that all women over the age of 18—or younger, if sexually active—should have regular pelvic examinations. Women over 65 should continue to have pelvic examinations to detect ovarian, cervical, and vulvar cancer, all of which increase in likelihood as women age. Pap tests (see entry) to detect abnormalities in the cervix do not need to be repeated annually in older women if they have previously had regular normal Pap tests and are not taking estrogen replacement therapy; they should have a Pap every 3 years. Women on ERT should continue to have the test annually. Women who have had a hysterectomy but whose ovaries remain should have periodic pelvic examinations to detect any signs of ovarian cancer; if the hysterectomy was done for cancer, a Pap test from the vagina should also be taken. In women who have had the uterus and both ovaries removed, the pelvic examination may be limited to an inspection of the vulva. Any woman who is sexually active and is using oral contraceptives, an intrauterine device, or a diaphragm as birth control should have a pelvic examination once a year, as should women with a family history of ovarian cancer and possibly other cancers of the reproductive organs. A woman whose mother took diethylstilbestrol (DES) when pregnant should have a pelvic examination at least once a year during her reproductive years.

Premenopausal women should try to schedule pelvic examinations for a time when they do not expect to be menstruating. If menstruation occurs on the day of the exam, the appointment will probably need to be rescheduled, since menstrual flow interferes with the reliability of some tests that may be conducted in conjunction with the pelvic exam—specifically the Pap test. It is important not to douche for at least 24 hours before the examination, since this can mask abnormal vaginal discharge which sometimes signals vaginitis (see entry). Having had sexual intercourse, however, does not interfere in any way with the examination, although spermicidal jellies or vaginal lubricants can affect a Pap test.

A woman should always urinate just before the examination. This not only makes the procedure more comfortable but also makes it easier for the clinician to detect any abnormalities.

How is the procedure performed?

Although pelvic examinations are rarely painful, their very nature means that they involve a certain inevitable loss of dignity. Some clinicians just seem to have a gentler or more sensitive approach than others or are more experienced at doing pelvic examinations. One option for women concerned about the violation of privacy or potential embarrassment, as well as for those who are frightened about the examination or who feel inhibited about asking questions, is to have a friend or patient advocate stay with them during the exam or to ask a male clinician if a female nurse can be present.

Relaxing the abdominal and pelvic muscles during the examination can be a great help to both the clinician and the woman being examined. Not only will relaxation make it easier for the clinician to perform each part of the examination, but often it also makes the whole procedure more comfortable for the woman. Many women also find that their anxiety diminishes if clinicians explain what they are doing at each step, giving advance warning if something will feel cold or if there will be a little pressure (a woman can specifically ask to be told these things beforehand). Some clinicians have an assistant hold up a mirror (or have one mounted at the correct angle) so that the woman can observe the examination as it proceeds. Often knowing what is happening helps promote relaxation.

Before the examination the woman will usually be asked to remove her clothing (or at least the lower half) and cover herself with either a large paper drape or a cloth gown. Sometimes the drape can block a woman's view of the clinician. If this is a problem, she should feel free to ask about removing or rearranging it. Before the examination begins, the woman should alert her clinician to any specific concerns she may have. If a woman finds pelvic examinations especially difficult, it is important to tell the clinician so that extra time for the examination can be taken.

When the clinician is ready to start the exam, the woman will be asked to lie on her back on the examining table, bend her knees, and put her feet into metal stirrups so that her knees are spread wide apart. There may be fleece or toweling over the stirrups to make the metal more comfortable; otherwise, it may help to wear a pair of socks. The woman is told to move her hips down to the edge of the table. This "dorsal lithotomy" position gives the clinician the best view of and access to the reproductive organs. Some women (such as those with scoliosis or arthritis of the hip) find this position painful or impossible, in which case other positions such as lying on the side with one leg supported in the air may be used.

A complete pelvic examination involves four separate parts, which together usually take only a few minutes to complete: an external examination, an internal (speculum) examination, a bimanual examination, and a rectovaginal examination. Not all clinicians perform the steps in the same order, and, depending on the reason for the examination, may not always need to perform each step.

The external examination. The external examination is usually the first and quickest part of the pelvic examination. The clinician visually inspects the vulva (the external genitalia) for any abnormal growths, irritations, skin lesions, discharges, or discolorations. Then the clinician palpates (feels) the Bartholin's glands and Skene's glands (which lie beside the vaginal entrance and under the urethra, respectively) for any lumps or abnormal discharges—which could signal cysts or infections.

The internal (speculum) examination. To inspect the vagina and the cervix (the opening to the uterus), the clinician needs to separate the vaginal walls and hold them open. This is accomplished with a two-bladed instrument made of metal or plastic called a speculum. After inserting the closed speculum into the vagina, the clinician positions it, opens up the blades, and locks them into position. Some clinicians warm a metal speculum before inserting it so that there is less shock to the skin. A woman may want to ask her clinician to do this.

The speculum is often slightly uncomfortable but rarely painful—even for women who have never had sexual intercourse or used a tampon. Some women, however, are bothered by the speculum pressing on the bladder or the rectum or simply find it painful. They should speak up if they would like the clinician to do the insertion more gently or to readjust the position of the speculum. Taking some slow deep breaths and making a conscious effort to relax the pelvic muscles can also help. If pain persists, trying a smaller speculum may help (they are available in graduated sizes).

Once the speculum is in place, the vagina and cervix can be inspected visually for swelling, discoloration, lesions, or abnormal discharge. Often the clinician will do a Pap test at the same time by inserting a cervical brush into the os (opening) of the cervix. By rotating this brush 360 degrees and then removing it, the clinician obtains a sample of cells from the cervix. Abnormal-looking discharge can also be collected and cultured for gonorrhea, or, if vaginitis is a possibility, it can be collected on a slide (a wet mount) and then examined under a microscope. If the woman is using an intrauterine device (IUD), its placement can be checked at this time.

At the end of the pelvic examination, a woman can also be

fitted for a diaphragm or have the fit of her existing one re-checked.

The bimanual examination. In the bimanual examination the clinician puts on a disposable plastic glove and then inserts two fingers into the vagina while pressing down on the lower abdomen with the other hand (see illustration). Usually the clinician starts by assessing the size, shape, firmness, and position of the uterus. Abnormalities may suggest the possibility of pregnancy or of uterine fibroids and other growths, as well as the existence of a prolapsed (fallen) or retroverted (tipped) uterus, though the latter is usually nothing more than a variation of normal. To check the strength of the pelvic muscles, the clinician sometimes asks the woman to bear down or strain for a few seconds. This part of the bimanual exam is almost always painless.

By moving the upper hand into various positions and pressing with the fingers in the vagina, the clinician can next assess the ovaries and fallopian tubes on each side of the pelvis and note if there are any lumps or unusual tenderness on them or in surrounding areas which might indicate abnormal growths, cancer, or infection. Locating the ovaries is generally the most difficult part of the examination for both the clinician and for the woman being examined. Not only can the ovaries be tricky to find (especially after menopause, when they usually shrink), but also they are more sensitive to pressure than the uterus. Sometimes the only way for a clinician to locate them definitively is to press to the point of discomfort. If a woman feels tenderness or pain, she should mention this to the clinician to see if it is abnormal.

The rectovaginal examination. In the rectovaginal examination the clinician inserts one gloved finger into the vagina and another gloved finger into the rectum. The purpose is to assess the pelvic organs from another angle as well as to make sure that the wall separating the vagina from the rectum is free from disease.

Sometimes the rectovaginal examination may be followed by a rectal examination (especially in women over 40). Here the clinician inserts a finger into the rectum to check for polyps and other abnormal growths, hemorrhoids, or blood. A woman who thinks or knows she has internal hemorrhoids, however, should mention this to the clinician, as it may help explain any blood detected in a stool test.

Although some women are repelled or embarrassed by the very idea of a rectovaginal or rectal examination, and many find it uncomfortable or awkward, the procedure is rarely painful. As with the other parts of the pelvic examination, relaxing the muscles can help alleviate discomfort. Some women find that bearing down a bit is helpful.

Related entries

Birth control, cervical cancer, colon and rectal cancer, cystocele/urethrocele/rectocele, diaphragms and cervical caps, diethylstilbestrol (DES), hemorrhoids, intrauterine devices, menopause, oral contraceptives, Pap test, physical examinations, prolapsed uterus, retroverted uterus, sexually

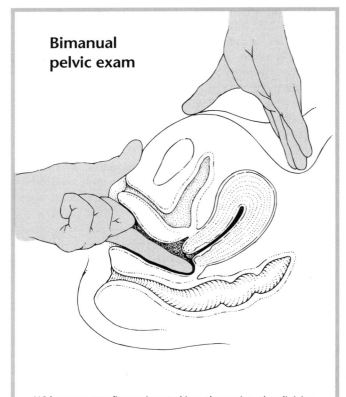

Bimanual pelvic exam

With one or two fingers inserted into the vagina, the clinician presses down on the abdomen to assess the size, shape, firmness, and position of the uterus. By moving the upper hand into various positions and pressing with the fingers in the vagina, the clinician can also assess the ovaries and fallopian tubes.

transmitted diseases, urinary tract infections, uterine fibroids, vaginal atrophy, vaginitis, vulvar disorders

Pelvic Inflammatory Disease

Pelvic inflammatory disease can affect the uterus, the fallopian tubes, or the ovaries. It is caused by bacteria, most often those responsible for sexually transmitted diseases (STDs) such as gonorrhea and chlamydia. More rarely, PID is acquired through other bacteria that travel up through the vagina and cervix via an intrauterine device (IUD) or an endometrial biopsy, or during miscarriage, abortion, or childbirth. Nearly a million American women develop PID every year. Countless others probably have the condition but are never diagnosed.

PID can lead to pelvic adhesions—scar tissue that develops between internal organs and often causes persistent pelvic pain. Without treatment, PID can lead to infertility when scars seal off the entrance to the fallopian tubes, making it difficult for eggs to enter, or distort the shape of the tubes, making it difficult for the egg to travel down toward the uterus. More than 1 of 5 women who acquire PID through an STD will eventually become infertile.

Distorted or partially blocked tubes associated with PID also increase the likelihood of an ectopic pregnancy, a sometimes life-threatening condition that occurs when the fertilized egg implants in the tube itself rather than in the uterus. Untreated PID can lead to chronic infection, which further increases the risks of infertility and ectopic pregnancy.

Sometimes PID produces a painful collection of pus (an abscess) on the uterus, ovaries, or fallopian tubes. In the rare cases when PID is not diagnosed early enough, this abscess may rupture, sometimes producing a life-threatening condition called peritonitis, in which the infection spreads throughout the pelvic and abdominal regions. In very rare cases blood poisoning (septicemia) may occur if the bacteria invade the bloodstream.

Who is likely to develop PID?

Although any woman can develop PID, sexually active women between the ages of 20 and 31 are most likely to acquire it through sexually transmitted bacteria. The infertility and ectopic pregnancy that eventually result from PID are seen most often in women aged 25 to 35. All sexually transmitted diseases are most common in young, poor city dwellers.

What are the symptoms?

PID sometimes remains undiagnosed because symptoms are mild enough to go unnoticed. Usually, however, PID causes diffuse pain and tenderness in the lower abdomen. If there is an abscess in one fallopian tube, the pain may be more severe on one side. There may also be increased, foul-smelling vaginal discharge and, in severe cases, fever, chills, and even nausea and vomiting. Some women experience pain during sexual intercourse.

Women with chronic PID may have a low-grade fever that lasts for months. Some notice no other symptoms, but others have persistent abdominal pain, backache, fatigue, heavy or irregular menstrual periods, and severe menstrual cramps.

How is the condition evaluated?

A woman who suspects that she may have PID should see her health care provider for a physical examination and laboratory tests. The practitioner will feel the woman's pelvic and abdominal area for tenderness and possible masses. Samples taken from the vagina and cervix will be sent to a laboratory for analysis to see if any sexually transmitted microorganisms are present. A blood test may be performed to check for an increased white blood cell count (which indicates the presence of an infection).

PID must also be distinguished from other causes of acute pelvic pain, which can include ectopic pregnancy, miscarriage, appendicitis, ovarian cysts, and urinary tract infections. Exploratory surgery may be necessary to eliminate some of these possibilities; this is usually done through lapa-

roscopy (see entry), in an ambulatory surgery or day surgery unit. An ultrasound examination can generally detect any suspected abscess.

How is pelvic inflammatory disease treated?

If there is evidence of gonorrhea or chlamydia, oral antibiotic treatment will be started immediately, usually before the results of the laboratory tests are ready. The woman's partner should be treated as well to prevent reinfection, even if there are no noticeable symptoms. Bed rest is a good idea until any fever has subsided, as is avoiding sexual intercourse or inserting any foreign objects (including tampons) into the vagina. Some women find that taking a hot bath several times a day or applying heat to the lower abdomen can relieve pain.

Severe infections may require hospitalization so that higher doses of antibiotics can be administered intravenously. If there is no improvement, or if symptoms worsen, surgery may be necessary. A conservative surgical procedure is to release some of the adhesions. More drastic measures involve removing infected organs—one or both tubes, uterus, and sometimes one or both ovaries—if the disease cannot be halted any other way.

Because antibiotic treatment cannot eliminate abscesses, these must be drained or removed through a surgical incision.

How is PID prevented?

Preventing PID involves keeping the causative bacteria out of the vagina. This is particularly important at times when the cervix is partially open, such as after childbirth, miscarriage, or an abortion. At such times sexual intercourse should be avoided until the cervix is fully closed, and foreign objects such as tampons should also be kept out of the vagina.

In addition, prevention of sexually transmitted disease is important. Although condoms, diaphragms, and spermicides may kill some bacteria, they alone are no guarantee against STDs. Any woman who suspects she may have been exposed to an STD should have a culture as soon as possible to allow early treatment. Women who use an IUD should be checked for symptoms of PID routinely.

Related entries

Abortion, adhesions, antibiotics, biopsy, birth control, chlamydia, condoms, ectopic pregnancy, gonorrhea, hysterectomy, infertility, infrequent periods, laparoscopy, menorrhagia, menstrual cramps, miscarriage, ovarian cysts, ovary removal, pain during sexual intercourse, pelvic pain, sexually transmitted diseases

Pelvic Pain

Pelvic pain is not clearly distinguished from lower abdominal pain. Many different problems can cause pain in this region of the body, particularly—in women—disorders having to do with the reproductive organs (see illustration). Quick identification of the cause is essential because some of these can have life-threatening complications. *Any sudden and severe pain in the lower abdomen or pelvis, especially if accompanied by nausea, vomiting, and rapid pulse, pallor, and faintness, should be considered a medical emergency.*

Pelvic pain is categorized as either acute, meaning that the pain is sudden and severe, or chronic, meaning that the pain persists for a long time (that is, for several months as opposed to several hours or several days). Reporting the timing, severity, and location of the pain, along with associated symptoms, can help the clinician distinguish one cause of the pain from another.

Below are described some of the more common causes of both acute and chronic pelvic pain in women, particularly disorders of the reproductive organs. Other serious conditions that may cause pain in this region of the body (such as appendicitis and bowel disorders) are described under abdominal pain.

Sources of acute pelvic pain

Ectopic pregnancy. Ectopic pregnancy occurs when a pregnancy grows outside the uterus. Warning signs of an ectopic pregnancy (see entry) in a woman of reproductive age include sharp or constant one-sided pain in the lower abdomen for more than a few hours with irregular bleeding or staining after a light or late menstrual period. Severe and steady pelvic pain may also signal a ruptured ectopic pregnancy, even if there is little or no bleeding. Because an ectopic pregnancy can be life-threatening, any woman who is pregnant (or thinks she could be pregnant) and who is experiencing pelvic pain should seek immediate medical attention.

Pelvic inflammatory disease. PID is an infection of the upper genital tract (the endometrium, or lining of the uterus, the fallopian tubes, and the ovaries). An invading organism produces inflammation, pus, and sometimes an abscess as the body tries to fight the infection. The pain from PID usually occurs in the lower abdomen on one or both sides, and can extend higher. If the abscess ruptures, a life-threatening

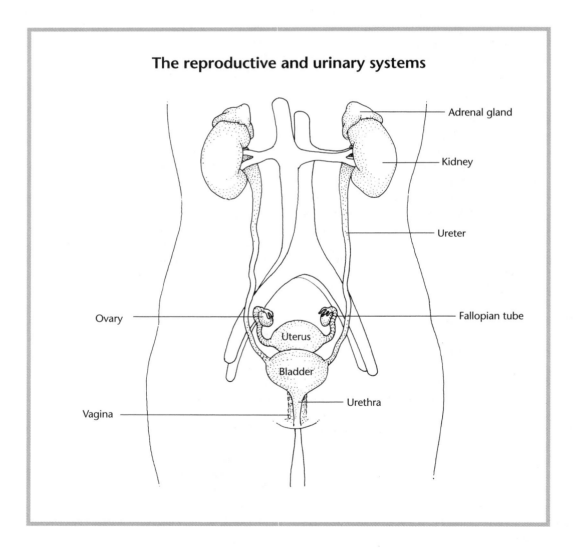

The reproductive and urinary systems

Adrenal gland

Kidney

Ureter

Ovary

Fallopian tube

Uterus

Bladder

Urethra

Vagina

condition called peritonitis may develop, in which the infection spreads throughout the pelvic and abdominal regions. In very rare cases blood poisoning (septicemia) may occur if the bacteria invade the bloodstream. Although PID itself usually causes only diffuse pain and tenderness in the lower abdomen and can go undetected for long periods of time, the pain tends to be much more severe if an abscess develops. Surgery and vigorous antibiotic therapy may be required to treat these conditions.

Twisted or ruptured ovarian cyst. Severe and steady pain with little or no bleeding may signal a ruptured ovarian cyst (see entry). An ovarian cyst is a fluid-filled growth on the ovary. If it twists, it can be extremely painful, and if it ruptures, fever, vomiting, and symptoms of shock may develop. Immediate medical attention is essential to remove the cyst. Extremely large ovarian cysts—or those that press on adjacent organs—can also cause pelvic pain.

Miscarriage or threatened miscarriage. Pelvic pain in any woman who might be pregnant can be due to an impending miscarriage (see entry). Pain may be either mild or severe but is usually in the middle of the pelvis and accompanied by bleeding from the vagina, sometimes preceded by a brownish discharge.

Cystitis. If bladder infection (cystitis) is causing pelvic pain, a burning sensation while urinating will be felt, as well as a need to urinate urgently and frequently. Sometimes a woman with cystitis may find blood in the urine as well (see urinary tract infections).

Sources of chronic pelvic pain

Pelvic pain that persists for weeks or months, whether intermittently or continuously, may be due to the same conditions that cause acute pain. Discussed below are additional sources of chronic pain which may be considered once the others have been ruled out.

Menstrual cramps. Many women experience crampy, spasmodic pelvic pain with each monthly menstrual period—a condition known as dysmenorrhea. Often this discomfort radiates to the hips, lower back, or thighs. Menstrual cramps (see entry) are sometimes accompanied by nausea, changes in bowel habits, and vomiting.

Endometriosis and adenomyosis. Both of these conditions occur when the tissue normally lining the uterus grows in other places. In contrast to the pain of menstrual cramps, which occurs during the first few days of a menstrual period, pain from either of these conditions generally begins a few days before menstruation and worsens as the period goes on. Sometimes women with endometriosis or adenomyosis (see entries) have particularly heavy menstrual flow as well.

Uterine fibroids. Uterine fibroids (see entry) are abnormal growths in, on, or within the uterine wall which can cause heavy or prolonged menstrual periods as well as chronic pelvic pain. Occasionally a fibroid may outgrow its blood supply, resulting in degeneration and acute pelvic pain. Many women with fibroids experience frequent urination and sometimes constipation.

Adhesions. Pelvic adhesions (scar tissue between the internal organs) can cause chronic pelvic pain that is intermittent or constant, sharp or dull. Some women may find that the pain occurs only with actions that put tension on the adhesions (see entry), such as intercourse, exercise, defecation, ovulation, or filling or emptying the bladder.

Endometrial polyps. Endometrial polyps are protrusions attached by a small stem which develop inside the uterine cavity (see polyps). In rare instances there may be pelvic pain and cramping if a very large polyp presses through the cervix (entry to the uterus). Some women with endometrial polyps also have unusually heavy menstrual periods or an abnormal vaginal discharge.

Cancers of the reproductive tract. In rare cases, chronic pelvic pain may be due to endometrial, ovarian, or vaginal cancer. Usually this occurs only in the later stages of the disease, when vague feelings of pelvic discomfort or fullness may result from the cancer pressing on adjacent organs.

How is pelvic pain evaluated?

A medical practitioner can usually distinguish the various causes of pelvic pain by asking the patient questions about her medical history and then conducting a physical examination and relevant laboratory tests. These tests often include blood tests, a pregnancy test, a urine test, a culture of cells from the cervix, and an ultrasound. Because pelvic pain can be caused by a variety of nongynecological conditions—including irritable bowel syndrome, kidney stones, and muscular pain—it is important for the clinician to consider these causes. Sometimes additional testing is performed if a nongynecological cause is suspected.

If the pain appears to arise from the reproductive system, and initial testing is unrevealing, exploratory surgery such as a laparoscopy may be necessary. Often when a diagnosis is made surgically—as with ectopic pregnancy, pelvic adhesions, or endometriosis—treatment can be performed at the same time.

If no physical disorder can be found, the pelvic pain may be diagnosed as a psychological defense or coping mechanism against some emotional trauma (see sexual abuse and incest, sexual assault, depression, domestic violence, posttraumatic stress disorder, psychosomatic disorders). Psychotherapy may help resolve some of these tensions; but if pelvic pain continues, a multidisciplinary approach may be more effective. In this approach a team of experts evaluates a woman's physical and psychological health and history and also considers environmental and nutritional factors that may be contributing to her pelvic pain. Over time, many women can often learn to adapt to their symptoms through a combination of counseling, drugs (such as nonsteroidal antiinflammatory drugs, antidepressants, or, if pain is cyclic, oral contraceptives), and relaxation techniques and exercises. Although such multidisciplinary teams are still not widely available, an individual clinician can approximate this approach by including psychological evaluation in initial assessments and referring the patient to physical therapists and nutritionists experienced in the treatment of chronic pelvic pain.

Occasionally hysterectomy (removal of the uterus, sometimes together with the ovaries and fallopian tubes) is used as a treatment for unexplained chronic pelvic pain. Nonetheless, between 5 and 20 percent of women who undergo the operation for this reason still have persistent pain more than a year after surgery. Thus, hysterectomy makes sense only after more conservative approaches have failed and after serious psychological disorders have been ruled out.

Related entries

Abdominal pain, adenomyosis, adhesions, antiinflammatory drugs, bowel disorders, depression, ectopic pregnancy, endometriosis, hysterectomy, laparoscopy, menstrual cramps, miscarriage, ovarian cysts, pelvic inflammatory disease, polyps, posttraumatic stress disorder, psychosomatic disorders, psychotherapy, sexual abuse and incest, sexual assault, urinary tract infections, uterine fibroids

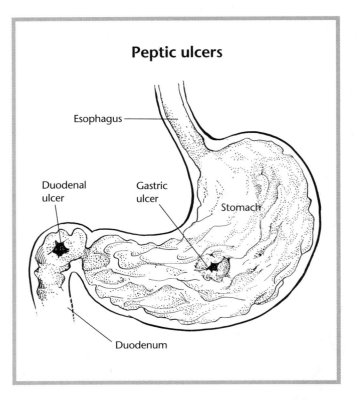

Peptic ulcers

Esophagus

Duodenal ulcer

Gastric ulcer

Stomach

Duodenum

Peptic Ulcer Disease

In peptic ulcer disease (PUD), holes (ulcers) develop in the inner lining of the esophagus, the stomach, or part of the small intestine closest to the stomach (the duodenum; see illustration). Digestive secretions that irritate the lining of the gastrointestinal tract have been considered the major culprit in PUD, but recent research has shown that a bacterial infection with an organism called *Helicobacter pylori* (see illustration) may set the stage for PUD in some cases.

Who is likely to develop PUD?

Older women with arthritis and others who take aspirin or nonsteroidal antiinflammatory drugs (NSAIDs) on a regular basis are particularly likely to develop peptic ulcers, as are women of all ages who smoke cigarettes and drink alcohol in excess. Caffeine may aggravate ulcers, and there is some evidence that a tendency to develop ulcers may be hereditary.

Among women who do shiftwork, peptic ulcers and other gastrointestinal disturbances such as gastritis (inflammation of the lining of the stomach) are common reactions to erratic schedules—changing frequently from a day shift to a night shift and back again. During a time shift, digestive juices are

secreted at the usual mealtimes, even when food is not present in the stomach. Without the neutralizing effect of food, digestive juices act against the stomach itself, causing damage to the lining that can lead to an ulcer.

What are the symptoms?

The primary symptom of PUD is a burning sensation in the upper middle abdomen. In the case of a duodenal ulcer, the pain usually occurs 1.5 to 3 hours after a meal and is relieved by eating. In the case of a stomach (or gastric) ulcer, the pain may become worse right after eating. The person with an ulcer may also develop other symptoms of indigestion, such as bloating, nausea, or vomiting.

If a blood vessel near the ulcer bursts, there can be bleeding. Usually the amount of blood loss will be slight and can be detected only in the stool. Sometimes, however, massive bleeding occurs, causing the patient to vomit blood, often in the form of small black particles. A bleeding ulcer is a medical emergency and requires immediate evaluation.

How is the condition evaluated?

The clinician will take a history that includes information about the timing, precise location, and nature of the pain and any associated symptoms. She or he will want to know, for example, whether eating, taking antacids, holding the breath, or sitting up make it better. The patient will be asked for details about her previous medical history, drugs being taken for other conditions, dietary habits (particularly use of alcohol and caffeine), smoking history, and work schedule.

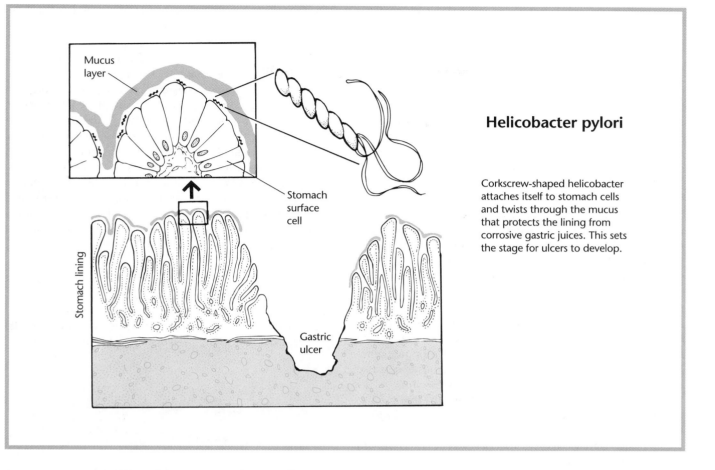

Mucus layer

Stomach surface cell

Stomach lining

Gastric ulcer

Helicobacter pylori

Corkscrew-shaped helicobacter attaches itself to stomach cells and twists through the mucus that protects the lining from corrosive gastric juices. This sets the stage for ulcers to develop.

A trial of antacid therapy or H_2 blockers (drugs that block the action of histamine on H_2 receptors in the gut, preventing acid secretion) may be started immediately, to strengthen the diagnosis as well as to treat the pain. A dramatic response is strong evidence of ulcers or gastritis. A series of x-rays, called an upper gastrointestinal (or GI) series, may be ordered, and an endoscopic examination may be performed. During endoscopy, a flexible fiberoptic tube is passed through the esophagus and into the stomach and duodenum to allow the physician to observe an ulcer directly. Using the endoscope, the physician may also perform a biopsy to check for helicobacteria. In other cases blood tests may be used in the diagnosis of bacterial infection.

How is peptic ulcer disease treated?

Bland diets including milk and excluding spicy or fatty foods were once the mainstay of ulcer therapy, but they are no longer believed to be particularly effective. Peptic ulcers and any accompanying gastritis can usually be treated with liquid antacids or H_2 blockers such as ranitidine (Zantac), cimetidine (Tagamet), or famotidine (Pepcid). Sometimes medications such as sucralfate (Carafate) or misoprostol (Cytotec) may also be given to protect the stomach lining.

If *Helicobacter pylori* infection is implicated, antibiotics may be prescribed. If there is massive bleeding, cautery may be

tried, and if that does not work, abdominal surgery may become necessary.

How can peptic ulcer disease be prevented?

Once an ulcer has healed, further damage may be prevented by avoiding aspirin and certain other antiinflammatory drugs, alcohol, caffeine, and cigarette smoking, all of which may promote acid secretion or otherwise irritate the lining of the gastrointestinal tract. Regularizing work schedules, if these seem to be a factor, may help prevent recurrence. In some cases clinicians recommend continuing the drugs used to treat an active ulcer, as a preventive measure.

High levels of stress (see entry) have been associated with a high level of peptic ulcers in some studies, although a firm cause-and-effect relationship has not been established. Because stress can lead to excess stomach acid secretion, can slow digestion, and, over time, can impair the immune system that fights off bacterial infections, it makes a certain amount of sense that stress may play some role in PUD. Women in stressful occupations or domestic situations who are also susceptible to peptic ulcers may want to think about ways to reduce their daily stress level.

Related entries

Abdominal pain, bowel disorders, chest pain, heartburn, occupational hazards, stress

Perimenopause

The term perimenopause has recently come into common parlance to describe the 5- to 10-year transitional state before menopause occurs. Technically, however, perimenopause also extends for a few years after the last menstrual cycle (*peri-* is the Greek word for "around" or "near"), a time when women may still have some vaginal bleeding due to occasional ovarian activity.

Experts by no means agree on just how long this period lasts, or when, precisely, it begins. In addition, considerable debate exists about whether this state deserves to have a name in its own right—or whether the state labeled "perimenopause" merely represents the first phase of the menopausal process (in which case it might be better called "the perimenopausal transition"). While the signs of approaching menopause rarely begin before women reach their 40s, perimenopausal symptoms—such as irregular periods—can begin as early as the mid-30s. That early age has led some cynics to conclude that giving this vague period its own status may merely be a means of extending the market for "perimenopause" and "menopause" products that previously appealed only to women who were in their late 40s or beyond.

Whatever the nomenclature, the fact remains that for 5 to 10 years before the cessation of monthly periods—as early as age 35—the body begins responding to various neuroendocrine and ovarian changes that will eventually result in menopause. Beginning in their mid- to late 30s, women often notice changes in their menstrual cycle such as shorter periods, irregular periods, shorter cycle length, heavy menstrual flow, or a combination of all of these that can differ from cycle to cycle. (Bleeding that is more frequent than every 21 days, lasts more than 8 days, or occurs between periods should be evaluated by a clinician.) As estrogen production declines, changes may be noticeable in body tissues that respond to this hormone, including the vagina, vulva, uterus, bladder, urethra, breasts, bones, heart, blood vessels, brain, skin, hair, and mucous membranes. The result may be vaginal atrophy (drying and thinning of tissues), a thickening waistline, accumulation of body fat around the abdomen, decreasing fertility, hot flashes (subjective feelings of warmth), and hot flushes (physiologically measurable changes in body temperature involving skin redness and sweating). Hot flashes and night sweats may also make sleeping difficult, which, in turn, can aggravate mood swings, feelings of depression, and general irritability. Depression and other mental changes may also be linked to falling estrogen levels, although the considerable research that has been conducted on this topic has thus far yielded contradictory findings.

Some women in the perimenopausal transition also notice a worsening in symptoms of premenstrual syndrome (PMS; see entry), while others may develop symptoms for the first time. Meanwhile, as estrogen declines, the bone loss that can precipitate osteoporosis (see entry) accelerates, and levels of blood fats, low-density lipoprotein (LDL) cholesterol, and triglycerides (all factors associated with an increased risk of coronary artery disease) may increase.

For most women, these gradual changes, if noticed at all, are only mildly uncomfortable. For more severe symptoms, however, various approaches can usually provide considerable relief. Oral contraceptives, for example, can help regulate menstrual periods and relieve hot flashes, vaginal dryness, and symptoms of PMS. As menopause itself approaches, estrogen replacement therapy (see entry) can help in similar ways, although individual women need to weigh risks and benefits in consultation with a clinician. Many women also find that lifestyle changes such as adopting a healthy diet, getting regular exercise, and practicing relaxation techniques (such as meditation) can minimize, if not alleviate, many of their symptoms as well.

Related entries

Cholesterol, coronary artery disease, depression, estrogen replacement therapy, infertility, menopause, menstrual cycle, menstrual cycle disorders, menstruation, osteoporosis, premenstrual syndrome, sleep disorders, vaginal atrophy

Personality Disorders

People who use certain kinds of inappropriate or maladaptive behaviors, emotions, and thoughts to cope with everyday life stresses are said to suffer from personality disorders. Although such thoughts and behaviors occur occasionally in almost everyone, they become inflexible and pervasive patterns in people with personality disorders. They are severe enough to keep a person from functioning effectively in either or both interpersonal or work settings, and yet people with personality disorders often think there is nothing wrong with them. The disorder may not cause dissatisfaction or unhappiness in the person who has the disorder, but it causes problems for the people with whom she lives or works. People with personality disorders are often at risk for other psychiatric disorders as well.

There is a great deal of controversy within the mental health and social science community about whether personality disorders are "illnesses" or just "coping styles." Considerable cultural and historical variation exists in what is defined as a personality disorder; a personality disorder may simply be a behavior that is maladaptive for the current cultural context.

Types of personality disorders

The American Psychiatric Association currently recognizes 10 separate personality disorders. These can be divided into 3 subgroups as follows:

- individuals who have odd or eccentric characteristics: paranoid, schizoid, and schizotypal;
- individuals who are overly dramatic or emotionally unstable: antisocial, borderline, histrionic, and narcissistic;
- individuals who have anxious and fearful characteristics: avoidant, dependent, and obsessive-compulsive.

Some people are diagnosed as having more than one of these disorders at the same time. Despite the name, the condition once designated as multiple personality disorder (see entry on dissociative identity disorder) is not a personality disorder as such but a separate category of psychiatric illness in which the person's identity is split between two or more alternating personalities.

Antisocial personality disorder. This disorder is marked by a disregard for the laws of society and for the rights of others. It occurs much more frequently in men than in women and peaks in prevalence between the ages of 24 and 44. It is particularly common in urban areas. Some psychiatrists believe that this disorder may develop in genetically predisposed people who grew up in emotionally deprived or inconsistent homes or whose parents exhibited antisocial behaviors.

People with antisocial personality disorder (popularly known as sociopaths) are typically irresponsible, amoral, and incapable of forming close relationships with others, although they are often outwardly witty and charming. They may violate the law, neglect duties to spouses or children, show financial irresponsibility, commit acts of physical aggression (such as domestic abuse), and act recklessly and impulsively. Typically they have a long history of lying, cheating, truancy, delinquency, vandalism, sexual promiscuity, homelessness, and substance abuse. People with antisocial personality disorder often abuse alcohol or attempt suicide, and they rarely feel guilt or loyalty. To them the world is a cold place to be exploited for personal gain.

Avoidant personality disorder. People with this disorder avoid people or situations that they think may result in failure or rejection. These people actually desire intimacy and success, but they are too preoccupied by worry and feelings of shyness and inadequacy to dare to attempt them. Some psychiatrists speculate that avoidant personality disorder may be caused by an inability to take criticism, a fear of losing control, or an exaggerated desire for acceptance. Sometimes people who have trouble facing or adapting to new situations eventually go on to develop avoidant personality disorder.

Borderline personality disorder. Three times more common in women than in men, this disorder is characterized by difficulties in regulating and tolerating negative emotions; unstable relationships, emotions, and self-image; and a fear of and intolerance for being alone. The result is often self-destructive behavior—including sexual promiscuity, substance and alcohol abuse, sadomasochistic relationships, and suicide attempts—as well as moodiness and feelings of emptiness and rage. Interpersonal relationships tend to be unstable and fluctuate between clinginess and withdrawal as the terror of being alone alternates with the terror of being dominated by another. People with this disorder often characterize others as either wholly good or wholly evil. They also commonly have coexisting forms of mental illness, including panic disorder, posttraumatic stress disorder, major depression, and somatization disorder (see psychosomatic disorders).

Borderline personality disorder is a highly suspect category for many feminist psychiatrists (see psychotherapy). According to their view, the diagnosis of borderline personality is often little more than a "sophisticated insult." Patients (usually women) who are diagnosed as having this disorder are often dismissed, suspected, or even frankly despised by caregivers. Behaviors that were once lumped together as hysteria are now frequently diagnosed as borderline personality disorder, multiple personality disorder, or somatization disorder, and all of them would be better understood, according to feminist psychiatrists, as variants of posttraumatic stress disorder (see entry). Indeed, borderline personality disorder is quite common in people who experienced childhood trauma, including incest and physical abuse. It is also more common in people with a family history of alcoholism. The earlier the onset of abuse and the greater its severity, the greater the chances of a person's developing borderline personality disorder later in life.

Dependent personality disorder. Also more common in women than in men, this disorder is diagnosed in people of normal intelligence who see themselves as helpless and inept, who avoid personal responsibility, and who rely on other people to make major decisions for them. Beset with a sense of their own inadequacy and a need for persistent acceptance, they may fear that expressing any aggressive or assertive impulses will result in unbearable rejection or criticism. Thus they typically subordinate their own needs to the needs of others, and as a result subtly bind others to them with guilt and indebtedness. Many people with this personality disorder also have problems with substance abuse, depression, and anxiety.

Dependent personality is a controversial disorder in feminist psychology circles because it is a depiction of extreme stereotypical femininity. From this perspective it simply represents a "pathologizing" of a cultural norm for women.

Histrionic personality disorder. People with histrionic personality disorder use extremely expressive, dramatic, and extroverted behaviors to attract and maintain the attention and appreciation of others. Perhaps because of inner insecurities about their worthiness of being loved or an unwillingness to recognize their own desires, these people are preoccupied with being the center of attention and attracting others. With their flamboyant or flirtatious clothing, intense or flighty speech, and exuberant mannerisms, they often exude superficiality and insincerity. Relationships with others are emotional but shallow and unsatisfying. Many people with histrionic personality disorder routinely attach sexual motivations to other people while denying any in themselves.

People who have relatives with a history of antisocial personality disorder or alcohol problems are particularly likely to develop this disorder. Women are much more likely than men to be diagnosed as having histrionic personality disorder. At least some of the explanation for this may be certain underlying cultural assumptions. Qualities such as "seductive," "emotional," and "charming," for example, are much more readily assigned to women in our society than to men. Some feminist critics have noted, too, that the sex of the clinician can have tremendous influence on these subjective judgments.

Narcissistic personality disorder. People with narcissistic personality disorder are characterized by an inflated sense of their own importance, uniqueness, and achievements. Typically, they are strikingly arrogant, carry a sense of entitlement, and constantly demand attention. Even trivial rejection is difficult for them and often results in either violent rage or deep shame. Regarding dependency as a sign of weakness, they generally have lasting relationships only when the other person is willing to reinforce their sense of superiority.

People with this disorder tend to lack empathy and have trouble seeing others as having both positive and negative qualities. Instead, they tend to rank others hierarchically, idealizing those they regard as superior to themselves and despising those they regard as less worthy. If they think someone else is more talented or powerful, they may become envious enough to resort to ruthless tactics, or else they may find a way to take credit for that person's achievements.

Obsessive-compulsive personality disorder. This disorder is sometimes called compulsive personality disorder, and is not the same thing as obsessive-compulsive anxiety disorder (see obsessive-compulsive disorder). People given this diagnosis (women somewhat more often than men) are preoccupied with control, rules, and orderliness. Rigid and inflexible, they are obstinate about not bending established patterns and generally fear new or intense situations or feelings (including interpersonal relationships) that may undermine their customary control. While often reliable and dependable, they can also be oddly ineffective—partly because they need to weigh all aspects of a problem before acting and partly because they are so preoccupied by details that they lose sight of larger goals. Also interfering with performance can be a sense of perfectionism, which makes it difficult to complete projects or delegate tasks to others for fear that they will not do a good enough job.

Typically people with this disorder are unjustifiably stingy with time and money, and often are workaholics, valuing productivity or possessions above other people. Find-

ing it difficult to express emotions, they seem cold and detached and can be excessively moralistic and judgmental about other people, for no apparent religious or ethical reasons.

Paranoid personality disorder. People with this disorder, which is more common in men than in women, tend to be suspicious and mistrustful of other people and frequently attribute hostile and malevolent motives to what others regard as neutral, trivial, or even kindly actions. Often this suspiciousness leads them to act aggressively, alienating other people and sometimes turning the suspicion into a self-fulfilling prophecy.

Nonetheless, people with paranoid personality disorder fail to recognize their own role in or responsibility for triggering the hostility of others and often develop a sense of righteous indignation. Apart from having problems with authority or with close interpersonal relationships, however, they are frequently conscientious and function relatively well. There is some evidence that paranoid personality disorder may be weakly linked genetically to schizophrenia and delusional disorders.

Schizoid personality disorder. The schizoid personality disorder, which is diagnosed more often in men than in women, is marked by a lifelong pattern of social isolation. People who are introverted and shy may be predisposed to this disorder, as may people who were ignored or neglected by their parents. Withdrawn, distant, and aloof, these people lack close friendships and generally seem to have little need for others. They often live by themselves and tend to favor solitary activities, especially those with theoretical or nonhuman—scientific, futuristic, or mechanical—subjects. Absorbed by their own daydreams and fantasies, they typically deny physical feelings and avoid close attachments, which they expect will be painful.

Despite the fact that many people with schizophrenia originally had schizoid personality disorder, the vast majority of people with this personality disorder never develop full-blown schizophrenia.

Schizotypal personality disorder. Schizotypal personality disorder—which can sometimes be hard to differentiate from schizoid or paranoid personality disorders—involves oddities of thinking, perception, and communication that suggest schizophrenia but are not severe enough to justify that diagnosis. For example, people with schizotypal personality disorder may have unorganized or superstitious thoughts, speak metaphorically or digressively, or be unjustifiably suspicious of other people. Work-related problems are common, as is social isolation.

There is some evidence that, for both genetic and environmental reasons, schizotypal personality disorder may be more common in people with relatives who are schizophrenic.

What causes personality disorders?

Many psychiatrists believe that personality disorders can be traced to childhood experiences, particularly in people with an inborn vulnerability to them. Many of the personality disorders most common in women in particular have been linked to childhood trauma, including sexual abuse, physical abuse, or both. Nevertheless, it is not uncommon for women to be diagnosed for years as having one or another personality disorder when in fact they are actually suffering from posttraumatic stress disorder.

In some susceptible women stressful issues that arise during pregnancy can serve as triggers for personality disorders. These issues include difficulty assuming adult roles, mixed feelings toward the fetus and toward motherhood, the resurgence of unresolved conflicts from childhood (such as differentiating the self from the mother), and changes in body image. Yet pregnancy can sometimes appear to be a solution to unresolved problems and therefore offers a reprieve—though temporary—from preexisting personality disorders.

Who is likely to develop a personality disorder?

It has been estimated that 15 percent of people in the general population have some form of personality disorder, and the rates seem to be higher among people from lower socioeconomic classes. These estimates are questionable, however, since they were based on idiosyncratic or outdated systems of diagnoses. In addition, some social scientists speculate that the rates are higher because people of lower socioeconomic class may be viewed differently by middle-class practitioners than middle- or upper-class people. Some of this problem will eventually be remedied as psychiatrists increasingly rely on the criteria for the 10 distinct categories of disorders established by the American Psychiatric Association.

How are these conditions evaluated?

Psychiatrists have traditionally been somewhat ambivalent about the personality disorders, partly because so many of them stood on rather shaky scientific ground. Even as better evidence accumulates, the existing categories are by no means etched in stone. Physicians and scientists as far back as Hippocrates in ancient Greece (who described "the four temperaments") have been trying to categorize human personality types, and today's psychiatrists are quick to admit that the current system is far from perfect. Although the personality disorder categories can be useful tools in differentiating one problem from another, they will continue to shift as we learn more about human attitudes and behaviors—and as we recognize some of the cultural biases that underlie our categories.

Masochistic personality disorder is a case in point. The subject of heated debate in the mid-1980s, this disorder was originally formulated to describe the personalities of women who were routinely abused by their partners. It ostensibly included people who kept returning to abusive or exploitative relationships that seemed to be avoidable.

Women's groups and feminist psychotherapists in particular strenuously opposed this category, arguing that it was simply a sophisticated way of blaming the victim. Citing new studies of victimization, they noted that it was the abuse itself that made victims passive, indecisive, cold, and self-loathing, and not some inherent personality flaw. Ultimately this disorder, renamed self-defeating personality disorder, was relegated to an appendix in the American Psychiatric Association's *Diagnostic and Statistical Manual*.

How are personality disorders treated?

Patients with personality disorders are notoriously difficult to work with—cantankerous, hostile, or resistant to help. Even more frustrating is the fact that, until recently, most psychiatrists have viewed treatment (which generally involves psychotherapy, sometimes supplemented with drugs) as a time-consuming and often futile undertaking. But, as progress continues in developing better definitions and providing scientific grounding for their validity, psychiatrists are becoming more optimistic about their ability to treat people with these disorders, often with long-term relational psychotherapy.

Related entries

Alcohol, anxiety disorders, body image, depression, dissociative identity disorder, domestic abuse, obsessive-compulsive disorder, panic disorder, phobias, posttraumatic stress disorder, psychosomatic disorders, psychotherapy, schizophrenia, sexual abuse and incest, substance abuse

Pesticides and Organic Foods

The possibility that pesticides and other toxic chemicals may be contaminating our nation's food supply is of particular concern to women. Not only have these substances been implicated in certain birth defects, but also some people fear that toxic chemicals may play a role in causing breast cancer and miscarriages as well. Television exposés about contaminated foods, reports of high cancer rates among certain farmers, and the emergence of organic produce in mainstream supermarkets all attest to a new caution about the food we eat, particularly produce. Many women now wonder how to balance these warning cries against the general admonition to eat 5 or more servings of fruits and vegetables a day in order to reduce the risk of cancer and heart disease.

To date, researchers understand very little about the extent to which pesticides damage human health. There is little doubt that many pesticides harm the environment by destroying valuable microorganisms that help protect the soil, but no one knows just how dangerous it is to eat the pesticide residues that remain on food after it has been washed or cooked. What we do know is that it is more healthful to eat fruits and vegetables with pesticide residues than not to eat fruits and vegetables at all (and that eating the amount of pesticide residues currently in our food supply is a lot less dangerous than smoking, eating too much fat, or drinking too much alcohol). But this knowledge has to be reconciled with evidence that pesticides do indeed cause cancer, damage the human nervous system, and affect reproduction in animals. It also has to be reconciled with the high rates of some cancers that occur in farm workers who work around pesticides and with the fact that pesticides can poison our drinking water, air, and soil.

What are the risks and benefits of pesticides in foods?

Currently most toxicologists do not believe that the levels of pesticides found in produce and meats present a significant risk to human health. Furthermore, the theoretical dangers posed by pesticides have to be weighed against their well-established utility—something all too easily forgotten. Synthetic pesticides have played an important role in ensuring an abundant and safe food supply in this country. In addition to increasing crop yields by reducing the incidence of contamination and infestation, pesticides have greatly reduced the number of food-borne illnesses caused by insects and molds. Without pesticides, fruits and vegetables would be far scarcer—and costlier—than they are today. The resulting decline in produce consumption would undoubtedly result in a rise in deficiency diseases—and probably the rates of certain cancers and other health problems—much greater than the level of potential (and at this point essentially theoretical) risks associated with pesticide residues.

Currently the Environmental Protection Agency (EPA) considers safe for human consumption one-hundredth of the largest dose of a toxic chemical that produces no adverse effects in laboratory animals, unless the chemical causes cancer. In the case of cancer, the safest dose is considered to be a level of intake expected to produce what the EPA calls "negligible risk," which is defined as no more than 1 case of cancer per 1 million people. When it comes to regulating agricultural pesticides, the EPA may use other standards. In particular, tolerance levels may be based not on toxicity studies but rather on the amount of a residue that might reach consumers after a farmer applies the highest dose needed to control pests. In most cases, however, if these levels exceed acceptable levels for human consumption, the pesticide will be banned or limited.

Numerous critics—including the prestigious National Academy of Sciences (NAS)—have called these standards into question. For one thing, the tolerance levels set by the EPA do not account for possible poisonous or cancer-causing breakdown products that pesticides may form during processing. Also, however safe the EPA limits are reputed to be, they do not explain the numerous studies linking pesticides to human disease. Several relatively small studies have shown that

women with breast cancer may have significantly higher levels of DDE (a by-product of the pesticide DDT) in their bloodstream than women without breast cancer. The evidence in these and other studies linking pesticides in food to human health is suggestive at best, but it does raise questions about safety.

Whatever the effects on the average adult, pesticides may have more serious repercussions for infants and young children, partly because of their relatively small body size and partly because their nervous, reproductive, and immune systems are still developing. According to the NAS, federal tolerance levels set for pesticide residues may be inadequate to protect infants, children, and fetuses.

The NAS and numerous other critics have questioned the process by which even the current tolerance levels are regulated. Theoretically at least, the tolerance levels are enforced through the efforts of two different federal agencies—the Food and Drug Administration (FDA), which checks levels of pesticide residues in produce shipped across state lines, and the U.S. Department of Agriculture (USDA), which checks residue levels in meat and poultry. According to government toxicologists, half of all fruits and vegetables shipped across state lines in the United States have no detectable levels of pesticide residues. They also report finding illegal residues in no more than 2 percent of domestically grown produce and no more than 4 percent of imported produce. And yet recent reports by the NAS and the Environmental Working Group (EWG) indicate that current testing methods used by the FDA are not sensitive enough to detect all the pesticide residues on produce. The FDA can—and sometimes does—use specific single-residue methods (SRMs) to screen for individual chemicals that may otherwise go undetected. But because growers are not required to tell the FDA which specific pesticides they use, SRMs are impractical when there are dozens of potential offending pesticides.

The solution to this problem is still uncertain. Some people have proposed requiring growers to report the specific pesticides used, or pumping more money into the regulatory system to help develop more sensitive means of detecting residues. Other experts believe that the only solution is a major overhaul of the regulatory system, including a reconsideration of tolerance levels which incorporates the potentially different amounts appropriate for children, the elderly, and pregnant women. Still other critics believe that energy would be better directed at modifying agricultural practices in the first place, banning the use of the most dangerous pesticides, and encouraging the growth and consumption of organic foods.

How can individual exposure to pesticides be minimized?

One step is to choose locally grown produce and meats whenever possible. These are less likely to have been sprayed with chemicals for preservation during shipment, whereas imported produce—which accounts for half of the American fruit and vegetable consumption during winter months—is often the worst offender. Not only are other countries less likely to enforce or monitor limits of pesticide residues, but also the FDA routinely inspects only a minuscule portion of imported shipments.

Women who are pregnant or trying to conceive should avoid eating fatty fish that may have been caught in polluted waters. Examples include striped bass, wild catfish, and bluefish, as well as salmon and trout from the Great Lakes.

No amount of washing or peeling can completely remove all pesticide residues, but the following steps may make a difference:

- Wash all produce well and rinse thoroughly. Immersing produce in a pot of water with a drop of mild dishwashing soap is more effective than using water alone.

- Scrub hard produce whose skin will be eaten (potatoes, carrots, sweet potatoes) with a vegetable brush.

- Chop produce that does not have a smooth surface (spinach, broccoli, cauliflower) before washing.

- Peel any fruit or vegetable with an obvious wax coating (cucumbers, apples, eggplants). Wax often seals in pesticides.

- Discard outer leaves of cabbage, iceberg lettuce, and other green, leafy vegetables. Trim leaves and tops of celery.

Are organic foods really safer?

Whether in the interest of health, nutrition, taste, or environmental protection, many Americans today seem willing to pay extra money for organic, ostensibly pesticide-free foods. Between 1990 and 1994, 3,000 additional certified organic farmers appeared in the United States. By 1994 organic foods accounted for $1.24 billion of sales per year, in contrast to $174 million in 1980.

Whether these foods are helping to prevent disease, however—or whether they are even tastier—is a matter of controversy. The most solid reason for eating organic foods—and supporting organic farming methods—is that reducing the use of pesticides could potentially help slow the depletion of valuable natural resources and the destruction of our environment. Advocates of organic farming maintain that reducing pesticide use by 50 percent or more could be accomplished without significantly affecting either crop yields or prices. Making these changes is not always so easy, however.

In addition to having to learn and incorporate new methods of farming into their lives, growers also face a number of institutional barriers that may decrease the motivation to change. For example, farmers would be ineligible for federal crop support programs, as well as for aid from some banks and insurance companies, if they stopped using pesticides. Some help is provided by integrated pest management (IPM), an alternative farming technique supported by the EPA, FDA, and USDA. IPM, which aims to reduce pesticide use by substituting helpful insects and crop rotation whenever possible, is already widely used in this country.

Beyond the issue of protecting the environment, however, the decision to eat organic foods is a matter of personal preference. If pesticide residues ultimately turn out to be a serious health hazard, then eating organic foods may indeed be the more healthful choice—but this remains to be established. As for nutrition, organic foods are no more likely to be nutritious than any other foods. A food's nutritive value is a product of many factors—including the quality of the soil it was grown in, weather conditions, the amount of fertilizer used, and shipping methods—but the use of pesticides is not one of these. As for taste, that is a matter of debate as well. Some people maintain that they can detect no flavor improvement whatsoever in organic foods or find the often blemished organic produce unappetizing. Advocates of organic eating regard these flaws as trivial or even as a sort of badge of honor.

There is also a question of just what "organic" means in the first place. This is because the very meaning of the term, as used in many markets today, is open to interpretation. "Organic" can mean that the food was grown without the use of any pesticides at all, or it can mean that the food was grown only with "natural" pesticides. In other cases it can mean that the food was grown with pesticides but has been found to be free of any pesticide residues. Other foods grown "organically" can still contain residues from soil contaminated with pesticides used years earlier or from pesticides used on neighboring farms.

The label "transitional organic" which appears on some produce grown in California means that the farmer claims to be using organic methods but that the produce has not yet been officially certified as organic. The label "integrated pest management" means that the farmer is using nonchemical methods of pest control, although sometimes in conjunction with the "judicious" use of pesticides. "No detected residues" means that independent inspection revealed minimal or no pesticide residues on the food, even if pesticides may have been used in the growing process. Finally, foods labeled "locally grown" may or may not have been grown organically, but they are less likely than imported foods to have been sprayed with preservatives or other chemicals. At present there are no federal standards differentiating one form of these "organic" foods from another, although some states and independent agencies offer their own certification programs.

Much of this problem should be resolved by the USDA's Organic Food Production Act. Under this law all foods labeled organic and shipped across state lines must be grown on farms that have followed organic practices for at least 3 years.

For the person who wishes to purchase only organically grown food, the best bet is to buy only foods labeled "certified organic." This label at least ensures that the food was inspected by a state or independent consumer group and met their standards—and eventually it will mean that the food meets federal standards as well. Another possibility is to shop at one of the retailers that claim to label foods organic only if they are purchased from a certified organic farm.

Related entries

Breast cancer, miscarriage, nutrition

Phobias

A phobia is an irrational, persistent fear and avoidance of an object, an image, or a situation. It is usually considered an anxiety-related disorder and often occurs as part of a panic attack. A phobia differs from free-floating anxiety in that it is focused on a specific object or circumstance such as cats, spiders, crowds, airplane travel, or confinement.

Many of the things feared by people with phobias do have genuinely dangerous aspects, but the odds of being harmed by them are extremely small. People with phobias fear these relatively harmless things to such an extent that they are compelled to avoid them or avoid even thinking about them—even though they are often able to admit that this compulsion is irrational. The need to avoid the object or circumstance of fear is often incapacitating and undermines the person's ability to lead a normal life.

Types of phobias

Phobias are generally divided into three basic types: phobias of situation, simple phobias, and social phobias.

Phobias of situation. These phobias are the most common of the three types. They involve specific circumstances that evoke anxiety. Among the better-known examples are a fear of enclosed spaces (claustrophobia) or a fear of heights (acrophobia). By far the most common phobia—and one that occurs in women 85 percent of the time—is fear of open places (agoraphobia).

Many episodes of agoraphobia begin when a person experiences a panic attack in public and subsequently avoids leaving home in order to prevent this unpleasant event from recurring. People with agoraphobia often spend years unable to venture into grocery stores, public parks, movie theaters, shopping malls, buses and subways, or even long lines. In extreme cases they are afraid to leave the confines of their own home for any reason. Some agoraphobics do have "obligatory companions"—specific close friends or family members only in whose company they are able to travel about in relative comfort.

Simple phobias. This second type of phobia involves fear of a specific object such as an animal or a form of transportation (airplanes, for example). Some psychologists also consider fears of very specific situations such as darkness, enclosed spaces, or heights to be simple phobias rather than phobias of situation.

Simple phobias are not always incapacitating. If the fear is of something rarely encountered (such as snakes), it is possible to go through most of life without having to face the object of one's fear too frequently. Occasionally, however, a simple phobia can be quite disruptive—as in the case of someone with a fear of flying who must take frequent business trips.

Social phobias. The least common type of phobia, social phobias (also called phobias of function), is evoked by the presence of other people. People with social phobias are deeply afraid of embarrassing or humiliating themselves in public and therefore avoid social situations as much as possible. Among the more common social phobias are fear of blushing (erythrophobia), fear of eating in front of other people, fear of using public restrooms, and fear of speaking in public.

What causes phobias?

Psychologists hypothesize that phobias, like other types of anxiety disorders, arise as a sort of defense reaction against certain traumatic or unpleasant experiences in the past. According to one theory, a young person anxious about having forbidden or embarrassing drives may repress memories of these feelings and then unconsciously disconnect or displace them from the original stimulus. Later these feelings are transposed or projected onto some specific external object or mental image which becomes the object of the phobia. Eventually the phobic person learns (or her autonomic nervous system is conditioned to the fact) that avoiding that object or image allows her to escape the unpleasant feelings of anxiety.

In contrast to these phobic responses, anxiety and panic attacks are usually seen as more purely biochemical events that have no particular relation to a past psychological experience. But that is not the whole story since a great deal of overlap exists between phobias, anxiety, and panic attacks. It is clear that more work must be done before the ultimate origins of all of these disorders—as well as the exact relationship between them—is fully understood.

Who is likely to develop a phobia?

Although it is common for children to have transitory phobias (such as fear of the dark or fear of dogs), most long-term phobias begin in early adulthood. Agoraphobia, for example, usually begins between the ages of 18 and 35. In addition, as many as a third of all people with panic disorders eventually develop agoraphobia, and many also develop irrational fears of specific events or situations (such as crossing bridges) that they think may provoke a panic attack. Phobias of all types are more common in women than in men.

What are the symptoms?

Often the only symptom of a phobia is the phobia itself—that is, an intense, persistent, and irrational fear of some specific object or circumstance and a compelling need to avoid it. If forced to confront the frightening object or circumstance, the phobic person may experience classic physical symptoms of an anxiety attack such as trembling, nausea, vomiting, sweating, dizziness, and heart palpitations. Even the very thought of confronting the object of fear can be enough to provoke these symptoms.

Some people with phobias also have feelings of depersonalization, as well as periods of depression. The depression, however, is not considered a symptom of the phobia itself but rather is seen as a secondary reaction to the lowered self-esteem that people with phobias often feel when they are unable to overcome their fears.

Occasionally phobias can be hidden behind "counterphobias," in which a person immerses herself in whatever activity she most fears. Thus, it is not unusual for rock climbers to have a secret fear of heights or for musical soloists to have to battle incapacitating stage fright. When phobias are overcome temporarily, there is often a sense of inner victory, resulting in feelings of mild euphoria and enhanced self-esteem.

Phobias of all sorts usually occur on a fluctuating basis for many years, with periods of remission sometimes interspersed with periods of exacerbation. They rarely go away altogether on their own, especially if symptoms have lasted over a year.

How are these conditions evaluated?

A phobia is usually easily diagnosed from the symptoms by a psychologist or psychiatrist. It is rarely confused with other illnesses. Very infrequently a phobia may be a symptom of a more serious psychiatric disorder such as schizophrenia, in which case it is probably accompanied by other symptoms such as delusions or hallucinations.

How are phobias treated?

Phobias are most successfully treated with a combination of behavior therapy and drug therapy. In the past, the psychotherapy for phobias was premised on the belief that they represented an unconscious defense mechanism against old conflicts. Thus, psychodynamic therapy was often used to help the patient uncover and eventually control the original sources of the anxiety. Research has shown that behavior therapy, which is focused on facing the fears without much concern for their origins, is more effective. In the form of behavior therapy known as systematic desensitization, the phobic person is incrementally exposed to the dreaded stimulus while using various relaxation techniques (such as hypnosis) to combat accompanying anxiety. Negative thoughts associated with the avoided situations are also restructured to be more adaptive and realistic.

Often the success of behavior therapy is enhanced with the use of antianxiety or antidepressant medications. Tranquilizers, for example, can reduce the intensity of the fear, allowing desensitization therapy to be used more effectively.

Related entries

Antianxiety drugs, antidepressants, anxiety disorders, depression, panic disorder, psychotherapy, schizophrenia

Physical Examinations

Not too many years ago an annual physical examination was considered the keystone of good health care. Today many clinicians no longer think that such frequent visits are cost-effective for all people, particularly for healthy adults under the age of 40. Even so, most clinicians still recommend that healthy young people have a regular physical checkup at least every 5 years so that problems can be detected in early and still treatable stages. Regular examinations also give the clinician a baseline picture of what is healthy and normal for each particular patient, so that new signs of trouble can be spotted more readily.

Adolescent women, whose bodies and concerns are changing quickly, may need to have somewhat more frequent physical examinations, perhaps every 2 years or so, and every year if they are sexually active. After the age of 40, and certainly after the age of 50, most clinicians recommend having an annual checkup. And many women in their 20s and 30s need to have pelvic examinations, which are often included as part of a regular physical examination, generally once a year.

Nothing is wrong with seeing a doctor more frequently if either the patient or the doctor feels that this is desirable; it is just that there is no evidence that more frequent visits are cost-effective for the population as a whole. Of course, any woman who is having specific symptoms or has other health concerns should consult a clinician promptly, whatever her age.

Although some gynecologists now provide a modified physical examination—and certainly many younger women rely on their gynecologist as their only source of medical care—a thorough physical examination by an internist, family practitioner, or general practitioner at least every 5 years is prudent. Both internists and family practitioners are trained to do gynecological procedures and tests as well as a more general examination. Having a relationship with a primary care physician (who takes responsibility for the patient's overall health) is important for those unexpected times when problems unrelated to the reproductive tract arise—for example, sinus infections or chronic headaches. And many of today's managed care insurance policies require a consultation

---

A patient questionnaire

Name _____ Date _____

What special concerns do you have today?

Below is a list of some health problems that many women have. How much pain or discomfort or worry does each of them cause you?

Problem	A lot	Some	None at all
Headaches	_____	_____	_____
Chest pain	_____	_____	_____
Abdominal pain	_____	_____	_____
Pelvic pain	_____	_____	_____
Back pain	_____	_____	_____
Pain in joints or muscles	_____	_____	_____
Menstrual problems	_____	_____	_____
Hearing or vision problems	_____	_____	_____
Nervousness (stress, anxiety, depression)	_____	_____	_____
Abuse (emotional, physical, or sexual)	_____	_____	_____
Coughing or breathing problems	_____	_____	_____
Sleeping problems	_____	_____	_____
Sexual concerns	_____	_____	_____
Urine problems	_____	_____	_____
Bowel problems	_____	_____	_____
Skin problems	_____	_____	_____
Worried about yourself, children, family	_____	_____	_____
Tiredness	_____	_____	_____
Medicines	_____	_____	_____
Eating problems	_____	_____	_____
Weight	_____	_____	_____
Smoking, alcohol, drugs	_____	_____	_____

---

with a primary care physician before a specialist (such as a gynecologist) can be seen.

The physical exam should include time for the patient to ask the clinician questions or to mention observations that may have a bearing on her health (such as sensitive areas or situations that seem to affect her symptoms). Sometimes, to help this process along, the patient will be asked to fill out a questionnaire (see chart) which indicates any special areas of concern. (Some women may want to copy this form and fill it out at home, when they have more time to think carefully about the health issues they want to discuss.)

It is best for patients to be actively involved in their own health care and to work together with the clinician to make decisions about various alternatives. During a physical examination a clinician who takes this patient-participation approach will explain what is happening and why, take time to answer questions, and at all times show respect for the patient as a participant in her own health care.

How is a physical examination performed?

Before a physical examination begins, the clinician (or an assistant) will ask the patient to provide a complete personal and family medical history. Besides being asked to describe any current problems or the reason for the visit, the patient

The leading causes of death and illness in women at different ages

Leading causes of death

Ages 13 to 18	Ages 19 to 39	Ages 40 to 64	Ages 65 and older
Accidents	Accidents	Cancer	Heart disease
Cancer	Cancer (malignant neoplasm)	Heart disease	Cancer
Homicide	Heart disease	Stroke	Stroke
Suicide	Suicide	Accidents	Chronic lung disease
	Homicide	Chronic lung disease	Pneumonia and influenza
	HIV infection	Diabetes	Alzheimer's disease
	Stroke	Liver disease	Diabetes
	Diabetes	Suicide	Accidents
			Kidney disease

Leading causes of illness

Ages 13 to 18	Ages 19 to 39	Ages 40 to 64	Ages 65 and older
Nose, throat, and upper respiratory conditions	Nose, throat, and upper respiratory conditions	Nose, throat, and upper respiratory conditions	Nose, throat, and upper respiratory conditions
Infections	Injuries	Osteoporosis or arthritis	Osteoporosis or arthritis
Sexual abuse	Infections	High blood pressure	High blood pressure
Injuries	Urinary conditions	Orthopedic impairments	Urinary incontinence
Ear infections		Hearing and vision impairments	Heart disease
Digestive system conditions			Injuries
Urinary conditions			Hearing and vision impairments

Source: Centers for Disease Control

will also be asked about previous illness, hospitalizations, and surgeries, as well as about serious diseases of other close family members (particularly cancer, heart disease, hypertension, and diabetes). Women will be asked about previous gynecological problems, any history of abnormal Pap tests, and whether the patient or her mother ever used diethylstilbestrol (DES).

If they are in their reproductive years, women will be asked about their menstrual cycle (regularity, associated pain, heavy bleeding), any pregnancies (number of children, miscarriages, complications), and, if relevant, the kind of birth control they are currently using and have used in the past. The clinician will also want to know about any medications the patient may be using and certain lifestyle habits (such as the use of cigarettes, alcohol, and illegal substances) and about any allergies or adverse reactions she may have had to medications. A doctor or nurse may ask these questions verbally and write down the answers. Or, alternatively, the patient may be given a printed form with questions on which she is asked to circle or fill in the answers.

Individual clinicians may vary slightly in the way they conduct a complete physical examination, but any thorough exam has certain common elements. The clinician measures and records height, weight, heart rate, blood pressure, pulse, and temperature, and uses a stethoscope to listen to the heart and lungs. Eyes, ears, nose, throat, skin, and nails are inspected for abnormalities; the back is pressed to see if there is any kidney pain; and the abdomen is felt to see if there is any abnormal swelling of the spleen, liver, or other internal organs.

The clinician will feel the neck to see if there is any swelling in the lymph nodes or thyroid gland and will check for swollen lymph nodes in the groin and armpits. Reflexes are evaluated by tapping the leg just under the knee with a lightweight hammer. Often adolescents have their vision and hearing checked. People over the age of 40 may have a rectal exam. Skin will be checked for abnormal moles or other conditions.

A breast examination, as well as a pelvic examination and Pap test (see entries) are included in a regular physical examination, along with instruction about performing breast self-examination (see entry) at home. Depending on the woman's age (see chart), her sexual activity, and her symptoms, other laboratory tests may be ordered: blood or urine tests, mammograms, tests for sexually transmitted diseases, or stool tests for occult (hidden) blood (see screening).

The sex of the clinician seems to have an influence on whether or not some of these tests will be done. One recent study indicates that male internists, family practitioners, and general practitioners were significantly less likely than female clinicians to do regular Pap tests and mammograms as part of a routine physical examination. Gynecologists of both sexes, however, were equally likely to do these tests.

What happens after the examination?

After the examination is over, the clinician will explain any abnormal findings and offer the patient another opportunity to ask questions. Sometimes it will be necessary to schedule a second appointment for further evaluation of a problem.

If a definitive diagnosis is made, the patient should ask for more information about the condition, including printed literature. She should get clear information about ▸ how to care for herself, ▸ the various treatment options, ▸ the treatment plan she and her clinician agree to pursue, ▸ any necessary referrals to specialists, ▸ medications being prescribed, and ▸

when to schedule another appointment. The patient should make sure she understands ▸ how and when to take her medications (with food or without, reactions with other medications, ▸ what to do if a dose is skipped), ▸ and what the common side effects and adverse reactions may be.

Related entries

Blood tests, breast self-examination, diethylstilbestrol (DES), immunizations, mammography, Pap test, patients' rights, pelvic examinations, screening, urine tests

Platelet Disorders

Platelets are a type of blood cell responsible for clotting. In certain conditions the body uses up the platelets (thrombocytes) too quickly, and this leads to a shortage of platelets (thrombocytopenia).

Who is likely to develop a platelet disorder?

Women are about 3 times more likely than men to develop forms of thrombocytopenia called immune thrombocytopenic purpura (ITP) and thrombotic thrombocytopenia purpura (TTP). Any form of thrombocytopenia can pose special problems for pregnant women.

About 8 percent of healthy pregnant women seem to develop abnormally low platelet counts for reasons still poorly understood. Infants born to these women are at no increased risk for complications, and few of the mothers have any bleeding problems or other complications. Generally platelet counts return to normal after pregnancy. Younger pregnant women in particular are also at increased risk for essential thrombocytosis (ET), a condition involving abnormally high platelet levels which more commonly occurs in both men and women between the ages of 50 and 70.

What are the symptoms?

In ITP a woman may notice small red spots called petechiae that result from bleeding under the skin, as well as a rash called purpura composed of these red spots. Other symptoms can include easy or excessive bruising, frequent nosebleeds, and heavy bleeding during menstruation. In severe cases there may be bleeding into the brain and digestive tract. Some women have no symptoms, however, and may not realize that they have ITP until a complete blood count (CBC) is done for unrelated reasons. ITP usually occurs when the spleen and lymph tissue produce antibodies that prematurely destroy the body's own platelets. This autoimmune process may be caused by a broader systemic illness such as lupus, by the use of certain medications, by HIV infection (see acquired immune deficiency syndrome), or for unknown reasons.

Symptoms of TTP include nausea and vomiting owing to

the presence of toxic products of protein metabolism in the blood (uremia), fever, and fluctuating neurologic changes.

How are these conditions evaluated?

ITP is usually diagnosed from an abnormal blood count. In women with TTP, blood counts will show a breakdown of red blood cells in addition to severe thrombocytopenia. The cause is unknown.

Women with essential thrombocytosis, which appears to be life-threatening in about a quarter of cases, have an elevated platelet count, as well as hemorrhage (severe bleeding) or the formation of a blood clot (thrombus) that blocks a blood vessel. Because platelet counts can also rise as a normal response to iron deficiency, chronic inflammation, infection, and the removal of the spleen, these possibilities must be eliminated before ET can be diagnosed.

In pregnant women with ITP, maternal antibodies can cross the placenta and affect the fetus, and this can put the infant at risk for internal bleeding when it passes through the birth canal. The only way to estimate the risk is to measure the infant's platelet levels. This usually involves obtaining fetal blood through a scalp vein after the head has engaged in the pelvis. Another procedure called percutaneous umbilical blood sampling can be done earlier in pregnancy (after 18 weeks) but is associated with a higher complication rate and is still not available at many centers.

If a pregnant woman has a low platelet count, she should be checked for more serious conditions. About 15 to 50 percent of pregnant women with preeclampsia will have low platelet counts, while others may develop the HELLP syndrome (hemolysis, elevated liver enzymes, low platelets), which is characterized by malaise, pain in the upper right quarter of the abdomen, and nausea. Since many women with HELLP also have protein in their urine and high blood pressure, HELLP is probably a form of preeclampsia.

How are platelet disorders treated?

ITP sometimes disappears on its own or goes into temporary remission. It may also produce only minor symptoms that require no treatment. Usually, however, women with ITP will be treated for the underlying condition or switched from the drug that may be causing the platelet shortage. Removal of the spleen and taking corticosteroid drugs such as prednisone can also help increase platelet levels. Pregnant women with ITP may require cesarean section.

Women with TTP can expect to recover following infusions or exchanges of normal blood plasma.

Pregnant women with both HELLP and preeclampsia-associated thrombocytopenia often require prompt delivery of the baby and blood transfusions to reduce the risk of maternal or fetal death. If the mother's thrombocytopenia is mild and she has not experienced any bleeding problems, most physicians are willing to have her go ahead with a vaginal delivery under close observation.

Although there is no definitive treatment for ET, drugs that lower platelet levels may be prescribed, or the physician may choose to observe the patient carefully for signs of worsening.

Related entries

Autoimmune disorders, blood tests, circulatory disorders, preeclampsia

Polycystic Ovary Syndrome (PCOS)

Polycystic ovary syndrome, or PCOS, is a common and complex condition affecting 4 to 10 percent of all women of reproductive age. It was once defined as a condition in which the ovaries develop tiny cysts, often becoming enlarged. All women with PCOS have other features in common, however: all are premenopausal, and all have high levels of the virilizing hormone androgen (see entry on hyperandrogenism), which interfere with the normal release of eggs from the ovaries (ovulation). As a result, they often have symptoms associated with high levels of male hormones, including masculinization, irregular menstrual periods, and fertility problems. In addition, these symptoms cannot be explained by or attributed to any other conditions.

Although historically PCOS has been associated largely with cosmetic changes and infertility, recent studies are showing how the hormonal abnormalities associated with PCOS put women with this condition at increased risk for various long-term health consequences, including obesity, endometrial hyperplasia (overgrowth of the lining of the uterus) and cancer, and Type 2 diabetes. Some of these risks suggest that women with PCOS might also be at increased risk for cardiovascular disease, but data so far have been conflicting.

Who is likely to develop PCOS?

PCOS is a common hormonal disorder in women, affecting up to 10 percent of premenopausal women. Although its cause remains unclear, growing evidence suggests that it may have a genetic basis. Other evidence suggests that it may be related to defects of insulin sensitivity or insulin secretion, or other hormonal defects.

PCOS usually develops within a few years of the first menstrual period (menarche), but it can first manifest itself in mid-life as well. A significant portion of women with PCOS are also obese, although it is still not clear whether PCOS predisposes women to obesity or vice versa. Women of Mediterranean descent are also at unusually high risk.

Many women with PCOS, particularly those who are obese, also have impaired glucose tolerance or Type 2 diabetes. And many, both obese and non-obese, also have insulin resistance, a condition in which levels of the hormone insulin in the blood serum after fasting or after a meal are higher than expected for age and weight. Whether or not this is associated with cholesterol or triglyceride abnormalities is controversial. Some studies do suggest that younger and leaner patients with PCOS may have higher total cholesterol and triglyceride levels and lower HDL levels than other women of their age and weight. Some researchers believe that these metabolic abnormalities may be present in all women with abnormally high levels of androgen, not just women with PCOS.

What are the symptoms?

Because women with PCOS have abnormally high androgen levels, they often develop acne, deepening of the voice, male-pattern baldness, or excess body hair, as well as the larger waist-to-hip ratios characteristic of males. Between 10 and 38 percent of women with PCOS are obese. Because ovulation is abnormal, absent or irregular menstrual periods are common as well, and women may have difficulty conceiving. Heavy to frequent dysfunctional uterine bleeding is also common. Some women with PCOS have very few if any symptoms, however, and may only be diagnosed during a workup for infertility. In general, younger women are most likely to develop cosmetic symptoms such as excess body hair, male-pattern balding, and acne, while women in mid-life are more likely to experience weight problems, infertility, or menstrual disorders.

Other symptoms of PCOS may include a thickening or darkening of the folds of skin at the nape of the neck, armpits, knuckles, knees, and elbows (a condition known as acanthosis nigricans).

How is the condition evaluated?

The physician will first want to exclude other conditions that can cause similar symptoms to those of PCOS, including pregnancy, diabetes, and abnormalities of the adrenal, thyroid, or pituitary glands. To do so, the clinician will do a thorough history and physical examination, including a review of the timing of the onset of symptoms, other associated symptoms, medication history, and family history.

A thorough physical examination will follow, often including blood tests to determine hormone levels, and possibly including a urine test for signs of Cushing's syndrome (see entry) as well. Ultrasound may be used to identify any abnormalities of the ovaries—although having cysts on the ovaries can signal several other conditions in addition to PCOS and may also be present in as many as one-quarter of otherwise healthy women.

How is PCOS treated?

Recently an experimental drug, D-chiro-iunositol, that normalizes the body's use of insulin has shown promise as a treatment for PCOS. A study by researchers from Virginia Commonwealth University published in the *New England Journal of Medicine* showed that this drug, found naturally in fruits and vegetables, can restore normal ovulatory cycles and reverse hormonal imbalances and related symptoms of PCOS. Even so, until more studies can be done to determine the safety and efficacy of D-chiro-iunositol, women with PCOS will have to rely on the more traditional treatments, which generally aim at alleviating symptoms of the disease rather than its underlying cause. If excess hair growth, acne, or absent periods are a problem, for example, antiandrogen drugs such as spironolactone (a diuretic) or finasteride (Proscar, Propecia) may be prescribed. Women with hirsutism should consider cosmetic approaches (such as tweezing, bleaching, shaving, or electrolysis) as well, since it usually takes at least 6 months before these drugs begin to alleviate excess body hair.

Women of reproductive age who are taking antiandrogens should use an effective contraceptive because the drugs can cross the placenta and block the normal development of a male fetus. Often oral contraceptives are recommended in conjunction with antiandrogens because they regulate menstruation and further reduce androgen levels, as well as provide excellent contraception. Women with irregular menstrual periods and few cosmetic symptoms (such as hirsutism and acne) may prefer cyclic progestin therapy (such as Provera) over daily oral contraceptives. Whatever the therapy, it is essential that menstrual bleeding occur regularly to prevent endometrial hyperplasia. Some women who have just been diagnosed as having PCOS may want to have a pelvic ultrasound to reassure them that the uterine lining has remained thin and is therefore unlikely to develop hyperplasia.

Some clinicians may also prescribe an insulin-lowering drug such as metformin (Glucophage) for women with PCOS to decrease insulin resistance and risk of diabetes. At present, however, this drug is not approved by the FDA for use in treating PCOS, and studies about its efficacy in treating PCOS remain equivocal.

Women with PCOS who want to become pregnant usually should see an endocrinologist or gynecologist. If they are not ovulating regularly, they may be prescribed clomiphene citrate (Clomid or Serophene), a fertility drug which induces ovulation. Effective in 4 out of 5 anovulatory women with PCOS, this drug slightly increases the chance of conceiving twins. Sometimes clomiphene may be combined with the diabetes drug metformin, which appears to increase the chances of conception even further. Infertile women will often need additional evaluation for other causes of infertility. If pregnancy occurs, women with PCOS will need to be monitored for signs of gestational diabetes, a condition for which they are at increased risk.

Another essential part of PCOS treatment involves taking steps to prevent, and monitor, health effects associated with excess levels of androgen. An initial evaluation will evaluate metabolic risk factors including body weight, blood pressure, and fasting lipid levels, and obese women with PCOS will be screened for impaired glucose tolerance and diabetes with a 2-hour glucose tolerance test. Women with irregular menstrual periods may be prescribed birth control pills or cyclic progestins to prevent endometrial hyperplasia, a thickening of the uterus that is sometimes a precancerous condition. In addition, they may be assessed for cardiovascular risk factors, including a family history of heart disease, high cholesterol in the blood, high blood pressure, and a history of smoking. And because many women with PCOS (and other forms of hyperandrogenism) are resistant to insulin, a doctor may also want to perform a blood test to look for early diabetes, particularly if a woman is obese or has other cardiovascular risk factors. Women with PCOS may also try to reduce risk factors for coronary artery disease by making dietary changes and/or embarking on an exercise program to promote weight loss. Because obesity tends to intensify the hirsutism, menstrual irregularity, and insulin resistance, too, healthy eating and exercise habits are particularly important.

Related entries

Acne, amenorrhea, birth control, cholesterol, coronary artery disease, Cushing's syndrome, diabetes, dilatation and curettage, diuretics, endometrial hyperplasia, endometriosis, galactorrhea, hair loss, high blood pressure, hirsutism, hyperandrogenism, hyperprolactinemia, infertility, infrequent periods, menstrual cycle disorders, obesity, osteoporosis, ovarian cancer

Polymyalgia Rheumatica

Polymyalgia rheumatica is a connective tissue disorder of unknown origin that causes sore muscles and joints. It is about as common as rheumatoid arthritis. Although this disorder generally clears up by itself after a couple of years and is easily treatable, around 15 to 30 percent of people with polymyalgia rheumatica also have a more serious condition called temporal arteritis (see entry), which involves inflammation of the medium-sized arteries of the scalp and head.

Who is likely to develop polymyalgia rheumatica?

Polymyalgia rheumatica usually develops after the age of 50. It occurs much more frequently among whites than in other ethnic groups, and about twice as often in women as in men.

What are the symptoms?

Stiff and sore muscles, particularly in the neck, shoulders, lower back, hips, and thighs, are the primary symptoms. Many people with the disorder find that they are so stiff in the morning, it is difficult to get out of bed. Unlike the similar condition polymyositis, however, polymyalgia rheumatica involves no muscle atrophy or weakness. Other symptoms can include fever, lack of appetite (anorexia), weight loss, anemia, and apathy. These symptoms can either appear suddenly or develop gradually.

If temporal arteritis is present, other symptoms can include a tender scalp, headache, blurred vision, and jaw pain when chewing. If not treated quickly, temporal arteritis can lead to irreversible blindness. Any women over 50 who develops these symptoms should seek medical attention right away.

How is the condition evaluated?

Diagnosing this rheumatic disorder requires a history, physical examination, and occasionally a radiological examination of the affected joints as well as various blood tests to rule out other possible causes of the symptoms. These may include rheumatoid arthritis, osteoarthritis, and polymyositis (see entries). Lab tests sometimes include an examination of blood for evidence of anemia (hematocrit level), erythrocyte sedimentation rate or ESR (which is elevated in polymyalgia rheumatica), and rheumatoid factor (associated with rheumatoid arthritis). Sometimes an artery may be biopsied to see if temporal arteritis is present.

How is polymyalgia rheumatica treated?

If polymyalgia rheumatica is suspected, corticosteroid drugs—which are antiinflammatory drugs (see entry) derived from adrenal hormones—are usually given. Relief of symptoms within 24 to 36 hours of taking the medication generally confirms the diagnosis.

The most commonly prescribed corticosteroid for this condition is prednisone, which can be taken in tablet form. As soon as symptoms subside, the dose should be decreased. The clinician may also use the ESR to monitor the drug's effectiveness. Since long-term steroid treatment suppresses the adrenal glands, a woman should never stop taking steroids suddenly unless advised to do so by a doctor. Treatment should continue for as long as any symptoms persist, which, for some people, may be years. In the meantime, symptoms may be relieved by taking aspirin and other nonsteroidal antiinflammatory agents (NSAIDs).

If any temporal arteritis (see entry) is present, higher doses of prednisone should be prescribed for at least a month. Because of the potential for vision loss, an ophthalmologist (a doctor who specializes in disorders of the eye) may be consulted.

Related entries

Anemia, antiinflammatory drugs, autoimmune disorders, blood tests, osteoarthritis, polymyositis and dermatomyositis, rheumatoid arthritis, temporal arteritis

Polymyositis and Dermatomyositis

Polymyositis is a connective tissue disorder in which muscles become inflamed and weakened. When areas of skin become inflamed as well, it is called dermatomyositis. These conditions have no known cause, but there is some speculation that they may be due to autoimmune reactions in which the body produces antibodies against itself.

Although polymyositis and dermatomyositis sometimes disappear spontaneously after a few months, they can be life-threatening, particularly if internal organs are involved. If throat muscles are weakened, for example, swallowing can become difficult. Occasionally the lungs, intestine, or heart can be damaged. About 10 percent of adult women with polymyositis and dermatomyositis develop malignancies within a year of the diagnosis. The most common are breast cancers, but cancers of the ovary and stomach are associated with this disease as well.

Who is likely to develop dermatomyositis or polymyositis?

Both dermatomyositis and polymyositis can develop at any age, but there is a peak in the number of cases between ages 10 and 14 and another larger peak in adults over 50. There are about 7 cases per million people annually in the United States. Adult polymyositis affects women about twice as often as men. The sex ratio is equal for dermatomyositis.

What are the symptoms?

Symptoms of polymyositis and dermatomyositis can appear suddenly or develop over months or years. The most common symptoms are progressive weakness in hip, shoulder, neck, pelvic, or throat muscles; pain and swelling in the joints; and skin rashes on the forehead, neck, shoulders, chest, back, wrists, knuckles, knees, or ankles. The classic skin rash of dermatomyositis is a lilac (heliotrope) rash on the upper eyelids and face, as well as a shawl-like rash on the chest.

Muscle weakness may be severe enough to prevent climbing steps, rising from a sitting position, or even raising the head, and some people become wheelchair-bound. There may also be fever, weight loss, and difficulty swallowing. Raynaud's phenomenon—a condition in which fingers or toes turn color, often from white to blue, after emotional stress or exposure to cold—sometimes occurs, especially when other connective tissue disorders are present.

How are these conditions evaluated?

To diagnose polymyositis and dermatomyositis, a doctor must first differentiate them from other conditions with similar symptoms, including scleroderma, lupus, myasthenia gravis, and other autoimmune disorders (see entries). Usually the doctor will do a physical examination and take blood samples to test for various muscle enzymes, autoantibodies, and a protein called rheumatoid factor. Although these substances are not unique to dermatomyositis and polymyositis, they are often present in these conditions, and measuring them can help show the progress of therapy. Tissue samples of affected muscles or skin may be removed for microscopic examination.

Often muscle activity will be measured with a test called electromyography (EMG). In this test a thin needle with a wire attached is inserted into the muscle being studied. The other end of the wire is attached to a device that measures electrical currents and then records patterns of electrical activity onto a film. Electromyography can be done on an outpatient basis and usually takes about an hour, with time varying according to the number of muscles studied.

How are polymyositis and dermatomyositis treated?

Polymyositis and dermatomyositis are usually treated with prednisone (a corticosteroid), together with antacids and potassium supplements. Corticosteroids are modified forms of adrenal hormones which reduce inflammation (see antiinflammatory drugs). Occasionally they can cause muscle weakness themselves, in which case a doctor may substitute a drug that suppresses the immune system (such as methotrexate, cyclophosphamide, azathioprine, or intravenous immunoglobulin). Many clinicians may choose the immunosuppressive agent methotrexate to use in conjunction with corticosteroids or by itself early in the disease. Specific exercises (suggested by a physical therapist) may help to strengthen muscles.

If cancer develops, removing the malignancy sometimes eliminates muscle weakness in nearby areas. It is extremely important for women with polymyositis to have regular breast exams, mammograms, pelvic exams, and thorough physical checkups.

Related entries

Antiinflammatory drugs, autoimmune disorders, breast cancer, breast self-examination, lupus, myasthenia gravis, ovarian cancer, Raynaud's phenomenon, scleroderma

Polyps

A polyp is a commonly occurring protrusion attached to mucous membranes by a small stem. Polyps are usually soft and spongy and can occur either singly or in clusters. They are almost always noncancerous, and they can occur in many parts of the body (see colon and rectal cancer).

The two types of polyps unique to women are cervical polyps and endometrial polyps. Cervical polyps result from an overgrowth of normal tissue in the cervical canal (the entrance to the uterus) or uterus and usually protrude from the cervix into the vagina. Endometrial polyps (also called intrauterine polyps or uterine polyps) develop inside the uterine cavity from a local thickening of the normal uterine lining. Endometrial polyps sometimes extend through the cervix and may even protrude into the vagina (see illustration).

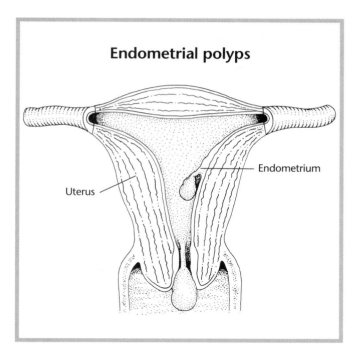

Endometrial polyps

Uterus

Endometrium

Who is likely to develop polyps?

Cervical polyps often occur after an injury to the cervix. During the healing process, new tissue sometimes becomes overgrown, resulting in polyps. Hormonal changes during pregnancy can also stimulate tissue overgrowth and polyp formation. But endometrial polyps are more commonly found in women at about the time of menopause.

What are the symptoms?

Both cervical and endometrial polyps often have no symptoms at all. Sometimes abnormal vaginal bleeding will occur, including bleeding or staining between periods, after intercourse, or after menopause. Occasionally there may be unusually heavy periods (menorrhagia) or a watery, bloody vaginal discharge. This discharge may be foul-smelling if a long endometrial polyp has become infected as a result of twisting or injury. There may also be cramping if a very large polyp pushes down through the cervical canal. Polyps that block the entrance to the cervix or interfere with cervical mucus production can sometimes cause infertility, but it is easily remediable by having the polyps removed.

How is this condition evaluated?

Cervical polyps and protruding endometrial polyps are usually easily detected during a pelvic examination. Many endometrial polyps, however, cannot be visualized unless a dilatation and curettage (D&C) or hysteroscopy is performed. These procedures also allow any polyps to be removed. Because the symptoms of both endometrial and cervical polyps resemble those of cervical cancer, a clinician will often do a Pap test or a biopsy of cervical tissue to rule out malignancy.

How are polyps treated?

Cervical polyps can be twisted or snipped off with a forceps under local anesthesia. This is a simple procedure that can be done either in a clinician's office or on an outpatient basis in a hospital or clinic. If polyps recur, a D&C may be necessary.

A hysteroscopy or D&C is usually required to remove endometrial polyps. Because additional polyps may be missed, it is sometimes necessary to repeat this procedure. If polyps recur or if abnormal vaginal bleeding persists, some doctors will recommend the removal of the uterus (hysterectomy). In premenopausal women hysterectomy is mainly a matter of convenience, to eliminate bothersome symptoms. Bleeding from polyps does not always resolve after menopause, however, and in postmenopausal women with recurrent bleeding, hysterectomy is recommended mainly because of concern about missing an underlying cancer. It is extremely rare for polyps themselves to go on to become cancerous, but the bleeding associated with them is hard to distinguish from bleeding that might be a symptom of an unrelated endometrial cancer.

Related entries

Biopsy, cervical cancer, dilatation and curettage, endometrial hyperplasia, hysterectomy, hysteroscopy, infertility, menopause, menorrhagia, Pap test, pelvic examinations, uterine fibroids, vaginal bleeding (abnormal)

Postpartum Issues

The postpartum period is often defined as the first 6 weeks after childbirth. At the end of 6 weeks a woman typically has a postpartum physical examination to make sure her body has recovered normally, after which she returns home to go on with the rest of her life as a mother. In reality, however, it takes many months or even longer (up to a year), depending on the individual woman, to work through all the physical, emotional, and social issues that arise after the birth of a baby.

Not all of these issues are problems, of course. The myth of the glowing new mother is not a complete fantasy: most mothers do experience intense and joyous feelings for their new babies, and many take pride in their ability to bear and nurture a child. Also, many women who have just had a baby feel a bond with other women for the first time in their lives or discover a new respect or love for their own mothers. For all the rewards of motherhood, however, having another person in the family almost always necessitates some changes in lifestyle, habits, and relationships. Though in the long run these changes are not necessarily for the worse, it is typical to experience some tension and turmoil until they are worked through.

Postpartum symptoms that should prompt a call to the doctor

Persistent or increasing perineal pain
Unusually heavy or foul-smelling vaginal discharge
Fever above 100.4° Fahrenheit
Hot, tender, or red breast
Nausea and vomiting
Painful, burning, or urgent urination
Pain or swelling in the legs
Chest pain or cough

The postpartum period can be a particularly vulnerable time for a woman's emotional and physical health. In the first weeks and months after birth, having sleep cycles interrupted, learning basic techniques of newborn care, and physically recovering from an arduous labor or a cesarean section (or both) virtually guarantee that no mother escapes fatigue. Breastfeeding, for all its virtues, makes additional demands on the mother's body and can contribute to fatigue, especially if she is not getting adequate nutrition and rest—which many new mothers are not. Even when the baby starts sleeping through the night and settles into a regular nap schedule (which may not happen for 6 months or more), taking care of the many needs of an infant or toddler continues to be physically draining. Women who already have one or more older children are likely to be even more exhausted: not only are opportunities to steal a nap few and far between, but also there are always more little people who need care.

The classic piece of postpartum advice—repeated again and again by doctors, nurse-midwives, health care manuals, and well-meaning relatives—counsels new mothers not to overlook their own needs. Nap when the baby naps, new mothers are told, let the housework go, accept all offers of help (casseroles, housecleaning, child care), eat nutritiously without worrying about recovering your figure for a while, get some exercise, take relaxing baths, and tend to your personal health. Although women preach to one another about the importance of these things, they rarely follow their own advice.

Instead, affluent moms sign their children up for baby gym but claim they have no time to join a postpartum exercise class. They spend half an hour cutting up cantaloupe and tofu for their toddlers but subsist themselves on potato chips and diet soda. They buy stimulating toys and puzzles for their kids but spend their own free time scrubbing the toilet bowl. They meticulously bring their infants to the pediatrician every 2 months for checkups but skip having their teeth cleaned because it is too time-consuming. Other mothers— less financially secure—are self-sacrificing because they have

little other choice: they have no safe and affordable child care, no adequate parental leave from work, no family health insurance. For new mothers in this situation, the postpartum period is particularly stressful.

Physical changes and discomforts

After delivery the changes that developed in the body over the previous 9 months rapidly begin to disappear. A postpartum examination (including a pelvic examination) should be scheduled for about 4 to 6 weeks after delivery (by which time all bleeding and any discomfort from an episiotomy should have stopped). Any woman who experiences unusual symptoms during the postpartum period should not wait for her scheduled checkup, however, but should arrange to see her clinician right away (see chart).

The postpartum checkup allows the clinician to make sure that the reproductive organs have returned to normal, and it gives the woman an opportunity to discuss any other physical, sexual, or emotional problems she may be having, as well as birth control or future childbearing plans.

Afterpains. The uterus, hard and round after delivery and protruding above the navel, will have shrunk back into the pelvis at the end of 6 weeks. The cervix closes even more quickly. In the first few days after delivery, many women (especially those having a second or subsequent baby) feel these changes in the form of afterpains—uterine contractions that resemble labor pains. These can occur spontaneously, as well as during breastfeeding, but usually subside after a couple of days.

Lochia. The lining of the uterus is shed over the 3 to 6 weeks after childbirth in the form of vaginal bleeding called lochia. Although it may start as bright red, heavy flow, sometimes containing small clots, it should gradually subside and change to a brown and then a creamy or yellow color. One sign that a mother is overexerting herself is a sudden increase in the flow, although this is normal after breastfeeding. Unusually heavy or foul-smelling discharge can signal an infection.

Normal menstrual periods generally return 7 to 9 weeks after delivery in women who are not breastfeeding, and may not reappear for months (or even until the baby is weaned) in nursing mothers. The absence of menstrual periods does not necessarily mean that the woman is not ovulating or cannot become pregnant, however. Women who do not wish to conceive right away therefore need to use some kind of birth control once they resume having sexual intercourse.

Breasts. For the first few days after delivery, the breasts secrete a thin yellowish fluid rich in antibodies called colostrum. It usually takes 3 to 5 days for the milk to come in, at which point the breasts may become painfully engorged. Frequent nursing, manually expressing or pumping, and warm compresses can help relieve engorgement in women who are breastfeeding. In women who choose not to breastfeed, engorgement will subside in several days. In the meantime it is often helpful to bind the breasts tightly, use pain relievers, decrease one's intake of fluids for a couple of days, and apply ice packs. Expressing milk from the breasts will only encourage additional engorgement.

Stitches, tearing, and hemorrhoids. Swelling in the perineal area (between the vagina and the anus) can be relieved with ice packs during the first day or so after delivery. After that, frequent warm sitz baths can help relieve hemorrhoids, tears in the perineum, or stitches from an episiotomy (a cut made by the clinician during delivery to prevent the perineum from tearing). Compresses of witch hazel (such as Tucks pads) can also provide relief. Hemorrhoids can be treated with over-the-counter sprays, ointments, or suppositories. It helps to avoid constipation by drinking plenty of juices and fluids and by eating high-fiber foods such as fresh fruits and vegetables, prunes, raisins, and whole grains.

Cesarean section. Women who have had a cesarean do not have to worry about perineal discomfort, but they do have the added burden of pain at the incision site—which will become noticeable as soon as the anesthesia wears off. Women having a second or subsequent cesarean often find that the pain is somewhat milder each time around. Pain relievers such as morphine or Demerol are usually given; the amounts that cross the placenta in breast milk are not thought to harm the newborn.

Another source of pain is intestinal gas—the result of a digestive system returning to normal. Some relief may come from walking, lying on the back or the left side, or drawing the knees up and breathing deeply. Otherwise, suppositories, an enema, or a tube inserted into the rectum may be used to help the gas to escape. Stitches or clips are usually removed 4 days after delivery (or resorb on their own). Until then, baths and showers should be avoided.

A woman who has had a cesarean section should be especially careful to get adequate rest, fluids, and nutrition during the postpartum period. A c-section is major abdominal surgery, and recovering from it imposes a serious drain on the body's resources. This drain is independent of—and added on to—the usual fatigue from a difficult labor, sleep interruptions, and the other stresses of caring for a newborn.

A breastfeeding mother should be especially careful to rest and eat well during the postpartum period if she has had a c-section, since her milk supply may be lowered somewhat by the stress of the surgery and recovery.

Fluid loss. The sudden withdrawal of estrogen leads many new mothers to drink, perspire, and urinate excessively, to have hot flashes or night sweats, or even vaginal dryness (especially during breastfeeding) similar to symptoms experienced during menopause. These disappear on their own after a few weeks. It is very important for new mothers to drink plenty of liquids (6 to 8 glasses per day), especially breastfeeding mothers and women who have had a cesarean.

Sleep and rest. In the weeks that follow delivery, getting enough rest is vital for a new mother's physical and emotional health. With prior planning (such as having a relative come to stay, allowing a spouse or friends to take on everyday household responsibilities or care for older children, availing oneself of hospital-provided home care, or, if budget allows, hiring outside help), it is possible for a new mother to focus her energy on her own health and the newborn's.

One advantage of a hospital birth is simply having some extra hands around so that the mother can rest as much as possible. As insurance companies continue to push for shorter and shorter hospital stays, however, this advantage is dwindling. Today women who give birth in a hospital will usually go home after 1 or 2 days (3 to 4 days after a cesarean section). This means that many women are now left on their own to take care of physical and emotional needs that were once monitored by the hospital staff.

Nutrition and exercise. Good nutrition and exercise are just as essential during the postpartum period as during pregnancy. Drinking extra fluids is important for all postpartum women, particularly those who are breastfeeding. Nursing mothers also need 500 to 1,000 calories a day more than they did before they became pregnant. Iron-rich foods are critical, since the rapid loss of blood volume during the first weeks after childbirth can increase the chances of developing anemia. New mothers should continue to take prenatal vitamins as long as they are breastfeeding.

Weight loss diets are never a good idea for the first couple of months after delivery, and women who are breastfeeding should avoid strict weight loss regimens until they have weaned their babies. The best way to restore muscle tone and regain pre-pregnancy shape is exercise. Women who have had an uncomplicated vaginal delivery can do gentle sit-up exercises beginning a couple of weeks after childbirth, followed gradually by leg lifts and pelvic tilts. Starting Kegel exercises soon after delivery can help restore slack pelvic floor muscles. Women can ask their clinicians to suggest appropriate exercises or sign up for a postpartum exercise class. Gentle exercises specifically for women who have undergone a cesarean section can begin within a day or two of surgery and can speed recovery.

Sex and family planning. Most clinicians recommend waiting until the postpartum examination (4 to 6 weeks) before resuming vaginal intercourse. In any case, a woman should wait until the lochia has stopped and the vagina and perineum have healed (usually 3 to 4 weeks). The desire for sex after childbirth varies greatly from one woman to the next: while some women find the whole childbearing experience sensual and feel aroused by their partners almost immediately after birth, others—plagued with perineal pain from tearing or stitches, the physical demands and presence of the baby, and, in many cases, a fervent desire to avoid becoming pregnant again while caring for an infant in diapers—have little interest in sex for many months. Ongoing fatigue and emotional tension commonly decrease sex drive in both parents. Lowered estrogen levels (particularly during breastfeeding) can dry out vaginal tissues, which makes intercourse physically painful for some women. Here a gentle and understanding partner can make a difference, as can the use of water-soluble vaginal lubricants. Alternatively, some couples temporarily choose other forms of sexual expression in lieu of intercourse.

Diaphragms need to be refitted, since size may change after childbirth. Women who do not want to become pregnant again immediately need to use birth control as soon as they resume having sexual intercourse. Breastfeeding (see entry) is not a reliable form of birth control. The long-term effects of birth control pills on breastfeeding babies have not yet been adequately studied, but combination pills can decrease the milk supply. Progesterone-only birth control pills do not decrease the milk supply and may be a good choice for contraception in breastfeeding mothers. For these reasons most clinicians recommend some other form of birth control prior to weaning.

Emotional adjustments

Adding a new person to a family and taking on the role of chief caregiver to that person can unleash a horde of unexpected and confusing feelings. In the first few days after delivery, inexplicable sadness and weepiness (the "baby blues") are as common as joy and exhilaration and are often attributed to the rapid readjustment of hormone levels. Some women develop postpartum psychiatric disorders (see entry) in the weeks and months after giving birth. These involve much more serious symptoms of depression and psychosis. But for most women, the emotional issues of new motherhood revolve around self-doubts, loss of a sense of identity, boredom, stress on relationships with other family members (particularly one's partner), and ambivalence or frustration around the question of returning to work.

Early fears and self-doubt. Much more common in the early weeks after childbirth are feelings of inadequacy, fear, or panic that come when a first-time mother realizes that she is responsible for all aspects of a new human life or suspects that she does not have natural maternal feelings. In traditional societies new mothers were helped in their unfamiliar role by older and more experienced caregivers or by some form of communal child-rearing arrangement. Today many women give birth hundreds or thousands of miles away from relatives, and few have the luxury of an accessible support system at their beck and call.

Today's mothers might take comfort in realizing that no human being is born knowing how to change a diaper, soothe the wails of colic, or give a bath to a slippery newborn.

These skills can all be learned and developed with practice, however.

Loss of self. Women having their first baby may also find it difficult to incorporate their new role as mother with their previous roles. For the first time in her life, a woman may find herself completely ignoring her personal needs (sleep, food, conversation) for those of another person—and doing this day after day after day. It is common to spend an entire day busily tending to the baby's needs, all the while feeling that nothing whatsoever has been accomplished. Tasks that used to be routine—reading the newspaper, taking a shower, cooking a meal—suddenly become the main activity of the day, if they are achievable at all. As career plans, jobs, and hobbies are submerged by the needs of the baby, a woman may lose a sense of her individuality and fear that she is becoming that generic thing, a mother. There are also many cultural pressures women confront about what "good" mothers are supposed to do. These pressures often entail the myth of total selflessness—devoting oneself completely to one's baby and ignoring one's own needs. These types of pressures may lead to feelings of guilt, inadequacy, and self-doubt on the part of many new mothers when they find that these ideals are impossible to live up to. Some of these feelings may eventually resolve, as the baby becomes more acclimated and the mother learns how to manage her time in new ways. In the meantime, sharing concerns with other new mothers can be beneficial.

Even the best, most organized mothers have occasional ambivalent or angry feelings toward their offspring because of the unceasing demands that come with motherhood. If a woman becomes seriously depressed or fears that she may harm herself or her infant, she needs to seek professional help as soon as possible.

Boredom. As the weeks go by, the mother who has tended the baby, cleaned the house from top to bottom, prepared the evening meal, and then finds herself with time to turn the mattresses may begin to notice that her initial fear and panic have been replaced by boredom. This is a problem especially for women who previously worked outside the home, but it can surface in any woman after the initial thrill of the new baby is gone. After the delivery truck stops arriving with gifts, and after friends stop popping in with casseroles, a new mother may begin to feel isolated from other adults. Accustomed to an outside job or regular social contact with peers, she may feel lonely spending all her time with a nonverbal little person whose needs are insatiable.

Many women find it helpful to join playgroups, where they can talk to other women in similar situations or, at the very least, express their feelings to close friends or relatives. If the budget allows, labor-saving tactics such as using disposable diapers or a diaper service, hiring an occasional babysitter, or paying for outside help with the housework can bring enormous relief. Sometimes it is possible to trade child care with friends or share the cost of a babysitter with a few other families.

Jealousy, distancing, and other problems with partners. If a woman for whatever reason has chosen to stay home and care for the baby while her partner works outside the home, she may find that her interests and her partner's are drifting apart. She may feel hurt when the father shows little reaction to her tales of the baby's bowel problems or their visit to the pediatrician, while she may find that his accounts of office politics have become trivial and irrelevant. At the same time, the father may find himself becoming jealous of his partner's sudden devotion to, passion for, and physical closeness with the newborn, while the mother may be jealous of his achievements, contacts, and rewards in the outside world.

Communication is the first step in handling these feelings. It is crucial that new parents express their concerns to each other and try to work out new patterns of living. Some couples find it helpful to discuss more gender-equal ways of sharing child care, at the very least dividing household chores or cooking differently than they did before a new family member entered the picture. It is also a good idea for the parents to get out alone together as adults (even just to take a walk) at least once a week. Finding a mature babysitter whom they trust and can call on for relief (without guilt) is one of the most important things new parents can do for their relationship during the postpartum period.

Managing older children. Although a woman having a second or subsequent baby may not find caring for a newborn particularly daunting (although it is amazing how quickly these skills can be forgotten) and will have adjusted already to her role as mother, she still faces her own set of challenges. Just trying to balance the needs of the baby with the needs of the rest of the family can be tiring and unnerving. Many mothers feel disloyal toward their older children for putting the baby's needs first—or, conversely, feel guilty for thinking that they can never love this anonymous new person as much as their engaging older child.

Just how these feelings work themselves out varies considerably, not only with the personalities involved but also with the spacing and ages of the children. A mother with a toddler at home, for example, may be torn between her older child's skinned knee and the newborn at her breast—especially if the older child's needs had previously been fulfilled on demand. The mother may also have to spend considerable time guarding the baby against the jealous overtures of an older sibling as well as managing the related regressions of the older child—who may lose skills just gained in toilet training, sleeping through the night, temper control, and the like.

Even if siblings are older and not overtly jealous of (or are even helpful with) the newborn, it may be harder for a household geared toward the older children's carpool, homework, and school schedule suddenly to have to accommodate a baby's nap, feeding, and early rising demands—or deal with the consequences when this sort of accommodation is impossible. And frequently older children, while not openly jealous of the baby, will reflect their feelings by fighting more with one another. This can occur, for example, when the younger of two older siblings, previously quite close to the older one, not only loses her place as baby of the family but also loses the undiminished affection of her big brother or sister.

Some of these problems can be minimized by preparing the older children for the new baby. For toddlers, this may involve reading them stories about other children with new siblings, bringing them along to obstetrician visits, and showing them pictures of themselves as newborns. Preschoolers and school-age children might benefit from attending one of the many older sibling courses offered by hospitals. Asking older children to help with the newborn—fetching or changing a diaper, holding the baby, or whatever is appropriate—can work wonders in subduing feelings of jealousy and rejection. Finally, having the father (or other relative) play an expanded role in family life can ease some of the mother's burden.

Work and child care. No blanket proclamations can be made about when (or if) a new mother should return to work. Physically, it is probably best for new mothers to stay home with the baby at least until the 6-week checkup—although some women bounce back to the daily routine within days of delivery. Depending on a woman's individual circumstances, her clinician may recommend a more extended period of time away from work. Of course, many women have no choice in this matter for financial reasons or because they do not have access to day care. Among women who do have a choice, some prefer to stay home for a few months so that they have a chance to savor this fleeting period with their newborn or so that they can finish breastfeeding before returning to work (although women can certainly continue to breastfeed while working outside the home, especially if they use supplemental formula or pump and freeze their own milk). Still other women may be able to make part-time, flextime, or job-sharing arrangements or may find ways to do part of their job at home.

Pregnant women should find out if they are eligible for maternity leave under the Family and Medical Leave Act (FMLA), which went into effect in August 1993. The act, which gave the United States the dubious distinction of being the last industrialized nation to provide family leave, gives workers of either sex the right to 12 weeks of unpaid leave in any calendar year to care for a new child or seriously ill family member, or to recover from personal illness. The employee is guaranteed her job and benefits back after the leave. One catch, however, is that employees are eligible for leave under this act only if their company has over 50 employees. The employee must also have worked for at least 1,250 hours in a single year at that company and can also be asked to cover the time away by giving up sick leave, personal days, and accumulated vacation days.

Needless to say, many people simply cannot afford to go 12 weeks without pay. Others fear that a request for leave may affect chances for promotion (or employment) somewhere down the line—which has been known to happen in spite of the law. This may be because, even though employers are theoretically required to provide eligibility criteria to their employees, very few employees or employers correctly understand their rights under this law, as shown in a study by 9 to 5 (the National Association of Working Women). To be fair, of course, many employers offer much more generous benefits than the bare minimum required by the FMLA, and it is worthwhile finding out just what they are well before the birth or adoption of a baby.

It is always a good idea to plan for child care before the baby is born. Not only should a working woman investigate the child care and maternity leave policies at her place of work (as well as actual experiences of co-workers), but also she should learn about other options for care, from live-in nannies and private babysitters to home day care and infant day care centers. Often arrangements for care must be made months in advance.

Even so, many women change their minds about work once the baby is born. An arrangement that looked good in the eighth month of pregnancy may take on a different aspect when the baby is suddenly a real person. The woman all set to return to work after 8 or 10 weeks' maternity leave may discover that she has fallen in love with her baby and cannot bear to tear herself away from the daily pleasures of mothering to go back to work. Other women, who vowed they would never leave their baby with a stranger, find themselves going crazy for lack of adult contact after only a month or two at home and may choose to look for a job or return to their former employment.

For all of these reasons, pregnant women and new mothers may want to keep their options about work and child care open whenever possible. Instead of quitting her job, a pregnant woman might try to arrange for an extended maternity leave; several months down the road, after the baby is born, she can then reassess her needs and make a more informed decision than she could have made earlier about either returning to work or resigning. This is why it is also a good idea for working women to make child care arrangements in advance of the birth, especially if high-quality infant care is scarce; a woman can always tell the day care provider later on that she has decided not to use the service. Finding good child care at the last minute is stressful at best and often impossible. Even the loss of a deposit later on may be worth the peace of mind that comes from planning in advance.

Related entries

Anemia, birth control, breastfeeding, cesarean section, childbirth, constipation, depression, dieting, estrogen, exercise, fatigue, hemorrhoids, Kegel exercises, laxatives, lubricants, mastitis, nutrition, pain during sexual intercourse, postpartum psychiatric disorders, stress

Postpartum Psychiatric Disorders

For women with a history of even mild emotional problems, pregnancy and childbirth can result in worsened or new psychiatric disorders, sometimes severe enough to endanger the woman's life or her baby's. The emotional and behavioral problems that arise after childbirth involve several distinct—though possibly overlapping—disorders, ranging from mild to severe.

The most common of these (and not really a disorder at all) is the so-called maternity (or baby) blues, which affects as many as 80 percent of all women soon after delivery. A separate disorder is postpartum nonpsychotic depression (also called postpartum neurotic depression, postnatal depression, or postpartum depression), which affects about 10 percent of women after delivery (there is some debate about prevalence because different researchers use different criteria to define this condition). Postpartum psychosis, a much rarer psychiatric disorder, is an often dangerous illness that carries a risk of infanticide and suicide and requires aggressive treatment in a hospital. Approximately 2 out of 1,000 new mothers (about 3,500 women each year in the United States) develop postpartum psychosis.

Less is known about other psychiatric disorders that may be linked to pregnancy or childbirth. Women who suffered from panic disorder before or during pregnancy may find that their symptoms worsen within the first 2 to 3 weeks after delivery. Similarly, women who were diagnosed as having obsessive-compulsive disorder before pregnancy may get worse both during pregnancy and in the months following delivery. Having a baby seems to induce this disorder in some women who have no previous history of mental illness.

Despite considerable effort, the cause and exact nature of all the postpartum psychiatric disorders remain unclear, although some researchers now suggest that they may have something to do with rapidly changing hormone levels. The lack of knowledge is partly due to a skepticism about the very existence of postpartum mental illness which has pervaded mainstream medicine for much of the last century. Even today the official position of the American Psychiatric Association (APA) is that postpartum psychiatric disorders are not distinct conditions but rather manifestations of standard psychiatric disorders (such as schizophrenia and manic depression) which happen to be brought on by the stresses of pregnancy, delivery, and child care.

For a decade or more, however, data have been accumulating which buttress what grassroots support groups maintain—and, indeed, what most doctors have believed since antiquity: that the timing and temporary nature of postpartum psychiatric disorders are not pure coincidence but rather an indication that these conditions require different treatment than do textbook cases of mental illness.

Who is likely to develop a postpartum psychiatric disorder?

Generally speaking, women in their childbearing years are particularly prone to depression and anxiety disorders, but just how these changes might be linked to menarche, the menstrual cycle, pregnancy, or menopause is still little understood. Until recently most investigators attributed the behavioral changes to social or psychological factors. Now it appears that these changes may ultimately stem from biochemical factors such as varying levels of hormones. This information has allowed researchers to begin identifying certain subgroups of women who may be more at risk of developing postpartum psychiatric problems than others.

So far it appears that the following factors put women at risk for some of these problems:

- a family history of depression, anxiety disorder, or alcohol abuse
- a personal history of mild depression or anxiety disorder (even if it was never brought to the attention of a health care professional)
- a history of postpartum depression
- a history of severe maternity blues
- a history of moderate to severe premenstrual mood changes

History of abuse of trauma

Stressful life situations—such as marital conflict, difficulties at work, concern about pregnancy complications, and physical or behavioral problems of the newborn—can increase the risk for women who, for whatever reason, are genetically or biologically vulnerable to postpartum psychiatric disorders. Another source of stress is a feeling of loss experienced by some new mothers—the loss of the woman's former life, roles, identity, and relationship with her partner. Some investigators think that postpartum depression which begins 4 or more months after delivery may be triggered by these "life event stressors"; depression that sets in earlier is less likely to be a reaction to these factors.

What are the symptoms?

Women with maternity blues have brief and self-limiting episodes of weeping, anxiety, mood changes, loss of appetite, and irritability. The blues begin 2 or 3 days after delivery and disappear within about 2 weeks. Although symptoms may occasionally continue for 4 or 5 weeks, some researchers suspect that women who have these longer-lasting blues may be prone to develop more severe psychiatric disorders in subsequent pregnancies.

Postpartum nonpsychotic depression may involve symptoms similar to maternity blues, but these generally begin at least a week or so after delivery. In fact, new mothers with this disorder may feel relatively well before symptoms begin, and some may not even develop symptoms for 6 to 8 weeks or even longer (there is still no consensus about whether depression that develops months after delivery should still be considered "postpartum"). Symptoms may last for over a year and may recur with subsequent pregnancies. Even though there is usually noticeable improvement from month to month, symptoms frequently flare up just before a menstrual period.

Common symptoms of postpartum depression are sleep disorders, panic attacks, poor concentration, and sometimes hostility or thoughts of suicide. Some new mothers have recurrent guilt feelings and blame themselves for being unhappy with motherhood, for not wanting to be left alone with the baby, for having fears about the baby's safety, for frequently calling the pediatrician, and even for their inability to be reassured. Sometimes there are physical symptoms as well, such as irregular menstrual periods, anemia, weakness, pallor, and gastrointestinal disorders.

Women with postpartum nonpsychotic depression have been known to harm themselves. This is a particular danger because so many people, including health care practitioners, assume that "the maternal instinct" guarantees that all mothers will protect themselves for the sake of the baby. In reality, many new mothers may be driven to desperate behavior because they feel insecure about their maternal abilities, especially if they have unrealistic expectations about what a good mother should be or do. This is particularly true of women from dysfunctional families. They may desperately want everything to be better for their newborn than it was for them but find such fantasies of perfection impossible to fulfill. A depressive disorder only fuels these feelings of failure.

Even more dangerous to both mother and child is postpartum psychosis, in which mothers actually lose touch with reality. This disease is often easily confused with the much milder maternity blues because for the first 48 hours after the baby's birth the only symptoms of psychosis are simple restlessness or insomnia, which hospital personnel and the new mothers themselves often chalk up to the excitement of having a new baby. Today, when the typical hospital stay for noncesarean births is 2 days or less, this means that the full-blown disease does not develop until after the woman goes home. Here she may still function normally most of the time or feel only slightly depressed; but she may suddenly experience periods of paranoia, confusion, disorientation, incoherence, irrationality, agitation, nightmares, delusions, delirium, hallucinations, or thoughts (and deeds) of harming herself or her infant. Appropriately treated, symptoms often disappear within 2 months, but there is a very high risk that the psychosis will recur after future pregnancies.

New mothers with obsessive-compulsive disorder may dwell obsessively on vivid thoughts of harming their babies—throwing them from a window, drowning them, or suffocating them. It is important to remember that thinking is still very different from doing, and, unlike women with postpartum psychosis, women with obsessive-compulsive disorder do not seem prone to act on their thoughts. Some may neglect their babies, however, perhaps in an attempt to keep from enacting their fantasies.

Women who suffered from panic disorder before pregnancy may find that their panic attacks increase or worsen after delivery. These attacks involve chest pain or tightness, tremulousness, sweating, palpitations, hyperventilation, tingling in hands and feet, numbness around the mouth, dizziness, feelings of unreality, a sense of being detached, a fear of losing control, or a sense of doom. The attacks generally begin within the first 2 or 3 weeks after delivery, often escalating to several attacks a day. This can lead to anxiety, inability to perform normal functions, and, sometimes, a depressive disorder.

How are these conditions evaluated?

More and more health care practitioners are beginning to look for risk factors as early as the first prenatal visit. Women found to be in a high-risk group may be given the name of a psychiatrist available to provide care after delivery if necessary. This is a lot easier than finding a psychiatrist later, when one is in the throes of a crisis.

As the pregnancy progresses, the health care practitioner may ask about any mood changes or swings, anxiety, irritability, tearfulness, and sleep difficulties. Some of these may be explained by the physical discomforts of pregnancy or frequent midnight trips to the bathroom during the first and third trimesters. If the patient's situation seems to warrant it, the obstetrician or midwife may recommend that the woman see a psychiatrist during the pregnancy, as these changes may be harbingers of a more severe depression or anxiety disorder.

Health care practitioners will also be on the lookout for signs of illness at the 6-week postpartum visit. A woman who has symptoms of these disorders should not let the practitioner focus only on physical recovery, nor should she be embarrassed to tell a doctor that things are "not that great."

Psychiatrists evaluating postpartum psychiatric disorders must first differentiate them from other psychiatric disorders such as manic depression which do not stem from pregnancy. In addition, they will do a test of thyroid function. This is because about 2 to 4 percent of women in the postpartum period develop hypothyroidism, the symptoms of which can resemble those of postpartum nonpsychotic depression. Women with depression will also be evaluated for the severity of symptoms and suicide risk.

How are postpartum psychiatric disorders treated?

Over the years, women with postpartum psychiatric disorders have gone from doctor to doctor looking for someone to give a name to their illness. If symptoms were particularly severe, they may have been diagnosed as having a chronic psychiatric condition requiring years of drugs, psychiatric care,

and sometimes institutionalization. In the past decade or so, however, various support and self-help groups have made it much easier for new mothers to find appropriate care and reassurance. These groups provide "warm lines" through which women can talk to fellow sufferers. They also recommend doctors who recognize that postpartum psychiatric disorders are temporary physiological illnesses related to pregnancy.

Reassurance and support are usually sufficient help for women with maternity blues. Often new mothers need the encouragement of others to give in to what they consider to be "selfish" needs. Many women feel they are "failures" as mothers if they accept help with meals, laundry, or errands, or if they let another family member give the baby a bottle so that they can get some sleep—vital to both mental and physical health. Hard as it is, new mothers must try putting these feelings aside and accept any and all offers of help during the vulnerable week or so after a birth (accepting, for example, that an occasional bottle is not detrimental to the breastfeeding relationship).

The more severe postpartum psychiatric disorders (depression, psychosis, obsessive-compulsive disorder, and panic disorders) are all treated not only with drugs and psychotherapy but also by taking precautions to promote the safety of both the mother and the baby. Depending on the specific symptoms, the psychiatrist may prescribe antidepressant, antianxiety, or antipsychotic medications. These are usually continued for at least a year and then tapered off to avoid relapse.

Selecting just the right drug or combination of drugs involves considering not only the health and safety of the mother but also the health, behavior, and development of the infant. Doses should be kept as low as possible to allow the mother to care for the baby. Nursing mothers should ask the doctor if there are any known ill effects of the drug on the baby. Because many of the drugs used to treat psychiatric disorders are considered unsafe for use during breastfeeding, it may be necessary to switch to bottle feeding. Women taking antidepressants should avoid taking birth control pills, since they can aggravate symptoms of depression. A woman who is being treated for depression and who wants to become pregnant should discuss her medications and plans with her clinician.

Despite frequent publicity and numerous studies, there is still no good evidence that progesterone suppositories have any effect on postpartum mental illness.

If drugs are ineffective in treating either depression or psychosis, electroconvulsive therapy is occasionally needed. Also helpful is psychotherapy for both the woman and her partner. Besides providing support and education, therapy can help open up communication between the couple at a time that is stressful for all parents of infants, even those who are not suffering from psychiatric disorders. Behavioral psychotherapy may be particularly helpful for women with postpartum panic disorders.

Ensuring the safety of mother and child is a vital part of treatment. When a woman with a serious postpartum psychiatric disorder cannot obtain supportive care at home, she may have to be hospitalized. One major drawback to this strategy is that most hospitals will not allow the baby to stay with the mother. This can actually hinder recovery by increasing the woman's guilt feelings and interfering with the mother-child relationship. For years the English (who have also been more ready to recognize postpartum psychiatric disorders as genuine and distinct conditions) have provided mother-baby units so that mothers can be treated without separation from their infants. A few pilot units are now being tried in various locations in the United States but are still not available to most women.

How can postpartum psychiatric disorders be prevented?

Lowering unrealistic expectations about postpartum experience is one way to reduce the risk of postpartum psychiatric disorders, especially the ones that are aggravated by life stresses. This can be done by reading about what to expect physically and psychologically, talking to other new mothers, and participating in childbirth education classes. New mothers should also strive to limit visitors, take frequent naps, and surround themselves with supportive friends and family.

Some researchers have hypothesized that giving estrogen to women just after delivery may stave off attacks of more severe psychiatric disorders, but this theory remains in the experimental stage.

Related entries

Antianxiety drugs, antidepressants, anxiety disorders, depression, manic-depressive disorder, menstrual cycle, obsessive-compulsive disorder, panic disorder, personality disorders, phobias, psychotherapy, stress

Posttraumatic Stress Disorder

Posttraumatic stress disorder is a mental illness that results after a trauma overwhelms normal biological and psychological defense mechanisms. It can develop in those who have experienced military combat, earthquakes, floods, fires, accidents, burns, abuse, kidnapping, torture, or concentration camps, and it is characterized by intense and alternating feelings of vulnerability and rage. The most common causes of posttraumatic stress disorder in women are sexual assault, incest, and domestic abuse. All of these traumatic events have the potential to "victimize" a person and produce a sense of helplessness, loss of control, and even the fear of annihilation.

Although psychiatrists and psychologists have been studying the psychological response to trauma for years, interest has waxed and waned depending on the contemporary polit-

ical climate. In the last two decades of the nineteenth century, Sigmund Freud, Pierre Janet, and Joseph Breuer linked symptoms of hysteria to psychological trauma. Freud's controversial finding that the specific traumatic experience was frequently sexual abuse and incest much earlier in life was dismissed by most of his colleagues, and eventually by Freud himself, since no one could accept that sexual trauma and violence against women were as prevalent as they turned out to be.

After World War I, interest in the "traumatic syndrome" was renewed when investigators began to notice that many veterans exhibited hysterical symptoms such as an inability to talk, see, feel, or move not caused by any physical injury. During World War II, some psychiatrists devised methods to help minimize this reaction to combat. It was only the efforts of disaffected veterans of the Vietnam War, however, that precipitated systematic large-scale studies of these symptoms and led to the American Psychiatric Association's recognition of posttraumatic stress disorder as a genuine psychiatric disorder.

Largely owing to members of the women's movement, who for over a decade had been documenting what they called the rape trauma syndrome and the battered woman syndrome, investigators after 1980 began to include in this category the responses to common but traumatic acts of violence against women.

Whatever the source of the traumatic stress, victims (or, as some prefer to call them, survivors) with posttraumatic stress disorder have an increased risk of developing major psychological problems such as depression, phobias, chronic pain syndrome, learning disorders, alterations in consciousness, memory changes, impaired concentration, sleep disturbances, and substance abuse. There is some evidence of immunological changes that reduce life expectancy, and people with posttraumatic stress disorder are at increased risk for committing suicide, homicide, child abuse, and incest.

The psychological symptoms of posttraumatic stress disorder, like those of many other mental illnesses, almost certainly have physiological roots (which, in turn, are brought on by environmental or social stresses). A growing body of evidence now suggests that the symptoms of posttraumatic stress disorder may be linked to an overactivity of certain neurotransmitters (substances that serve as messengers between nerve cells).

Who is likely to develop posttraumatic stress disorder?

Although posttraumatic stress disorder can develop in anyone—and may be almost inevitable after certain particularly traumatic experiences—it occurs most frequently in people who are psychologically or physiologically vulnerable, have suffered physical injury (especially to the head) during the trauma, or who lack social support systems. For this reason, children and the elderly are the most frequent victims. Children are particularly vulnerable because neither their physiological nor their psychological functions are fully developed and are therefore more likely to be permanently damaged.

What are the symptoms?

People with posttraumatic stress disorder tend to numb themselves to all thoughts, feelings, or actions that remind them of the traumatic event. Often they show signs of depression, losing interest in the world around them, taking no pleasure from previously enjoyable activities including sexual contact, and estranging or isolating themselves from family and friends. They have an overall sense of hopelessness about the future. Young children may regress from previous achievements such as talking or toilet training.

Part of this numbing reaction is the development of a "learned helplessness," in which the person becomes extremely passive and stops believing that she has any control over her own life. This can result in further social isolation or excessive clinginess to family, mental health professionals, or other caregivers. Often people also tend to dissociate themselves from, or become unconscious of, what is going on around them because they find associated emotions too hard to bear (see entry on dissociative identity disorder).

It is also common for people with this disorder to deny the trauma or to intellectualize it as something under control. Later they may relive the trauma in the form of hallucinations or flashbacks that can induce the same fear and lack of control as the original event. The survivor may actually believe that she is reexperiencing it.

Punctuating the "background" numbness of a person with this disorder is a state of hyperarousal in which survivors perpetually expect danger. They are frequently irritable, anxious, moody, and agitated and are easily startled by the slightest provocation. They may develop phobias to situations that remind them of the original traumatic event. Vivid nightmares distressing enough to produce insomnia are also common. Many survivors become fixated on the trauma and have intrusive recollections of their experience that disrupt daily functioning. The anniversary of the trauma can be particularly distressing, and survivors who outlived other people who died during the same trauma, or who believe they had to commit a morally unconscionable act to survive, may be haunted by "survivor guilt."

Violent outbursts of temper are common, especially in survivors who have not acknowledged their experience. Some evidence suggests, however, that male and female survivors of child abuse and incest may handle their anger in different ways. Whereas males tend to deal with their anger by becoming physically aggressive or abusive themselves, females tend to direct their anger inward, engaging in self-destructive behaviors. Rather than taking out their anger on other people, women are more likely to become depressed or purposely avoid intimacy with others.

All of these symptoms may appear within days of the traumatic event, or they may take many months to develop. Often mild symptoms or symptoms that appear early may resolve spontaneously within about 6 months as the person integrates the trauma into the totality of her life experiences instead of feeling that it is the sole defining event of her existence. Symptoms that develop more slowly, however, tend to become chronic or recurrent and can be extremely disabling.

Sometimes people with posttraumatic stress disorder may perform acts of self-mutilation or become trauma addicts, since physical stress can trigger the release of the body's built-in painkillers (which temporarily relieve their chronic pain). Many traumatized persons cope with their passivity, hyperarousal, fear, or chronic pain by resorting to chemicals, and often end up dependent on alcohol or other substances of abuse.

How is the condition evaluated?

Posttraumatic stress disorder includes symptoms of other mental illnesses: depression, anxiety, cognitive disorders, and phobias. But if these symptoms are linked to a specific traumatic event and are accompanied by numbing, hyperarousal, nightmares, fixation on the trauma, and violent outbursts of temper, a clinician will most likely diagnose the problem as posttraumatic stress disorder. To rule out a physical cause such as a brain injury, however, the clinician will perform a thorough neurological examination.

How is posttraumatic stress disorder treated?

The most prominent symptoms of posttraumatic stress disorder can be treated with behavioral modification techniques such as relaxation training or progressive desensitization (see panic disorder). Stress management techniques are particularly useful in helping people to overcome learned helplessness, social isolation, and depression and to increase their mastery of the environment.

In addition to behavioral techniques, cognitive psychotherapy can help the survivor come to see the trauma as just one part of a multifaceted life story. Once the survivor learns to feel safe, the psychotherapist can help her reconstruct the story of the trauma. This process of remembrance and mourning is based on the belief that symptoms can be alleviated by putting intense feelings and traumatic memories into words. With the support and encouragement of the psychotherapist, the survivor accepts that she has been a victim and acknowledges the effects of the victimization. Slowly, she decides to recover a sense of control over her own life and to restore connections with the rest of the community. By doing so, she eventually recreates the damaged psychological coping mechanisms and returns to ordinary life.

Some therapists recommend that their clients put themselves in positions of controlled risk, such as self-defense classes or wilderness trips. At this point group therapy with other people who have experienced similar trauma—for example, an incest survivors' or rape victims' support group—can be helpful. Some survivors eventually develop a sense of mission in which they want to turn their tragedy into something positive for the rest of the world. They may become active in rape crisis or domestic violence centers, for example, or become involved in some other kind of social action. It is important to remember, however, that survivors never completely transcend the impact of their experience and may find that their symptoms are reawakened during periods of stress, significant life-cycle events, or anniversaries of the trauma.

A relatively new and controversial therapy is EMDR (eye movement desensitization and reprocessing). This therapy involves stimulating the left and right hemispheres of the brain with eye movement, tapping, or auditory tones while traumatic memories are imagined.

Related entries

Anxiety disorders, depression, dissociative identity disorder, domestic abuse, insomnia, phobias, psychosomatic disorders, psychotherapy, sexual abuse and incest, sexual assault, sleep disorders, stress, substance abuse

Preconception Counseling

A baby's health can be determined by factors set in motion long before conception. For this reason, many couples today are seeking preconception counseling to discuss their pregnancy plans and to identify and minimize risks to future offspring. The counselor—who may be an internist, family physician, obstetrician, nurse-midwife, or genetic counselor—will emphasize what a couple can do before conception as well as during pregnancy to ensure the health of the baby. Preconception counseling should take place routinely during complete physical examinations for all women who are contemplating pregnancy.

What happens during preconception counseling?

During a preconception visit the counselor asks questions about the couple's medical and pregnancy history, lifestyle and personal habits, interpersonal relationship, and living and working conditions. The counselor will want to know if there is a family history of certain inherited conditions such as muscular dystrophy, hemophilia, cystic fibrosis, Tay-Sachs disease, sickle cell anemia, abnormally short stature, mental retardation, or birth defects so that the odds of having a child with one of these conditions can be assessed. Both partners will be asked to consider possible risk factors associated with their home and work environment, including exposure to radiation, insecticides, or other toxic chemicals.

The counselor will also want to know if the woman has been immunized against rubella or if she has a history of certain medical disorders that may complicate pregnancy, such as diabetes, hypertension, epilepsy, asthma, anemia, and sexually transmitted diseases (including possible exposure to HIV, the virus that causes AIDS). She will be questioned about her diet, exercise, and medication habits, as well as her use of cigarettes, alcohol, and illicit drugs, since using any of these substances during pregnancy can affect the growing fetus. Usually there is also a discussion of any

psychological or interpersonal factors that may have an impact on a pregnancy. These include readiness for children, job security, or signs of significant stress, depression, or anxiety. All of this information is kept strictly confidential.

Once potential risks have been assessed, the counselor will offer information about proper nutrition, weight control, and exercise. Another topic of discussion will be good prenatal care (see entry). If necessary, advice will be given about the importance of controlling certain underlying conditions—such as hypertension or diabetes—before attempting a pregnancy. Depending on the couple's particular situation, issues such as pregnancy spacing and contraception may be discussed, and advice may be given about various social, financial, and vocational assistance programs.

If necessary, the counselor may offer ways to reduce any known risks. Some interventions are relatively simple: for example, a woman planning a pregnancy may need to be immunized against rubella (at least 3 months before attempting conception) or hepatitis (the series of 3 shots can be started anytime), have an intrauterine device (IUD) removed, avoid prolonged exposure to elevated temperatures (for example, hot tubs), or get someone else to change a cat's litter box (to help prevent toxoplasmosis; see entry). Another simple intervention advocated by most physicians and preconception counselors involves taking 400 micrograms of folate (folic acid) every day from at least 1 month before conception until at least 6 weeks afterward to help prevent neural tube defects such as spina bifida. This is most easily taken in the form of an over-the-counter multivitamin. Higher does of 4 milligrams per day are often prescribed to women known to be at increased risk for offspring with neural tube defects.

What happens after the visit?

Other risks may take longer or be more difficult to modify. If some occupational hazard known to affect sperm, eggs, or a growing fetus has been identified during the counseling, the affected partner may need to find a way to change jobs before attempting conception (see occupational hazards). This can sometimes lead to job loss and related financial and interpersonal problems that in and of themselves may complicate a pregnancy.

In the case of complex or long-term problems, the preconception counselor will often refer women or couples to psychotherapists, social workers, nutritional counselors, genetic counselors, family planning centers, community mental health centers, home health agencies, or other medical or housing assistance programs. Women with preexisting medical conditions may be referred to doctors trained in managing high-risk pregnancies, while other women may be referred to substance abuse centers or other programs that can help them modify harmful health behaviors.

Related entries

Genetic counseling, hepatitis, occupational hazards, pregnancy over age 35, prenatal care, rubella, sexually transmitted diseases, stress, toxoplasmosis

Preeclampsia

Preeclampsia is a complication of pregnancy characterized by high blood pressure, protein in the urine, and a number of other symptoms such as headache, visual disturbances, and abdominal pain. Fluid retention is also part of the syndrome, but this is so common that it is not considered a symptom of preeclampsia in and of itself. Untreated, preeclampsia can rapidly progress to eclampsia (see entry), a life-threatening condition that involves convulsions and coma.

Various theories have been proposed to explain preeclampsia, but none have been proved conclusively. For this reason, and because we still know so little about the nature of this condition, it often goes under a number of descriptive names, including pregnancy-induced hypertension, toxemia, or preeclamptic toxemia.

About 6 percent of all pregnant women will develop preeclampsia sometime after completing 20 weeks of gestation. Eclampsia is much less common, occurring in only about 0.1 percent of pregnancies. Complications from eclampsia are a leading cause of maternal death in the United States, second only to pulmonary embolism (a blood clot lodged in an artery supplying the lung). They also are a leading cause of fetal growth retardation, fetal death, and complications owing to the necessity of premature delivery. Major risks to the mother include strokes, seizures, ruptured liver, and failure of the heart, liver, lungs, or kidneys. It is not clear whether having preeclampsia during pregnancy predisposes a woman to developing chronic high blood pressure later in life.

Who is likely to develop preeclampsia?

This condition most often occurs in women having their first baby, but once a woman has had preeclampsia, she has a 25 to 50 percent chance of developing it again in a subsequent pregnancy. Other women at risk are those at the extremes of age such as (teenagers and women over 45), as well as women with various underlying medical problems, including high blood pressure, kidney disorders, autoimmune disorders, and diabetes (see entries). A multiple pregnancy, as well as a molar pregnancy (an abnormal pregnancy in which the embryonic tissue develops into a grapelike cluster of cells instead of a fetus; see entry), also increase the likelihood of preeclampsia.

What are the symptoms?

Symptoms of preeclampsia usually appear in the third trimester of pregnancy. Women with mild forms may have only a slight elevation in blood pressure and levels of protein in their urine. A woman is said to have hypertension if—in 2 measurements made at least 6 hours apart—her blood pressure is at least 140/90 or if it has risen significantly (by more than 30 mm systolic or 15 mm diastolic) since her first trimester of pregnancy. A woman is said to have proteinuria if, in 2 random urine samples taken 6 hours apart, she has at least 0.3 grams of albumin per liter of urine.

Another symptom of preeclampsia is rapid weight gain (more than 2.2 pounds per week), which may include fluid retention. Swelling of the face and hands was once thought to signal preeclampsia, but it occurs so often in normal pregnancies that it is no longer considered a cause for concern by itself. The same is true for swollen legs and ankles, which develop in about a third of pregnant women whether or not they have preeclampsia.

In severe preeclampsia, hypertension and proteinuria increase even more, and urine output may decrease. Other symptoms include blind spots, blurred vision, headaches, pulmonary edema (fluid in the lungs), abdominal pain, seeing tiny flashing lights (scotomata), and exaggerated reflexes.

How is the condition evaluated?

If a pregnant woman is found to have either high blood pressure or protein in her urine, and she is past her 20th week of gestation, her clinician will suspect mild preeclampsia. Severe preeclampsia is associated with dysfunction of other organs or slow growth of the fetus. If severe preeclampsia develops, various laboratory tests of blood and urine may be done to look for elevated levels of liver transaminases, bilirubin, uric acid, and creatinine, and low levels of platelets—all of which are common in preeclampsia.

Preeclampsia is sometimes misdiagnosed as an acute illness that has nothing to do with pregnancy. Liver disease, kidney disorders, inflammation of the gallbladder, severe bleeding (hemorrhage), immune thrombocytopenic purpura (see platelet disorders), and heart failure can all be confused with preeclampsia if the disorder has atypical features.

How is preeclampsia treated?

The only definitive cure for preeclampsia is delivery of the baby. Since the disorder usually develops late in pregnancy, this can often be accomplished without compromising the fetus's chances of survival (that is, after 36 weeks' gestation). If the fetus is not ready to be born, the decision to deliver can be difficult, but many obstetricians recommend inducing labor because the risks to both mother and child from preeclampsia usually outweigh the risks of premature delivery. Among those risks are acute kidney failure, bleeding disorders, and eclampsia in the mother, as well as the premature separation of the placenta from the uterine wall and fetal death. If seizures occur, they may be treated with anticonvulsants. In some instances the mother's condition can be managed with bed rest and intravenous medication in the hope of giving the fetus a few more weeks to mature.

If preeclampsia is relatively mild, it may be possible to delay delivery with careful monitoring of both mother and fetus. Sometimes this involves hospitalization and bed rest, but some women may instead be able to visit their obstetricians every couple of days for frequent tests of blood pressure and urine. Lying on the left side is recommended because it keeps the uterus from resting on a major vein (the inferior vena cava) and thus improves blood flow. The fetus will also be monitored for problems, as well as for signs of lung maturity, which indicate readiness for delivery.

During delivery fetal heart rate will be monitored constantly. At the same time, the obstetrician will probably administer magnesium sulfate to the mother to prevent seizures from eclampsia. Her fluid levels will be watched closely, and any hypertension that develops will be controlled with blood pressure medicine such as hydralazine or labetalol administered intravenously. Because the risk of seizure can persist after delivery, magnesium sulfate may be given for at least 24 hours following the birth, and fluid intake and output will be measured as carefully as during labor and delivery. Usually symptoms and signs of preeclampsia begin to lessen within a day or two of delivery and disappear completely within a week or so. If hypertension persists, the woman may need to take blood pressure pills such as beta blockers until her blood pressure returns to a normal level (which can sometimes take a couple of months).

How can preeclampsia be prevented?

Doctors used to try to prevent preeclampsia by limiting a pregnant woman's salt intake or by prescribing diet pills (amphetamines) to prevent weight gain or diuretic drugs to prevent fluid retention. It is now known that these steps are actually quite dangerous in themselves and can lead to protein deficiencies, electrolyte imbalance, and, in the case of amphetamines, drug dependence.

There is no way to prevent preeclampsia, but it can be kept from progressing to eclampsia with good prenatal care. This involves frequent checkups during the last trimester of pregnancy, including routine checks of blood pressure and urine. Newer studies have shown promise in preventing preeclampsia in future pregnancies.

Related entries

Eclampsia, edema, headaches, high blood pressure, platelet disorders, prenatal care

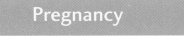

Pregnancy

Pregnancy is a state in which a woman is carrying a fertilized egg, embryo, or fetus inside her body. It is dated from the beginning of the last menstrual period (LMP), and a full-term pregnancy can last anywhere from 37 to 42 weeks beyond this time. A good way to estimate the due date is to subtract 3 months from the LMP and add 7 days. Thus, a woman whose last menstrual period began on May 7 would have a due date of February 14. Most women deliver their babies within 2 weeks of their due date.

Normal physical changes

Pregnancy is divided into 3 trimesters, each lasting a little over 13 weeks. During the first trimester some women may hardly notice they are pregnant except that there is no monthly menstrual period. (Light spotting may occur, and

though this can be normal, it should be evaluated by a clinician.) Other women experience distinct physical changes that can begin within a week or two of conception. These include fatigue, dizziness, morning sickness, breast tenderness, and frequent urination. About 6 in 10 women develop shortness of breath because of increased production of progesterone. Some or all of these symptoms may abate during the second trimester, a time when the uterus has still not grown large enough to be particularly uncomfortable.

Many women describe the second trimester as the easiest part of pregnancy, although some develop constipation, headaches, excessive salivation, sweating, nasal and sinus congestion, and nosebleeds at this point if not before.

Some women develop cholestasis of pregnancy during the last 2 trimesters. This disorder is characterized by intense itching; while it does not pose much risk to the mother, it does pose additional risks to the fetus, and for that reason the clinician will want to monitor the condition and prescribe medications for the itching. The condition improves immediately after delivery.

During the third trimester new symptoms may arise as a result of the added weight of the uterus and the size of the fetus (see illustration). These can include renewed fatigue, Braxton-Hicks contractions (false labor pains), frequent urination (after lightening—or the dropping of the fetus into the pelvis—has occurred), hemorrhoids, backaches, varicose veins, stretchmarks, edema, shortness of breath, heartburn, abdominal and leg cramps, and sleep disturbances. By contrast, headache symptoms sometimes improve as the pregnancy progresses.

Possible danger signals

A pregnant woman with any of these symptoms should contact her clinician immediately.

- vaginal bleeding
- continuous headaches during the last 3 months of pregnancy
- severe, unrelenting abdominal pain
- persistent vomiting
- marked or sudden swelling of eyelids, hands, or face during the last 3 months
- dimness or blurring of vision during the last 3 months
- decreased fetal movement after 24 weeks
- rupture of the "bag of waters" (amniotic membranes)

Normal emotional changes

Many women undergo dramatic emotional changes during a pregnancy as they begin to foresee potential alterations in their lifestyle, job, finances, living arrangements, health, and relationship with the father. Pregnant women are reputed to have a "glow" about them, and indeed many women love being pregnant and feel vibrant and even enchanted throughout the entire experience. Numerous women, however, find

Pregnancy month by month

Fetus

First month

By the end of this month, the embryo has a head and trunk, as well as limb buds, which will grow into arms and legs. The liver and digestive system are developing, and the heart starts to beat on the 25th day. The embryo is nourished and excretes wastes through vascular structures that connect it to the uterine wall. These are called the umbilical cord and placenta. The embryo is only about 1/5 of an inch long.

Second month

Early this month the foundation is established for the entire nervous system, including the brain and spinal cord. By the end of 8 weeks, the arms and legs have begun forming, facial features are more defined, and the fetus has a complete skeleton of cartilage. Toward the end of the month, true bone cells replace cartilage, marking the transition from embryo to fetus. All major internal organs have begun to form, and the heart is pumping blood. The fetus is now nearly an inch long and weighs under an ounce.

Third month

The fetus is growing rapidly, and the face becomes more "human" looking as ears and eyelids form and features become more distinct. Fingers and toes are formed and have soft nailbeds. All major organs are now in at least initial stages. The kidneys are secreting urine into the bladder, the palate which will form the roof of the mouth is closing, the heart is forming four chambers, and major blood vessels are near completion. By the end of this month the fetus is about 4 inches long and weighs just over an ounce.

Mother

First month

The uterine lining is thickening, and the body produces increasing amounts of estrogen and progesterone. Many women do not notice any physical changes, although most will miss a menstrual period or have unusually scanty bleeding or spotting. Some women notice that their breasts are swollen or tender or that tiny bumps around their nipples have become more prominent. Some women also need to urinate more frequently.

Second month

Blood volume and output of blood from the heart are increasing rapidly. Changes are occurring in the function of many internal organs, including the kidneys, lungs, gastrointestinal tract, liver, thyroid glands, adrenal glands, and skin. Many women find that their breasts are still tender or that they have developed other discomforts such as constipation, fatigue, frequent urination, nausea, and vomiting.

Third month

If they haven't already, most women notice some physical signs of pregnancy. Weight begins to increase, and while it may be possible to get by without maternity clothes for another month or two, it may be necessary to let out clothes or choose pants or skirts with elastic waistbands.

---

pregnancy miserable, either physically, psychologically, or both. Some have trouble adjusting to their expanding body and may feel that they are no longer sexually attractive (a feeling that can be either reinforced or assuaged by their partner).

Other women may fear losing their job, not being able to afford a family, hurting or losing the baby, having a baby that is abnormal, or experiencing the pain of childbirth. Some women feel unsure about whether they really want to have a baby in the first place. Women having their first baby may be confused, scared, or overwhelmed by the realization that they will be taking on responsibility for another human be-

ing. Or they may feel that they are becoming distant from a partner whose level of interest in the pregnancy is less intense than theirs.

Most pregnant women have some of these feelings on occasion. Joining a childbirth education class or merely talking to a friend who has recently had a baby can be reassuring. Communicating feelings to her partner can also help a woman bridge many misunderstandings and ease anxieties, as can extra planning with older children or in preparing the home for the new baby. A woman who feels overwhelmed by negative emotions or worries, however, should talk to her clinician or childbirth educator about them.

Fetus

Fourth month

As this month begins, all organs are formed and need only now grow for the remainder of the pregnancy. The fetus becomes increasingly active, moving, kicking, and swallowing, although most women still cannot feel this activity. The fetus can also sleep, wake, swallow, pass urine, and hear. It now has eyebrows, a bit of hair on the head, and transparent skin. By the end of the month, the fetus is 6–7 inches long and weighs over a quarter pound.

Fifth month

A growth spurt occurs this month, and the fetus becomes more active so that it is easier for the mother to feel movements. Internal organs mature, and fingernails develop. A clinician can now hear the fetus's heartbeat with a stethoscope. By the end of the month the fetus is about 8–12 inches long and weighs between 1/2 and 1 pound.

Sixth month

The fetus's organs continue to develop, and growth is rapid. The skin appears red and wrinkled and is covered with downy, fine hair called lanugo. Although the lungs are still not fully developed, a fetus born at the end of this month could potentially survive if given extremely specialized care. It is now 11–14 inches long and weighs between 1 and 1.5 pounds.

Seventh month

This is another period of rapid fetal growth. As calcium is stored, the bones begin to harden. The fetus may now open its eyes at times and can suck its thumb. Its chances of survival if born at this time have improved, although special care would still be required. By the end of the month it weighs between 2.5 and 3 pounds and is about 15 inches long.

Mother

Fourth month

As the second trimester progresses, many women find the early symptoms of pregnancy disappear. This is often the month that women notice their abdomen swelling as the uterus enlarges to accommodate the fetus. Often the nipples and areola darken, and some women notice a dark line called the linea nigra running from the navel to the top of the pubic hair. Women with dark hair and fair skin especially may develop chloasma (also called mask of pregnancy or melasma). This condition, which often worsens in the sun, involves brownish patches that appear on the face and usually disappear or fade after delivery. Women who are very thin or who have had children before may notice some fetal movements (quickening) toward the end of this month (at about 16 weeks after the last menstrual period but possibly even earlier). These often feel like the fluttering of butterfly wings or gas bubbles.

Fifth month

The uterus now reaches up to the navel, and the overlying skin becomes more taut. By 20 to 22 weeks after the last menstrual period most women can feel fetal movements.

Sixth month

This is usually the month of maximum weight gain for the mother. Her abdomen continues to enlarge. Many women can feel the fetus kicking and notice vigorous fetal movements. Various symptoms of later pregnancy become more common after this month. These include heartburn, backache, varicose veins, hemorrhoids, or a stitch-like pain down the side of the groin or lower abdomen.

Seventh month

As the fetus grows and the uterus expands, some women begin to feel increasingly uncomfortable. Some women develop stretchmarks on the breasts and abdomen. Others notice false labor pains called Braxton-Hicks contractions. Other problems common in the latter part of pregnancy include insomnia, leg cramps, and numbness or tingling in the extremities.

Fetus

Eighth month
As the due date approaches, the fetus continues to grow and its skin becomes somewhat less wrinkled. Many babies go into the head-down position, from which they will be born. The bones of the head are soft and flexible outside, so that they will be able to fit through the birth canal. Movements become more restricted since there is less free space available for flips. The fetus now weighs 4–5 pounds and is between about 16 and a half and 18 inches long.

Ninth month
In this last month, the fetus gains about 1/2 pound a week and readies itself for birth. Often it will "drop" lower into the abdomen, curled up with its knees against its nose. Full-term delivery can occur anytime between 37–42 weeks after the mother's last menstrual period. Most babies weigh 6–9 pounds and are about 20 inches long.

Mother

Eighth month
The top part of the uterus now lies just under the diaphragm, and some women feel short of breath. Fetal movements can be seen along the surface of the woman's skin, and it may be possible to recognize distinct body parts. Braxton-Hicks contractions are often stronger, and symptoms related to the increasing weight of the uterus may be exacerbated. Colostrum, a yellowish fluid secreted before breast milk, may begin to leak from the breasts.

Ninth month
Shortness of breath may abate as the fetus drops lower into the abdomen, but it may be necessary to urinate more frequently. The navel may protrude as the skin over the abdomen becomes extremely taut. Many women are very fatigued and need to take frequent naps. It is also common for ankles to swell, especially at the end of the day. As the cervix softens in preparation for childbirth, contractions may increase. Colostrum leakage may become more noticeable.

Related entries
Abortion, childbirth, eclampsia, ectopic pregnancy, exercise, genetic counseling, hemorrhoids, miscarriage, morning sickness, nutrition, postpartum issues, preeclampsia, preconception counseling, pregnancy over age 35, pregnancy testing, prenatal care, vaginal bleeding during pregnancy, varicose veins

Pregnancy over Age 35

In the United States today there is a virtual epidemic of delayed childbearing. While the number of women aged 30 to 44 rose by 60 percent over the last three decades, the number of women in this age group giving birth to their first child rose by 460 percent. By 1998, 23 percent of first births and 13 percent of all births occurred in women over the age of 35. This trend was expected to continue until at least the year 2010, when the youngest of the baby boom generation will have reached menopause.

There are numerous reasons for this trend. Many women are marrying later, waiting for children until they have had a chance to complete their education or establish a career, or deciding to have smaller families and thus starting them later in life. Some women over 35 are also deciding to have children as single parents, sometimes through artificial insemination. Prenatal tests such as chorionic villi sampling, amniocentesis, and ultrasound have reduced the risks of bearing a child with a genetic abnormality, at least for the many women who consider abortion an option. In addition, better and more freely available methods of birth control and treatment for infertility, improved access to child care facilities, and the increased longevity and improved health of the population in general have all allowed more and more women to extend their childbearing years.

The good news is that most women having either first or later babies after the age of 35 can have successful pregnancies. Age 35 is not some kind of magic number at which women suddenly become high-risk: the chance of various pregnancy complications increases gradually from the age of 20 on, but the risks for most women at any age are extremely low.

Nevertheless, women who wait until they are 35 or older to have children must recognize that the odds of developing certain medical problems are high enough to warrant special considerations. Older mothers have no increased risk of giving birth prematurely, but they do have higher than normal risks of infertility, miscarriage, chromosomal abnormalities, low birth weight babies (owing to decreased uterine growth), stillbirth, and various medical complications.

Any woman over 35 who is considering pregnancy can improve her odds of having a healthy baby by learning about

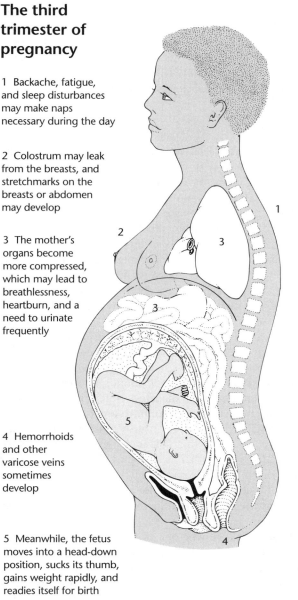

The third trimester of pregnancy

1 Backache, fatigue, and sleep disturbances may make naps necessary during the day

2 Colostrum may leak from the breasts, and stretchmarks on the breasts or abdomen may develop

3 The mother's organs become more compressed, which may lead to breathlessness, heartburn, and a need to urinate frequently

4 Hemorrhoids and other varicose veins sometimes develop

5 Meanwhile, the fetus moves into a head-down position, sucks its thumb, gains weight rapidly, and readies itself for birth

which suggests that the simple fact of aging eggs is responsible for much of the infertility in older women.

Although most physicians recommend an infertility evaluation in younger women after a full year of trying to become pregnant, older women concerned about the "biological clock" should probably start an infertility workup after just 6 months.

Miscarriage

Since a woman's eggs age with her, the chances of their developing chromosomal abnormalities increase with age. And because over half of the miscarriages that occur in the first trimester of pregnancy seem to be due to chromosomal abnormalities, it is no surprise that the miscarriage rate also rises with maternal age. What remains unclear is whether older women have a higher risk than younger ones of miscarrying chromosomally normal fetuses or if their higher rate of miscarriage is attributable to the fact that their fetuses are already genetically damaged.

Miscarriage can be particularly traumatic to the older woman, who may have had trouble conceiving or who may worry about the time left to her to conceive and carry another child. If grief is particularly severe or does not subside after a few months, support groups such as RESOLVE (see infertility) or short-term therapy with a professional counselor may be of help.

Chromosomal abnormalities

Chromosomal abnormalities of the fetus can lead to conditions such as Down syndrome, a birth defect caused by the presence of an extra chromosome and characterized by mental retardation as well as certain distinctive physical traits: slow growth, broad hands and feet, small head, flat nose, slanting eyes, and a predisposition toward serious heart defects. Many other chromosomal abnormalities are so severe that the fetus cannot survive the pregnancy. The risk of giving birth to a child with a chromosomal abnormality increases with age. At the age of 24 only 1 woman in 1,250 gives birth to a baby with Down syndrome, whereas at the age of 30 the odds rise to 1 in 952, and by age 35 the risk is 1 in 378 (see chart). By the age of 40 nearly 1 woman in 100 will give birth to a baby with Down syndrome. Of course, even for a woman of 40 the chances of bearing a baby without Down syndrome are still 99 percent—a comforting statistic, though not, of course, to the woman who bears a baby with a chromosomal defect.

For these reasons most pregnant women over the age of 35 are offered either amniocentesis or chorionic villi sampling (see entries). Both of these allow the chromosomes to be examined while the fetus is still nonviable (incapable of surviving outside the mother's body). Even a woman who would not consider terminating the pregnancy through elective abortion may want to have these tests so she can prepare herself and her family for the arrival of a child with special needs.

the various risks and by making sure to get good prenatal care. Women with preexisting medical conditions such as high blood pressure or diabetes should seek individual counseling (see preconception counseling).

Infertility

Women over the age of 35 are 3 times more likely to have difficulty conceiving than women aged 20 to 29. When women in their 40s have undergone in vitro fertilization using eggs donated by younger women, their chances of carrying a pregnancy to term were comparable to those of younger women,

Risk for chromosomal abnormalities		
Age of mother at delivery	Risk of Down syndrome	Risk of any chromosomal abnormality
20	1/1667	1/526
22	1/1429	1/500
24	1/1250	1/476
26	1/1176	1/476
28	1/1111	1/455
30	1/952	1/385
31	1/909	1/385
32	1/769	1/322
33	1/602	1/286
34	1/485	1/238
35	1/378	1/192
36	1/289	1/156
37	1/224	1/127
38	1/173	1/102
39	1/136	1/83
40	1/106	1/66
41	1/82	1/53
42	1/63	1/42
43	1/49	1/33
44	1/38	1/26
45	1/30	1/21
46	1/23	1/16
47	1/18	1/13
48	1/14	1/10
49	1/11	1/8

Low birth weight babies

There is some evidence that maternal age increases the chance of insufficient uterine growth, leading to low birth weight babies. Whether this effect is due to age alone or to factors such as high blood pressure (which is more common in older mothers) or cigarette smoking (which more profoundly affects older mothers) remains uncertain. A practitioner who suspects a problem in the fetus's growth rate may want to check it using an ultrasound or other test.

Stillbirth

The risk of stillbirth doubles for babies born to women in their late 30s in comparison with younger women, and quadruples by the age of 45. Part of the explanation lies in the increased number of older mothers who have preexisting medical conditions such as hypertension and diabetes, either of which can lead to abnormal fetal growth, increasing the chances of death within the uterus. Other stillbirths may be attributable to chromosomal abnormalities.

Genetic counseling and prenatal diagnosis can eliminate the increased risk of stillbirth for women who are found not to have preexisting medical conditions, since for older mothers whose blood pressure and weight are normal, there does not appear to be any excess risk of stillbirth. Even so, some clinicians feel that all older women ought to have electronic fetal monitoring during labor to keep a continuous record of the infant's heart rate and signal any fetal distress.

Medical complications

Numerous studies indicate that pregnant women over the age of 35 have at least twice the usual risk of developing complications from high blood pressure—chronic hypertension, pregnancy-induced hypertension, and preeclampsia. Preeclampsia is most common in first pregnancies, and in subsequent pregnancies in women who had preeclampsia in their first pregnancy. For women bearing a second or later child after the age of 35, there is an increased risk of hypertension, especially if they are obese. Women who are being treated for hypertension should discuss with their clinician the medications they are taking before they conceive, since some medications for high blood pressure may cause birth defects and will need to be changed.

Like hypertension, diabetes mellitus also becomes more prevalent with age. The risk of developing this disease is even higher among women who are obese or who have had previous babies weighing over 9 pounds at birth. Women who had insulin-dependent diabetes before they became pregnant have an increased risk of stillbirth and of having babies with congenital abnormalities or birth injuries. It is still unclear, however, whether this risk increases in women with gestational diabetes (that is, diabetes developed during pregnancy). What is known is that gestational diabetes increases a woman's chance of having an abnormally large infant, and this in turn can lead to difficult labor, increasing the chance of birth injury.

Older mothers, whether or not they have had other children, are obese, or have diabetes, also tend to have excessively heavy babies (over 8.8 pounds), and this too can complicate delivery. Pregnant women over 30 are often screened for gestational diabetes using an oral glucose challenge test (which measures the body's response to sugar) at some time between 24 and 28 weeks of gestation.

Abnormal vaginal bleeding during the third trimester seems to occur about twice as frequently in older mothers. And women who have had multiple births seem to be at increased risk for postpartum hemorrhage—heavy, uncontrollable bleeding from the vagina—either because the uterus retains part of the placenta or fetal tissue or because it does not contract sufficiently.

The risk of maternal death also increases with age. Maternal death rates among women aged 35 and older are double those for 25-year-old women and quadruple by age 45. This is largely an indirect result of underlying medical problems or of complications that result from bearing many children. Even so, the risk of maternal death is still extremely low, with fewer than 8 maternal deaths for every 100,000 live births in this country. Thus, there is little reason for a healthy woman over 35 to worry about an increased risk of dying.

A question of balance

A decision to have children at any age cannot be based solely on medical concerns. Financial, social, and personal factors must also be balanced against the physical ones. When a decision to have a baby is examined from all these perspectives, it is clear that there is no perfect time to begin or extend a family.

Whereas some women prefer having children early in life because they have more stamina then or because they picture a carefree existence by the time they are in their 40s, other women find child rearing a welcome respite after a decade or two of "the rat race." Many couples are better off financially in their 30s and early 40s than they were at 20 or are psychologically better prepared to become parents. Still others have more stable partnerships at that point in life. Older mothers, too, often have the perspective and self-awareness to appreciate the experience of child rearing—and to understand the sacrifices involved. And because many more mature women have already fulfilled themselves through personal accomplishments, they are less likely than their younger counterparts to look for fulfillment through their children.

Nonetheless, after decades of independence, adjusting to the demands of motherhood can be difficult. Some women over 35 with a newborn feel isolated from friends who have teenagers or grown children. Many women in this age group also have to weigh the demands of child rearing against the demands of caring for aging parents.

A woman with older children will also want to consider the changes in the family's lifestyle that a new baby will bring and the impact it will have on her other children. If she has returned to a full-time job, she must consider whether she will leave the work world once again or stay there and spend less time at home with this child than she did with her older ones. Though always difficult, this type of decision can sometimes be easier for the older mother, who has years of experience juggling schedules and priorities.

Women in their late 20s and early 30s who are on the fence about whether to postpone pregnancy or to go ahead with it may want to take into account their decreasing fertility. Many 30-year-old women are marginally fertile but have problems that can be readily corrected with medication or surgery. As time passes, these fertility problems tend to respond less readily to treatment. If having a biological child is high on a couple's list of priorities, they should think carefully about starting their family at a time when they have the best possible chance of success.

Related entries

Abortion, alpha-fetoprotein screening, amniocentesis, chorionic villi sampling, diabetes, genetic counseling, high blood pressure, infertility, miscarriage, obesity, preconception counseling, preeclampsia, pregnancy, prenatal care

Pregnancy Testing

Not too many years ago women who suspected that they were pregnant had to wait a couple of months for confirmation. For those who desperately desired the pregnancy, as well as for those who desperately did not, these weeks of waiting could be extremely stressful.

Today sophisticated, sensitive tests conducted in clinic laboratories can confirm conception even before a menstrual period has been skipped, and home pregnancy tests—available without prescription in drugstores—can detect conception as early as 1 day after a woman has missed her period.

Generally women (and their clinicians) confirm a pregnancy shortly after a skipped period. As soon as a woman knows she is pregnant, she can make an appointment for a first prenatal visit (which is usually scheduled at 12 weeks of pregnancy) and can start practicing good prenatal care by eating well, taking prenatal vitamins, getting adequate rest, and avoiding drugs (including cigarettes and alcohol). Many of the most vital fetal developments take place in the first 3 months of pregnancy; knowing that she is pregnant during this time can sometimes make a big difference in a woman's behavior and in the outcome of her pregnancy.

Women who are thinking of terminating the pregnancy benefit from early diagnosis, too, since abortions done early in a pregnancy are generally safer and less physically painful than later ones. Whatever her intentions, any woman who tests positive with a home pregnancy kit should make an appointment to have the results confirmed by a clinician.

What are the signs of pregnancy?

The classic sign of pregnancy is a missed menstrual period. There is enormous variation from woman to woman and from pregnancy to pregnancy, however. Some women continue to bleed at the time of their normal menstruation, and many women skip their periods for reasons other than pregnancy (see menstrual cycle disorders). Moreover, the symptoms of early pregnancy are sometimes similar to those of an approaching period. But in general a woman should suspect she is pregnant if she notices any of the following symptoms (even if she is using birth control):

- a missed menstrual period
- an unusually short or scanty menstrual period; this symptom, combined with abdominal pain, can be the sign of an ectopic pregnancy, which is a medical emergency
- unusual tingling, throbbing, or aching in the breasts
- unusual fatigue
- nausea or vomiting just prior to the time that a period is expected
- unusual bloating or cramping
- more frequent urination than usual

- a basal body temperature (see birth control) that does not drop around the time that a period is expected

How do pregnancy tests work?

All pregnancy tests work by detecting the presence of human chorionic gonadotropin (hCG), a hormone produced by the developing placenta and detectable in the mother's blood and urine. Urine tests are done in doctors' offices, private laboratories, and clinics at a small cost (about $10 to $15). In many communities family planning organizations (such as Planned Parenthood) offer free pregnancy tests as well. Women used to be asked to provide a sample of the first urine passed in the morning because it contains the highest concentrations of hCG. This is no longer necessary since tests are now powerful enough to detect hCG in urine passed at any time of day.

All pregnancy tests work by seeing if hCG contained in the woman's urine or blood can displace hCG that is locked into antibodies in a test solution. The formation of a characteristic ring at the bottom of a test tube, the formation of clumps on a slide, or some kind of color change in a bead or solution is a sign of a positive test.

Some blood tests (radioimmunoassay and radioreceptorassay) using radioactively labeled hCG as markers can detect pregnancy as early as 7 days after conception. Unless the woman is at high risk for having an ectopic pregnancy or missed abortion (a type of miscarriage) or has a medical condition (such as heart disease, diabetes, hypertension, or a kidney disorder) which can cause pregnancy complications, these expensive early tests are not usually ordered.

How accurate are the results?

A false-positive pregnancy test is one that indicates a woman is pregnant when she is not. A false-negative test indicates that a woman is not pregnant when she is. Though generally quite accurate, no pregnancy test is foolproof, and occasionally there are false positives and negatives, as well as inconclusive tests that need to be repeated. Some tests can yield false-positive results because luteinizing hormone (LH), a hormone that soars around the time of ovulation, is chemically similar to hCG and can sometimes displace the test for hCG. The urine of women nearing menopause also contains high levels of LH and can produce false-positive results on a pregnancy test. Newer tests that use monoclonal antibody technology such as the enzyme-linked immunoassay (which can test either blood or urine) or the radioimmunoassay avoid this problem because they test only for a uniquely shaped part of the hCG molecule (the beta subunit).

Other reasons for false positives include the use of marijuana, methadone, methyldopa (used to treat hypertension), some tranquilizers and antidepressants, and even large doses of aspirin. Occasionally some rare cancers, trophoblastic disease (abnormal cell growth, including hydatidiform moles; see molar pregnancy), ovarian cysts, and thyroid disorders can yield false-positive results. In addition, a pregnancy test will remain positive for about 10 days after a miscarriage or abortion, sometimes longer.

False-negative results can occur if the urine is too dilute or has sat too long at room temperature, if the collection jar was contaminated, or if the test is done too early or too late in the pregnancy (hCG levels start to dwindle a couple of months after conception). A false-negative result can also occur if a pregnancy is developing abnormally or if a miscarriage is about to occur. Occasionally an ectopic pregnancy will also lead to a false negative in a urine pregnancy test.

When can home pregnancy tests be used?

Once available only in the clinician's office, pregnancy testing can now be done by a woman in the privacy of her own home with a kit available without prescription. In recent years these tests have become quite sensitive (if directions are followed exactly)—that is, they respond to extremely low levels of hCG. A positive test conducted about 2 weeks after a woman has skipped a period almost always means that she is pregnant (except in cases where the woman has a rare medical condition or is taking a medication that can yield a false-positive result).

If the test is conducted sooner, the result may be positive, but it can lead to disappointment later for a woman who is eager to have a child. In perhaps 50 to 75 percent of all conceptions, the fertilized egg never implants or else spontaneously aborts shortly after implantation. These conceptions can nevertheless yield a temporarily positive pregnancy test, since the blastocyst (a very early form of the embryo) produces hCG which can be detected in the blood as early as 6 days after conception. At least half of these blastocysts will not implant.

A negative test very early in a pregnancy does not necessarily mean that the woman is not pregnant. About 20 percent of women obtaining negative results in home pregnancy tests may simply have miscalculated the date of their expected period or may not have quite enough hCG in their urine to yield a positive result. In these cases the test should be repeated after another week if the woman still thinks that she is pregnant. If results are again negative, she should consult her clinician, who may repeat the urine test or do a blood test.

There are a number of different brands of home pregnancy tests (such as EPT, Clear Blue Easy, First Response, and Answer Plus), and most give results within a few minutes. Some of the tests call for mixing the urine with a test solution, following several mixing steps, and then waiting for a bead to change color. Other tests merely require urinating on a chemical-coated stick, which changes color if the woman is pregnant. Home tests cost about as much as a test in a clinician's office (ranging from about $7 to $14 a test). Some tests with different brand names and prices are in fact identical products made by the same manufacturer, and higher price is no guarantee of superior accuracy.

Related entries

Abortion, chorionic villi sampling, diabetes, ectopic pregnancy, genetic counseling, miscarriage, molar pregnancy, pregnancy, prenatal care, vitamins

Premenstrual Syndrome

Many clinicians define premenstrual syndrome as some combination of physical, mood, or behavioral changes which occur consistently and predictably before or during each menstrual period and which are severe enough to interfere with some aspects of a woman's life. A woman who starts feeling weepy, "headachy," and bloated about 5 to 15 days before her period is due each month may be said to have PMS. The same is true for a normally calm woman who becomes so overwhelmed by feelings of anger in the days before her period that she screams at her children and cannot concentrate on her work. Having just a few isolated symptoms, such as a craving for chocolate, moodiness, or cramps, before or at the beginning of menstruation is not the same as having premenstrual syndrome, unless these symptoms are severe enough to interfere with normal activity.

Given the enormous hormonal changes associated with the menstrual cycle, it is no wonder that many women experience changes in physical functioning, mood, or behavior over the course of the month. Most women probably go through at least some kind of noticeable physical or psychological changes during the week before menstruation begins. What is more mysterious is why these changes become disabling in some women. There do not seem to be differences in daily levels of various hormones in women with and without PMS. There does seem to be some evidence that changes in ovarian hormones may modify circadian rhythms (the body's precisely timed physiological response to light-dark cycles over 24 hours), decrease sensitivity to endorphins (the body's natural painkillers), or decrease the levels of the neurotransmitter serotonin in the brain (which can lead to irritability and depression). But precisely how or why is still unclear. It may also turn out that there is more than one form of PMS, each associated with a different underlying mechanism.

Who is likely to develop PMS?

Many clinicians, and many more women, have observed anecdotally that PMS symptoms worsen for some women as they approach menopause. There has been so little well-designed research in this area, however, that these observations have not yet been proven conclusively. The most serious cases of PMS, affecting 1 to 5 percent of all women, seem to occur most often in women who are between the ages of 26 and 35, who have cycle lengths of 25 to 28 days, and who report having experienced stressful life events in the preceding year. Other factors associated with severe PMS are a personal or family history of depression, a history of migraine headaches or postpartum depression, having several children, and a higher than average intake of alcohol or chocolate.

Some other psychiatric disorders are a risk factor for PMS. Two thirds of women who suffer from depression also have premenstrual syndrome, and 45 to 70 percent of women with PMS have a past history of depression. About a third of women with PMS who also have children have a history of mild to severe postpartum depression, which is twice the rate in the general population. If a woman has an underlying psychiatric illness, chances are these symptoms will worsen during the premenstrual phase of her monthly cycle. For example, many women who have panic attacks find that the frequency of attacks increases in the premenstrual phase. The rate of PMS in women with personality disorders does not seem to be any higher than in the general population of women.

What are the symptoms?

Like seasonal affective disorder and postpartum psychiatric disorders (see entries), PMS is primarily characterized by the timing of symptoms. There are literally hundreds of symptoms that may occur in PMS, but what makes them distinctive is that they are severe enough to disrupt daily activity and that they begin during the last 5 to 15 days of each menstrual cycle and stop during menstruation. Among the most frequent symptoms of PMS are acne, anger, anxiety, appetite changes, bloating, breast pain, depression, difficulty concentrating, fatigue, headaches, joint swelling, mood swings, nausea, nervousness, pelvic pain, sleep disorders, sweating, vomiting, and weight gain.

The American Psychiatric Association also has specific diagnostic criteria for what it has termed premenstrual dysphoric disorder, which may or may not be the same as PMS. The symptoms of this disorder largely involve the mood changes (as opposed to the physical symptoms) that may occur cyclically in women. To be diagnosed as having this disorder a woman must have at least 5 of the following symptoms: mood swings, anger or irritability, anxiety or tension, depressed mood, decreased interest in usual activities, fatigue, difficulty concentrating, increase or decrease in appetite, sleep disturbance, and physical symptoms such as breast pain, bloating, or headaches. These symptoms must occur cyclically and during most of the woman's menstrual cycles, and they must be serious enough to interfere with activities.

How is the condition evaluated?

In evaluating premenstrual syndrome, a clinician will take a careful history that includes information about the nature, timing, and severity of the symptoms. Before an effective treatment plan can be made, the clinician will need to understand the woman's living situation, diet, and exercise habits, and determine if the woman or her family has any psychiatric problems or history of alcohol or substance abuse.

A thorough physical and pelvic examination, and possibly certain laboratory tests as well, will be done to see if there are

Monthly record of premenstrual experiences

Cycle day 1 is the day that bleeding starts. Enter the dates of the cycle (for example, 3/15) in the second row. Record your daily weight (taken first thing in the morning, no clothing) in the third row. Then, throughout the cycle, indicate the severity of any symptoms, using 0 (not present), 1 (noticeable but not troublesome), 2 (interferes with normal activities), or 3 (intolerable). In the fourth row use these numbers to record bleeding.

Cycle day	1	2	3	4	5	6	7	8	9	10	11	12	13	14	15	16	17	18	19	20	21	22	23	24	25	26	27	28	29	30	31
Date																															
Weight																															
Bleeding																															
Acne																															
Bloatedness																															
Breast tenderness																															
Dizziness																															
Fatigue																															
Headache																															
Hot flashes																															
Nausea																															
Diarrhea																															
Constipation																															
Palpitations																															
Swelling																															
Angry outbursts																															
Anxiety																															
Difficulty concentrating																															
Crying easily																															
Depression																															
Food cravings																															
Forgetfulness																															
Mood swings																															
Overly sensitive																															
Wish to be alone																															

any underlying systemic disorders such as hypothyroidism or anemia which may mimic PMS or if there are any anatomical disorders such as endometriosis or uterine fibroids which may be contributing to pelvic pain.

The clinician will also ask the woman to record her symptoms on a daily basis for at least two complete menstrual cycles (see chart). This is the best way to see just how—and if—symptoms are linked to the menstrual cycle.

How is PMS treated?

Because of the variety of symptoms found in PMS, there is no one, universally effective treatment. Among the many different approaches are changes in lifestyle, support groups and other stress management techniques, vitamin supplements, and drugs aimed at relieving specific symptoms or groups of symptoms. With information about PMS treatments still so limited, it remains difficult to predict which women will respond to which therapies. Thus, treating PMS often requires trial and error, and it may take several months, even a year, to arrive at the optimal treatment.

Usually the first line of attack involves modifying diet and exercise habits. Many women find that eliminating caffeine, alcohol, and sugary foods, eating frequent small meals, and ensuring adequate protein and complex carbohydrate intake help control PMS symptoms. Regular aerobic exercise for 20 to 45 minutes a day at least 3 times a week seems to benefit some women with PMS. Others find that eating carbohydrate-rich meals in the evening during the second half of the menstrual cycle also helps, possibly because this diet may raise levels of the neurotransmitter serotonin (which, when low, has been linked to depression). One randomized trial suggested that a strict low-fat diet (less than 15 percent of calories from fat) reduces premenstrual breast pain.

Joining a support group, especially one led by a leader trained in group psychotherapy, can be helpful. Often members of the group keep daily records of their symptoms and discuss any relationship they may have with the menstrual cycle, as well as with any changes made in diet or exercise habits. Support groups can provide new ideas about effective relaxation and stress management strategies and generate discussion about other lifestyle changes that may ease symptoms. The peer support available in these groups can make it easier to implement these changes. And simply meeting other women who have similar symptoms can make a woman with PMS feel less alone and help affirm that her condition is not "all in her head."

Admittedly, the rationale for the diet, exercise, and stress management approaches comes more from trial and error than from randomized clinical trials (the gold standard in scientific studies). Still, they are certainly worth trying, given the minimal risk and cost involved, as well as the fact that many women have found them effective.

If symptoms persist, another approach may be to try various vitamin or mineral supplements. Among the most promising of these are calcium (1,000 mg each day), magnesium (200 mg taken during the last half of the cycle), vitamin B_6 (50 to 200 mg each day), and vitamin E (150 to 400 IU each day). These recommendations are based on only a handful of studies and may not work for all women. Still, at least when it comes to vitamin B_6, there seems to be a verifiable mechanism for action. This vitamin plays a role in the metabolism of serotonin, and there are some studies showing that it can alleviate the depression associated with the use of birth control pills. Women should take care not to exceed the recommended dosage of vitamin B_6, since nerve damage from overdose (2,000 mg or more daily) can occur. Many clinicians prescribe vitamin E to relieve breast pain, although there is no scientific proof that this vitamin actually does any good. But, as with lifestyle modifications, the cost and risk of vitamin and mineral supplements (in recommended amounts) is low enough to justify giving them a try.

Some symptoms of PMS may also be amenable to drug therapy. One of the problems plaguing the research on these treatments is the lack of a universally accepted definition of PMS and a universally accepted method of measuring symptoms. What this means is that studies are apt to involve a diverse group of women, many of whom may not actually have PMS or may have different forms of PMS—not all of which respond well to whatever medication is being tested. In addition, there is a considerable placebo effect in many of the drug studies—that is, the women taking "sugar pills" do just as well as the women taking the drug.

The few randomized clinical trials of medications published to date do afford some promise. Some of these trials involve drugs that treat specific symptoms of PMS. For example, taking nonsteroidal antiinflammatory drugs (such as ibuprofen or naproxen) can help relieve pelvic pain and may also reduce fatigue, mood swings, and headache. The diuretic drug spironolactone seems effective in relieving bloating and edema if taken during the luteal (second) phase of the menstrual cycle. Taking low doses of bromocriptine during this phase of the cycle seems to relieve severe breast pain.

Hormonal therapy can be effective, although the side effects may make it impractical. Drugs called GnRH (gonadotropin releasing hormone) analogs (such as Lupron or Synarel), for example, seem to relieve both physical and psychological symptoms of PMS. But, besides being very expensive, they cannot be used for more than 6 months without seriously compromising bone density; in the future it may be possible to overcome some of this effect by taking supplements of estrogen and progesterone. Bothersome side effects, including excess hair growth, acne, and hot flashes, also limit the use of danazol, a synthetic antiestrogenic hormone.

For years researchers in the field have had high hopes for progesterone supplements, but the results of the many studies so far are conflicting. Some studies indicate that taking progesterone may actually worsen premenstrual symptoms. As for birth control pills, these seem to affect only a small number of premenstrual symptoms. Yet, if a woman with PMS chooses to use the pill for contraception, she may be pleasantly surprised to find that some of her PMS symptoms disappear at the same time.

Finally, some psychotropic agents seem to relieve certain premenstrual symptoms. For example, using an antidepressant such as fluoxetine (Prozac), citalopram (Celexa), or sertraline (Zoloft) appears to be beneficial, probably because it alters serotonin levels. Another drug that affects serotonin, D-fenfluramine, also seems to reduce depression and stem calorie, fat, and carbohydrate consumption in women with PMS. This drug is not currently available in the United States.

The antianxiety drug alprazolam (Xanax) seems to alleviate both anxiety and depression, as well as physical symptoms, whether it is taken during the luteal phase or throughout the menstrual cycle, although the chances of becoming dependent on this medication can be reduced by restricting its use to the luteal phase. There is also some limited evidence that the beta-blocking drug atenolol may help relieve premenstrual irritability and reduce premenstrual migraine headaches.

Other treatment alternatives on the horizon may one day make it possible to avoid drug therapy. There has been some success, for example, in alleviating depression with bright light treatments or late sleep deprivation (awakening at 2 A.M.) as soon as symptoms begin.

If all else fails, and if symptoms are intolerable, hysterectomy (including the removal of both ovaries) is another option. This is a drastic solution that should not be undertaken without a second opinion from a physician experienced in the care of women with PMS.

Related entries

Acne, alcohol, anemia, antiinflammatory drugs, anxiety disorders, birth control, breast pain, coffee, depression, diuretics, edema, endometriosis, estrogen, exercise, fatigue, headaches, hirsutism, hypothyroidism, hysterectomy, menstrual cycle, ovary removal, panic disorder, pelvic pain, postpartum psychiatric disorders, psychotherapy, sleep disorders, stress, substance abuse, uterine fibroids, vitamins

Prenatal Care

Prenatal care is a term that includes all the preventive measures followed during pregnancy to maximize the health of both the mother and the baby. Involving both early and regular medical checkups and self-care practiced by the pregnant woman, good prenatal care also makes possible the early detection of various complications of pregnancy. These include gestational diabetes, preeclampsia, anemia, urinary tract infections, genetic abnormalities, abnormal fetal presentation or growth, and cholestasis of pregnancy (intense itching attributable to the suppression of bile secretion from the liver).

Much of the improvement in both maternal and fetal health in this country in recent decades is almost certainly attributable to improvements in prenatal care. For example, federal health researchers have speculated that lack of adequate prenatal care may help explain why African American women are more than twice as likely as white women to deliver low birth weight infants. A recent survey by the National Center for Health Statistics showed that black women were 20 percent more likely than white women to say that their doctor never told them about the dangers of smoking during pregnancy and 30 percent more likely to say that they were never counseled about alcohol consumption.

A study conducted at the Madigan Army Medical Center in Tacoma, Washington, indicated that short spacing between pregnancies may also account for some of the differences in outcome between ethnic groups. The study concluded that women need at least 9 months between pregnancies to build up the nutritional reserves optimal for a growing fetus. Despite equivalent economic and educational circumstances, the black women in the study were much more likely to have babies close together and also to have higher rates of premature delivery.

Prenatal visits

Early and regular medical checkups by an obstetrician, family practitioner, general practitioner, or nurse-midwife are the cornerstone of good prenatal care. Women who have the option of choosing their own clinician should consider not only the cost and convenience but also the hospital at which the clinician delivers (if applicable), the backup physician available (in the case of a midwife), and the personality of the clinician.

Above all, a woman should find out the clinician's philosophy about prenatal screening, natural childbirth and the use of anesthesia, and fetal monitoring and cesarean sections, so that she can make sure the clinician's attitudes about when and how to intervene during the course of pregnancy, labor, and delivery match her own intentions. When it is not possible to choose her clinician, a woman should make a point of expressing her own values and desires early in the process of prenatal care so that a mutually agreeable plan can be made.

The first prenatal visit should be scheduled as soon as a woman learns (or suspects) she is pregnant. For most women, this visit is scheduled for the 12th week of pregnancy.

The first prenatal visit is usually the longest. The woman is asked for a personal and family medical history and then has a thorough physical examination, often including a pelvic examination, to determine her overall state of health and to confirm the pregnancy. The clinician estimates the baby's due date and evaluates the woman's pelvis—in a process called pelvimetry—to see if an uncomplicated vaginal delivery seems possible. A Pap test may be done if the woman has not had one recently. Blood samples are taken for various laboratory tests, including a complete blood count, an identification of blood type, and a check for Rh factor, gonorrhea, syphilis, and antibodies that indicate whether the woman has already had German measles (rubella) and whether she has been exposed to hepatitis. A urine sample is taken to see if it contains protein or sugar and to find out if the woman has a urinary tract infection. Many clinicians now screen for chlamydia (see entry) and HIV (the virus that causes AIDS) as well.

If the woman is over 35, has a family history of genetic defects, or is a member of an ethnic group susceptible to certain genetic diseases, the clinician may suggest that she consider genetic counseling and ultrasound, amniocentesis, or chorionic villi sampling (see entries). The clinician will also briefly describe what to expect during pregnancy, discuss nutrition and exercise guidelines, and will give information about what medications and other substances to avoid. Often the clinician will recommend practicing especially vigilant dental hygiene and scheduling an appointment with a dentist, since gum problems are common during pregnancy. Many clinicians prescribe prenatal vitamins at this time as well. (Women who received preconception counseling will already be taking prenatal vitamins, particularly folate, during this critical period.)

After this first appointment the woman will be seen every 4 to 6 weeks until the eighth month of pregnancy, when appointments are usually scheduled every 2 weeks. In the ninth month, most clinicians want to see the woman every week. Women with underlying medical conditions such as hypertension, heart disease, or diabetes will need to be seen more often and start the care earlier. At all examinations the woman's weight and blood pressure will be measured, her urine will be checked for sugar and protein, the size of her uterus will be assessed, as will the size, position, and heart rate of the fetus. Many clinicians routinely take a blood sample at about 16 weeks' gestation for an alpha-fetoprotein test (or the triple screen test, which is more sensitive) to screen for neural tube defects such as spina bifida and for Down syndrome. Pregnant women are routinely screened for gestational diabetes by 30 weeks of pregnancy, with special attention paid to women with risk factors such as hypertension and obesity. Some clinicians do a blood test to check for anemia between weeks 28 and 32.

Weight gain

Pregnant women have traditionally claimed to be eating for two. This was a particularly difficult stance to take 30 or 40 years ago, when these same women were also warned not to gain more than 10 or 15 pounds lest they deliver huge babies, develop preeclampsia, or lose their figure. Current thinking is that pregnant women do not need to eat vast quantities of food—most women, in fact, need to add only about 300 extra calories per day—but rather need to select foods more carefully, with the goal of eating a diet rich in protein, fresh fruits and vegetables, whole grains, and dairy products (see nutrition). Previous exhortations to cut out protein and salt (supposedly to prevent preeclampsia as well as to keep weight down) are now considered not just pointless but actually dangerous.

Most pregnant women who are eating appropriately will find that they naturally gain between 22 and 27 pounds—the recommended gain for a woman who starts out at normal weight. Underweight women ought to gain a little more and overweight women a little less. This gain includes not only the weight of the fetus but also the weight of the amniotic fluid and placenta, as well as the increased weight of the mother's uterus, breasts, blood supply, and body fluids. A good rule of thumb is to aim at gaining about a quarter of the total weight between weeks 12 and 20, about half between weeks 20 and 30, and the final quarter between weeks 30 and 40. A good diet supplies enough of virtually all necessary nutrients, with the exception of folic acid, iron, and sometimes calcium. Taking prenatal vitamins can make up for this deficiency.

Exercise, activity, and travel

Mild to moderate exercise is not only permissible but desirable during pregnancy. It is probably not a good idea for pre-viously sedentary women to start jogging or swimming a mile a day, but there is usually no reason for a woman not to continue doing the same exercises she was doing before she became pregnant. The exception may be activities associated with a risk of dangerous falls or those that increase the pulse rate to over 140. Walking is particularly healthful, as are exercise classes designed specifically for pregnant women; often a clinician can recommend a class taught by a qualified instructor. Pregnant women should also get in the habit of practicing Kegel exercises regularly to help prepare the pelvic muscles for childbirth.

Most healthy pregnant women can plan to continue working until a short time before their due date, although some find it easier to cut back on activities in the last month or so, especially if they are feeling fatigued. Some forms of work involving heavy lifting or long periods of standing may be inadvisable, as well as work involving exposure to certain chemicals or ionizing radiation (see occupational hazards). There is no evidence that video display terminals are dangerous to pregnant women or their fetuses in any way. Women who think that conditions in their workplace might be harmful to their fetus should check with their clinician. In these cases they may want to consider requesting a temporary transfer to a safer job.

Travel—whether by car, boat, train, or plane—is also usually safe during pregnancy, though certain precautions and advance planning may be necessary. Women traveling by car or boat in the first trimester, for example, may be particularly prone to nausea and should consult a clinician before taking any anti–motion sickness medications. Seatbelts should always be worn during car travel, with the lap belt placed snugly above the upper thighs (never above the abdomen) and the shoulder belt running between the breasts. Pregnant women traveling at any point in pregnancy should think about where they would seek emergency medical care should it become necessary (especially in the case of foreign travel). During the last 6 weeks of pregnancy, any woman who travels should accept the possibility that she may have to deliver the baby in an unfamiliar setting with an unfamiliar clinician.

Travel in unpressurized airplanes at very high altitudes is not advisable, but this is not a concern for women who use only commercial airlines. There is no evidence that the radiation from airport metal detectors poses any risk to the fetus.

Medications and other risks

Virtually any drug taken by a pregnant woman can affect the fetus and should be approached with caution. This does not mean that pregnant women should abandon medications prescribed to them by physicians. In some cases the benefits of the drug to the mother outweigh by far the risks to the fetus. Nevertheless, a pregnant woman should always consult her clinician before taking any prescription medication or (with some exceptions, see chart) over-the-counter drug, and she should alert her clinician to any other medical conditions she may have. Also, if she is seeing a specialist for some

Medications that are safe to use during pregnancy

Symptom	Acceptable medication	Comment
Pain or fever	Acetaminophen (Tylenol)	Avoid aspirin and nonsteroidal antiinflammatory drugs except under a doctor's orders
Colds or coughs	Actifed, Sudafed, Co-Tylenol for congestion, or any Robitussin cough syrup	
Infections	Antibiotics such as penicillin and penicillin derivatives. Women allergic to penicillins can use erythromycin. Sulfa drugs (sulfonamides) are generally considered safe until the third trimester.	Avoid tetracyclines, which can discolor the baby's teeth. Avoid Ciprofloxacin (quinolones), which can cause severe bone abnormalities
Constipation	Some stool softeners and laxatives including Metamucil, Milk of Magnesia, Peri-Colace, Colace, Senokot, Surfak	
Heartburn or indigestion	Antacids including Maalox, Mylanta, Riopan	
Diarrhea	Kaopectate or Pepto-Bismol	

condition not related to the pregnancy (including a dentist who wants to take x-rays), she should mention that she is pregnant. Many other substances can potentially harm the fetus and should be avoided by pregnant women when possible (see chart).

Preparation for the birth

Childbirth education classes help prepare a woman (and usually her partner) for labor and delivery. There are several different methods and sets of values guiding these classes. All, however, share a general belief that knowing something about the childbirth process in advance and learning certain breathing and relaxation exercises can help take some of the fear and pain out of labor, and may reduce the need for anesthesia, forceps, and other medical interventions that may pose a risk to the fetus. Many classes also cover topics such as infant care, breastfeeding, and postpartum adjustments.

Usually these classes meet for an hour or two a week for about 8 weeks, starting early in the third trimester of pregnancy. Often they are covered by insurance and may also be tax deductible. There are refresher classes available for women who have already had babies, as well as sibling preparation classes and repeat c-section classes. Some centers even offer intensive weekend courses for busy couples who do not have time for 8 separate sessions.

In addition to learning more about childbirth itself, women in the last trimester of pregnancy should start thinking about securing medical care for the newborn. For some women this simply involves making the acquaintance of a pediatrician or primary care provider in their health maintenance organization and making arrangements for care after the delivery. Women who have more choice may want to ask their clinician, as well as friends who already have children, to recommend pediatricians, family practitioners, or other clinicians who provide pediatric care. Many of these professionals are happy to talk with a pregnant woman who wants to know more about their philosophy, personality, and policies.

Related entries

Alpha-fetoprotein screening, amniocentesis, cesarean section, childbirth, chorionic villi sampling, exercise, Kegel exercises, midwifery, miscarriage, morning sickness, nutrition, occupational hazards, postpartum issues, preeclampsia, pregnancy, prenatal genetic counseling, Rh disease, rubella, toxoplasmosis, ultrasound

Drugs and chemicals that can adversely affect a pregnancy

Medication	Effects
Amphetamines (diet pills)	Heart defects; blood vessel malformations
Androgens	Genital abnormalities
Anticoagulants, such as warfarin (Coumadin) or dicumarol	Eye, bone, and cartilage abnormalities, including cleft lip, cleft palate; central nervous system defects
Anticonvulsants, such as valproic acid (Depakene), phenytoin (Dilantin), paramethadione (Paradione), and trimethadione (Tridione)	Neural tube defects; abnormal development; growth and mental retardation
Aspirin in large doses	Miscarriage; hemorrhage in newborn
Birth control pills	Arm and leg malformations; defects in internal organs; masculinization of females
Chemotherapeutic agents, such as methotrexate	Miscarriage; various fetal abnormalities
Cortisone	Various fetal and placental abnormalities, including cleft lip and stillbirth
Diethylstilbestrol (DES)	Numerous abnormalities in cervix and uterus of female fetuses; possible infertility in both males and females
Diuretics	Blood disorders; jaundice
Isotretinoin (Accutane)	Miscarriage; severe birth defects, including heart defects, cleft palate, ear deformities
Lithium	Congenital heart disease
Nasal decongestant sprays	Reduce oxygen and nutrition to fetus by contracting blood vessels in placenta
Quinolones	Severe bone abnormalities
Tetracycline	Underdevelopment of tooth enamel; incorporation of tetracycline into bone
Thalidomide	Growth deficiency and other abnormalities
Chemical	
Lead	Miscarriage; stillbirths
Organic mercury	Brain disorders
Pesticides	Depends on specific chemical. Pregnant women should have someone else ventilate their home if extermination is necessary

(continued)

Other	Effects
Alcohol	Growth and mental retardation; fetal alcohol syndrome
Cat litter boxes	Toxoplasmosis
Herbs, including blue or black cohosh, pennyroyal, mugwort, tansy, slippery elm	Miscarriage
Illicit drugs	Numerous effects depending on the specific drug, including miscarriage, stillbirth, developmental abnormalities, growth and mental retardation, premature delivery, low birth weight, addicted newborns
Raw or undercooked meat	Toxoplasmosis
X-rays	Growth and mental retardation
Smoking cigarettes	Miscarriage, stillbirth, premature delivery, low birth weight, sudden infant death syndrome (SIDS). Smoking also increases the mother's risk of complications, including vaginal bleeding

Prenatal Genetic Counseling

Genetic counseling has become a routine part of prenatal care for many women at increased risk of carrying a congenitally abnormal fetus. The process usually starts with a woman's primary care physician or obstetrician, who will review the family medical histories of the woman and her partner—as well as their ethnic backgrounds, vocations, and habits—to identify the risk of various abnormalities. If the couple desires more in-depth information (possibly because of a family history of chromosomal abnormalities), or if there was a previous problem pregnancy, the physician will refer the couple to a counselor specially trained in genetics. Oftentimes, the couple has a session with a genetic counselor if the woman is pregnant and over 35.

Some genetic abnormalities are life-threatening or else will result in disabilities so severe that the offspring will experience pain and suffering, will require costly medical care that may not improve the quality of life, or will never be able to live self-sufficiently. Other abnormalities will result in only minor dysfunction, readjustment, or expense. Determining which is pertinent in their case and then deciding what to do with the information is influenced by the couple's religious, moral, philosophical, social, and economic circumstances. A session with a genetic counselor can facilitate this process by helping them elucidate their values and constraints. Some

couples will choose to terminate a pregnancy in which the fetus is malformed or carries a serious genetic defect, while others will use the advance information to plan for the birth and care of a child with a disability.

A genetic counselor will also explain the tests available to screen for genetic abnormalities, as well as the risks and limitations of these procedures. Should a test reveal a problem, the counselor will review options such as abortion or adoption. If counseling occurs prior to conception, assisted reproductive techniques (see infertility) that can reduce the risks of some genetic disorders may be an option.

Who should have prenatal genetic counseling?

Prenatal genetic counseling is often recommended for women who will be 35 or older at the expected date of delivery. Other women at increased risk of bearing genetically abnormal children are those with a family history of genetic disease such as hemophilia, Tay-Sachs, sickle cell anemia, thalassemia, or cystic fibrosis. Counseling may also be recommended for women who have been exposed to certain environmental toxins or contagious diseases during pregnancy, as well as to women who have had multiple miscarriages.

In women of any age, if an ultrasound suggests malformations, further genetic screening and counseling may be advisable. Even some minor malformations found in ultrasound examination such as abnormal length of the leg and arm bones, size of kidneys, and thickness at the back of the neck have been linked to Down syndrome.

Down syndrome. The risk of some genetic defects—especially Down syndrome (see illustration)—increases with the mother's age. The risk of having a baby with Down syndrome is 1 in 1,250 at the age of 24, but by the age of 36 the risk rises to 1 in 289—higher than the risk of miscarrying as a result of amniocentesis, the procedure most commonly used to screen for genetic defects (see illustration). By age 40 the risk of bearing a child with Down syndrome is about 1 in 100. It should be remembered, however, that 80 percent of Down syndrome babies are born to women under 35 since so many more babies are born to these women in the first place.

Hemophilia and other sex-linked disorders. Genetic screening will be recommended for couples at high risk for a sex-linked disorder such as hemophilia. Normally, women have two X chromosomes (one of each is inherited from their parents) and men have one X (inherited from their mother) and one Y (from their father). In sex-linked disorders the mother has one defective X chromosome, but her other, normal X chromosome protects her from having symptoms. Her sons, however, who will inherit only one of her two X chro-

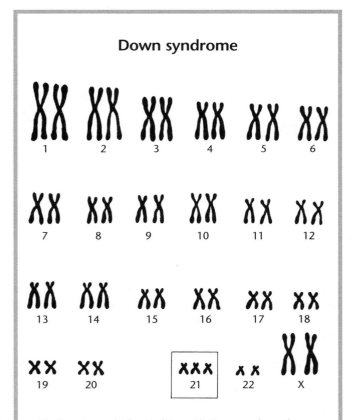

Down syndrome

The karyotype of a female fetus with Down syndrome has an extra chromosome number 21. This condition most often results from an incomplete separation of the chromosomes when the egg is formed in the ovary.

mosomes and have no second X chromosome to protect them, have a 50 percent chance of inheriting the defective X and therefore developing the disease. Often, prenatal diagnosis allows the presence or absence of the disease, as well as the sex of the fetus, to be determined.

Tay-Sachs disease. Approximately 1 in 22 people of Ashkenazi (eastern European) Jewish descent carry a recessive gene for Tay-Sachs disease, a degenerative neurologic condition which almost always results in a child's death by the age of 4 (see illustration). Descendants of French Canadians also have an increased prevalence of the Tay-Sachs gene. Because the disease manifests itself only in people with two copies of the gene, "carriers" do not show any symptoms. If a carrier has children with another carrier, however, each offspring has a 1 in 4 chance of inheriting both defective genes and therefore developing the disease. Any couple that suspects they may carry the Tay-Sachs gene can be screened with a blood test before conception to determine if they are at risk. Prenatal diagnosis of the fetus can be undertaken with amniocentesis.

Sickle cell anemia. This disease results from a mutation in the gene responsible for producing part of the hemoglobin molecule; hemoglobin is the component of red blood cells that carries oxygen to body tissues. A person who inherits two copies of the defective gene will develop sickle cell anemia. In people with this painful condition, the abnormal hemoglobin molecules cause the red blood cells to take on a crescent or sickle shape, and the person becomes anemic. The patient may also have episodes of pain—and may develop infections, jaundice, and leg ulcers—because sickle cells are poor transporters of oxygen, and they tend to clog up capillaries in vital organs, further reducing their oxygen supply (see anemia).

Approximately 1 in 10 African Americans carries a single copy of the sickle cell gene, making that person a carrier of the genetic defect while not having the disease itself. People of Hispanic, Central American, Greek, Italian, Arabic, Cuban, Puerto Rican, and Haitian descent also have a higher frequency of this gene than the rest of the population, as do people from certain parts of India and Pakistan. If two carriers have a child together, the risk that the child will develop the disease is 1 in 4. If a couple are both carriers and the woman becomes pregnant, prenatal diagnosis with amniocentesis can be offered.

Thalassemia. Other inherited blood disorders include the thalassemias, which involve various structural abnormalities in hemoglobin molecules (see anemia). At about 3 months of age, babies with a variant of the disease called beta thalassemia start to develop chronic anemia and require frequent blood transfusions, leading to other serious complications. A different genetic defect results in alpha thalassemia minor, a less severe condition that involves mild anemia and is often confused with iron-deficiency anemia.

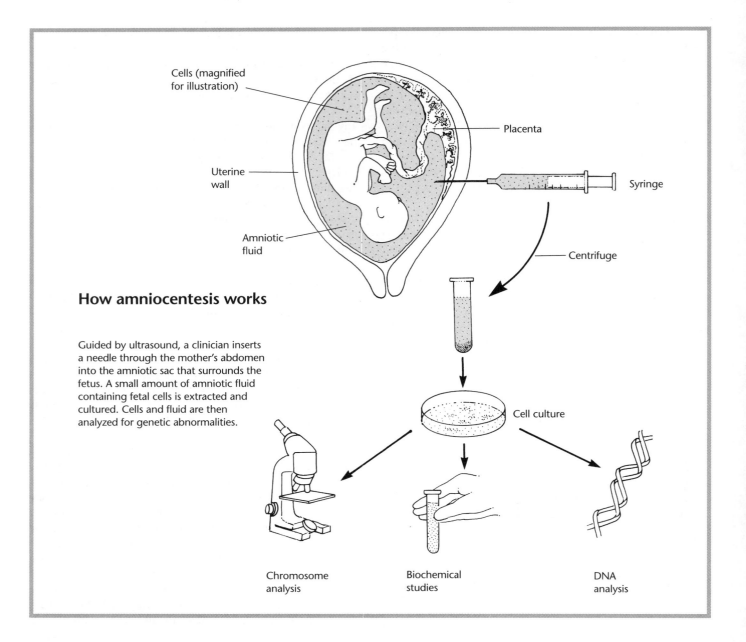

Cells (magnified for illustration)

Placenta

Uterine wall

Syringe

Amniotic fluid

Centrifuge

How amniocentesis works

Guided by ultrasound, a clinician inserts a needle through the mother's abdomen into the amniotic sac that surrounds the fetus. A small amount of amniotic fluid containing fetal cells is extracted and cultured. Cells and fluid are then analyzed for genetic abnormalities.

Cell culture

Chromosome analysis

Biochemical studies

DNA analysis

Couples at high risk for carrying a thalassemia gene are those of Greek, Italian, Turkish, Middle Eastern, Hispanic, Vietnamese, Laotian, Cambodian, Filipino, Southern Chinese, North African, Pakistani, or Indian descent. There is a 1 in 4 chance that a baby conceived by two carriers will inherit thalassemia. Screening involves a blood test followed by prenatal diagnosis by amniocentesis if necessary.

Cystic fibrosis. Whites are at the highest risk of carrying a gene for cystic fibrosis, another genetic disease which results when the baby inherits two copies of the cystic fibrosis (CF) gene. In this disease, in which thick and sticky mucus clogs the respiratory system and pancreas and promotes bacterial infection, life expectancy is 28 years. Approximately 1 in 25 whites carries the CF gene, although other groups are also at

relatively high risk (1 in 45 Hispanics, 1 in 60 African Americans, and 1 in 150 Asians). Screening for this condition involves a blood test to identify CF mutations by looking at DNA.

What prenatal genetic tests are available?
New techniques often allow couples at risk to see if one or both are carriers even before conception. Although the specific technique varies for each condition, all involve taking a blood sample from the potential parents so that their chromosomes can be analyzed.

Currently only 85 percent of carriers for cystic fibrosis can be determined, since 15 percent of carriers have not yet been linked to a specific genetic mutation on the chromosomes. If, after genetic screening, only one parent is known to be a car-

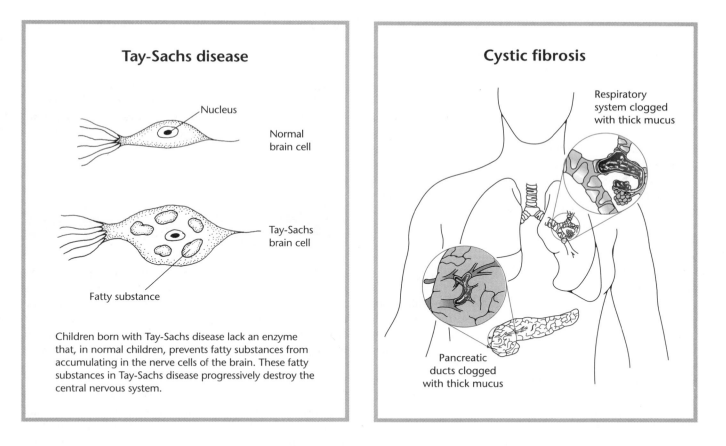

Tay-Sachs disease

Nucleus

Normal brain cell

Tay-Sachs brain cell

Fatty substance

Children born with Tay-Sachs disease lack an enzyme that, in normal children, prevents fatty substances from accumulating in the nerve cells of the brain. These fatty substances in Tay-Sachs disease progressively destroy the central nervous system.

Cystic fibrosis

Respiratory system clogged with thick mucus

Pancreatic ducts clogged with thick mucus

rier, there is still a very small chance that the other parent is a carrier as well and that the offspring will be affected with the disease. If both parents are known to be carriers, however, the risk to the child is much greater: 1 in 4.

Once carrier status is determined, a couple will be better equipped to decide whether to pursue further genetic counseling and prenatal screening through a technique such as amniocentesis or chorionic villi sampling (CVS), should a pregnancy occur. Such tests can screen for Down syndrome, as well as less common and more severe genetic defects in which there are three rather than two copies of a specific chromosome. They can also determine Turner syndrome, Klinefelter syndrome, and other conditions that result from defective numbers of sex chromosomes. In Turner syndrome (see entry), female fetuses have only one sex chromosome, an X. As adults they are short in stature and do not develop secondary sex characteristics; they are also infertile and have a constellation of other organic problems. In Klinefelter syndrome, male fetuses have an extra X chromosome, making them XXY. As adults they are infertile and tend to be unusually tall, with small testes, enlarged breasts, and poorly developed secondary sex characteristics.

High-risk couples who would consider aborting an affected fetus sometimes prefer CVS even though in many medical centers it remains a slightly riskier procedure than amniocentesis. This is because CVS allows women the option of knowing the genetic status of their fetus as early as 9 to 12 weeks of pregnancy, a time when termination is somewhat easier, psy-

chologically as well as physically. Another option is early amniocentesis, done at 10 to 12 weeks' gestation. There is less associated pregnancy loss than with CVS, and the recovery of cells appears to be the same as with amniocentesis done between 16 and 20 weeks. Women at lower risk, such as those over 35 without any known genetic abnormality, may also choose CVS because of the timing, although most still prefer amniocentesis.

For couples at risk for sex-linked disorders, a newer technique called preimplantation biopsy may soon be used after in vitro fertilization to determine the sex of the embryo before it is placed in the uterus. In humans, though, this remains a difficult procedure to carry out. In the case of genetic disorders such as cystic fibrosis and hemophilia, even before in vitro fertilization the genetic material in the tissue known as the "polar body" (which is produced at the same time as the egg and is its genetic equivalent) can be analyzed to see if the egg carries a defective gene.

Another technique that is available (though only rarely appropriate) is called percutaneous umbilical cord blood sampling (PUBS). Performed from about 18 weeks' gestation until the end of pregnancy, PUBS involves checking the fetus's blood for some diseases and evaluating reasons for slow fetal growth. Results generally take about 4 days, depending on what is being measured. Certain blood disorders, for example, take only a couple of hours to diagnose. PUBS is relatively risky (with a fetal loss rate of 1 to 2 percent), but for some indications it is the standard of care, including when the decision to have genetic testing is made so late in the pregnancy that rapid results are necessary.

Less invasive techniques to help determine the genetic status of their offspring may be appropriate for many women. Ultrasound imaging, though still limited in its ability to detect genetic abnormalities, can at least suggest whether or not further screening might be desirable, especially when used in conjunction with the triple marker test (see alpha-fetoprotein screening). On the horizon are improved tests of the fetal cells that appear in the mother's blood. The result of advances in molecular genetics, these tests can now separate fetal from maternal cells and identify minute quantities of fetal DNA (genetic material). Eventually these techniques may allow fetuses with genetic defects to be identified with less risk to the fetus than current methods.

What are the risks and complications of prenatal counseling?

Genetic counseling can be costly and time-consuming, but this expense must be contrasted to the cost, time, and pain involved in bearing, raising, and perhaps losing a child with a genetic abnormality. Even couples who would not consider terminating a pregnancy may find that genetic counseling prepares them and their family for the arrival of a child with special needs. Information obtained through genetic screening can also signal the need for delivery at a hospital that has the facilities to care for such a child.

One aspect of prenatal testing that is often overlooked relates to the negative side of knowledge. Although it is true that prior knowledge of a defect obvious at birth—such as Down syndrome—may help a family make advance preparations, knowing about a less obvious defect may actually be detrimental to both the family and the potential child. In the case of various sex chromosome anomalies, for example, in which the fetus has extra or missing X or Y chromosomes, the associated conditions may not be obvious until the child reaches puberty—or even later. A parent who learns through amniocentesis or CVS that a fetus has one of these conditions will nonetheless be told that the child has a high probability of having certain learning disabilities or behavioral traits, although studies are still extremely limited.

Some parents may view this knowledge as an opportunity to begin early intervention—or to terminate the pregnancy. But others will see it as a serious blight on their relationship with the child. They may end up expecting less of this child than of their other children, or interpreting every action in light of the chromosomal makeup. If they had not had the testing, they might never have thought that anything at all was wrong with the child.

When considering genetic testing, therefore, each couple needs to be aware that, instead of getting advance warning of a rare fatal, painful, or expensive condition, they may end up learning something about their child which they might prefer never to have known. In the process of deciding whether to undergo genetic testing, a couple needs to examine carefully their personal feelings about these issues, in light of the information and recommendations that a clinician can provide.

Related entries

Abortion, alpha-fetoprotein screening, amniocentesis, anemia, chorionic villi sampling, infertility, miscarriage, preconception counseling, pregnancy over age 35, prenatal care, testicular feminization syndrome, Turner syndrome, ultrasound

Prolapsed Uterus

A prolapsed uterus occurs when the uterus drops down into the vagina (see illustration). It is due to the weakening of the muscles and tissues that normally support the uterus. Sometimes in women with a prolapsed uterus, other internal organs—the bladder, the urethra, the rectum, or part of the intestine—may also bulge into the vagina, for the same reason.

Who is likely to develop uterine prolapse?

Uterine prolapse (also called a fallen uterus or uterine descensus) is generally a by-product of aging, injury to vaginal tissues, or both. It is most common in women who have delivered babies vaginally, particularly if they have had many children or experienced long or difficult labors or deliveries (which increase the chances of permanent damage to the pelvic support structures). Symptoms usually do not occur until after menopause, however, when a deficiency of the hormone estrogen weakens the supporting tissues further and decreases their blood supply.

In addition to childbirth, excessive abdominal pressure or stress can weaken pelvic support. For this reason, some jobs requiring heavy lifting can predispose women to uterine prolapse, as can being obese or wearing tight corsets or girdles. Disorders that cause long periods of coughing—including chronic bronchitis, asthma, and emphysema—can also put undue pressure on the abdomen and increase the chances of developing a prolapsed uterus.

Uterine prolapse often runs in families, so that a woman with an affected mother, sister, grandmother, aunt, or other female relative may be more likely than other women to develop it.

What are the symptoms?

Although it is possible to have a severely prolapsed uterus without having any symptoms, most women with this condition sense a sort of heaviness or bearing-down feeling in the pelvic region. Others may have a backache or find that they leak urine whenever they cough, sneeze, or laugh (this problem is known as stress incontinence; see incontinence). In severe prolapse, simply walking can become difficult because the uterus and cervix actually bulge through the vaginal

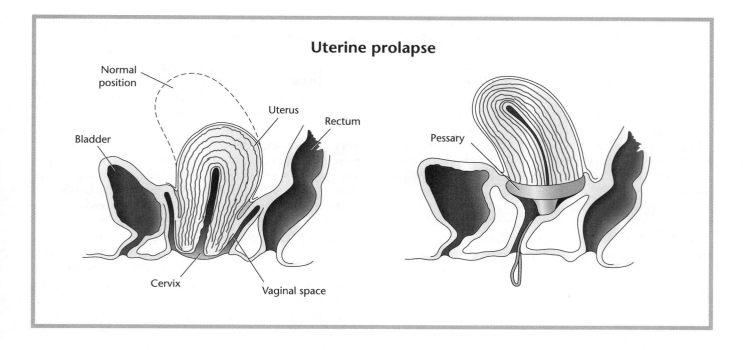

Uterine prolapse

Normal position

Uterus

Rectum

Bladder

Cervix

Vaginal space

Pessary

opening, possibly even bringing with them the bladder and the rectum. Because of gravity's pull, symptoms are usually worse while the woman is standing, increase as the day goes on, and may be relieved by lying down.

How is the condition evaluated?

A clinician will first do a thorough physical examination and a pelvic examination to determine all sites of damage. The woman will be asked to strain or bear down, usually in both a prone and a standing position, to see if this makes the uterus descend further into the vagina.

How is uterine prolapse treated?

Treatment for a prolapsed uterus depends on the degree of the prolapse, as well as the woman's age, overall health, and childbearing intentions. Mild forms of prolapse may require no treatment at all or may be remedied by doing exercises to strengthen the pelvic muscles (Kegel exercises). Women who are obese may find that losing weight helps relieve symptoms.

If the symptoms are more severe, several other options are available. For women who want to preserve childbearing potential or whose health puts them at too high a risk for surgery, the uterus can be supported with a rubber device called a pessary. Before fitting this device, a clinician will usually prescribe estrogen replacement therapy to postmenopausal women to help restore the vaginal tissues. This may involve weekly applications of an intravaginal cream or systemic estrogen supplements given in either tablet or patch form. The pessary should be rechecked 2 or 3 weeks after insertion to make sure it is not eroding vaginal tissue or causing any problems with urination.

Pessaries require a lot of maintenance (regular cleaning,

frequent checks for fit) and, because they are foreign bodies, can predispose a woman to vaginal irritation and infection (see vaginitis).

One way to reduce the chances of abrading vaginal tissue is to learn how to remove and replace the pessary at home. This allows a woman to take out her pessary each night, preventing round-the-clock contact and making sexual intercourse more feasible, since pessaries may shorten the vagina and interfere with penetration. If a woman removes her pessary herself, she should also clean it on a regular basis. A woman who feels uncomfortable removing and maintaining her own pessary, however, should see her clinician every 8 to 12 weeks so that the device can be cleaned and refitted.

Surgery is another option, especially for women past childbearing age, and it is the only permanent cure. It is an option for women who cannot retain a pessary, who dislike the meticulous care required, or who find that pessaries lose their effectiveness over the years. The surgery involves repairing any damaged support structures and is usually done through the vagina, although it may occasionally be performed through the abdomen. Any associated cystoceles, urethroceles, rectoceles, or enteroceles (bulging into the vagina of the bladder, urethra, rectal, or intestinal wall, respectively) can be repaired at the same time.

Many surgeons recommend a hysterectomy to remove a prolapsed uterus if symptoms are very bothersome, and especially if it protrudes through the vaginal opening. Although some women object to removing a perfectly healthy uterus, the repair of pelvic muscles (necessary to prevent other types of hernia) is often much easier and more effective once the uterus is gone. Women who want to preserve their uterus should discuss this matter with their surgeon—and seek a second opinion—before making any decisions.

Like any form of major surgery, repairing a prolapse carries certain risks (adverse reactions to anesthesia, infection, bleeding, scarring), but they are relatively low for women in reasonably good health. Putting off the surgery until advanced age only increases these risks.

How can uterine prolapse be prevented?

Women who think they may be prone to uterine prolapse may be able to prevent or reduce problems by regularly doing Kegel exercises. This is particularly true for pregnant women or women whose female relatives have had a prolapsed uterus.

Related entries

Asthma, breathing disorders, cystocele/urethrocele/ rectocele, estrogen replacement therapy, hysterectomy, incontinence, Kegel exercises, menopause, occupational hazards, vaginitis

Psychosomatic Disorders

People with psychosomatic disorders—called somatoform disorders by psychiatrists—show physical symptoms of disorders that cannot be linked to any identifiable disease process or injury. Instead, the symptoms seem to be triggered, amplified, or nurtured by social or psychological crises or stress. This process of developing a physical symptom as an expression of an emotional or mental state is called somatization.

It is easy for most people to accept that physical problems can affect the emotions. No one questions the connection between having incapacitating arthritis and feeling depressed, for example, or the connection between a diagnosis of terminal cancer and feeling afraid. The idea that emotions can affect the body, however, is less acceptable to many people. And yet anyone who has ever had stage fright knows very well the havoc wrought on the body by the mind. Producing tears when we feel sad or turning red when we feel embarrassed are other everyday examples of the mind's control of the body.

Researchers still do not fully understand just how the mind exerts power over the body (or, for that matter, how the body exerts power over the mind). The connection clearly has much to do with the many different brain chemicals called neurotransmitters. Emotions may somehow alter the levels of these chemicals and in turn alter the functioning of other parts of the body.

Types of psychosomatic disorders

Among the many forms of psychosomatic disorders are somatization disorder, conversion disorder (formerly called hysteria), hypochondria, and chronic pain syndrome. Some of these disorders have overlapping syndromes and may not be completely distinguishable. Sometimes physicians, frustrated with an inability to diagnose symptoms owing to limitations in the current state of medical knowledge, will tell women that their physical symptoms are psychological, which can be extremely frustrating. The distinction between a psychosomatic disorder and a difficult-to-diagnose underlying physical disorder can be a very gray area indeed.

Somatization disorder. People with this disorder have numerous physical complaints, none of which can be traced to any specific physical defect, or if there are physical causes, they are insufficient to account for the severity or duration of the distress. This does not make the symptom or the discomfort any less real, and people with somatization disorder may remain convinced (sometimes correctly) that there is a physical cause underlying their complaints, even if current medical science seems unable to uncover it. People with somatization disorder spend many frustrating years going from doctor to doctor without obtaining a satisfactory diagnosis. As they make the rounds, they are in danger of developing a substance abuse disorder as they are given numerous prescriptions for psychoactive medications.

Somatization disorder often begins in the teenage years but rarely after the age of 30. It occurs much more commonly in women than in men, and the risk of developing it is far higher in women who have first-degree relatives with somatization disorder or who have male relatives (either biological or adoptive) with histories of substance abuse or antisocial personality disorders.

Symptoms can involve gastrointestinal complaints, chest pain, headaches, breathing problems, weakness, or urinary problems. Women with somatization disorder sometimes have symptoms of the reproductive system that are unusually frequent or severe. These can include painful menstruation, irregular menstrual periods, excessive menstrual bleeding, and vomiting throughout pregnancy.

As with all psychosomatic disorders, somatization disorder often includes symptoms that indicate depression, including insomnia, poor appetite, and lack of interest in sex. Symptoms of both anxiety disorder and panic disorder are quite common, although they alone do not account for the physical complaints.

Conversion disorder. Previously called hysteria, conversion disorder involves a loss or alteration in some physical function that seems to have a physical origin but that is actually caused by specific psychological factors. It differs from somatization disorder (which sometimes includes symptoms of conversion disorder) because the physical problems are directly linked to some identifiable psychological conflict or need. A woman with violent feelings toward a husband who is cheating on her, for example, might develop amnesia as a way of keeping herself from acting on these feelings. A young girl with an alcoholic mother who neglects or abuses her might develop paralysis in the hand she might otherwise have used to strike back.

People with this disorder are not consciously producing the symptoms. The pain sometimes involves female reproductive organs or sexual dysfunction, but there are other symptoms in nonsexual areas as well. Among the most common are amnesia, blindness, partial or total paralysis, numbness, seizures, false pregnancy, excessive vomiting during pregnancy, and an inability to talk or swallow. Oddly enough, people with conversion disorder often maintain a striking serenity, termed *la belle indifférence* (the beautiful indifference), despite these dramatic problems.

Although conversion disorder is probably more common in women, it can occur in either sex. Its former name, hysteria, was coined by the ancient Greeks to describe a disease that supposedly resulted from a "wandering womb" (*hysterikos* is the Greek word for "uterus"). For many centuries hysteria was thought of as a physical disease linked to the uterus or, later, the female reproductive organs in general. A woman might go blind, for example, because excessive menstrual bleeding deprived her brain of nourishment. In the eighteenth and nineteenth centuries the nervous system replaced the uterus as the presumed source of the disease, but hysteria was still thought of as a woman's disorder.

Eventually psychiatrists such as Sigmund Freud turned the definition on its head by viewing mental states (usually involving sexuality) as the cause rather than the effect of the physical problems. From this perspective hysterical blindness might result because a woman was repressing a deep-seated conflict: she became blind to avoid having to see something she both desired and feared.

Discarded now by both psychiatrists (because it does not refer to a specific disease) and feminists (because it connotes misogyny, that is, hatred of women), the term hysteria has been replaced by the term conversion disorder. Today the psychiatric community no longer views the physical symptoms of conversion disorder as real in any objective way. Although a woman with conversion disorder may truly be unable to see, the thinking goes, her "blindness" cannot be accounted for by a recognizable defect in the visual system. The root of the symptoms is not physiological but rather psychosomatic: people with this disorder unintentionally convert psychological or sexual conflicts into physical symptoms.

Conversion disorder most commonly appears in adolescence or early adulthood. People with other psychiatric illnesses—in particular, major depression—or certain personality disorders (such as dependent and histrionic types) are particularly likely to develop it. Some investigators regard conversion disorder as analogous to combat neurosis in men, viewing it as a posttraumatic stress disorder, which in women most commonly occurs as a result of sexual assault, incest, or domestic abuse.

Hypochondria. People with hypochondria are preoccupied with the belief or fear that they have a serious illness despite medical reassurance to the contrary. Like people with other psychosomatic disorders, hypochondriacs have genuine physical complaints—probably triggered or amplified by some kind of emotional stress—for which no underlying physical defect can be found. The distinction is that people with hypochondria involuntarily let their lives revolve around these symptoms, which they can describe in excruciating detail. Despite reassurance from health care practitioners, these people remain convinced that they have a serious illness. This conviction is not delusional, however, and people with hypochondria can acknowledge the possibility that their fears or beliefs may be unfounded.

In women, hypochondria tends to develop in mid-life, later than the onset of most other psychosomatic disorders. It is particularly common in people with symptoms of an obsessive-compulsive disorder—a kind of anxiety disorder characterized by persistent and repetitive thoughts or actions. Sometimes a transient period of hypochondria may also occur as part of an acute grief reaction. Like other psychosomatic disorders, hypochondria frequently includes symptoms associated with depression, such as insomnia, loss of appetite, and lowered sex drive. Often people with hypochondria also have symptoms of anxiety and substance abuse.

Chronic pain syndrome. Chronic pain can be the result of a number of medical conditions such as back injury or cancer. But people with chronic pain syndrome (also known as somatoform pain disorder and formerly as psychogenic pain disorder) experience pain that is incompatible with their physical abnormalities. In some cases people have an actual injury or disease, or have recently had surgery, but their pain is much more severe or long-lasting than would normally be expected. Others feel relentless pain with no identifiable physical defect at all. Chronic pain syndrome involves pain anywhere in the body which has lasted at least 6 months.

Whatever its source, chronic pain often wreaks havoc with people's lives, leaving them debilitated, jobless, angry, demoralized, alienated from friends and family, and frequently dependent on narcotic painkillers. In at least half the people with this syndrome, the first symptoms develop suddenly following some specific physical trauma. In the next weeks or months the pain becomes more severe. It can be so unrelenting that basic functioning becomes a challenge, and many people stop working, seek disability compensation, and visit doctor after doctor, perhaps undergoing numerous ineffectual surgical operations along the way and taking larger and larger doses of narcotic painkillers for relief. Because these drugs become less effective over time, drug dependency results.

Many people with chronic pain syndrome believe that their pain can be traced to a physical injury or disease still not understood by medical science. In some cases they may be right, since our understanding of the human body continues to evolve. Still, there is ample evidence that psychological factors often contribute to the pain. This does not mean that the pain is any less real or that the patient is purposely faking it. It does mean, however, that, without the patient's being aware of it, the pain may be a way of coping with some psychological or emotional stress. A woman who feels guilty about putting her mother in a nursing home may develop chest pains after her mother dies of a heart attack, for example.

Chronic pain syndrome can begin at any age but most often starts in the middle years. It occurs about twice as often in women as in men and is extremely common in people who were physically or sexually abused as children. In fact, over half of all patients treated for this syndrome have a history of being abused as children. Often people with chronic pain syndrome also have symptoms of depression such as insomnia, lack of appetite, and loss of interest in sex. In addition, they may have symptoms of fibromyalgia (see entry), which can have a sudden onset following an injury.

What causes psychosomatic disorders?

Exactly how and why psychosomatic disorders occur has been explained from a variety of viewpoints. In many cases psychosomatic disorders may be symptoms of other psychiatric disorders, including major depression, panic disorder, other anxiety disorders, and personality disorders. In other cases psychosomatic symptoms may be better interpreted as symbolic expressions of some underlying conflict. Some individuals with psychosomatic disorders may simply feel bodily sensations more intensely than others. This extreme perception of pain may be attributable to an underlying abnormality of the central nervous system in the sensory pathways to the brain.

It is also possible to see somatization as an abnormal behavior learned during childhood and reinforced by people and events throughout life. Some women have grown up in families in which the only time they received attention or concern was when they were sick. Some model their behavior on that of another family member who used complaints of illness to control others. Through these kinds of situations people learn—usually unconsciously—that to get attention, support, or power, their only option is to be physically ill.

For similar reasons, it is not unusual for any invalid to discover quickly the joys of extra attention and solicitousness, as well as freedom from responsibility, and unconsciously continue illness behavior well beyond the anticipated healing period. Such scenarios are especially common when the direct expression of emotion is discouraged or when having a psychiatric disorder such as depression or anxiety is stigmatized.

Who is likely to develop a psychosomatic disorder?

Somatization is particularly common in women who suffered from sexual abuse during childhood. It is also common in elderly women who emphasize physical rather than emotional symptoms, possibly because our society still stigmatizes mental illness. In addition, it is a more common expression of distress in women from certain cultural groups (e.g., among those with Asian or Hispanic backgrounds).

Sometimes psychosomatic disorders are transient reactions in times of distress. A person who develops a serious or chronic illness, for example, or who is grieving over the loss of a loved one may become temporarily fixated on bodily processes and physical sensations.

Psychiatrists have suggested that people with certain personality disorders may have a "somatasizing personality" that predisposes them to psychosomatic disorders. People with a passive-aggressive personality style may harbor unfocused hostility which produces an illness consistent with their feelings of having been deprived and wronged by the world. People with a dependent personality style may use illness behavior to maneuver themselves into the position of needing and receiving care. Psychosomatic disorders are also common in people with a borderline personality, which is characterized by instability in a number of areas including interpersonal relationships, behavior, mood, and self-image.

How are these conditions evaluated?

A primary care provider may suspect a psychosomatic disorder in a patient who complains about having seen many doctors without being taken seriously or who has a history of many medical tests and procedures for the same complaint. A patient with more than 10 complaints at any given time will also be suspected of having a psychosomatic disorder. Although it is vital to distinguish psychosomatic symptoms from those with a distinct organic basis, often a clinician can do so without subjecting the patient to more poking and probing. This requires listening carefully and taking a thorough history of the symptoms and any interpersonal stresses or other life crises that may underlie them.

At the same time, the clinician will want to make sure that the patient is not consciously creating the symptoms through malingering, factitious illness, or Münchausen syndrome. Malingerers knowingly fake their symptoms for some clear benefit—perhaps to avoid imprisonment or collect disability payments. People with factitious illness—more often women than men—create physical evidence of a symptom, such as a false reading on a thermometer, so that they can take on the sick role. People with Münchausen syndrome, which is quite rare and occurs mainly in men, typically go from hospital to hospital with well-rehearsed and convincing medical histories that serve as tickets to frequent invasive procedures or surgeries. People with Münchausen syndrome and factitious illness often have severe psychiatric problems and should be evaluated by a psychiatrist.

Once a psychosomatic disorder has been diagnosed, the clinician will want to determine if the patient has a history of childhood sexual abuse so that appropriate therapy can be initiated. An evaluation will be done to see if the patient may be simultaneously suffering from any other emotional disorder.

How are psychosomatic disorders treated?

People with psychosomatic disorders are notorious for going from doctor to doctor without finding satisfactory care. This is often distressing not only to the patient but to her doctors as well, who may feel aversion, fear, guilt, inadequacy, and even malice when they realize they are incapable of helping. If the patient also has a personality disorder, these negative reactions may be even stronger. So long as these feelings are guarded against, however, supportive and effective care is possible.

A woman with a psychosomatic disorder should seek a physician who will take her symptoms seriously and work with her as a partner to help relieve—but not necessarily cure—them. While accepting the presence or severity of symptoms, this doctor will also provide reassurance that there does not appear to be any degenerative or life-threatening disease underlying the symptoms.

Psychosomatic disorders are not usually treated with psychotherapeutic drugs unless they are associated with some other clearly defined mental or emotional disorder (such as major depression, generalized anxiety disorder, obsessive-compulsive disorder, or panic disorder) that requires this treatment. If necessary, drugs may help relieve specific physical symptoms. In most cases, however, psychotherapy is the treatment of choice if the patient can accept the association between emotions and physical complaints.

If the disorder developed following a recent psychological crisis, the patient will probably respond well to reassurance and education about how to handle emotional reactions to life stresses. Recovery usually occurs quickly. It is more difficult to treat women who have a lifelong history of somatization; but the value in having an objective, caring person to listen empathetically to problems cannot be overemphasized. Therapists generally strive to help the patient learn to live with the symptoms, improve function at home and at work, and avoid unnecessary surgery as well as dependence on potentially addictive medications (such as narcotics and benzodiazepines) that may be prescribed to treat some of the symptoms of these disorders. In addition, the therapist will help hone coping and socialization skills and provide insight into the connection between emotions and physical symptoms.

Usually hypochondria, like other psychosomatic disorders, is treated with psychotherapy rather than drugs. Perhaps because hypochondria may be a form of obsessive-compulsive disorder, antidepressants such as fluoxetine (Prozac), sertraline (Zoloft), paroxetine (Paxil), or clomipramine (Anafranil) can also be successful in treating it.

Because so many people with chronic pain syndrome have symptoms of depression, they are often treated with antidepressant medications as well. Most physicians do not prescribe narcotic painkillers because their use can lead to dependency, and over time they become ineffective at relieving the pain. Certain anticonvulsant drugs are also often used to relieve chronic pain. Both cognitive and behavioral psychotherapy can sometimes help alter the perception and response to pain.

In recent years numerous pain management centers and clinics have opened throughout the United States which al-

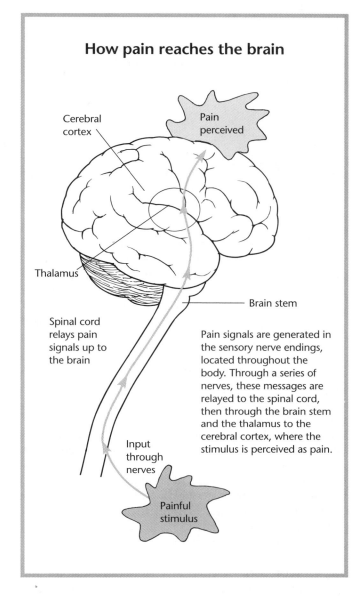

How pain reaches the brain

Cerebral cortex

Pain perceived

Thalamus

Brain stem

Spinal cord relays pain signals up to the brain

Input through nerves

Painful stimulus

Pain signals are generated in the sensory nerve endings, located throughout the body. Through a series of nerves, these messages are relayed to the spinal cord, then through the brain stem and the thalamus to the cerebral cortex, where the stimulus is perceived as pain.

low people with chronic pain to work with a multidisciplinary team of specialists. In addition to traditional psychotherapy, pain centers offer physical and occupational therapy as well as medical procedures to help control pain. For example, researchers have had some success in reducing chronic pain with electrical stimulation. In this procedure a neurosurgeon inserts an electrode into the part of the brain called the thalamus and moves it around until the patient feels vibrations in the painful body part. Then the electrode is implanted in that specific place and attached to a small pulse generator implanted under the collarbone. By waving a magnet past this pulse generator, the patient can initiate a pulse of electricity at any time, apparently providing considerable relief. Alternative techniques to manage stress and control pain, including biofeedback, relaxation therapy, hypnosis, and acupuncture, are often available at pain centers as well.

Related entries
Alternative therapies, antidepressants, anxiety disorders, depression, domestic abuse, obsessive-compulsive disorder, pain management, panic disorder, personality disorders, posttraumatic stress disorder, psychotherapy, sexual abuse and incest, stress

Psychotherapy

Psychotherapy is a form of treatment for psychological and emotional disorders that involves communication—through words and behavior—between a psychotherapist and a patient. Although there are dozens of forms of psychotherapy, some of which have overlapping philosophies, they can be divided into two basic kinds: psychodynamic and behavioral. Depending on the disorder, therapists may combine aspects of both approaches in treatment.

Psychodynamic therapies
Psychodynamic therapies are forms of "talk therapy" in which the psychotherapist and patient together attempt to uncover emotions and motivations and dysfunctional interpersonal interaction patterns assumed to underlie a psychological or emotional disorder. The aim is to develop insight about conflicts that may produce recurring maladaptive patterns in a person's work life and personal relationships—and then to use this new understanding to bring about positive changes. Conflicts often stem from early childhood events or relationships with parents.

Psychodynamic therapy may continue for an indefinite period of time. Although it may involve a one-to-one relationship between therapist and patient, as in individual therapy, its principles are also used in many forms of group therapy, including some family and couples therapy and self-help/support groups (which may, but do not necessarily, include a psychotherapist as facilitator).

Psychoanalysis is a highly specialized form of psychodynamic therapy based in the work of Sigmund Freud and his successors, who have extended and modified his ideas. Freud theorized that psychological problems could be alleviated by putting traumatic memories and emotions into words, as well as through a process known as transference, in which a person projects feelings about significant others onto the therapist.

Some therapists still practice classical psychoanalysis, which delves into the patient's unconscious thought and past experience in three to four 50-minute sessions per week to achieve a major deconstruction and reconstruction of the personality. The trend today, however, is toward using psychoanalytic techniques less stringently to uncover insights into the patient's current life situation, with meetings taking place less frequently (perhaps once a week). To be effective, this form of psychotherapy often requires long hours of work over many years and can be quite costly.

Behavioral therapies
In contrast to psychoanalysis and other psychodynamic forms of psychotherapy, behavioral therapies are concerned with the problem behavior itself rather than its psychological roots in the past or the unconscious. Using specific techniques from learning theory (such as classical conditioning, which originated in Ivan Pavlov's research on dogs), the behavioral therapist helps people learn to change undesirable responses (either actions or feelings) to a particular situation or stimulus.

A behavioral therapy such as systematic desensitization, for example, can help people overcome phobias or panic disorder through repeated and deliberate exposure to whatever stimulus provokes the symptoms. Over time the person learns to substitute feelings of relaxation for feelings of fear or anxiety. Similarly, in assertiveness training a person learns to substitute clear and direct expressions of anger for feelings of anxiety or fear.

Other types of behavioral therapy include training in social skills such as listening and starting a conversation, and biofeedback, which is used to treat stress-related conditions such as headache (see alternative therapies) and to manage anxiety. Sex therapy (see sexual dysfunction) also relies on techniques of behavioral psychotherapy in addressing a particular couple's needs.

Cognitive therapy, a major form of behavior therapy, is premised on the belief that negative or distorted patterns of thinking underlie various psychological problems. A depressed woman, for example, may consider herself worthless, and consistently interpret other people's responses as negative and judgmental—a pattern of thinking that becomes a self-perpetuating cycle of self-denigration. After helping to identify such patterns, the therapist guides the patient in adopting more functional and positive alternatives.

Feminist therapy
Practitioners of more mainstream psychotherapy—regardless of whether their basic approach is psychodynamic, behavioral, or both—frequently incorporate principles of what is called feminist therapy into their practice. These principles include the idea that the therapist is not the healer but rather the facilitator of the woman's recovery, that the woman is a client rather than a patient, that the woman has the means of recovery within herself, and that women in general are not only active and independent in their own right but also equal to, if in many ways different from, men.

It is the centrality of these feminist ideas that characterizes a feminist therapy or therapist. In addition, for feminist therapists, societal and cultural conflicts (especially power imbalances between women and men) are just as important as—if not more so than—internal conflicts as the sources of women's psychological problems. It is not surprising, then, that feminist therapists were pioneers in recognizing the relationship between psychological problems such as depression, anxiety, and personality disorders and events in a woman's past such as domestic abuse, rape, incest, or alcohol and substance abuse. For example, a major focus of feminist therapy with a lesbian client would be to acknowledge how damaging it is to live in a homophobic society, rather than to explore the origins of the woman's sexual orientation.

Finding a psychotherapist

Psychotherapy can be a tremendous help in treating many psychological and emotional disorders, but practiced improperly, it can result in tremendous harm. For this reason it is important to select a psychotherapist with care. Not only should the person chosen have training and experience appropriate for treating the particular disorder, but also patient and therapist should have compatible styles and values. In fact, the rapport between patient and therapist is often much more essential to success than is the therapist's specific philosophy.

This is not to say that a person seeking a psychotherapist should not learn as much as possible about a potential therapist's philosophy, approach, and training, as well as about the cost of each session and whether it is covered by insurance. The therapist should be asked to estimate how long therapy will continue (months or years) and to set up a specific timetable for evaluating progress. Response varies so much from patient to patient, however, that it is unreasonable to expect a therapist to predict exactly how many sessions will be required.

Because today's managed care health programs restrict most patients' access to long-term therapy, goals and realistic short-term expectations need to be established at the outset. In recent years short-term behavioral therapy has been found to be effective in treating clinical depression, anxiety, and phobias, as well as other immediate areas of emotional conflict. The success of any therapy depends on the patient's basic motivation, her willingness to mobilize her own resources, and the degree of trust and esteem that exists between her and her therapist.

It is also worth thinking about which type of psychotherapist is appropriate for treating a given psychological disorder. A great deal of confusion exists about the differences between the many types of specialists who practice psychotherapy. Many people, for example, confuse psychiatrists, psychologists, and psychoanalysts.

- Psychiatrists are physicians who have undergone 4 years of medical school as well as 4 years of a psychiatric residency, which includes training in psychotherapy. They are the only psychotherapists who can prescribe drugs or perform physical examinations in most states.

- Licensed psychologists have specialized training (usually a doctorate) in treating emotional problems, performing psychological tests, and practicing psychotherapy.

- Psychoanalysts (who can be either psychiatrists or psychologists) also have additional training in the practice of psychoanalysis.

Among the many other specialists who may practice psychotherapy are psychiatric nurses, MSWs (people holding a master's degree in social work), other social workers, marriage and family counselors, ministers, rabbis, priests, and other members of the clergy, as well as individuals trained in specific approaches such as Gestalt therapy, transactional analysis, family therapy, couples counseling, and Jungian psychoanalysis. The training, experience, and philosophy of these disciplines varies greatly.

Interviewing therapists to evaluate their training and philosophy can seem overwhelming, but few people have to do it on their own. Most of the time a short list of eligible psychotherapists can be garnered from friends, clinicians, school counselors, community health centers, or support groups. Women's health clinics and feminist organizations may also be able to provide names of feminist therapists.

Choosing the treatment setting

A careful initial diagnostic assessment of a patient's situation is necessary before she and a therapist can determine together which approach and which therapeutic setting will be most appropriate and effective. These decisions influence how active a role the therapist will play in the therapeutic relationship—or alliance—with the patient and whether treatment will take place in an individual or a group setting.

Individual therapy, a one-to-one interaction between therapist and patient, is a familiar model, but a group structure has also proven helpful in many instances and is sometimes the only form of treatment available or the only one covered by an individual's health insurance. The goal of group therapy is to offer a context that encourages group members to work on underlying conflicts and move toward a more autonomous self through mutual support and interaction. Issues such as inclusion and acceptance, power and independence, and equality and sharing characterize group evolution. Group therapy may involve one therapist and a number of patients, or several therapists and large or small groups.

Family therapy—a variation on group therapy which has emerged over the last several decades—focuses on the individual's problems within the context of family dynamics. The therapist meets with the patient—a woman with anorexia, for example—and other family members to probe long-established patterns of interaction and role playing. These may have served to maintain the emotional and psychological equilibrium of the family unit, but at the expense of the individual family member. Without taking sides, the therapist seeks to clarify family processes in order to open up channels of communication and create a space for movement and growth.

Couples therapy, another form of family intervention, addresses problems in interactions between partners. Understanding that their negative exchanges are mutually reinforcing helps couples clarify their difficulties and begin to resolve them through improved communication.

Psychodrama, or group dramatization of situations that embody underlying conflicts, feelings, and tensions, is a useful approach for those who have difficulty expressing themselves in words. Through their actions, patients bring to awareness and express those parts of themselves they cannot talk about directly.

It can take a fair amount of time (and sometimes money) to choose a compatible therapist and an appropriate treatment setting. It may be necessary for a person to meet with several candidates before she finds one with the right style. Ultimately, it is up to the patient to decide within the first two or three sessions if things feel right. This can be particularly difficult for someone living with emotional pain at the same time. Still, leaving the decision about compatibility up to the therapist is, in the end, counterproductive.

Related entries

Anxiety disorders, depression, domestic abuse, multiple personality disorder, panic disorder, personality disorders, phobias, postpartum psychiatric disorders, posttraumatic stress disorder, psychosomatic disorders, schizophrenia, sexual abuse and incest, sexual assault, sexual dysfunction, sexual orientation, stress, substance abuse

Pubic Lice

Pubic lice are yellow-gray insects with crablike claws which live off human blood (see illustration). They can survive only about a day on their own. Once settled into a warm, hairy part of the body (usually, but not always, the pubic area), the female lays small eggs called nits which cling to the base of the hairs. These take about 7 to 9 days to hatch.

Although lice are not a serious threat to health, they can cause agonizing itching and often require a good deal of time and effort to eliminate.

Who is likely to develop pubic lice?

Pubic lice (also known as crabs or pediculosis pubis) are usually passed from one person to another during intimate physical contact (not necessarily intercourse), though they are occasionally acquired from contaminated linens, clothing, or toilet seats.

What are the symptoms?

It is possible to have pubic lice without noticing them, but most people experience itching so intense that it cannot be relieved by scratching. Scratching itself can irritate the pubic region, leading to vulvitis (see entry), and can also spread the lice to other hairy areas of the body, including the underarms, scalp, eyelashes, and eyebrows. Sometimes people with pubic lice notice a bluish gray "rash" (lice) or dark brown specks in undergarments (excrement from the lice). They may also notice tiny white, translucent nits at the base of the hair. These look something like crystalline dandruff but cannot be easily dislodged from the hair shafts.

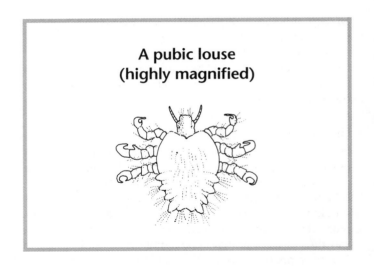

A pubic louse (highly magnified)

How is the condition evaluated?

The only way to diagnose pubic lice is to find actual lice or, more likely, their nits attached to pubic hairs.

How does one get rid of pubic lice?

Various commercial treatments that readily kill lice and their nits are available over the counter in the form of creams, shampoos, and lotions. The safest and most effective of these, which has become available without prescription, is Nix (permethrin). Available as a cream rinse, this product kills both lice and their nits with a single application. Some other products, including Kwell (lindane) and RID (pyrethrin with piperonyl butoxide), may require a repeat treatment a week later if any live lice remain.

Because these are very strong medications that can irritate underlying skin or cause allergic reactions, it is important to follow directions on the label carefully and avoid unnecessary application. Pregnant women should consult their doctor before using any of these treatments.

All clothing, towels, and bed linen recently used by the infected person, as well as items used by any sexual partners, should be washed in hot water and machine dried for at least 20 minutes, or dry-cleaned. Nonwashable items can be stored away in a plastic bag for at least 2 weeks—long enough to give any remaining nits time to hatch and die. If there is any chance that upholstery or mattresses contain lice or nits, they can be sprayed with special pesticides for lice available at most drugstores.

How can infestation with pubic lice be prevented?

Preventing pubic lice infestation is similar to preventing all sexually transmitted diseases (see safer sex). In addition, because pubic lice are occasionally acquired through intermediate objects, avoiding other people's towels or (at least in theory) covering public toilet seats with tissue may help prevent their spread.

Related entries

Safer sex, sexually transmitted diseases, vulvitis

Radiation Therapy

Radiation therapy involves the treatment of disease, primarily cancer, with high-energy x-rays or other sources of ionizing radiation such as radioactive cobalt, radium, or iodine. Also called radiotherapy, irradiation, or x-ray therapy, radiation therapy kills cells by damaging the DNA (genetic material) within them. It is particularly effective in killing rapidly dividing cells, including cancer cells. Unlike chemotherapy (see entry), it has little effect on cells outside the area (field) of treatment.

Radiation therapy is often used alone as the primary treatment in many forms of cancer, such as cancers of the cervix, vagina, bladder, skin, lymph nodes, and vocal cords, including certain inoperable cancers. It is increasingly being used, too, in conjunction with chemotherapy to kill any errant cancer cells after surgery. For example, after a lumpectomy for breast cancer, radiation is almost always used to destroy cancer cells that may still be present in the remaining breast tissue. In advanced incurable cancers, radiation therapy may be used to shrink tumors in the hope of alleviating pain, pressure, or bleeding.

How is radiation therapy performed?
The experience of having radiation therapy is much the same (and just as painless) as having a diagnostic x-ray, except that it takes longer. As with all x-rays, parts of the body not being irradiated are covered with a lead shield to prevent unnecessary exposure and to protect them from long-term side effects. In most cases the x-ray treatments are delivered in a matter of minutes, daily, 5 times per week for a period of several weeks.

Radioactive substances can also be placed near or into cancerous cells within the body and are often left in place for several days. This more direct means of delivery allows higher doses of radiation to be focused directly on the cancer while minimizing the amount of radiation to sensitive surrounding organs such as the rectum and bladder.

What happens after the procedure?
Like chemotherapy, another common treatment for cancer, radiation is often associated with a number of side effects. Depending on the dosage and site of radiation, the skin around the site of therapy can become red, sore, itchy, sensitive, or even blistered, in which case a clinician can prescribe soothing ointments or powders.

Some people experience difficulty swallowing, dry mouth, loss of appetite, fatigue, or excessive sleepiness as well. Temporary hair loss usually occurs on irradiated skin, although most people can expect their hair to begin growing again a few months after therapy ends. Radiation to the abdominal or pelvic area may result in nausea, vomiting, or diarrhea.

What are the risks and complications?
Radiotherapy occasionally weakens bones to the point where they are susceptible to sudden fractures. Thus, women who are receiving radiation treatments for breast cancer may in rare cases experience rib fractures. The treatments also carry a very small risk of causing another tumor in the same location. This risk depends to a great extent on the dosage of radiation given and the area of exposure.

Related entries
Breast cancer, cervical cancer, chemotherapy, colon and rectal cancer, endometrial cancer, lumpectomy, melanoma, ovarian cancer, vulvar cancer

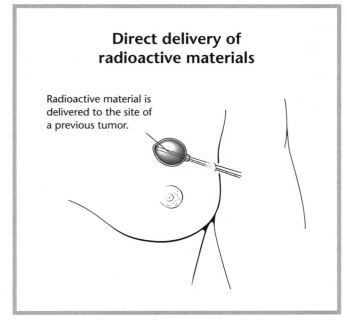

Direct delivery of radioactive materials

Radioactive material is delivered to the site of a previous tumor.

Raynaud's Phenomenon

In Raynaud's phenomenon fingers or toes turn temporarily white and blue after exposure to cold or sometimes after emotional stress (see illustration). This is often an independent occurrence (in which case it is referred to as Raynaud's disease), but Raynaud's phenomenon can occur in conjunction with a connective tissue disease or other conditions. Few people (only about 5 percent) with Raynaud's phenomenon ever develop a connective tissue disease, however. Such disease is especially unlikely if the phenomenon persists independently for several years.

Who is likely to develop this condition?
Occurring in about 5 percent of Americans, this phenomenon is much more likely to occur in women than in men. The most common connective tissue problems associated with Raynaud's phenomenon are scleroderma and related

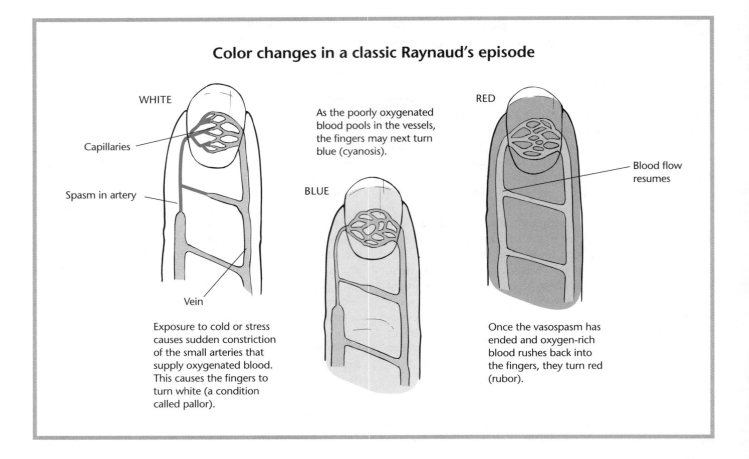

Color changes in a classic Raynaud's episode

WHITE

Capillaries

Spasm in artery

Vein

As the poorly oxygenated blood pools in the vessels, the fingers may next turn blue (cyanosis).

BLUE

RED

Blood flow resumes

Exposure to cold or stress causes sudden constriction of the small arteries that supply oxygenated blood. This causes the fingers to turn white (a condition called pallor).

Once the vasospasm has ended and oxygen-rich blood rushes back into the fingers, they turn red (rubor).

disorders. Women with lupus, rheumatoid arthritis, polymyositis and dermatomyositis (see entries), and atherosclerosis are also more likely than other women to have episodes of Raynaud's.

Exposure to certain drugs and toxins can trigger Raynaud's phenomenon. These include beta blockers (used to treat heart disease, high blood pressure, and migraine headaches); ergots (used to treat migraine headaches); certain anticancer drugs such as bleomycin, cisplatin, and vincristine/vinblastine; nicotine (which decreases blood flow); pseudoephedrine (an over-the-counter decongestant); phenylpropanolamine (found in certain cold remedies and diet pills); and exposure to chemicals such as polyvinylchloride (PVC). Birth control pills can sometimes decrease circulation and promote attacks, as can the long-term use of vibrating tools such as jackhammers or chain saws.

What are the symptoms?

Raynaud's phenomenon usually occurs in three phases. First, the ends of the fingers or toes turn white or pale; next they become bluish; and finally, as circulation is restored, they become red before returning to their normal color. Sometimes the color changes are accompanied by numbness or pain. Occasionally the nose, earlobes, or even tongue may also be affected. Attacks may last from a few minutes to hours. In some cases, ulcers and skin breakdown may develop as well.

Other vascular disorders more common in women have symptoms similar to Raynaud's phenomenon. In the condition called acrocyanosis, for example, fingers or toes almost always feel cold, whatever the outside weather. In the condition called livedo reticularis, the skin of the lower extremities, hands, and arms becomes mottled and bluish red, and during the winter feet and legs may become cold and achy or even develop ulcers.

How is the condition evaluated?

A doctor will want to determine if the symptoms indicate an isolated disease or if they are associated with some other condition. Usually this can be determined through a physical examination and consideration of the woman's medical history.

How is Raynaud's phenomenon treated?

Prevention of exposure to cold is a key part of treatment. It is advisable always to wear gloves or mittens, a hat, and a vest in cold or cool weather. During an attack, waving the affected arm or leg can be helpful. Drugs called calcium-channel blockers (such as nifedipine), generally used to treat chest pain from coronary disease and hypertension, may also be prescribed. Most doctors advise people with Raynaud's phenomenon to avoid cigarette smoke and cold temperatures as well as beta blockers and other drugs that may lead to the phenomenon. Biofeedback (see alternative therapies), a technique in which patients learn how to regulate ordinarily involuntary body functions, is often beneficial in preventing future episodes of Raynaud's phenomenon.

If Raynaud's phenomenon appears to be due to some underlying disease, the woman may be referred to a rheumatologist for evaluation and treatment appropriate to the specific condition.

Related entries

Alternative therapies, autoimmune disorders, circulatory disorders, lupus, rheumatoid arthritis, scleroderma, smoking

Retinal Detachment

A retinal hole—a rip or tear in the retina, the transparent membrane in the back of the eye which processes light—can be caused by age-related changes or trauma to the eye. Retinal holes can be dangerous because vitreous fluid (the gel-like substance that fills the eye between the lens and retina) can flow through the hole and force the retina to peel away, or detach, from underlying blood vessels (see illustration). These vessels provide essential oxygen and nutrients without which the eye cannot function. Retinal detachment can be quite sudden or it can develop over a number of years. In rare cases, it may result from inflammation or tumors in the eye.

Who is likely to develop this condition?

Retinal detachment is most likely to occur among whites and among people who are nearsighted, and it tends to run in families. It may occur after cataract surgery, but this complication is less common now than in past years because of advances in the technology of this surgery.

What are the symptoms?

Although detachment of the retina itself is painless, certain changes in vision can indicate a possible problem. For example, a sudden burst of flashing white lights or sparks, blurry vision, or numerous small floaters—the familiar spots, squiggles, and specks that occasionally drift across the visual field—may signal a shrinking vitreous fluid, which in turn can tug on the retina and contribute to holes and detachment. Generally, if the visual aura of flashing lights lasts longer than a couple of seconds or minutes, and especially if it affects both eyes, it may be caused by some other problem, such as a migraine headache. In most cases floaters do not signal anything serious, but an ophthalmologist (eye specialist) should be consulted if they are a frequent problem. If part of the retina has already become detached, there may also appear to be a dark curtain moving over a portion of the visual field.

How is retinal detachment evaluated?

Anyone with symptoms of retinal detachment requires immediate medical attention by an ophthalmologist. Vision

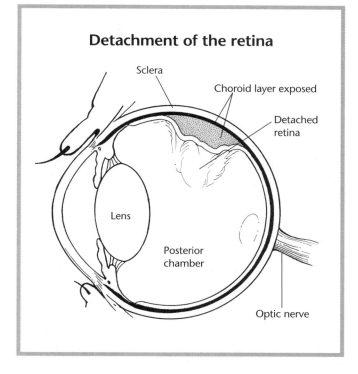

Detachment of the retina

Sclera

Choroid layer exposed

Detached retina

Lens

Posterior chamber

Optic nerve

can be permanently lost if the detachment, whether partial or complete, is not quickly repaired. To diagnose the condition, an ophthalmologist will examine the eye in detail, determining whether a retinal hole is present and if so whether detachment (partial or complete) has occurred. Ultrasound may be used to elucidate structures in the eye more thoroughly.

How is retinal detachment treated?

With prompt attention, a retinal hole without detachment can be treated with surgery to prevent any vision loss. If some of the retina has already detached, vision is easier to save if the part responsible for central vision (the macula) remains attached. Even if the retina totally detaches, microsurgery can usually reattach it, although central vision is at greater risk if there is macular detachment.

Often a form of laser surgery called photocoagulation is used to prevent detachment of a retinal hole. A laser beam directed at the detached area results in scar formation, which in turn causes the retina to adhere to the underlying blood vessels and tissue. Alternatively, another approach called cryopexy can be used to produce a scar that serves the same function. A special probe freezes the wall of the eye overlying the hole and induces inflammation, which in turn leads to scarring and sealing of the hole. Both of these surgeries can be done on an outpatient basis.

If the retina is already detached, more intensive surgery will be necessary.

How can retinal detachment be prevented?

Because trauma to the eye is one cause of retinal detachment, wearing protective eyegear during sports is an important preventive measure. Prompt medical attention for symptoms of retinal detachment (such as sudden flashes of light) can minimize the risk of visual loss.

Related entries

Cataracts, dry eye, eye care, glaucoma, laser surgery, macular degeneration, ultrasound

Retroverted Uterus

In most women the uterus rests on the bladder and tilts slightly forward so that it is at a right angle to the vagina. In about 1 woman in 5, the uterus tilts backward, away from the bladder (see illustration). This is called a retroverted uterus, or a tipped uterus. Once blamed for a host of medical woes—ranging from backaches to infertility—a retroverted uterus is considered today to be a variation of normal anatomy which rarely causes problems. In fact, many women may never even know that they have one unless a clinician happens to mention it in passing during a pelvic examination.

A retroverted uterus does not seem to have any detrimental effect on conception, pregnancy, or childbirth. In fact, the uterus may temporarily move into a forward position during pregnancy, and then return to its retroverted position after delivery. If the uterus does not move forward, however, the cervix—the bottom part of the uterus, which points forward when the uterus tips back—may occasionally lock into the pubic bone and block the outlet to the bladder. This problem,

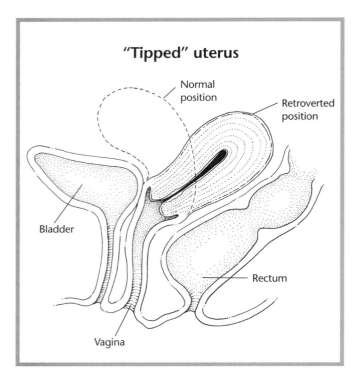

"Tipped" uterus

Normal position

Retroverted position

Bladder

Rectum

Vagina

called an incarcerated uterus, usually occurs during the late first or early second trimester of pregnancy. As a result the woman has great difficulty urinating, and in rare cases an acute kidney infection may result. A clinician can sometimes correct an incarcerated uterus by exerting pressure on the back of the uterus through the vagina. Otherwise, a catheter is placed through the urethra into the bladder to drain it, and is kept in place until the uterus grows out of the pelvis as the pregnancy progresses.

Who is likely to develop a retroverted uterus?

Most of the time a retroverted uterus is something that a woman is born with. Occasionally it may develop after a pregnancy stretches the ligaments that normally hold the uterus in place. Sometimes adhesions (scar tissue) related to pelvic inflammatory disease or endometriosis can pull the uterus back into a retroverted position. It is also possible for the uterus to be displaced by a particularly large uterine fibroid or ovarian tumor or cyst.

What are the symptoms?

The vast majority of women with a retroverted uterus have no symptoms whatsoever. Some may experience a mild lower backache, particularly during their menstrual periods. In most cases, however, backaches will turn out to be due to some source other than the retroverted uterus. Additional symptoms—such as irregular menstrual bleeding and painful periods—may develop if the uterus is fixed into position by adhesions.

If the cervix is directly in line with the vagina, it may account for painful sexual intercourse, although this occurs only rarely.

How is the condition evaluated?

Most of the time a retroverted uterus is discovered by a clinician doing a routine pelvic examination, sometimes because it is difficult to do an adequate Pap test.

How is a retroverted uterus treated?

Most women require no treatment since a retroverted uterus is not a disease and usually causes no problems. If a woman is bothered by backache or pain during intercourse, however, the clinician may insert a plastic ring or rubber cap called a pessary into the vagina to help push the uterus forward. Pessaries require meticulous cleaning and maintenance (either by the woman herself or at regular intervals by her clinician), and sometimes can cause vaginitis. In rare instances a clinician may suggest a uterine suspension—a surgical procedure in which the uterus and any stretched ligaments are stitched into a forward position and any adhesions are removed. This surgery used to be a standard treatment for retroverted uterus but is rarely done today.

Related entries

Adhesions, back pain, endometriosis, infertility, kidney disorders, menstrual cramps, ovarian cancer, ovarian cysts, pain during sexual intercourse, pelvic examinations, pelvic inflammatory disease, pregnancy, uterine fibroids, vaginitis

Rh Disease

In Rh disease antibodies produced by a pregnant woman break down the fetus's red blood cells, causing anemia and sometimes serious illness or even death of the fetus.

This disease can develop when the fetus's blood contains Rh factor, an antigen commonly present on the surface of red blood cells. An antigen is a protein that can bring on an immune response. Human blood is typed according to the antigens it contains so that blood containing an antigen will not be mixed with antigen-free blood (such as during a transfusion). If blood is mixed, the blood without the antigen may produce an antibody to the antigen, resulting in dangerous and sometimes lethal effects.

Blood commonly contains the A antigen (in which case the person is said to have type A blood), or the B antigen (type B), or both the A and B antigens (type AB). People with neither A nor B antigens are said to have type O blood. If a person's blood also contains the Rh factor, the person is said to be Rh-positive. If the Rh factor is missing, the person is Rh-negative. Thus, A-negative blood contains the A antigen but does not contain the Rh factor; O-positive blood has neither the A nor B antigen but does contain the Rh factor.

The biggest significance of the Rh factor for women arises during pregnancy. Problems can occur if an Rh-negative mother is carrying an Rh-positive fetus—as often happens if the father of the baby is Rh-positive. If the fetus's blood mixes with the mother's, the mother's body may begin to produce antibodies against the Rh factor in a process called sensitization. This can result in Rh disease.

Who is likely to develop Rh disease?

Rh disease is much more common in second and subsequent pregnancies because fetal and maternal blood usually do not mix until delivery. It can develop in a first pregnancy, however, if fetal blood enters the mother's body through the placenta or during an amniocentesis. Some Rh-negative women who have never been pregnant before may also have become sensitized to the Rh factor if they were given Rh-positive blood during an earlier blood transfusion.

How can Rh disease be prevented?

Rh disease can be prevented in women whose blood does not already contain antibodies to the Rh factor. This is usually accomplished using injections of Rhogam (Rh immune globulin), which prevents the formation of antibodies to the Rh factor. Women who do not already know their blood type will have it typed as a part of routine prenatal care. Rhogam is usually administered at about 28 weeks of pregnancy—even in first-time mothers, since there is a small chance that fetal

and maternal blood may have mixed already. Another injection is given within 72 hours of delivery if the baby is found to have Rh-positive blood. This treatment must be repeated with each pregnancy because protection lasts only about 12 weeks. It is also necessary after every miscarriage, ectopic pregnancy, amniocentesis, or elective abortion as well, since all of these events can stimulate the production of antibodies in the mother.

Rhogam appears to be safe for use during pregnancy. Although it is made from blood, the method of preparation kills bacteria and viruses that might have been present. Occasionally fever or soreness develops at the injection site, but these are temporary reactions.

How is Rh disease treated?

Rhogam is useless if the mother's blood already contains antibodies to the Rh factor. The blood of pregnant women in this situation is tested regularly throughout the pregnancy to assess the level of the antibodies it contains. If the levels are high, an amniocentesis may be done to detect the level of bilirubin in the amniotic fluid. This indicates the degree of damage done to the fetus's blood cells.

If the fetus is anemic, a blood transfusion will be necessary to replace the fetus's blood supply with Rh-negative blood, which cannot be damaged by the mother's antibodies. A generation ago many babies died of Rh disease because this transfusion could not be done until after delivery. It is now possible to give a transfusion through the umbilical cord while the fetus is still in the uterus, from 18 weeks of pregnancy on. This procedure is somewhat risky, however, so many clinicians prefer to induce labor and treat the baby after delivery if problems are detected late enough in the pregnancy.

Related entries

Abortion, amniocentesis, anemia, ectopic pregnancy, miscarriage, pregnancy, prenatal care

Rheumatoid Arthritis

Rheumatoid arthritis is a chronic, progressive disease that involves inflammation of the connective tissue or membranes that line the joints. Because RA is a systemic disease, it not only causes red, swollen, and painful joints but also can affect internal organs such as the heart, lungs, kidneys, and eyes. Overgrowth of the synovial membranes in the joints can erode surrounding supportive tissue such as ligaments, muscles, and bones, thereby immobilizing the joints (see illustration).

The origins of this often lifelong, expensive, and disabling disease remain unclear, but there is some evidence suggesting that it may be due to an infection or to an autoimmune reaction in which the body attacks some of its own tissues,

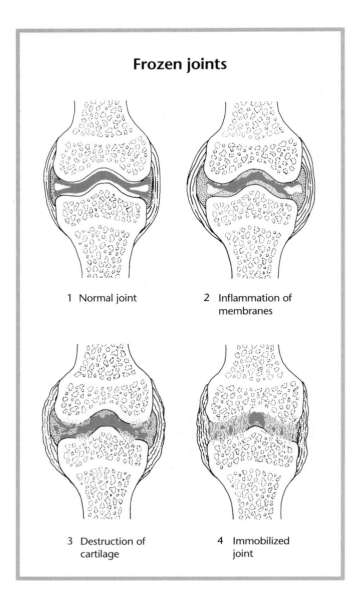

Frozen joints

1   Normal joint

2   Inflammation of
    membranes

3   Destruction of
    cartilage

4   Immobilized
    joint

abate or even go into complete remission during pregnancy, and there seems to be no adverse effect in babies born to mothers with RA. But the disease sometimes flares up again within about 6 to 9 months after delivery. Women with RA should be counseled regarding the use of medications during pregnancy.

What are the symptoms?

Although symptoms of RA tend to vary in nature and severity and may come and go over time, persistent joint inflammation lasting more than 6 weeks is a hallmark of the disease. Inflamed joints are painful, swollen, and warm to the touch, usually on both sides of the body. Wrists and knuckles are most commonly affected, but the disease often progresses to other joints, including the elbows, shoulders, jaw, hips, knees, ankles, and feet. Eventually joints may become permanently deformed. Many people find that their joints are particularly stiff and achy for over an hour after waking in the morning or after inactivity of any sort. Symptoms usually develop slowly over weeks to months.

Often people with RA experience fatigue, malaise, lack of appetite, and depression, as well as a low-grade fever and mild anemia. Other conditions that frequently are associated with RA include Sjögren syndrome, carpal tunnel syndrome, and Raynaud's phenomenon (see entries). About one-quarter of people with RA develop small lumps under the skin called rheumatoid nodules. These lumps are usually not painful unless they become ulcerated or infected.

The symptoms of elderly-onset RA are similar to those in RA that develops at an earlier age. People with elderly-onset RA are particularly likely to have pain and stiffness in the shoulder region.

How is the condition evaluated?

A doctor who suspects RA will first perform a thorough examination of the joints, heart, and lungs, as well as a search for rheumatoid nodules. If RA is still considered likely, other conditions that might account for the symptoms must be eliminated. These include other connective tissue disorders such as lupus, polymyositis and dermatomyositis, scleroderma, polymyalgia rheumatica, and fibromyalgia (see entries), as well as viral illnesses and rheumatic fever. (Rheumatic fever sometimes develops after strep throat and is characterized by arthritis, inflammation of the heart, fever, and skin changes.) RA must also be differentiated from other forms of arthritis (see entry), from other systemic inflammatory diseases such as inflammatory bowel disease (see bowel disorders), and from infections.

Results from various tests can be combined with the physical findings to help eliminate some of these other possibilities. One of these is a blood test for rheumatoid factor. The mere presence of this antibody does not necessarily mean that the patient has RA, since it is also present in various other conditions as well as in 5 to 10 percent of healthy individuals. It is also frequently absent in elderly-onset RA. Still, rheumatoid factor is present in about 80 percent of people

or a combination of the two causes. Although there is still no cure, appropriate therapy overseen by a multidisciplinary team of health care practitioners can help most people with RA avoid becoming severely crippled or bedridden with joint deformity and pain.

Who is likely to develop rheumatoid arthritis?

RA occurs about 2 to 3 times as often in women as in men, and afflicts about 20 percent of all women in the United States. It can begin anytime from adolescence to old age, but the peak years of onset are between age 25 and 50. The disease tends to run in families.

When symptoms of RA begin after the age of 60, the condition is called elderly-onset rheumatoid arthritis. Elderly-onset RA tends to be less severe and to have a better outcome than forms that develop earlier in life.

RA seems to have no effect on the menstrual cycle or fertility. In fact, most women with RA find that their symptoms

with RA, especially in those at increased risk for more severe forms of the disease.

Another blood test that can be used to diagnose RA is a measure of the erythrocyte sedimentation rate (ESR, or "sed rate"), that is, the rate at which red blood cells settle to the bottom of a container. The ESR is often elevated in people with rheumatoid arthritis (as well as in various other disorders).

Samples of synovial fluid (which lubricates the joint) from a hot, red, swollen joint are often "tapped" for laboratory analysis to see if there are any signs of inflammation (suggestive of RA), infection, or crystals (suggestive of other inflammatory arthritic conditions such as gout and pseudogout). This procedure, which requires that a needle be guided into the joint after lidocaine is injected locally into the skin, is generally done in the physician's office.

Other tests may be performed to see if there are any associated lung, heart, neurological, or blood disorders. X-rays are rarely helpful in diagnosis but may sometimes differentiate RA from osteoarthritis and other forms of inflammatory arthritis. More commonly they are done to evaluate the progression of the disease and to guide therapy.

How is rheumatoid arthritis treated?

There is currently no cure for RA. Controlling the symptoms of this disease involves a delicate, individually determined balance between drug therapy, lifestyle changes, physical and occupational therapy, and surgical interventions. Alternative or "complementary" therapy such as acupuncture, and behavioral modification are increasingly tried as a part of an overall treatment plan as well, although success with nutritional supplements has been dubious to date. No single drug or other therapy works best for all people with RA, or even in the same individual at all times. Decisions about the specific treatments should therefore be made by the physician and patient together after considering factors such as the stage of the disease, specific signs and symptoms, and any other illnesses the patient may have.

Nondrug treatments. In managing this disease, it can be very useful to consult a multidisciplinary team of health care specialists, including an internist, a rheumatologist (a specialist in RA), a physiatrist (a doctor specializing in the treatment of disease with physical or mechanical agents), a physical and occupational therapist, a nurse specialist, an orthopedist, and an orthotics technician (a person trained in the use of appliances that correct bone and joint deformities). The challenge is to find an appropriate balance between rest and exercise in order to reduce pain and inflammation, while restoring and maintaining range of motion, strength, and the capacity for work and for going about one's daily life.

Generally exercise should be minimized during flare-ups of the disease and increased during periods of remission. Various heat treatments can reduce joint pain, and massage may relieve muscle tension and pain. Inflamed joints may be protected with splints.

Medications. Many of the drugs used to treat rheumatoid arthritis take weeks or months before they have any noticeable effect, and several may have to be tried before an effective one is found. Generally, a doctor will first prescribe medication to treat flare-ups of pain and inflammation and recommend others that actually interfere with the disease process itself if symptoms persist.

A regimen of aspirin and other nonsteroidal antiinflammatory drugs (NSAIDs) is often prescribed for symptom relief as soon as a diagnosis of RA has been made. Using buffered or coated aspirin can reduce the chances of stomach upset from NSAIDs (see antiinflammatory drugs). The newer COX-2 inhibitors (such as Celebrex or Vioxx) also tend to be easier on the stomach, although they still need to be used cautiously in people who have a history of ulcers.

While it was once standard to wait and see if merely treating the symptoms with these drugs (sometimes together with occupational or physical therapy) would provide sufficient relief, more and more clinicians are now supplementing these antiinflammatory drugs with second-line agents (also called slow-acting antirheumatic drugs, or SAARDs, and disease-modifying antirheumatic drugs, or DMARDs). These drugs, at least in theory, modify the underlying process leading to rheumatoid arthritis but generally take from 6 weeks to 6 months to act. Often the drug of choice is methotrexate (a drug used in cancer treatment). This drug is highly effective and begins to work relatively quickly, although it can lead to side effects such as mouth sores and hair loss. Methotrexate (which is taken in much lower doses than are used in cancer treatment) should never be mixed with alcoholic beverages or sulfa antibiotics.

Other second-line agents also include antimalarials (Plaquenil), gold salts, sulfasalazine (an antiinflammatory drug), and occasionally antibiotics such as minocycline and other drugs that suppress the immune system. Newer treatments include the immunosuppressant leflunomide (Arava), a drug related to thalidomide that can be very effective either alone or in combination with methotrexate. Women using leflunomide or methotrexate who have any chance of becoming pregnant need to use reliable contraception because this drug can cause malformations in a growing fetus.

A new class of slow-acting drugs called tumor necrosis factor (TNF) blockers work to block chemicals called cytokines that can cause inflammation; they are usually taken together with methotrexate. The two TNF blockers approved for treating RA are entanercept (Enbrel) and infliximab (Remicade).

Once any second-line agent starts to work, the rheumatologist may suggest tapering off or even stopping the NSAIDs completely. Anyone taking these medications needs to see a doctor regularly so that side effects can be monitored.

If symptoms persist despite the use of the slower-acting drugs, various experimental medications or oral corticosteroid therapy (such as prednisone tablets) may be prescribed. Because corticosteroids (which are modified forms of adrenal hormones that reduce inflammation) can have many side effects, they should be used cautiously. Long-term risks of corticosteroid therapy include atrophy of the adrenal glands, weight gain, acne, water retention, osteoporosis, mood swings, insomnia, and, at high doses, depression and other serious mental disturbances. During severe flare-ups, corticosteroids may be injected directly into individual joints.

Unless her symptoms are quite mild, any woman with RA who becomes pregnant should consult both a rheumatologist and an obstetrician-gynecologist to discuss potential problems and appropriate care before and after delivery. Because neither NSAIDs nor SAARDs have been proven safe for use during pregnancy, SAARDs are usually not prescribed for a woman who becomes pregnant or is thinking of becoming pregnant. Acetaminophen (Tylenol) and low-dose corticosteroids are generally used instead to relieve pain and inflammation. This strategy works well for most pregnant women because it usually takes several months for symptoms to flare up after SAARDs are stopped (with the notable exception of methotrexate).

Although many women find that their symptoms abate somewhat during pregnancy, most doctors advise restarting antirheumatic drugs shortly after delivery to help prevent the flare-ups that often occur in the postpartum period. They also advise bottle-feeding the baby, since most antirheumatic drugs are secreted to some extent in breast milk. None has been approved by the Food and Drug Administration for use while nursing, although the American Academy of Pediatrics states that prednisone is safe to use.

Surgery. Orthopedic surgery is sometimes performed to relieve pain or restore damaged joints. In early stages of RA, the most common procedures performed are synovectomies (removal of the inflamed synovium) from the hand or wrist, and severing a ligament to free the trapped median nerve in the case of people with carpal tunnel syndrome (see entry), a condition that results from compression of the nerve that runs through a narrow passageway in the wrists, when tissues surrounding it become swollen. Joint fusion (arthrodesis) may help relieve pain and stabilize motion in wrists and ankles. In more advanced cases, damaged joints may be repaired by removing part of the adjacent bone (osteotomy) or by inserting an artificial hip or knee (a procedure called arthroplasty; see entry).

People with RA may want to consult the Arthritis Foundation, which issues pamphlets regarding the course and treatments of RA, conducts self-help groups, and provides listings of rehabilitative services, exercise classes, and an information and referral service.

Complementary approaches. Despite the considerable hype, solid data proving that various nutritional supplements can relieve the symptoms of rheumatoid arthritis are still lacking. Some studies have shown that fish oils may modestly improve symptoms, but only when ingested in amounts large enough to cause numerous side effects. The newer cartilage supplements such as chondroitin sulfate and hyaluronic acids have been shown to help relieve the pain of osteoarthritis in a few studies, but to date there is no evidence of their efficacy in treating rheumatoid arthritis.

Despite the paucity of solid evidence, the fact remains that many patients with rheumatoid arthritis have turned to nutritional supplements and other forms of complementary remedies. These include herbal remedies, chiropractic manipulations, and high doses of vitamins. Some of these approaches, if used with due caution (see entry on alternative therapies) and in conjunction with standard treatments, may play a role in relieving symptoms.

Related entries

Antiinflammatory drugs, arthritis, arthroplasty, autoimmune disorders, carpal tunnel syndrome, depression, fibromyalgia, lupus, osteoarthritis, osteoporosis, polymyalgia rheumatica, polymyositis and dermatomyositis, Raynaud's phenomenon, scleroderma, Sjögren syndrome

Rhinoplasty

"Nose job" is the colloquial term for rhinoplasty, a form of plastic surgery that reshapes the nose. It is most often performed for the sake of altering appearance, either by reducing or enlarging the nose or straightening out bumps or bends. It is also sometimes used to correct an injury or to improve breathing difficulties that may result from a broken nose or a deviated septum (the septum is the flexible cartilage that separates the nostrils).

Just what constitutes an attractive nose varies from culture to culture and to some degree is a matter of personal taste. For this reason a plastic surgeon will often spend a good deal of time with a patient before surgery to determine her exact expectations and to see if they are compatible with realistic outcomes.

In most cases the decision to have the nose altered is made much earlier in life, although it is often laden with the potential to provoke considerable family tension. For example, a daughter's decision to alter the shape of her nose may be viewed as an insult to other family members who share the same profile, or as a rebellion against the family's heritage or ethnic group. In some families, however, having a nose job is a sort of rite of passage or "sweet sixteen" present, which an adolescent daughter may either welcome or view as an assault on her already fragile body image.

Whatever the particular feelings evoked, it is generally not a good idea to have a nose job before the age of 16 or 18, by which time the bones of the face have developed to adult proportions and the nose has taken on its adult contours.

How is the procedure performed?

The surgery itself can be performed under either local or general anesthesia, depending on the preferences of both patient and surgeon. Just where the surgeon will make incisions depends on a variety of factors. Although some surgeons make the incisions from outside the nose, which allows a direct view of underlying structures, many cut from within the nostrils to minimize visible scarring. External cuts may also have to be made if the shape of the nostrils themselves is to be altered.

Once the incisions are made, the surgeon proceeds to separate bone and cartilage from the soft tissue above it and then breaks and repositions some of the nasal bones so that they will heal into a new shape. In the case of a deviated septum, the central cartilage may be cut and reshaped as well. Sometimes excess cartilage is chiseled away to shorten the nose or alter a curve. If the goal is to elevate the bridge or increase overall length, the surgeon may implant cartilage or bone from elsewhere in the body (or, rarely, synthetic material such as silicone) between the bone and overlying skin. Sometimes chin surgery is performed at the same time, especially if a small chin magnifies the apparent size of the nose.

What happens after surgery?

After surgery both nostrils may be packed with gauze, which is kept in place for a few days. Often an external cast or splint may be applied as well and kept in place for up to 2 weeks. This helps hold the nasal bones in their new position until healing is complete and also limits swelling and protects the nose from injury. Significant pain is rare, though many patients are bothered by some numbness and dislike having to breathe through their mouth until the gauze is removed.

Another unpleasant but almost universal aftereffect is the swollen, discolored "raccoon eyes" which usually last for a couple of weeks. Most of the numbness and swelling disappears within 2 or 3 weeks, and women can generally resume normal activities—including exercise—after that time. Contact sports are best avoided for 6 months.

What are the risks and complications?

Nose jobs, like any form of surgery, can result in serious complications—including excess bleeding, infection, or unexpected reactions to anesthesia. Also, it is not always possible to predict just which patients will develop excessive scar tissue that distorts the contour of the new nose or results in undesired asymmetry. About 5 to 8 percent of patients will need to have corrective surgery.

More rarely the septum may be perforated during surgery, or the bridge of the nose may collapse. Some people develop frequent nosebleeds because of crusting at incision sites or find themselves with pinched or partially closed nostrils.

Although most rhinoplasty yields excellent results, any woman considering such surgery for purely cosmetic reasons should factor these possible complications into the equation.

Related entries

Anesthesia, body image, cosmetic surgery, keloid scarring, otoplasty

Rosacea

Rosacea is a chronic inflammatory disorder in which the central areas of the face become reddened—probably because of enlarged blood vessels under the skin. Although rosacea sometimes resembles acne (and was once known as acne rosacea or adult acne), the absence of either blackheads or whiteheads marks it as a distinct condition. It appears more often in women than in men.

Who is likely to develop rosacea?

Rosacea is particularly common in fair-skinned people. It usually begins in middle age or later and tends to flare up and then improve for a time. There appears to be a genetic predisposition to developing this skin disorder.

What are the symptoms?

Rosacea almost always involves reddened or inflamed cheeks, nose, forehead, eyelids, or chin. More rarely the trunk, arms, and legs may be affected as well. The redness is sometimes accompanied by spider veins (telangiectasia), pimples, or pustules. If rosacea goes untreated, there can be tissue overgrowth in the nose (rhinophyma), although the resulting red, bulbous nose is more common in men with rosacea than in women.

How is the condition evaluated?

Before diagnosing rosacea, a clinician will want to rule out other conditions that may produce similar symptoms. These

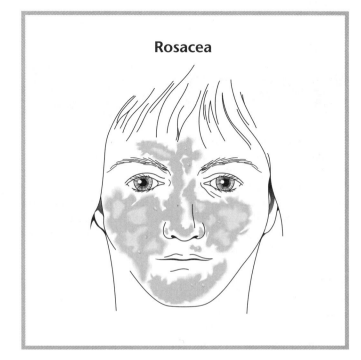

Rosacea

include acne, drug reactions, lupus, and other forms of skin inflammation.

How is rosacea treated?

The only really effective treatment is long-term antibiotic therapy. This usually involves either a topical cream (such as metronidazole, an antibiotic) or oral tetracycline—which is the antibiotic prescribed most frequently because it has minimal side effects with long-term use. Dosages are gradually reduced until, once the condition is under control, the medication can eventually be stopped altogether. Pregnant and breastfeeding women should consult their clinicians about alternative treatment plans. Tetracycline taken after the second month of pregnancy can damage the bones and teeth of a fetus.

If antibiotics are ineffective, 13-cis-retinoic acid (Accutane), a drug sometimes used to treat severe acne, may be prescribed. This drug is quite costly, and it is associated with a number of side effects. It should also never be used by a woman who is pregnant or planning to become pregnant.

If spider veins are a problem, they can be vaporized with laser surgery. More conventional surgery may be required to correct a red, bulbous nose.

How can rosacea be prevented?

Rosacea cannot be prevented, but very hot liquids, spicy foods, alcohol, and any other substances or behaviors that make a person flush should be avoided, since flushing worsens symptoms and may cause the disease to progress more rapidly. When the skin is exposed to sunlight, a potent sunscreen should be used, even in winter months.

Related entries

Acne, antibiotics, laser surgery, lupus, varicose veins

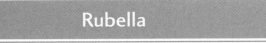

Rubella

Rubella—also called German measles or three-day measles—is a relatively mild disease in a child or adult, but it can have devastating effects on a fetus if it is contracted by the mother during pregnancy, particularly during the first trimester. About half of all fetuses whose mothers are infected during the first month of pregnancy will be severely affected, as opposed to only 10 percent of all fetuses whose mothers are infected during the third month.

What are the symptoms and effects of rubella?

Symptoms usually develop 2 to 3 weeks after exposure and, in adults, begin as a rash of raised pale pink spots on the face and neck. These fade within a day or so, although similar spots may appear on the trunk, arms, and legs. Other symp-

toms may include fever, swollen lymph glands, or runny nose.

The most common effects of rubella during pregnancy include miscarriage, stillbirth, and a number of birth defects (such as cataracts, deafness, and heart defects) collectively known as the congenital rubella syndrome. Later in life other disorders may develop, including diabetes. Babies born with rubella may have severe internal bleeding, and many do not survive a full year.

How can rubella be prevented?

The association between rubella and birth defects has been known for many years, and since 1969 a vaccine against rubella has been routinely administered to preschool and school-age children. Most children are vaccinated against rubella (along with measles and mumps) at the age of 15 months, and many schools require evidence of rubella immunization for admission. The purpose of this immunization is both to protect the children being vaccinated and to prevent them from bringing the disease home to mothers who may be pregnant and who may not have antibodies to the virus.

Because immunization (or previously having the disease) generally gives lifelong protection, about 75 to 80 percent of women in this country are protected against rubella by the time they reach childbearing age. Even so, because the dangers are so great for the remaining 20 to 25 percent of unprotected women, any woman who is contemplating pregnancy should have a rubella test, unless she is absolutely positive that she has already had the disease or received a vaccination for it. All that is required is a simple blood test that can detect antibodies to the rubella virus. Many states require rubella testing before a marriage license is obtained.

Any woman without antibodies should be vaccinated not less than 3 months before she attempts to become pregnant—during which time she should be using an effective form of birth control. Although the chances of the vaccine's harming a fetus are slim (there have been no reported cases), the fact that it is made from an attenuated (weakened) virus means it is theoretically possible for the virus to infect the fetus. It is also important for a woman who has older children to make sure that they have been vaccinated against rubella. Antibodies can be lost after radiation therapy, so any woman who has been treated for cancer with radiation should be revaccinated.

Rubella testing should be a routine part of prenatal care. Although the vaccine is not considered safe for administration during pregnancy, a pregnant woman who learns she is not immune can take special precautions to avoid infection—and to watch for any symptoms of the disease if she is exposed to the virus. She should also plan to be vaccinated after delivery.

How is rubella treated?

If a woman who is already pregnant seems to have developed rubella or has been exposed to it, rubella testing will be repeated. If she has indeed been infected, she may want to consider terminating the pregnancy, especially if the symptoms developed during the first trimester. An option for women who will not have an abortion is an immunoglobulin (gamma globulin) injection. This cannot prevent the fetus from becoming infected but may decrease the length of time that it is exposed to the virus.

Related entries

Abortion, birth control, diabetes, miscarriage, pregnancy, prenatal care

Safer Sex

Admonitions about "safe" or "safer" sex are so commonplace today that many Americans can repeat them almost like a mantra. Public health educators for years have routinely offered advice to sexually active people about ways to minimize the spread of sexually transmitted diseases (STDs), but until the AIDS epidemic the idea of "safe sex" usually had more to do with preventing pregnancy than preventing serious disease or death. True, for much of human history, sex, disease, and death were intimately associated, but the emergence of penicillin in the 1940s temporarily took the bite out of the most deadly STDs. When AIDS arrived on the scene, however, the old dread returned.

Because of AIDS and its deadly implications, the tone and intensity of the familiar rules have been transformed. If you want to save your life, say these new warnings, never have sex with anyone who has not been tested for HIV and make sure you and your partner are tested regularly—unless you are in a mutually monogamous, long-term relationship. Even if both partners have tested negative, the warnings continue, safe sex still means never having intercourse without a condom, refraining from oral-anal contact, and using a latex square or condom to separate you from your partner during oral-genital contact.

These often repeated rules, while well intentioned, are turning out to be self-defeating in many cases. They are based on two inconsistent assumptions: on the one hand, the rules urging regular testing except in mutually monogamous relationships assume that people can trust HIV testing and also that they can trust their partners. At the same time, however, people are admonished to observe other rules premised on the assumption that each and every partner should be presumed to be infected—regardless of negative testing or protestations of faithfulness.

Some sociologists and psychologists have observed that these absolutist rules have ended up encouraging rather than discouraging unsafe sexual practices. The reason is simple: many people take one look at the rigid rules—which usually do not differentiate between truly risky practices and only slightly risky practices—and realize that they are not willing

to go that far in modifying their lifestyle and sexual behavior. The result for some people is a sense that if they are at high risk of disease anyway owing to certain behaviors that they refuse to modify, all caution can therefore be thrown to the wind, since all behaviors are seemingly of equal risk.

The truth is that there are indeed ways to practice "safer" (if not absolutely safe) sex and to weigh relative risk. Apart from complete abstinence, of course, there is no such thing as 100 percent risk-free sex. Even people who believe that they are in a mutually monogamous relationship run some degree of risk—first, because a partner may have been infected years earlier (for some diseases, through a nonsexual source) without knowing it and, second, because not every relationship believed to be monogamous actually is. Also, tests for sexually transmitted diseases (including tests for HIV) are not infallible. Thus, it always makes sense to err on the side of caution when assessing the risk posed by a potential partner.

Still, by knowing some basic facts about risk and modes of transmission, sexually active people can continue to enjoy passion and intimacy while still minimizing their chances of transmitting or acquiring AIDS, chlamydia, gonorrhea, herpes, syphilis, or any other STD.

What sexual behaviors are "safer"?

Some so-called safer sex is little more than common sense. For example, sexual intimacy with multiple or unknown partners, or with people known to be at high risk for infection, is risky behavior. The better partners know each other, and the more open the communication between them, the lower the risks of STD infection.

People who inject themselves with drugs (for any medical or nonmedical reason) and who share needles are at very high risk for infection. This is because some of the microorganisms that can be transmitted sexually (such as HIV and hepatitis B) can also be transmitted through direct contact with an infected person's blood.

Finally, abusing alcohol or drugs when engaging in sexual activity is risky, since these substances can impair judgment and lead to dangerous decisions.

Sexual behaviors that are risky for one STD may not be risky for another, but most practices can be ranked in terms of their overall riskiness (see chart). It is important to emphasize that risk is near zero for any kind of sexual intimacy between partners who are free of infection and involved in a mutually monogamous relationship.

How can risk be reduced?

Even people who engage in risky sexual behaviors (such as having sex with multiple partners or with people whose infection status is unknown) can reduce the risks considerably by using protective devices such as new (never reused) latex condoms. Not all condoms are alike in their capacity to prevent transmission of HIV, so it is important to choose one with a label that says it can be used for disease prevention.

Risk of acquiring or transmitting sexually transmitted diseases

Behaviors are listed in order of riskiness. Risk becomes considerably less if protective measures are used, and is near zero for uninfected partners in a mutually monogamous relationship.

Extremely high risk

Receptive anal intercourse
Insertive anal intercourse

Latex condoms can reduce the risk of both acquiring and transmitting STDs during anal intercourse. To reduce the possibility of breakage (which is higher in anal than in vaginal intercourse), using water-based lubricants is highly recommended. If a finger or hand with open sores or cuts is inserted into the anus (or vagina), it is also a good idea to wear a latex glove. Disposable latex gloves are available at minimal cost from many pharmacies.

High risk

Receptive vaginal intercourse
Insertive vaginal intercourse

Latex condoms significantly reduce the risk of both acquiring and transmitting STDs during vaginal intercourse. Condoms should also be used on dildos or other sex toys inserted into the vagina (or anus) if they are used by more than one person.

Risky

Oral sex on a man with ejaculation
Oral sex on a man without ejaculation

The risk of transmitting HIV (the virus that causes AIDS) during unprotected oral sex is believed to be very low, but risk for other STDs (including gonorrhea and herpes) is considerably higher.

Low to medium risk

Oral sex on a woman
Oral-anal contact

Chances of acquiring HIV through oral sex on a woman (cunnilingus) are very low—and may be virtually nil. There is some unproven speculation that risk may be somewhat increased during menstruation. Unprotected cunnilingus carries a moderate risk of acquiring other STDs, however, such as gonorrhea and herpes. Oral-anal contact (rimming) also seems to carry a low risk of HIV infection but may easily transmit other microorganisms unless a barrier method (cut-open condom, latex square, or dental dam) is used correctly.

Latex (rubber) condoms are generally more effective in this respect than natural skin ones.

For greater protection, condoms can be used together with a water-based lubricant to reduce the chances of breakage. Even better is a spermicidal cream, foam, or gel, which not only doubles as a lubricant but also contains nonoxynol-9, a chemical that seems to provide some degree of protection against HIV and certain other sexually transmitted microor-ganisms. If intercourse is repeated, it is important to use a fresh condom and additional spermicide. Vaseline or other oil-based lubricants should never be used on condoms because they can weaken the latex.

Women whose partners refuse to wear a condom should consider using a female condom (see condoms). Condoms can also be used for fellatio (mouth-penis contact), but a fresh one should be used before having intercourse. Cunni-

Extremely low risk

Intimate kissing
Casual kissing
Touching, massage
Mutual masturbation

The risk of mutual masturbation increases if there are cuts or sores on the hands. There is no evidence that deep kissing spreads HIV.

No risk

Masturbation
Talking
Fantasizing
Abstinence

lingus (mouth-vagina contact) is believed to carry only a very small risk of HIV transmission from the woman to the man (and almost none from the man to the woman).

Related entries

Acquired immune deficiency syndrome, bacterial vaginosis, chancroid, chlamydia, condoms, diaphragms and cervical caps, gonorrhea, hepatitis, herpes, lubricants, sexually transmitted diseases, spermicides, syphilis, trichomonas

Salpingectomy

Salpingectomy is the surgical removal of one or both fallopian tubes. Bilateral salpingectomy, which involves the removal of both tubes, is most commonly performed during surgery to remove the ovaries or uterus (or both). Unilateral salpingectomy, which involves the removal of only one tube, is usually done after a fertilized egg is found to have implanted in that tube—if newer methods to save the tube, such as treatment with the drug methotrexate, are unsuccessful (see ectopic pregnancy). Women with one tube are still able to conceive and carry a pregnancy to term.

How is the procedure performed?

Often salpingectomy can be performed through a laparoscope. The procedure involves making a small cut just under the navel and through the abdominal wall. When salpingectomy is done with a laparoscope, regional or general anesthesia is used, and the hospital stay is 1 to 2 days. When salpingectomy is necessary because of chronic pelvic infection, often an abdominal incision (laparotomy; see entry) is

required to allow the surgeon to see and remove all scar tissue. In this case, a horizontal (bikini) incision 4 to 6 inches long is made across the pubic hairline, or, less commonly, a vertical (midline) incision from the pubic bone toward the navel is used.

What happens after surgery?

Often some discomfort in the incision area is felt for the first few days after a salpingectomy. Most women are up and walking by the third day, and gradually resume normal activities—including driving, exercising, and working—over the next month or two.

What are the risks and complications?

As with other forms of major surgery, certain initial risks are involved, including the risks of infection, hemorrhaging, abnormal scarring at the incision site (see keloid scarring), and adverse reactions to anesthesia. Almost all pelvic surgery results in some internal scar formation (adhesions), which can, in rare cases, cause discomfort years after the surgery.

Related entries

Ectopic pregnancy, fallopian tube cancer, hysterectomy, keloid scarring, ovary removal

Scabies

Scabies is a highly contagious parasitic infection. It occurs when microscopic mites called *Sarcoptes scabiei* burrow under the skin and deposit their eggs and feces. The result is often raised, irregular lines on the skin and agonizing itching, particularly at night. Scratching can lead to broken skin, which can become infected with other microorganisms. Infestations are particularly common between the fingers and on the wrists, armpits, soles of feet, breasts, labia, and buttocks.

When scabies is transmitted through sexual contact, it is considered to be a sexually transmitted disease. Though not generally a serious condition, scabies can be extremely annoying and, if untreated, can persist for years.

Who is likely to develop scabies?

Anyone whose skin comes in contact with infested sheets, towels, clothing, or furniture can develop scabies. It is sometimes transmitted through sexual contact with an infected partner.

What are the symptoms?

The first time a person is infected with scabies, it may take as long as a month before symptoms develop. Later infestations manifest themselves more quickly—sometimes in as little as a day.

The first sign of an infestation is a small, raised, wavy line on the affected area which soon begins to itch. Itching is particularly intense at night. Often the area becomes red and inflamed when a secondary infection develops.

How is the condition evaluated?

The symptoms of scabies may be similar to those of a number of skin conditions, including eczema, poison ivy, and allergic reactions. One way to differentiate these conditions from scabies is to have a clinician examine a scraping of the affected skin under a microscope to check for microscopic mites (one-sixtieth of an inch), eggs, or larvae.

How is scabies treated?

Various prescription commercial creams, lotions, and shampoos such as Kwell (lindane) can be used to kill the scabies parasite. Many physicians recommend Nix (permethrin), which is available without a prescription, and is effective with only a single application. Because many of these treatments can be irritating or provoke allergic reactions, it is a good idea to get a definite diagnosis of scabies from a clinician before starting treatment.

Most of the medications for scabies need be applied only once or twice and left on overnight, although itching from secondary infection may persist for days. In the meantime, applying a calamine or aloe vera lotion—or taking an antihistamine—can provide some relief. After a couple of weeks it may be necessary to repeat the treatment if symptoms do not seem to be subsiding. Pregnant women should consult their clinician before attempting to treat an infestation.

All clothing, towels, and bed linen recently used by the infected person, as well as any used by a person with whom she has had intimate contact, should be washed in hot water, machine dried for at least 20 minutes, or dry-cleaned. Some clinicians recommend treating the entire household with medication, even if there are no obvious signs of infestation.

How can scabies be prevented?

Preventing the sexual transmission of scabies involves practicing the same safer sex measures that can help prevent the spread of all sexually transmitted diseases. In addition, because scabies can be easily transmitted through intermediate objects, avoiding other people's towels and covering public toilet seats with tissue may help prevent its spread.

Related entries

Safer sex, sexually transmitted diseases

Schizophrenia

The most chronic and disabling of all mental illnesses, schizophrenia is a complex and still poorly understood condition that involves severely disturbed moods, thoughts, and behaviors. It can take a variety of forms, leading many investigators to speculate that the term schizophrenia may encompass several distinct disorders with different causes. In all cases, however, schizophrenia is characterized by psychotic episodes in which a person loses touch with reality or is incapable of distinguishing real from unreal experiences. The National Institute of Mental Health estimates that nearly 3 million Americans will develop schizophrenia during the course of their lives and that about 100,000 schizophrenic patients are in public mental hospitals on any given day.

Some people with schizophrenia have only one psychotic episode, while others have many but lead essentially normal lives in between. Still others with chronic (continuous or recurring) schizophrenia may require long-term treatment and may never be able to function independently. Without treatment, these people can lose the ability to manage basic needs and often end up on the streets or in jail. People with schizophrenia also appear to have a higher rate of suicide than the population at large. Over the past quarter century, however, improved therapies and a better understanding of the biological and psychosocial factors underlying mental illness have allowed increasing numbers of people with schizophrenia to lead independent lives.

Who is likely to develop schizophrenia?

Schizophrenia appears equally often in men and women. Men usually develop the first psychotic symptoms in their teens or early 20s, whereas women are more apt to develop them about a decade later.

There is strong evidence that the potential to develop schizophrenia is inherited, possibly because of a biochemical abnormality (such as an enzyme defect) or a subtle neurological deficit. Studies of identical twins (who have identical genes) separated at birth and raised in different families indicate, however, that some type of environmental factor or factors must also be involved, since in some cases one twin will develop schizophrenia while the other does not.

Whatever the exact relationship between genetics and environment turns out to be, there is no doubt that close relatives of schizophrenic patients have a higher than average chance of developing the disorder. In fact, a child who has a schizophrenic parent has a 1 in 10 chance of becoming schizophrenic, as opposed to the 1 in 100 chance for a child in the general population.

About 1 out of 1,000 pregnant women develop a schizophrenia-like (schizophreniform) disorder soon after delivery. This form of postpartum psychiatric disorder (see entry) does not appear to be inherited but does occur more often in women with a history of manic-depressive disorder or who have close relatives with manic-depressive disorder (see entry). In addition, about 1 in 4 women with a history of schizophrenia will develop postpartum psychosis.

What are the symptoms?

Before developing psychotic symptoms, some people with schizophrenia may become withdrawn or socially isolated, or show marked changes in speech, thinking, or behavior. The psychotic episodes themselves can vary greatly from person to person and can range from mild to severe. Generally, however, these episodes involve distorted perceptions of reality that can lead to feelings of anxiety and confusion. These feelings in turn may lead a person to sit rigidly for hours without moving or speaking. Alternatively, these feelings may lead her to pace the room or rock back and forth.

Hallucinations (particularly hearing voices), bizarre delusions of grandeur or persecution, illogical thinking, or reduction in emotional expressiveness are all common symptoms of schizophrenia, as are displays of emotion inconsistent with the person's words or thoughts—such as laughing while claiming to be besieged by space aliens. Contrary to popular belief, however, schizophrenia does not involve having a "split personality" or dissociative identity disorder.

Women who develop schizophreniform disorder following childbirth may have similar symptoms, although these tend to disappear after a couple of months of appropriate treatment. Symptoms are apt to recur after subsequent pregnancies, however.

How is the condition evaluated?

Displaying psychotic symptoms does not necessarily mean that a person has schizophrenia. Usually a clinician will do a physical examination and run various laboratory tests to rule out any medical disorders that may account for the symptoms. Because some people with symptoms of schizophrenia may have episodes of elation or depression, the possibility of other mental illnesses such as manic-depressive disorder or depression also needs to be eliminated. Occasionally a person who has both a mood disorder and psychotic symptoms and does not fit neatly into any other categories will be diagnosed as having a schizoaffective disorder.

How is schizophrenia treated?

Given that schizophrenia may not be a single condition, and that its causes remain unknown, current methods of treatment are based on the ability to reduce symptoms and minimize the chances of relapse. Despite the success of these methods for many people with schizophrenia, far too many others still suffer from frequent recurrences and live with chronic disabilities that interfere with school, work, and interpersonal relationships. Also, because there is still no cure for schizophrenia, even people who find an effective treatment must continue to use it on a long-term or even indefinite basis.

Antipsychotic medications (neuroleptics) such as haloperidol (Haldol), risperidone (Risperdal), and clozapine (Clozaril) are the most commonly used treatments for schizophrenia. They are particularly effective at relieving hallucinations, delusions, and confusion, and allow many people with schizophrenia to function more effectively. They do not help all people, however, and are no guarantee against relapse: about 40 percent of people using antipsychotic medications will have a relapse within 2 years of discharge from the hospital. Even so, this rate compares favorably with an 80 percent chance of relapse in people who do not use the drugs. For this reason, antipsychotic drugs should never be discontinued without the advice and supervision of a clinician.

Occasionally people who use antipsychotic medications for many years develop a condition called tardive dyskinesia. This irreversible neurological condition involves involuntary movements, usually of the mouth, tongue, and lips. The potential for the disabling effects of tardive dyskinesia must be weighed against the disruptive effects of schizophrenic symptoms. During pregnancy and breastfeeding, too, the benefits of controlling the schizophrenia should be taken into account along with risks to the fetus or nursing infant.

Lobotomy, a brain operation that was once used to treat people with severe schizophrenia, is now extremely rare. There is no evidence that hemodialysis (a blood-cleansing method used in some kidney disorders) or large doses of vitamins are useful treatments for schizophrenia.

The emotional, interpersonal, and job-related problems that accompany schizophrenia can often be helped with various psychosocial treatments, particularly once the psychotic symptoms are under control. These include vocational counseling, problem-solving and money management training, social skills training, individual psychotherapy, family therapy, group therapy, and self-help groups, though not all of these services are available for treating schizophrenia in all regions. More information can be obtained by contacting national mental health associations and advocacy groups. For example, the National Mental Health Consumers' Association, a network of self-help organizations, operates a Self-Help Clearinghouse. The National Alliance for the Mentally Ill (NAMI), which has statewide affiliate organizations, also offers patient resources, information, and support groups for mentally ill individuals and their family members.

Today most people with schizophrenia can live at home with their families and visit a clinic, occupational therapist, or doctor's office frequently for treatment. Hospitalization is usually necessary during acute or severe episodes, but prolonged hospital stays are becoming less common. In fact, there is a trend against institutionalization based on a documented lack of efficacy and the negative effects of prolonged hospitalization on the mentally ill. People who cannot live at home are likely to avail themselves of halfway houses or other short-term residential care facilities. These offer a protective atmosphere and close monitoring without completely disrupting a person's contact with family and community.

Related entries

Depression, manic-depressive disorder, multiple personality disorder, personality disorders, postpartum psychiatric disorders, psychotherapy

Scleroderma

Scleroderma is a disease of a connective tissue called collagen which is found in bones, skin, ligaments, and cartilage. In this condition (also called progressive systemic sclerosis), which appears more frequently in women than in men, overproduction of collagen in the skin causes a thickening and hardening of the dermis (inner layer of skin) and a thinning of the epidermis (outer layer of skin). Sweat glands and hair follicles are greatly diminished, and affected skin becomes permanently tight and shiny (see illustration). Sometimes internal organs may be involved as well. The cause is unknown, but scleroderma is probably an autoimmune disorder (see entry), in which the body attacks itself by producing antibodies against its own tissues.

Although rarely life-threatening and sometimes mild enough to be only a minor nuisance, for some women scleroderma can have profound effects on quality of life owing to cosmetic changes or reduced limb or lung function.

Who is likely to develop scleroderma?

Scleroderma usually develops between the ages of 30 and 60, although it can occur at any age. It is more common in African Americans than in whites.

What are the symptoms?

Symptoms of scleroderma usually take a couple of years to develop. Skin on the arms, face, or hands thickens and tightens; hands and feet become puffy; and joints may become stiff and painful. In limited scleroderma only the skin of the hands and face, and sometimes the lungs, is involved. Sometimes heartburn, sores on the fingers, and Raynaud's phenomenon (see entry), a condition in which fingers and toes turn white and blue after exposure to cold or emotional stress, occur. In diffuse scleroderma skin damage is more extensive and internal organs may be affected, sometimes leading to hypertension, lung problems, kidney damage, and malnutrition resulting from a damaged intestinal tract. In rare instances these developments can be life-threatening.

How is the condition evaluated?

A doctor evaluating scleroderma will do a thorough physical exam, paying special attention to the skin of the hands, feet,

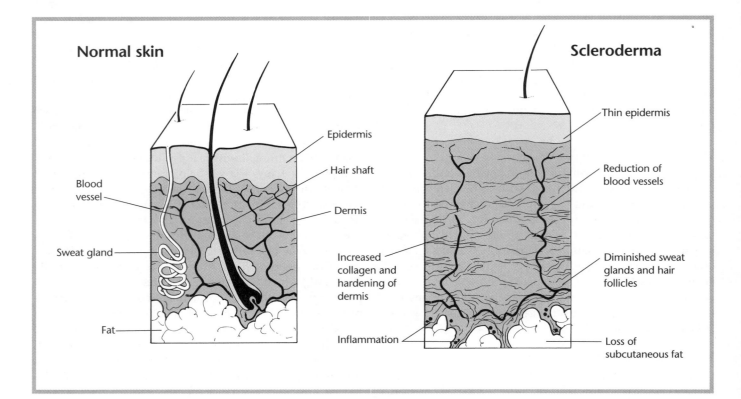

face, and arms and asking questions about accompanying symptoms such as Raynaud's phenomenon. Blood testing may be done to see if certain antibodies characteristic of this condition can be detected, and other tests will be done to distinguish it from other connective tissue diseases. Additional tests may be ordered to determine damage to internal organs. These may include kidney or liver function tests, an assessment of muscle enzymes, and urine testing.

How is scleroderma treated?

There is no cure for scleroderma, although numerous drugs and high-tech treatments are being studied by 30 U.S. medical centers involved in the Scleroderma Clinical Trials Consortium. Anyone with this condition may want to ask her clinician or a scleroderma support group about the possibility of getting into one of these trials.

Until a cure becomes available, specific symptoms can be treated as appropriate with antihypertensive medications, corticosteroids (antiinflammatory drugs), antacids, and painkillers. If Raynaud's phenomenon develops, it is advisable to avoid exposure to cigarette smoke, since nicotine can cause blood vessels to contract, and to wear gloves against exposure to cold. Some patients find that exercising affected areas reduces stiffness.

Related entries

Autoimmune disorders, heartburn, high blood pressure, kidney disorders, musculoskeletal disorders, nail care, Raynaud's phenomenon, skin care and cosmetics, skin disorders

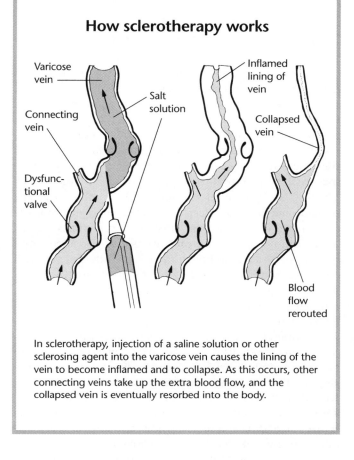

How sclerotherapy works

In sclerotherapy, injection of a saline solution or other sclerosing agent into the varicose vein causes the lining of the vein to become inflamed and to collapse. As this occurs, other connecting veins take up the extra blood flow, and the collapsed vein is eventually resorbed into the body.

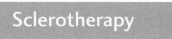

Sclerotherapy

Sclerotherapy is a procedure used to eliminate spider veins, hemorrhoids, and other superficial varicose veins. Used for decades in Great Britain, this relatively noninvasive procedure has only recently become accepted in this country, mainly because of a better understanding of how to prevent complications. Given the relative novelty of this procedure—as well as the promotion it often receives from vein clinics—it is a good idea to get the name of an experienced and competent practitioner from a primary care clinician before undergoing sclerotherapy. If the procedure is done for purely cosmetic reasons—as it usually is—chances are that it will not be covered by insurance.

How is the procedure performed?

Sclerotherapy is usually performed in a clinician's office by either a licensed physician or a registered nurse. A highly concentrated saline (salt) solution is carefully injected into the affected veins (see illustration). This solution irritates and inflames the blood vessel, causing the lining to swell and close off the vessel. Eventually the blood-deprived vein col-

lapses and is absorbed into the body. The blood that formerly flowed through it is merely rerouted into nearby veins.

If a relatively large vein is involved (that is, if the problem is more than spider veins), the clinician sometimes also uses Doppler ultrasound, a noninvasive imaging technique, to find the precise trouble spot and help direct the injection to it.

It usually takes only a few minutes to treat each vein, although if veins in both legs need to be treated, the procedure will probably be done on two separate days. The area around the injection site may itch or burn as the irritant is being injected, and sometimes nearby muscles may cramp. Occasionally hives develop as an allergic response to the solution, but these usually disappear within an hour and can be relieved with antihistamines.

What happens after sclerotherapy?

After the procedure an elastic bandage is wrapped from the base of the toes to the highest injection site and kept in place for at least 24 hours, after which support stockings should be worn for at least 3 weeks. The injection site remains sore or tender for a few days after the procedure, and it is a good idea to avoid aerobic exercise until the pain goes away. After the pain stops, walking as much as possible can activate the calf muscle to pump blood and help keep blood from pooling in the lower leg. The discoloration associated with varicose veins starts to fade within a week and is usually gone completely after about a month.

What are the risks and complications?

There is no guarantee that varicosities will not develop in other, previously healthy veins—particularly if the patient has certain attributes that predispose her to varicose veins, such as obesity, a sedentary lifestyle, or a job that requires long periods of standing.

One out of three people who have sclerotherapy develop yellowish-brown streaks or spots near the injection site. These probably result from blood and sclerosing fluid that have escaped from the ruptured vessel, and they generally clear up by themselves after 6 to 9 months. Of greater concern may be small ulcers that occasionally develop near the injection site and then crust over, sometimes leaving scars. Thin networks of purplish veins may also appear near the injection site, and though these sometimes fade on their own, laser surgery may be necessary to eradicate them completely.

In rare cases sclerotherapy may result in serious side effects, such as potentially fatal shock from an allergic reaction or inflammation of a vein caused by a blood clot (thrombophlebitis; see circulatory disorders). These side effects have become much less common with the use of saline solution, particularly as clinicians use less concentrated solutions. Even so, sclerotherapy is not advisable for anyone with a history of diabetes or circulatory disorders (other than varicose veins, of course), including thrombophlebitis, temporal arteritis, and other blood vessel inflammations (vasculitis).

To avoid the possibility of blood clots, women should stop taking birth control pills for at least 6 weeks before the procedure and use another means of contraception. Like all surgery for varicose veins, sclerotherapy should be postponed until at least 6 months after a pregnancy.

Related entries

Circulatory disorders, diabetes, exercise, hemorrhoids, laser surgery, obesity, pregnancy, temporal arteritis, ultrasound, varicose veins

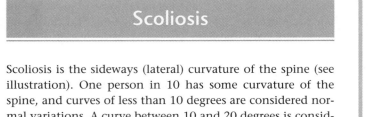

Scoliosis

Scoliosis is the sideways (lateral) curvature of the spine (see illustration). One person in 10 has some curvature of the spine, and curves of less than 10 degrees are considered normal variations. A curve between 10 and 20 degrees is considered mild. Although small degrees of curvature progress in 2 to 4 percent of the U.S. population of both sexes, women are apt to have more serious curvature. Approximately two-thirds of scoliosis patients are adolescent women. Most girls undergo a growth spurt during the 12 months before their first menstrual period, and this is the time when many curves progress.

In the not too distant past scoliosis was believed to progress inevitably to serious medical and physical problems and was routinely treated with braces to keep the curve from worsening. For many young women the cure was worse than the disease; however much they regretted their asymmetrical hips or their unevenly hanging skirts, it often seemed worse to have to wear a rigid, unattractive, uncomfortable brace which only called attention to the deformity. At a stage of life when many young women are insecure about their appearance and have a tenuous body image, such experiences often left lifelong emotional scars.

Added to the problem of back braces was the exposure of many young girls to large doses of radiation—required both to diagnose the scoliosis and then to monitor the progression (worsening) of the curve. The school screening programs which began in the 1940s across the United States were a mixed blessing. Although they certainly brought many

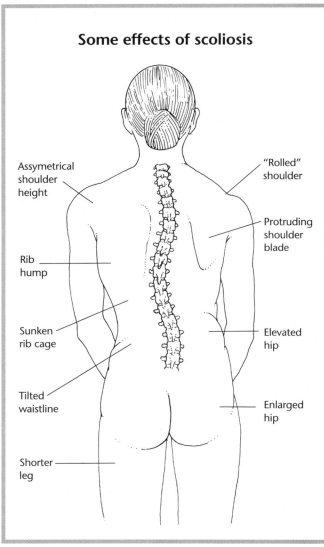

Some effects of scoliosis

Assymetrical shoulder height

"Rolled" shoulder

Rib hump

Protruding shoulder blade

Sunken rib cage

Elevated hip

Tilted waistline

Enlarged hip

Shorter leg

young girls in for treatment before their curves had progressed to the point of disability, they also yielded a large crop of children whose curves turned out to be insignificant—or nonexistent—but who ended up exposed to relatively high levels of radiation. Even among children who actually did turn out to have scoliosis, radiation dosage was probably unnecessarily high. It was not at all uncommon to have the curves first diagnosed at the age of 10 and then to have one or two x-rays every 6 months for many years to come—that is, until the end of skeletal growth.

A leap forward in knowledge about the natural history of scoliosis and the best way to manage it has made this kind of experience less common. Most researchers now believe, for example, that many scoliotic curves will never progress to the point of causing serious damage. In fact, most mild curves may not even progress at all. Unless there is significant pain or a cosmetic problem, therefore, braces may be unnecessary. Even when the curve is moderate (deviating more than 30 degrees from the spinal column) or shows signs of definite progression, treatment options are now available that make it possible to treat scoliosis in a less traumatic fashion. As for concerns about radiation, improved technology (such as special filters and x-ray film) and efforts to minimize exposure (including the use of breast shields) have made this much less of a problem.

Even so, scoliosis can occasionally lead to disabling pain and disfigurement. And when it does, treatment can be long-term, extensive, and often quite upsetting to both patients and their families. Pregnancy and the ability to bear children usually are not affected, and the spinal curves of pregnant women do not progress any more quickly than the curves of women who are not pregnant. In some cases, though, scoliosis may increase the chances of needing a cesarean section.

Who is likely to develop scoliosis?

In most cases—referred to as idiopathic scoliosis—the cause is not well understood, although there is good evidence that genes are involved to some extent. Some investigators think that balance and coordination deficits, perhaps regulated by a genetic mechanism, may play a role. Whatever the cause, the problem usually does not develop to a point where it is noticeable until a girl is between 10 and 16 years old.

Scoliosis occasionally appears in women with eating disorders such as anorexia. This is probably because skeletal abnormalities can result from the extremely low levels of estrogen that result when the proportion of body fat falls below a certain critical level (see osteoporosis). Because a high proportion of female athletes suffer from eating disorders and have a low ratio of fat to lean tissue, they are particularly likely to suffer from scoliosis.

What are the symptoms?

Scoliosis is visible to the untrained eye in the form of a protruding shoulder blade, rib hump on one side of the back, asymmetrical rib cage (visible from front and back), uneven hip height and size, shoulders that roll forward, or lopsided gait. In most girls and women it is the rib hump in particular that causes the most concern.

Untreated curves may progress to the point where the spinal column rotates toward the convex side of the curve, separating the ribs on one side of the body and compressing those on the other. Another part of the spine may compensate for the first curve by bending in the opposite direction, creating an S curve. If these bends are severe enough—and particularly if they involve the upper (thoracic) portion of the spine—the curves can even contract the ribs to the point where the lungs and heart are compressed, impairing breathing and circulation. The resulting respiratory problems are of particular concern when women with severe scoliosis become pregnant. A pregnant woman with scoliosis should be carefully monitored by a clinician.

A dramatic curve or spinal rotation can cause considerable back pain. Some investigators have observed, however, that the rate of back pain associated with scoliosis is no higher than the rate of back pain in the general population.

How is the condition evaluated?

Scoliosis is often first suspected by parents who notice that their daughter's spine looks crooked when she is wearing a bathing suit or that she has trouble finding clothes that fit. They often have difficulty hemming their daughter's pants and skirts. School screening programs detect a large number of cases, as do pediatricians doing routine physical examinations. These screenings may also detect cases of two related conditions, kyphosis (round back) and lordosis (swayback).

A clinician usually begins with a physical examination, asking the patient to bend over and looking to see if there is a visible deviation in the spine. More extensive testing is necessary to confirm the curve and determine its extent. Until recently this almost always meant having a number of spinal x-rays, but today there are several noninvasive alternatives that have made it possible to diagnose and monitor mild curves without exposure to radiation. These include moiré shadow photography, a technique in which the contours of shadow patterns from the spine are used to assess asymmetries, and Integrated Shape Investigation System (ISIS), a technique in which the contours are measured with computerized images of several different planes of the spine. X-rays become necessary only if these other techniques show significant changes in the curve.

The clinician may also perform a test for bone age or spinal maturity, usually by taking an x-ray of the wrist. The patient's x-ray is then compared to wrist x-rays in a special atlas to determine how mature her bones are and how much more her spine may be expected to grow. A pelvic x-ray or menstrual history may also help the clinician determine bone age. A patient with a curve around 25 degrees who has not yet menstruated is at greater risk for future deformity and pain than a girl who has reached menarche.

How is scoliosis treated?

One of the frustrating aspects of treating scoliosis is that researchers do not know what would happen in many cases if curves were left untreated. The fear is that many young women are being (or have been) forced to endure expensive, onerous, distressing, and even risky therapy when their curve might have remained stable on its own—or, at the very least, never progressed to the point of serious concern. What is now known with relative certainty is that the vast majority of mild curves do not progress, and therefore probably do not require correction. All that is needed is regular monitoring to make sure the curve remains stable.

Nonetheless, the consensus at this point is that curves that have progressed beyond 25 to 30 degrees in a child whose skeleton is still growing require some form of correction—even though the efficacy of this correction remains controversial. In most cases the treatment of choice remains some kind of spinal brace to keep the curve from progressing.

Throughout the centuries a variety of corsets, casts, and braces have been used to correct spinal deformities, but the first successful device for treating scoliosis was the Milwaukee brace. This device, originally developed in 1946 to support the spine after surgery, consists of a rigid metal frame extending to the throat and containing a customized pelvic girdle, together with pads that are fitted to the frame near the apex of the curve and pull the spine laterally. Widely used between the mid-1950s and early 1970s to keep curves from progressing, this cumbersome device probably accounted for a great deal of the adolescent misery associated with scoliosis. And although long-term follow-up studies indicated that the Milwaukee brace was indeed successful in stemming the progression of curves, some orthopedic surgeons regard the findings as somewhat specious, given that no one really understands which curves might have stabilized without a brace. Moreover, many young women simply were not willing to wear the contraption for the required period of time—usually 23 hours a day.

Then the 1970s saw the arrival of a variety of lower-profile devices such as the Boston Bracing System (BBS). Though still somewhat cumbersome and uncomfortable, these newer braces were at least less conspicuous. Of even more help was the discovery in the late 1980s that part-time bracing was just as effective as full-time. Today it is necessary to wear most braces for only 16 to 18 hours a day—which means it is possible for a girl to attend school without the brace and still obtain its full benefits. There is even some evidence that nighttime bracing alone may be effective.

Bracing tends to be most successful when there is sufficient commitment on the part of the patient and her family. Regular monitoring and emotional support from a team of health care professionals can help. This team usually consists of an orthopedic surgeon, who assesses and monitors the curve; an orthotist, who builds and adjusts the brace; a nurse, who coordinates care and gives instruction in using and living with the brace; and a physical therapist, who designs individualized exercises.

The role of exercise in treating scoliosis remains somewhat controversial. Although some investigators have claimed that exercise alone may stabilize curves, the more general opinion is that it cannot be used as a substitute for bracing. When used in conjunction with a bracing program, however, exercise can help correct posture and maintain proper breathing, muscle strength, range of motion in the joints, and spinal flexibility.

Transcutaneous electrical nerve stimulation (also known as TENS) was once viewed as a promising alternative to bracing. In this therapy, electrodes were placed at key points on the patient's back each night and an intermittent electric current was passed through them as she slept, ostensibly to keep the spine in place. It was hoped that TENS treatments would dispense with the need for a cumbersome brace during the day. Recent studies have shown, however, that patients who received electrical stimulation fared about the same as patients who received no treatment for their scoliosis.

If the curve continues to progress despite other efforts, or if it is severe (over 40 degrees in an adolescent and 50 degrees after growth has ended), spinal fusion or some other form of surgery may be necessary to reduce the curve, stabilize the spine, and balance the trunk. Scoliosis in adults may also require surgery, particularly if there are signs of progression (which is now known to occur in some patients even after skeletal maturity), pain, or breathing difficulties.

New types of instrumentation have greatly improved these operations (although correction remains more difficult in adults) and have reduced the number of complications. For example, many patients whose scoliosis was corrected with Harrington rods—the standard instrumentation for many years in correcting scoliosis—ended up with a problem known as flat back syndrome. This occurred when the spinal disks collapsed below the point of fusion, making it difficult to stand erect without either flexing the knees or leaning forward.

Newer instrumentation systems have made this syndrome much less likely. Monitoring spinal cord function throughout surgery and other preventive tactics have greatly reduced the risk of nerve damage (including paralysis). And physical therapy both before and after surgery—including training in deep breathing and in deep, effective coughing—have reduced the number of surgical complications. Today most patients can expect to walk independently within 4 to 7 days of the operation and usually have hospital stays of no longer than about 7 to 10 days.

Surgery for scoliosis is not without its share of uncertainties. Most distressing is that some of the correction may be lost within a few years after the operation. If the back pain and breathing difficulties turn out to be caused by some problem other than the scoliosis (or in addition to it), the surgery, while successfully correcting the curve, may not eliminate the symptoms that prompted it.

How can scoliosis be prevented?

Most scoliosis cannot be prevented, but early detection can limit its effects through careful monitoring by a clinician and intervention in severe cases. Screening techniques now used in school programs are reducing the number of unnecessary referrals, making the program more cost-effective. In addition, parents—in particular parents of girls between the ages of 10 and 16—should be aware of the signs of scoliosis; and if a curve seems to be developing, it should be called to the attention of a physician.

For girls who show signs of scoliosis, learning body awareness when standing, walking, and sitting, practicing proper posture, and choosing clothing styles that do not accentuate asymmetries may make mild curves less noticeable and boost a young person's self-image. Above all, a supportive parent can help a teenage daughter with scoliosis maintain a positive body image, so important to her psychological development during this period of dramatic physical, emotional, and sexual growth.

Related entries

Anorexia nervosa and bulimia nervosa, back pain, body image, exercise, mitral valve prolapse, musculoskeletal disorders, osteoporosis

Screening

Screening is the practice of assessing people for the presence of a disease before the disease has a chance to develop. The idea behind any screening program is that early detection of disease can save lives and eliminate unnecessary suffering. The annual physical examination is a good example of a screening procedure, and from its inception at the turn of the century until quite recently, it had been upheld as one of the fundamental tenets of good health care. As the years go by, ever more powerful diagnostic tools and techniques continue to emerge—including the x-ray, the Pap test, ultrasound, CT scanning, MRI scanning, chromosomal analysis, and mammography—and with them grows the temptation to identify hidden abnormalities in apparently healthy people.

On the surface, of course, the goal of detecting a disease before it manifests itself seems laudable. This is not always the case, however. First of all, many people would prefer not to know about a disease if there is nothing that can be done to treat it, and so universal screening for such conditions makes little sense. That is why—at least so far—being tested for conditions such as multiple sclerosis or Huntington's disease remains an individual decision.

Universal screening is also hard to justify if only a relatively few people suffer from a particular disease, if the disease has relatively trivial effects on health, if the test is very expensive, or if treating the disease once symptoms appear is just as effective as therapy begun earlier. Furthermore, the value of a screening procedure is severely limited if it yields a high percentage of false positives (that is, positive results for people who do not have the disease) or false negatives (negative results for people who do have the disease).

In recent years health care authorities have started to reconsider the rationale for many kinds of screening procedures, from the most sophisticated scanning procedure right on down to the annual physical examination. Not only have more rigorous scientific tests failed to demonstrate the overall efficacy of many once-routine screening procedures, but also the refusal of third-party insurers to pay for some of them has forced clinicians to be more careful about using them indiscriminately.

What are the risks and complications?

Even the best tests carry certain risks, as well as pain, inconvenience, and cost. A false-positive result may not only cause unnecessary anxiety but also necessitate additional expensive and risky diagnostic procedures. A false-negative result can build a false sense of security and possibly delay subsequent detection of and treatment for a serious disease. To prevent an inordinate number of false positives and false negatives, many screening tests are recommended only for groups of people known to have a high prevalence of the disease, such as people who fall within a certain age range or have certain risk factors for that specific condition.

In recent decades, various health authorities have made a concerted effort to evaluate the usefulness of individual preventive tests and develop screening guidelines based on more scientific data. These authorities include the Canadian Task Force (CTF), the U.S. Preventive Services Task Force (USPSTF), the American College of Physicians, and the American Cancer Society. Because research is still limited, however, these groups often disagree about the appropriate use of any given screening test. The chart on pages 532 and 533 reflects what is probably the majority but by no means the universal opinion at present. Given the high cost of screening, as well as the high cost of treating preventable disease, it is clear that considerably more research needs to be done to evaluate screening procedures more thoroughly. Undoubtedly these guidelines will be modified accordingly.

Related entries

Blood tests, breast self-examination, colon and rectal cancer, mammography, Pap test, pelvic examinations, physical examinations, sexually transmitted diseases, urine tests

Seasonal Affective Disorder

Seasonal affective disorder is a recurrent form of depression which develops during the fall and winter months and disappears during the spring and summer. Much more severe than the "winter blahs" or the "holiday blues," SAD makes people go into a sort of hibernation during the dark and dreary months, which involves long periods of sleep, withdrawal from the world, and stocking up on high-calorie sweets and carbohydrates.

Screening guidelines for women

Test	Purpose	Recommended frequency
Comprehensive history and physical	Establish clinician-patient relationship; opportunities for immunization and counseling, promote preventive care	Ages 18–40: Annual physical exam no longer recommended, although a baseline exam is recommended so that there is a record of the patient's medications, allergies, current and past medical history, health habits, and social and family history. For women in this age group, physical exams are recommended no less frequently than every 3 years. Age 40+: For women, an annual physical exam is recommended to ensure a yearly breast exam.
Counseling on diet, smoking cessation, safe sexual practice, alcohol abuse, seatbelt use, and other preventive measures	Prevent subsequent health problems and accidents	Should be available during any clinician visit
Mammography	Detect breast cancer	Ages 35–39: Baseline exam no longer recommended. If family history of breast cancer or other high risk factors, some authorities recommend beginning yearly mammograms at age 35 or 5 years before a first-degree relative developed breast cancer. Ages 40–49: Highly controversial. American Cancer Society recommends mammography every 1–2 years, but many other authorities say not necessary for women at average risk. Ages 50–70: Yearly, according to most authorities. Age 70+: No more than every 2 years if desired. Efficacy still not proven.
Breast self-examination	Detect breast cancer	Monthly
Clinical breast examination	Detect breast cancer	Ages 20–40: Every 3 years, but more often if a family history of breast cancer. Yearly after age 35 if high risk. Age 40+: Yearly

(continued)

In the past decade or so psychiatrists and other members of the medical community have come to recognize SAD as a legitimate diagnostic category. Some investigators estimate that as many as 10 million Americans suffer from this disorder, and as many as 25 million—or 1 in 5 Americans—may suffer from a mild form. Most of these people are women.

Researchers still do not know just what causes SAD, although there is increasing evidence that it may have something to do with the effect of light on levels of melatonin. Melatonin is a hormone produced by the pea-sized pineal gland in the brain, which is thought to be involved in the way the body regulates its circadian (daily) sleep-wake cycle.

Test	Purpose	Recommended frequency
Pap test	Detect cervical cancer	Recommendations vary somewhat. In general:
		Ages 18–65: Every 1–3 years after 3 consecutive years of normal tests. Sexually active women under age 18 should also follow these guidelines. Women with multiple sexual partners or onset of intercourse at an early age (before 16) should have annual tests.
		Age 65+: Can be performed every 3 years if consistently normal in past.
Pelvic examination	Detect cancers of the female reproductive tract	No clear guidelines, but generally the same as for Pap test
Rectal examination	Detect colorectal cancer	Age 40+: Yearly
Stool occult blood testing	Detect colorectal cancer	Age 50+: Yearly
Sigmoidoscopy	Detect colorectal cancer	Age 40+: Every 3 to 5 years in people with a first-degree relative with colorectal cancer, personal history of ovarian or breast cancer, or adenomatous polyps (which are potentially cancerous).
		Age 50+: Every 3–5 years.
Colposcopy	Detect cervical and vaginal abnormalities	Women whose mothers took DES while pregnant with them should have regular exams.

This, in turn, may be related to the relatively longer periods of darkness that occur during the fall and winter months. Because periods of darkness stimulate melatonin production, some investigators have theorized that people with SAD may be overproducing melatonin or may simply be hyperresponsive to normal amounts of melatonin produced during the winter months. It is also possible that circadian rhythms in people with SAD are disrupted because they secrete melatonin abnormally late in the day.

Other evidence suggests that decreased levels of neurotransmitters (chemicals that transmit signals between nerve cells) such as serotonin or dopamine may also play a role in triggering SAD. Low levels of serotonin in particular have been associated with carbohydrate cravings in people with SAD, and with sleep disorders and depression in the population at large.

Who is likely to develop SAD?

Approximately 80 percent of people with seasonal affective disorder are women. Why SAD is more prevalent in women remains a mystery, although there is speculation that the disorder may have some connection with female reproductive

hormones. At least some of the prevalence in females may also be due to the fact that women are more likely than men to seek medical attention in the first place, and are thus more likely to be diagnosed as having SAD.

Symptoms of SAD usually begin when a person is in her late teens or early 20s and often—though not always—disappear later in life, particularly after menopause in women. The farther a person lives from the equator, the more likely she is to develop SAD.

What are the symptoms?

Like some other disorders that exclusively or predominantly affect women—such as premenstrual syndrome and postpartum psychiatric disorders—SAD is defined not by specific symptoms but rather by the specific timing of the symptoms. Unlike clinical depression or bipolar affective disorder (manic depression), for example, which can occur at any time of year, SAD affects people on a seasonal basis (although some researchers wonder if SAD may be an atypical form of manic depression without the manic phase). During the rest of the year people with SAD tend to be happy, outgoing, and productive. Because until recently the timing of symptoms was not a standard way of differentiating one disease from another, many people with SAD were misdiagnosed as suffering from other conditions.

Many of the symptoms of SAD are similar to those of depression or hypothyroidism (see entries)—except that they occur only during the fall and winter. These include fatigue, a tendency to sleep more, irritability, poor concentration, apathy, crying spells, a desire to withdraw from social contacts, and a change in eating habits—in particular, irresistible cravings for carbohydrates. It is typical for people with SAD to gain about 10 pounds every winter and then to lose weight with ease every spring. Other people with SAD suffer from headaches, lethargy, and restless sleep.

How is the condition evaluated?

SAD is essentially a diagnosis of exclusion. This means that it is diagnosed only after a psychiatric evaluation reveals no other obvious psychological, emotional, or social factors that might account for the symptoms. To be diagnosed with SAD a person must have had at least one major depression or a history of at least two consecutive fall-winter depressions.

How is SAD treated?

Recently there has been a great deal of success treating SAD with light therapy (phototherapy). This is based on the theory that light suppresses the secretion of melatonin—and that people with SAD may develop symptoms because of diminished exposure to light. The simplest form of phototherapy is a temporary relocation to the tropics, but of course this is not always practical. Instead, most people undergoing phototherapy bask in the artificial light from one of various devices called light boxes. These boxes, some of which are portable, rest on tables or desks and emit a broad spectrum of fluorescent light that is 5 to 20 times brighter than ordinary indoor lighting and is free of ultraviolet rays. Treatment lasts between 15 and 120 minutes a day, and often can be done at home—although it should be undertaken only by people who are under the care of a qualified clinician.

Another option still under investigation is using full-spectrum lightbulbs in household lamps. There is some evidence that phototherapy—or any regular exposure to light—may relieve symptoms in as many as 4 out of 5 people with SAD, often within a few days.

None of the devices currently in use has been formally sanctioned by the federal Food and Drug Administration (FDA), which still labels the treatment as experimental. A light box costs between $300 and $500, an expense not covered by many insurance policies (although patient pressure is changing this in some cases). There may also be side effects, most notably hypomania—a mild increase in excitement—as well as insomnia, irritability, eye strain, and headaches. People whose skin is particularly sensitive to light or who are taking drugs that increase light sensitivity cannot use phototherapy, nor can those who have recently had eye surgery.

Other treatments for SAD—sometimes combined with phototherapy—include antidepressant medications and psychotherapy. Most clinicians encourage people with SAD to make sure that they eat a balanced diet and get adequate exercise. Generally, the newer antidepressants called selective serotonin reuptake inhibitors (SSRIs, which include Prozac, Zoloft, and Paxil) are preferable to the more traditional tricyclic antidepressants. This is because the tricyclics tend to exacerbate some of the symptoms of SAD, such as increased appetite and sleepiness. The SSRIs have just the opposite effect. Also, investigation is now under way to see if taking a melatonin supplement at a critical time of day may help people with SAD by resetting the body's internal clock.

Related entries

Antidepressants, depression, exercise, fatigue, headaches, hypothyroidism, insomnia, manic-depressive disorder, menopause, nutrition, psychotherapy, sleep disorders

Sexual Abuse and Incest

Incest (sexual contact between blood relatives) and sexual abuse of children (sexual contact between an adult and a minor) are considered by most psychiatrists to be acts of violence in which the perpetrator asserts power and control over someone who is defenseless, dependent, and trusting. Occurring in families of every race, educational background, and income level, sexual abuse is most commonly inflicted by fathers, brothers, stepfathers, or stepbrothers, although it is not unknown for mothers to abuse their children sexually (with boys abused by their mothers about twice as often as girls). Fathers who commit incest often have histories of childhood sexual or physical abuse themselves, as well as emotional deprivation, personality disorders, alcohol abuse, and unemployment. Their own low self-esteem, feelings of powerlessness, and anger often turn them into victimizers of even more helpless family members. The mothers of these abused children also often have a history of being abused as children, and may be victims of domestic abuse, or emotionally unavailable owing to depression or physical illness. Such backgrounds also predispose women to physical abuse of their own children.

One out of every 4 adult women reports having been involved in a nonvoluntary sexual encounter before the age of 18, making women 2 to 4 times more likely than men to have been sexually abused as children. Some investigators estimate that between 15 and 40 percent of all children under 14 in the United States are sexually abused, with 10 percent of that abuse involving incest and the rest involving close friends of the family, teachers, babysitters, or health care professionals—or, much more rarely, strangers.

It is not clear whether cases of sexual abuse and incest are increasing or whether social workers, teachers, and health care professionals are simply looking for them more. Skeptics have argued that leading questions by professionals can cause children to manufacture incidents that never actually occurred, and undoubtedly there have been some false accusations. Nonetheless, reports of incest and sexual abuse of children are too prevalent to be dismissed as pure fiction.

Who is likely to be a victim of sexual abuse or incest?

Although incestuous activity can begin even in infancy, it typically begins with genital fondling or oral-genital stimulation when the child is between 8 and 12 years of age. When the victim reaches puberty, the incest may proceed to sexual intercourse. Being the eldest or the only daughter seems to increase a girl's risk of being sexually abused.

What are the aftereffects?

Sexual abuse of young children can lead to scarring and permanent damage to the genitals, rectum, mouth, and throat, and even, in severe cases, death. Abused girls and young women are at high risk for acquiring sexually transmitted diseases, particularly bacterial vaginosis, trichomonas, chlamydia, and AIDS. Because many abused children are prevented from receiving routine medical attention, these problems are often neglected until they become quite serious. After puberty, sexually abused young women also risk becoming pregnant.

The long-term effects of childhood sexual abuse and incest generally correlate with the amount of force used and the amount of physical violation involved, as well as with the nature of the relationship and the age difference between the victim and the abuser. Many women with a history of childhood sexual abuse are not aware of any long-term damage, though for others physical and emotional scars can last a lifetime and spark a chain of abuse that may continue for generations.

Women who were sexually abused as children develop high rates of depression, substance abuse, self-destructive behaviors, eating disorders, and dissociative identity disorder. Many develop posttraumatic stress disorder as children and live in a state of constant fear and anxiety: some develop learning disabilities or specific delays in speech and motor functions or social skills. Many abused children grow up thinking of themselves as "bad" because a person they loved and trusted treated them so badly. Reflecting on their childhood, many women feel worthless and guilty and persist in the belief that somehow they were at fault for permitting, promoting, reporting, or not reporting the abuse.

Adult sexual dysfunction is common among victims of childhood sexual abuse, usually involving aversion to sex, distrust of men, and anxiety about intimate relationships. It may also involve difficulty setting sexual boundaries, with the result that some victims of childhood sexual abuse become promiscuous teenagers, prostitutes, or participants in pornography. As many as 4 out of 5 girls who are severely sexually abused will end up as sexually abused women, usually by spouses or other sexual partners. Prone to "revic-

timization," these women are also more likely than other women to be sexually abused by health care providers.

Even as children, victims may have a hard time knowing the boundaries of intimacy and may develop what psychiatrists call a "disorder of hope" in which they either idealize or despise new acquaintances. The result, in either case, is disappointment and a confirmation of their own helplessness in facing the rest of the world.

Psychosomatic disorders such as conversion disorder (hysteria) and somatization disorder are common in women with a history of childhood incest and sexual abuse. These often manifest themselves as chronic pelvic pain, abdominal pain, or other gastrointestinal problems.

How is sexual abuse evaluated?

Legislation in almost all states requires that any health care professional, teacher, child care provider, social worker, or other person who cares for children must report known cases of child abuse. The child is usually put into a protective environment immediately and given a medical and psychological examination as soon as possible so that effective intervention can be taken.

Anyone who becomes aware of someone who sexually abuses a child—including the abuser's private therapist—is also required to report the abuser. Some professionals question the efficacy of this law, feeling that it will keep abusers from seeking help for fear of being reported. Still, the majority opinion is that reporting, handled sensitively, is beneficial for both victim and abuser. The mental health community, which once maintained that family therapy could effectively alleviate incest, now believes that the abuser must be arrested before any other therapy can be effective.

How is sexual abuse treated?

Many women who were sexually abused as children have kept this knowledge a deep, dark secret for years. Some do not come to realize the full extent of the crime until they are adults and begin to talk to other women who had more normal childhoods.

Often women find it therapeutic to tell their stories to other women, usually in the form of psychological counseling or support groups for survivors of incest or childhood sexual abuse. Many also seek psychotherapy or other psychiatric attention for specific psychological problems that often result from childhood abuse. Long-term psychodynamic therapy (see psychotherapy) has proven quite helpful for some sexual abuse survivors, as has a therapy called EMDR (eye movement desensitization and reprocessing; see entry on posttraumatic stress disorder).

Related entries

Acquired immune deficiency syndrome, alcohol, anxiety disorders, bacterial vaginosis, chlamydia, depression, domestic abuse, dissociative identity disorder, pelvic pain, personality disorders, posttraumatic stress disorder, psychosomatic disorders, psychotherapy, sexual assault, sexual dysfunction, sexually transmitted diseases, substance abuse, trichomonas,

Sexual Assault

Sexual assault is nonconsensual sexual penetration—including but not limited to sexual intercourse—achieved with physical force or the threat of physical force. Motivated by the desire to dominate or humiliate, it is an act of violence rather than an act of sexuality. Sexual assault is commonly referred to as rape, although technically this is a legal term with a definition that varies from state to state.

Sexual assault is more likely to be committed by someone the victim knows than by a stranger—thus the terms date rape, acquaintance rape, and marital rape. Sexual assault by a known person is also more likely to result in physical injury. Most assaults are planned in advance, and over half occur in the victim's own home.

In the past two decades or so, the number of reported sexual assaults has been increasing faster than any other crime of violence. This is partly because women are more willing to report such assaults now that some of the stigma associated with rape has been lifted, largely owing to the efforts of the women's movement and the victims of crime movement. But since the mid-1970s an explosion of research has confirmed the pervasiveness of sexual assault and incest against women and children in the United States.

Formerly it was common to assume that women provoked rape or even that they enjoyed it. Law enforcement officials, academic investigators, and health professionals typically minimized the trauma that the victim experienced or blamed her for the assault. Although this kind of thinking is by no means extinct, grassroots support services (such as local rape crisis centers), rape reform legislation, and even financial compensation for victims is now available in many parts of this country.

Who is likely to be sexually assaulted?

Anyone (including babies, males, and the elderly) can be a victim of sexual assault, but being female, young, married or formerly married, and living in a city all increase the chances. Somewhere between 6 and 25 percent of women in this country have been victims of a completed rape, and up to 50 percent of women have been threatened with rape at least once in their lives. Marital rape has been reported to occur in 3 to 14 percent of marriages.

High as these numbers are, they undoubtedly underestimate the extent of the problem, given the reluctance of many women to report rape, especially marital rape. It is generally believed that only about 1 sexual assault in 10 committed by a stranger is reported, and the percentage is even lower when the victim knows the attacker.

Women hesitate to report sexual assault, or actually decide not to report it, for a number of reasons. They may not wish to turn in an acquaintance or spouse because they do not want to see that person prosecuted and jailed. Other women are reluctant to report an assault because they feel ashamed, embarrassed, or polluted, and prefer to withdraw rather than face what they fear will be (and often is) public humiliation and exposure. Even with increasing public support for victims and widening discussion of sexual assault, until recently it was common for defense attorneys to impugn a victim's character and personal life. Some women—even if they have been victimized—may feel that their personal life is not the business of the state.

Despite many improvements in training people in police departments and hospital emergency rooms to respond sensitively, the treatment a victim gets still varies according to her race, sexual orientation, degree of affluence, marital status, and relationship to the rapist. Only half of all alleged rapists are ever arrested. Of these arrests, only 3 in 5 result in prosecution, and only half of the cases that are prosecuted are strong enough to be brought to trial. In the end, fewer than 1 in 6 of the cases that do eventually go to trial result in conviction. Knowing that prosecuting a rape often means being interrogated by hostile defense attorneys and accused of seduction in a court of law and that few rape trials end in conviction discourages many women from reporting this crime in the first place.

What are the physical and psychological effects of sexual assault?

Because sexual assault generally involves force, it frequently results in physical injuries. These usually involve the violated area (genital tract, mouth, or anus), as well as cuts and bruises on other parts of the body. Nausea and abdominal pain are common.

Women who have experienced sexual assault are at future risk for chronic pelvic pain, abdominal pain, irritable bowel syndrome, and sexual dysfunction. Memories of the assault combined with actual physical injury can result in a variety of gynecological complaints. In addition, women who have been raped face the risk of contracting a sexually transmitted disease, including HIV. Women in their reproductive years may be at risk for pregnancy.

Almost all women who have been sexually assaulted experience some degree of emotional or psychological disturbance, even if at first they numb themselves to the trauma, deny their feelings, and try to go on with life as if nothing had happened. At some point most women experience anger, fear, insecurity, depression, insomnia, nightmares, aversion to sexual contact, and feelings of violation and loss of control. These can last for months or even years. An event that reminds the woman of the assault or makes her feel that she has no control over her life can trigger these feelings even after she thinks she has recovered.

Many women feel that they were somehow responsible, that they should not have flirted with the man in a bar, or that they should have made sure the bedroom windows were locked, or that they should have avoided being alone in the house with the perpetrator, or that they should not have walked down a deserted street after dark. As a result, they may feel guilty and worthless.

It is common for rape victims to develop posttraumatic stress disorder (see entry), which results when the mind and body are overwhelmed by a traumatic experience. Sexual assault has also been associated with other psychiatric conditions, including major depression, obsessive-compulsive disorder, and alcohol or substance abuse.

Frequently problems develop with marital or other sexual partners. Men from certain backgrounds may reject a woman who has been sexually assaulted as "fallen" or "polluted," while other men, though sympathetic, may involuntarily respond with rage or anger directed at the victim, when in fact the woman needs love and support. Other partners may feel helpless and prefer to ignore the trauma by continuing as usual once the obvious physical problems have been resolved, oblivious to the woman's need to talk through her feelings.

What should a woman do after a sexual assault?

The first step to take after a sexual assault is to seek medical attention for any physical injuries that may have been sustained. This can usually be done in a hospital emergency room. Besides evaluating the woman's physical health, the examiner will try to collect physical evidence of the assault in case the woman later decides to prosecute. For this reason—and because of the risk of acquiring a sexually transmitted disease or becoming pregnant—it is important even for women who feel they are fine physically to have a thorough medical examination.

Most emergency room staff are trained in examining sexual assault victims and familiar with the local laws regarding the collection of physical evidence. Many emergency rooms also have nurses on staff with special training in helping victims of sexual assault. Evidence of the assault will be more convincing if it is obtained as soon as possible after the incident. Evidence of sperm, for example, can disappear after only about 8 hours. Hard as it may be for the woman, it is important, too, to be examined before taking a shower, bathing, or douching, since these can wash away evidence that may turn out to be crucial in obtaining a conviction.

Besides evaluating and treating injuries and recording them in detail, the examiner will look for physical evidence such as blood or hair from the rapist on the woman's body or clothing. The woman's clothing may be kept as evidence, so if possible she should take an extra change of clothes with her to the emergency room or doctor's office. If the assault was vaginal, the examiner will do a pelvic examination and a Pap test to look for any evidence of sperm cells. These can also be used to determine the rapist's blood type. The cervix and vaginal walls will be examined for the presence of sperm or acid phosphatase, a substance produced by the prostate gland and ejaculated in the seminal fluid. If the assault was

anal or oral, specimens will also be taken from the rectum or mouth.

How is a victim of sexual assault treated?

Although some tests will be done for sexually transmitted diseases at the time of the initial examination, not all of these diseases can be diagnosed after initial exposure. For this reason, some of the tests will need to be repeated later. For example, a woman must wait at least 2 weeks for another gonorrhea test, 3 months for syphilis, and 6 months for HIV. In the meantime, the doctor may prescribe antibiotics to be taken as a preventive measure. She will also probably be tested for HIV every 3 months for a year after exposure.

If the woman is in her reproductive years, not using birth control pills or some other form of contraceptive, and near mid-cycle, the chance of a pregnancy is considerable. For that reason she should consider taking a morning-after pill. This medication, taken orally or by injection within 72 hours of unprotected intercourse, usually consists of a high dose of estrogen such as is found in some birth control pills.

In the emergency room of some larger hospitals, there may be a social worker trained to support women who have been sexually assaulted. If the hospital does not provide such services, women should consider contacting a local rape crisis center either before or after the medical examination. Often these centers, which are available across the United States and in many places are open 24 hours a day, can be contacted by the hospital if the woman has not already called. These crisis centers can send someone to act as the woman's advocate—that is, a person who will provide support and assistance—at the hospital and the police station. They can also provide counseling on getting medical care, as well as instructions on how to report a sexual assault to the police and how to handle the legal process if the woman decides to press charges. Later, advocates may accompany the woman to the lawyer's office and courthouse as well, working at all times to ensure that she is treated respectfully. Similar information may also be available from programs for victims of domestic abuse, women's self-help clinics, or the district attorney's office, as well as through attorneys specializing in family law or personal injury.

An advocate from a rape crisis center can also help the woman find psychological counseling should she need it. This is often available through rape victims' groups sponsored by the center itself, other community organizations, or hospital psychiatric departments. If necessary, the advocate can also help the woman find a professional psychotherapist experienced in working with rape victims. Teenage and younger victims of sexual assault are especially likely to require this additional counseling.

Whether or not a woman eventually decides to press charges, she should carefully consider reporting the assault to the police as soon as her medical needs have been met. At the police station she will be asked to describe in detail what happened and to describe and identify the attacker as specifically as possible so that he can be arrested. Prompt reporting will greatly improve the woman's case should she decide to press charges.

For those women who may not be willing to have an acquaintance or partner arrested, or who for whatever reason do not wish to make the assault a matter of public record, many states now allow women to report a rape anonymously. This allows police to keep records of the crime and provide support for the victim but still gives her time to decide if she wants to identify herself and the rapist and press charges against him. More specific information on local provisions can be obtained through a local rape crisis center.

How can sexual assault be prevented?

The notion of preventing sexual assault is specious in the sense that it implies that rape can be avoided and that victims are somehow to blame if it is not. Because the majority of assaults are committed in the home by someone the victim knows, many of the safety measures routinely suggested are of little value. Still, the realities of modern life demand that women take certain precautions. While no guarantee against sexual assault, they do restore to women a degree of control over their own bodies.

Thinking about one's options (screaming, fighting back, talking, yelling "Fire!") if a rape is attempted is one way to be prepared, and taking some courses in self-defense makes sense as well, if only to bolster a woman's self-confidence and make her appear less vulnerable. But there is no one "right" way to deal with a rapist. Some evidence suggests, however, that resisting may increase the risk of physical injury, and what makes sense in one situation may be pointless in another.

Women living alone should keep entrances well lit and outside doors deadbolted, and should consider using initials instead of a first name on mailboxes and in telephone listings. Windows should be locked and, whenever possible, covered with iron grids (especially in urban areas or on the ground floor of an apartment building). It should be routine to find out the identity of a visitor before opening a door.

Walking in dark parking lots alone, taking strolls through dangerous streets in the wee hours of the morning, and getting into a car before checking the back seat are risky behaviors for all women. Many colleges provide free shuttle bus services so students can avoid walking back to the dormitory alone late at night. Some women always keep keys, Mace, ammonia, or a police whistle ready for use whenever they have to walk alone at night. Others work out commuting arrangements with friends or set up houses of safety where they know they can stop in anytime they feel afraid.

Related entries

Abortion, acquired immune deficiency syndrome, depression, domestic abuse, gonorrhea, obsessive-compulsive disorder, Pap test, pelvic examinations, pelvic pain, posttraumatic stress disorder, psychosomatic disorders, psychotherapy, sexual abuse and incest, sexual dysfunction, sexually transmitted diseases, substance abuse, syphilis

Sexual Dysfunction

The exact incidence of sexual dysfunction in the general population is not known, but a recent survey ranked sexual difficulties fourth among the top problems facing heterosexual American couples, after rapid social change, domestic abuse, and money. Sexual problems appear to be more prevalent in females, affecting 43 percent of adult women and 31 percent of adult men. Nonetheless, most research about both the physical and psychological nature of sexuality has involved males, and even today most knowledge of female sexuality is based primarily on our knowledge of males. Following the approval of sildenafil (Viagra) for the treatment of impotence in men, however, there has been a surge of interest in female sexual dysfunction as well.

There are three basic types of sexual dysfunction. The first type, disorders of desire, takes the form of inadequate sexual desire (libido) in both sexes. The second type, disorders of excitement (or arousal), involves insufficient vaginal lubrication (wetness) in women and, in men, impotence (failure to attain or maintain an erection through the completion of the sexual act). Some women may also experience vaginismus, a disorder in which the muscles in the entrance to the vagina contract involuntarily, making intercourse difficult and painful, if not impossible. The third type of sexual dysfunction, disorders of orgasm, includes difficulty achieving orgasm, and, in men, premature ejaculation (orgasm that occurs before the man wishes it to occur).

These disorders often appear together, and problems in one partner can affect the other. Lack of sexual desire in a heterosexual woman, for example, may ultimately affect her partner's ability to achieve an erection. Similarly, a man who experiences premature ejaculation or who does not engage in adequate foreplay may make it difficult or impossible for his partner to achieve orgasm.

A host of factors, both physical and psychological, may underlie these problems. Male sexual dysfunctions (such as impotence) once thought to be purely psychological have now been shown in many cases to have a physiological basis. Far less is known about the physiological roots of female sexual dysfunction, but many diseases, disabilities, and surgical procedures (as well as premenstrual syndrome) have been linked to sexual problems in women; in addition, various medications can also significantly alter sexual functioning (see charts).

Sexual pleasure in humans is as much a product of the mind as of the body. Depression, anger, anxiety, and fear can interfere with a person's ability to enjoy sexual activity. Many women find that their sexual response is inextricably linked to other, nonsexual feelings they have for their partner. Mundane squabbles, lack of communication, basic incompatibility, arguments over money, and marital infidelity all impinge on sexual response. A man or woman exhausted from stress at work or other responsibilities may simply have no energy

Disorders and surgeries that can affect sexual response in women

Endocrine problems	Associated sexual dysfunction
Diabetes	Reduced vaginal lubrication; vaginal infections
Thyroid, adrenal, or pituitary gland disorders	Reduced vaginal lubrication
Vascular problems	
Sickle cell anemia	Decreased arousal and orgasm
Heart disorders such as heart attack or angina	Fear of death leading to reduced frequency of sexual activity
Neurologic problems	
Spinal cord damage or multiple sclerosis	Decreased arousal, orgasm, and vaginal lubrication
Gynecologic problems	
Vaginitis, pelvic inflammatory disease (PID), or endometriosis	Vaginismus; pain during sexual intercourse
Prolapsed uterus or uterine fibroids	Decreased arousal and desire
Kidney problems	
Kidney failure (using dialysis)	Decreased arousal and desire; electrolyte and hormone imbalance
Musculoskeletal problems	
Arthritis	Chronic pain; limited motion
Sjögren syndrome	Decrease lubrication
Surgical procedures	
Oophorectomy or episiotomy	Decreased estrogens and lubrication; tightness of vaginal opening
Mastectomy or colostomy	Loss of self-esteem and fears of discomfort that may interfere with any phase of sexual function

left to engage in the flirtation or seduction behavior necessary for enjoyable sex.

Sometimes sexual dysfunction can be traced to a lack of information about sexuality and sexual response—such as not knowing the importance of adequate foreplay or the fact that females generally require much more time than males to reach orgasm. Even women aware of these things may feel uncomfortable expressing their needs to their partner. Other women, afraid of feeling vulnerable, may have problems "letting go" or losing control. They may also worry about what their partner is thinking about them or fear that they are not doing the right thing to give and experience pleasure.

Medications that can affect sexual response in women

	Side effect
Antihypertensives	
Methyldopa, reserpine, clonidine, propranolol, or spironolactone	Decreased libido; difficulty having orgasms
Anticholinergics	
Propantheline or methantheline	Decreased lubrication
Hormones	
Estrogen, progesterone, or steroids	Decreased libido (sometimes)
Androgens	Increased libido
Psychotropics	
Sedatives, such as alcohol or barbiturates	Various sexual problems at high doses
Antianxiety medications, such as diazepam and alprazolam	Difficulty having orgasms
Antipsychotics, such as thioridazine	Difficulty having orgasms
Antidepressants, including	Difficulty having orgasms
MAOIs, such as phenelzine	
Tricyclics, such as imipramine, clomipramine	
SSRIs, such as Prozac (fluoxetine), Zoloft (sertraline), and Paxil (paroxetine)	
Trazodone	Increased libido (sometimes)
Lithium	Decreased libido
Opiates	
Morphine, codeine, methadone	Decreaseed libido; difficulty having orgasms
Miscellaneous	
Phenytoin, indomethacin, clofibrate, cimetidine, or carbamazine	Decreased libido

Growing up in a family with negative attitudes about sex can interfere with a woman's enjoyment of her sexuality, as can earlier traumatic sexual experiences such as sexual assault or incest, which may lead a woman to equate sex with impropriety, danger, or pain.

Disorders of desire

Sex drive ebbs and flows in the course of a relationship, and one partner often desires sex more often than another. Al-though these problems may be temporarily troublesome and require better communication, they are not considered dysfunctions per se. In contrast, women whose sexual desire is low (a condition called hypoactive sexual desire disorder or, more simply, low libido) persistently have little or no interest in sex and rarely if ever have sexual fantasies. (The term frigidity, formerly used to describe this disorder, has been discarded because of its vague meaning and derogatory connotations.) Low libido usually goes hand in hand with disorders of arousal and orgasm, but some women can go on to experience orgasm despite having little desire for sexual intercourse. About half the people who see doctors about sexual disorders say that lack of desire is their main problem (most people who complain of this are men).

Physical health, attractiveness of the partner, sensory stimulation, thoughts, and emotions all play a role in creating sexual desire. Whereas some women have never had any interest in sex, for others a reduced sex drive is a temporary response to an alteration in lifestyle, health, or relationships. Lifestyle changes after the birth of a child, for example, may diminish a woman's sex drive. After full days tending children or balancing child care and job-related duties, a new mother may find herself uninterested in sex with a partner she no longer has much of a relationship with outside the bedroom. Sexual interest is also bound to decline in a woman who believes that her partner does not listen to her or appreciate her, who resents her partner's lack of help with housework, child care, cooking, and shopping, or who feels that her partner does not make enough effort to please her sexually.

Low libido is also a characteristic symptom of depression and may occur as a side effect of numerous medications. It can be a logical consequence of painful intercourse, which is common in many gynecological infections and disorders. In some older women painful intercourse can result from thinning vaginal walls (vaginal atrophy) and inadequate natural lubrication, and this may reduce the desire for sex, as may the hormonal changes of menopause. New studies also suggest that numerous hormones that vary on a daily and monthly basis—including testosterone, estrogen, and progesterone—may also play a role. While the relationship among these hormones is complex, increasing evidence suggests that testosterone, together with other androgens such as DHEA, promote sex drive in women and also affect mood and the overall sense of well-being.

Because so many different factors are involved, a disorder of desire can be difficult to treat in women. Simply having more positive sexual experiences can help. Other women find that their libido revives after they are treated for some underlying illness or after they switch medications or discontinue the one that was causing their symptoms. If a woman has a history of menstrual irregularity or other physical disorders, her doctor may want to check levels of various hormones in her blood and treat any underlying imbalances. Postmenopausal women often find that supplementary testosterone or estrogen can enhance libido. So far, however, studies of Viagra's effectiveness in boosting women's sexual desire have been disappointing, although research is still under way.

If the cause of low libido appears to be nonphysical, certain exercises advocated by sex therapists often help. These include sensate focus exercises—a series of "pleasuring" techniques developed by the sex therapists William Masters and Virginia Johnson in the 1960s to enhance enjoyment without any pressure to perform in some predetermined way.

Many therapists also encourage the use of erotic materials, as well as training women to masturbate while fantasizing so that they can become aware of conditions necessary for a positive sexual experience. Women who have a life history of low libido may need further counseling to discover if they have a history of trauma as well or a deeper aversion to pleasure in general.

Women with the rarer but still fairly common condition called sexual aversion disorder are so repulsed by the idea of sex that they avoid genital sexual contact with a partner. Often people with this disorder have phobias, or deep-seated fears, about sexual activity or even the thought of sexual activity. Typically people with this disorder have intercourse only once or twice a year, but they often have a fairly natural sexual response once they get past their initial dread and anxiety. Men with sexual aversion disorder tend to have it from an early age, while women more frequently develop it after years of normal sexual desires.

About a quarter of people with sexual phobias and aversions also have panic disorder (see entry). When sexual aversion disorder is related to panic attacks, it is relatively easy to treat by taking antipanic medications such as tricyclic antidepressants (imipramine) or benzodiazepines (alprazolam) for about 3 or 4 months. Otherwise, the treatment is similar to that for hypoactive sexual desire.

Disorders of excitement
During sexual excitation the vaginal lining secretes a lubricating fluid and the inner lips and clitoris become engorged with blood. When women have problems attaining or maintaining this response through the completion of sexual activity, they are said to have excitement phase disorder. Many women with this disorder also have problems with sexual desire and feel pain during intercourse.

Arousal problems can occur for mundane reasons. Sexually inexperienced women, for example, may for the first few times focus more on how they perform than on how they feel. Similarly, women who are afraid of becoming pregnant at certain times of the month may have problems with arousal, as may women who attempt intercourse without adequate foreplay or stimulation.

Often hormonal deficiencies account for these symptoms. In women nearing or past menopause, for example, a deficiency of estrogen can dry the lining of the vagina. Vaginal lubrication also tends to be sparser during menstruation and for the first few days afterwards, as well as after childbirth and during breastfeeding. If the excitement phase disorder is due to a deficiency of estrogen, it can be easily treated by applying topical estrogen cream to the vagina and by using water-based lubricants such as K-Y Jelly, Transi-Lube, or Replens. (Petroleum jellies such as Vaseline should be avoided, since they do not dissolve in the vagina and can foster bacterial growth.)

More frequently, however, some psychological problem, including depression or stress, underlies the disorder. Women who feel long-standing anger or hostility toward their partner may have problems becoming aroused. For these women most doctors advise psychotherapy or marital therapy to help alleviate the underlying problem.

Disorders of orgasm

That women often "fake" orgasms has become a cliché. This is probably because having an orgasm is a difficult feat for many women. Some of the problem lies in unrealistic expectations. The belief that the only "real" orgasms occur during sexual intercourse, that simultaneous orgasm with a partner is essential to sexual fulfillment, or even that having an orgasm every time is necessary for sexual satisfaction can contribute to a woman's feelings of inadequacy.

Some women cannot relax because of distrust and fear of vulnerability, while others feel guilty about sexual pleasure and do not allow themselves to experience it. Any kind of discord in the relationship can also lead to difficulties with orgasm.

But much of the problem with orgasm can be traced to physiological factors. Most women require much more foreplay and stimulation than do most men before reaching orgasm. And at least 30 to 40 percent of women require direct clitoral stimulation (manual or oral) and are unable to have an orgasm with intercourse alone. This is perfectly normal, but unless a woman learns to communicate her needs to her partner and the couple tries to modify their sexual activity to fit them, orgasmic problems are almost inevitable.

Between 5 and 8 percent of women are unable to achieve orgasm during intercourse, even with direct clitoral stimulation. Some women can have orgasms during masturbation but not with a partner, while others do not have orgasms under any circumstances. When a woman cannot have an orgasm with a partner, despite normal desire and excitement phases, she is said to have orgasmic dysfunction.

For some women the solution to this problem is a matter of practice and experience. For others, a variety of specific exercises and techniques have been highly successful. For women who have never had an orgasm, a doctor or sex therapist will usually provide education about female sexual response and then encourage self-exploration, including masturbation and use of fantasy material. In addition, practicing Kegel vaginal exercises can help develop muscles in the vagina called the pubococcygeus muscles, which are involved in orgasm. Through these techniques about 90 percent of women being treated eventually achieve orgasm.

Women who have trouble having orgasms with a partner are given sensate focus exercises to help discover or rediscover what is pleasurable. These usually begin with nongenital stimulation (with intercourse and orgasms prohibited) to take away performance pressure. If a woman wants to experience orgasm during intercourse, many sex therapists advocate the "bridge technique," in which the clitoris is stimulated manually or with a vibrator while the penis is inserted into the vagina. Other couples find it helpful to have sex in a "back protected" position (in which the partner sits with the woman between the partner's legs and her back against

the partner's chest). This allows the woman to control stimulation without unnecessary self-consciousness. Heterosexual couples are also encouraged to explore pelvic thrusting in a nondemanding way, beginning with female superior position, followed by a lateral (side-by-side) position which allows both partners to move freely.

Success of these techniques depends greatly on the nature of the couple's relationship. About 30 to 50 percent of women who try these techniques eventually learn to have regular orgasms during intercourse. About 70 to 80 percent will be able to experience orgasm with a partner, but not necessarily during intercourse.

Sadomasochism

Sadomasochism is a highly controversial form of sexual expression in which sexual excitement is enhanced through an unequal power relationship between the partners. It is a combination of sadistic behavior in one partner (inflicting pain on another person to heighten one's sexual pleasure) and masochistic behavior in the other (experiencing pain, suffering, or humiliation to heighten one's sexual pleasure). S/M often involves a fantasy situation in which each partner takes on a role. One partner may be the teacher while the other is the student, for example, or one may be the master while the other is the slave. Ideally, this playacting comes to a stop when either partner wants it to.

Defenders of sadomasochism argue that S/M is a healthy form of sexual expression because it allows consenting partners to express the power issues that are a natural, if hidden, part of sexuality. Moreover, particularly in homosexual relationships, the roles can be reversed at will, allowing each partner an opportunity to be dominant and subordinate. But many critics, including feminist critics of mainstream sexuality, have expressed concern about the practice of S/M. They argue that, in heterosexuals, this behavior reinforces traditional male-female relationships and, in all relationships, it may encourage or mask dangerous situations such as domestic abuse or rape.

If a woman involved in an S/M relationship believes her partner may suffer from true sexual sadism, she should seek help from her clinician or from a battered women's shelter. Sexual sadism is a kind of paraphilia, that is, a gross impairment of a person's ability to engage in affectionate sexual activity. Paraphilias occur almost exclusively in men. In contrast to most rapists, who are motivated more by violent than by sexual impulses, sexual sadists derive sexual excitement and pleasure from brutally hurting their partners. Many people fantasize about inflicting pain, but sexual sadists actually enact their fantasies and sometimes inflict extensive or even mortal injuries. Long-term psychotherapy can sometimes help people with this problem.

Sexual dysfunction in lesbians

The nature and extent of sexual dysfunction in lesbians has been investigated even less extensively than in heterosexual women. The limited studies that do exist, however, indicate that most lesbian women, like most heterosexual women, highly value interpersonal relationships. Like heterosexual women, too, lesbian women tend to equate sexual attraction with love and often feel uncomfortable with sex outside the context of a relationship. Lesbians, however, seem to be generally more sexually responsive and more satisfied with sex than heterosexual women, although they report having less sex and fewer partners than homosexual men.

Lesbians also appear to have fewer problems achieving orgasm than do heterosexual women, probably because of sexual technique. For the same reason, they are less likely to experience pain during sexual intercourse. Sexual dysfunction in lesbians is more likely to take the form of low sexual desire and of low rates of sex, especially in the context of long-term committed relationships. A common complaint is a low frequency of genital sex in contrast to hugging and other nongenital physical contact. In one study, half of the couples who reported that they had genital sex infrequently also reported dissatisfaction with their sex lives. Often this dissatisfaction led one partner to have an affair and, eventually, end the relationship.

How is sexual dysfunction treated?

Some sexual problems can be worked through with the help of good books and a caring partner, whereas others might call for professional help. For many women, turning to friends or women's support groups may provide valuable ways of dealing with sexual dysfunction. This is particularly true for lesbians or women with disabilities, who tend to have trouble finding health care professionals attuned to their particular needs. Many popular books on the subject of sexuality offer valuable suggestions for overcoming sexual dysfunction.

Women who suspect that they may have more serious physical, psychological, or marital problems may want to seek help from a health care provider trained in sex counseling or from a sex therapist. If there is an underlying physical problem, the solution involves treating that problem or changing a medication. Most problems will entail additional changes, however, and these often require the cooperation of both partners.

A thorough gynecological examination can help determine if any physical problems play a role in sexual dysfunction. In cases of vaginal dryness, the clinician may do additional tests to check hormone levels and to determine if menopause is approaching. The clinician will also want to rule out underlying conditions that may be causing the symptoms. For example, pain during sexual intercourse can sometimes signal pelvic inflammatory disease, endometriosis, adhesions, or growths—either cancerous or noncancerous—on the reproductive organs. If low sexual desire is a problem, the clinician may also do blood tests to determine hormone levels. Some women, particularly those past menopause, find that either estrogen replacement and/or supplementary testosterone (androgen replacement) can restore sex drive.

More sophisticated tests originally designed for male sexual disorders are now being considered for women. Research is currently under way in women to measure genital blood flow, vaginal pH, and the status of nerves in the vagina, and eventually these findings may underlie new methods for treating female sexual dysfunction.

The techniques of sex therapy, a relatively new form of short-term psychotherapy which emphasizes behavioral changes in contrast to elucidating underlying causes of a problem, have helped some couples. A sex therapist (or doctor trained in sex therapy) usually takes a history of the woman or the couple, provides information about sexual anatomy and response, and then offers specific suggestions and exercises that both partners can attempt at home to try to heighten sexual pleasure. Sex therapists emphasize increasing communication between partners, decreasing performance anxiety by changing the goal of the sexual activity from emphasis on orgasm toward feeling good, and encouraging sexual experimentation.

Although sex therapy is frequently effective—especially in treating disorders of excitement and orgasm—some couples may need more intensive psychotherapy or couples counseling as well. This is particularly true for people with inadequate sexual desire, since this dysfunction tends to stem from more complex (and often cognitive) factors and cannot usually be remedied with short-term behavioral techniques.

Because anyone can hang up a shingle as a sex therapist, finding a competent and reputable one can be a challenge. Sex therapy is rarely effective unless it is practiced by a person also trained in more broadly based couples and family therapy, and who is also capable of assessing and treating individual psychological problems that may have nothing to do with sexual dysfunction per se. Anyone seeking a sex therapist should be wary of therapists who suggest genital surgery as the solution to sexual dysfunction. And they should avoid any so-called sex therapist who asks them to engage in sexual exercises in the office or to observe sexual activities there or who offers to serve as a "sex surrogate." A good source of certified sex therapists is the national register put out by the American Association of Sex Education Counselors and Therapists.

Related entries

Anxiety disorders, depression, fatigue, galactorrhea, headaches, Kegel exercises, pain during sexual intercourse, panic disorder, phobias, psychotherapy, sexual assault, stress, vaginal atrophy

Sexual Harassment

Sexual harassment is any unwanted sexual attention in a situation where there is a difference in power between the harasser and the person being harassed. The term has been a part of the common vocabulary ever since 1991, when the Senate Judiciary Committee reviewed Anita Hill's charges of sexual harassment against Supreme Court nominee Clarence Thomas. Captivated by these hearings, women from many walks of life declared that this problem was ubiquitous in workplaces and schools across America and voiced concern that men "just don't get it"—that is, despite all the outcry, men simply do not understand why sexual harassment is so troubling to women.

One of the reasons why many people may have trouble "getting it" is that it is not always obvious just which behaviors constitute sexual harassment. Virtually everyone would agree that there has been sexual harassment when a women's refusal to grant sexual favors to her boss results in her being barred from job advancement, demoted, or fired. Equally clear is the case of a college student who must sleep with a professor to obtain a recommendation for graduate school, or the office worker who is subjected to obscene propositions on a regular basis from a co-worker. But most women—and most courts of law—consider less egregious actions to constitute sexual harassment as well. A woman who works in a small factory whose walls are covered with nude pin-ups, the secretary who must endure endless pinches and pats from her boss, the student who has to listen to off-color jokes in an auto mechanics class: all of these women are being sexually harassed as well.

Just why some of these behaviors constitute sexual harassment seems to baffle many men—and even some women. The reason why unwanted sexual attention is so troubling to women has to do with the power differential, perceived or real, between men and women in our culture. A woman who is sexually harassed often feels that she has no option but to endure the mistreatment because she might lose her job, flunk a course, or anger the harasser to the point of physical harm. This power differential means that sexual harassment can occur even when a woman is not in an officially subordinate position. For example, in one oft-cited case, a female surgeon and tenured professor at Stanford University Medical School ended up resigning her position after receiving clandestine caresses and being called "Honey" by her colleagues for many years. Similarly, many a waitress has to put up with the leers and lewd remarks of her customers day after day, and these women are being harassed as well—even though the customers are not her employers in any formal sense. Whether a woman is harassed by a boss, a co-worker, or a client, any sexual attention that makes the work environment hostile or pressured is clearly sexual harassment.

Because many men consider sexual advances and remarks flattering, however, or belong to a generation or an ethnic tradition in which such behaviors are accepted, they fail to understand why many women find them degrading or even frightening. Differing perspectives about what constitutes sexual harassment can lead even the best-intentioned people to feel that they are walking on eggshells as they try to determine an appropriate way to entertain clients, travel with colleagues of the other sex, or express gratitude to their subordi-

nates. As women continue to join men in the workplace—working, traveling, and socializing with male colleagues—the old rules about acceptable behavior between the sexes become increasingly outmoded and subject to a great deal of misinterpretation. Lesbian and minority women may be at particular risk for sexual harassment because they are members of stigmatized groups who are often in a position of lesser status and power than heterosexual and white women.

What are the physical and emotional symptoms?

Sexual harassment not only makes women feel afraid and powerless but also creates emotional stress. This can manifest itself as anxiety, anger, fear, and helplessness, as well as in frequent headaches or problems with drug or alcohol abuse. A few women develop symptoms reminiscent of the posttraumatic stress disorder (see entry) sometimes experienced by victims of sexual assault or domestic abuse. Some women miss days of work because of these symptoms or find that their job performance suffers along with their motivation and their confidence in their abilities.

A now classic random survey of government employees conducted by the U.S. Merit Systems Protection Board in 1981 found that 42 percent of over 10,000 women responding said that they had been sexually harassed on the job. This study estimated that sexual harassment had resulted in significant amounts of job turnover, absenteeism, and a cost to taxpayers of $189 million in health benefits over a two-year period.

How can a woman protect herself against sexual harassment?

Regulatory protections. A set of guidelines issued in 1980 by the Equal Employment Opportunity Commission (EEOC), the federal agency that handles cases of sexual harassment, defined sexual harassment as "unwelcome sexual advances, requests for sexual favors, and other verbal or physical conduct of a sexual nature" when employment decisions hinge on submission to or rejection of this conduct, or when this conduct substantially interferes with a person's work performance or creates an "intimidating, hostile, or offensive working environment." Six years later the U.S. Supreme Court ruled that sexual harassment in the workplace was illegal because it violated the antidiscrimination laws under Title VII of the 1964 Civil Rights Act.

Charges of sexual harassment in the workplace can be filed with the Federal Equal Employment Opportunity Commission or with a state's Human Rights Commission. In a school or university setting, sexual harassment is defined as a form of sexual discrimination under Title IX of the Education Amendment of 1972.

Whether or not a woman wants to press charges, her first step in handling sexual harassment should ideally be to let the harasser know in no uncertain terms that his or her behavior is unacceptable. This is not always possible, of course. Some women sense that if they confront the harasser di-

rectly, the repercussions will far outweigh any possible benefits. Other women have difficulty with direct confrontation,
and may find themselves smiling and apologizing even as
they chastise. This kind of behavior is easily misinterpreted
and does not hold up very well as evidence in court.

If filing a lawsuit is a possibility, it is best to document all
incidents and confrontations in as much detail as possible,
and to save copies of any written correspondence either to or
from the harasser. Repeated harassment should be reported
to a supervisor or personnel officer (if possible), and information should be obtained about the company's sexual harassment policy (if one exists). Since the Supreme Court's 1986
decision, many companies have found it in their own best interest to institute such policies, since they are liable for sexual
harassment that occurs in the workplace and may have to
pay the damages, attorney's fees, and even lost wages of any
employees who are sexually harassed. The EEOC also encourages employers to raise the subject of sexual harassment actively, issue statements or handbooks to increase employees'
awareness, develop appropriate sanctions against it, and educate employees about their rights under Title VII. Sometimes
companies that do not have a sexual harassment policy can
be induced to institute one on these grounds.

Nonlegal recourse. For all the talk about sexual harassment
and recent legal protections, very few women actually press
charges and follow through. The reasons are similar to the
reasons why many women do not prosecute the perpetrators
of sexual assault or domestic abuse. Some women are held
back by concern for the harasser; as troubled as they are, they
cannot justify embarrassing the harasser or "ruining his life"
by prosecuting him publicly. Other women hesitate to file
charges because they are afraid of emotional, occupational,
or even physical consequences. In addition, many women
know that victims of sexual harassment end up being cross-
examined by a defense attorney as if they themselves were on
trial: their behavior in the workplace, their social life, and
their style of dress are often held up to scrutiny, as if they had
somehow brought the harassment on themselves.

There are a number of jobs in which pressing charges is not
really practical. Not all women have the means or opportunity to fight their way through all the red tape involved in
alienating an employer, hiring a lawyer, and going to court. It
is also harder to press charges when the harassment comes
from customers—patrons at a restaurant, clients at a travel or
real estate agency—rather than employers.

There are some private steps that can be taken by any
woman who is being harassed in the workplace. One is to remember that, whatever others may say, women do not bring
sexual harassment on themselves; they are not to blame for
being victims. It can also be helpful to talk to other women in
the same environment, who often will have experienced a
similar problem. At the very least this can result in a support
network; at best it may generate some form of collective action against the offender. Sometimes, however, co-workers
isolate themselves from a woman who claims to have been
sexually harassed, to protect either their jobs or their own
sense of security. In such cases it may be better to turn to a
women's advocacy organization or local rape crisis center for
support and guidance.

Related entries
Anxiety disorders, domestic abuse, headaches, occupational
hazards, posttraumatic stress disorder, sexual assault, stress,
substance abuse

Sexual Orientation

Not so long ago anyone whose sexual orientation was other
than purely heterosexual—that is, anyone who was ever attracted to a member of the same sex—was universally considered deviant. Homosexuality was believed to be a form of disease (mental or physical) of which people could and should
be cured. In 1973, however, the American Psychiatric Association (APA) declared that preference for a person of one's
own sex is neither a psychiatric disorder nor a disease but
merely one of several normal forms of sexual expression. Although there is still considerable debate about whether sexual orientation is determined primarily by culture or by biology (which can include prenatal development as well as
genetic endowment), very few authorities still believe that
people consciously choose to be homosexual or heterosexual.

Newer research on sexual behavior and feelings indicates
that a person's sexual orientation is not as clear-cut as was
once believed. Instead, most researchers today regard sexual
orientation as best measured along two continuums: the degree of attraction to the same sex (0 to 100 percent) and the
degree of attraction to the other sex (0 to 100 percent). Bi-
sexuals might have an equally high degree of attraction for
same-sex and other-sex partners, while heterosexuals would
be highly attracted to the other sex and only minimally attracted to the same sex. Homosexuals and lesbians would be
highly attracted to same sex-partners and only minimally attracted to partners of the other sex, while asexual individuals would be minimally attracted to both the same and the
other sex.

Just where a person falls on these sexual orientation continuums is not always immediately obvious. Not only do
many teenagers experiment with both heterosexual and homosexual behavior before learning what is most natural to
them, but also women in particular (many of them married,
with children) are apt to discover a lesbian leaning well into
life, only when they have enough time, confidence, and experience for that self-awareness. Other women know that
they have homosexual feelings at an early age but do not
choose to act on these feelings until much later.

Various studies suggest that as many as 20 percent of all
American women have had some kind of intimate relation-

ship with another woman, either exclusively or in addition to relationships with men. These numbers would be much higher if they included women who are attracted to other women but never act on (or even acknowledge) these feelings. Increasing awareness about, and acceptance of, homosexuality among the American public (as reflected in laws upholding basic rights regardless of sexual orientation) has gone a long way toward encouraging more and more homosexuals of both sexes to come out of the closet. Even so, there is still a pervasive taboo about homosexuality which leads to various forms of discrimination—including difficulties adopting or gaining custody of children and getting or keeping jobs, particularly jobs involving children. Homosexuals often find themselves ridiculed, chastised, or ostracized by peers and family members—and this treatment results in considerable stress and feelings of loneliness, isolation, depression, and low self-esteem. Because the homosexual community provides some support against homophobia, for many lesbians homosexuality becomes a matter of personal identity and lifestyle as well as sexual orientation.

What special health issues do lesbian women face?

Although anecdotal evidence abounds on this subject, scientifically convincing studies comparing the health of lesbians with that of other women are still extremely limited. Some of the paucity of information is attributable to limited interest in and funding for research—and to the fact that lesbians are too often just lumped in with "single women" in general—but there are also some inherent obstacles. Lesbians do not necessarily reveal their sexual orientation to health care professionals who are studying these issues, so any data common to lesbians in particular may be invisible.

Even so, there is general agreement among medical professionals and lesbian advocacy groups that the nature and prevalence of certain health problems differ between lesbian and heterosexual women.

Sexually transmitted diseases. Lesbians are much less likely than heterosexual women to acquire certain sexually transmitted diseases (STDs)—particularly syphilis, gonorrhea, and AIDS. This is probably because many of the organisms that cause these diseases are not easily spread through mouth-to-vagina contact (cunnilingus) and other forms of sexual behavior common between lesbians. It is also possible that these microorganisms are simply less prevalent in the lesbian community than in society at large. Other STDs—including herpes and trichomonas—occur just as frequently in lesbians as in heterosexual and bisexual women.

It is important to remember, however, that sexual orientation and sexual identity are not the same as sexual behavior. Many self-avowed lesbians occasionally engage in sexual behavior with men, which puts them at the same risk for STDs as heterosexual women.

Cancer. Most epidemiologic evidence on the incidence and mortality rates of cervical, breast, and other cancers in lesbi-

ans is still speculative at best. Nevertheless, it is often suggested that at least some lesbians may be less susceptible to developing cervical cancer than other women, since they lack a major risk factor for this disease—frequent sexual intercourse with men at an early age.

As for breast cancer, because lesbians are less likely than heterosexual women to have given birth, it has been suggested that they are at increased risk for breast cancer. Giving birth before age 30 and breastfeeding both seem to lower the risk of this disease.

The statistical evidence that exists at present cannot tell us whether or not either of these notions about lesbians is true. In any event, there does seem to be general agreement that lesbians who do develop breast, cervical, and perhaps other cancers are more likely to die from these diseases than are other women. Part of the reason may be that lesbians as a group are less likely to have routine checkups (including Pap tests and breast examinations) than other women—who are more apt to consult clinicians about issues of birth control and pregnancy. As a result, these cancers, as well as other serious diseases, tend to be detected at later—and less easily curable—stages.

Mistrust of the mainstream health care community also seems to run high among lesbians, partly in response to past insensitivity toward—or even overt condemnation of—their particular needs and lifestyles. This mistrust probably keeps many lesbian women from seeking regular health care. And when they do consult a clinician, those who reveal their sexual orientation may be less likely than other women to receive routine gynecological care such as STD screening and Pap tests. They are also less likely to be asked if they have problems with domestic violence (which the clinician may mistakenly assume does not occur among lesbians).

Mental and emotional disorders. Lesbians are more likely than women in the general population to attempt suicide and to have problems with alcohol, tobacco, and substance abuse (see entries). These facts suggest a higher rate of depression (often untreated) among this group of women.

Pregnancy, adoption, and child rearing. Having and raising children can present particular challenges—medical and otherwise—for lesbian and bisexual women, whether they are single or involved in long-term partnerships.

Women who come out as lesbian after a conventional marriage with children may face obstacles gaining or keeping custody of their children after a divorce. And lesbian partners who are raising children often find themselves in uncharted waters, where, with very little guidance (or legal recognition of their parenthood), they must continually redefine what it means to be a parent, a mother, or a stepmother.

Most of the time a homosexual woman's decision to have children is by necessity a very conscious one, often involving years of uncertainty and planning. Women in long-term relationships may find that the issue of having children produces considerable conflict: there is the question of whether or not there should be a child at all, and also perhaps debate about which partner should become pregnant, and by what method.

The time, effort, and expense involved in becoming pregnant are almost always greater for lesbians than for women in long-term heterosexual relationships. Many lesbians choose to be artificially inseminated, a process that entails numerous medical, legal, social, and emotional complications for any woman (see infertility). Finding a reputable facility willing to inseminate a single and/or lesbian woman can be a special challenge, and using donor sperm from a sperm bank can be expensive. Many lesbian women, like many heterosexual women with fertility problems, dislike having conception turned into a sterile, medicalized procedure over which they feel they have little control.

Some women prefer to use a known donor—such as a friend or relative of either partner. Should a lesbian couple decide to include this father in the child's life, all parties will have the additional complication of raising a child in an unconventional situation for which society provides few positive guidelines. They may also have to deal with the possibility that the biological father will one day decide he wants custody, since the courts may give him preference over a lesbian household. This is true even for a woman who uses several donors to avoid potential legal problems, since sophisticated tests can frequently determine the biological father.

Some women prefer to try home insemination, especially if they live in areas where clinics are not available or if they want to save money or have more control over the process. Without professional assistance and the routine tests that would normally be conducted by any reputable medical facility or sperm bank (including a sperm count and various tests for allergies and STDs, including AIDS), home inseminations are somewhat riskier and less likely to succeed than professional insemination.

Adoption—another option for lesbian couples—has its own share of challenges. Not only is adoption costly and frustrating (as it often is for married heterosexual couples), but also single lesbian women and lesbian couples have difficulty finding an agency that is willing to consider them as adoptive parents. Private adoption arrangements can be uncertain and prohibitively expensive.

Finally, whether a child arrives through adoption, artificial insemination, or otherwise, many lesbian parents worry about how prejudices regarding their sexuality will affect their children. There is currently no evidence that children raised by lesbian couples have any more psychological problems than children raised in more traditional settings. Even so, women with these concerns—as well as concerns about other issues unique to lesbian mothers—may find it helpful to join one of the many support networks for lesbian mothers that have developed in recent years, or to consult the growing literature on the subject.

Related entries
Alcohol, anorexia nervosa and bulimia nervosa, body image, breast cancer, cervical cancer, depression, domestic abuse, infertility, mammography, Pap test, pelvic examinations, pregnancy, sexual harassment, sexual response, sexually transmitted diseases, stress, substance abuse

Sexual Response

Sexual response in humans is as much a function of the mind as of the body. Feelings for the partner, the physical surroundings, fears about pregnancy or AIDS, and personal morals and values about sexuality can all shape a person's sexual satisfaction. There is also considerable individual variation—and variation in the same person at different times—in the types of sexual stimulation that bring pleasure.

For all people, however, the physiology of sexual response is remarkably similar—whether it occurs during masturbation, during heterosexual relations or homosexual relations, in men or in women. In both sexes the physical aspects of sexual response result from increased muscle tension and increased blood circulation in certain parts of the body.

Part of the similarity between the sexes may lie in the embryological origins of the male and female reproductive organs. Both sexes start life with a basically female blueprint, and it is only the production of certain hormones (under genetic direction from the Y chromosome) in male embryos that eventually shapes the penis, testes, scrotum, and seminal vesicles which would otherwise become the vagina, vulva, uterus, ovaries, and fallopian tubes in a female fetus. Because female reproductive organs originate from the same tissue as male organs, some of the female structures correspond to the male ones and respond to the same stimuli. Both the clitoris and the penis, for example, are extremely sensitive to touch (especially at the glans, or tip) and play a central role in sexual pleasure. Both are covered with a hood or foreskin and become engorged with blood during sexual arousal.

Phases of human sexual response
During the 1960s the large-scale scientific studies of William Masters and Virginia Johnson divided human sexual response into a four-phase cycle: excitement, plateau, orgasm, and resolution. Although there is no hard-and-fast barrier between these phases, and sexual fulfillment does not necessarily require experiencing all four of them, this cycle remains the foundation for our understanding of the physical side of human sexual response.

The excitement phase. In the excitement (or arousal) phase, heart rate and blood pressure increase, skin flushes, and nipples become erect in both men and women. The arteries in the genital area become engorged with blood, causing an erection of the penis in men and of the clitoris in women. In women, the labia become engorged with blood and darken in color. Meanwhile, the vaginal lining begins to secrete a lubricating fluid, wetting the vaginal lips.

Various stimuli—physical, mental, emotional, even aesthetic—can trigger the excitement phase. Some women are aroused when their breasts, nipples, thighs, or genitals are touched, while others can be stimulated when less "sexual" areas of the body are caressed or massaged. Fantasies, daydreams, music, colors, thoughts, expressions of affection or desire, or conversation often play a powerful role in arousal.

The plateau phase. This occurs when the muscle contraction and congestion in the pelvis near their peak. In both men and women heart rate and blood pressure increase even more and breathing rate accelerates. In women, the breasts increase in size, the clitoris lifts and retracts under its hood, the vaginal opening swells, and the uterus moves up higher into the pelvis.

The orgasm phase. Also called climax (or, in slang, "coming"), this phase involves sudden rhythmic contractions of the pelvic muscles and genitalia, accompanied by intense feelings of pleasure and a release of tension. In women the contractions occur in the vagina, clitoris, and uterus. In men the contraction of the urethra inside the penis causes ejaculation, the expulsion of seminal fluid (semen). The intensity or pleasurability of an orgasm can vary considerably from one sexual experience to the next.

Claims that stimulation of a sensitive area on the front wall of the vagina called the "G spot," or Grafenberg spot, will trigger female orgasm have never been substantiated. Another myth (one that has persisted since it was proposed by Sigmund Freud) is that women can have two different kinds of orgasms: clitoral and vaginal. Clitoral orgasms, which supposedly result from direct clitoral stimulation, were thought to be less mature and less satisfying than vaginal ones, which supposedly occur only during sexual intercourse. Masters and Johnson showed conclusively that, even though they may be produced or perceived differently, from a physiological perspective all orgasms are alike and involve both the clitoris and the vagina.

For many women, having an orgasm (particularly with a partner) is a learned behavior that becomes easier with age and experience. Many women require direct clitoral stimulation to reach orgasm, and most women cannot become adequately excited without foreplay preceding intercourse. Even after penetration women require much more stimulation than do men to reach orgasm. It has been estimated that at least half of heterosexual American women do not regularly have orgasms during sexual intercourse.

Often this situation can be remedied by working together with a partner (sometimes with the help of a sex therapist) to find positions and techniques that are mutually satisfying. This is particularly important if a woman feels inadequate or frustrated because she cannot have an orgasm, or if she has pain or discomfort because of regularly congested pelvic tissues. Despite the women's movement and the explosion of sexuality in American culture, many women still feel shame or guilt about their own sexual needs. Problems with orgasm can sometimes be resolved by learning to acknowledge these sexual needs and communicating them to partners. Often couples need to explore ways of making love that go beyond penis-vagina intercourse.

Many women, however, feel sexually fulfilled (at least some of the time) with the emotional or sensual pleasure that comes from hugging, kissing, being held, or satisfying a partner, and they should not be pressured into trying to have an orgasm. The same is true for women who cannot experience genital sensations because of a disease, disability, or injury but who may be able to receive sexual pleasure from other parts of the body.

The resolution phase. In the last phase of sexual response, the body goes back to its original, unaroused state except that there is a feeling of general well-being. Congestion and erection subside, and respiration, heart rate, and blood pressure return to normal. The time this process takes varies considerably between the sexes. Some (but by no means all) women stay aroused after one orgasm and can continue to have one orgasm after another without passing through the resolution phase. This is called having multiple orgasms. Men generally need a recovery period (called the refractory period) before they can have another orgasm. The refractory period increases with age and can range in any individual from a few minutes to half a day.

Related entries
Sexual dysfunction, sexual orientation

Sexually Transmitted Diseases

Sexually transmitted diseases are infectious diseases acquired primarily through sexual contact with an infected partner. STDs are caused by bacteria, viruses, fungi, protozoa, mycoplasma, and parasites that thrive on the warm, moist mucous membranes of the genital area, mouth, and throat.

Types of STDs
STDs that commonly affect women include acquired immune deficiency syndrome (AIDS), chancroid, chlamydia, genital warts, gonorrhea, hepatitis B, herpes, pubic lice, scabies, syphilis, and trichomonas (see entries).

Acquired immune deficiency syndrome. AIDS is caused by the human immunodeficiency virus (HIV), which weakens the body's ability to fight lethal infections and cancers. People with AIDS are prone to "opportunistic infections," that is, infections caused by bacteria, viruses, parasites, and fungi that normally would not be a threat to healthy people. AIDS also affects the central nervous system and can cause mental deterioration and paralysis.

Although drugs can alleviate for a time some of the symptoms and opportunistic infections that arise from AIDS, no person who has developed full-blown AIDS has recovered normal immune system function. There are currently 20,000 women with AIDS in the United States, and 140,000 American women are known to be HIV-infected. Most of them seem to have acquired their infection through sexual intimacy with infected partners (see acquired immune deficiency syndrome).

Chancroid. This STD, caused by a bacterium, is most common among people who live in tropical climates, but its prevalence is increasing in North America. Chancroid (see entry) can develop in anyone who has sexual or skin-to-skin contact with an infected person, even if that person has no symptoms. Most women with chancroid (also known as soft chancre) have no noticeable symptoms, and they are often unknowing carriers of the organism. If symptoms do develop, they usually involve a small, raised, painful sore surrounded by a reddish border which develops 3 to 7 days after initial infection, most often on the vulva, vagina, urethra, cervix, or inner thighs. The condition is treatable with antibiotics.

Chlamydia. This is the most common sexually transmitted disease (STD) in the United States today. Four million cases are diagnosed each year, but because this disease often produces no symptoms—particularly in women—it frequently goes undiagnosed.

Chlamydia (see entry) currently accounts for between a quarter and a half of all cases of pelvic inflammatory disease (PID), which in turn increases a woman's risks of infertility, abdominal adhesions (scarring), chronic pelvic pain, and ectopic pregnancy. Chlamydia also underlies about half of all cases of cervicitis (see vaginitis) and up to a fifth of all cases of urethritis (inflammation of the urethra). It is highly curable with antibiotics.

Genital warts. These are generally benign growths in the genital and anal area caused by the human papilloma virus (HPV), but some types have been associated with cervical cancer. Genital warts (see entry) result from sexual contact with an infected partner, although they can be spread by touching the genitals with wart-infested hands.

Some warts are unnoticeable, but others are over 3 inches around and interfere with the ability to sit or to walk. Sometimes the warts itch or burn, and scratching them can cause irritation. They are highly contagious and hard to eradicate.

Gonorrhea. "The clap" is the second most common STD in the United States. About 80 percent of women infected with gonorrhea have no symptoms, and many suspect a problem only when symptoms arise in a male partner—a thick, milky discharge from the penis and a burning sensation during urination. Gonorrhea (see entry) in women is likely to go untreated. It is believed to cause 20 to 40 percent of all cases of pelvic inflammatory disease (PID), which in turn can result in infertility, ectopic pregnancy, and chronic pelvic and abdominal pain as a result of adhesions (scarring). Gonorrhea is usually spread from one person to another through sexual contact—vaginal, anal, or oral—and is caused by a bacterium. This disease can be halted readily with antibiotics.

Hepatitis B. This type of liver inflammation accounts for 9 percent of all deaths worldwide. The virus that causes hepatitis B (HBV) is about a hundred times as contagious as the AIDS virus (HIV), and though it is spread mainly through sexual intercourse, it can be passed through any bodily fluid (including blood, sweat, tears, saliva, semen, and vaginal secretions), as well as through contaminated needles. HBV can be acquired through kissing or sharing toothbrushes as well as more intimate contact.

Symptoms resemble those of intestinal flu: nausea, vomiting, diarrhea, lack of appetite, headache, muscle aches, abdominal pain, and low-grade fever. Often the skin and eyes become yellowed. The great majority of people infected with HBV recover within a few months and after recovery have a lifelong immunity to hepatitis B. About 10 percent, however, become carriers of the virus, with the potential to infect others although they have no further illness themselves. About 3 to 5 percent of all people with hepatitis (see entry) go on to develop chronic hepatitis and cirrhosis. There is no known drug or other specific treatment that can cure hepatitis B.

Herpes. Genital herpes affects 10 million Americans. Its primary symptoms are recurrent outbreaks of painful sores in the genital region. The disease is caused by the herpes simplex virus, which enters the body through mucous membranes and travels into nerve endings, where it can remain dormant. Outbreaks may continue intermittently for years—particularly during illness or stress—but they are self-limiting. Recurrences tend to be less severe and more infrequent as time goes by.

The virus is most contagious when a person has obvious sores, but it can also be spread through secretions and breaks in the skin or mucous membranes even during the latent periods. Although there is no cure for herpes (see entry), the antiviral drug acyclovir is often successful in treating outbreaks and reducing the frequency of recurrences.

Pubic lice. Also known as "crabs," these creatures live in pubic hair and, while not a serious threat to health, cause agonizing itching. Pubic lice (see entry) are usually passed from one person to another during close sexual contact (though not necessarily intercourse), and are occasionally acquired from contaminated linens, clothing, or toilet seats. They require a good deal of effort to eliminate, but various over-the-counter treatments in the form of creams, shampoos, and lotions are effective in killing lice and their nits.

Scabies. Scabies (see entry) is a highly contagious infection caused by tiny mites that burrow under the skin and deposit their eggs and feces. The result is raised, irregular lines on the skin and agonizing itching, particularly at night. Scabies can be transmitted through sexual contact, but anyone who touches infested sheets, towels, clothing, or furniture can become infected. Though not generally a serious condition, scabies can be extremely annoying and, if untreated, can persist for years. Various nonprescription commercial creams, lotions, and shampoos can kill the scabies parasite.

Syphilis. This STD is caused by a spiral-shaped bacterium known as a spirochete. It is transmitted through sexual contact, although occasionally it can be acquired through a blood transfusion or skin contact. In the first stage of syphilis (see entry) an open sore, pimple, or blister (chancre) appears at the site of infection—usually in the cervix, vagina, rectum, or other genital areas—and then goes away. In the second phase malaise, fever, sore throat, joint pain, and headache develop.

The most characteristic symptom is a rash on the palms of the hands and the soles of the feet. Secondary syphilis can also result in meningitis (an inflammation of the lining of the brain) or uveitis (an eye inflammation characterized by pain and redness). After these symptoms go away, the person may have no outward signs of disease for decades, but the spirochete continues to damage the heart, brain, spinal cord, blood vessels, and bones. The final (or tertiary) stage of syphilis results in heart disease, blindness, dementia, and death. If caught early, syphilis is highly treatable with antibiotics.

Trichomonas. "Trich" is caused by a one-celled protozoan that can live for years in the male reproductive tract without producing any symptoms. It is the third most common form of vaginitis in the United States, affecting 3 million women, some of whom have no symptoms. Most of the time, however, a copious, green, frothy, and foul-smelling vaginal discharge is present, along with vaginal or vulvar itching, redness, or swelling. Some women experience a burning sensation during urination and the need to urinate frequently and urgently, while others may develop pain during sexual intercourse. Trichomonas (see entry) is almost always acquired through sexual contact with an infected partner. It is highly treatable with antibiotics.

Who is likely to contract a sexually transmitted disease?

With the exception of gonorrhea, the number of cases of virtually every STD has been increasing in the past decade or so—and even gonorrhea still afflicts Americans in epidemic proportions. Each day an estimated 33,000 persons in the United States (12 million annually) contract one or more STDs. Most of these (86 percent) occur in people between the ages of 15 and 25, the age group just entering their reproductive years.

At any age, the risk of contracting an STD is higher for women with a history of multiple sexual partners, a previous STD, and illicit drug use, as well as women whose sexual partners have had other partners in the past 3 months and do not use condoms. Risk for some STDs is lower among lesbian

women (see sexual orientation). STDs are diseases primarily of the young, the poor, and the urban, although no woman who is sexually active is immune. Many women have more than one STD at the same time, and unlike some other infectious diseases, STDs can recur many times in a person's life. Having had a particular disease once is no guarantee against acquiring it again.

What are the symptoms?

Some STDs have symptoms no more severe than mild discomfort or irritation, and women often have no symptoms of infection at all. So unless women have regular screening tests, they are at risk for developing a number of complications from "hidden" infections, including infertility, pelvic inflammatory disease (PID), abdominal pain, and cervical cancer (see entries). STDs such as gonorrhea, syphilis, and AIDS can damage nonreproductive organs, including the eyes, heart, and brain. Because infection is particularly likely in women who are still in their early reproductive years, women under the age of 25 who have had at least one sexual encounter should seriously consider appropriate screening tests even if they have no symptoms. These would include a gonorrhea culture, a chlamydia swab, a blood test for syphilis, and possibly an HIV test. And regardless of age, any woman with a sexual history that puts her at risk for STDs should also seek regular screening; this can be done at the time of an annual gynecological checkup.

Often a clinician will want to screen for other STDs in a woman who has symptoms of a specific STD, since these conditions so often coexist. It is important to remember, however, that symptoms such as pelvic pain (see entry) can stem from nonsexual causes. Some critics of the current STD screening program claim that the symptoms of African American women are frequently assumed to arise from any STD that is detected during screening, when in fact these women may actually have some additional disease such as endometriosis (see entry) that does not receive careful diagnosis or treatment.

How are sexually transmitted diseases treated?

With some notable exceptions (AIDS, hepatitis B, and herpes), even the more serious STDs are treatable with antibiotics. There is currently no cure for hepatitis B, herpes, or AIDS, which are caused by viruses that can remain dormant in the body for years. But some medications can relieve symptoms, and in the case of AIDS, drug treatment can slow the progression of the disease.

How are STDs prevented?

Even when appropriate tests are done, screening is no panacea. Because of shame or embarrassment, many people avoid seeking medical care for STDs until they develop severe and often irreversible symptoms. Also, no matter how early screening is sought, there are simply no reliable diagnostic tests for some of these diseases, and several are incurable even if diagnosed early.

The best way to avoid the consequences of STDs is to avoid

getting the infections in the first place. Practicing safer sex (for example, using condoms and spermicides)—though no guarantee against infection—can greatly reduce risks.

Women who are diagnosed as having an STD should also inform all recent sexual partners so that they can be evaluated and treated before spreading the disease further.

Related entries
Abdominal pain, acquired immune deficiency syndrome, antibiotics, bacterial vaginosis, cervical cancer, chancroid, chlamydia, condoms, diaphragms and cervical caps, endometriosis, genital warts, gonorrhea, hepatitis, herpes, infertility, pelvic inflammatory disease, pelvic pain, pubic lice, safer sex, scabies, spermicides, syphilis, trichomonas

Shingles

This common condition is due to the reactivation of the *Varicella zoster* (herpes zoster) virus, which causes chicken pox and then becomes dormant in the nerves for many years. Reactivation first produces a sensitivity or tingling in the affected nerves and then sometimes progresses to excruciating pain.

Who is likely to develop shingles?
Shingles are most likely in people over the age of 50 or those experiencing ill health or severe stress.

What are the symptoms?
Often the first sign of shingles is pain along one side of the chest, although pain can also develop in the abdomen and face. Several days later, fluid-filled blisters develop along the path of the affected nerves. The blisters crust and scab over within a few days, and both the pain and rash are usually gone within weeks.

But about 10 percent of all people with shingles, and about 50 percent of those over the age of 60 or those who have a weakened immune system, continue to have pain in the affected area for months or even years, a condition called postherpetic neuralgia. This pain syndrome is particularly common in women. It usually resolves after a few months, but in some people it develops into a chronic pain syndrome (see psychosomatic disorders).

How are shingles evaluated?
The pain caused by shingles can easily be confused with many other conditions because the exact location of the pain depends on which nerves are affected (see chest pain and abdominal pain). Several days later, however, characteristic blisters erupt along the nerve path and make the condition unmistakable.

If parts of the face, particularly around the eye, are involved, the clinician may recommend a consultation with an ophthalmologist. If intractable pain develops, the patient may be referred to a physician who specializes in chronic pain or to a pain clinic (see psychosomatic disorders).

How are shingles treated?
The antiviral agents acyclovir (Zovirax) and famcyclovir (Famvir) can sometimes lessen the severity of an attack if prescribed early. These drugs will almost always be prescribed if skin around the eye is affected. Oral corticosteroids taken near the beginning of the attack were once thought to lower the chances of chronic pain later, but controlled studies have shown no convincing evidence of their benefit. Cool compresses or lotions can often help soothe the pain, as can aspirin and other nonprescription painkillers.

In the case of chronic pain, low doses of antidepressants such as amitriptyline (Elavil) and transcutaneous electrical nerve stimulation (TENS) have helped some sufferers. In TENS, electrodes are placed at key points on the patient's body and an intermittent electric current is passed through the electrodes to alleviate the pain.

Related entries
Abdominal pain, chest pain, eye care, psychosomatic disorders

Sjögren Syndrome

Sjögren syndrome is a common but often misdiagnosed inflammatory disorder involving the eyes, mouth, and other mucous membranes. It occurs when white blood cells called lymphocytes infiltrate the tear ducts and salivary glands and impair the secretion of saliva and tears. A systemic disorder, Sjögren syndrome can also involve inflammation of other organs such as the kidneys, lungs, thyroid, heart, and pancreas. The cause remains unknown, but it is suspected to be an autoimmune disorder.

Who is likely to develop it?
Sjögren syndrome occurs most often in women in their 40s and 50s. It can be associated with certain other connective tissue (rheumatic) diseases including rheumatoid arthritis, lupus, polymyositis and dermatomyositis, and scleroderma, all of which are also autoimmune disorders. But it often occurs as an isolated disorder of tears and saliva, without these other diseases.

What are the symptoms?
Sjögren syndrome is marked by extremely dry eyes, mouth, and lips. The eyes are generally red and painful and often feel gritty as if they contained some foreign object. In more advanced cases, the cornea of the eye can become severely damaged. Diminished saliva production can make it hard to chew and swallow and can promote tooth decay. Some people with

Sjögren syndrome also lose their ability to taste and smell. Symptoms of connective tissue disorders, particularly painful and inflamed joints (arthritis), occur in about a third of the people with this condition.

How is the condition evaluated?

A doctor may suspect Sjögren syndrome in a patient with dry eyes and mouth, especially if arthritis is present as well. A physical examination may reveal enlarged salivary glands. Various laboratory tests can then be performed to see if these glands are functioning normally, as well as to measure the quantity of tears secreted by the tear ducts. The doctor may also order various blood tests to look for certain antibodies and other qualities such as a high erythrocyte sedimentation rate (ESR or "sed rate"), that is, the rate at which red blood cells settle to the bottom of a container. This test is a nonspecific marker for inflammatory and rheumatic disorders. A lip biopsy may be done to check for the presence of lymphocytes in the salivary glands, a sign of Sjögren syndrome.

How is Sjögren syndrome treated?

Because there is no cure for Sjögren syndrome, treatment involves alleviating the symptoms. Usually eyedrops containing methylcellulose or polyvinyl alcohol can relieve dry, red eyes, although some people find relief only from using soft contact lenses and wetting them often with saline drops.

Analgesics (painkillers) can be used to relieve any pain that may result from the sudden enlargement of salivary glands, and tablets of pilocarpine (an analog of the neurotransmitter acetylcholine) may be prescribed to stimulate salivary flow. Another analog of acetylcholine, cevimeline, has recently been shown to alleviate both dry mouth and dry eye. This drug can cause major side effects, however, including excessive sweating, nausea, runny nose, diarrhea, and visual disturbances and should not be used by anyone with asthma or certain eye disorders (narrow-angle glaucoma or iritis). Dryness in the mouth and risk of tooth decay may also be reduced by drinking many fluids, using a solution of methylcellulose as a mouthwash, applying a topical fluoride gel to the teeth, and chewing sugarless gum. It is also a good idea to avoid drugs that can decrease saliva flow, such as antihistamines and certain antidepressants. People with Sjögren syndrome should have regular dental care to make sure that deposits of tartar (calculus) are promptly removed.

Corticosteroids (modified forms of adrenal hormones that relieve inflammation) are sometimes prescribed to help relieve arthritis or other symptoms of connective tissue disease. These are usually unnecessary, however, because symptoms of these diseases in people with Sjögren syndrome tend to be relatively mild.

Related entries

Antiinflammatory drugs, arthritis, autoimmune disorders, blood tests, dry eye, lupus, polymyositis and dermatomyositis, rheumatoid arthritis, scleroderma

Skin Care and Cosmetics

The skin is the body's largest organ. It serves many different functions: protecting vital organs, regulating body temperature, providing a barrier against infectious microorganisms, excreting a small proportion of waste products, transforming sunlight into vitamin D, and, through the production of melanin, helping reduce exposure to the sun's damaging ultraviolet rays. The skin is also packed with specialized nerve endings that send messages of touch, pressure, heat, cold, pain, and sexual arousal to the brain. The skin's texture, color, and tone are a major part of a person's attractiveness and, as a result, her overall sense of well-being, and they also give the clinician clues to a woman's general health.

Skin consists of two layers: the outer epidermis and the underlying dermis (see illustration). The epidermis is a thin, relatively transparent layer which itself can be divided into three layers—the basal cells on the bottom (just next to the dermis), the squamous cells, and, on the outer surface (stratum corneum), dead skin cells made of a protein called keratin which is also found in hair and nails. These outer cells are regularly sloughed off (both from washing and from everyday pressure and friction) and replaced by newer skin cells, which have been manufactured in the blood-enriched base layers of the epidermis. The new skin cells rise to the outer surface in the course of a month or so, gradually dying as

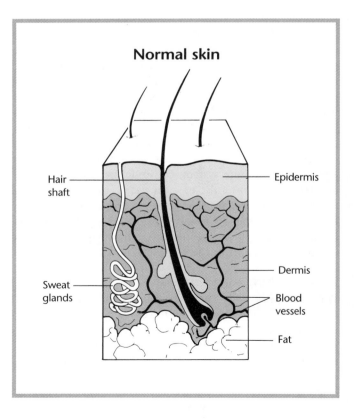

Normal skin

Hair shaft

Sweat glands

Epidermis

Dermis

Blood vessels

Fat

they become increasingly thinner and flatter. In this way the skin is a naturally replenishing organ. Turnover takes a bit longer in areas subject to the most friction and pressure—such as the soles of the feet and the palms of the hands—which also tend to be thicker than other areas of the skin. A small percentage of the cells in the epidermis produce melanin, the dark pigment that is responsible for skin color and that helps protect the skin from ultraviolet light. The more melanin a person has, the darker her skin will be.

Just beneath the epidermis is the much thicker dermis. It consists of proteins called collagen and elastin, which together give skin its strength, as well as its supple, stretchy properties. Running through the dermis are hair follicles, sweat glands, oil-secreting (sebaceous) glands, blood vessels, muscle cells, nerve fibers, and lymph ducts. The oil glands are particularly prevalent in the face, scalp, genitals, and chest. They secrete a waxy oil (sebum) that rises through hair follicles and lubricates and protects the outer skin.

Below the dermis is a layer of fat which helps insulate the body against temperature extremes and also gives shape to the face and other parts of the body. Muscle fibers, blood vessels, and nerves also run through this subcutaneous fat, as do the roots of the oil and sweat glands.

Some dermatologists—and cosmetologists—find it useful to divide skin into categories depending on its degree of oiliness. Ideal skin—that is, skin that is neither too oily nor too dry—falls into the balanced category. Adolescents are more likely to have oily skin, which is particularly susceptible to problems associated with overactive sebaceous glands—acne in particular. As women age, their skin tends to become drier and less elastic. This occurs in part because of a decline in the production of oil and sweat by the glands, as well as a general decline in the whole skin renewal process. For this reason oily skin is much less common once a woman gets beyond her mid-20s. At that point dry skin and combination skin (that is, skin that is dry in some places and oily in others) predominate. Dry skin is much more prone to irritation and wrinkles than to blemishes.

After menopause the outer layer of skin cells takes longer to renew itself. This intrinsic factor, combined with extrinsic factors such as the cumulative effects of ultraviolet light exposure, result in thickened skin which often feels leathery. In women with lighter complexions it may also appear to yellow. At the same time, the collagen and elastin in the dermis become disorganized, resulting in a thinner dermis and the development of furrows, wrinkles, and easy bruising. The layer of subcutaneous fat tends to disappear, and the skin becomes more transparent, with blood vessels appearing more prominently. Often small liver spots (areas of darker pigmentation) develop on the face and hands, particularly in light-skinned women. The changes associated with aging can develop in younger women who smoke cigarettes or who have had excessive sun exposure.

Although dermatologists urge women not to neglect functional but unglamorous areas of the skin—such as the soles of the feet—there is no question that the vast majority of skin care effort goes into the face and hands. Not only are these generally the most visible areas of skin, but they are also most frequently exposed to harsh soaps and detergents, drying environments, and—most damaging of all—ultraviolet light.

Avoiding sun exposure, eating a balanced diet, exercising regularly, getting adequate rest, and avoiding cigarette smoking, excessive alcohol consumption, and rapid and frequent weight fluctuations are the best things a woman can do to take care of her skin in the long run. But in the short run, a multimillion-dollar cosmetic industry is supported by the belief among women that special soaps, moisturizers, antiperspirants, deodorants, facial treatments, and makeup can make their skin look, smell, and feel more attractive.

Soaps and cleansing

Generally skin needs to be cleaned only once a day—or when obviously dirty. Bathing too much tends to dry out the skin; women with dry skin may want to take showers in lieu of long soaks in the bathtub (unless, of course, they find a moisturizing bath oil that works). Women with oily skin, by contrast, may want to cleanse 2 or 3 times a day; excessive cleansing, however, can stimulate oil production.

To protect the delicate tissues around the eyes, eye makeup should be rubbed off gently with cotton balls. The rest of the skin can be safely cleaned with a terry washcloth or sponge. Most dermatologists recommend using lukewarm water to wash the face, together with a mild soap, which helps emulsify oils and foreign particles on the skin. Because soaps are alkaline preparations, however, they may disrupt the normally acidic skin and can cause chapping and irritation. For this reason women with dry skin may want to use special moisturizing ("superfatted") soaps or "beauty bars," which have lower pH values than regular soaps. One caveat here is that soaps labeled "mild," "superfatted," and "nondrying" are not necessarily so. Only trial and error will tell.

Another option for dry skin is to limit soap use to face, underarms, hands, feet, and genitals and to apply a moisturizer after every bath or shower—particularly during winter months.

Sunscreens

Ultraviolet light not only wrinkles, dries, and burns the skin but also significantly increases the odds of developing skin cancer, including the often deadly melanoma. Although dark skin can tolerate more sun than lighter skin, no one is immune to the deterioration wrought over time by ultraviolet light. Dermatologists recommend that even women with dark skin, those who live in cloudy climates, and those who work indoors get into the habit of applying a sunscreen every day, in all seasons. In fact, one of the most intense exposures to sun occurs on sunny days when the ground is covered with snow.

The rays from the sun come in two major forms, the "burning" ultraviolet B (UVB) rays and the longer-wave ultraviolet A (UVA) rays. Although UVB rays make up only about 10 percent of the energy that reaches the earth on a bright, sunny day, they are about 1,000 times more powerful than UVA rays. UVA rays can cause long-term damage because they are able to penetrate beyond the epidermis into the dermis layer of skin. UVA rays can also pass through glass—which is why a woman who spends all day near a window needs to wear sunscreen just as much as a woman who spends all day outdoors.

The majority of sunscreens protect only against UVB, which is why the skin will still tan from the UVA rays. It is important to find a sunscreen that protects the skin from both UVA and UVB rays. Many people who use sunscreens stay out in the sun all day, never realizing that their skin is still absorbing the UVA rays that can dry, wrinkle, and age their skin, as well as increase the odds of developing skin cancer. Sunscreens that protect against UVA have not been as well researched as UVB sunscreens.

The sun protection factor (SPF) indicates the multiple by which the sunblock extends the safe period of exposure— that is, the amount of time a person can stay in the sunlight without becoming slightly sunburned. If a woman could normally stay out for 15 minutes (0.25 hours) without burning, using a sunblock with an SPF of 15 would extend the safe exposure time to 3.75 hours (15 × 0.25 hours). Sunscreens and sunblocks need to be reapplied after swimming or excessive sweating. Most women should use a sunscreen with a minimum SPF of 15 to 30.

A variety of sunscreen products are available in lotion, cream, oil, and lip protector forms, and many makeup products also contain sunscreens. Some people are allergic to the ingredient para-aminobenzoic acid (PABA), but many effective sunscreens are now advertised as "PABA-free." Even so, certain people experience sensitization reactions to sunscreens. This may lead to a vicious circle of irritation because, when the sensitized skin becomes red, the person assumes she is getting sunburned and applies even more sunscreen. Her skin then becomes more inflamed and irritated than ever (see cosmetic safety).

Moisturizers

There are two basic strategies for moisturizing skin: putting moisture in and keeping it in. The first turns out to be extremely difficult. While various products claim to pour moisture into skin, the chances are slim that any moisturizing product can penetrate the outer epidermis to transform the living, actively growing layer of skin cells.

Since it is so difficult to put moisture into the skin, most products are designed to keep in any moisture that is already there. These products—usually skin lotions—are best applied right after a bath or shower, when the skin is still slightly damp. Hands should be moisturized more frequently, especially after they have been immersed in water.

Many moisturizers on the market disappear into the skin almost immediately and have effects lasting a half hour or less. Heavy ointments such as petrolatum (Vaseline) or lanolin are longer-lasting and are best for very dry skin, unless a woman is allergic to them. Many dermatologists also recommend glycolic acid preparations for dry skin. These are available from dermatologists, aestheticians, and some pharmacies. Lighter lotions, made from a mixture of both oil and water emulsions (including Eucerin, Nivea, Keri, Lubriderm, and Nutraderm), are also effective, since the water evaporates after the product is applied. They are usually recommended for normal to dry skin. There is some evidence that products containing urea and lactic acid (such as Aquacare HP, Carmol Ten, Lacticare, Nutraplus, and Purpose) may help soften and moisturize skin. Women with very oily skin may want to use oil-free lotions.

Another way to moisturize dry skin is to soak in a bathtub full of water and bath oil. Many bath oils are dispersed into the water, presumably so some portion of the oil (along with a surfactant) will be absorbed into the skin. Other bath oils coat the surface of the bath water and then coat the body as it emerges from the tub (they also make the tub very slippery, which can cause accidents). These oils certainly make skin feel smooth and may also help prevent water from evaporating. Some women, however, find that their skin feels drier and itchier after they use these products. Ultimately, a woman choosing a moisturizing product has to experiment to find what works best for her. Sometimes a product that moisturizes well will also promote acne on the face or produce an allergic reaction.

When a woman is choosing a moisturizer, price is not a very good guide to quality. The most expensive ingredients may not be any more effective than baby lotion or lanolin. Among those for which there is little if any scientific backing are liposomes (microscopic spheres made out of a variety of fatty substances, including natural components of cell membranes), yeast extract (which supposedly refines and concentrates yeast cells to a point where they can smooth lines and wrinkles), collagen (a protein found in connective tissue and often used in moisturizers), and cerebrosides (a type of glycolipid produced by basal epidermal cells and then secreted to the outside of cells). Aloe vera is another much touted component of moisturizers and other skin care products. Taken from a plant in the lily family, this natural substance has anti-irritant effects which have been recognized for millennia. The amount of aloe vera necessary to produce these effects is far greater than the amount available in today's cosmetics, however, and some people turn out to be allergic to aloe vera.

Dry skin can be helped with much less costly measures than using expensive moisturizers. These include hydrating the skin from the inside out by drinking plenty of fluids. Also, during the winter months it may be helpful to use a vaporizer or humidifier to counteract the dryness of indoor heating systems, or to place pans of water over radiators. Merely reducing the amount of time spent in the bath or shower can be helpful as well, as can using only gentle, nonsoap, nondrying cleansers. It also makes sense to avoid hot water baths and showers altogether, since they can strip skin of vital moisture. And since sleeping under a hot electric blanket is basically equivalent to baking the skin slowly all night long, women who dislike getting into a cold bed may want to preheat the bed before getting in, and then turn the blanket off for the night.

Dry skin needs extra protection from the wind—which pulls water right out of the skin. In cold weather, the skin should be covered as much as possible with hats, scarves, gaiters, gloves, and mittens. When the wind-chill factor is very low, face or ski masks are in order. Any skin exposed to severely cold temperatures should be coated with petroleum jelly. This is especially true for skiers and other winter athletes. In windy weather, walkers, joggers, and bikers may want to begin their route facing into the wind in order to avoid heading back into it while covered with sweat.

Antiperspirants and deodorants

There are two types of sweat glands: eccrine and apocrine. The eccrine glands are packed into the underarms, forehead, palms, and soles, and scattered less densely throughout the rest of the body. The apocrine glands are densest under the arms and around the genitals and nipples; at puberty they enlarge to produce an oily, colorless perspiration that may leave stains on the clothing. This perspiration is odorless until it accumulates bacteria, which produce a strong body odor as they metabolize the body's secretions (see body odors). Both excess heat and emotional stress (including sexual arousal) can trigger the apocrine glands to secrete perspiration.

For many people antiperspirants are the answer to undesirable wetness, and deodorants are the answer to odor. Antiperspirants reduce sweating, while deodorants help mask odor without inhibiting the amount of perspiration. Many products combine both an antiperspirant and a deodorant. Most nonprescription antiperspirants contain aluminum compounds, which reduce (but do not eliminate) sweating in most people. These are available in various forms, although creams and roll-ons are generally preferable to aerosol sprays, which can irritate the lungs.

Women with more resistant perspiration might want to try a prescription preparation called Drysol. This consists of a saturated solution of aluminum chloride in alcohol which is held in place overnight with an airtight wrap. For some women the only solution is to have the sweat glands surgically removed from the armpits.

Because armpit odor is caused predominantly by bacteria that grow in the warm, moist environment of the armpit, deodorants that simply coat the armpit with a pleasant aroma are only temporary weapons. To be effective, deodorants have to be able to inhibit bacterial growth. This is accomplished to some extent by the aluminum compounds in antiperspirants. Some people find these compounds irritating, however, particularly after shaving. Alternatives include using antibacterial soaps or solutions or applying topical antibiotics.

Facials, antiwrinkle creams, and makeup

Just how much the cheeks sag or the eyes bag is largely determined by a woman's genes combined with the amount of time she has spent in the sun. This does not stop many women from spending large amounts of money for various creams, lotions, and facial treatments in the hope of removing wrinkles and preventing other ravages of age.

The best that can be said for many of these investments is that they may leave a woman feeling pampered and refreshed. Take facial masks, for example. Whether they are made of mud, cucumber, or avocado oil, applied at home or lavished on at a beauty parlor, facial masks do little more than cleanse the skin—and perhaps increase the blood flow to it temporarily. As a result, they may leave the skin looking healthier for a short while. When it comes to long-lasting effects on dryness or wrinkles, facial masks are no more effective than a moisturizing cream or lotion. The same can be said for costly antiwrinkle creams (other than tretinoin, or Retin-A), collagen implants, and electrical stimulation. A series of collagen injections, however, can sometimes "plump up" the surface skin, thus obscuring superficial wrinkles for several months. Collagen used in injections is extracted from cows, and about 3 percent of people are allergic to bovine collagen. A skin test should be performed before the injections.

Drugs containing tretinoin (including the acne medication Retin-A and the emollient cream Renova) have shown considerable promise in smoothing out wrinkles associated with dry skin. Increasing evidence suggests that this vitamin A acid may help smooth fine lines and improve skin texture by restoring the skin's ability to produce collagen (see wrinkles). The emollient cream Renova, which contains a 0.05 percent concentration of tretinoin, is currently approved by the Food and Drug Administration (FDA) for the treatment of wrinkles. Alpha-hydroxy or fruit acids can also reverse pigmentation changes and fine wrinkling and, in sufficient concentrations, may increase the density of collagen as well.

Abrasive facial masks and body scrubs which exfoliate the skin by removing the top layer of dead cells can actually do more harm than good. Even without these products, the skin already sheds millions of cells every day. When the rate of shedding is increased, the result can be increasingly sensitive skin, scaly patches, and graying skin tones.

Makeup that transforms the skin's appearance and modifies its features is always an option for many women. Dermatologists recommend matching makeup to skin type. Thus, women with dry skin should use an oil-based foundation, and women with oily skin a water-based one. Many women choose products that contain a sunscreen and are noncomedogenic—which means that they will not clog the pores and promote acne.

Cellulite

Despite the vast number of miracle products and systems marketed to remove it, the stubborn fat sometimes called cellulite is just like all other body fat except that it is deposited in places that may give it a dimpled or bulging appearance. Fat cells that lie between connective tissue—especially in the hip, thighs, and buttocks—often push up against the tissue to create a dimpled look. Although advertisements often portray cellulite as abnormal or unsightly, this effect is perfectly normal. It is particularly apparent in women whose fat tends to be deposited in their hips and thighs, as well as in people with relatively thin skin. Skin thickness is partly a product of genetics, and partly a product of age (the skin tends to thin over time), and therefore are outside of anyone's control. As with any other excess fat, however, removing "cellulite" is a matter of following the inescapable laws of physics—use up more calories through exercise than are consumed through diet.

Cosmetic surgery

For women willing to spend a lot more money and go through the inconvenience and discomfort, cosmetic surgery, particularly face lifts and eyelid surgery (see entries), can tighten sagging skin. Dermabrasion and chemical peels (see entry) can remove deep scars resulting from acne or injuries, but these procedures need to be performed by a skilled technician and are not appropriate for the changes caused by everyday aging. New laser techniques are being developed that may be able to remodel or resurface facial wrinkles.

Related entries

Acne, body image, body odors, cosmetic safety, cosmetic surgery, dermabrasion and chemical peels, exercise, eyelid surgery, face lifts, hair care, melanoma, nail care, nutrition, skin disorders, smoking, stress, wrinkles

Skin Disorders

Skin tends to change its properties with age, as well as with changing hormone levels associated with different stages of the life cycle. These changes are not disorders, but they can lead to skin conditions that sometimes require treatment. In adolescents, for example, increased levels of androgens (virilizing hormones) tend to encourage the production of excess sebum by the sebaceous glands, often resulting in oily skin and acne (see entry).

Oral contraceptives containing certain forms of the hormone progesterone can lead to acne or skin rashes. The high levels of estrogen associated with pregnancy, some birth control pills, and estrogen replacement therapy may change the skin's pigmentation, producing irregular brown patches (melasma) on the face or darkening preexisting freckles. Pregnant women may also develop a dark line (linea nigra) extending from the navel to the top of the pubic area, or may find that their nipples have darkened in color. These changes often fade after delivery.

Some skin disorders can result from sexually transmitted diseases (see entry). STDs are acquired primarily through sexual contact with an infected partner, and are caused by bacteria, viruses, fungi, protozoa, mycoplasma, and ectoparasites that thrive on the warm, moist mucous membranes of the genital area, mouth, and throat. Many of them can also produce sores, rashes, or other disorders of the skin. STDs include chancroid, genital warts, gonorrhea, herpes, HIV infection, pubic lice, scabies, and syphilis.

Types of skin disorders

Among the many other skin disorders that affect women are acne, atopic dermatitis (eczema), rosacea, scleroderma, psoriasis, lichen planus, dermatomyositis, lupus erythematosus, liver spots, moles, melanoma, stretchmarks, keloid scars, and tears and bruises from aging skin (see also vulvar disorders; vulvitis).

Acne. This skin condition is characterized by a collection of blackheads, whiteheads, pimples, pustules, and sometimes cysts on the face, chest, and back. It is common in adolescents but can appear for the first time in adult women because of a genetic predisposition or hormonal fluctuations. In certain women it appears during the week before a menstrual period and may worsen around the time of menopause; it often improves during pregnancy. Severe acne seems to be hereditary, although why certain individuals develop worse cases than others remains unknown. Acne (see entry) can also result from reactions to cosmetics and hair treatments, as well as to many drugs.

Atopic dermatitis (eczema). Dermatitis means skin irritation, and atopic dermatitis—also known as eczema—is a kind of skin irritation that results from an allergic reaction. In this condition, the skin appears dry, red, itchy, cracked, scaly, or oozy. Atopic dermatitis often begins in infancy or childhood and is particularly common in people with asthma, hay fever, or allergies. While atopic dermatitis often clears up spontaneously before adolescence, many women remain susceptible. Women allergic to nickel, for example, often develop atopic dermatitis on their earlobes, wrists, or back due to nickel-containing jewelry or bra hooks, and those allergic to latex gloves may develop itchy patches on their hands and wrists. In adults, rashes on the face and hands often become hardened and leathery, as well as extremely itchy, if untreated. Repeated scratching can also result in painful sores and skin infections. Atopic dermatitis can be controlled with anti-itching medications such as oral antihistamines and H_2 blockers and, often, antibiotics to fight infections. Avoiding harsh soaps and applying unscented emollient creams after baths or showers can also be helpful.

Rosacea. Although rosacea sometimes resembles acne, the absence of either blackheads or whiteheads marks it as a distinct condition. It is a chronic inflammatory disorder in which the central areas of the face become reddened—probably because of enlarged blood vessels under the skin. Rosacea (see entry) appears more often in women than in men and is particularly common in fair-skinned people. It usually begins in middle age or later.

Scleroderma. Scleroderma (see entry) is a disease of a connective tissue called collagen that is found in bones, skin, ligaments, and cartilage. Affected skin becomes permanently tight, shiny, and hardened, and sometimes internal organs may be involved. The cause is unknown, but scleroderma is probably an autoimmune disorder, in which the body attacks itself by producing antibodies against its own tissues. It appears about 4 times as frequently in women as in men. Although rarely life-threatening and sometimes only a minor nuisance, scleroderma can affect the quality of life of some women by causing changes in their appearance or reduced use of their limbs.

Psoriasis. People with psoriasis develop characteristic scaly, red patches when new skin cells are produced at a more rapid rate than normal and do not mature (see illustration). Inflammation and growth of new blood vessels redden the affected areas. People with psoriasis sometimes develop psoriatic arthritis, in which the inflamed areas of skin are accompanied by painful finger, toe, knee, or elbow joints. This condition is more common in women than in men.

Lichen planus. Lichen planus is a recurrent inflammatory skin disease that can cause pain and itching, particularly in the mouth or vulva (see vulvar disorders). Distinct patches of shiny, itchy violet spots appear on the skin of the legs, wrists, trunk, and genitals, or there may be gray-white spots on the inner cheeks, lips, and tongue. Some people develop ridges on their nails.

Lichen planus can occur in either sex, and most frequently

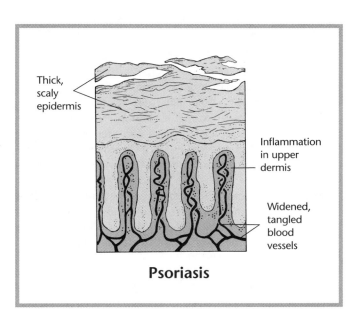

Thick, scaly epidermis

Inflammation in upper dermis

Widened, tangled blood vessels

Psoriasis

develops in people aged 30 to 60. Usually the first attack lasts for weeks or even months, and recurrent attacks may occur sporadically for many years. The cause of this skin disorder is unknown, but stress may lead symptoms to flare up. Certain drugs (including quinacrine, arsenic, blood pressure medications, and gold) can produce symptoms in some people identical to those seen in lichen planus. If symptoms are troublesome, a clinician can prescribe a high-potency topical corticosteroid to be applied directly to the sores.

Dermatomyositis. In the connective tissue disorder called polymyositis, muscles become inflamed and weakened; when areas of skin become inflamed as well, the condition is called dermatomyositis. The classic skin rash for dermatomyositis is a lilac (heliotrope) rash on the upper eyelids and forehead, but it may also appear on the neck, shoulders, chest, back, wrists, knuckles, knees, or ankles. Although polymyositis and dermatomyositis (see entry) sometimes disappear spontaneously after a few months, they can be life-threatening, particularly if internal organs are involved. About 10 percent of adult women with these conditions develop malignancies within a year of the diagnosis. Polymyositis and dermatomyositis have no known cause, but there is some speculation that they may be due to autoimmune reactions in which the body makes antibodies against itself.

Lupus. The term *lupus* is Latin for "wolf," and refers to a rash or mask over the nose and cheeks (referred to as a malar rash) that frequently appears in people with this disease. When the term is used by itself, it usually refers to systemic lupus erythematosus, or SLE, which is an autoimmune disease that affects many body systems (see lupus). Another form of lupus is discoid lupus erythematosus (DLE), which can exist as an independent condition or as one symptom of SLE. Both forms of lupus share this distinctive rash.

In DLE round, red scaling patches appear on the skin, usually on the cheeks, bridge of the nose, scalp, or ears and sometimes on the upper trunk and extremities. In many patients these symptoms appear after exposure to the sun. Sores may develop inside the mouth. About 10 percent of people with DLE eventually develop more internal and systemic inflammatory symptoms, sometimes resulting in full-scale SLE (see entry on lupus).

Liver spots. Liver spots (see entry) are patches of increased pigmentation that frequently appear on the face and hands of people over 40. They seem to result from cumulative ultraviolet light exposure.

Liver spots are generally harmless and require no treatment. If they are bothersome for cosmetic reasons, it is possible to lighten them with skin bleaching products which inhibit pigmentation, cover them with special cosmetic creams, or have them frozen off with liquid nitrogen (cryosurgery). Lasers are an alternative (and expensive) method for removing liver spots, and are about as effective as cryosurgery. Long-term use of Retin-A has been shown to lighten these spots over the course of months (see wrinkles).

If a new growth on the skin seems suspicious, especially if it suddenly feels sore, changes color, or thickens, a dermatologist or other clinician should be consulted to make sure that it is not skin cancer.

It may be possible to prevent new liver spots by applying a sunscreen (with a sun protection factor, or SPF, of 15 or greater) to areas routinely exposed to the sun, such as the hands and lower arms. Sunscreens should be applied in all seasons, not just summer, to be effective. Some liver spots develop for reasons that are not well understood but are apparently unrelated to sun exposure.

Moles. Moles (see entry) are dark spots that can appear on any part of the skin and are generally brown, blue, or black. In light-skinned people they may also be flesh-colored. Some moles also contain hairs or rough yellow bumps. Moles may be present from birth, but they also frequently appear or disappear spontaneously later in life. Moles that have been present since childhood often darken at puberty.

Generally moles pose no health hazard whatsoever but should be watched carefully because certain changes may signal a potentially fatal form of skin cancer called melanoma. Moles that one is born with (congenital moles) carry a slightly increased risk of melanoma over a lifetime.

Melanoma. This is the least common but most lethal form of skin cancer. Involving skin cells that produce pigment (melanin), a melanoma (see entry) is usually painless but burrows into the skin and, if untreated, can rapidly spread to distant organs via either the blood or lymphatic system. Occasionally melanomas appear in the eye, on the vulva, in the vagina, or in some parts of the central nervous system. In women, melanomas are more likely to appear on the legs than on the torso.

Stretchmarks. Stretchmarks are pinkish, silvery, or reddish-brown streaks that appear on skin that is stretched, usually by weight gain. They most commonly appear during the later months of pregnancy, particularly on the enlarging abdomen and breasts but also sometimes on the thighs and buttocks. Stretchmarks (see entry) are primarily a cosmetic problem.

Keloid scars. These elevated, fleshy, ridged scars occur when the skin produces excess scar tissue. True keloids do not conform to the dimensions of the original wound but take on a size and shape of their own. In susceptible people they can develop after any kind of skin trauma—including surgery, injury, vaccination, or skin infection. They have also been known to occur for no apparent reason, especially on the face, neck, or chest. People with dark skin are much more susceptible to keloid scarring (see entry). Trying to remove keloids with surgery results in yet another keloid in 50 percent of cases, but occasionally a keloid scar will recede on its own.

Tears and bruising. As skin ages, the dermis shrinks and becomes less firmly attached to the epidermis. Consequently, in an elderly person, even a slight bump can cause the two skin layers to tear apart (see illustration). And because blood vessels in older skin are closer to the surface, they are more prone to break as well with even the slightest impact. The result is a sore and discolored bruise. Aspirin and oral corticosteroids taken regularly for such conditions as arthritis can make these bruises even worse.

Older people can protect themselves from some skin tears and bruises by modifying their environment—moving or getting rid of hard-edged chairs and any other pieces of furniture that cause injuries, and padding any sharp corners that cannot be moved. Wearing long sleeves, long pants, and gloves when injuries are most likely to occur can also cut down on the number of skin tears and bruises, as can keeping the skin moist and supple (see skin care). Younger people can slow down the aging of skin somewhat (but not prevent it indefinitely) by being vigilant about sun protection and by not smoking.

When skin tears occur, the wound should be washed and disinfected with mild soap (not iodine, hydrogen peroxide, or alcohol, all of which can damage skin cells and slow healing). A topical antibiotic ointment to prevent infection and a dressing that holds in moisture but lets air through are very beneficial. These "hydrocolloid dressings" include DuoDERM, Actiderm, and Omniderm.

Related entries

Biopsy, cosmetic safety, cryosurgery, foot care, keloid scarring, laser surgery, lupus, melanoma, moles, polymyositis and dermatomyositis, rosacea, sexually transmitted diseases, skin care and cosmetics, varicose veins, vulvar disorders, vulvitis, wrinkles

Sleep Disorders

The best-known sleep disorder is insomnia (see entry), the inability to fall or stay asleep. But there are many others, including restless legs syndrome, leg cramps, sleep apnea, narcolepsy, bruxism, sleepwalking, and night terrors. According to the National Commission on Sleep Disorders, 20 to 30 million Americans have some kind of sleep-related problem, at least intermittently.

Sleep disorders are usually brought on by underlying physical conditions, emotional stress, or certain sleep medications or other drugs. Lack of sleep is a common problem for women who are under stress from balancing the responsibilities of career, home, and children or who deliberately cut back on their hours in bed as they put the needs of others before their own. It is particularly prevalent during pregnancy and menopause and often occurs as a symptom of certain disorders common in women, such as depression, anxiety, tension headaches, and thyroid disorders.

Sleep normally occurs in a series of approximately 90-minute cycles, each of which can be divided into three stages of progressively deeper sleep and then into a final stage called REM (rapid eye movement) sleep. In REM sleep the brain becomes quite active, the eyes move rapidly under the lids, and dreaming probably occurs. As the night goes on, periods of REM sleep gradually lengthen. It takes an average of four complete cycles to allow a person to awaken feeling refreshed.

Just what can be considered a normal sleep pattern varies considerably from one person to the next (see illustration). A newborn baby's sleeping pattern provides the most obvious example. A young infant can spend 20 hours of the day asleep, waking and going back to sleep five or six times, and this is considered perfectly normal. Brain wave studies also show that infants fall into deep REM sleep almost immediately and spend as much as half their total sleeping time in this stage of sleep. As a baby grows, the need for sleep typically dwindles, while at the same time naps are gradually replaced by one single long sleep. By late childhood the need for sleep has dropped to about 8 or 9 hours a night, and then increases temporarily during adolescence. Adults average between 7.5 and 8.5 hours per night, although some people need as few as 4 or as many as 10 hours to function well during the day. In later life most people need considerably less sleep, which explains why many older people find themselves rising much earlier than they did as young adults. People past mid-life may also find that they wake up several times during the night and may need to resume taking daytime naps. Brain wave studies show that as people age, a smaller proportion of sleep is spent in the non-REM stages.

These patterns are all considered part of the normal human life cycle and not signs of sleep disorders. Still, some of the "average" sleep patterns—particularly the amount of time we spend sleeping—may reflect changes in our lifestyle more than changes in our bodies. For example, the National Commission on Sleep Disorders estimates that the average person in America today sleeps 1.5 hours less each night than the average person did at the turn of the last century. Just what effects, if any, this decrease has or will have is unclear. Perhaps our great-grandparents were sleeping too much, perhaps we are sleeping too little, or perhaps everyone was getting just as much sleep as they needed, given their particular set of life circumstances. No one really knows just how much sleep people need for good health, much less how much sleep any one individual needs.

For that matter, no one really understands the exact function of sleep. One of the most widely accepted theories at present is that sleep somehow serves to recharge the body and brain. Another theory holds that the REM phase of sleep in particular helps the brain learn and remember by processing the events of the day. Whatever theories ultimately pan out, it is already clear that a good night's rest is essential for normal physical functioning and emotional stability. Fur-

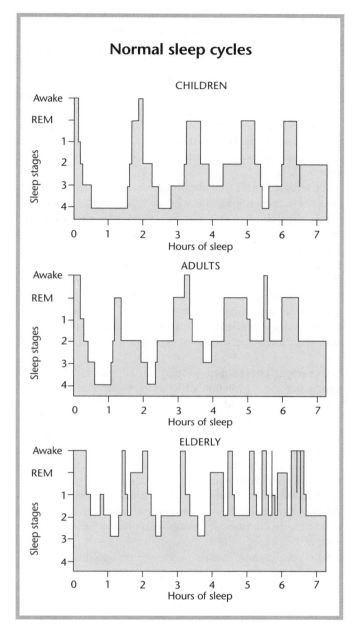

thermore, excessive sleepiness, difficulty working and concentrating, and unusual irritability during the day can all be signs that a person is not sleeping adequately and may well warrant a search for a specific sleep disorder.

Types of sleep disorders

Restless legs. Also known as nocturnal jerking movements, restless legs are a much more common problem than once thought. As many as 10 percent of all Americans may suffer from this sleep disorder at some point, although it is most common after middle age. In most cases restless legs do not seem to be the sign of more serious disease.

As people with this disorder begin to fall asleep, they are

aroused by a creepy, disturbing sensation deep inside their legs (usually the calves but also sometimes the feet, thighs, or even arms) as if worms or insects were crawling under their skin. This sensation can last for an hour or more and soon leads to an almost irresistible need to move the legs. This provides only temporary relief, since after moving, shaking, or walking out the problem, one finds that it almost always returns. Symptoms are often worse during times of emotional stress or anxiety, or after heavy caffeine intake. Besides disturbing bed partners, restless legs lead to drowsiness the next day.

Some people find that simple self-help measures such as a warm bath before bed or muscle relaxation exercises can help reduce symptoms of this disorder. Cold or hot packs on the legs may also provide some relief. For more severe cases, a physician might prescribe a benzodiazepine tranquilizer. These medications can be used safely only for a short period of time, however, and may disrupt sleep in and of themselves. Low doses of certain anti–Parkinson's disease medications can also be effective. Occasionally restless legs may be related to vitamin deficiency, in which case it may clear up once the underlying condition is diagnosed and treated.

Leg cramps. These sharp, sudden muscle pains in the calves during the night probably afflict almost half of all adults under the age of 50 and as many as 70 percent of adults over that age. Unlike restless legs, they are not associated with the irresistible urge to move, but they do cause enough discomfort to interfere with sleep. Many people find that massaging the calf, straightening the leg, or flexing the toes can provide quick relief. Hot baths and heating pads may also be helpful, although some people find that ice packs work even better. Again, though, in severe cases it may be necessary to have a physician prescribe some kind of tranquilizer or other sleep aid.

Often leg cramps can be prevented by avoiding dehydration, sleeping with the feet flexed, or doing leg-stretching exercises to strengthen the calf muscles. Some people report that taking a daily dose of vitamin E (400 IU) helps ward off nightly leg cramps. Another promising and relatively inexpensive possibility involves taking 200 to 300 mg of the nonprescription drug quinine each day. This often stops cramps within a week, after which it may only be necessary to take the quinine intermittently. Quinine is not safe for use during pregnancy, nor is it safe for women who have a glucose-6-phosphate deficiency (G6PD).

Sleep apnea. Of the 30 million Americans who snore, about 2.5 million have a sleep disorder known as sleep apnea (absence of breathing). People with this disorder have 30 or more periods during the night in which they stop breathing for up to 10 seconds or so. Although sleep apnea is particularly common in men of middle age or older (especially if they are overweight and have hypertension), women become increasingly prone to this disorder after they reach menopause.

The most common form of sleep apnea, called obstructive sleep apnea, occurs when a flap of muscle or other flabby structure in the upper airway partially blocks the flow of air. Less often, sleep apnea occurs because the respiratory muscles stop working temporarily, possibly because something is interfering with breathing signals from the brain. As carbon dioxide levels in the blood rise, the brain is stimulated to increase air intake. The result is often extremely loud snoring, violent grunting, and wild gasping, after which the person returns to a more peaceful slumber, until carbon dioxide levels rise again.

Besides keeping people from reaching deep levels of sleep, severe sleep apnea can trigger cardiac arrhythmias or even heart attacks, particularly in people who also have coronary artery disease (as many people with sleep apnea do). Risk of death is even higher during an apneic episode if the person is using alcohol or sleep medications.

Many people with sleep apnea never realize the trauma they have been through hundreds of time during the night (although their bed partners are generally aware of the problem). Excessive daytime sleepiness the next day (including falling asleep at the wheel), however, may suggest that something is not right. Other signs of sleep apnea are sleep attacks during the day, irritability, and possibly shortened attention span, slowed thinking, and limited short-term memory. A person who thinks she may have sleep apnea should be evaluated at a sleep disorders center or by a clinician with the equipment to measure brain waves and breathing patterns during sleep.

Treatment for sleep apnea usually involves some combination of lifestyle changes and surgery. Losing weight is almost universally advised, but it rarely eradicates the problem and, of course, is often quite difficult to achieve. More effective may be treating any coexisting medical problems that may be aggravating the apnea. There are some mechanical devices such as the CPAP machine that can be strapped over the face to help promote airflow during the night, and, though inconvenient and uncomfortable, they can sometimes provide relief.

If all else fails, surgery is a possibility. Usually this involves a tracheotomy (an opening made directly into the trachea, or windpipe), so that air can easily enter the passage beneath the point of blockage. This hole can be plugged during the day to allow normal breathing and speaking. Given the cost and potential complications of surgery—not to mention the threat of a tracheotomy to a person's body image—the surgical approach should be considered only after less drastic measures have been tried.

Narcolepsy. Narcolepsy—a tendency to have sudden and unpredictable sleep attacks in the middle of the day—is a much more common problem than was once suspected. People with this disorder often drop into REM sleep in the middle of a dinner party, class, conversation, car trip, or even sexual encounter, and continue to sleep anywhere from a few seconds to half an hour. They then reawaken feeling alert until another attack overtakes them. The alert reawakening is what distinguishes narcolepsy from the excessive daytime sleepiness associated with sleep apnea. Some people with narcolepsy continue to function during their sleep attacks, walking across a room, putting things away, or even engaging in conversation, only to awaken with no memory whatsoever of their actions.

About three-quarters of all people with narcolepsy also experience temporary muscle paralysis during their sleep attacks, a condition known as cataplexy. In the middle of a conversation—or sometimes simply after a strong emotional reaction such as anger, amusement, or astonishment—the person's jaw will suddenly drop and her shoulders will slump as she falls into a deep sleep. If the person is standing or driving, this can obviously be quite dangerous or even life-threatening. People with cataplexy often awaken from sleep while having dreamlike hallucinations which last for several minutes until their sleep paralysis wears off.

The cause of both narcolepsy and cataplexy remains elusive. Some researchers think these disorders may be due to a genetic predisposition combined with an alteration in the biological clock that was, in turn, provoked by shift work or other environmental causes. Others believe that it represents some kind of neurological problem involving the part of the brain that governs REM sleep. Whatever the explanation, narcolepsy often first appears during young adulthood and is equally common in both sexes, although some recent evidence suggests that women may be more likely to have a different form of a gene linked to this disorder. It can be diagnosed in a sleep laboratory by measuring brain waves and eye movements during sleep.

It may be possible for people with narcolepsy to prevent embarrassing sleep attacks by napping briefly before important social or work-related events. Avoiding heavy meals and using caffeinated beverages in moderation can also help ward off drowsiness. Occasionally a physician may prescribe amphetamine drugs such as methylphenidate (Ritalin), which increase alertness by stimulating the brain. Antidepressant medications such as Prozac also seem to be helpful in preventing cataplectic symptoms. And a newer drug, modafinil (Provigil), can also be helpful, with fewer side effects and without the addictive potential of amphetamines. Some new evidence suggests that women with narcolepsy may respond to lower doses of this drug than their male counterparts.

Bruxism. Bruxism means grinding the teeth during sleep. As many as 15 percent of all Americans have this problem, especially people who are anxious or tense or who are suppressing anger. It often worsens after heavy alcohol use and seems to run in families. While nocturnal gnashing, clenching, and grinding may sometimes be violent enough to disrupt sleep, the more common adverse effects involve damage to the teeth and jaw. Besides wearing down tooth enamel, bruxism can also lead to temporomandibular joint syndrome (see entry), a particularly common problem in women.

Treatment for bruxism depends on its cause. If the prob-lem is largely psychological, stress reduction techniques (see stress), relaxation exercises (see alternative therapies), or psychotherapy (see entry) may be warranted. If alcohol seems to exacerbate the problem, cutting down on its use can help. In other people bruxism may result from misalignment between the upper and lower jaw, a problem that can be fixed by orthodontia (see entry). If necessary, a dentist can also provide a plastic mouth guard to help protect the teeth while the underlying problem is being corrected.

Sleepwalking. Sleepwalking occurs when a sleeping person opens her eyes, gets out of bed, and begins to take a stroll about the house (or yard). Sometimes sleepwalkers open and close drawers, use the toilet, change their nightclothes, or even leave the house entirely. Contrary to popular belief, sleepwalkers are not magically protected from danger and can become seriously hurt or even killed if they trip, fall down the stairs, or attempt to drive an automobile. If awakened during a midnight stroll, a sleepwalker is usually confused and disoriented.

Although sleepwalking is most common in children, it can afflict adults who are undergoing significant anxiety or other psychological problems. Although there is no specific treatment, avoiding the use of alcohol and other drugs that depress the central nervous system can sometimes reduce the number of sleepwalking episodes. Benzodiazepine tranquilizers may help some people. In any case, bolting the bedroom door, gating the top of the stairs, clearing the floor of obstacles, and hiding car keys before bed can at least minimize the possibility of serious danger.

Night terrors. A person who wakes from sleep screaming or shaking without coming into full consciousness and with no concrete memory of a bad dream is said to have had a night terror. Unlike nightmares, night terrors are more apt to occur during the first part of the night and are rarely remembered the next morning, although sometimes the person retains a single terrifying vision. Night terrors can last for as long as 20 minutes.

Most common in children between the ages of 3 and 5, night terrors can also occur in adults who are undergoing deep emotional or psychological disturbances. Alcohol use can exacerbate them. Adults who experience night terrors often benefit from psychotherapy to help alleviate the underlying tension.

Sleepwalking and night terrors are both considered disorders of REM sleep. This may explain why many pregnant women undergo marked exacerbations or remissions of these disorders during the later stages of pregnancy, a period when the amount of time spent in REM sleep becomes disproportionately small.

Related entries

Alcohol, alternative therapies, anemia, anxiety disorders, body image, coffee, coronary artery disease, depression, headaches, high blood pressure, insomnia, obesity, orthodontia, personality disorders, psychotherapy, stress, temporomandibular joint syndrome, thyroid disorders

Smoking

Cigarette smoking is the leading preventable cause of death for both men and women in the United States. It has been blamed for an estimated 419,000 deaths per year in this country (or 1 in every 5 deaths) from cardiovascular disease (including heart attacks and sudden death), stroke, and cancers of the lung, mouth, larynx, esophagus, trachea, bladder, pancreas, and stomach. Smokers have higher rates of peptic ulcer disease, are more susceptible to upper respiratory infections, and are more likely to develop cataracts than nonsmokers.

Most of what we know about the ill effects of smoking is based on large-scale studies in men. But the evidence is becoming increasingly clear that a woman who smokes like a man can expect to get sick and die like a man. In fact, today women account for 39 percent of all smoking-related deaths, a proportion that has more than doubled since the mid-1960s. Since 1980, over 3 million women have died from smoking-related causes.

Which women are likely to smoke?

Before World War II smoking was relatively rare among women (it had begun to increase substantially in men about 3 decades earlier). Even in 1965, a peak year for smoking in this country, only 32 percent of adult women smoked, in comparison with 50 percent of adult men. After 1965 smoking rates fell 4 times faster among men than among women as young women began taking up smoking at far greater rates than young men.

In both sexes the childhood and teenage years are the peak times for starting to smoke. But between the mid-1970s and the mid-1980s the number of female smokers aged 12 to 18 doubled, and since then the prevalence of smoking among adolescent girls has exceeded that among boys. In one recent survey 30 percent of high school senior girls said they had smoked in the previous month. Observers have attributed this phenomenon to a number of factors. For one thing, adolescent girls are particularly susceptible to peer pressure—which too often links cigarettes and alcohol with popularity, maturity, and independence. Often sensitive to physical appearance, teenage girls are easily swayed by arguments that smoking can help them lose weight or stay slim or make them as attractive and desirable as the models in cigarette advertisements.

The more education a woman has had, the less likely she is to start smoking cigarettes as an adult or to continue smoking once she has started. As a result, the problems associated with smoking are increasingly concentrated among young and disadvantaged women. In 1992 only 13 percent of female college graduates smoked cigarettes, as opposed to 27 percent of women who were high school dropouts.

The result of this trend has been a narrowing of the gender gap between male and female smokers. By 1992, 24 percent of adult women and 28 percent of adult men were cigarette smokers. Some investigators fear that, as a result, the much-touted female advantage in life expectancy may begin to diminish. The latest surgeon general's report says that smoking can cut short a woman's life by an average of 14 years.

What are the health effects of smoking?

Changes in women's smoking habits have led to substantial increases in smoking-related disease and death among women. Most striking is the increase in lung cancer rates among women in the past 3 or 4 decades, but the list of other health effects is long. Women smokers of any age are more than 10 times as likely as nonsmoking women to die of cancers of the larynx and esophagus and of chronic obstructive lung disease, including emphysema (see breathing disorders). Cancer risk rises even more if cigarette smoking is combined with alcohol use or with occupational exposure to toxic substances such as asbestos (see occupational hazards).

Each year smoking accounts for 25 percent of all deaths among American women, accounting for approximately 106,000 deaths per year. The specific risk of developing any of the many conditions that have been linked to cigarette smoking depends on how long a person has smoked, how many cigarettes she has smoked altogether, and how deeply she inhales.

Damage to the respiratory system. Between 1960 and 1986 the rate of lung cancer increased more than 4 times among women smokers, surpassing breast cancer as the leading cause of cancer death in women. In 1991 cigarette smoking was implicated in 79 percent of all lung cancer deaths in women and 21 percent of cancer deaths in women overall (including cancers of the mouth, throat, and cervix). Lung cancer now claims 27,000 more women's lives per year than does breast cancer.

There is preliminary evidence that women run about twice the risk of developing lung cancer from smoking that men do, because of relatively greater injury to the DNA in women's lung cells. Damage to the lungs can be traced to the dozens of toxic gases and particles of tar and nicotine that enter the lungs with each inhalation. In addition to lung cancer, women who smoke suffer more from bronchitis, emphysema, asthma, tuberculosis, pneumonia, influenza, colds, and coughs than women who do not smoke.

Damage to the cardiovascular system. In general, a middle-aged woman who smokes is 3 times more likely to die of coronary artery disease and 5 times more likely to die of a stroke than a nonsmoking woman of the same age. Women smokers over the age of 35 who use birth control pills have an increased risk of both heart attack and stroke.

Even women who smoke as few as 1 to 4 cigarettes per day have a higher risk of cardiovascular death than nonsmoking women. Contrary to common belief, reduced tar and nicotine cigarettes do not seem to afford any protection against these risks. No level of tobacco use is known to be safe.

Effects on the reproductive system. Women who smoke run the risk of developing a number of health problems not shared by male smokers. For example, smoking during pregnancy has been clearly linked to low birth weight in infants—that is, a weight of less than 5.5 pounds at birth, which increases the chances of infant death during the first month of life by a factor of almost 40.

Although some of this risk occurs because smoking increases the chances of a premature delivery, the primary cause of low birth weight among babies born to mothers who smoke is that smoking slows the fetus's rate of growth inside the uterus. This may be related to the fact that cigarette smoke in the mother's bloodstream crosses the placenta and introduces harmful chemicals into the fetus's blood. Carbon monoxide in particular reduces the amount of oxygen that can be carried in the blood of both the mother and the fetus, and nicotine can cause the fetus's blood vessels to constrict so that even less oxygen and fewer nutrients reach the fetus.

Smoking during pregnancy has been linked to increased rates of miscarriage, stillbirth, and neonatal death, as well as various bleeding problems, including placenta previa (a condition in which the placenta covers the cervix and is prone to bleeding) and placenta abruptio (a condition in which the placenta abruptly separates from the endometrium). Sudden infant death syndrome—the unexplained death of an apparently healthy infant—is 2 to 4 times more common among babies whose mothers smoked while they were pregnant, and children of mothers who smoked during pregnancy have a higher than average rate of brain damage, cerebral palsy, and behavioral disorders.

Smoking seems to accelerate the onset of menopause by a year or so, possibly because tobacco alters the metabolism of estrogen or has a direct toxic effect on the ovaries. But premenopausal women who give up smoking tend to go through menopause at the usual time. Infertility in both men and women is more common among smokers.

Women who smoke have relatively higher rates of cervical cancer, and components of tobacco smoke can be isolated from the cervical mucus of women smokers. Cervical cancer rates are much lower in ex-smokers than in current smokers.

Damage to the musculoskeletal system. Some studies have linked cigarette smoking with reduced bone mass and osteoporosis in women. This link may be due to some component of cigarette smoke itself, but it could also be due to the fact that women who smoke cigarettes tend to be thinner than nonsmokers and have an earlier menopause—both of which are risk factors for osteoporosis. One other possibility is that smoking may undo the positive effects of estrogen on the body. A large study of women in Framingham, Massachu-

setts, showed that estrogen replacement therapy protected nonsmokers but not smokers from hip fractures related to osteoporosis.

Damage to the skin. Women who smoke tend to experience more severe skin wrinkling than nonsmokers, no matter how much lifetime sun exposure they have had.

Damage to the health of family members. Smoking accounts for the majority of fatal residential fires, which often claim children and the elderly as victims. Children of parents who smoke have on average more serious respiratory infections, more respiratory symptoms, and more ear infections and asthma than the children of nonsmokers. In 1993 the Environmental Protection Agency blamed secondary smoke for approximately 3,000 lung cancers per year among nonsmokers in the United States. Exposure to cigarette smoke also seems to increase the risk of coronary artery disease in nonsmokers. Women appear to be at particularly high risk. While secondhand smoke increases a nonsmoker's risk of heart disease by 25 percent in the general population, findings from the Nurses' Health Study, a long-term study of over 30,000 nonsmoking women, suggested that this risk nearly doubles in females.

What are the benefits of quitting?

Many people continue to smoke despite all of this knowledge because they feel—or hope—that they are personally immune to these problems, because they believe that the benefits (pleasure, relief from stress and anxiety, or weight maintenance) outweigh the risks, or—more often than not—because quitting is difficult.

Many of the risks associated with cigarette smoking—including lung and other cancers, heart attack, stroke, chronic lung disease, and peptic ulcer disease—can be reversed or substantially reduced by quitting. Ten to 15 years after stopping, an ex-smoker's overall risk of death from these diseases is close to that of a person who has never smoked. This is true no matter how old a woman is or how long or heavily she has smoked. It is even true for women who stop smoking after they have developed some smoking-related symptom—although it has recently become clear that certain changes which occur with prolonged heavy smoking can never be reversed. In addition, the more damage that has been done, the longer it will take to reverse even what can be undone.

Some of the risks fall faster than others. An ex-smoker's excess risk of dying from cardiovascular disease, for example, is eliminated in the first year after quitting, while 30 to 50 percent of her excess risk of dying from lung cancer remains as long as 10 years after quitting. Even 15 years after quitting, an ex-smoker still has some excess risk of dying from lung cancer. But, all in all, former smokers have a significantly longer life expectancy than do continuing smokers.

The biggest gains come to smokers who quit when they are young, when they have been exposed to relatively few cigarettes, and when they are still free of smoking-related disease. The health hazards associated with the small amount of weight that many women gain after stopping smoking are minuscule compared with the hazards associated with smoking.

A pregnant woman who smokes can completely reverse the hazards to her unborn child by stopping smoking during the first 3 or 4 months of gestation. Abandoning cigarettes at any time up to the 30th week of pregnancy can help bring the birth weight of the newborn up to average. Simply cutting back on cigarettes—rather than quitting altogether—does not seem to be of much help in preventing low birth weight, however.

What is the best way to quit?

For the most part, awareness of health risks is not enough to motivate people to quit. Over 90 percent of current smokers know full well that smoking is harmful to health, and yet a vague fear of some future disease is not enough to keep them from smoking. What does seem to motivate many smokers to quit, however, is the development of a smoking-related symptom such as persistent cough, breathlessness, or chest pain in the smoker herself or in a close family member or friend. These symptoms may or may not be related to the cigarette smoking, but they often scare a smoker into seeing herself as personally vulnerable. Social pressure also plays a role in evoking the desire to quit.

Most smokers today say they would like to stop and have made at least one concerted attempt to do so. It often takes two or three serious efforts before this mission is accomplished. That is because quitting is more than a matter of willpower. Smoking cessation is often a learning process in which mistakes made in the first attempt help improve the odds of success in the next one. In fact, most smokers go through a slow series of psychological stages before they are able to stop smoking. The first is characterized by an initial lack of interest in quitting. Next the smoker begins to think about the health risks associated with cigarettes and contemplates quitting—someday. Eventually something—whether the development of a symptom or pressure from peers or health professionals—will stimulate active plans to quit within the next month. At last the actual "quitting day" arrives, and the person stops smoking. The final stage arrives when nonsmoking is maintained permanently.

One thing that makes quitting difficult is that many smokers are both physically and psychologically dependent on cigarettes. When smoking is abandoned, withdrawal symptoms may make life difficult. Symptoms of nicotine withdrawal include ▸ cravings for a cigarette; ▸ irritability, anxiety, impatience, and anger; ▸ difficulty concentrating; ▸ excessive hunger; and ▸ sleep disturbances. These symptoms usually start within a few hours of the last cigarette. They are strongest during the first 2 to 3 days of abstinence but gradually diminish over 2 to 3 weeks. Just how severe these symptoms are depends on the smoker's prior level of nicotine intake. Since most of these symptoms (except the craving for cigarettes)

are not specifically related to smoking, many people do not recognize them for what they are.

Despite some evidence that nicotine withdrawal symptoms are more severe during the luteal phase (the second half) of a woman's menstrual cycle, quitting earlier in the cycle does not seem to improve the chances of success. A better solution to overcoming nicotine withdrawal symptoms involves behavioral methods. These methods help smokers identify cues to smoking and let them break the link between the trigger and the behavior and learn how to handle urges to smoke. Such skills can be learned at home from booklets or videotapes (these can be recommended by a clinician) or in a formal group program. If necessary, a doctor may also recommend nicotine gum or skin patches to ease the transition from smoking to nonsmoking. These are both readily available over the counter. Nasal and oral inhalers can be prescribed but may not be as effective.

Anyone trying to quit smoking should be aware of the insidious effects of coffee and alcohol—drugs that are more commonly used by smokers than nonsmokers. Many clinicians advise ex-smokers to avoid alcohol temporarily after quitting, since drinking alcoholic beverages seems to induce relapses in cigarette smoking. As for coffee, smoking tends to increase the rate at which caffeine is excreted from the body. When cigarettes are abandoned, therefore, the amount of caffeine left in the blood after the customary intake of coffee is higher than before, and the result is unaccustomed jitteriness.

Because smokers use cigarettes to relax or relieve negative emotions such as anger, anxiety, and frustration, quitting often makes it difficult to get through their daily routine. Losing this coping tool may be particularly difficult for women, many of whom find it hard to express anger directly. Abandoning cigarettes can also be difficult for the many smokers conditioned to light up a cigarette whenever they wake up in the morning or whenever they have a cup of coffee. Despite the best of intentions in the person trying to quit, these activities trigger the desire for a cigarette the way the ringing of a bell triggered Pavlov's dog to salivate. Again, behavioral modification strategies are often the best way to circumvent these psychological and behavioral barriers to quitting.

Another reason why so many smokers continue to use cigarettes is that they have a certain ambivalence about abandoning the habit. This is particularly true of women smokers. Although women are about as likely as men to quit smoking successfully, there are certain issues that complicate the process for them. Chief among these is concern about weight. The truth is that for about a year or two smokers who quit do temporarily weigh on average 5 to 10 pounds more than people of comparable age and height who never smoked. This transient weight gain probably occurs because the metabolic rate decreases when nicotine is withdrawn, although it may also have something to do with a tendency among ex-smokers to substitute food for cigarettes. Whatever the explanation, approximately 4 out of 5 smokers do experience a transient weight gain after abandoning cigarettes, and women who quit smoking seem to gain more weight than men. Given the cultural pressure on women to be slender, this fact certainly discourages many women smokers from abandoning the habit.

Nonetheless, given all the risks of smoking, the best approach might be a change in attitude about carrying a few excess pounds. After all, in the grand scheme of things, 5 to 10 pounds of excess weight does not represent a serious health risk. Only about 1 in 10 women ex-smokers gains more than 25 pounds, although heavier smokers (more than 25 cigarettes per day) do gain somewhat more weight than lighter smokers. In most cases a woman should expect only a small increase in weight, which can be shed—if she wishes—once the attempt to stop smoking has been accomplished. Using nicotine gum may also delay weight gain—at least until the gum use stops. Avoiding high-calorie snacks and increasing physical activity can also help. But trying to diet and give up cigarettes at the same time is almost always counterproductive on both counts.

Another obstacle to quitting is the frequent lack of social support. The evidence is abundantly clear, for example, that smokers whose efforts are bolstered by partners, family, and friends are more likely to succeed than smokers without such support. Moreover, smokers with a nonsmoking spouse are more likely to quit than smokers with spouses who smoke. And yet women smokers are less likely than men smokers to have spouses or partners who actively support their effort to quit. For these reasons, women trying to give up cigarettes have to find ways to ask family and friends to restrict smoking to outdoor areas or to limited areas indoors in order to ensure a smoke-free area in the home or workplace. Sometimes it can also help to seek additional social support in a formal smoking cessation program.

A final obstacle to quitting that plagues women in particular involves mood disorders—especially depression. It now appears that smokers have more symptoms of depression and are more likely to have a history of major depression than nonsmokers. Some researchers also suspect that quitting may actually precipitate depression in smokers with a history of major depression, and that resuming smoking may elevate mood. Also, depressed smokers are less likely to stop smoking than smokers who are not depressed. Since depression is about twice as common in women as in men, all of these observations are particularly relevant to women who smoke. It is important to have symptoms of depression treated before one attempts to stop smoking. In addition, any woman who is trying to stop smoking should be alert for symptoms of depression (see entry).

In all cases, anyone trying to quit smoking should not be discouraged by temporary setbacks. If "going cold turkey" is too difficult, it may help to start by gradually cutting down or switching to cigarettes low in tar and nicotine. If quitting on her own is impossible, a woman can join a nonsmoking pro-

gram or support group or enlist the help of a clinician. Contacting a local chapter of the American Lung Association or the American Cancer Society (listed in the phone book) is another good way to find smoking cessation programs and other helpful information. Many of these programs not only provide intensive training in behavioral techniques but also offer social support from a counselor and other group members, and this may be particularly valuable to women who smoke.

Does nicotine replacement therapy work?

Giving up cigarettes involves two separate challenges: the addiction to nicotine has to be overcome, and the habit of smoking cigarettes has to be broken. Nicotine replacement therapy—in the form of either nicotine gum or nicotine patches—can help separate these two challenges by allowing the smoker to focus on breaking the smoking habit before dealing with the nicotine addiction. Although many smokers are able to overcome the addiction on their own, a doctor may suggest either of these aids, available over the counter, to patients who experience severe nicotine withdrawal symptoms.

Both nicotine gum and nicotine patches can be quite safe and effective—even in smokers with coronary artery disease—if used properly. They work even better if used in conjunction with a behavioral counseling program that teaches the smoker how to break the cigarette habit. All forms of nicotine therapy work by replacing nicotine in amounts just large enough to block the symptoms of nicotine withdrawal but too small to reproduce the pleasure of smoking. In contrast to smoking, which leads to fluctuating levels of nicotine in the bloodstream, both the gum and the patch produce relatively constant blood levels of nicotine.

Women who have recently had a heart attack or who have unstable angina or serious arrhythmias (irregular heartbeat) should not use any form of nicotine replacement, nor should women who continue to smoke cigarettes. Researchers still do not know if either product is safe for use during pregnancy.

Nicotine patches. A nicotine patch is applied to a hairless spot on the upper arm or torso on the first morning that the smoker plans to quit. It contains a fixed amount of nicotine which is released continuously and absorbed through the skin throughout the day. Three of the four brands of patches now on the market are worn for 24 hours and replaced the next morning; the fourth product is removed before bedtime so that there is a patch-free period. Most patches need to be used for about 2 to 3 months, during which time the dose of nicotine contained in them can be gradually tapered off.

Local skin irritation is the most common side effect of the nicotine patch, but this can usually be treated with topical steroid preparations. The patch is inappropriate for women with widespread skin eruptions. Occasionally people using the patches find they have vivid dreams, insomnia, and nervousness. To control these side effects, it often helps to remove the patch at bedtime or reduce the dose of nicotine in the patch. In all cases, however, anyone using a nicotine patch should see a clinician after the first week so that the level of withdrawal symptoms can be assessed and proper use of the patch can be ensured.

Nicotine gum. Nicotine gum is somewhat more difficult to use correctly. Available in two different strengths, it is not chewed like regular gum. Instead, each piece should be chewed only long enough to release the nicotine, which produces a peppery flavor, and then parked between the cheek and gums for a few minutes, or until the peppery taste or tingling has disappeared. At this point the gum should be chewed a few more times until the nicotine is released, and then parked between the cheek and gums once again. This entire process should be repeated for about half an hour or until no more peppery taste is released. It is important not to drink any liquid while the gum is in the mouth and to avoid drinking any acidic beverages such as coffee for at least an hour or two before using the gum.

Most people need to chew between 9 and 12 pieces of gum a day (it helps to try chewing 1 piece every hour) to prevent withdrawal symptoms, although some heavy smokers may need as many as 30 pieces. After 3 months of use, the number of pieces can be gradually reduced.

Nicotine gum use often produces a number of minor side effects. Many of these—such as nausea, dyspepsia, hiccups, and dizziness—are related to nicotine withdrawal. Others are related to chewing, and include sore jaw and mouth ulcers. About 5 to 10 percent of nicotine gum users develop a long-term dependence on the gum.

Nicotine gum should not be used by women with temporomandibular joint syndrome (see entry).

What about non-nicotine medications?

A relatively new alternative to nicotine products is Zyban (buproprion hydrochloride), which has been sold for many years as an antidepressant. Some evidence suggests that this drug increases the neurotransmitters dopamine and norepinephrine in much the same way as nicotine. Zyban is taken once daily for 3 days and then twice daily for about 7 to 12 weeks. Smokers set a quit date and can continue smoking for up to 2 weeks after starting to take the pills. Side effects are few, and usually mild, but may include dry mouth and insomnia, as well as a small risk of seizures. Zyban can sometimes also minimize the weight gain that can occur during smoking cessation.

While Zyban is a safe, easy-to-use, and relatively inexpensive (if covered by an insurance plan) alternative to nicotine replacement for many smokers, it is not for everyone. Besides the fact that using it requires visiting a clinician for a prescription, this medication is considered unsafe for people who have epilepsy or other seizure disorders, as well as those with a history of stroke or serious head injury. Anyone taking monoamine oxidase inhibitors (MAOIs) or other drugs containing buproprion for depression should also avoid Zyban, as should people with eating disorders.

Combined approach

A new—and extremely effective—approach to smoking cessation involves a combination of steps that can help many smokers overcome the traditional obstacles, both physical and psychological, to quitting. This triple-pronged approach calls for: the antidepressant buproprion; gradually declining doses of nicotine delivered via nasal spray, patches, or inhalers; and individually tailored counseling. Recent studies suggest that this combination raises the success rate from less than 5 percent to approximately 40 to 60 percent after a year of treatment.

Related entries

Abdominal pain, alcohol, alternative therapies, angina pectoris, anxiety disorders, asthma, birth control, breast cancer, cervical cancer, chest pain, coffee, colds, coronary artery disease, depression, estrogen replacement therapy, infertility, insomnia, menopause, menstrual cycle, miscarriage, obesity, occupational hazards, osteoporosis, stress, stroke, substance abuse, temporomandibular joint syndrome, wrinkles

---

Social Anxiety Disorder

Social anxiety disorder is an extreme form of shyness that may afflict as many as 17 to 19 million Americans (many of them undiagnosed).

People with this form of anxiety disorder (see entry) are deeply afraid of embarrassing or humiliating themselves in public and, as a result, avoid social situations as much as possible. Sometimes this disorder takes the form of a generalized fear of social situations; in other cases it involves deep-seated fears (phobias; see entry) of specific public actions such as blushing (erythrophobia), eating in front of other people, using public restrooms, and speaking in public.

As with many other anxiety disorders, social anxiety disorder can significantly impair the quality of life and may interfere with educational attainment, job advancement, and the ability to have a healthy family or social life. This disorder has also been associated with other health problems and an accompanying increase in the utilization of health care services.

Who is likely to develop social anxiety disorder?

While many surveys suggest that social anxiety disorder may be more common in women than in men, men seem to be much more likely to seek help for the problem. This difference may be attributable to societal expectations and gender roles, since shyness is more acceptable among women and girls than among men and boys.

As many as 70 percent of all people with social anxiety disorder also suffer from depression. In addition, this disorder is more common in people who suffer from other anxiety disorders, as well as those who abuse alcohol; whether or not any of these conditions are causes or effects of one another has not yet been established.

What are the symptoms?

Social anxiety disorder is characterized by fears of embarrassment, humiliation, criticism, or scrutiny in any of a number of social and performance situations. Some women may experience these fears only when speaking in public or performing on stage—in which case they are said to have "performance anxiety." Feelings of fear may also develop in the context of many different kinds of social situations, whether it be attending parties, participating in group meetings, being the center of attention, interacting with authority figures, engaging in confrontations, eating or drinking in public, or even using a public restroom. Although many people have some kind of fear about many of these situations, the "social phobias" associated with social anxiety disorder are excessive and often incapacitating, leading victims to avoid the fear-provoking situations altogether.

In addition, fears can be so extreme in people with social anxiety disorder that physical symptoms develop, including blushing, sweating, tremulousness, and palpitations. These symptoms often exacerbate—and draw attention to—the fears.

How is the condition evaluated?

A clinician evaluating a woman for social anxiety disorder will first want to rule out any medical problems that may underlie the physical symptoms (e.g., sweating and palpitations) that often occur during social encounters. They will also try to differentiate patients who are embarrassed in public because of body image concerns (see entry), including those with eating disorders and those who are obsessed with the belief that a part of their body is ugly or distorted as part of body dysmorphic disorder, a condition in which people have a negatively skewed perception of their physical appearance.

Women diagnosed as having social anxiety disorder should also be evaluated for depression, which occurs in up to 70 percent of all people with this anxiety disorder.

How is social anxiety disorder treated?

In most cases treatment for social anxiety disorder includes a combination of psychotherapy (see entry) and antianxiety medications. Psychotherapy usually involves cognitive-behavioral therapy that focuses on recognizing and delineating the fears and learning to replace maladaptive with adaptive thoughts.

Because depression is often a part of social anxiety disorder, antidepressant medications are often used as a first-line mode of treatment. The antidepressants most commonly used in treating anxiety disorders are the selective serotonin reuptake inhibitors, or SSRIs (including citalopram, fluoxetine, fluvoxamine, paroxetine, and sertraline). Of these, fluoxetine appears to be the safest for use during pregnancy. A sizable number of patients with anxiety disorders experience troubling side effects such as jitteriness, insomnia, nausea, and even anxiety with SSRIs, however. For this reason, most clinicians will start out by prescribing these drugs in low doses, only gradually increasing them as tolerated. Ultimately these doses may have to be higher than those used to treat depression, however, and the drugs must be continued even after symptoms have resolved, according to the clinician's recommendations.

Antianxiety medications are usually tried only after the SSRIs have failed. These drugs include high-potency benzodiazepines (such as alprazolam and clonazepam). Because these drugs may lead to psychological and physiological dependence, however, they should be avoided by patients with a history of alcohol or substance abuse. If these drugs are used, it may be necessary to take other medications as well to treat any accompanying depression.

On the horizon are various new antidepressants (including venlafaxine, nefazodone, and mirtazapine) that show some promise in treating social and other anxiety disorders. In addition, beta blockers—drugs sometimes used to treat coronary artery disease—appear to be effective in treating performance anxiety in particular, although they do not seem to be helpful in treating more generalized forms of social anxiety disorder. Finally, the anticonvulsant drug gabapentin (neurontin) has shown promise in controlling symptoms of anxiety, either alone or as a supplement to SSRIs. While this drug is readily eliminated by the kidneys and has not been associated with any serious side effects, its safety for use during pregnancy has not yet been established.

Related entries

Antianxiety drugs, anxiety disorders, body image, depression, obsessive-compulsive disorder, phobias, psychosomatic disorders, psychotherapy, stress, substance abuse

Spermicides

Spermicidal foams, creams, and jellies are chemicals that are placed into the vagina close to the cervix before sexual intercourse in order to kill sperm. Creams and jellies come in tubes together with a plastic applicator. They are differentiated primarily by color and consistency: creams are white and somewhat less gloppy than jellies, which are clear. Foams come in aerosol cans along with an applicator and look and feel a lot like shaving cream. Spermicides are also available as suppositories (such as the Encare Oval, Semicid, and Intercept) and films (VCF) which are inserted directly into the vagina.

In addition to killing sperm, the active ingredient in most spermicides—nonoxynol-9—is believed to help reduce (though not eliminate) the chances of acquiring a sexually transmitted disease, including AIDS, during sexual intercourse.

Spermicides are often used together with barrier methods of contraception such as diaphragms, cervical caps, sponges, and condoms. They may also be used as a backup method of contraception during the first few months in which a woman is using oral, injectable, or implanted contraceptives or an intrauterine device (see birth control).

How are spermicides used?

If the spermicide is to be used alone, a full applicator should be injected into the vagina no more than 15 minutes before penis-vagina contact. Some brands of spermicide require 2 full applicators for each act of intercourse. The applicator is twisted onto the end of the tube of cream or jelly, which is then squeezed until the plunger on the other end of the applicator has moved all the way out. To fill an applicator with foam, the can needs to be shaken to make sure that the spermicide is well distributed. The applicator is then placed on top of the can and either tilted or pushed down until the foam pushes the plunger fully up. It is also possible to buy spermicide in the form of preloaded applicators.

Suppositories and contraceptive films should be inserted into the vagina no more than half an hour before penis-vagina contact, and they remain effective for no more than an hour. Contraceptive films are wrapped over a finger, which is then pushed up against the cervix to cover it. Neither the suppositories nor the film should be removed for at least 6 hours.

Many women find insertion easiest in the same position they use to insert a tampon—for example, lying in bed with the knees up, sitting on a toilet, or squatting. The plunger should be pushed gently toward the cervix—that is, angled back and up into the vagina. It is important to remove the applicator without withdrawing the plunger, since this could result in the removal of some of the spermicide. Later, the applicator should be washed in mild soap and warm water.

After ejaculation, another full plunger (or suppository or sheet of film) needs to be inserted before any additional intercourse occurs. It is not necessary (and probably not desirable) to douche or otherwise wash the spermicide from the vagina, and in no case should the spermicide be removed before at least 6 to 8 hours have passed.

The lowest expected failure rate for spermicides used alone is only 3 percent, but the more typical failure rate is as high as 21 percent—which means that 21 out of 100 (or more than 1 in 5) women who rely only on this method in any given year can expect to become pregnant in that year. Spermicides are much more effective when used in conjunction with other forms of contraception. There is some evidence that foams and suppositories used alone may be somewhat more effective than other forms, possibly because of the way they coat the vaginal walls. Even so, it is definitely safest to use all spermicides together with a barrier method of contraception.

Although spermicides are somewhat messy (especially if used without a diaphragm) and disruptive to sexual intercourse, foams tend to be less drippy than creams, and creams less drippy than jellies. Another inconvenience of spermicides is the need to keep a ready supply available. This can be particularly problematic in the case of foam, since it is not always easy to tell when the can is nearing depletion.

Some couples are bothered by the feel, taste, or smell of spermicides, although sometimes this problem can be solved by switching brands or choosing one of the tasteless, odorless versions.

On the positive side, spermicides are readily available without a prescription. The yearly cost of using spermicides depends on the frequency with which a woman has sexual intercourse. A 3.8-ounce tube of spermicidal cream or jelly usually costs somewhere in the neighborhood of $7 to $10.

What are the risks and complications?

At present it does not appear that the spermicides on the U.S. market pose any potential dangers other than an occasional allergic reaction. Any irritation that occurs can often be alleviated by switching to another brand or form of spermicide. Using spermicides does not appear to reduce a woman's fertility, and conception can be attempted as soon as a woman stops using the product. A few years back there was some concern that spermicides might increase the risk of certain birth defects, but the data on which these fears were based have since been discredited.

Related entries

Abortion, acquired immune deficiency syndrome, birth control, condoms, diaphragms, cervical caps and sponges, douching, hormonal contraception, intrauterine devices, lubricants, natural birth control methods, nonsurgical abortion, oral contraceptives, pregnancy testing, safer sex, sexually transmitted diseases, tubal ligation, urinary tract infections, vacuum aspiration

Sports Injuries

In health clubs and community centers, and on college and community playing fields, bike trails, and jogging paths across America, the number of women who actively participate in sports is at an all-time high. Much of this activity can be traced to the passage of Title IX of the 1972 Education Amendments Act, which prohibits federally funded educational programs and activities in all secondary and postsecondary institutions from discriminating by gender. As a result of Title IX, there is a growing number of women who started playing soccer or other sports in grade school and who have been active in sports over their entire lifetime. In addition, increasing numbers of older women—inspired sometimes by their daughters and/or by mounting evidence that regular exercise is essential to long-term health—take up sports and exercise programs later in life.

Along with increased participation in sports come a number of sports-related injuries, many of them unique to women. Women who stay active during pregnancy, for example, may develop certain problems associated with gestation-related changes in the joints and ligaments. A woman who has recently given birth often has temporary weakness of the pelvic floor, and her exercise routines must be altered to accommodate the accompanying back and pelvic pain and urinary incontinence. Hormonal changes and bone density loss may put middle-aged women athletes at increased risk of overuse injuries. And older women may have to adjust patterns of movement to avoid injury due to age-related degenerative changes of the spine and limbs.

While the female body may require certain gender-specific changes in routine, however, the injuries that women athletes are prone to develop are similar to those of male athletes in the same sport (see the sections on specific injuries below). Women who participate in contact sports, for example, are at risk for injuries related to the transfer of force to body tissues. Women who participate in sports such as tennis or golf are prone to "overuse injuries" due to the repetitive nature of practice and competition. Women who participate in gymnastics, soccer, basketball, field hockey, volleyball, lacrosse and softball are at particularly high risk of ankle injury. It is important to remember, however, that there is no typical injury for either a male or a female athlete, and that each individual has her own unique set of strengths and vulnerabilities that cannot be predicted based on the nature of the sport alone.

Nevertheless, unique biochemical, hormonal, and training issues do make women athletes susceptible to several specific interrelated health problems, termed the "Female Athlete Triad" by the American College of Sports Medicine (ACMS): menstrual irregularities, eating disorders, and premature osteoporosis (see entries). All three disorders are interconnected: insufficient caloric intake, common in female athletes, can alter the ratio of body fat to lean muscle mass enough to produce menstrual irregularities or stop periods altogether, sometimes leading to reduced fertility. Low levels of the female hormone estrogen associated with low ratios of body fat to muscle mass can result in premature osteoporosis, leaving women with this triad of conditions at particularly high risk for musculoskeletal injuries, including stress fractures (see below). The Female Athletic Triad also has long-term implications for bone health because, at least according to some studies, the reduction in bone density may persist even after hormone replacement and resumption of normal menstrual periods. To help prevent this trio of conditions, female athletes must be particularly careful to drink plenty of fluids, eat nutritiously, and seek medical attention at the first sign of an eating disorder and/or menstrual irregularity.

The sections below give brief descriptions of some of the most common sports injuries experienced by women, followed by a general discussion of treatment options.

Head injuries

The most common head injury in athletes is concussion, a temporary loss of consciousness following a blow to the head. Women who play softball, soccer, and lacrosse are most susceptible. There has also been some concern that repetitive minor impacts from "heading" the ball in soccer may lead to temporary or even permanent brain damage. Most research in this area has been done on male athletes, however, and findings so far have been inconclusive; final conclusions will have to await newer studies, including some currently under way that include female soccer players.

Any head injury that occurs during a game should be evaluated by a clinician as soon as possible, preferably on the sidelines. If a player sustains a head injury without losing consciousness, it may be safe to return to the field, but the more conservative guidelines recommend sitting out the duration of the game.

Back injuries

Neck (cervical spine) injuries. Male football players often complain about "burners" or "stingers," referring to the acute pain that travels down the arm after a neck injury. As women participate increasingly in sports such as wrestling and hockey, they too are experiencing these sensations. While burners and stingers usually abate on their own, they may require medical attention to prevent them from recurring or worsening.

Other pain or stiffness in the neck in a female athlete should be evaluated by a clinician and may require magnetic resonance imaging (MRI) or an electromyogram (a test to measure electrical activity in a muscle) to check for nerve damage.

Mid-spine (thoracic) injuries. The most common sports injuries to the mid-spine in female athletes are compression fractures of the vertebra. These fractures occur when one vertebra presses against another to the point that the bone breaks. Compression fractures of the middle region of the spine occasionally occur in women who participate in activities such as cheerleading, which can place excessive loads on the flexed spine.

A woman who has a compression fracture should have her bone health checked by a clinician. The examination should consider factors such as menstrual history, nutritional status, and any eating disorders—all of which play a role in bone strength.

Lower back (lumbar spine) injuries. Low back pain in a woman athlete can be due to conditions that affect non-athletes as well—including mechanical low back pain, internal disc derangement, and disc herniation (see entry on back pain). Whether these conditions are unusually common in athletes remains unclear. What is clear, however, is that repetitively placing loads on the spine put women athletes, particularly gymnasts, at risk for certain lower back problems, including spondylolysis. This condition—which is thought to result from a stress fracture that never healed—occurs when a part of the vertebra that protects spinal nerves becomes detached.

Occasionally in women with spondylolysis, one vertebra slips forward on the one beneath it, creating a condition called spondylolisthesis. In teenagers this kind of slipping sometimes becomes severe because the upper vertebra slips off the lower one completely. In most women, however, there is only a small amount of forward slipping. X-rays, CAT scans, or MRI scans may be necessary to differentiate spondylolysis and spondylolisthesis from other causes of low back pain. The conditions are usually treated similarly to other causes of low back pain, often without surgery.

Upper body injuries

Shoulder injuries. Women athletes appear to be unusually vulnerable to shoulder injuries. For one thing, they tend to have shorter arm length and shorter body length than men; as a result, the amount of exertion involved in completing the same task may be greater. For example, women swimmers require more strokes to swim the same distance as their male counterparts. Women also historically have poorer conditioning than men, although this conditioning gap may be narrowing as girls become increasingly athletic at younger ages. Using resistance training equipment designed primarily for the male body may also put women at unusually high risk for shoulder injury. It is possible—though not confirmed—that joint laxity, more common in females, may play a role as well. Men also tend to have a much greater differential in upper to lower body strength than women, although this difference is virtually eliminated when fat-free weight is taken into consideration.

The shoulder is especially prone to injury because the very same design that allows its freedom of moment also necessitates a certain amount of instability. The shoulders are vulnerable to both direct and overuse injuries. As a result, shoulder pain and stiffness are common problems for many athletes. One of the most common experiences occurs when the bursa (a lubricated sac of tissue that protects muscles and tendons as they move against one another) becomes inflamed, a condition called bursitis.

One of the major causes of bursitis is a condition called impingement syndrome. Each time the arm is raised, the tendons—which connect the muscles to the shoulder bone—and bursa are rubbed against the top of the scapula, one of the three bones that make up the shoulder. The result is a rubbing or pinching called impingement. Because many sports—particularly swimming and sports involving swinging a racquet or throwing a ball—require repeated raising and lowering of the arms, bursa in the shoulder often become irritated and swollen, resulting in bursitis. The classic sign of impingement syndrome is pain when the arm is raised out from the side or in front of the body. This pain can be sharp when trying to reach to the back of the body and can be severe enough to interfere with sleep. Over time, bone spurs (sharp outgrowths) may develop underneath the joint, worsening symptoms.

Lifting or catching heavy objects, especially with the arm extended, can also lead to the inflammation of the rotator cuff, a condition known as rotator cuff tendinitis and another common cause of bursitis. The rotator cuff is a group of four tendons that are attached to the four muscles of the shoulder and that together help raise and rotate the arm. If the rotator cuff becomes inflamed, the shoulder area feels week and painful. If the tendons in the rotator cuff are torn (a condition known as a rotator cuff tear), raising the arm may be difficult or, if the tear is complete, impossible. The tendons in the rotator cuff have a relatively poor blood supply that keeps them from healing and maintaining themselves as well as many other body parts and makes them vulnerable to degeneration with age. Because rotator cuffs often become weakened with age, middle-aged and older athletes are particularly likely to experience rotator cuff injuries.

Women who repeatedly raise the arm over the head (as in serving a tennis ball) may also develop a condition called shoulder instability, another leading cause of bursitis in the shoulder. This condition involves a loosening of the fit between the upper arm bone (humerus) and the socket (glenoid). A shoulder that has slipped out of the socket completely is said to be dislocated. Eventually untreated shoulder dislocations can result in joint inflammation—arthritis (see entry).

Elbow injuries. Women who engage in tennis, golf, rowing, softball, or any other activities that involve repetitive rotation of the forearm may develop epicondylitis, a condition often referred to as "tennis elbow" or "golfer's elbow." This condition is probably caused by numerous small tears in the tendons that attach the lower arm muscles to the elbow. The characteristic symptom of epicondylitis is recurrent pain on the outer, upper part of the forearm which may radiate down to the wrist. Usually moving the elbow or wrist worsens the pain. Symptoms generally develop gradually (see tendinitis and tenosynovitis).

Wrist, hand, and finger injuries. Falling on an outstretched hand or catching a forcefully thrown object can all result in a break of the wrist, hand, or fingers. Symptoms of a broken hand may include feelings of pain or tenderness when the affected area is pressed. A broken wrist (Colles fracture) usually causes severe pain when the wrist is moved or pressure is put on the hand. Other signs of a break in the wrist, hand, or fingers include swelling around the injured area, wrist pain, and difficulty moving the fingers.

In addition to fractures, injuries to the wrist, hand, and fingers can include tears of tendons and ligaments. One of the most common tears involves the tendons that help straighten the fingertip. These can be torn if a ball strikes an outstretched finger—as may happen in a basketball game, for example—and the result is a "mallet finger" (also known as a "jammed finger" or a "baseball finger"). Not only is a mallet finger impossible to straighten, but also its top joint will be swollen and painful. Treatment usually involves splinting for about 6 weeks.

Lower body injuries

Stress fractures and "shin splints." The term "shin splints" refers to pain in the lower leg that occurs during exercise. This pain can have many causes, including stress fractures (hairline cracks in bones that result from small but repetitive force). Particularly common among runners and dancers, stress fractures are most likely to occur in the lower leg, the back of the foot, or behind the knee. Wearing inadequate footwear, changing to a new kind of training surface, or suddenly increasing the intensity and/or duration of training without an adequate warm-up period all raise the chances of experiencing a stress fracture—and can intensify lower leg pain, whatever its cause.

Symptoms of a stress fracture usually involve tenderness, warmth, and swelling over the affected area, and pain that intensifies when the foot on the affected side is hopped on. The pain usually improves with rest.

Another common cause of shin splints is posterior tibial syndrome, or PTS. The pain associated with this syndrome—which occurs on the inside of the shin bone—usually dissipates as a person warms up but then intensifies once exercise is over. It is particularly common in beginning runners, as well as in any athlete who changes running surfaces, footwear, or the intensity or duration of exercise.

Pelvic and sacral injuries. Occasionally, stress fractures can also occur in the pelvis or the sacrum (the 5 fused vertebrae in the lower part of the spine just above the 4 fused vertebrae of the coccyx). Pain in these areas, however, can be difficult to diagnose because they are susceptible to a variety of injuries, many of which are characterized only by pain. Among possible sources of this pain are muscle strains, bursitis, and tendinitis. Pain in the spine and pelvis can also sometimes be traced to a discrepancy in leg length.

Skaters, golfers, and gymnasts—or participants in any sport that involves assymetrical movement of the lower extremities—are particularly susceptible to pain in the joint that connects the sacrum to the pelvis (the sacroiliac, or SI, joint). Pregnant women are also susceptible to SI joint pain because ligaments typically loosen during pregnancy. Using stair-steppers and elliptical trainers may exacerbate this kind of pain.

Hip injuries. Occasionally women experience a "snapping" sensation in the hip as they exercise. The source of this problem is usually some underlying joint problem in the hip, bursitis, tendinitis, or muscle tears, sprains, or strains. Long distance runners are particularly susceptible to tendinitis in the hip area and may need injections of corticosteroid medications if rest, NSAIDs, and stretching exercises do not help. They may also develop stress fractures in the thighbone that can also result in hip pain.

Pain in the hip or pelvic regions can also be a sign of disease in internal organs such as the ovaries (a phenomenon known as "referred pain"). If hip pain is associated with the menstrual cycle, abnormal bleeding, or other pelvic symptoms, a woman should consult her physician about non-athletic sources of the problem.

Knee injuries. Women athletes are more vulnerable to knee injuries than their male counterparts. In addition to underlying differences in muscle strength and joint laxity, women use their bodies differently than men; when women land from a jump, for example, they tend to use their quadriceps muscles to stabilize the knee. Anatomical and postural differences also make women more susceptible to tears of the ligaments that hold the knee in place. If the supporting ligaments are torn, the kneecap deviates to the side of the thigh bone. Pain is usually felt in the front of the knee or just behind the kneecap and frequently intensifies during kneeling, squatting, or walking downstairs. Over time excessive tension can break down the cartilage (fibrous connective tissue) in the joint.

Another common knee injury in female athletes—particularly runners and volleyball players—is patellofemoral pain syndrome. This problem is often attributed to the turning out of the feet and "knock knees," which are particularly common in women who repeatedly flex and extend the weight-bearing knee joint.

Occasionally women athletes may also tear cartilage in a knee (meniscal tears), although they are no more susceptible to this problem than male athletes. The menisci are wedges of crescent-shaped cartilage cushioning the thigh and lower leg bones and stabilizing them against rotational forces. An athlete with a meniscal tear will feel that her knee is "giving way" or "locking" into a fixed position. Often there is a painful click when the knee is bent or the leg is rotated.

Ankle injuries. Of all body parts, the ankle is the most vulnerable to sports injuries—with sprained ankles being by far the most common injury of all. A sprain occurs when a ligament, tendon, or muscle is stretched or torn—usually because the ankle is rolled over and subjected to the full weight of the body. Symptoms of a sprained ankle include pain, redness, swelling, bruising, and loss of mobility, and they vary in intensity depending on the severity of the sprain. Athletes who frequently sprain their ankles should tape or brace the ankles before sporting activities.

Breast injuries

Breast pain is a relatively common problem among female athletes, particularly those with large breasts and/or those who participate in sports during the premenstrual phase of the menstrual cycle. Sports bras with strong back support and non-stretch straps can alleviate this discomfort to some degree.

Padded sports bras can also help protect breasts from injury. If breasts do become injured, they should be treated like any other bruised body part with ice, painkillers, and support (see next section).

Occasionally runners develop a condition known as "runner's nipples," in which clothing irritates or abrades the nipples. The best way to prevent this condition is to cover the nipples with petroleum jelly or tape, wear a seamless bra, and wear a windbreaker that covers the chest during exercise in cold weather.

Treating sports injuries

Treating and preventing other sports-related problems generally involves treating the specific symptoms involved, as well as identifying (and, if possible, alleviating) any factors that predispose the athlete to that particular type of injury.

Once serious injury (e.g., fracture, underlying disease, or concussion) have been ruled out, many minor sports injuries can be treated with self-help measures. Just about any minor injury will respond to the classic "RICE" treatment (rest, ice, compression, and elevation) in the first 24 hours. The affected area should be rested ("R") to minimize bleeding and swelling, and an icepack ("I") or equivalent should be applied to the injury to limit pain and inflammation. The ice should ideally be kept in place for 10 minutes at a time, alternating with about 10 minutes without ice, with the pattern repeated for an hour or so. This routine should be followed several times in the first 24 hours after an injury—or as long as swelling and bruising continue. Gently compressing ("C") the injured area with an ace bandage (without restricting blood flow) and elevating ("E") it can also help minimize swelling.

Many sports injuries also respond to some kind of supportive bandaging or splinting to prevent painful movements, control swelling, and reduce stress on the injury as it heals. Splints and bandages should be loose enough, however, to permit blood flow. Taking pain-relieving medications, particularly nonsteroidal antiinflammatory drugs (NSAIDs), is often helpful. In some cases, special stretching and strengthening exercises can relieve pain and improve function in affected joints or muscles as well.

After the first 24 hours have passed, heating pads or other heat sources can help speed recovery by drawing blood to the site of the injury, relieving muscle tension, and promoting relaxation. At this stage in recovery, too, healing creams may be helpful, if laid gently on the skin and allowed to soak in. Rubbing in these creams can promote internal bleeding and damage torn muscle fibers.

Various alternative approaches may also be helpful if more conventional means of self-help aren't working. Certain forms of massage therapy and other forms of bodywork, for example, can improve muscle function, expand range of motion, and increase coordination and balance, and acupuncture may relieve some kinds of pain and speed healing if performed by a skilled therapist soon after the injury occurs.

Some injured joints and muscles, particularly those in the lower back, may respond to chiropractic treatment. And even some traditional Chinese remedies, as well as other forms of herbal and remedies, may help as well: bromelain and extremely diluted forms of arnica applied externally, for example, may help reduce pain and inflammation. Some people swear that homeopathic remedies also relieve pain and perhaps even speed the healing of tendons and ligaments.

If pain persists despite these simple self-help measures, a clinician should be consulted. Serious sports injuries often require weeks or months of rehabilitation therapy. The goal (and challenge) of sports rehabilitating medicine is to return the athlete to participation and/or competition as soon as possible, without risking ongoing injury. Usually rehabilitation requires a team approach, with different specialists involved, possibly including physicians, physician assistants, nurse practitioners, nurses, physical therapists, occupational therapists, chiropractors, trainers, and complementary medicine practitioners.

Related entries

Antiinflammatory drugs, arthritis, back pain, eating disorders, exercise, infertility, knee pain, menstrual disorders, musculoskeletal disorders, nutrition, osteoporosis

Stress

Strictly speaking, stress is any kind of force or pressure. This pressure can be physical, such as the stress of exercise or the stress of a debilitating disease, as well as emotional or situational, such as the stress of a high-pressure, low-freedom job. Today the term stress is loosely applied to virtually any event or situation that can evoke frustration, anger, or anxiety.

Whatever its source, true stress triggers a characteristic physiological response known as the fight-or-flight response (also called physiological stress). In this response the brain sends signals to the adrenal glands which lead them to secrete the "stress hormones" epinephrine and norepinephrine. These hormones cause muscles to tense, heart rate and blood pressure to increase, and breathing to accelerate. The fight-or-flight response originally evolved to prepare animals to respond to danger, and in this sense stress was a very positive factor that helped preserve and protect life.

Many forms of stress are positive. The stress triggered by regular exercise, for example, can be invigorating, as can the mental stress posed by a challenging work or school assignment. The same stress that may frustrate one person may motivate or relax another. We all know people who are tense and miserable on the beach, for example, but who appear to thrive when tackling a project at work. Nevertheless, for many people modern life is fraught with all sorts of frustrations and threats to which the only acceptable response is internalized misery. In the case of women the sources of stress may be boring and low-paying jobs, sexual discrimination or harassment, sexual and domestic abuse, lack of empathy from a partner, the strain of balancing work and family life, or sometimes the boredom and frustration of staying at home with children while partners and neighbors develop stimulating careers. The result often can be prolonged negative stress.

Classic research on the impact of negative *and* positive life events on health has produced a scale of life stressors (see chart). These studies show that positive events (such as getting married or having a baby) as well as negative ones (death of a spouse, divorce, job loss) temporarily increase the chance of becoming physically ill.

Psychologists have tried to develop strict definitions for "stress" and "anxiety" and other behavioral terms in order to allow scientific study of their effect on emotional health and physical well-being. But most of the studies on these risk factors so far have used subtly different definitions; thus, it is hard to compare results. Furthermore, many studies rely on self-ratings, asking subjects questions such as, "Do you feel upset when . . . ?" or "Do you find this stressful?" Yet the way people rate their own emotions is subjective: what one woman calls anxious, another might call normal. This lack of objective measurements makes it hard to compare one subject with the next, much less compare studies.

Finally, the theories relating behavior and emotions to physical health sound just a little too pat. Society always has a tendency to blame the victim when there is no obvious physical explanation for a problem, and the psychosocial-behavioral findings sound judgmental: they imply that people would not have heart disease or other health problems if they were not so obsessed with their work, anxious, easily upset, or (fill in the blank). If people just changed their behavior, they would not be sick. Thus, having a stress-related illness is not the same as being inadvertently exposed to a bacterium or hit by a car. There is always a subtle implication that we are more to blame for our behavioral and attitudinal failings than our physical ones, perhaps because people assume that these basic emotions are more easily controlled.

Even so, the accumulation of evidence implicating stress as a risk factor in physical health cannot be denied. Although recent findings suggest that the role of emotions and behaviors in disease is probably more complex than previously believed, it is hard to dismiss the many studies suggesting that people who experience anxiety, depression, sleep disturbances, emotional drain, or a tendency to express emotional problems as bodily complaints may be more prone to various physical diseases and disorders than the general population.

Stress and heart disease

According to highly popularized reports some years back, people tagged as having the infamous high-stress "Type A" personality—characterized by high levels of competitiveness, ambition, hostility, impatience, abruptness, and obsessiveness—were particularly susceptible to heart disease. Although

newer studies indicate that at least some people with such personality types may thrive (particularly if they are successful), many doctors still feel that chronic troubling emotions, interpersonal conflicts, and depression—as well as plain old stress and anxiety—may indeed be risk factors in heart disease.

Several animal experiments and clinical observations of humans have suggested some plausible physiological mechanisms that help explain why and how emotions and behaviors can affect the heart. For example, even minimal stimuli such as casual conversation can provoke acute elevations in blood pressure. Blood pressure will rise even more—and for a longer time—when emotions such as anger or fear are aroused. Anxiety seems to evoke the greatest increase in women's blood pressure, whereas anger evokes the greatest rise in men's. According to some researchers, such brief elevations, occurring many thousands of times, may damage vulnerable blood vessel walls (see high blood pressure).

Furthermore, mammals under stress show physiological changes that encourage blood clotting (to protect the animal against blood loss from a potential injury) and increase blood flow to vital organs and to muscles necessary for fighting or fleeing. Increased blood clotting and greater demands placed on the heart caused by these changes can set the stage for a heart attack (see circulatory disorders). Other studies show that emotional changes can influence the autonomic nervous system, which in turn regulates the heart's rate and rhythm (see arrhythmia). Sustained stress may lead people to overeat, smoke more, or neglect exercise, and these poor health habits have a negative effect on the heart (see obesity, smoking, and exercise).

Of course, none of this necessarily means that people with Type A personalities should try to transform themselves into calmer, less ambitious Type B's. So far there is no convincing evidence that changing emotional responses can actually prevent heart disease or other serious disorders, and "personality" may be almost impossible to change anyway. And given that Type A behavior often leads to great rewards in our society, trying to change it may provoke even greater anxiety in many people.

A person already at risk for any stress-linked disease may nevertheless want to think about ways she can change her behavior or attitude so as to reduce frustration, stress, and anxiety, especially if doing so will result in a more enjoyable life. More important, anyone experiencing considerable stress would be wise to pay special attention to eliminating other habits or conditions more closely linked to disease—such as smoking or high blood pressure.

Who is likely to develop high levels of stress?

The modern woman is said to be drowning in a sea of stress. In addition to the traditional sources—such as the demands of young children and aging parents—many women today also face considerable stress in the workplace. Since the late 1960s, 300 hours of work—including time spent on paid employment as well as time spent caring for a household—

Social readjustment rating scale

Life event	Life-change units	Life event	Life-change units
Death of one's spouse	100	Trouble with in-laws	29
Divorce	73	Outstanding achievement	28
Marital separation	65	Spouse beginning or stopping work	26
Jail term	63	Beginning or ending school	26
Death of a close family member	63	Change in living conditions	25
Personal injury or illness	53	Revision of personal habits	24
Marriage	50	Trouble with one's boss	23
Being fired	47	Change in work hours or conditions	20
Marital reconciliation	45	Change in residence	20
Retirement	45	Change in schools	20
Health change in a family member	44	Change in recreation	19
Pregnancy	40	Change in church activities	19
Sex difficulties	39	Change in social activities	18
Gain of a new family member	39	Mortgage or major loan	17
Business readjustment	39	Change in sleeping habits	16
Change in one's financial state	38	Change in family get-togethers	15
Death of a close friend	37	Change in eating habits	15
Change to a different line of work	36	Vacation	13
More arguments with one's spouse	35	Christmas	12
Taking out a mortgage	31	Minor violations of the law	11
Foreclosure of a mortgage or loan	30		
Change in responsibilities at work	29		
Son or daughter leaving home	29		

The SRRS, developed by Holmes and Rahe in 1967, assigned "life-change units" to several dozen stressful events and linked the number to risk for medical problems.

have been added to a working woman's annual schedule. "Working moms" are the major breadwinners in many two-parent families, and the only breadwinner in the vast majority of single-parent families. Although both men and women often feel stressed from repetitive, unstimulating work, stress for women is compounded by pay inequity (women's pay is still on average only 71 percent that of men with comparable training and responsibilities), the lack of adequate health insurance and other benefits (especially in parts of the service sector where the majority of women work), a "glass ceiling" and "mommy track" that prevent women from rising to positions of authority as often or as rapidly as men with comparable abilities, and, above all else, the difficulty of balancing work and family responsibilities.

A report by the U.S. Department of Labor has revealed that working women rank stress as their greatest everyday problem. The largest number of complaints came from women in their 40s who had professional and managerial jobs, and from single mothers who said that their biggest problem is balancing family and work, including finding affordable child care.

Interpersonal conflict seems to be particularly stressful to

women, whereas competition and intellectual challenge are more stressful to men. Studies have shown that competitive challenges lead to greater than average elevations in blood pressure—even during sleep—in men with Type A personalities. Such findings suggest that difficult work permanently damages the circulatory system (or, alternatively, that men with Type A personalities or high blood pressure tend to choose high-pressure jobs). But when it comes to women, the pressures of work seem much less likely to affect blood pressure. The only exceptions are women in top management jobs.

What does seem to send women's blood pressure soaring are interpersonal conflicts and strains at home, especially problems with partners and children. These findings make things look particularly bleak for young women in upper management who go home to children and other family responsibilities. Men tend to relax after leaving a high-pressure job, but women with equivalent jobs often get no relief. This unremitting stress of the "second shift" is what ultimately sends many women around the bend, emotionally and, eventually, physically.

During their reproductive years, these young women may

have a built-in buffer against the physical effects of stress because of the protective effects of estrogen—particularly on serum cholesterol levels. In one study, for example, even Type A women had serum cholesterol levels similar to those of less competitive (and less stressed) women and much lower than those of Type A men. Although LDL cholesterol levels (which have been linked to heart attack risk) were higher in women managers, protective HDL levels also remained high in all women, regardless of the nature of their job or their personality type.

How can women alleviate stress?

Some women may handle the stress in their lives better than men because they are better able to identify and deal with it. By venting their frustrations with friends or even allowing themselves a good cry, women may be dispelling some of the most toxic effects of stress. Aware that their lives are stressful, women may purposefully adopt a healthier lifestyle, perhaps choosing foods more carefully, losing weight, cutting out cigarettes, getting enough sleep, or embarking on an exercise plan—which often helps relieve frustration in and of itself.

Women who feel overwhelmed by stress may want to try adopting some of these stress-resistance strategies (see chart). Delineating specific sources of stress, prioritizing demands, and learning to find satisfaction in less frustrating areas of life can work wonders. Establishing a stable daily routine, actively seeking social support, and believing in one's personal ability to solve problems can help some women better manage stress. Taking steps to make home and work environments as safe and comfortable as possible—though not always easy to accomplish—can also work wonders. For extremely compulsive women, stress can be reduced by accepting the necessity, sometimes, of a temporary disruption in one's daily routine, or realizing that one cannot solve all of one's problems at the same time.

Consciously and systematically changing attitudes about life's inevitable burdens can make an immense difference in everyday perception of stress. Little reminders—ubiquitous in the many books and articles on managing stress—that it is not necessary to be perfect or to be a superwoman can instantaneously relieve self-imposed pressure. So can replacing phrases such as "I have to" or "I must" with "I hope I can." Even making a list of stresses and unfulfilled obligations can paradoxically reduce pressure. Taking some time every day to push aside what didn't get done or what went wrong and list what was accomplished and what went right can also be helpful. And even without learning formal meditation techniques, many women find that in just a few minutes a day they can stop stress in its tracks by focusing on the present—pushing thoughts of responsibilities out of one's mind even for a few minutes—or physically walking away from the source of the stress.

Relaxation exercises can also often undo some of the stresses of everyday life. Transcendental meditation and yoga, practiced over many months or years, have been credited with lowering elevated blood pressure and with making people feel less anxious and out of control, as has hypnosis (see alternative therapies). In some situations becoming more assertive can alleviate stress: it may be helpful to speak up about job frustrations, or to investigate a company's grievance procedures. Taking a course in time management or in meditation techniques has given many women relief during periods of unusual stress, as can formal stress-reduction and assertiveness training programs.

Related entries

Alternative therapies, anxiety disorders, cholesterol, depression, domestic abuse, estrogen, exercise, fatigue, headaches, high blood pressure, psychosomatic disorders, sleep disorders, smoking

---

Stress-reducing techniques

Change your environment

Reduce external stress such as noise and pollution
Reduce stimulation at home when possible
Reduce stimulation at work when possible
Reduce threats to your physical safety

Change your behavior

Eat a balanced diet
Get enough sleep
Get adequate exercise
Learn relaxation techniques or meditation
Cut back on alcohol and caffeine consumption
Reduce exposure to situations that involve conflict
Take a time-management course
Undergo hypnosis

Develop a new attitude

Set limits for yourself and others
Become more aware of other options
Become more aware of what you are feeling
Be more willing to express what you are feeling
Become more confident about your own perceptions
Become more aware of the possibility of internal change

Stretchmarks

Pinkish, silvery, or reddish brown streaks that appear on skin that is stretched, usually by weight gain, are called stretchmarks. They most commonly appear on the abdomen and breasts during the later months of pregnancy, but also sometimes on the thighs and buttocks (see illustration). Stretch-

Stretchmarks

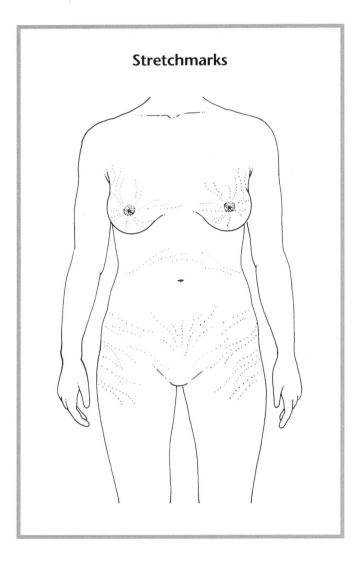

marks (also called striae) are primarily a cosmetic problem, though occasionally they may itch.

Who is likely to develop stretchmarks?

The tendency to develop stretchmarks is determined by a woman's heredity, skin type, and weight gain. But at least half of all pregnant women develop them. Women with Cushing syndrome (see entry) may also develop stretchmarks, particularly on the abdomen. Adolescents who experience a very rapid growth spurt may develop stretchmarks on hips and thighs.

How are stretchmarks treated?

Generally stretchmarks fade to a white, silvery, or fainter color and, since they pose no medical risk, require no treatment. Lipectomy (the surgical removal of fat from under the skin), an operation that some women choose to have after pregnancy or a large weight loss to tighten skin, can minimize stretchmarks. Some of them may be cut away along with the extra overlying skin; and the ones that remain usu-

ally appear less conspicuous once the defatted skin becomes tauter. Lipectomy is a serious surgical procedure, however, whose risks and benefits should be weighed carefully (see lipectomy and liposuction).

How can stretchmarks be prevented?

Stretchmarks that appear during pregnancy or normal adolescent growth cannot be prevented. There is no evidence that taking vitamins, eating a high-protein diet, maintaining erect posture, wearing support undergarments, or rubbing moisturizing creams or lotions on the skin can prevent or even minimize stretchmarks. For healthy women, avoiding rapid weight gain and yo-yo dieting is the only preventive measure that works.

Related entries

Dieting, exercise, lipectomy and liposuction, pregnancy, skin care and cosmetics, skin disorders

Stroke

A stroke is one of several potentially fatal disorders that occur after the blood supply to the brain is disturbed. Overall, women have fewer strokes than men in every age group with the exception of those few cases occurring in people younger than 45. Even so, roughly 42 to 49 percent of all strokes occur in women, and women who have strokes are twice as likely to die of them. This may be because women have a longer life expectancy than men and tend to have strokes at later ages. In addition, certain conditions unique to or more common in females—such as pregnancy and mitral valve prolapse (the ballooning out of the valve linking the upper and lower chambers of the heart; see entry)—may predispose certain women to strokes.

Strokes fall into two basic categories depending on the cause: infarcts and cerebral hemorrhages.

Infarcts. These are similar to heart attacks in that some of the brain's nerve tissue dies when its blood supply is reduced. Like coronary artery disease, infarcts result most often from atherosclerosis, a condition in which arteries are clogged with fatty deposits and scar tissue that eventually enlarge and harden into plaque. In people with atherosclerosis, a blood clot (thrombus) may form in the narrowed channel and block blood flow to the brain, a condition called cerebral thrombosis. In other cases, called cerebral embolism, a piece of plaque or a blood clot dislodges from the heart or a blood vessel and travels to block the flow of blood in an artery supplying the brain.

Cerebral hemorrhage. Strokes in this category occur when an artery leaks blood into or around the brain, eventually resulting in tissue death. In women many strokes occur because an aneurysm (bulge) in an artery in the head ruptures.

Who is likely to have a stroke?

The risk of having a stroke rises with age, with the chances doubling for each decade beyond the age of 35. Atherosclerosis, hypertension, diabetes, and smoking all increase the risk of stroke in both men and women.

Certain inherited or acquired conditions can increase the likelihood of blood clots and therefore strokes. These conditions include cancer, immobilization in bed, and certain blood disorders, as well as the presence of antibodies in the blood that are sometimes found in women with lupus and certain blood abnormalities (a condition known antiphospholipid syndrome that also increases the risk of spontaneous abortion, blood clots, and migraine headaches). In addition, people who have already had temporary deficiencies in the blood supply to the brain (called transient ischemic attacks) owing to a narrowing of the small arteries in the brain circulation or of the larger carotid arteries in the neck are prone to strokes.

Certain forms of heart disease such as a recent heart attack, deformities of the heart valves, or heart rhythm problems (called atrial fibrillation; see illustration) are associated with embolic strokes. In younger women with mitral valve prolapse (which is three times more common in women than in men), the risk of stroke rises fourfold—although because a young woman's chances of having a stroke are so low in the first place, even a fourfold rise means the risk of having a stroke is still quite low. Obesity—particularly abdominal obesity—appears to increase risk of stroke as well. Abnormally high cholesterol levels and migraine headaches have also been linked to strokes, but more studies need to be done before these links are clearly established.

Hemorrhagic strokes are a rare complication of pregnancy, but they remain a leading cause of maternal death (which is also rare). In pregnant women blood often has an increased ability to coagulate, and so blood clots or emboli may develop during the last trimester of pregnancy. The increased cardiac output and blood volume in the second and third trimesters of pregnancy may also lead to the rupture of preexisting aneurysms. Even more rarely eclampsia (see entry) in a pregnant woman may lead to stroke, as may significant blood loss during delivery.

Federal regulators recently asked manufacturers to remove a number of prescription and nonprescription drugs from the market because they contained an ingredient linked to a slight risk of hemorrhagic stroke in young women. This ingredient, phenylpropanolamine, or PPA, was commonly contained in the appetite suppressants Acutrim and Dexatrim, as well as in certain formulations of the cold remedies Alka-Seltzer, Contac, Dimetapp, Robitussin, and Triaminic. New rules were being drafted to effectively ban PPA.

Contrary to earlier belief, there is no convincing evidence that using oral contraceptives increases most women's risk of stroke. Even so, many doctors advise women who smoke,

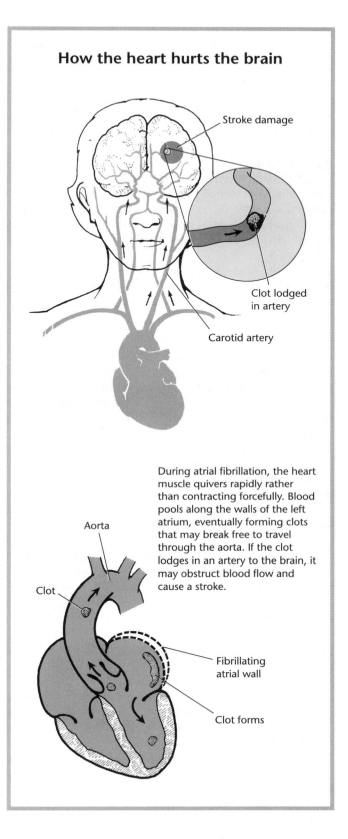

How the heart hurts the brain

Stroke damage

Clot lodged in artery

Carotid artery

Aorta

Clot

During atrial fibrillation, the heart muscle quivers rapidly rather than contracting forcefully. Blood pools along the walls of the left atrium, eventually forming clots that may break free to travel through the aorta. If the clot lodges in an artery to the brain, it may obstruct blood flow and cause a stroke.

Fibrillating atrial wall

Clot forms

abuse substances such as cocaine or amphetamines, or have a history of blood clots to use oral contraceptives cautiously.

What are the symptoms?

Symptoms of a stroke, as well as its long-term effects, depend on how much and which parts of the brain are affected. Common symptoms include a sudden loss of consciousness, dizziness, confusion, or rapid deterioration in vision (including double vision), speech, or sensation. One or more limbs or part of the face (often on one side of the body) may become rapidly weakened or paralyzed. The person may also experience headache, vomiting, or difficulty in swallowing. Symptoms last at least 24 hours but may fluctuate in severity over the first day or two, after which the stroke is said to be "complete."

Symptoms of stroke in pregnant women include severe headaches, nausea, vomiting, lethargy, seizures, or diminished vision.

How is the condition evaluated?

If a stroke is suspected, a doctor will first do a detailed neurological examination and blood tests to distinguish a stroke from infections that can be treated with antibiotics, as well as tumors, multiple sclerosis, hypoglycemia and hyperglycemia (low and high blood sugar, respectively), seizures, sudden confusion caused by drugs, or other metabolic processes.

If it is determined that the woman is having a stroke, treatment will depend on its type and location. Usually a CT scan of the head will be done to see if there has been hemorrhage. If the CT scan does not show blood, the stroke is probably due to an infarct, and tests such as an echocardiogram (which uses reflected sound to create an image of the heart), a portable electrocardiogram (which uses electrodes attached to the body to monitor heart rate and rhythm), ultrasound of the carotid arteries (which supply blood to the brain), and blood cultures may be used to help identify heart disease that might have resulted in an embolism. A lumbar puncture (also called spinal tap)—in which a needle is inserted into the space around the spine so that fluid can be removed for analysis—often helps the physician evaluate the patient's condition.

An MRI scan may be done to look for abnormalities in blood vessels; and in major medical centers, new radiologic tests are available to study the flow of blood in the brain. These include single photon emission computed tomography (SPECT) and positron emission tomography (PET) scans.

If a pregnant woman experiences a stroke, a doctor will first want to see if it was the result of some condition unrelated to pregnancy. She will usually be evaluated with an MRI or CT scan and, if necessary, an angiogram—an x-ray lasting 1 to 3 hours in which injected dye allows a doctor to see blood circulating within the vessels of the brain. To protect the developing fetus from the hazards of radiation, the pelvic area is shielded.

How is stroke treated?

Emergency treatment for a person having a stroke involves calling an ambulance and having the person lie down, with any paralyzed parts protected from movement. No food or drink should be given, and if vomiting occurs, the woman's head should be turned to one side. If she has difficulty breathing, it may help to raise her head and shoulders; if breathing stops completely, cardiopulmonary resuscitation (CPR) should be started. Except in the case of extremely mild strokes involving a day or two of weakness or dizziness, most people who have had a stroke will need to be admitted to the hospital. Often intensive care may be required to maintain basic functions.

Time is of the essence in getting a patient with a suspected stroke to a hospital for evaluation. That is because—in some cases—injecting recombinant tissue plasminogen activator (t-PA) directly into the brain through a catheter can limit and even reverse damage due to infarcts. Called thrombolytic therapy, this approach must be done within 3 hours of the onset of symptoms. An experimental drug called recombinant pro-urokihnase (r-proUK) can be effective up to 6 hours after the onset of symptoms, and so far has been used to treat strokes caused by clots in the middle cerebral artery, the site of as many as a third of all infarct-based strokes. While life-saving in many cases, these "thrombolytic" approaches carry a significant degree of risk (particularly bleeding into the brain) and should be attempted only after consultation with a highly skilled neurologist.

Although no drug can revive dead nerve tissue, certain medications can prevent further damage even if thrombolytic therapy was not or could not be used. For women whose strokes are not due to hemorrhage and who do not have high blood pressure, simply taking one aspirin tablet per day seems to be quite effective in reducing the risk of subsequent strokes. This is probably because aspirin inhibits blood clotting; often a cause of stroke is a blood clot that gets stuck in an artery already partially obstructed by plaque. Studies so far have involved mostly men, however, and there is some evidence that aspirin, at least in higher doses, is more effective in men than in women.

If a woman using aspirin continues to have stroke symptoms or cannot tolerate the side effects, the drug clopidogrel (Plavix) may be used. Like aspirin, Plavix inhibits the blood's ability to clot. In addition, it appears to be just as safe as aspirin. Because Plavix is very expensive, however, most clinicians still recommend aspirin as a first line of therapy.

Sometimes surgery is required to remove blood from brain tissues after a hemorrhagic stroke or to correct an underlying aneurysm.

Pregnant women who have had strokes are usually treated with bed rest, plenty of fluids, and drugs that prevent subsequent convulsions and blood clotting. About a quarter of strokes during pregnancy result in death; survival depends on where the stroke occurs and the degree of damage. If the damaged area is limited, there may be few lasting effects.

Physical, occupational, or speech therapy is often essential after a woman has had a stroke. These programs can help educate patients and their families about stroke and teach prevention of common complications such as limb contractures and bedsores. Physical therapy, including speech therapy, can sometimes help "train" other areas of the brain to take over functions once performed by the dead tissue. To be most effective, rehabilitation therapy should be started as soon as possible after the stroke.

How can strokes be prevented?

Preventing stroke involves eliminating or reducing as many risk factors as possible. Avoiding cigarette smoking and normalizing blood pressure offer the biggest payoff in stroke prevention. In women with a history of certain forms of heart disease, the risk of embolic stroke can be reduced with long-term anticoagulation therapy. This usually involves taking a drug called warfarin (Coumadin). Women with severely narrowed carotid arteries can also reduce their risk of stroke or its recurrence through the surgical removal of plaque. One large study indicates, however, that women are less likely than men to benefit from this surgery. Researchers at the National Institute of Neurological Disorders and Stroke (NINDS) are trying to determine why this is so.

Pregnant women with heart failure or irregular heartbeat (arrhythmia) should be treated with bed rest, digoxin (a heart drug), and diuretics (pills that increase the volume of urine and keep blood pressure down). Drugs that reduce the coagulability of the blood may also be necessary. The anticoagulant with the least risk to the fetus is heparin, which does not cross the placenta.

Related entries

Arrhythmia, cholesterol, circulatory disorders, coronary artery disease, diabetes, eclampsia, headaches, heart disease, high blood pressure, hypoglycemia, lupus, mitral valve prolapse, multiple sclerosis, obesity, smoking, substance abuse

Substance Abuse

Substance abuse involves the use of drugs or other chemicals to the point where physical, psychological, or social functioning is impaired. Although the term is often associated with the use of illegal drugs such as marijuana and cocaine, it can also mean excessive reliance on legal substances such as alcohol or nicotine, prescription medications, and even certain over-the-counter products. Prescription medications such as minor tranquilizers, painkillers, and diet pills are much more commonly abused by women than is either alcohol or street drugs.

Types of substance abuse

The federal government classifies all drugs with the potential for abuse under the Controlled Substances Act. There are five separate categories (schedules) of drugs, grouped by likelihood that the drug will cause dependence and other harmful effects.

Schedule I includes drugs (such as heroin) with the highest risk and which have no accepted medical use (even for research) or accepted level of safe use.

Schedule II drugs also have a high potential for abuse but are sometimes acceptable for use in medical research. These drugs include codeine and morphine (derived from opium), cocaine, marijuana, and phencyclidine (PCP, or angel dust).

Schedule III drugs are legally available by prescription to treat specific medical problems. Examples include diet pills, certain hypnotic-sedative drugs, and medications that combine narcotics with other drugs (Percocet and Percodan, for example).

Schedule IV includes barbiturate sleeping pills such as pentobarbital (Nembutal) and minor tranquilizers, including the benzodiazepines (Xanax, Valium, Klonopin).

Schedule V, the group of drugs with the lowest potential for abuse, includes certain drugs containing small amounts of codeine used to treat coughs or pain (such as Tylenol with codeine) or containing small amounts of paregoric to treat diarrhea (such as Parepectolin).

Abuse of illegal drugs

The National Comorbidity Survey found that 6.6 percent of all women—in contrast to 8 percent of all men—had been diagnosed as having problems with substance abuse or dependence in the past year. These numbers are clearly underestimates, since most substance abusers do not receive professional treatment. The highest prevalence of use was reported in women of childbearing age, 8 percent of whom had used illegal drugs, marijuana being the most common. An estimated 3 to 17 percent of pregnant women use cocaine.

Higher than average levels of use are reported among women who live in the inner city or who have criminal records, as well as among lesbians and women in the military. It should be pointed out, however, that these are women who (unlike middle-class homemakers) are at greatest risk of being "caught" abusing drugs. In some inner cities more women than men use crack, a highly purified and fast-acting form of cocaine. Women with college degrees are more likely to use cocaine than are those with only a high school degree. The illegal drugs most commonly abused by women are cocaine and other stimulants, heroin, and marijuana. In addition, abuse of anabolic-androgenic steroids to enhance athletic performance and improve physical appearance—while still most common among male adolescents—is growing rapidly among young women. In women side effects include growth of facial hair, male-pattern baldness, menstrual cycle changes, clitoral enlargement, and deepened voice. In addition, women who abuse steroids are at risk for developing liver tumors and cancer, jaundice, fluid retention, high blood pressure, adverse changes in cholesterol levels, kidney tumors, severe acne, and trembling. In addition, using non-sterile techniques to inject these or other drugs puts abusers at risk for viral infections such as HIV or hepatitis B or C, as well as bacterial infections such as endocarditis or skin abscesses.

The risk of acquiring a sexually transmitted disease, including acquired immune deficiency syndrome (AIDS), is increased in women who abuse illegal substances. Intravenous (IV) drug abuse has been involved in 80 percent of the AIDS cases that have occurred in women. Although occasionally women acquire AIDS through direct infection by a contaminated needle, most of the cases occur because women under the influence of drugs or alcohol tend to engage in risky sexual behaviors—including sex with a male IV drug user infected with the AIDS virus. Some investigators have linked the recent rise in the incidence of syphilis to the use of cocaine and other drugs.

Abuse of opiates, cocaine, and some other illegal substances can produce various forms of sexual dysfunction. Contrary to the common perception that certain drugs such as cocaine, heroin, or amphetamines (uppers or pep pills) enhance sexual functioning, chronic use of these drugs can inhibit orgasm and decrease sexual desire (libido). Dependence on heroin can also suppress ovulation (the monthly release of an egg from an ovary). Although menstrual periods often return to normal after a few months of maintenance treatment with methadone (a substitute narcotic used to treat heroin addiction), methadone itself depresses sexual interest and response. Some tests indicate that marijuana use may also cause irregular menstrual cycles and a temporary loss of fertility.

Using cocaine while pregnant increases the risk of certain complications of pregnancy, including placenta previa (a condition in which the placenta covers the cervix and is prone to bleeding), placenta abruptio (a condition in which the placenta abruptly separates from the endometrium), intrauterine growth retardation, premature labor, and stillbirth. There is evidence linking cocaine use during pregnancy to numerous birth defects, including neural tube defects and malformations of the genitourinary, gastrointestinal, and cardiovascular systems of the fetus. The effect of cocaine on the neuropsychological development of children is less clear because studies so far have not ruled out nutritional, social, or other factors that might explain these developments.

One dangerous myth about cocaine use during late pregnancy has led some young women to use this drug in the hope that it will shorten their labor and make it less painful. This false belief stems from cocaine's stimulant and vasoconstrictive properties. Rather than facilitating labor, these properties have been linked to sudden death in pregnant women and to premature rupture of membranes, premature labor, and fetal distress (see chart).

Another illegal drug increasingly popular among young women in particular is MDMA, also known as Ecstasy. Widely used among young adults and college students, particularly at all-night dance parties (raves), this drug is becoming increasingly popular among older groups as well. MDMA is usually taken as a tablet or capsule but is also sometimes snorted and occasionally smoked in powder form. MDMA has both stimulant and psychedelic (hallucinogenic) properties. Popular mythology has it that MDMA is much safer than its chemical cousins MDA and methamphetamine ("ice"), both of which are known to cause brain damage, and extols its ability to heighten the sense of closeness, trust, and intimacy between people. MDMA also is believed to increase the sense of pleasure and self-confidence, and it can boost alertness to the point where users can dance or party for extended periods of time. Psychedelic effects, which can include feelings of peacefulness, acceptance, and empathy, are also re-

Known effects of substance abuse during pregnancy

Type of drug	Growth retardation	Behavior changes	Birth defects	Increased fetal or newborn death	Withdrawal in newborn	Premature birth
Opiates	Yes	Yes	No	Yes	Yes	No
Alcohol	Yes	Yes	Yes	Yes	Yes	Yes
Nicotine	Yes	Yes	No	Yes	No	Yes
Cocaine	Yes	Yes	Yes	Yes	Yes	Yes
Barbiturates	No	Yes	No	No	Yes	No
Stimulants	No	Yes	No	No	No	Yes
Hallucinogens	No	Yes	No	No	No	No
Marijuana	No	Yes	No	No	No	No
Minor tranquilizers	No	No	No	No	Yes	No
Major tranquilizers	No	No	Yes	No	No	No

putedly milder than those associated with other hallucinogens such as LSD (see below) or mescaline.

The reality, however, is that using MDMA can be just as dangerous as using cocaine or amphetamines. Besides increasing heart rate and blood pressure (particularly dangerous in people with circulatory or heart disease), the stimulant properties of MDMA can lead to dehydration, hypertension, and heart or kidney failure—especially under the hot, crowded conditions that frequently characterize raves. Nausea, faintness, blurred vision, teeth clenching, muscle tension, rapid eye movement, and chills or sweating are other common reactions. In high doses, body temperature can increase to the point of potentially fatal muscle breakdown and kidney, heart, and lung failure (malignant hyperthermia). Heart attacks, strokes, and seizures may also occur. Heavy use of MDMA may result in long-term and possibly permanent brain damage, including damage to both the visual and verbal memory. Heavy users may experience serious psychological problems such as confusion, depression, drug cravings, anxiety, and paranoia, sometimes for weeks after taking the drug.

Abuse of prescription drugs

A major substance abuse problem for women involves prescription mood altering drugs, particularly sedatives and minor tranquilizers. Mood altering drugs are prescribed at an earlier age in women than in men, and prescribed more frequently. This is partly because women are more likely to suffer from depression and anxiety than are men, because they may be more likely to seek help for psychological and emotional problems, and because some physicians tend to resort to medications for personal problems that might be better treated with psychotherapy or other forms of social support. Among women alcoholics, 30 to 70 percent are also dependent on other drugs, including sedatives and minor tranquilizers.

Women are also at risk for dependency on analgesics (painkillers). Analgesics fall into two categories—narcotic and nonnarcotic. The nonnarcotics are not addictive and include drugs such as aspirin and acetaminophen (Tylenol). The narcotic drugs, which include opium derivatives such as codeine and morphine, are addictive and therefore have a much higher risk of abuse, especially among those who suffer from chronic pain syndrome—a problem more common in women than in men (see psychosomatic disorders).

The pervasive concern with weight among women in our culture sometimes leads them to take diet pills (amphetamines) without regard for their huge potential for addiction—and extremely limited potential for long-term weight loss. Women also commonly take these drugs for chronic fatigue and other sleep disorders. Although low doses can suppress the appetite and increase alertness, tolerance to the drug develops within weeks. As larger doses are taken to produce the same effects, women may become irritable, anxious, or overconfident, and various physical symptoms may occur, including blurred vision, dizziness, and insomnia. Chronic use of amphetamines can permanently damage the heart and blood vessels and result in a number of health problems, including various psychiatric symptoms, malnutrition, and an increased susceptibility to infection.

Prescription drug abuse is a particular problem for elderly women because aging makes people more sensitive to drugs. A dosage that poses no problem in younger women becomes "overmedication" in older ones and leads to significant side effects. Even more pervasive in older women is the problem of multiple drug use, which occurs when people take several medicines at once. Tranquilizers and sedatives, frequently used by older people, can be especially dangerous if mixed with other drugs that depress the central nervous system. (A high rate of hip fractures in older women, for example, has been linked with overuse of minor tranquilizers, which can cause falls.) The problem of multiple drug use is compounded by the fact that many older women who see more than one physician hesitate to ask questions about possible drug interactions for fear of seeming to question the doctor's authority.

Virtually any drug taken during pregnancy (or breastfeeding) has the potential for some effect on the growing fetus (or infant). This does not mean that pregnant or nursing women should not take the medications they need to care for their own health; often the benefits will be found to outweigh the risks. But it does mean that any woman who is pregnant should consult her clinician before taking any drug—even seemingly harmless over-the-counter medications.

Who is likely to abuse drugs and other substances?

Women with family members who abuse substances, women who started using drugs or alcohol early in life, and those who have been prescribed a mood altering drug (such as a tranquilizer, antidepressant, or sedative) are at risk for developing a substance abuse problem. Other risk factors include living in a high crime/high drug abuse environment, nicotine dependence, eating disorders, and a history of sexual assault, incest, or physical molestation during childhood. Younger women who abuse drugs are also more likely than other women to be victims of domestic abuse and sexual assault.

Women who abuse substances have a high rate of psychiatric illness such as depression and of attempted suicide, although no one knows if these are causes or effects of the substance abuse. Female substance abusers are also more likely than other women to have family and marital problems, whereas for men, substance abuse more commonly leads to high rates of legal and job-related problems. Women substance abusers frequently end up divorced after seeking treatment.

What are the symptoms?

People who are dependent on drugs develop a tolerance to them, that is, they require larger and larger doses to create the same effect. They also become addicted, which means that they experience physical or psychological symptoms of

Symptoms of drug abuse and withdrawal

Type of drug	Common symptoms of overuse or abuse	Common symptoms of withdrawal
Minor tranquilizers (such as Valium, Librium, Xanax)	Drowsiness Incoordination Confusion Rashes Constipation Menstrual changes Reduced sex drive	Nausea Headache Jitteriness Insomnia
Amphetamines (pep pills, diet pills, stimulants)	Overconfidence Excitability Irritability Anxiety Sweating Insomnia Blurred vision Dizziness Diarrhea	Suicidal depression Lethargy Fatigue Anxiety Nightmares
Barbiturates (sleeping pills, including Amytal, Butisol, Nembutal, Seconal)	Grogginess Headache Impaired motor function	Seizures Anxiety Weakness Insomnia Sweating
Alcohol	Lack of coordination Stupor Coma Impaired judgment Memory loss Blackouts Release of inhibitions	Headache Nausea, vomiting Anxiety Malaise Tremors Panic attacks Confusion Delirium tremens Hallucinations Seizures

(continued)

withdrawal when they stop or reduce their intake of the substance.

In addition to the symptoms of tolerance and withdrawal, other behavioral indications that a person may have a problem with substance abuse include being unable to reduce usage, feeling guilty about the habit, or denying that there is a problem even when the effects on work or interpersonal relationships are obvious. Defensiveness when a friend expresses concern about drug use, using the drug in order to deal with interpersonal or work problems, changing doctors to get a prescription for the drug, mixing drugs and alcohol, or needing the drug to get going in the morning or to get to sleep each night are other signs of dependence.

Common physical symptoms of substance abuse—which vary according to the substance (see chart)—include anxiety, heart palpitations, depression, insomnia, fatigue, sexual dysfunction, abdominal pain, unexplained weight loss, bloodshot eyes, sweating, skin flushing, and, in women, a variety of menstrual complaints. Substance abuse can also underlie mood swings, loss of appetite, apathy, or a distant de-

Symptoms of drug abuse and withdrawal

Type of drug	Common symptoms of overuse or abuse	Common symptoms of withdrawal
Marijuana, hashish	Increased pulse Relaxation Mild euphoria Diarrhea Chest pains Panic attacks Slowed reaction time Apathy Impaired judgment Disorientation Delirium Hunger Dry mouth, throat Feeling of unreality Confusion Paranoia	Tremors Sweating Nausea, vomiting Diarrhea Irritability Sleep disturbances Decreased appetite Tremor Chills
Cocaine, crack	Sense of euphoria Increased alertness Dilated pupils Rapid heart rate Rapid breathing Temperature increase Paranoid hallucinations Confusion Slurred speech Anxiety Agitation Chest pain Seizures	Depression Confusion Irritability Seizures
Hallucinogens (such as LSD, mescaline)	Altered perceptions Increased heart rate Hypertension Impaired memory Shortened attention span Impaired thinking Excitability Incoordination Analgesia Insomnia Lack of appetite	None

(continued)

Symptoms of drug abuse and withdrawal

Type of drug	Common symptoms of overuse or abuse	Common symptoms of withdrawal
Phencyclidine (PCP)	Hallucinations Euphoria or mood swings Lack of coordination Slurred speech Jerky eye movements Feeling of weightlessness Sweating Muscle rigidity Disorganized thinking Drowsiness Stupor Coma Apathy Violent behavior Paranoia Breathing difficulties Convulsions	Lethargy Craving Depression
Narcotics (addictive analgesics or painkillers such as opiates—morphine, methadone, heroin)	Confusion Drowsiness Sedation Dizziness General weakness Sweating Lack of coordination Euphoria Decreased sex drive Coma Seizures Slowed breathing	Diarrhea Tremor Nervousness Drop in blood pressure Muscle pain Insomnia Nightmares Nausea Yawning Dilated pupils
Inhalants (such as amyl nitrite, room deodorizers, Freon, benzene, nitrous oxide, glue)	Headaches Dizziness Increased heart rate Nasal irritation Cough Muscle weakness Vomiting Abdominal pain Confusion Paralysis of nerves Itching	None reported
Laxatives	Chronic constipation	Constipation

meanor. Some people who abuse substances have no obvious symptoms.

How is the condition treated?

Treating substance abuse is usually a long-term process that involves changing deeply rooted habits and confronting complex emotional or social problems. Because abuse is a disease that occurs in people with a biological predisposition, the afflicted person usually must learn how to avoid the abused substance for the rest of her life. Programs offered by rehabilitation centers, residential treatment facilities, and outpatient clinics can help facilitate the process of detoxification—the systematic and gradual withdrawal of the drug—and also provide support and education about drug use. The ideal program is tailored to a woman's individual circumstances and includes psychotherapy to address any issues of self-esteem, sexual abuse, and interpersonal relationships that may underlie the substance abuse problem. Many women also find that self-help fellowships such as Cocaine Anonymous, Narcotics Anonymous, or Nar-Anon (for families of substance abusers) are helpful in providing long-term support and preventing relapses.

All of these resources are greatly underused by women, especially pregnant women. Part of the problem stems from the failure of many clinicians to recognize substance abuse in women; symptoms are attributed instead to depression or anxiety. Also playing a role is a lack of child care in many treatment facilities. A few programs are starting to admit both mothers and children, but they are still few and far between. Cost and lack of adequate insurance coverage can also make many facilities inaccessible to women, particularly those who are single, unemployed, or employed in low-wage jobs.

Another problem that keeps women from seeking help is the fear of losing custody of their children, especially if they have to involve a public agency in their care. Infants have been removed from mothers who had a single positive drug test, even before any effort was made to diagnose or treat the problem. Owing to misplaced concern about the effects of illegal drugs on a fetus, women have been arrested and jailed for "delivering controlled substances to a minor." Instead of preventing substance abuse (which cannot be accomplished simply through an act of will), these efforts have kept other women—many of whom are already suspicious of the medical care system—from seeking the prenatal and postnatal care that could help both themselves and their children. Efforts are now being made in a few states to promote treatment of chemical dependency in lieu of this counterproductive prosecution.

Related entries

Acquired immune deficiency syndrome, alcohol, antianxiety drugs, antidepressants, anxiety disorders, breastfeeding, depression, diuretics, domestic abuse, fatigue, insomnia, laxatives, menstrual cycle disorders, personality disorders, pregnancy, psychosomatic disorders, psychotherapy, sexual abuse and incest, sexual assault, sexual dysfunction, sexually transmitted diseases, smoking, syphilis, vaginal bleeding during pregnancy

Syphilis

For several decades it looked as though syphilis—a potentially life-threatening sexually transmitted disease—was no longer the scourge of humanity it had been for centuries. With the advent of penicillin, it became possible to cure syphilis in the early stages, which not only reduced the number of debilitating complications but also helped prevent the disease from spreading. Syphilis, however, seems to be on the rise once again, with 40,000 to 50,000 cases reported annually—the highest incidence rate in this country since 1949. Much of the increase is attributable to rising rates of infection among women and heterosexual men. Syphilis is also common among people infected with HIV, the virus that causes acquired immune deficiency syndrome (AIDS).

Untreated, syphilis can eventually lead to paralysis, lack of coordination, dementia, and death. Caused by the *Treponema pallidum*, a spiral-shaped bacterium known as a spirochete, the disease is generally transmitted through sexual contact, although occasionally it can be acquired through a blood transfusion or skin contact.

An infected mother can pass syphilis on to a developing fetus through the placenta after about 16 weeks of pregnancy, resulting in congenital syphilis, a condition associated with serious deformities or stillbirth. The more recently the pregnant woman has acquired the disease, the more likely she is to pass it to a developing fetus, and the more serious the congenital syphilis is likely to be. As the number of cases of syphilis among women of childbearing years and among heterosexual men has increased, so has the number of cases of congenital syphilis. Today this condition afflicts 1 in every 10,000 infants born in this country.

Who is likely to develop syphilis?

People most at risk for developing syphilis are also those at risk for acquiring other sexually transmitted diseases (STDs)—that is, young, poor city dwellers. At highest risk are those whose sexual partners have symptoms of the disease. The chances of being infected after a single sexual encounter with an infected person are 30 percent. Although a person remains infectious for about 4 years after acquiring the disease, chances of infection are particularly high during the initial stages of the disease when there are open sores or rashes. Because the spirochete thrives in the warm, moist mucous membranes of the human body—such as the genitals, urethra, anus, eyes, or mouth—it is possible to be infected from deep kissing, although this mode of transmission is probably rare. Occasionally a person develops syphilis after receiving a contaminated blood transfusion or after touching the mucous membranes of an infected person with broken skin. People infected with HIV seem to be particularly likely to be infected with syphilis.

What are the symptoms?

Syphilis is a disease of stages, the last of which can take many years to develop. In the first, or primary, stage an open sore, pimple, or blister (chancre) emerges at the site of infection—usually in the cervix, vagina, rectum, or other genital area. This usually painless sore generally appears between 10 and 90 days after exposure. In most cases there is only a single chancre, although occasionally multiple chancres develop and may be mistaken for herpes simplex infection. Women are much more likely than men to overlook the chancre, since painless sores within the labia or on the vaginal walls or cervix are less obvious than those on the penis or scrotum. Sometimes surrounding lymph nodes may become enlarged, although this seems to be more common in men. The chancre and swelling disappear on their own within about 5 weeks, even without treatment.

The secondary phase of infection develops after the spirochete has had a chance to spread through the bloodstream—generally about 2 to 8 weeks after the chancre appears, and sometimes while the chancre is still present. Many symptoms of secondary syphilis are easily mistaken for the flu: malaise, fever, sore throat, joint pain, and headache. Occasionally there may be some hair loss from the scalp, but the most characteristic symptom is a rash on the palms of the hands and the soles of the feet, as well as various other parts of the body. Depending on where the spirochete takes hold, secondary syphilis can also result in meningitis (an inflammation of the lining of the brain) or uveitis (an eye inflammation characterized by pain and redness).

The symptoms of secondary syphilis clear up spontaneously within 2 to 10 weeks, at which point a latent stage begins. During this stage, which can last for a decade or more, the person will test positive for syphilis if a blood test is done but has no outward symptoms of disease. Within the first 4 years of the latent stage, some people have relapses in which a chancre or rash recurs. And throughout the latent stage the spirochete continues to spread in the body, doing insidious damage to the heart, brain, spinal cord, blood vessels, and bones.

The final (or tertiary) stage of syphilis occurs when manifestations of this damage begin to appear—including cardiovascular disorders (such as coronary artery disease, aortic aneurysms, and aortic insufficiency), blindness, nervous system disorders (neurosyphilis), and death. Tertiary syphilis is rare today because most cases are treated long before they have a chance to develop. Recently, however, there has been an increase in the number of cases of neurosyphilis—including dementia, lack of coordination and vibration sensation (tabes dorsalis), and syphilitic meningitis, which can lead to stroke.

How is the condition evaluated?

Anyone with a sore in the genital area should be evaluated for syphilis, as should anyone at risk for syphilis who has suspicious symptoms. Because sores on the genitals are associated with an increased risk of HIV infection, the possibility of AIDS testing should be discussed with a clinician. And because syphilis so frequently coexists with other STDs, syphilis screening makes sense in a woman with any sexually transmitted infection.

Women with multiple sexual partners should be screened at health examinations. Syphilis screening is already routine in people who want to obtain a marriage license in certain states, join the armed forces, or give blood. To prevent congenital syphilis, pregnant women—whatever their sexual history—are screened for syphilis early in the first trimester of pregnancy. This allows the disease to be treated before the spirochete can cross the placenta and infect the fetus—which is usually impossible until the 16th week of pregnancy. Women at high risk for syphilis may be retested later in the pregnancy, since damage to the fetus—while not reversible—can be halted with prompt treatment.

If there are genital sores or swelling, these need to be distinguished from those of herpes, lymphogranuloma venereum (see chlamydia), and genital warts. This can sometimes be accomplished by removing some pus from the chancre and examining it under a microscope for the presence of spirochetes. A careful examination and consideration of other symptoms can also help distinguish syphilis from other conditions. Further testing may be done to determine if a rash is due to some other problem—such as a drug allergy, viral illness, or skin condition—rather than syphilis.

Once the spirochete has entered the bloodstream, various blood tests can be used to screen for syphilis. Usually the first test done is a nonspecific screening test—that is, it detects a group of antibodies that can arise when a person has syphilis but also can arise in a number of other diseases, including lupus and tuberculosis. The most commonly used screening tests are the VDRL (named for the Venereal Disease Research Laboratory of the U.S. Public Health Service, where the test was developed), an RPR (for rapid plasma reagin), or an ART (for automated reagin test). If any of these tests comes out positive, more expensive and time-consuming—but also more specific—tests can be done to confirm the diagnosis.

How is syphilis treated?

Syphilis is usually treated with an injection of penicillin, ideally a type (such as benzathine penicillin) that takes a long time to break down in the body. Women who are allergic to penicillin and who are not pregnant can use other antibiotics such as doxycycline, tetracycline, or erythromycin.

Pregnant women should be treated with penicillin before the 16th week of pregnancy if possible. If treatment begins later than this, the spirochete may already have passed to the fetus. It still makes sense to be treated as soon as possible, however, to minimize the amount of damage to the fetus. If a pregnant woman has a history of penicillin allergy, her clinician may suggest skin testing to pinpoint whether she is truly allergic to the drug. If she is, hospitalization and special care may be necessary. Doxycycline and tetracycline are not prescribed because they can cause birth defects, and erythromycin is not prescribed because it cannot eradicate infection in the fetus.

After primary or secondary syphilis has been treated with antibiotics, a follow-up blood test should be done every 3 months for at least 2 years. This helps ensure that the spirochete has been eradicated. A person with latent syphilis needs to have a follow-up test every 6 months, while pregnant women should have the test repeated each month throughout the pregnancy.

Finally, no treatment for syphilis can be effective unless all sexual partners of the infected person are evaluated for the disease and, if necessary, treated. Even if their tests come out negative, anyone who has been exposed within 90 days of the diagnosis of either primary or secondary syphilis should be treated with antibiotics anyway. Over 90 days, only those who are diagnosed as being infected require treatment, since the blood test should come out positive if infection has indeed occurred.

How can syphilis be prevented?

With the entire genome of the *Treponema pallidum* finally sequenced in the late 1990s, efforts to develop a vaccine for syphilis have become considerably more promising. For the time being, however, the key to preventing the spread of syphilis is still the same as for all other STDs: receive prompt diagnosis and treatment and inform all sexual partners of the disease so that they too can be diagnosed and treated. Practicing safer sex—such as using condoms and limiting the number of sexual partners—can minimize the chances of acquiring syphilis in the first place. Relying on a condom alone, however, is not enough to avoid syphilis, since infection can result from contact with any uncovered chancre or mucous membrane.

Related entries

Acquired immune deficiency syndrome, antibiotics, chlamydia, condoms, coronary artery disease, genital warts, hair loss, headaches, herpes, lupus, safer sex, sexually transmitted diseases

Temporal Arteritis

Temporal arteritis is a vascular disorder involving inflammation of the large blood vessels throughout the body. Although the cause is unknown, some researchers think it may be due to an autoimmune reaction which somehow damages arteries. As a result blood supply is blocked to certain parts of

the body, particularly the head and neck. Without prompt diagnosis and treatment, temporal arteritis can lead to irreversible blindness in one or both eyes.

A rare form of immune arteritis, which can occur with temporal arteritis, is Takayasu's arteritis, also known as pulseless disease. This often fatal condition tends to involve the arteries of the heart, lungs, and abdomen rather than those in the head and neck. Takayasu's arteritis can result in hypertension and stroke, and only a quarter of those afflicted live more than 2 years after the onset of symptoms. The cause of this condition remains little understood.

About half of patients with temporal arteritis have polymyalgia rheumatica (see entry), a connective tissue disorder in which neck, shoulder, and sometimes lower back, hip, and thigh muscles become stiff and painful.

Who is likely to develop temporal arteritis?

Temporal arteritis (also called giant cell arteritis, cranial arteritis, or granulomatous arteritis) occurs more frequently in women than in men, with 65 being the average age of onset. It rarely occurs under the age of 50, and is rare in African Americans at any age. Takayasu's arteritis, which affects women 8.5 times more often than men, is particularly common in women of Asian or African descent, usually occurring between the ages of 15 and 30.

What are the symptoms?

The most common symptom of temporal arteritis is a severe headache, often but not always in the temples. The pain sometimes intensifies after exposure to cold or when hair is brushed or the head rests on a pillow. Other symptoms may include a tender scalp, blurred vision, and jaw pain while chewing or swallowing. Some people also lose weight or develop a fever, anemia, malaise, or abnormal liver function. If temporal arteritis is not promptly treated, it can lead to irreversible blindness.

Common symptoms of Takayasu's arteritis are fever, joint and muscle aches, loss of appetite, visual disturbances, and general malaise.

How is the condition evaluated?

A physician may suspect temporal arteritis in any patient over 50 who has a headache as well as several other symptoms associated with the disorder. A blood test will be done to measure the erythrocyte sedimentation rate (ESR), which is almost always elevated in both temporal arteritis and polymyalgia rheumatica, as well as in Takayasu's arteritis. The ESR measures the rate at which red blood cells settle to the bottom of a container.

If the ESR is elevated and if other signs suggest temporal arteritis, a biopsy of a temporal artery will also be done as soon as possible (preferably within a few days of the initial examination) to look for cell changes associated with temporal arteritis. This is a relatively safe and simple procedure that can be done by a surgeon in an outpatient facility. After the scalp hair is shaved, a local anesthetic is used to anesthetize the skin, and then a piece of artery about 5 to 10 mm long is removed for laboratory study. The entire procedure takes about half an hour, although sometimes it may need to be repeated several times before the diagnosis can be confirmed.

If Takayasu's arteritis is suspected, the clinician will use an imaging procedure such as magnetic resonance imaging (MRI) or magnetic resonance angiography (MGA) to delineate the extent and anatomic location of obstructions.

How is temporal arteritis treated?

Temporal arteritis is initially treated with high doses of a corticosteroid (an antiinflammatory drug derived from adrenal hormones), usually prednisone. This drug can be taken in tablet form. After 4 to 6 weeks the physician (usually in consultation with an ophthalmologist) will begin to reduce the dosage gradually for as long as the ESR continues to fall. After about 2 years medication can be discontinued completely, and symptoms can be relieved by taking aspirin and other nonsteroidal antiinflammatory agents (NSAIDs).

Steroid treatment should never be stopped abruptly, however, because acute adrenal gland failure can occur. This can lead to severe vomiting, diarrhea, dehydration, loss of consciousness, and (rarely) death.

In the early stages, symptoms of Takayasu's arteritis can also be relieved with corticosteroids. Occasionally methotrexate, an immunosuppressive drug, is used to treat this disorder. There is no actual cure for the disease.

Related entries

Antiinflammatory drugs, autoimmune disorders, blood tests, circulatory disorders, polymyalgia rheumatica, stroke

Temporomandibular Joint Syndrome

TMJ is a common disorder of the joint that connects either side of the jawbone to the skull (see illustration). In this condition the disk of cartilage that cushions the temporomandibular joint slips out of position, resulting in a malfunctioning or dislocated jaw.

Who is likely to develop TMJ?

Between 70 and 90 percent of people experiencing symptoms of TMJ are women. The syndrome develops in 1 of 5 people with rheumatoid arthritis and is also common in people who have suffered from whiplash, trauma to the face, or emotional stress that leads them to grind their teeth or clench their jaw, particularly during sleep (see sleep disorders). In rarer cases, symptoms can appear in people who have a "bad bite" (malocclusion of the teeth) or a tumor in a nearby area of the skull. People with osteoarthritis may experience some of the symptoms of TMJ (such as clicking or snapping jaw sounds) but tend not to have any associated pain.

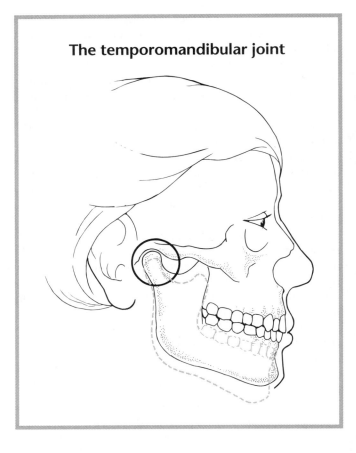

The temporomandibular joint

What are the symptoms?

Symptoms of TMJ include sinus or jaw pain and tenderness, limited jaw movement, dull and diffuse earache, ringing in the ears, dizziness, headaches, and a clicking or popping sound while chewing (a common occurrence which alone is not a sign of TMJ). Pain may also involve the eyes, teeth, head, neck, shoulders, and back and often worsens during or after eating or yawning.

How is the condition evaluated?

TMJ is often confused with conditions that have similar symptoms, including rheumatoid arthritis, tinnitus (ringing in the ears), neuralgia (nerve pain), migraine headache, sinus headache, earache, and chronic ear pain. To differentiate these conditions, as well as pinpoint a specific cause of the problem, a dentist or doctor will usually examine the patient's bite and the wear on the teeth (from grinding teeth during sleep), and consider associated symptoms. Often an x-ray or magnetic resonance imaging (MRI) of the skull will be done to see if there are any structural defects in the temporomandibular joint.

How is TMJ treated?

The vast majority of people with TMJ improve with mild pain medication (such as aspirin or acetaminophen) and other nonsurgical treatments. Muscle relaxants, tranquilizers, or a topical spray of ethyl chloride may relieve or mask muscle pain, as can applying moist heat to the affected area. When TMJ is due to inflammation of the temporomandibular joint, aspirin or nonsteroidal antiinflammatory drugs are often effective, as well as injections of corticosteroids into the joint (see antiinflammatory drugs).

To prevent nighttime grinding and clenching of teeth, some dentists or oral surgeons will prescribe a plastic mouth guard to separate the jaws during sleep. People with TMJ should avoid chewing hard or sticky foods or ice. If emotional stress is playing a role, as it often is, physical or behavioral therapy is very helpful, as well as alternative techniques such as biofeedback and relaxation therapy.

Abnormalities in tooth alignment that cause symptoms of TMJ can sometimes be corrected with a plastic bite plate (splint) worn over the teeth. Some abnormalities can also be corrected by smoothing the biting surfaces or replacing missing teeth, fillings, and crowns. If symptoms persist, more expensive and invasive surgery or orthodontics may be necessary to reposition the jaw. Adhesions in the temporomandibular joint that may be interfering with movement can also be removed through a tiny incision with the aid of a viewing instrument called an arthroscope (see knee pain).

Related entries

Alternative therapies, antiinflammatory drugs, dentures/bridges/implants, headaches, knee pain, orthodontia, osteoarthritis, psychotherapy, rheumatoid arthritis, sleep disorders, stress

Tendinitis and Tenosynovitis

Tendons are the cordlike tissues connecting muscles to bones. Tendinitis is a general term to describe inflammation in a tendon. With repeated or excessive use of a muscle, the tendon that connects it to the bone sustains tiny tears. The inflammation results from the body's normal mechanisms to heal these microinjuries. Tenosynovitis is an inflammation of the protective sheath or membrane surrounding each tendon (the synovium).

Tennis elbow, a form of tendinitis usually having nothing to do with playing tennis, typically produces pain in the back of the elbow, near the site of the sensitive area sometimes called the funnybone. Extending the wrist back, as occurs during a backhand stroke in tennis, aggravates the pain. This condition (also called lateral epicondylitis) probably stems from small tears in the tendons that attach the lower arm muscles to the elbow, and it is particularly common in women.

A form of tenosynovitis that occurs 9 times more often in women than in men is deQuervain's tenosynovitis. In this condition tendons in the thumb become inflamed and the

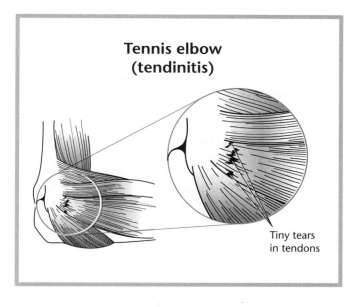

Tennis elbow (tendinitis)

Tiny tears in tendons

sheaths surrounding them narrow. People with deQuervain's cannot flex their thumb fully or else require external force to straighten it once it is flexed.

Who is likely to develop tendinitis or tenosynovitis?

Tennis elbow most often results after activities or exercises that involve repetitive rotating motion of the forearm. These can include various sports such as tennis, bowling, or badminton; painting; or using tools such as a screwdriver or wrench.

DeQuervain's tenosynovitis occurs most frequently after activities involving repeated forceful extensions, pinches, or twists of the thumb—such as prolonged use of a screwdriver, typing, or lifting a baby or child by the armpits.

What are the symptoms?

The characteristic symptom of tennis elbow is recurrent pain in the outer, upper part of the forearm which may radiate down to the wrist. Usually moving the elbow or wrist worsens the pain. Symptoms generally develop gradually.

People with deQuervain's have pain in the affected thumb which usually worsens during movement. Attempts to straighten the thumb may have no effect for a few moments and then the thumb will suddenly jerk or snap into position.

How are these conditions evaluated?

Tennis elbow can usually be diagnosed during a physical examination in which the doctor checks the elbow and forearm for tenderness and asks the patient to extend and flex the wrist to see if there is any pain. If symptoms continue after treatment, x-rays may be taken to rule out more serious conditions.

To diagnose deQuervain's tenosynovitis, a physician will check the thumb for tenderness and then ask the patient to fold the thumb into the palm, curl the fingers around the thumb, and bend the wrist inward. People with deQuervain's will find this motion painful because it pulls on the already inflamed tendons.

How are tendinitis and tenosynovitis treated?

The initial treatment for tennis elbow involves modifying activities that may be causing symptoms and taking antiinflammatory drugs such as aspirin to relieve pain and swelling. Often symptoms will resolve after about 6 months to a year. In the meantime, ice packs, massage, and protective straps or braces can help. Injecting corticosteroids (antiinflammatory agents derived from adrenal hormones) can sometimes reduce pain as well, but the effects are often only temporary. Surgery is rarely necessary.

The best treatment for any form of tendinitis or tenosynovitis is to modify the activities that produce the symptoms. Sometimes antiinflammatory drugs such as aspirin can provide relief, as can immobilizing the joint. For deQuervain's, immobilization can be accomplished with a splint. For tennis elbow, a forearm strap can be used to absorb force against the tendons. An exercise program supervised by a physical therapist can strengthen forearm and wrist muscles, preventing recurrence in many cases.

Injecting corticosteroids (a form of antiinflammatory agent derived from adrenal hormones) around the tendon sheath is also effective in many patients. Steroid injections relieve symptoms in 60 to 90 percent of patients with deQuervain's. In tennis elbow, injections have a short-term success rate of up to 90 percent, but relapse is common.

When none of these methods works, surgery may be necessary to release the tightened tendon sheath. For deQuervain's this surgery can be done in an outpatient setting under local anesthesia. Surgery is rarely performed for tennis elbow.

Related entries

Antiinflammatory drugs, arthritis, carpal tunnel syndrome, hypothyroidism, musculoskeletal disorders, osteoarthritis, rheumatoid arthritis

Testicular Feminization Syndrome

Also called androgen insensitivity syndrome, this congenital condition develops in women who have XY (male) chromosomes rather than XX (female) chromosomes. Infants born with testicular feminization syndrome lack a uterus and fallopian tubes and have internal genital organs that resemble testes. Although masculine organs begin to form in the fetus, they never fully develop because cells in the fetus lack the ability to respond to virilizing hormones called androgens. Reproductive organs in both males and females develop out of the same rudimentary tissue in the fetus, and therefore the final appearance (male or female) of the reproductive system depends on hormonal influences as well as the fetus's chromosomal status.

What are the symptoms?

Girls and women with testicular feminization have essentially normal-looking external genitals and breasts, absent or sparse pubic hair, and an abnormally short vagina. They may have a small lump in each groin. Women with this syndrome never menstruate and are infertile.

How is the condition evaluated?

A woman with primary amenorrhea (failure to begin to menstruate by the age of 18) will probably be examined for testicular feminization syndrome as well as various other conditions that can interfere with menstruation. If a physical examination shows that there is no uterus, a blood test will be done to measure levels of testosterone, a form of androgen hormone that is normally much higher in males than in females. If testosterone levels are abnormally high, the doctor will then perform a karyotype, or study of the chromosomes, to see if the woman has XY chromosomes characteristic of testicular feminization syndrome.

How is testicular feminization syndrome treated?

Women with testicular feminization syndrome should have the testes removed because they are prone to develop cancer. After surgery, estrogen replacement therapy is recommended. In addition, women with testicular feminization can have plastic surgery to lengthen the vagina, thus permitting sexual intercourse. Without a normal uterus, however, they are unable to bear children.

Related entries

Amenorrhea, estrogen replacement therapy, genetic counseling, Turner syndrome

Thyroid Cancer

Cancer that originates in the thyroid gland (see illustration) is relatively rare, but when it does occur it is 3 to 4 times more common in women than in men.

There are four basic types of thyroid cancer: papillary, follicular, anaplastic, and medullary carcinomas. Of these, papillary carcinomas are by far the most common, with follicular carcinomas a distant second. Both of these cancers are almost always slow-growing, although papillary cancers can spread to the lymph glands and follicular cancers to more distant organs through the bloodstream.

Anaplastic and medullary carcinomas are more lethal, but they account for only 5 percent of all thyroid cancers. In anaplastic cancer the malignant lump enlarges rapidly and painfully. In medullary cancer the tumor produces excessive

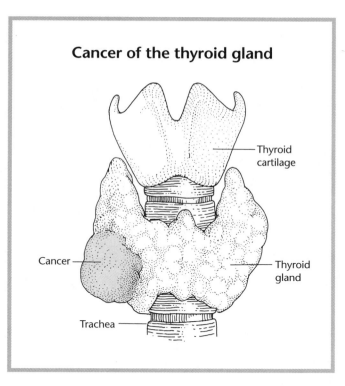

Cancer of the thyroid gland

- Thyroid cartilage
- Cancer
- Thyroid gland
- Trachea

amounts of a hormone called calcitonin, which can make diagnosis possible even when no lump can be felt.

Who is likely to develop thyroid cancer?

The risk of developing one of the various types of thyroid cancer is age-dependent. Whereas papillary cancers develop most often in younger people, the elderly are particularly prone to both follicular and anaplastic cancers. Medullary cancers are rare, but occur in children and sometimes run in families.

People who have had radiation therapy to the head or neck (to treat disorders such as Hodgkin's disease) are more likely to develop papillary or follicular thyroid cancer. This can develop as much as a decade or more after treatment. People with a history of thyroid underactivity or other hormonal problems, however, are no more likely to develop thyroid cancer than people with no history of thyroid problems.

What are the symptoms?

Thyroid cancer is generally symptom-free, except for the appearance of a painless lump at the base of the throat. Occasionally people with medullary cancer may have diarrhea. The rapidly enlarging lump of anaplastic cancer can lead to throat pain, hoarseness, difficulty swallowing, and spitting up blood.

How is the condition evaluated?

Any person who develops a thyroid nodule (an enlargement of part of the thyroid gland) should be screened for thyroid cancer, even though approximately 95 percent of these nodules will turn out to be noncancerous. Screening often begins

with a thyroid scan using radioiodine to see if the nodule is "hot," that is, producing excessive amounts of thyroid hormone, and a blood test to measure levels of thyroid stimulating hormone. Since hot nodules are almost always benign, these results can eliminate the need for additional testing.

In a thyroid scan the patient first swallows or has an injection of radioactive iodine and then returns the next day. A special camera produces an image of the thyroid, based on the amount of radioiodine that has collected at various sites. Since iodine is a key component of thyroid hormones, nodules with high levels of radioactivity will be assumed to be synthesizing large amounts of these hormones. Thyroid scans are done on an outpatient basis.

If the nodule is "cold," cancer remains a possibility, though still a small one, since most nodules turn out to be benign adenomas (growths) or cysts. Even the few nodules that do turn out to be cancerous will most often be relatively non-aggressive papillary or follicular carcinomas. For these reasons some doctors choose to treat them conservatively, testing them for malignancy about 6 months later only if the lump continues to grow. Sometimes an ultrasound examination is done so that the progress of the lump can be followed over time.

Some doctors may choose to do a definitive test for cancer right away, particularly in elderly patients, who have a greater chance of having anaplastic cancer, or to relieve any anxiety about malignancy. Tissue from the nodule is removed (in a procedure called a fine-needle aspiration) for evaluation under a microscope. Fine-needle aspiration can be done in a doctor's office with only local anesthesia. When tissue is analyzed by an experienced pathologist, it usually provides enough information to distinguish cancerous from noncancerous nodules.

How are thyroid cancers treated?

Papillary and follicular thyroid cancers are treated with surgery to remove part or all of the thyroid gland (thyroidectomy), as well as any affected lymph nodes. After surgery some patients may need to take radioiodine to help prevent further spread of the cancer, especially if it has invaded other tissue. The oral thyroid hormone levothyroxine (Synthroid) is prescribed to suppress the remaining thyroid tissue, in order to reduce the likelihood that a tumor will recur. Treatment of anaplastic cancers is individualized, since surgery is not helpful if the cancer is advanced.

Once anaplastic cancer has spread, death usually occurs within 6 to 12 months.

How can thyroid cancers be prevented?

People who have received radiation to the head and neck should have a thyroid scan or ultrasound of the thyroid every 2 to 3 years. If any nodules are present, they should be evaluated. Growth of any benign nodules should be suppressed with levothyroxine.

When medullary thyroid cancer runs in a family, careful

periodic screening of all family members is an essential part of prevention.

Related entries

Acne, goiters and thyroid nodules, hyperthyroidism, radiation therapy, thyroid disorders

Thyroid Disorders

The thyroid is a two-lobed gland that bridges the windpipe, or trachea, at the base of the neck (see illustration). It secretes the hormones thyroxine (T4) and triiodothyronine (T3). Normal growth and metabolism depend on having the proper amount of these hormones circulating throughout the body. This is achieved through a "negative feedback loop" (similar to the one regulating the hormones of the menstrual cycle) in which hormones from the pituitary gland and the hypothalamus help keep the thyroid hormones in check.

Falling levels of T3 and T4 trigger the pituitary to release more thyroid stimulating hormone (TSH), which, in turn, stimulates the thyroid to secrete more T3 and T4. As T3 and T4 levels rise, TSH secretion falls again, eventually reducing secretion of thyroid hormone.

Types of thyroid disorders

Various disorders can result if hormones circulating in the blood are not maintained at appropriate levels. Both an excess of thyroid hormone and a deficiency can affect the menstrual cycle and impair fertility, as well as adversely affect other organs.

Hyperthyroidism. Excessive thyroid hormone leads to a state in which the body's metabolic rate is increased. Symptoms such as weight loss, heart palpitations, heat intolerance and sweating, mood swings, muscle weakness, diarrhea, and, in many cases, protruding eyes may result. The most common form of hyperthyroidism is Graves disease. It occurs when an abnormal antibody stimulates the thyroid to secrete excessive amounts of thyroid hormone.

Other sources of too much thyroid hormone are toxic nodules and toxic goiters. Toxic nodules are one or more discrete lumps which develop in part of the thyroid gland and manufacture excessive amounts of thyroid hormone. Toxic nodules are almost never cancerous. Toxic goiters are enlargements of the thyroid gland which are associated with an excess production of thyroid hormone.

DeQuervain's thyroiditis and silent (or painless) thyroiditis (a form of autoimmune disease) are two other forms of hyperthyroidism which occur when part of the thyroid gland becomes inflamed and destroyed, resulting in the release of large amounts of stored thyroid hormone. Occasionally exposure to excess iodine can also result in hyperthyroidism.

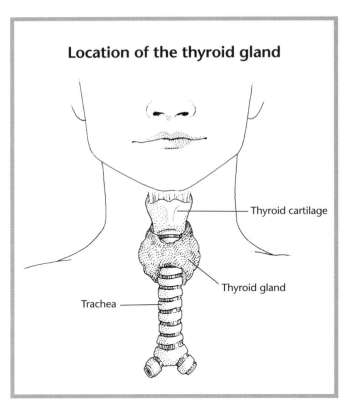

Location of the thyroid gland

Thyroid cartilage
Thyroid gland
Trachea

Hypothyroidism. Deficient levels of thyroid hormone slow the metabolic rate, producing a state called hypothyroidism. It is characterized by weight gain, fatigue, constipation, intolerance of cold temperatures, muscle cramps, and, if untreated, possibly life-threatening coma. Almost all hypothyroidism in the United States is due either to Hashimoto's disease (an autoimmune disorder in which an abnormal antibody destroys the thyroid gland) or to prior treatment for an excess of thyroid hormone. Women who have had part of their thyroid gland removed because of cancer or during a biopsy for potentially cancerous nodules are at risk for hypothyroidism.

Diffuse goiter and thyroid nodules. People with diffuse goiters have uniformly and symmetrically enlarged thyroids and may have visible swelling at the bottom of the throat. If thyroid hormone levels are normal, diffuse goiters may be no more than cosmetic problems unless they obstruct the windpipe or esophagus, in which case swallowing may become uncomfortable. Nontoxic thyroid nodules do not produce excess thyroid hormone, and they are generally harmless. Since about 5 percent of them are cancerous, however, they must be screened for thyroid cancer.

Thyroid cancer. Thyroid cancers are rare and occur in several types, which tend to appear at different ages. Cancer of the thyroid is generally symptom-free, except for the appearance of a painless lump at the base of the neck, and the majority are slow-growing. In some cases, however, symptoms such as hoarseness and difficulty swallowing can occur.

Who is likely to develop a thyroid disorder?

Women are more likely than men to develop virtually all forms of thyroid disorder. From 4 to 7 percent of women develop thyroid disorders in the months following the birth of a baby.

How are thyroid disorders evaluated?

Thyroid function is most reliably evaluated by measuring the levels of thyroid stimulating hormone (TSH) in the blood. Abnormally high levels of this hormone ordinarily indicate hypothyroidism, while abnormally low levels of TSH indicate hyperthyroidism. In women with galactorrhea or amenorrhea (or other disorders caused by dysfunction of the pituitary or hypothalamus), however, TSH levels can be normal even when the thyroid function is disturbed. Galactorrhea is a condition in which a woman who has not recently given birth can express milk or a milky discharge from her breasts, and amenorrhea is an absence of menstrual periods; both can be caused by an underfunctioning thyroid gland. For these women it is necessary to do an additional test to measure levels of T4 in the blood.

How are thyroid disorders treated?

Treatment varies from condition to condition (see entries under the various conditions), and some disorders such as goiter and thyroid nodules often require no treatment.

Related entries

Amenorrhea, galactorrhea, goiters and thyroid nodules, hyperthyroidism, hypothyroidism, menstrual cycle, menstrual cycle disorders, thyroid cancer

Toxic Shock Syndrome

Toxic shock syndrome is a rare disease affecting many systems of the body. It is caused by a toxin from the *Staphylococcus aureus*, a bacterium that is often present in the vagina and other parts of the body but usually causes no harm.

Although TSS can occur in people of any sex, age, or race, most cases reported in recent years have involved menstruating women who were using tampons. This fact came to light in the 1980s after a number of otherwise healthy young women suddenly developed life-threatening symptoms associated with TSS and some even died of the disease.

Since late 1979 and early 1980 when this small epidemic of cases was first reported to the Centers for Disease Control (CDC), the number of cases of TSS has declined substantially. Some observers have attributed this decline to increased awareness of this syndrome on the part of both the public

and professionals, as well as the exclusion of cases that would have been counted as TSS in earlier years but that do not meet the strict new CDC criteria for the disease. Above all, though, the decline in the incidence of TSS is probably due to steps on the part of tampon manufacturers to discontinue using materials previously added to tampons to increase absorbency—particularly polyester foam, carboxymethylcellulose, and polyacrylate rayon. The brand of tampon associated with most cases of TSS was removed from the market. Nonetheless, TSS still occurs in about 17 out of every 100,000 menstruating girls and women per year, and over half of these cases are attributable to tampon use.

Who is likely to develop TSS?

Although cases of toxic shock have occurred in women who use all brands and styles of tampons, they are most common among users of "super absorbent" and other high-absorbency styles. Researchers still do not understand why this occurs, although it probably has something to do with both the absorbency itself (which may make the tampon a good breeding ground for bacteria) and the chemicals used to increase the absorbency (which may irritate the vagina and allow bacteria or toxins to enter the bloodstream). Teenagers and women under 30 seem to be at the highest risk, as are women who have had TSS before. TSS has also developed in women who left contraceptive sponges or diaphragms in the vagina for over 24 hours.

About 30 percent of TSS cases occur in men and children, as well as in women who do not use tampons. Most cases develop after surgery or infection.

What are the symptoms?

TSS often begins with symptoms such as high fever (over 102°F), sunburn-like rash (often on the hands and feet), headache, muscle aches, bloodshot eyes, vomiting, diarrhea, dizziness, and fainting. Some of the early symptoms can be confused with those of the flu, but TSS can quickly progress to life-threatening complications. Blood pressure may drop rapidly, for example, and result in serious shock (a reaction to severe injury which involves symptoms such as rapid pulse, pallor, clammy skin, and sometimes unconsciousness). Kidney and liver failure may develop as well.

How is the condition evaluated?

Any woman using tampons (or who has recently been using tampons) who develops symptoms suggesting TSS should remove the tampon at once and contact a clinician. The clinician will probably want to examine the vagina for signs of inflammation. Other tests may be done to rule out gonorrhea and chlamydia, since these sexually transmitted diseases sometimes produce symptoms that mimic those of TSS.

How is TSS treated?

Toxic shock syndrome is treated with antibiotics after the vagina has been cleansed with an antiseptic solution (Betadine) to decrease the colonization of the bacteria producing the toxin. To prevent dehydration and restore lost electrolytes, intravenous fluids may be necessary, and therefore the patient may have to be admitted to the hospital.

How can TSS be prevented?

The risk of developing TSS can be minimized by alternating tampons with sanitary napkins and by using the lowest-absorbency tampon that controls menstrual flow. Since flow varies from one day to the next, this may mean using 2 or 3 different absorbencies on different days of the menstrual period. In the past, choosing the minimally absorbent tampon was more difficult for women because of inconsistent labeling of absorbency among different brands. Now, largely because of grass-roots efforts by women's health activists, the Food and Drug Administration has mandated standardized absorbency ratings on all tampon boxes to guide consumers.

One way to evaluate absorbency is to examine the tampon after keeping it in for about 4 hours (removing a tampon more frequently than this can be difficult or irritating to the vagina). If the tampon has white areas or is still dry when it is pulled out, or if it is difficult to remove, it is probably more absorbent than necessary.

Related entries

Antibiotics, birth control, chlamydia, gonorrhea, sexually transmitted diseases

Toxoplasmosis

Toxoplasmosis is an infectious disease caused by *Toxoplasma gondii,* a kind of parasite common in undercooked meat (especially lamb and mutton) as well as in cat feces. Generally a relatively harmless condition which may not even produce symptoms, it is a concern for pregnant women since about a third of women infected during pregnancy will pass the parasite on to the fetus through the placenta, and about a third of infected fetuses will develop the disease.

Who is likely to develop toxoplasmosis?

Between 20 and 40 percent of the public have already been exposed to toxoplasmosis without necessarily realizing it, and they carry antibodies to the parasite in their blood. Fetuses are affected, however, only if a woman who has never previously been infected acquires the infection during pregnancy.

What are the symptoms?

Adults infected with toxoplasmosis may have no symptoms at all, or they may have a rash as well as flulike symptoms: fatigue, fever, sore throat, and muscle pain.

Occasionally toxoplasmosis can result in miscarriage during the first trimester. Infected babies are often born underweight and premature, and develop fever, jaundice, eye problems, and other long-term neurological disorders. Although the risk that the fetus will be infected is highest during the last 3 months of pregnancy, the risk of severe complications is greatest if infection occurs during the first 3 months. Approximately 1 fetus in every 1,000 pregnancies is infected with the toxoplasmosis parasite.

How is the condition evaluated?

The American College of Obstetricians and Gynecologists does not recommend routine blood testing of pregnant women for toxoplasmosis. Problems occur only when the mother acquires the infection during the course of her pregnancy, and if she has few symptoms, there is no way to know if infection is recent, since so many women already have antibodies from previous exposure. The only way to confirm newly acquired toxoplasmosis infection would be to test all women for antibodies just before they become pregnant, and then, over the course of the pregnancy, to retest those who previously tested negative. Such a procedure is not cost-effective or practical.

How is toxoplasmosis treated?

If a woman becomes infected with toxoplasmosis during her pregnancy, antibiotics (pyrimethamine and sulfadiazine plus leucovorin) can be used after 14 weeks' gestation. The safety of these drugs for use earlier in pregnancy has not been established, however, so prevention should be the goal.

How can toxoplasmosis be prevented?

The best way to avoid acquiring toxoplasmosis is to cook all meats thoroughly and always wash hands with soap and water after touching raw meat and vegetables, soil, or cats. Pregnant women in particular should avoid changing cat litter boxes. If that is not possible, they should change the litter box daily—since feces do not become infectious until 24 hours have passed—and wear gloves whenever changing them or gardening in areas to which cats have access. Pregnant women should also avoid acquiring new cats, holding outdoor cats close to their face, or allowing them to sit on beds or bed linens. Cats should be fed only commercial cat food and should be prevented from eating mice, which often carry the parasite.

Related entries

Antibiotics, miscarriage, pregnancy

Trichomonas

Trichomonas vaginitis (also known as "trich" or trichomoniasis) is a sexually transmitted disease caused by a quickly moving one-celled protozoan called *Trichomonas vaginalis.* This microorganism can live for years in the male reproductive tract without producing any symptoms. Although trichomonas is the third most common form of vaginitis in the United States, affecting 3 million women each year, the incidence is decreasing, probably because a specific antiprotozoal medication can cure most cases quickly and effectively.

Who is likely to develop trichomonas?

Trichomonas is almost always acquired through sexual contact with an infected partner. Although there have been scattered reports that the organism can be acquired from contaminated toilet seats, washcloths, water, clothing, and the like, these reports have never been confirmed in any scientifically convincing study. There does not seem to be any solid evidence that emotional stress can cause symptoms of trichomonas to flare up or recur.

What are the symptoms?

Some women harbor the organism for years without developing symptoms. Most of the time, however, a copious green or gray, frothy, and foul-smelling vaginal discharge is present, along with vaginal or vulvar itching, redness, or swelling. Some women experience symptoms of urinary tract infection, including a burning sensation during urination and the need to urinate frequently and urgently, while others may develop pain during sexual intercourse.

How is the condition evaluated?

A clinician who suspects trichomonas will first do a pelvic examination, looking for the characteristic "strawberry" cervix, that is, small red dots on the entrance to the uterus which result from tiny areas of bleeding. The vaginal secretions will be examined under a microscope or cultured to detect the organism. Sometimes trichomonas is detected incidentally in women with no symptoms on the basis of an abnormal Pap test during a routine pelvic examination.

How is trichomonas treated?

Nine out of 10 cases of trichomonas can be successfully cured with a single dose (2 grams, in tablet form) of the drug metronidazole (Flagyl, Protostat). This is taken by both the infected woman and her partner, since up to a quarter of women will be reinfected if their partner is not treated. People who become nauseated with this large dose of metronidazole can take a lower dose 3 times a day for 7 days. Because trichomonas affects not only the vaginal tissue but also the urethra and nearby glands under the skin, topical gels or suppositories such as metronidazole gel (Metrogel) are much less effective as treatments.

Metronidazole has been linked to cancer in laboratory mice and rats, but there is no evidence that it causes cancer in human beings. The risks from a single treatment dose are believed to be vanishingly small. Alcohol consumption should be avoided for at least 24 hours after using metronidazole, since the combination of the drugs can lead to abdominal cramps, nausea, vomiting, headaches, and skin flushing. Metronidazole is considered unsafe for use during pregnancy, particularly during the first trimester because of its theoretical potential to cause birth defects. It should also be avoided by breastfeeding mothers since it can pass into the breast milk.

In the rare cases when trichomonas does not respond to metronidazole, treatment can be repeated. If symptoms persist, higher doses may be tried. These stronger treatments seem to be more successful if used in conjunction with intravaginal gels or washes made of acetic acid such as Aci-Jel. Homemade vinegar washes can be made by mixing 1 tablespoon of white vinegar into a quart of water for use once or twice a week. Povidone-iodine douches (such as Betadine, available without prescription) may also help relieve symptoms. There are some reports—though still unproven—that saltwater douches alone can provide relief. Vinegar washes and Aci-Jel are probably safe, although studies still must be done before they are proved safe and effective for use during pregnancy. Povidone-iodine douches are definitely not safe for use during pregnancy because iodine absorption by the fetus can lead to hypothyroidism.

Women with an infection that continues to be difficult to treat should consult a specialist experienced in dealing with severely resistant trichomonas.

How can trichomonas be prevented?

Trichomonas can be prevented in the same ways as other sexually transmitted diseases—including using male condoms or female condoms (see safer sex). There is some evidence that the chemical nonoxynol-9, present in spermicidal creams, foams, and jellies, may help protect against trichomonas and other sexually transmitted diseases.

Related entries

Condoms, douching, hypothyroidism, pain during sexual intercourse, safer sex, sexually transmitted diseases, urinary tract infections, vaginitis

Tubal Ligation

Tubal ligation is a means of female sterilization in which the fallopian tubes are tied, cauterized, cut, or clipped, thus blocking access of sperm to a fertilizable egg (see illustration). This means of contraception is frequently used by women who do not wish to bear children in the future and who do not want to be bothered by other cumbersome birth control methods.

How is the procedure performed?

Tubal ligations are often performed in an ambulatory surgery or day surgery unit of a hospital. Two of the most common techniques are laparoscopic surgery and minilaparotomy.

Laparoscopic surgery. This is by far the most prevalent technique. It involves making a small cut just under the navel and through the abdominal wall, and inserting an instrument to grasp and then surgically interrupt the tubes.

With the woman under regional or general anesthesia, the surgeon first pumps either carbon dioxide or nitrous oxide gas into the abdominal cavity through a needle in order to lift the abdominal wall away from the intestine. This makes it easier to locate the fallopian tubes, and it minimizes the chances of accidental injury to other internal organs. When only regional anesthesia is used, some women feel bloating or moderate discomfort as the abdominal area is filled with the gas.

Next an electrically nonconductive sleeve is inserted into the abdomen with the aid of a large metal instrument called a trocar. The laparoscope, a high-powered fiberoptic instrument, is then inserted through this sleeve, along with a forceps. Some surgeons who are using electrocautery (see entry) to seal off the tube also make a second incision lower in the abdomen for the electrocautery device. This can also be uncomfortable to a woman under only regional anesthesia.

Using light from the laparoscope as a guide, the surgeon locates each fallopian tube, pinches it with the forceps, and closes it off (see illustration). After the tube has been clipped, coagulated with electrocautery, or tied off, the gas is evacuated from the abdomen. All instruments are then removed, and the incision is sutured.

Minilaparotomy. This simpler and generally less painful means of tubal ligation can be accomplished in as little as a few minutes by either a surgeon or a trained technician. In this procedure, which can be performed under general, regional, or local anesthesia, the surgeon or technician inserts a speculum into the vagina and inserts a blunt instrument called an elevator through the cervix into the uterus. A one-inch incision is made just above the pubic bone, and the surgeon or technician guides the elevator so that the uterus moves up near the opening and the fallopian tubes become accessible. Each fallopian tube is pulled through the incision, closed off, and then returned to the body, after which the incision is stitched together.

What happens after surgery?

With laparoscopic surgery the entire operation takes about half an hour, and most women can expect to leave the hospital the same day. If the incision site is somewhat tender or red, soaking it in warm water several times a day is often helpful.

Many women can go home within hours of a minilaparotomy, and there is generally less tenderness and discomfort than after a traditional laparotomy. Normal activities can usually be resumed within a day or so.

Tubal ligation is immediately effective. Once the surgery is over, a woman can have sexual intercourse freely without worrying about becoming pregnant. It is over 99 percent effective in preventing pregnancy. If a woman does eventually change her mind and decide that she would like to bear another child, tubal ligation is occasionally reversible—although no one should have a tubal ligation if she thinks she may someday change her mind. Not only is the microsurgery required for reversal extremely expensive (and usually not covered by insurance), but also it is unsuccessful in approximately half of all attempts.

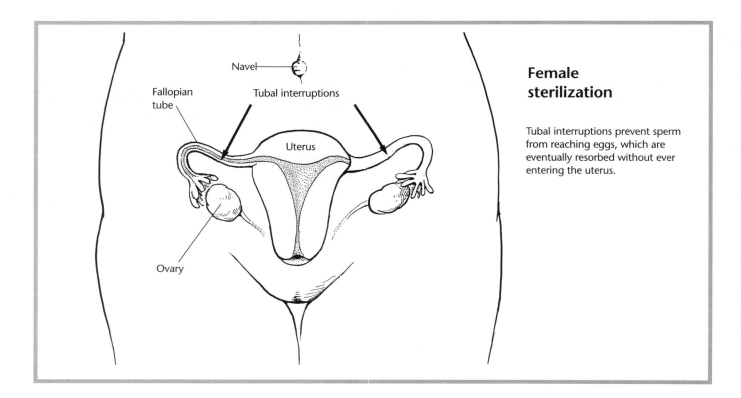

Navel

Fallopian tube

Tubal interruptions

Uterus

Ovary

Female sterilization

Tubal interruptions prevent sperm from reaching eggs, which are eventually resorbed without ever entering the uterus.

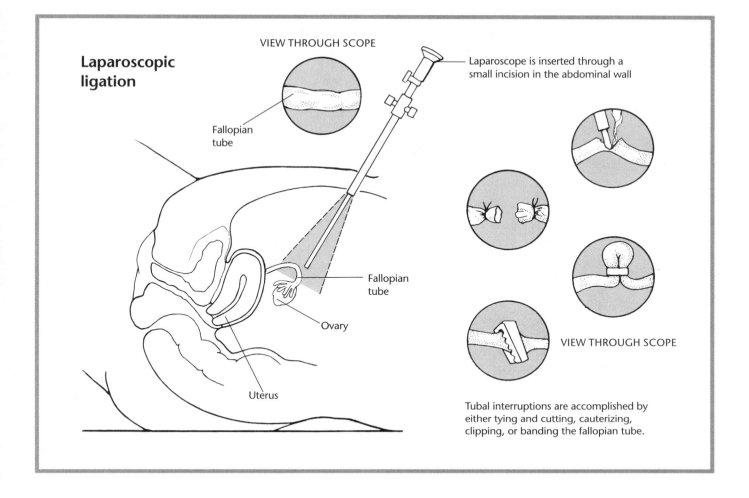

Laparoscopic ligation

VIEW THROUGH SCOPE

Laparoscope is inserted through a small incision in the abdominal wall

Fallopian tube

Fallopian tube

Ovary

Uterus

VIEW THROUGH SCOPE

Tubal interruptions are accomplished by either tying and cutting, cauterizing, clipping, or banding the fallopian tube.

What are the risks and complications?

Tubal ligation is considered a relatively safe procedure, but like any form of surgery it carries a certain degree of risk, including hemorrhaging, infection, and reactions to anesthesia. About 1 in 1,000 women will experience one of these or another more specific complication of surgery, including puncture or perforation of internal organs or blood vessels, skin burns, or (with the laparoscopic procedure) a carbon dioxide embolism (a pocket of gas that escapes into the circulation, causing tissue death in the lung). Occasionally, a surgeon may have great difficulty locating the fallopian tubes in a woman who is obese or has pelvic adhesions (that is, internal scarring from previous surgery, infection, or endometriosis). In general, women who choose a surgeon with considerable experience in doing tubal ligations can expect a lesser chance of complications.

Controversy exists about whether tubal ligation has any long-term complications. There are some reports of heavy, irregular, or painful menstrual periods developing years later in women who have had tubal ligations. Also, several studies have shown that women who have undergone this procedure are more likely than other women to have a hysterectomy later on.

Many women decide to have their tubes tied right after childbirth. This is an optimal time for the surgery because, with the uterus still enlarged, the fallopian tubes are easily accessible, and surgery can often be performed without gas and with minimal anesthesia. If a woman is planning to have a cesarean section for some other reason, performing a tubal ligation during the same operation is an even simpler procedure since no new incision needs to be made.

Women who are obese or who have adhesions, abdominal cancer, or endometriosis should probably not have a mini-laparotomy because they run a higher than normal risk of developing complications.

Although very unlikely, it is possible to become pregnant after a tubal ligation, and about 40 percent of these pregnancies are ectopic (that is, the embryo implants in the tube itself or in some part of the abdomen other than the uterus). Some physicians believe that the failure rate is higher when the surgery is done just after giving birth. In light of the very rare possibility of an ectopic pregnancy (see entry), which can be life-threatening if untreated, a woman who has undergone tubal ligation should see a clinician promptly if she ever develops pelvic pain and vaginal bleeding.

Related entries

Adhesions, anesthesia, birth control, cesarean section, ectopic pregnancy, electrocautery, endometriosis, laparoscopy

Turner Syndrome

This chromosomal defect, also called gonadal dysgenesis, is usually due to the absence of, or a defect in, one of the two X chromosomes normally found in females. Women and girls with Turner syndrome have underdeveloped or missing ovaries and therefore do not produce the hormones necessary for normal sexual development and fertility. This rare syndrome occurs in about 1 out of every 3,000 female newborns.

What are the symptoms?

Signs of Turner syndrome may include unusually short stature, webbed neck, abundant pigmented moles, childlike female genitals, wide-set eyes, absent breast development, and a low hairline on the back of the neck, as well as certain heart, kidney, gastrointestinal, and blood vessel defects.

Although it is sometimes obvious at birth, Turner syndrome often is not recognized until the teenage years when signs of puberty such as breast development and menarche fail to occur. Most people with Turner syndrome have normal verbal intelligence, but spatial disorientation may impair mathematical performance.

How is the syndrome evaluated?

A woman with primary amenorrhea (failure to begin to menstruate by the age of 18) will probably be examined for Turner syndrome as well as various other conditions that can interfere with menstruation. Usually the clinician will do a physical examination for signs of the syndrome and then a blood test to check hormone levels. If hormone levels are abnormal, a karyotype, or study of the chromosomes, will be performed.

Turner syndrome can be detected through amniocentesis or a chorionic villi sampling procedure during gestation.

How is Turner syndrome treated?

Estrogen replacement therapy can be used to produce normal breast development and menstruation. Growth hormone is usually given before estrogen to increase height. Women with Turner syndrome who take ERT can sometimes achieve pregnancy with donor eggs (see infertility).

Related entries

Amenorrhea, amniocentesis, chorionic villi sampling, estrogen replacement therapy, genetic counseling, infertility, menarche, moles, testicular feminization syndrome

Ultrasound

Ultrasound is a diagnostic procedure in which high-frequency sound waves are bounced off certain internal structures of the body. The reflections or echoes of these sound waves are then recorded on a video screen to form a picture, or sonogram, of the internal structure (see illustration).

In pregnancy, ultrasound can help determine the size of the uterus or fetus, confirm the due date, detect the presence of a multiple pregnancy, reveal certain anatomical defects in the fetus, or locate an ectopic pregnancy. It is also useful in guiding the needle safely in prenatal screening procedures (amniocentesis and chorionic villi sampling). A study suggests, however, that routine ultrasound is not cost-effective in women under the age of 35 who are not at unusually high risk for bearing a child with a genetic abnormality.

In addition to assessing development during a pregnancy, ultrasound is used to measure the flow of blood and to help diagnose ovarian cysts, uterine fibroids, and pelvic pain. Ultrasound is also used to diagnose various cancers and to examine a wide variety of organs, including the breast, thyroid gland, pancreas, and kidneys.

How is the procedure performed?

An ultrasound can be done on an outpatient basis at a hospital, laboratory, or doctor's office and usually takes about 15 minutes. Unless she is in an advanced stage of pregnancy, a woman about to undergo a pelvic ultrasound may be asked to drink copious fluids and to avoid urinating for about an hour before the test so she can arrive with a full bladder, which allows a better view.

During the procedure itself, the woman lies on an examination table and her abdomen (or other area to be examined) is coated with mineral oil or jelly-like material, which improves the transmission of sound waves. A hand-held scanner (transducer) which produces the sound waves is gently rubbed over the skin. The woman can see the black and white sonogram on the screen, which can be photographed for subsequent examination. In a newer technique called vaginal ultrasound, the transducer is inserted into the vagina to allow a better view.

What are the risks and complications?

To date there are no known harmful effects from ultrasound to the patient or to a fetus.

Related entries

Amniocentesis, chorionic villi sampling, computerized axial tomography scans, ectopic pregnancy, genetic counseling, magnetic resonance imaging, mammography, ovarian cysts, pelvic pain, prenatal care, uterine fibroids

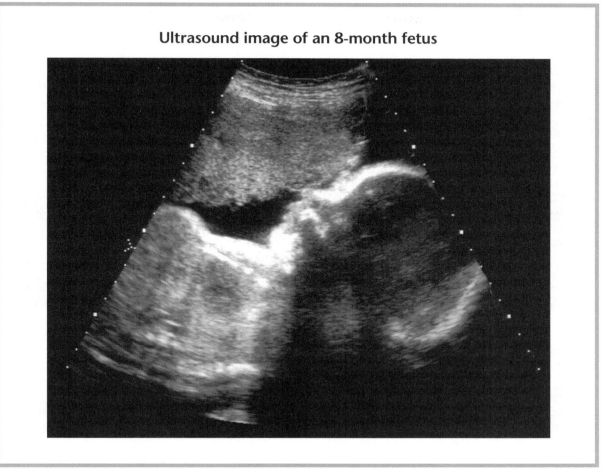

Ultrasound image of an 8-month fetus

Umbilical Hernia

An umbilical hernia is a protrusion of the abdominal wall through the navel. A condition much more common in women than in men, these hernias are often harmless but occasionally may constrict and interfere with blood circulation. A loop of bowel can sometimes become trapped within the hernia, causing a bowel obstruction.

Who is likely to develop an umbilical hernia?

Umbilical hernias appear most often in women who have given birth to many children, although they seem to have no effect on subsequent pregnancies. Women who are obese may also develop an umbilical hernia. They are even more common in newborn babies of both sexes, and may protrude when the baby cries or coughs.

What are the symptoms?

Most of the time the hernia appears as an enlargement around the navel. Some women may notice only vague and sporadic pain and tenderness in this region.

How is the condition evaluated?

Although a hernia is usually obvious to a clinician, occasionally it can be felt only if the woman lies down and coughs with her head raised.

How are umbilical hernias treated?

Umbilical hernias can be surgically repaired if a clinician suspects they may interfere with blood circulation. In infants, however, they almost always heal themselves and require no treatment.

How can they be prevented?

There is no known way to prevent an umbilical hernia.

Related entries

Childbirth, obesity

Urethral Syndrome

Urethral syndrome is a chronic, relatively common problem which produces the same symptoms as a urinary tract infection but which does not appear to be caused by bacteria. It is also known as dysuria-pyuria syndrome and chronic urethritis. As the ability to culture microorganisms improves, investigators are finding that many women who were previously diagnosed as having urethral syndrome actually have urinary tract infections caused by anaerobic bacteria (bacteria that do not require oxygen to grow) or chlamydia (a bacterium that causes the sexually transmitted disease of the same name). Even so, there is still a sizable group of women with urethral syndrome whose symptoms cannot be linked to any obvious cause.

What are the symptoms?
Urethral syndrome has symptoms that mimic those of urinary tract infections—painful urination, the need to urinate frequently and urgently, and pelvic pain—but in the case of urethral syndrome these symptoms can continue for months.

How is the condition evaluated?
A clinician diagnosing urethral syndrome will do a physical examination to see if the urethra (the tube that connects the bladder to the outside of the body) is tender. Urethral syndrome will be diagnosed only after the clinician has eliminated other possible causes of the symptoms—including urinary tract infections, vaginitis, gonorrhea, chlamydia, herpes, and allergic reactions. This usually involves doing a urinalysis, which in the case of urethral syndrome will show low levels of bacteria but may show high levels of pus (white blood cells).

How is urethral syndrome treated?
With no known cause, urethral syndrome has no specific treatment, and many of the treatments that have been tried have never been proven effective. The classic treatment for this disorder has involved stretching the urethra with a special instrument (a procedure called urethral dilatation), but it still is not known whether this procedure really helps. The clinician may also suggest taking sitz baths to relieve pain or may prescribe the bladder anesthetic phenazopyridine (Pyridium).

If symptoms persist, the patient will probably be referred to a urologist, who will evaluate the function of the urinary tract with an instrument called a cystoscope. Cystoscopy is often performed in the urologist's office under local anesthesia, although sometimes regional or general anesthesia is used in a day surgery setting. The urologist inserts a lighted tube through the urethra into the bladder, looking for signs of interstitial cystitis (see entry) or other abnormalities.

If a clinician suspects that symptoms may in fact be due to a bacterial infection (especially a sexually transmitted disease) which for some reason is hard to confirm, appropriate antibiotic drugs will be prescribed.

Related entries
Antibiotics, chlamydia, cystocele/urethrocele/rectocele, gonorrhea, herpes, interstitial cystitis, kidney disorders, pelvic pain, prolapsed uterus, sexually transmitted diseases, urinary tract infections, urine tests, vaginitis

Urinary Tract Infections

Urinary tract infections (UTIs) occur when a large number of bacteria grow in the urethra (the tube leading from the outside of the body into the bladder), the bladder itself, the ureters (the tubes that carry urine from the kidneys to the bladder), or the kidneys (see illustration). The most frequent cause of UTIs is the *Escherichia coli* bacterium, commonly found in the intestinal tract.

Infection in the urethra (urethritis) generally coexists with infection of the bladder (cystitis). Although these lower-tract infections can be annoying and painful, they are usually easily treated with antibiotics. In rare cases, undiagnosed or improperly treated urethritis and cystitis may lead to kidney damage.

Female anatomy predisposes women to UTIs because the urethral opening is located very close to the anus, a common source of bacteria. In addition, because a woman's bladder is only about an inch from her urethra, while a man's is 6 inches away, bacteria introduced into the urethral region have a much shorter distance to travel before infecting the bladder.

Some women have recurrent UTIs owing to reinfection by new bacteria. Other women experience a relapse within a week or two of completing treatment if the original bacteria were not completely eradicated. Occasionally these recurrences are caused by an anatomical defect or injury in the urinary tract. Relapses and recurrent infections may also signal a more serious infection of the upper urinary tract known as a silent kidney infection (subclinical pyelonephritis). These infections can be difficult to distinguish from infections of the lower urinary tract (cystitis and urethritis) but usually respond to similar treatment. Perhaps 30 percent of women with painful urination turn out to have these silent kidney infections. When back pain, vomiting, fever, or chills occur, however, there may be a full-fledged kidney infection (pyelonephritis; see kidney disorders), a condition that requires immediate medical attention.

Although mild cases of urethritis and cystitis can disappear without treatment, a woman who has symptoms for over 2 days or who has symptoms suggesting kidney infection should consult her physician.

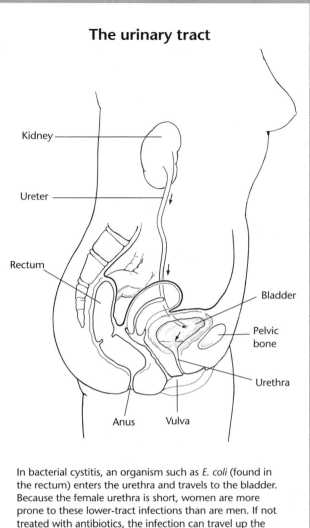

The urinary tract

Kidney

Ureter

Rectum

Bladder

Pelvic bone

Urethra

Anus   Vulva

In bacterial cystitis, an organism such as *E. coli* (found in the rectum) enters the urethra and travels to the bladder. Because the female urethra is short, women are more prone to these lower-tract infections than are men. If not treated with antibiotics, the infection can travel up the ureters and invade the kidneys, causing more serious disease.

Who is likely to develop a UTI?

Most women will develop UTIs at some point in their lives. Poor hygiene, sexual intercourse, withholding urination, childbirth, and gynecological surgery can all introduce bacteria into the urethral area and eventually lead to cystitis. Hormonal changes after menopause increase the risk of UTIs. Pregnant women are particularly prone to cystitis because the fetus pressing on the bladder can impede complete emptying. For the same reason, a cystocele (a condition in which the bladder bulges into the front of the vagina) can lead to UTIs. Certain forms of birth control such as spermicidal foams and jellies and condoms have been linked to UTIs, if only because they may irritate the urethra and thus make infection more likely. Diaphragms compress the urethra, making it difficult to empty the bladder completely, and this can

set the stage for a UTI. Some women seem genetically prone to recurrent infection.

Silent kidney infections seem to occur most frequently in poor inner-city women. They are also common in women who have underlying defects of the urinary tract, diabetes mellitus or other conditions that depress the immune system, or a history of urinary infections in childhood. Also at risk are women who have experienced relapsing UTIs in the past, have had 6 or more previous UTIs in the past year, or who have had a kidney infection in the past year. Any woman whose symptoms have persisted for 7 to 10 days may also have a silent kidney infection, although another possibility is chlamydial urethritis (irritation of the urethra resulting from a sexually transmitted disease; see chlamydia), or infection by some other sexually transmitted organism.

Perimenopausal and postmenopausal women are particularly susceptible to urinary tract infections. As the hormone estrogen decreases, tissues in the urinary and reproductive tracts thin out and become more easily irritated.

What are the symptoms?

A painful, burning sensation during urination is often the only symptom of a UTI. Many women also find that they need to urinate frequently although little urine comes out, and some notice blood or pus in the urine. The area just above the pubic bone may feel particularly tender, and the urine may have a strong smell.

Silent kidney infections (infection of the upper urinary tract), which occur in about 30 percent of women with painful urination, usually have the same symptoms as cystitis and urethritis.

How is the condition evaluated?

Between 60 and 70 percent of women with painful urination turn out to have an infection of the lower urinary tract. If a UTI is suspected, a urinalysis (or urine dipstick) test is performed in the office to check for pus (white blood cells). If the urinalysis is positive, a urine culture is usually done in the laboratory to identify the bacteria. Urine is collected using a "clean catch" procedure, in which the vulva is first washed thoroughly with a disinfectant, then the urine is collected midstream in a sterile container. This procedure prevents contamination of the urine by bacteria on the body.

Although urine culture is still performed routinely, recent studies indicate that up to half of all women with the symptoms of cystitis do not have enough bacteria to yield a positive culture (see urethral syndrome). If no bacteria are found, a clinician will try to eliminate other causes of painful urination such as sexually transmitted disease, vaginitis, or yeast infections.

Sometimes—if symptoms are pretty straightforward—a clinician might omit the culture and simply prescribe antibiotics (even over the phone). If the clinician suspects a silent kidney infection, however, a urine culture will be necessary to determine levels and types of bacteria so that appropriate antibiotic therapy can be administered. Currently there is no simple laboratory test to differentiate silent kidney infections from cystitis and urethritis.

Women who have had a relapsing infection with the same organism (often *E. coli*) or who have had 3 or more infections in the past year with the same organism (suggesting persistent infection) may undergo further tests to see if there are any defects in their urinary tract predisposing them to infection. These defects can include abnormal passages (fistulas), pouches (diverticula), or blockages (strictures) in the urethra, as well as interstitial cystitis, cancer of the bladder, and kidney stones.

Often the urologist will have a radiologist do an intravenous pyelogram (IVP), in which a dye is injected into the veins prior to an x-ray of the kidney and bladder. To avoid the risk of an allergic reaction to the dye, as well as the risks associated with radiation, some clinicians recommend using cystoscopy instead of an IVP; in this procedure a telescope-like instrument is used to visualize the bladder directly. An ultrasound may be done to study the kidney and urinary system more thoroughly. All of these tests can be performed in a doctor's office or in the radiology department of a hospital on an outpatient basis.

The vast majority of women who have recurrent UTIs, however, turn out to have no identifiable problem.

How are UTIs treated?

For years UTIs were almost always treated with an antibiotic administered for a full 7 to 14 days. Many studies have now demonstrated that, for most UTIs, a single dose of antibiotics by mouth is nearly as effective as the traditional course. Slightly more effective is a 3-day course of treatment, and occasionally a physician will recommend a 5-day course. Not only is shorter treatment less expensive, but also it lowers the risk of side effects commonly associated with antibiotic treatment such as yeast infections, rash, and diarrhea. Symptoms usually disappear within a day or two of the first dose, but medication should be taken for the length of the prescription, whatever that may be. Although a follow-up urine exam after treatment is sometimes recommended, it is not always necessary in uncomplicated UTIs if symptoms resolve. Short-course therapy is not appropriate for pregnant women, women with diabetes, or elderly women, since these groups are at high risk for kidney infection.

Sometimes women with chronic UTIs develop resistance to the standard drugs (sulfa drugs for *E. coli,* for example) and require stronger antibiotics such as ciprofloxacin and norfloxacin. These medications can also be taken in a short course.

Clinicians who suspect a silent kidney infection may prescribe antibiotic treatment even before results of the urine culture become available. These infections require 10 to 14 days of treatment. Patients who have experienced relapsing kidney infection (with the same bacteria) may require even longer treatment. Because about 10 to 15 percent of women with silent kidney infections can expect their symptoms to recur, having a follow-up urine culture 2 to 4 days after treatment ends is particularly important.

Pregnant women who are found to have bacteria in their urine during a prenatal exam should be treated promptly—even if they have no symptoms of a urinary tract infection. This is because without treatment about a third of them can expect to go on to develop a serious kidney infection later in the pregnancy. Usually all that is necessary is taking an antibiotic for about a week and having a follow-up urine culture to make sure the bacteria have been eliminated.

If some physical defect is found to underlie the symptoms, it can often be corrected with surgery. Women whose symptoms do not respond to antibacterial drugs may be referred to a specialist to make sure they do not have urethral syndrome (see entry), a disorder that has the symptoms of a urinary tract infection but does not appear to be due to bacterial infection.

Some women find that acidifying the urine by drinking cranberry juice or taking 500 mg of vitamin C a day helps alleviate the symptoms of UTI. Others find relief by soaking in a hot tub or placing a heating pad on their abdomen or back—although medical attention should be sought if symptoms do not resolve within a day or two. Herbal remedies are often suggested by popular health guides, but there are as yet no formal scientific studies proving their effectiveness.

How can UTIs be prevented?

Emptying the bladder before and after sexual intercourse and changing sanitary napkins frequently can help prevent the recurrence of UTIs in susceptible women, as can wiping from front to back after a bowel movement (to avoid spreading bacteria from the intestinal tract into the urethra). Drinking 10 ounces of cranberry juice each day seems to reduce a woman's chances of developing a UTI significantly, perhaps because the juice contains a substance that stops bacteria from invading the bladder lining. Drinking large quantities of water to dilute the urine and make it less favorable to bacterial growth may also keep the number of infections down.

Women prone to recurrent infections may want to avoid bubble baths, chlorinated swimming pools, and other irritants. If they are currently using a diaphragm, spermicide, or condom, they may also want to consider changing their form of birth control to one that does not irritate the urethra. Diaphragm users can have their diaphragm refitted to the smallest effective size or to a type with a softer rim which exerts less pressure on the urethra.

Women who have recurring infections may be given prophylactic (preventive) doses of antibiotics to be taken each day or after sexual intercourse. Other women may want to ask their clinician about obtaining an antibiotic to keep in their medicine cabinet for use as soon as symptoms recur. This method of treatment should be pursued only when a clinician is confident that the woman understands her condition and the importance of reporting any unusual symptoms.

Related entries

Antibiotics, birth control, chlamydia, cystocele/urethrocele/rectocele, diabetes, diaphragms and cervical caps, interstitial cystitis, kidney disorders, sexually transmitted disease, urethral syndrome, urine tests, vaginitis, yeast infections

Urine Tests

A urinalysis at each visit to the doctor is a regular part of prenatal care. It is no longer done routinely during physical examinations in nonpregnant women, but in those with symptoms of diabetes, urinary tract infections, and certain other conditions, a urine test can help the clinician make the correct diagnosis.

Among the many substances that are frequently checked for in urine are protein (particularly albumin), ketones, glucose (sugar), bilirubin, red blood cells, white blood cells, and bacteria. The presence of protein in the urine, for example, can be a sign of damage to or inflammation of the kidneys, bladder, or ureters, and, in a pregnant woman, may signal preeclampsia. If ketones (by-products from breakdown of proteins) are present in the urine (ketonuria), the problem may be uncontrolled diabetes mellitus, starvation, or alcohol intoxication. Glucose in the urine (glucosuria) is sometimes a sign of diabetes mellitus, especially if it is detected consistently; in a pregnant woman it may signal gestational diabetes. Bilirubin, a breakdown product of aged red blood cells, sometimes appears in the urine if there is some dysfunction of the liver or bile ducts. The presence of red blood cells in the urine (hematuria) suggests a urinary tract infection, kidney infection, kidney stones, kidney failure, or possibly a tumor of the bladder or kidneys. White blood cells in the urine (pyuria) usually mean there is some kind of infection.

The specific gravity of the urine—that is, the weight of the urine compared with the weight of the same volume of normal urine—can indicate how effective the kidneys are in maintaining the body's overall balance of fluids. The urine's pH (acidity or alkalinity) can give clues about the presence of disease and how well the kidneys are excreting acids.

How is urine testing performed?

All urine testing requires that a sample of urine be collected in a clean, dry container. Some procedures, particularly those that screen for infections, require the urine to be collected by the "clean catch" method to ensure that the sample is not contaminated by menstrual fluids, vaginal discharge, bacteria on the outside of the body, and the like. Women asked for a clean catch sample are usually given a disinfectant-soaked towelette with which to wipe the vulvar area before urinating. They are then told to urinate a few ounces into the toilet before starting to collect the remainder of the stream, and to avoid touching the lips of the collection cup to the vulva or the pubic hair. The easiest way to accomplish this is to hold the vaginal lips open with one hand while holding the cup several inches below them with the other.

The simplest form of urine testing, the dipstick test, can be done within seconds in a clinician's office. In this test various sticks of chemically coated paper are dipped into the urine sample. Depending on which chemical the dipstick has been treated with, a change in the color of the paper can indicate the presence of abnormal levels of protein, ketones (acetone), glucose, bilirubin, or blood in the urine, as well as the urine's relative acidity.

A more complex urinalysis may be performed if a dipstick test reveals an abnormality or if there is any suspicion of infection. Urinalysis is usually done in a laboratory, although some clinicians are equipped to perform it in the office. The procedure begins by putting the urine sample into a test tube and spinning it in a centrifuge until the liquid and solid portions separate out. The solid sediment is collected and examined under a microscope for the presence of pus (white blood cells), red blood cells, bacteria, and other abnormal cells.

If any abnormalities are detected, additional testing may be done to look for infections, tumors, or other disorders of the urinary tract or kidneys. For example, if the presence of bacteria or white blood cells (as well as the patient's symptoms) suggest infection, a urine culture may be done in a laboratory to determine the exact nature of the bacteria involved so that an appropriate antibiotic can be prescribed. To do a culture, the urine is spread onto a nutrient plate and heated until the bacteria multiply into a colony large enough to be examined. Usually the results of a urine culture are available within 48 hours.

If a urinalysis shows protein in the urine, the clinician may want to do a 24-hour test to measure the total amount of protein voided over a 24-hour period. A woman undergoing this test needs to collect an entire day's worth of urine for analysis. A 24-hour test may also be done to test the urine for calcium and other substances if there are symptoms suggesting kidney stones (such as flank pain, persistent urge to urinate, and blood in the urine).

What are the risks and complications?

There are no risks or complications associated with urine testing, other than the possibility of a false positive, which could lead to further (unnecessary) testing.

Related entries

Blood tests, diabetes, physical examinations, preeclampsia, pregnancy testing, prenatal care, screening, urethral syndrome, urinary tract infections

Uterine Fibroids

Uterine fibroids are tumors that grow outside, inside, or within the wall of the uterus, sometimes changing its shape (see illustration). Composed of muscular and fibrous tissue, these growths may enlarge over time but do not become cancerous. Although their cause remains unclear, fibroids seem

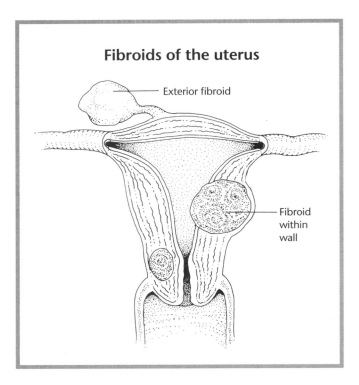

Fibroids of the uterus

Exterior fibroid

Fibroid within wall

to be related to the production of the hormone estrogen; recent research suggests that progesterone may play a role as well.

Who is likely to develop fibroids?

Uterine fibroids (also known as myomas, fibromyomas, myofibromas, and leiomyomas) are the most common pelvic tumors in women; as many as 1 woman in 4 will be diagnosed with them during her reproductive years. Recent evidence suggests that over a lifetime between 40 and 75 percent of women may develop fibroids, often without realizing it. Fibroids are most frequently found in women between the ages of 30 and 50 and only rarely occur before the age of 20 or after menopause. Some studies suggest that African American women may be more likely than white women to develop them, for reasons not yet understood.

What are the symptoms?

Symptoms vary according to the number, size, and location of the fibroids. The majority of women with fibroid tumors experience no symptoms or complications. Fibroids inside the uterus or within the uterine wall, however, may cause heavy or prolonged menstrual periods, while large fibroids that press on nearby pelvic organs can produce pelvic pain, frequent urination, or, less frequently, constipation. Occasionally, fibroids within the uterus or uterine wall may lead to problems with pregnancy, labor, or delivery such as infertility, miscarriage, and premature birth.

How is the condition evaluated?

Women often learn they have fibroid tumors when an enlarged or irregular uterus is discovered during a routine pelvic examination (see entry). A clinician who suspects fibroids may order an ultrasound test to differentiate them from other causes of uterine changes, including ovarian cysts, pregnancy, or various forms of cancer. To help rule out malignancy or determine the cause of heavy or prolonged menstrual periods, a clinician may also perform outpatient procedures such as endometrial biopsy or dilatation and curettage (D&C), in which cells lining the uterus are removed and studied.

Although fibroids themselves are not cancerous, a rare form of uterine cancer (a leiomyosarcoma) may mimic a fibroid, particularly in a postmenopausal woman. This occurs in fewer than 3 out of every 1,000 women with suspected fibroids. Nevertheless, if a mass thought to be a fibroid grows rapidly, or develops in a postmenopausal woman, laparotomy (see entry) may be necessary to rule out cancer.

How are fibroids treated?

Women today have many more treatment choices than they did a decade or two ago, when removal of the uterus (hysterectomy) was the most frequent recommendation for uterine fibroids. These choices often involve weighing a desire to keep the uterus against the risk that fibroids and associated symptoms will return. A woman's proximity to menopause also plays a role in the decision, since most symptoms from fibroids generally resolve after menopause.

A woman who has minor or no symptoms may need only to visit a doctor periodically to see if the fibroids have grown or if the symptoms have worsened. In the past, the standard approach was to do a hysterectomy in women with asymptomatic fibroids once they reached the size of a 12-week pregnancy. This was done because gynecologists were concerned about the difficulty of examining the ovaries in the presence of a large fibroid, and about the potential for surgical complications if hysterectomy later became necessary. Research now suggests that it is just as safe to leave the fibroid and uterus intact as long as a woman has regular checkups to monitor the development of symptoms or of problems in other organs.

If there has been no rapid increase of fibroid size or symptoms, a woman will have to be seen once or twice a year so the size and shape of the fibroids can continue to be monitored. Ultrasound is useful in detecting uncommon (and otherwise hidden) problems, such as blockage of the ureters from an enlarging fibroid. Because in rare cases rapidly enlarging uterine growths, particularly in postmenopausal women, can be a sign of malignancy, regular checkups are vital.

If a woman has more severe symptoms (mainly bleeding or pain) or anemia from excessive blood loss, she may require drug treatment or surgery. Hysterectomy remains an option for any woman who wants to eliminate symptoms permanently, especially if she is over 35 and no longer wants to bear children. Indeed, fibroids account for nearly half of all hysterectomies performed in women in this age range and are the single most common reason for hysterectomies among all women, accounting for 175,000 annually. Unless she is near or past menopause, a woman who has a hysterectomy for fibroids will probably have her ovaries left intact.

Although hysterectomy is the only guarantee of complete freedom from fibroids, it is also a major surgical procedure that requires 4 to 8 weeks for full recovery. And, as with any major surgery, there are certain risks, including infection and bleeding. Despite widespread concerns, there is no convincing evidence that hysterectomy causes long-term mood disturbance or depression. Sexual drive or responsiveness often improves after hysterectomy, particularly if symptoms have been severe; up to 25 percent of women, however, report a decrease in sexual function after a hysterectomy.

Uterine myomectomy is another option for a woman who wants to retain childbearing capacity or to preserve her uterus for other reasons. A surgical procedure with risks similar to those of hysterectomy, myomectomy involves removing fibroids while leaving the uterus in place. This procedure can help alleviate some of the menstrual and pregnancy-related symptoms associated with fibroids.

Usually the fibroids are removed through an abdominal incision called a laparotomy because it can be difficult to remove large fibroids through the vagina. Sometimes doctors may use a procedure called hysteroscopy, especially when smaller fibroids within the uterus produce excessive bleeding or reproductive problems. In this procedure, which circumvents the need for an abdominal incision and shortens hospitalization time, fibroids are removed through a thin telescope-like instrument that has been inserted through the vagina and into the uterus. Only certain fibroids are amenable to this approach.

In as much as a quarter of women, fibroids recur after myomectomy. Although myomectomy is sometimes preferred for treating infertility related to fibroids, in some cases scarring after myomectomy may actually impair fertility. Women who have had an abdominal myomectomy and later become pregnant may require delivery by cesarean section.

An even less invasive approach is uterine fibroid embolization (UFE), a technique used for years to control heavy bleeding after childbirth but only recently applied to the removal of uterine fibroids. In this procedure, usually performed by a radiologist, small particles of plastic or gelatin are injected into the uterine arteries to cut off the blood supply that feeds the fibroids. These particles are injected through a thin tube (a catheter) that has been guided through the leg and up into the uterine artery.

UFE is quick—usually taking only about an hour—and rarely involves more than an overnight stay in the hospital. Pain and cramping after the procedure can almost always be controlled with narcotics, and it is usually possible to go back to work about a week or so after surgery. Risks, while small, include uterine infection or damage. More studies need to be done, however, to determine the effect of UFE on future pregnancies, as well as the possibility that the fibroids will recur.

A nonsurgical option for women with fibroids involves drugs called GnRH agonists (gonadotropin releasing hormone agonists), which suppress estrogen production and produce a temporary (reversible) "artificial menopause." By shrinking fibroids and reducing or eliminating menstrual flow, GnRH agonists (Lupron, Synarel) can help reduce excessive blood loss and alleviate pelvic pain. They may also reduce some of the risks of subsequent surgery.

GnRH agonists often have side effects similar to those of menopause, such as hot flushes, insomnia, thinning of vaginal tissue, and decrease in bone mass, and thus are generally used for no more than 6 months. Fibroids usually return after a woman stops taking these drugs unless she is approaching menopause, a time when fibroids may continue to shrink as estrogen levels decline naturally.

Other medical treatments are sometimes tried prior to surgery. Although the birth control pill has traditionally been thought to aggravate bleeding from fibroids by stimulating their growth, recent research shows that women with fibroids who were taking the pill for other reasons had an overall decrease in their bleeding over time. More research is needed to determine whether oral contraceptives have some role in treating women whose fibroids cause significant bleeding or discomfort.

Other drugs sometimes used to treat fibroid symptoms are progestins and danazol—both hormonal treatments that block the effects of estrogen. There is little research on their effectiveness, however. Nonsteroidal antiinflammatory drugs (NSAIDs) can help relieve pain or discomfort associated with fibroids but have little or no effect on bleeding.

For women whose heavy bleeding causes anemia, increasing iron intake through diet or iron supplements may be sufficient. Iron-rich foods include liver, prune juice, red meat, beans, raisins, and molasses. Iron supplements are available as ferrous sulfate or ferrous gluconate, which should be taken in doses of 300 mg 2 or 3 times a day.

How can fibroids be prevented?

Fibroids cannot be prevented. But because they sometimes seem to grow in response to estrogen, women with fibroids who choose to use birth control pills (which contain synthetic estrogen) should be followed by their physicians to make sure the condition does not worsen. The relatively low doses of estrogen provided by estrogen replacement therapy have recently been shown to have no significant effect on fibroids in most women, despite earlier concerns.

Related entries

Anemia, antiinflammatory drugs, biopsy, cesarean section, dilatation and curettage, endometrial cancer, estrogen replacement therapy, hysterectomy, hysteroscopy, iron, laparotomy, menorrhagia, menopause, oral contraceptives, vaginal bleeding (abnormal)

Vacuum Aspiration

Vacuum aspiration is a surgical procedure in which a syringe or a mechanical pump is used to suction tissue out of the uterus. In addition to being the most common method of first trimester abortion, vacuum aspiration is often performed to biopsy the endometrium (uterine lining) for diagnosing possible causes of abnormal vaginal bleeding, other menstrual irregularities, and infertility.

Sometimes a pregnant woman will start to bleed early in the first trimester and, through ultrasound, her clinician will determine that the fetus is not viable. In those cases, rather than waiting for the miscarriage to follow its natural course, the clinician and patient may choose vacuum aspiration.

The procedure is also occasionally used to remove menstrual fluid just before a normal period is due in order to circumvent menstrual cramps or bothersome menstrual flow. This practice (sometimes called menstrual extraction), which was developed by feminist self-help groups in the 1970s, is by no means widely accepted as safe or justifiable by the mainstream medical profession.

How is the procedure performed?

When used to biopsy endometrial tissue, vacuum aspiration is usually a brief and relatively painless procedure. Sometimes called endometrial aspiration, vacuum curettage, or Vabra, this procedure can be performed in either a doctor's office or a clinic and generally requires no anesthesia. The doctor first inserts a speculum into the vagina, steadies the cervix with a metal clamp (tenaculum), and then inserts a plastic tube (cannula or vacurette) through the cervix and into the uterus. This tube is attached to a syringe or a pump, which suctions out the uterine lining by creating a vacuum. Usually there is no need to dilate (widen) the cervix before inserting the tube, and discomfort is often limited to mild and brief uterine cramping during the suction.

The procedure is essentially the same when vacuum aspiration is used to abort an early pregnancy, although the terminology can be confusing. When vacuum aspiration is done before about 6 weeks of pregnancy (that is, within 6 weeks of the woman's last menstrual period), it is also sometimes called menstrual extraction, minisuction, miniregulation, or miniabortion, or, if the pregnancy has not yet been confirmed, preemptive abortion or endometrial aspiration. Performed after 7 weeks' gestation, it may be called suction abortion, vacuum abortion, or early uterine evacuation. Whatever the name, all of these procedures involve evacuating the contents of an at least potentially pregnant uterus with the aid of vacuum suction.

After 7 weeks of pregnancy it is usually necessary to dilate the cervix to some extent with a series of metal rods of progressively increasing diameter (this procedure is sometimes called dilatation and evacuation, or D&E). Because dilating the cervix can be painful, a local anesthetic (paracervical block) may be used to numb the cervix and surrounding areas. Sometimes a woman may be given the option of having an intravenous tranquilizer to offset her anxiety, particularly if the procedure is being performed on a woman whose pregnancy is not viable and who is distraught about her impending miscarriage.

The fetal tissue and other products of conception are suctioned out of the uterus along with the endometrial lining. The uterus may also be scraped with a curette following the suction to make sure all fetal tissue has been removed, although the need for such a precaution in first trimester abortions remains debatable. A first trimester abortion done by vacuum aspiration usually takes under 10 minutes, although the further the pregnancy has progressed, the longer the procedure.

What happens after the procedure?

Vacuum aspiration can usually be performed in one visit. The woman recuperates for about an hour and then can be discharged to go home. She may gradually resume her normal activities over the next few days but should refrain from intercourse, swimming, bathing, and inserting any objects (such as tampons) into the vagina for 2 weeks.

What are the risks and complications?

The risks of the procedure include uterine perforation and cervical incompetence (a condition in which the cervix does not stay closed during pregnancy), but these risks are very low if the procedure is performed by an experienced surgeon. There is no significantly increased risk of spontaneous miscarriage, preterm delivery, or low birth weight in future pregnancies.

Related entries

Abortion, anesthesia, biopsy, dilatation and curettage, infertility, menstrual cycle disorders, miscarriage, vaginal bleeding (abnormal), vaginal bleeding during pregnancy

Vaginal Atrophy

Vaginal atrophy occurs when decreased levels of the hormone estrogen make the vaginal walls thinner, drier, and less elastic. Often the urethra and vulva are involved as well. These tissues become increasingly sensitive to irritation and susceptible to urinary tract and vaginal infections. Vaginal atrophy is a chronic condition that can sometimes make sexual intercourse uncomfortable or impossible.

Because vaginal irritation is not a symptom unique to vaginal atrophy, it is easily confused with other conditions. When a woman experiences itching in the vulva or the vagina, for example, she and her clinician may simply assume that the problem is caused by a yeast infection. After several futile attempts to treat this "infection" with antifungal drugs, the woman may end up mistakenly labeled as having "recurrent yeast infections."

Who is likely to develop vaginal atrophy?

Vaginal atrophy develops after menopause to some extent in most if not all women. Women who are breastfeeding, using birth control pills, or taking certain drugs to treat endometriosis or fibroids may also develop vaginal atrophy because of unusually low estrogen levels.

What are the symptoms?

Vaginal atrophy often develops so slowly that many women do not notice any changes until 5 or 10 years after menopause. Over time, however, the vaginal walls become perceptibly thinner, smoother (as the ridges—or rugae—flatten out), and lighter in color. As the outer lips and vagina shrink, the urethra, clitoris, and vagina all become more exposed, the vagina becomes shorter or narrower, and pubic hair becomes sparser.

Often these changes predispose women to a form of vaginitis called atrophic vaginitis. Its chief symptoms are itching, dryness, and discomfort in the vaginal and vulvar areas. Some women also notice a watery vaginal discharge. Depending on the amount of thinning that has occurred, sexual intercourse can be mildly to severely painful, and there may be bleeding afterwards.

How is the condition evaluated?

A clinician can usually diagnose vaginal atrophy during a routine pelvic examination. Sometimes a Pap test of vaginal (as opposed to cervical) cells will be done so that cells can be examined more closely. Tissue from affected areas may also be removed and biopsied to help rule out other conditions with similar symptoms, such as lichen sclerosus (see vulvar disorders), vaginal cancer, or precancerous cellular changes.

Postmenopausal women who bleed after intercourse may need to have an endometrial biopsy, since clinicians cannot always tell precisely where the bleeding is coming from. On the chance that it is coming from the uterus rather than the irritated vaginal walls, an endometrial biopsy is necessary to rule out endometrial cancer.

How is vaginal atrophy treated?

The most effective treatment for vaginal atrophy is estrogen replacement therapy. Oral supplements and intravaginal creams are equally effective in alleviating the physical problems associated with this condition. If a postmenopausal woman chooses not to take systemic estrogen for other reasons, she may use an estrogen cream. Inserting the cream into the vagina twice a week is usually effective, although some women find that once a week is sufficient. Estring, a ring containing estrogen that is inserted into the upper third of the vagina and left in place for three months at a time, may be more convenient, though it is also prohibitively expensive for some women. These products should generally be avoided during breastfeeding, although some doctors believe that use of small amounts is safe.

Systemic (oral) estrogen is usually not prescribed for women with a history of breast cancer, but some clinicians are rethinking this restriction on estrogen replacement therapy—particularly for vaginal estrogen, since there are few data linking its use to recurrence of breast cancer.

There are no particularly effective alternatives for women who cannot or choose not to use supplemental estrogen. For women who have only mild symptoms—such as those who have recently undergone menopause, or those who are breastfeeding—water-based vaginal lubricants can relieve vaginal dryness and pain during intercourse, and acidifying agents (such as Aci-Jel) can help reduce the risk of infection and vaginal sensitivity. Many of these products are available without prescription, and some (such as Replens and Astroglide) combine both lubricating and acidifying properties. Generally, however, these products do not work well for moderate or severe atrophy because they have only a negligible effect on the underlying estrogen deficiency. What may help is regular sexual stimulation, which counters some of the dryness by promoting vaginal secretions.

Related entries

Biopsy, estrogen replacement therapy, lubricants, menopause, pain during sexual intercourse, Pap test, pelvic examinations, urinary tract infections, vaginitis, vulvar disorders, yeast infections

Vaginal Bleeding (Abnormal)

Abnormal vaginal bleeding in a woman who is not pregnant can occur for a wide variety of reasons, ranging from normal physiological events to serious life-threatening illness. It can include any spotting or bleeding from the vagina in a postmenopausal woman, irregular or unpredictable bleeding in an adolescent, and heavy or irregular bleeding in a mature woman.

The causes of these problems vary according to both the symptoms and the woman's reproductive stage (see menstrual cycle disorders). In any woman, using medications such as anticoagulants can sometimes produce abnormal vaginal bleeding, as can physical injury to or cancer of the reproductive tract (see cervical cancer, endometrial cancer, fallopian tube cancer, ovarian cancer, vulvar cancer).

Irregular vaginal bleeding in adolescents

Irregular menstrual periods are common for the first 5 years following menarche (the first menstrual period). Although abnormal bleeding in any woman can sometimes signal injury to the reproductive tract or cancer, in adolescents the most frequent cause is anovulatory periods, that is, periods that do not involve the release of an egg from the ovary.

Anovulatory periods are sometimes called dysfunctional uterine bleeding. They are most common in adolescents and in perimenopausal women (premenopausal women over the age of 40). The normal menstrual cycle involves a finely tuned feedback system between the hormones of the hypothalamus, pituitary gland, and ovaries, which works to produce an egg for fertilization and an endometrium (uterine lining) that is receptive to implantation by the fertilized egg.

Normally the pituitary secretes follicle stimulating hormone (FSH), which in turn stimulates several ovarian follicles (cystlike structures which surround the eggs) to develop and secrete estrogen. Estrogen stimulates the endometrium (uterine lining) to thicken, prompts FSH levels to fall, and induces the pituitary to produce increasing amounts of luteinizing hormone (LH), a process known as the "LH surge." Large amounts of LH stimulate the remaining follicle (the Graafian follicle) to mature and release an egg. The ruptured follicle becomes the corpus luteum, a yellow structure that secretes both progesterone and estrogen.

If the egg is not fertilized, these two hormones inhibit the production of FSH and LH, and, as LH levels drop, the corpus luteum atrophies, estrogen and progesterone levels fall, and the thickened endometrium is shed through menstruation.

Often at both ends of the reproductive years, this intricate feedback mechanism does not work properly, and ovulation does not occur. Without ovulation, no corpus luteum forms and so no progesterone is secreted. Constant estrogen secretion by the ovarian follicle thickens the endometrium so that it eventually sheds, resulting in the irregular bleeding that is common in the first years following menarche.

Irregular vaginal bleeding in perimenopausal women

In some ways the menstrual cycle physiology of the perimenopausal woman mirrors that of the adolescent. In the later reproductive years most women find that their menstrual pattern changes. The average length of a menstrual cycle of a woman in her early 20s is 32 days, but many women over the age of 35 have cycles of 28 days or less. The cycles shorten because of inadequate production of progesterone by aging corpora lutea, leading to a shortened luteal phase (the second part of the menstrual cycle).

Eventually, poorer quality and diminished numbers of follicles reduce estrogen production until finally there is not enough estrogen to produce the LH surge and ovulation. Continuous low-level stimulation of the endometrium by estrogen in the absence of progesterone results in endometrial hyperplasia, an overgrowth of the uterine lining that will be shed at irregular intervals. Therefore, women at this stage of the reproductive life cycle, like adolescents, usually go through a phase of dysfunctional uterine bleeding before menses stop altogether and menopause begins.

Abnormal vaginal bleeding in mature women

Abnormal bleeding in mature women (including perimenopausal women) may result from anatomical abnormalities, systemic illnesses, or certain contraceptives. Pregnancy is also a common cause of abnormal bleeding in this age group (see vaginal bleeding during pregnancy).

Anatomical abnormalities. These can occur in the vagina itself (such as a laceration, vaginal cancer, or vaginal atrophy); in the cervix (polyps, cervical cancer, or cervicitis); the uterus (endometrial cancer, adenomyosis, uterine fibroids, endometriosis, or endometritis, a form of pelvic inflammatory disease in which the uterine lining is infected); fallopian tubes (ectopic pregnancy or fallopian tube cancer); or the ovary (ovarian cancer or corpus luteum cyst, a form of ovarian cyst).

Abnormal bleeding may be the only symptom of some of these conditions, but women with endometrial polyps may notice some cramping between menstrual periods. Degenerating uterine fibroids, endometritis, corpus luteum cysts, and adenomyosis can also cause pain.

Any woman who has vaginal bleeding after sexual intercourse should be evaluated for cervical polyps and cervical cancer. Such bleeding may also be due to vaginal atrophy or cervicitis.

Bleeding that occurs between menstrual periods (called breakthrough bleeding) is often a normal and harmless part of ovulation. But bleeding between periods is also a characteristic symptom of endometritis and may also occur in endometrial cancer or after an incomplete miscarriage (when parts of the placenta, fetus, or fetal membranes are retained in the uterus) or ectopic pregnancy (which is a medical emergency; see entry).

Another anatomical cause of abnormal bleeding, which is often self-limiting and requires no treatment, is a persistent corpus luteum. In this condition the corpus luteum survives longer than the usual 10 to 16 days. As a result, the menstrual period is delayed beyond expectation (pregnancy can be ruled out with a blood test for hCG).

Systemic illnesses. Many systemic illnesses are associated with abnormal vaginal bleeding. Hypothyroidism (underproduction of thyroid hormone) and hyperprolactinemia (overproduction of prolactin) can lead to luteal phase defects that increase the frequency of menstruation (resulting in cycle lengths of 16 to 22 days), or to anovulatory bleeding. Stress, anxiety, kidney failure, and anorexia nervosa can all reduce the frequency of menstruation or stop it altogether. Polycystic ovary syndrome, which involves elevated levels of virilizing hormones called androgens (see hyperandrogenism), can produce absent or infrequent periods (see amenorrhea, infrequent periods), along with other symptoms such as obesity, excess hair growth (hirsutism), and enlarged ovaries. Excessive menstrual flow (menorrhagia) may be due to bleeding disorders (see platelet disorders), hypothyroidism, or lupus.

Contraceptives. Using an intrauterine device (IUD) often increases the length of the menstrual period and thus increases the amount of blood lost. Oral contraceptives, by contrast, usually reduce menstrual bleeding, since the low estrogen content of most preparations causes the endometrium to be thinner than in women who ovulate so that there is less of it to be shed. Using an intrauterine device or oral contraceptives can sometimes cause bleeding between menstrual periods as well. Oral contraceptives that produce abnormal bleeding beyond the first 3 cycles of use should be replaced by others with a higher dose of either progesterone or estrogen.

Bleeding or spotting in postmenopausal women

Abnormal bleeding in the postmenopausal woman can be caused by many conditions, including all of the anatomical abnormalities listed above. Most clinicians, however, assume vaginal bleeding in a postmenopausal woman to be caused by some cancer of the reproductive tract until proven otherwise. The more benign causes include obesity, physical trauma to the vagina, and certain medications, including estrogen replacement therapy.

Older women with vaginal atrophy may bleed after sexual intercourse. And obese women often have excess estrogen levels (because fat cells transform androgen hormones from the adrenal glands into estrogen), which in turn promote endometrial hyperplasia, a condition that not only can result in irregular bleeding but also in older women is sometimes a precursor to endometrial cancer.

Women taking estrogen replacement therapy may experience irregular bleeding when treatment first begins. Taking daily estrogen together with a low dose of progesterone may produce irregular, unpredictable bleeding for 3 to 6 months. If this persists beyond 6 months, however, an evaluation for anatomical causes of bleeding should be pursued. In women taking daily doses of estrogens and then adding progestin 10 to 12 days per month, it is normal for light withdrawal bleeding to occur around the time the progestin is stopped.

How is abnormal vaginal bleeding evaluated?

Any nonpregnant woman who is experiencing abnormal vaginal bleeding or spotting should see her primary care practitioner or gynecologist. After first ensuring that the bleeding is from the reproductive tract (and not the rectum or urethra), the practitioner will do a focused pelvic and physical examination and review the woman's medical history and the specific timing and severity of other symptoms. This often helps differentiate many of the causes of vaginal bleeding.

Premenopausal women with even a remote possibility of pregnancy will be given a pregnancy test, as well as tests to see if ovulation is occurring. These tests may involve filling out a basal body temperature chart, measuring serum progesterone levels, or performing an endometrial biopsy. Some women may also need blood tests, cervical cultures for chlamydia and gonorrhea, a Pap test, liver function tests, thyroid function tests, and tests that measure the levels of various hormones. A pelvic ultrasound may also be done to look for fibroids as a cause of bleeding.

A postmenopausal woman who has any kind of vaginal bleeding (with the exception of those who have just started hormone replacement therapy) should have an endometrial biopsy to rule out endometrial hyperplasia or cancer. If these tests are negative, the clinician will want to rule out estrogen- or androgen-producing tumors of the ovary and adrenal glands.

How is abnormal vaginal bleeding treated?

Treatment for abnormal vaginal bleeding depends on its cause. Bleeding that occurs as a result of systemic illnesses such as thyroid, kidney, and liver disorders can be expected to improve once the underlying disease is treated.

Treatment for anovulatory bleeding not due to some underlying condition varies with the age of the woman. In adolescents, observation alone is usually enough. Heavy bleeding (which may lead to iron-deficiency anemia) can usually be controlled with oral contraceptives, which should be discontinued in about 6 months to see if the cycles have normalized. Abnormally frequent periods owing to a shortened or inadequate luteal phase can be treated with oral contraceptives or with progestins or natural progesterone suppositories beginning the day after ovulation. Frequent menstruation that results from a shortened follicular phase (first half of the cycle) usually corrects itself over time.

Anovulatory periods or other dysfunctional uterine bleeding in more mature women may be treated with either progesterone supplements, oral contraceptives (in women who do not wish to become pregnant), or clomiphene citrate (Clomid) in women who are having difficulty becoming pregnant. In perimenopausal women, the progesterone may be supplemented with estrogen until natural menopause occurs. If this is ineffective, a surgeon may consider endometrial ablation. Under the guidance of a hysteroscope (a telescope-like instrument inserted into the uterus through the vagina), parts of the uterine lining are removed through either laser surgery or electrocautery. Hysterectomy (removal of the uterus) may be considered if bleeding cannot be controlled with other treatments.

Related entries

Adenomyosis, anorexia nervosa and bulimia nervosa, biopsy, cervical cancer, dilatation and curettage, electrocautery, endometrial cancer, endometrial hyperplasia, endometriosis, estrogen replacement therapy, hyperandrogenism, hyperprolactinemia, hysterectomy, hysteroscopy, infertility, kidney disorders, laser surgery, menopause, menstrual cycle, menstrual cycle disorders, miscarriage, obesity, ovarian cancer, ovarian cysts, Pap test, pelvic inflammatory disease, platelet disorders, polyps, sexually transmitted diseases, stress, thyroid disorders, uterine fibroids, vaginal atrophy, vaginal bleeding during pregnancy

Vaginal Bleeding during Pregnancy

Most vaginal bleeding that occurs in women of reproductive age at any time except during menstruation is due to a pregnancy-related problem. A pregnant woman should consult her physician promptly if she notices any vaginal bleeding. Although many pregnancies continue successfully despite episodes of bleeding, bleeding can also signal more serious problems that require immediate medical attention.

Who is likely to develop vaginal bleeding during pregnancy?

Over half of pregnant women experience vaginal bleeding during the first trimester (first 3 months) of pregnancy. About half of these women will eventually have a miscarriage (see entry), especially if the bleeding is heavy and associated with cramping. Bleeding can also occur after the implantation of the fertilized egg, or because of an ectopic (tubal) pregnancy or a molar pregnancy (see entries).

Although most women experiencing vaginal bleeding during pregnancy have some problem related to the pregnancy itself, there are many other reasons that can account for bleeding. These include vulvitis, vaginitis, polyps, vaginal or cervical cancer, a foreign body in the uterus, thrombocytopenia (abnormally low levels of platelets, the blood cell responsible for clotting; see platelet disorders), and other diseases or medical treatments that can interfere with blood clotting.

Vaginal bleeding in late pregnancy (third trimester) can merely be "bloody show," the passage of the bloodstained mucus which has kept the cervix closed during the pregnancy; this bleeding occasionally precedes the beginning of labor. Bleeding may also simply result from inflammation of the cervix. Sometimes, however, bleeding in the third trimester signals a more serious disorder, such as placenta previa, placenta abruptio, or premature labor.

In placenta previa, the placenta is located over or near the opening (os) of the cervix. When the cervix begins to dilate, the placenta may detach from the uterine wall and disrupt nearby blood vessels, which leads to heavy though sometimes painless vaginal bleeding. The result can be premature labor. In placenta abruptio, the placenta becomes prematurely detached from the uterine wall, which can deprive the fetus of essential oxygen. Bleeding is often accompanied by constant and severe abdominal pain.

Pregnant women over the age of 35 are about twice as likely to suffer from placenta previa or placenta abruptio as younger women. These conditions are more common in women who have had several previous children or who have had these problems in previous pregnancies. Placenta abruptio is also unusually common in women with hypertension, as well as in women who use cocaine during pregnancy.

In rare instances, vaginal bleeding in the final trimester may be caused by factors unrelated to the pregnancy, such as abnormal tissue growth or trauma to the reproductive tract.

How is the condition evaluated?

Any woman of reproductive age who is experiencing vaginal bleeding between periods will be given a pregnancy test to see if the bleeding is pregnancy-related. If she is not pregnant, other diagnostic tests will be performed to determine the cause of the bleeding (see vaginal bleeding, abnormal).

If she is pregnant, determining the date of the last menstruation will help distinguish bleeding that is due to implantation (which occurs about day 21 of the menstrual cycle) from a possible ectopic pregnancy (which usually does not become symptomatic until 6 to 8 weeks' gestation). A physical examination will help differentiate many of the causes of vaginal bleeding, as can a review of the specific timing and severity of other symptoms such as pain and cramping. If the pregnancy is 6 weeks along, ultrasound can be performed to look for a fetal heartbeat; if none is found, miscarriage is usually inevitable, or the dates may be inaccurate. Most vaginal bleeding early in pregnancy will turn out to be due to either a threatened or an inevitable miscarriage (see entry).

If an ectopic or molar pregnancy is suspected (see entries), blood will be tested for levels of human chorionic gonadotropin (hCG), a hormone produced by the placenta. Levels of hCG fail to rise appropriately in ectopic pregnancy, whereas abnormally high levels of hCG in combination with vaginal bleeding can indicate a molar pregnancy (although occasionally a multiple gestation may also account for the high levels). The diagnosis can be confirmed with ultrasound. In a molar pregnancy the uterus may be larger than it should be at that particular gestational age.

If the serum hCG level is below a certain level (less than 1,500 mU/ml), however—as it may well be in early pregnancy—an ultrasound will not be able to detect a gestational sac. If the woman has severe pain, low blood pressure, and massive bleeding, she should have a laparoscopy to rule out ectopic pregnancy. If her symptoms are less severe, the woman should be observed and her hCG level measured again after 48 hours. If bleeding and pain continue, a dilatation and curettage procedure (D&C; see entry) may be performed to check the uterus for chorionic villi, microscopic fingerlike projections that surround the outermost membrane of a fertilized egg in the early stages of a pregnancy. Villi would be present in the case of a miscarriage, and no further treatment would be required except for monitoring hCG levels until they reach zero. If no villi are found and hCG does not go down, however, an ectopic pregnancy is likely. This can be treated with the drug methotrexate or, if necessary, laparoscopic surgery. If bleeding occurs in late pregnancy, an ultrasound may help determine if placenta previa or placenta abruptio is causing the problem.

How is vaginal bleeding during pregnancy treated?

Treatment of vaginal bleeding depends on its cause. Polyps and other benign lesions of the cervix are often removed in the first trimester; polyps discovered later in pregnancy can usually be watched and removed after delivery, provided that bleeding remains under control. In the case of infections such as vulvitis, vaginitis, or cervicitis, antibiotics appropriate for use in pregnancy are generally prescribed. In the case of an inevitable miscarriage (or a "missed abortion"), a vacuum aspiration or a dilatation and curettage (D&C) may be performed.

Women who are diagnosed as having a molar pregnancy will need to undergo a D&C, sometimes in combination with chemotherapeutic drugs that kill cells—unless the mole is expelled spontaneously, which often occurs near the end of the fourth month of pregnancy. Almost all such moles are noncancerous, but they have the potential to give rise to a cancer called choriocarcinoma.

If bleeding is due to cervical dysplasia (premalignant cervical lesions), cells from the cervix should be evaluated via colposcopy. If cervical cancer is suspected, a gynecologic oncologist, who specializes in cancer of the female reproductive organs, should biopsy the cells.

Placenta previa may require several weeks of hospitalization to prevent premature labor or massive blood loss in the mother. If the baby is sufficiently developed, labor may be induced soon after the bleeding begins. Often a cesarean section will be performed, especially if bleeding is heavy or if there are any signs of fetal distress. In severe placenta abruptio, labor will almost always be induced immediately (or a cesarean section performed), regardless of the fetus's state of development. Sometimes mild or moderate abruptions are simply watched carefully, with steroids given to speed up the maturation of the fetus. This prevents extensive blood loss in the mother as well as oxygen deprivation in the fetus. The mother may need transfusions to replace lost blood and antibiotics to prevent infection.

Related entries

Biopsy, cervical cancer, cesarean section, dilatation and curettage, ectopic pregnancy, laparoscopy, miscarriage, molar pregnancy, platelet disorders, pregnancy, pregnancy over age 35, ultrasound, vacuum aspiration, vaginitis, vulvitis

Vaginitis

Vaginitis literally means inflammation of the vagina. In practice, most clinicians use the term more specifically to mean various conditions in which there is an abnormal vaginal discharge accompanied by vaginal irritation.

Normally, all women produce a slight vaginal discharge, which varies in amount and quality depending on the time in the menstrual cycle. Unlike the discharge of vaginitis, this discharge is odorless, nonirritating, and clear, milky, whitish, or sometimes clumpy. It typically increases as ovulation approaches, when it becomes thin and clear, like egg white. Discharge typically increases during pregnancy, sexual arousal, and stress, or after birth control pills are discontinued.

The discharge that occurs in vaginitis, in contrast, appears gray, greenish, frothy, cheesy, smelly, or particularly profuse. The vagina and vulva burn, itch, or swell (see chart). There may be pain during urination, but unlike the internal burning felt during a urinary tract infection, the urinary pain associated with vaginitis is usually sharp and external because it results from urine hitting the irritated vaginal lips (labia).

Vaginitis is a common and often frustrating problem that can occur whenever something happens to upset the normal balance of organisms that live in the vagina. The vagina is a delicate ecosystem consisting of helpful bacteria called lactobacilli as well as various other microorganisms. The lactobacilli keep potentially dangerous microorganisms in check by breaking down glycogen (the stored form of glucose, or sugar) into lactic acid. This keeps the vagina acidic (pH 3.8 to 4.2) and inhospitable to disease-causing bacteria, fungi, and protozoa.

When the vaginal defenses are down, the way is cleared for various infections, including pelvic inflammatory disease and vaginitis. Women can have more than one type of vaginitis at a time. Among the many factors that can alter the vaginal environment are antibiotics taken to treat another infection, birth control pills, estrogen replacement therapy, douching, diabetes, and pregnancy. Lack of sleep, inadequate diet, poor hygiene, and stress may also lower a woman's resistance to vaginitis. Having sexual intercourse with a partner infected with a sexually transmitted disease is a risk factor as well.

Common types of vaginitis

Bacterial vaginosis. This is the most prevalent form of vaginitis in the United States. It was formerly known as nonspecific vaginosis, hemophilus vaginitis, corynebacterium vaginitis, and Gardnerella vaginitis. Bacterial vaginosis (see entry) is now thought to be caused not by any one specific bacterium but rather by a number of different ones that produce similar symptoms. These include a homogeneous gray,

Common types of vaginitis

Condition	Symptoms	Amount of discharge	Appearance of discharge	Odor of discharge
Normal vagina	None	Usually 4–5 cc per day but increases around time of ovulation and during pregnancy; decreases after menopause	Clear or white	None
Bacterial vaginosis	None or irritation	Increases	Homogeneous, gray	Fishy, especially after intercourse or washing with soap
Yeast infection	Itching, burning	Usually increases	Cottage cheesy, white	Sweet or breadlike
Trichomonas	Itching	Increases	Frothy, green, or gray	Foul
Atrophic vaginitis (in women with vaginal atrophy)	Irritation, itching, pain during sexual intercourse	None or increases	Watery, yellow, or green	None
Cytologic vaginosis	Burning, itching; irritation, pain during sexual intercourse; symptoms may worsen during second half of menstrual cycle	Increases	Clumpy, white	None
Retained foreign bodies (tampons, diaphragms, sponges, pessaries)	None or discharge	Profuse	Watery or bloody	Foul

fishy-smelling discharge (especially after intercourse or washing with soap). There may or may not be irritation.

Yeast infections. These are the second most common form of vaginitis in this country and are caused by a yeast or fungus called Candida. Sometimes they are confused with cytolytic vaginosis (see below). The symptoms of a yeast infection (see entry) include itching and burning, along with a cottage-cheesy discharge that may smell sweet or bread-like.

Trichomonas. The third most common form of vaginitis in the United States is trichomonas (see entry), a sexually transmitted disease caused by a one-celled parasite. The symptoms are itching and a foul-smelling, frothy green or gray discharge.

Cytolytic vaginosis. If there is burning, itching, and irritation of the vulvar area, pain during sexual intercourse, and a clumpy white discharge—and especially if symptoms worsen during the second half of the menstrual cycle—cytolytic vaginosis (see entry) may be the correct diagnosis. The organism causing this newly described condition has not been identified, and the condition may result simply from an overgrowth of lactobacilli.

Other organisms. Occasionally vaginitis can result from overgrowth of other bacteria, including *Streptococcus* (which commonly colonizes the vagina without causing inflammation) or *E. coli* (which normally resides in the gastrointestinal tract). Vaginitis can also result from *Shigella* bacteria infections. A clinician may suspect this rare infection in a postmenopausal woman who has diarrhea as well as symptoms of vaginitis. Occasionally women who have recently visited an undeveloped part of the world may acquire amoebic vaginal infections. Symptoms include a foul-smelling and often bloody discharge, as well as sores on the vagina.

Atrophic vaginitis. Itching, irritation, and a watery yellow or green discharge can occur in postmenopausal women or others with low levels of the hormone estrogen (including breastfeeding mothers). This is due to vaginal atrophy, the thinning of the tissue in the vaginal walls, which makes women more susceptible to infections. The condition can make sexual intercourse painful.

Retained foreign bodies. Occasionally a forgotten tampon, diaphragm, or pessary (a device inserted into the vagina for medical purposes) can result in vaginitis. The discharge will usually be watery or bloody, profuse, and very malodorous.

Psychological or emotional problems. Clinicians may diagnose "psychosomatic vaginitis" when there is no apparent infection or other physical abnormality but there is a long history of symptoms (often including pain during sexual intercourse) which have not responded to treatment. This diagnosis does not make the symptoms any less real or painful, however (see psychosomatic disorders).

How is vaginitis evaluated?

It is often difficult to differentiate one form of vaginitis from another. Part of the problem is that the three most common forms—bacterial vaginosis, yeast infections, and trichomonas—often have overlapping symptoms. Also, some women with vaginitis have unusual symptoms while others may have none at all. And because vaginitis is often regarded as a relatively trivial medical problem, some clinicians tend to make quick diagnoses—which, when inaccurate, only make treatment more frustrating. For example, women are often diagnosed as having yeast infections as soon as they complain of vulvar itching and the clinician sees a thick white vaginal discharge. Similarly, when women who originally had a yeast infection return to the doctor with the same symptoms, they are assumed to have a "recurrent" problem, when in fact this time around they may actually have bacterial vaginosis, or vice versa. As a result women are often falsely labeled as having "recurrent yeast infections" or "chronic bacterial vaginosis."

With a little extra time, accurate diagnosis can be relatively simple and inexpensive. After performing a routine pelvic examination, a clinician usually needs only to test vaginal acidity (pH) and inspect vaginal secretions under a microscope to distinguish one form of vaginitis from another. Occasionally it may be necessary to culture cells from the secretions in a laboratory to see what kinds of microorganisms are involved. A clinician must rule out cancers of the reproductive organs (endometrial cancer, cervical cancer, and vaginal cancer), which can also cause an abnormal vaginal discharge.

When painful sexual intercourse is a symptom, the clinician will want to make sure the problem is not vulvar vestibulitis, a physical disorder that sometimes can be treated with local injections or surgery (see vulvar pain). Several other skin conditions of the vulva can cause symptoms that mimic vaginitis (see vulvar disorders). If no physical cause can be determined, the clinician may ask questions to see if the symptoms are perhaps psychosomatic.

How is vaginitis treated?

For vaginal infections the standard treatment is a specific medication (such as an antimicrobial cream or pill) which kills the responsible microorganism. Sometimes the woman's sexual partner may need to take the drug as well.

Some women prefer treating themselves, at least initially, with sitz baths or Betadine douches (available premixed from pharmacies). Quick relief can also come from applying an acidifying gel (such as Aci-Jel) or a nonprescription corticosteroid cream to painful or itchy areas. It is important to consult a clinician if symptoms do not clear up within a couple of days, to make sure the vaginitis is not due to a sexually transmitted disease that requires prompt medical attention.

Vaginitis caused by a foreign object in the vagina is usually relieved soon after the object is removed. Inserting estrogen creams and acidifying agents (such as Aci-Jel) into the vagina can alleviate any discharge associated with a pessary. Finally, if the vaginitis appears to be psychosomatic, psychotherapy may be necessary.

How can vaginitis be prevented?

Some basic health and hygiene practices may help prevent both vaginitis and vulvitis (irritation of the vulva). Getting enough rest, eating a nutritious diet, and finding ways to cope with stress can increase resistance to vaginal infections. In addition, keeping the vulva as clean, dry, and cool as possible can prevent the overgrowth of harmful microorganisms, as can wiping from front to back after a bowel movement so that bacteria from the gastrointestinal tract do not spread into the vaginal area.

Douching can actually predispose a woman to vaginal infections by changing the acidity of the vagina and encouraging the growth of potentially harmful microorganisms. Similarly, tampons and sanitary napkins that contain deodorants, and feminine hygiene sprays, may do more harm than good by killing some of the protective lactobacilli.

Many women prone to vaginitis and vulvitis advocate avoiding undergarments made of synthetic fabrics and tight jeans, probably because these increase heat and moisture and therefore foster bacterial growth. There is also some evidence suggesting that spermicidal jellies, creams, or foams that contain the chemical nonoxynol-9 may help prevent the spread of certain sexually transmitted microorganisms. Spermicides themselves, however, can sometimes cause vaginal irritation.

If vaginal atrophy is a problem, or if sexual intercourse is painful, using a water-soluble lubricant (such as Astroglide) can help prevent unnecessary irritation to vaginal tissues.

Some women douche once or twice a week with a solution of 1 or 2 tablespoons of white vinegar per quart of warm water, a method that is probably safe but has not been proved effective in any scientific study. In addition, douching may interfere with the growth of normal vaginal flora. Boric acid capsules are also sometimes used to acidify the vagina.

The common advice to cut back on coffee, alcohol, sugar, and refined carbohydrates is not supported by actual evidence (although a woman may want to cut down on such things for other reasons). Nor is there any evidence that diets high in sugar or any of these other substances radically alter the normal acidity of the vagina.

Related entries

Alternative therapies, antibiotics, bacterial vaginosis, birth control, cytolytic vaginosis, douching, estrogen replacement therapy, pain during sexual intercourse, pelvic inflammatory disease, psychosomatic disorders, psychotherapy, sexually transmitted diseases, stress, trichomonas, urinary tract infections, vaginal atrophy, vulvar pain, vulvitis, yeast infections

Varicose Veins

Varicose veins are enlarged, twisted, or swollen veins. Although any vein can become varicose, the veins most frequently affected are the ones lying just under the skin on the back of the legs and the inner part of the calves (see illustration). These include the veins in the saphenous system (the saphenous veins are the two large superficial veins in the leg), and the veins in the perforator system (a system of veins connecting the deep and the superficial veins of the legs). When veins of the rectum or anus become varicose, they are called hemorrhoids (see entry).

Varicose veins occur when the valves inside the veins malfunction. Veins are thin-walled blood vessels which carry deoxygenated blood back to the heart and lungs. Blood in the leg veins has to pulse upward toward the heart against the force of gravity. The valves in the veins help keep the blood from flowing back down between pulses, opening up only when pressure from below becomes irresistible. When the walls of a vein stretch out or the valve weakens, however, blood starts to pool up behind the valve. As a result, the vein beneath the valve becomes enlarged and increasingly distorted over time.

Frequently the varicosities can be seen through the skin in the form of unsightly dark blue networks of twisted, raised, or ropey veins. These may also be accompanied by spider veins (telangiectases), a mild and common form of varicose veins which form a hair-thin network of bluish-purple lines near the surface of the skin.

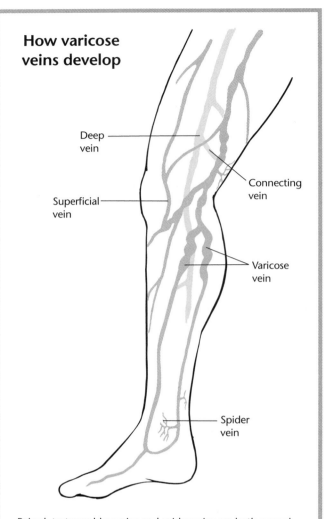

How varicose veins develop

Deep vein

Connecting vein

Superficial vein

Varicose vein

Spider vein

Raised, tortuous blue veins and spider veins are both caused by a defect in the valve of a vein that causes blood to back up and distort the shape of the vein. When saphenous or other large veins near the surface of the leg develop valve failure, they start to resemble knotted blue twine. Spider veins are about the diameter of a hair and occur most commonly on the thigh and ankle.

Who is likely to develop varicose veins?

Varicose veins occur in about 1 in 4 Americans of both sexes, but they are about twice as likely to appear in women as in men. This may be because pregnancy seems to promote the development of varicose veins in many women, in both the legs and the vulva. This, in turn, may be related to hormonal changes in early pregnancy, as well as to the restriction of blood flow from the leg veins to the pelvis by the enlarging uterus. Many women find that varicose veins appear earlier and are more noticeable with each pregnancy.

In addition to pregnancy, simply being a woman or being over 40 increases the likelihood of developing varicose veins.

Other risk factors include congenital weakness of the valves, previous thrombophlebitis (see circulatory disorders), obesity, wearing garments that restrict blood flow in the pelvis and calves, and jobs that involve long periods of standing. Varicose veins tend to run in families, for reasons still little understood.

What are the symptoms?

There are no specific symptoms associated with spider veins beyond the appearance of the spider-like patterns through the skin of the leg. Many women with varicose veins report that their legs become swollen or feel heavy, achy, or tired, particularly at the end of the day. Some women also find that their symptoms are particularly noticeable during menstruation.

In more severe forms of varicose veins, the legs may develop a brownish-gray discoloration, itching, or scaling, particularly around the ankles. Increased pressure from above can produce skin ulcers in the same area. This is more likely if some of the veins farther below the surface (the deep veins) are affected. In rare instances, varicose veins can become inflamed (a condition called phlebitis), develop blood clots (thrombophlebitis), or bleed.

How is the condition evaluated?

Women often diagnose their own varicose veins simply from appearance, but looks alone do not always indicate the extent of the problem. To judge this accurately, a clinician will often feel the legs and look for swelling while the woman is standing. If elevating the legs above the level of the heart relieves leg pain, there is a good chance that the problem is varicose veins.

For a more precise diagnosis the clinician may do additional tests, including Doppler ultrasound, a noninvasive test that measures blood flow in the veins, and venography, which allows visualization of the veins by x-ray after they have been injected with a contrast dye. The clinician may also ask some questions or conduct several tests to rule out other conditions that may account for the swollen veins. These may include various nerve disorders (which may be caused by diabetes or alcohol abuse), osteoarthritis of the hip or knee, and other circulatory disorders.

How are spider veins and varicose veins treated?

No treatment is medically necessary for spider veins since they never pose any medical problems. If the cosmetic problems begin to interfere with a woman's enjoyment of life, however, covering them with makeup is a possible option. Spider veins can also be treated with laser surgery or sclerotherapy.

Once a vein has become varicose, there is no way to return it to its original state. For this reason most treatment merely involves relieving the symptoms. For many women, wearing elastic support hosiery (from the time they get out of bed in the morning until they go to sleep at night) seems to do the trick. Store-bought support hose usually suffice for mild

symptoms, but if symptoms persist, a clinician can prescribe fitted stockings that are heavier and put more pressure on the lower legs. Pantyhose are preferable to below-the-knee stockings since they provide uniform pressure along the entire course of the vein. Women with arthritis or certain other conditions that make it difficult to get into pantyhose might ask their clinician to prescribe a special kind of zippered pantyhose.

Another simple way to relieve the symptoms of varicose veins is to elevate the legs above the level of the heart. Exploiting the force of gravity, this position makes it easier for blood to flow in the right direction through the veins without the help of the valves. Women with varicose veins should spend some time at the end of each day in this position. It is also a good idea to prop up the legs and feet on a stool or chair when sitting. Regular exercise, walking, or flexing the feet and ankles frequently when sitting helps propel the blood toward the heart and prevent further swelling.

If varicose veins are causing severe pain, inflammation, bleeding, skin ulcers, or serious cosmetic concerns, surgery may be necessary. Unless symptoms are severe, surgery of any sort should be postponed until after delivery in pregnant women with varicose veins. Many varicosities clear up spontaneously within 6 months of childbirth.

Vein stripping. In this procedure the surgeon ties off the upper end of the vein to stop backflow of blood from any defective valves and then makes an incision in the skin above the lower end of the vein. Next a plastic or metal wire is threaded from the bottom of the vein up through the groin, and defective tributary veins are tied off. Then the larger vein is lifted away. Depending on the number of veins involved, this procedure can be done under either local or spinal anesthesia either in the hospital or as outpatient surgery. Afterwards the leg must be kept elevated for 6 to 8 hours and then wrapped with elastic bandages or stockings for at least 6 weeks.

The most frequent complication of vein stripping is bleeding under the skin, but this is rarely serious. The loss of a few veins is generally no problem either, since circulation is merely rerouted to nearby veins, and the vast majority of women who have had this procedure experience excellent long-term benefits. Stripping one vein, however, is no guarantee that other, formerly healthy veins will not become varicose at a later time. And despite its effectiveness, stripping veins has become less popular since the advent of coronary bypass surgery, which generally requires the use of one of the large superficial leg veins (saphenous veins). A woman who has coronary artery disease (see entry)—or a family history that puts her at high risk for coronary artery disease—should think twice before sacrificing a saphenous vein. Of course, if a saphenous vein is varicose from ankle to groin, stripping it makes more sense, since it will hardly be of value in some later surgical procedure.

Sclerotherapy. This alternative to vein stripping is a technique that only recently became available in the United

States. It involves injecting a solution of highly concentrated saline (salt) into the affected veins until they collapse. Circulation is unaffected because blood simply reroutes itself into one of the many other available veins in the leg. Sclerotherapy (see entry) works for spider veins as well as varicose veins.

How can spider veins and varicose veins be prevented?

There is no known way to prevent the formation of spider veins. Keeping weight within normal limits, exercising regularly (particularly walking, swimming, and bicycling), avoiding long periods of sitting or standing, and keeping the legs elevated when sitting may keep varicose veins from appearing or from becoming worse. Constrictive garments such as girdles, garter belts, or socks with tight elastic cuffs, which cut off the blood flow by squeezing off a limited area of the vessel, should be avoided. Women with a family history of varicose veins might also try wearing support hose as a preventive measure, particularly during pregnancy.

Related entries

Circulatory disorders, coronary artery disease, hemorrhoids, pregnancy, sclerotherapy, ultrasound

Vitamins and Minerals

Technically known as micronutrients, vitamins and minerals are a group of chemicals essential to the smooth operation of many normal body processes. In general, the body must obtain these essential nutrients from foods, dietary supplements, or other outside sources.

Vitamins not only help in the breakdown of foods but also play a crucial role in the production of cells, hormones, and genetic material. Only small amounts of vitamins are sufficient to facilitate these processes, but their absence can produce serious deficiency symptoms. Although the body (and bacteria inside the intestinal tract) can synthesize some of the vitamins on its own, at least in small amounts, the chief source is still a balanced, varied diet.

There are two basic groups of vitamins: fat-soluble (A, D, E, and K) and water-soluble (B vitamins and C). When fat-soluble vitamins are abundant, they can be stored in the liver and drawn upon for up to 6 months. By contrast, excessive amounts of water-soluble vitamins are generally excreted in the urine.

The minerals needed in the human diet (essential minerals) are chemicals found in nonliving substances. These minerals are usually categorized as either major minerals or trace elements. The major minerals (calcium, phosphorus, magnesium, sulfur, sodium, potassium, and chloride) are needed in relatively large amounts, whereas the trace elements (iron, zinc, iodine, selenium, copper, manganese, fluoride, chromium, and molybdenum) are needed only in small amounts. (See entries on calcium, iron, and zinc).

What are the recommended levels of vitamins and minerals?

Currently, specific recommendations about vitamin and mineral intake come in three different forms—dietary reference intakes (DRIs), reference daily intakes (RDIs), and daily reference values (DRVs). These recommendations continue to be modified as new research comes in but are still generally good guidelines.

Recently developed by the National Research Council's Food and Nutrition Board, the DRIs are a set of reference values that designate daily intake of each of various vitamins and minerals. These values vary depending on age, reproductive status, sex, and other factors. They are meant to replace and expand earlier standards issued by the Food and Nutrition Board (Recommended Dietary Allowances, or RDAs), which also vary by age and sex (see tables on pages 354–357) and are intended to incorporate new findings about the role nutrients play in preventing nutritional deficiency diseases and in reducing the risk of chronic diseases.

Reference daily intakes were developed separately by the Food and Drug Administration. Unlike the values set by the National Research Council, the RDIs recommend only one dosage of vitamins and minerals regardless of age, gender, or reproductive status. Because they were established to help prevent deficiency disease in people with the greatest needs, they are usually set at the highest level recommended for that vitamin by the National Research Council—except for pregnant and breastfeeding women. As a result, the RDIs tend to err on the side of generosity.

An even newer term used to describe vitamin and mineral content on food labels is "daily reference value." This value indicates the amount of a nutrient provided by a single serving of the food in question—specifically, the percentage of the recommended daily intake for a given nutrient provided by a serving of this food, assuming a 2,000-calorie-per-day diet. Women who require fewer or more calories per day will need to modify the daily values accordingly. For some nutrients, daily value is represented in terms of the weight of the nutrient found in one serving of the food, but for most vitamins and minerals it is merely the percentage of the nutrient contained in a single serving.

It is important not to regard any set of recommendations as some kind of quota that needs to be reached on a daily or even near-daily basis. These standards are used not just for assessing any individual's diet but also to help professionals assess the nutritional standards of the American population as a whole. The recommendations are also used to set standards for school lunch and food stamps programs as well as to establish guidelines for feeding in nursing homes and other health care facilities.

The RDAs in particular are generally more useful in assessing the average food intake of a large group of people than in determining the adequacy of any individual woman's diet. A woman who is ill, taking medications, or undergoing unusual stress may need more or less of a vitamin than the amount set down as an RDA. For example, there is some evidence that cigarette smoking may decrease the body's ability to maintain normal levels of vitamin C; these levels also seem to fall with the use of birth control pills, as do levels of folic acid and vitamin B_6. And women who are trying to prevent osteoporosis by taking high doses of calcium usually need to increase their vitamin D intake to 800 mg, since vitamin D facilitates the absorption of calcium. Differences in body size, percentage of body fat, metabolism rate, and heredity can also alter an individual woman's needs in a way the RDAs simply cannot take into account. No individual woman should regard an RDA as anything more than a general guideline.

Many critics, in both the mainstream and alternative health professions, maintain that the RDAs and other recommended levels of nutrients may sometimes be too low because they are based on typical rather than optimal intake of vitamins. Thus, recent recommendations for folic acid intake were reduced because most women found it difficult to consume large amounts, not because there were any objective data showing that smaller amounts were preferable.

Critics also contend that the RDAs do not take into account new research and thinking about the possible role certain vitamins may play in preventing and even curing disease. In recent years researchers have claimed, for example, that large doses of vitamins C, E, and A (in the form of beta carotene) in particular could help prevent the common cold and reduce the risk of cataracts, cardiovascular disease, and even certain cancers (although there is equally convincing evidence negating their findings). Some women find that higher than recommended doses of vitamin E are helpful in relieving menopausal hot flushes.

What are the risks of dietary supplements?
Without question, eating a healthy, balanced diet is the best way to ensure adequate intake of these vitamins and minerals. But because many women eat irregular meals or subsist on low-calorie diets, taking multivitamins, which balance the RDA dosages in 1-to-1 ratios, may be advisable.

For the most part, individual decisions to supplement specific vitamins and minerals must be made with great caution. Until there are better data available about the role of these substances in disease prevention, there is no reason to think that ingesting a higher than recommended level will miraculously guarantee long and healthy life or compensate for a lifetime of unhealthy habits. In fact, sometimes megadoses of vitamins or minerals can be downright dangerous or even fatal. This is particularly true of fat-soluble vitamins, which are not eliminated in the urine when taken in higher than needed doses. But it now appears that even the water-soluble vitamins (with the possible exceptions of vitamins B_2, and B_{12}) can be dangerous if taken in larger than needed doses.

Even the promising antioxidant vitamins such as vitamin E and beta carotene should generally be obtained through foods rather than supplements. This is because most of the research suggesting an association between greater intake of these vitamins and health benefits has so far involved consumption of antioxidant-rich foods and therefore has not shown that the health benefits were *directly* linked to the antioxidant vitamins per se. In some cases (particularly beta carotene), increased intake of dietary supplements was actually associated with negative health effects (i.e., an increase in lung cancer risk among male smokers). Until more studies address these issues, therefore, the American Heart Association continues to recommend consuming a diet high in fruits, vegetables, and grains in lieu of taking supplements of vitamin E, beta carotene, or other antioxidants.

Furthermore, it is becoming increasingly clear that vitamins and minerals, like other nutrients, work synergistically with other vitamins and minerals—which means that dosing up on a single nutrient can be counterproductive if it interferes with the absorption of some other, equally vital nutrient. Nutrients do not seem to work in any kind of simple, black and white manner. At least for now, therefore, the best way to ensure adequate vitamin and mineral intake is to eat a balanced diet that emphasizes variety and moderation. In addition to the vitamins and minerals themselves, whole foods also contain other substances (phytochemicals), some of them still unidentified, which may be involved in producing some of the health benefits attributed to vitamins and minerals alone.

Related entries
Alternative medicine, anemia, anorexia nervosa and bulimia nervosa, calcium, cholesterol, coronary artery disease, iron, nutrition, osteoporosis, smoking, zinc

Vulvar Cancer

Cancer of the vulva is relatively rare, accounting for just 3 to 5 percent of all tumors of the female reproductive organs. The vulva includes all of a woman's external genitalia: the pubic mound, the labia majora, the labia minora, the vaginal opening and nearby glands, the urethral opening, and the clitoris. Preinvasive disease is called vulvar intraepithelial neoplasia (VIN), which is confined to the skin of the vulva. VIN is not cancer but rather a precancerous change in the vulvar skin that may go away on its own, or may eventually develop into cancer. Early invasive cancer—stage 1 (less than 2 cm in size) and stage 2 (greater than 2 cm)—is confined to the vulva. But if not treated it can eventually extend to nearby tissues or spread (metastasize) through the lymphatic system to other organs.

The most common type of vulvar cancer, accounting for 90 percent of all cancers that originate in the vulva, is squamous cell carcinoma, a type of skin cancer. About 5 percent of vulvar cancer is melanoma (see entry), another type of skin cancer.

Who is likely to develop vulvar cancer?

Invasive cancers occur most commonly in postmenopausal women, with a peak occurring at age 70 to 79. In contrast, VIN occurs more frequently in women in their 20s and 30s, probably because of an association with the human papilloma virus (HPV), which causes genital warts and has been implicated in cervical cancer, or with herpes simplex virus II. Both of these infections are sexually transmitted (see sexually transmitted diseases). Clinicians are seeing an increasing number of HPV-related invasive vulvar cancers in women in their 40s.

There is some inconclusive evidence that women who take drugs that suppress the immune system or have diabetes are at increased risk of developing cancer of the vulva. Vulvar cancer is three times more common in white women than in African American women.

About 10 percent of women with vulvar cancer also have another separate cancer in some other part of the lower genital tract, usually the cervix (see cervical cancer).

What are the symptoms?

All too often women and health care providers ignore vulvar abnormalities and symptoms, with the result that diagnosis and treatment of vulvar cancer is delayed for up to a year. The most common symptom of vulvar cancer is persistent itching in the vulva. Often there will be white, dark, red, raised, or warty lumps or sores on the outer lips of the vulva (labia majora), and, less frequently, on the inner lips (labia minora), clitoris, or perineum (the area between the inner lips and the anus). There may also be vulvar burning, pain, discharge, or bleeding. If the cancer has advanced to the invasive stage, there may be a large mass on the vulva or groin.

How is the condition evaluated?

Diagnosing vulvar cancer requires both a careful physical examination and a vulvar biopsy. Usually a punch biopsy (see biopsy) can be done in a clinician's office with local anesthesia. Sometimes a special type of microscope called a colposcope may be used to examine any abnormalities not visible to the naked eye. Since vulvar cancer often occurs simultaneously with other genital cancers, a Pap test and complete pelvic examination will usually be done during the same visit.

How is vulvar cancer treated?

Although readily curable, vulvar cancer is often neglected for years or assumed to be vulvitis (an inflammation of the vulva) and treated with creams and lotions. The type of treatment that is appropriate depends on the extent of the cancer. For VIN, treatment is designed to eradicate the affected area while preserving as much of the original appearance and sexual function of the genitals as possible. If the area is small, applying a topical cream containing the chemotherapy agent 5-fluorouracil (Efudex) may be helpful, although complications can include burning and ulceration. Using this drug can also alter cell appearance so that a biopsy may falsely indicate cancer.

Larger noninvasive lesions may require a simple vulvectomy. In this operation, skin from the clitoris, the labia, and the surrounding vulvar area is removed. New skin usually grows over the area, although skin grafts may be required to close the wound. Alternatively, skin may be removed with laser surgery. Although it is associated with more postoperative pain, laser surgery generally leads to less scarring and faster healing.

Since the 1940s the standard procedure for treating invasive vulvar cancer has been a radical vulvectomy, an operation involving the removal of the vaginal lips, clitoris, underlying glands in the groin, part of the vagina, and skin between the lymph glands and the tumor. This procedure can be done under general or regional anesthesia and a hospital stay of 1 day to 2 weeks. Although a very successful procedure in terms of prolonging life, radical vulvectomy leads to complications including scarring and wound breakdown and, eventually, swelling in the lower legs, vaginal stricture (stenosis), and weakened pelvic muscles that can lead to a fallen bladder (cystocele) or bulging of the rectal wall into the vagina (rectocele). Thus, in recent years there has been more effort to individualize treatment by removing only as much tissue as is necessary to ensure a cure rate similar to that of radical vulvectomy.

If the cancer has spread to the lymph nodes, radiation therapy is usually given after surgery. In addition, women who are not good candidates for surgery because of exceptionally large tumors or involvement of adjacent organs may receive more radiation therapy and chemotherapy. This may shrink tumors enough to allow surgery with fewer potential complications.

How can vulvar cancer be prevented?

Vulvar cancer can be prevented or detected early by careful physical examination and biopsies of skin changes, and by avoiding sexually transmitted diseases. Limiting sexual contacts and using condoms may lower risk for VIN.

Related entries

Biopsy, birth control, cervical cancer, chemotherapy, condoms, cystocele/urethrocele/rectocele, diabetes, laser surgery, melanoma, Pap test, pelvic examinations, radiation therapy, safer sex, sexually transmitted diseases, vulvar disorders, vulvitis

Vulvar Cysts

Various types of cysts—enclosed sacs that usually contain a liquid or semisolid material—often develop on the external female genitalia. The most common ones are Bartholin's cysts, which appear on one or both of the Bartholin's glands. These are a pair of small, normally unnoticeable mucus-secreting glands located in the vestibular bulbs on either side of the vaginal opening. If some obstruction near the opening of these glands blocks mucus secretion, a cyst can develop. This cyst is usually painless and does not require treatment, but it is prone to infection by various microorganisms, including the gonococcus (responsible for gonorrhea), in which case a painful abscess (collection of pus) may form (see illustration).

Benign (noncancerous) lesions or small abscesses also often develop in the outer lips of the vulva (the labia majora). Sometimes these are infections of the hair follicle which disappear on their own after a few days. More often they are sebaceous cysts. These are slow-growing, fluid-filled growths which develop when the sebaceous (oil) glands become obstructed. Sebaceous gland cysts are common in other parts of the body as well, including the breasts, face, ears, scalp, and back. They are generally harmless but may become infected and painful.

Who is likely to develop vulvar cysts?
Anything that obstructs the ducts to the Bartholin's glands—such as a vaginal infection or trauma to the vulva—can increase the risk of developing a Bartholin's cyst or abscess.

What are the symptoms?
Bartholin's gland cysts are usually soft but not tender swellings that appear on the inner lips of the vulva, or just inside the vaginal entrance. Large cysts can extend under the outer

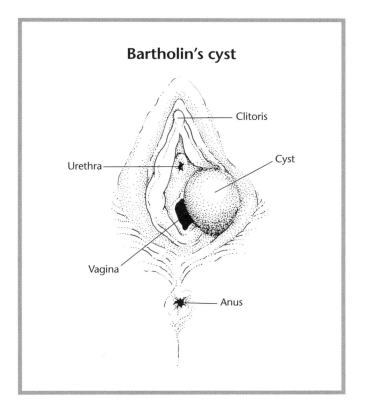

Bartholin's cyst

lips as well. If an abscess has formed, the lump will be red, hot, and extremely tender.

Both sebaceous cysts and infections of the hair follicle occur under the skin. Cysts resulting from a hair follicle infection can vary in size from about one-eighth of an inch to over an inch in diameter. They are usually solitary and tender. Sebaceous cysts range from about one-eighth of an inch to over half an inch and are usually soft, smooth, and yellowish in color. Sometimes they have a small black dot in the middle.

How is the condition evaluated?
Usually a clinician evaluating a vulvar cyst will do a punch biopsy so that the tissue can be examined in a laboratory. This is done not only to distinguish the various types of cysts but also to rule out the rare cancer of the vulva (especially if the woman is postmenopausal) and other medical conditions. If a Bartholin's gland abscess is suspected, a culture will probably be done to test for gonorrhea.

How are vulvar cysts treated?
Small Bartholin's cysts can generally be left untreated unless they cause discomfort. Larger ones may have to be surgically opened and drained. If an abscess has formed, surgery is imperative, as is aggressive therapy with antibiotics. Usually this surgery can be done in a doctor's office with local (if any) anesthesia, although some doctors may want to hospitalize the patient and operate using regional or general anesthesia in order to make a more thorough evaluation of the growths. Often the patient goes home with a small catheter inserted into the swollen gland to drain excess fluid. This drain may have to be left in place for several weeks.

Although this surgery quickly relieves pain, Bartholin's cysts and abscesses often recur. This is because scar tissue from the first infection serves as a new obstruction to mucus secretion. Usually recurrences are treated through a process called marsupialization. In this procedure, which can be done under local anesthesia in a doctor's office, the cyst is removed and the gland is cut and stitched into a pouch so that fluid can drain from it. There may be some tenderness and swelling in the vulva for several weeks afterward, which can be relieved by soaking in a sitz bath. If gonorrhea is present, it needs to be treated promptly with antibiotics.

Sebaceous cysts should generally be left alone. In fact, aspirating fluid from them may introduce bacteria that can result in a painful abscess. If a cyst does become infected, sitz baths or other applications of moist heat may stimulate drainage. Otherwise the cyst can be lanced and drained on an outpatient basis with local anesthesia. The wall of the cyst may need to be removed to prevent the cyst from recurring.

Inflamed hair follicles generally drain on their own without any medical or surgical attention. Many women find that hot baths relieve the pain from these and other vulvar cysts.

Related entries
Anesthesia, antibiotics, biopsy, gonorrhea, vulvar cancer, vulvar disorders, vulvitis

Vulvar Disorders

The vulva is a woman's external genitalia. This includes the pubic mound (mons pubis), the outer lips (labia majora), the inner lips (labia minora), the vaginal opening and nearby glands, the urethral opening, and the clitoris (see illustration). It is subject to a number of varying disorders involving different degrees of pain, itching, burning, irritation, redness, and swelling.

Types of vulvar disorders

Among the most common vulvar disorders are lichen sclerosus, lichen planus, vulvitis, vulvar pain, vulvar cysts, vulvar cancer, pubic lice, and genital warts. Vaginitis (see entry) can also involve the vulva.

Lichen sclerosus. Lichen sclerosus is one of a group of conditions that involve abnormal skin changes in the vulva. Although it is not usually serious, it can cause annoying itching and, in rare cases, may be a precursor of vulvar cancer. Up to 5 percent of women with lichen sclerosus go on to develop malignancies of the vulva, while about 10 percent of women who already have vulvar cancer also have lichen sclerosus.

The cause of this condition is still not fully understood, but recent evidence suggests that it may have something to do with a defect in the immune system. Lichen sclerosus (also known in the past as atrophic vulvar dystrophy) can appear at any age but is most common in women who are past menopause. Some investigators think it may run in families.

Lichen sclerosus usually begins as an isolated itchy white patch on the vulva. Over time it may extend over the entire vulva as well as to the area around the anus. If the woman scratches to relieve the often unbearable itching, the tissue may become red, painful, and eroded. Isolated thickened areas also may develop from scratching, sometimes accompanied by tiny blue or purplish patches where bleeding has occurred under the skin. The labia and clitoral hood take on a glistening, paper-like appearance and appear to be shrinking (although they are not). This gives the illusion that the vaginal opening is narrowing.

Because lichen sclerosus occasionally occurs together with vulvar cancer, a biopsy of the vulva is particularly important for correct diagnosis. A woman who has had this condition for years and then develops vulvar pain also needs to be investigated for vulvar cancer—especially because persistent fiery red areas can mask underlying cancer. Vulvar biopsies usually involve a punch biopsy, which can be done in the clinician's office with local anesthesia. At the same time, abnormalities in the vulva and vagina can be examined with the aid of a special type of microscope called a colposcope.

Itching can usually be relieved by applying corticosteroid creams (usually in prescription strength) to the affected area. When symptoms are more severe, the standard treatment

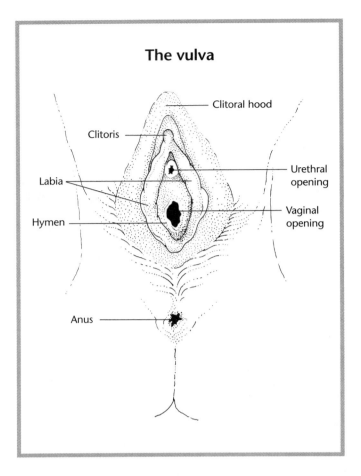

The vulva

Clitoral hood

Clitoris

Labia

Hymen

Urethral opening

Vaginal opening

Anus

has been a testosterone cream rubbed into the skin twice daily until there is some improvement and then used twice weekly on a maintenance basis. This topical cream rarely leads to any side effects except, on occasion, enlargement of the clitoris.

Some newer drugs are becoming the preferred treatment for this condition. These include superpotent topical steroid drugs such as temovate (Clobetasol), which do not produce the serious side effects usually associated with systemic oral steroids. Symptoms eventually recur after treatment has stopped, however, perhaps because there has been some permanent change in the structure of the vulvar tissue. Some investigators have successfully treated lichen sclerosus with cyclosporine, a drug that suppresses the immune system.

In subsequent years any woman who has been treated for lichen sclerosus needs to have follow-up biopsies and examination by a specialist familiar with this condition to make sure a cancer does not go undetected.

Lichen planus. This recurrent inflammatory skin disorder (see skin disorders) can cause pain and itching in the vulva. Pimples often form a white, raised, lacy network that can be quite painful, causing the labia to stick together and narrowing the entrance to the vagina so that it bleeds on contact. Intercourse is extremely painful, and it is impossible for a clinician to insert a speculum into the vagina to do a pelvic examination. Topical corticosteroid creams can help relieve symptoms in most cases, but if the vaginal canal has narrowed, it may be necessary to take systemic corticosteroid drugs (in tablet form) or undergo reconstructive surgery.

Vulvitis. Vulvitis—a general term meaning inflammation of the vulva—can result from a number of different diseases, infections, injuries, allergies, and external irritants. Stress, poor hygiene, insufficient rest, and inadequate diet can increase a woman's susceptibility. Prepubescent girls and postmenopausal women sometimes develop vulvar itching and inflammation, possibly because of inadequate levels of estrogen. Vulvitis (see entry) is usually not life-threatening except in the rare cases when it is associated with vulvar cancer, but it can be agonizing to the woman and frustrating to her clinician because of the frequent difficulty in pinpointing the cause.

Vulvar pain. Pain and discomfort in the vulva can be caused by sexually transmitted diseases (see entry), other infections, physical trauma to the vulva, or allergic reactions to undergarments, soaps, or vaginal douches. Some women experience vulvar pain during sexual intercourse (see entry).

When vulvar pain (see entry) occurs independently of any other known disorder, the syndrome is called vulvodynia. Vulvar vestibulitis—one form of vulvodynia—is characterized by tenderness of the area just inside the labia minora. A growing group of investigators within the mainstream medical community now believe that vulvodynia is a distinct medical condition with as yet unknown physical causes, and that it afflicts between 150,000 and 200,000 American women, often to the point where their work and family lives are disrupted.

Vulvar cysts. Various types of cysts—enclosed sacs that contain a liquid or semisolid material—can develop on the vulva. The most common are Bartholin's cysts, which appear on one or both of the Bartholin's glands—a pair of small mucus-secreting glands located in the vestibular bulbs on either side of the vaginal opening. This usually painless cyst is prone to infection, in which case a painful abscess (collection of pus) may form. This requires immediate medical attention. Small abscesses often develop in the outer lips of the vulva and disappear on their own after a few days, though sometimes they may become infected and painful (see vulvar cysts).

Vulvar cancer. Cancer of the vulva is relatively rare, accounting for just 5 percent of all tumors of the female reproductive organs. By far the most common is squamous cell carcinoma, a type of skin cancer. About 5 percent of vulvar cancer is melanoma (see entry). Even more rarely, other cancers may arise from areas of chronic inflammation in the vulva, mostly in postmenopausal women. In its early preinvasive stages vulvar cancer (see entry) is usually easy to treat, but if left un-

treated it can eventually extend to nearby tissues or spread through the lymphatic system to other organs.

Pubic lice. Pubic lice (see entry) are yellow-gray insects with crablike claws which settle into the pubic area and live off human blood. The female lays small eggs called nits which cling to the base of hairs and take about 7 to 9 days to hatch. Pubic lice are not a serious threat to health, but they can cause agonizing itching in the vulva and often require a good deal of time and effort to eliminate.

Genital warts. Vulvar pain can be caused by genital warts which appear on the labia. These benign growths are a common form of sexually transmitted disease, caused by one of various forms of the human papilloma virus (HPV). Although they are easily spread and hard to eradicate, genital warts (see entry) are generally no more than an annoyance. Warts caused by certain types of the HPV, however, have been associated with cervical cancer.

The warts start as pink, tan, or red swellings about the size of rice grains but often merge together to resemble small cauliflowers. Some warts are so minute and painless that they are unnoticeable. Others are over 3 inches around and interfere with the ability to sit or to walk. Sometimes the warts itch or burn, and scratching them can cause irritation.

How are vulvar disorders evaluated?

A clinician evaluating vulvar disorders may sometimes need to do a biopsy by taking a tissue sample for laboratory analysis. Biopsies are necessary because it can be difficult to differentiate these disorders through visual inspection or symptoms alone, and vulvar disorders are occasionally signs of vulvar cancer or its precancerous changes. Biopsies of the vulva can usually be done in the office with local anesthesia.

How are vulvar disorders treated?

The majority of vulvar disorders are readily treated once they have been diagnosed correctly. The type of treatment undertaken depends on the diagnosis.

Related entries

Anesthesia, antiinflammatory drugs, biopsy, genital warts, pain during sexual intercourse, pubic lice, sexually transmitted diseases, vulvar cancer, vulvar cysts, vulvar pain, vulvitis

Vulvar Pain

Pain and discomfort in the vulva—the region surrounding the vaginal opening and the urethra—can have numerous external causes, including sexually transmitted diseases, other infections, physical trauma to the vulva, or allergic reactions to undergarments, soaps, or vaginal douches. Sometimes there may also be pain during sexual intercourse (see entry) as well. But when vulvar pain occurs independently of any other known disorder, the syndrome is called vulvodynia. Vulvar vestibulitis is one form of vulvodynia characterized by tenderness of the vulvar vestibule (the area just inside the labia minora, the inner vaginal lips), sometimes accompanied by redness. The cause has not been established, but microscopic examination of tissue from the affected area reveals signs of chronic inflammation without evidence of allergy.

For years unexplained vulvar pain was often dismissed as "all in the head" because it had no obvious physical cause or cure. Many women spent years going from doctor to doctor in search of a diagnosis for this "nameless" disease. Sometimes they were misdiagnosed as having other vulvar disorders, and as a result underwent many expensive, painful, and ineffective procedures including electrocautery, removal of the Bartholin's glands (soft but not tender glands that appear on the inner lips of the vulva, or just inside the vaginal entrance), antimicrobial treatments, and laser surgery. At other times these women were dismissed as being "frigid" or unhappy in their role as a woman. Even today, some women with unexplained vulvar pain are referred to psychiatrists on the presumption that the symptoms are emotionally based. Accumulating evidence suggests, however, that a great deal of vulvar pain probably has a physical—if as yet unidentified—basis.

Furthermore, there is now a growing—though still small—group of investigators within the mainstream medical community who believe that vulvodynia is a distinct medical condition that may have been described in the medical literature back in the 1880s and again in the 1930s. These investigators estimate that somewhere between 150,000 and 200,000 American women suffer from this condition, often to the point where their work and family lives are disrupted.

According to these investigators, vulvodynia is probably a complex condition that may stem from one of a number of different physical roots. Among the causes under investigation are abnormally high levels of calcium oxalate crystals in the blood and urine, chronic infections with the herpes simplex virus, an autoimmune response to yeast or human papilloma virus (HPV), and disturbances of chemicals in the brain called neurotransmitters.

Research on causes of vulvar vestibulitis has shown that recurrent yeast infections and genital warts are more common in women with vulvar vestibulitis than in other women. One hypothesis is that a yeast or HPV infection triggers an autoimmune response in susceptible women, leading to vulvar inflammation.

Who is likely to develop vulvodynia?

By definition vulvodynia cannot be traced to any obvious source. Some evidence suggests, however, that it may be particularly common in women who suffer from chronic pain syndrome (see psychosomatic disorders), as well as those who have interstitial cystitis (see entry), a chronic and often misdiagnosed condition involving bladder damage.

Vulvodynia occurs most often (though not exclusively) in white women in their 20s and 30s. Although the condition sometimes develops after childbirth, it is much more common in women who have never had children.

What are the symptoms?

Women with vulvodynia have burning, painful, stinging sensations in the vulvar region, which is often dry, irritated, or raw. Whether or not itching is a symptom of this particular condition remains controversial. Symptoms can be so intense that sexual intercourse becomes impossible, and even sitting, walking, or wearing tight pants can be unbearable. The pain is not restricted to any one event, however—such as touching or sexual activity—but tends to be present almost all the time.

The hallmark of vulvar vestibulitis is that specific areas of the vulva feel tender when a clinician lightly touches them with a cotton swab. It is common for women with vulvodynia to be depressed and even to consider suicide. But the relation of depression to vulvodynia is a chicken-and-egg problem. The investigators who argue that vulvodynia has a physical origin hypothesize that chronic pain and misery, often combined with many years of misdiagnosis and dismissal as a hypochondriac, is a logical source of depression. They attribute marital, family, and job problems to the physical and emotional miseries of this disorder. At the same time, it is equally possible that women who are already depressed are prone to develop chronic pain syndromes, including vulvodynia.

Ultimately, it may turn out that both of these theories are correct, depending on individual circumstances, but further investigation needs to be done before any definitive conclusions can be drawn.

How is the condition evaluated?

Vulvodynia is diagnosed by excluding other possible causes of vulvar pain, including easily remediable infections or allergic reactions and vulvar cysts. A clinician familiar with vulvar vestibulitis may evaluate a woman who complains of vulvar pain or painful intercourse by testing for the "focal" points of pain. In addition, a pelvic examination and additional appropriate tests may be done to eliminate other causes of vulvar pain.

Investigators who believe that calcium oxalate may play a role in causing vulvodynia advocate testing a urine sample to see if it contains elevated levels of this substance. In addition, some clinicians may want to order a CT scan or magnetic resonance image (MRI) of the lower vertebrae to make sure that no tumors or cysts are compressing a nerve.

How is vulvodynia treated?

Sometimes vulvodynia disappears on its own without treatment. Other women adapt to the condition by finding sexual

Oxalate in foods

High	Moderate
Baked beans in tomato sauce	Apples
Beans	Apricots
Beer	Asparagus
Beets	Black currants
Berries	Broccoli
Berry juices	Carrots
Beverage mixes	Chicken soup
Black pepper	Coffee
Celery	Corn
Chard	Cornbread
Chocolate	Cranberries
Citrus peel	Cucumbers
Cocoa	Grapes
Collards	Green peas
Concord grapes	Iceberg lettuce
Dandelion greens	Lima beans
Eggplant	Oranges
Escarole	Orange juice
Fruit cake	Parsnips
Green peppers	Peaches
Grits	Pears
Kale	Pineapples
Leeks	Plums
Mustard greens	Sardines
Okra	Spaghetti sauce
Ovaltine	Sponge cake
Parsley	Tomato sauce
Peanuts	Tomatoes
Pecans	Turnips
Rhubarb	
Rutabagas	
Spinach	
Summer squash	
Sweet potatoes	
Tangerines	
Tea	
Tofu	
Vegetable and tomato soups	
Watercress	
Wheat germ	

medical specialist knowledgeable about the physical aspects of vulvodynia before seeking psychiatric care.

Even if a woman shows no evidence of depression, vulvodynia can often be successfully treated with low doses of antidepressants, such as amitriptyline (Elavil), which are often used for other "neuropathic" pain syndromes. These usually need to be taken for long periods of time.

If vulvar pain is due to some physical cause, therapy will usually aim at reversing or eliminating that cause. For example, if a nerve root is compressed, surgery can be done to decompress it. There is some preliminary evidence that this can provide immediate and long-lasting relief from vulvar pain.

For vulvar vestibulitis, the most successful treatment has been surgical excision of the affected area (a procedure called perineoplasty or vestibulectomy). These operations involve cutting out the tender areas in the vulva and then sewing together the surrounding skin. Although this is often successful in relieving pain and preventing recurrence after subsequent childbirths, healing can be slow. In the studies done to date, sexual function has returned to normal in 75 percent of women treated surgically. Also fairly effective are local injections of interferon alpha 2b, which is approved by the FDA only for treating genital warts. These injections can cause local pain and mild flulike symptoms.

If vulvar vestibulitis seems to be linked to high levels of calcium oxalate, medications (such as calcium citrate) that reduce calcium oxalate levels may help relieve symptoms. It may also help to eliminate foods that contain oxalic acid (oxalate), although doing so may mean changing a good part of the customary diet (see chart). If a woman is trying to reduce her intake of high-fat, high-cholesterol, or high-calorie foods at the same time, she may find herself with virtually nothing "safe" left to eat.

Related entries
Alternative therapies, antidepressants, autoimmune disorders, depression, electrocautery, genital warts, herpes, interstitial cystitis, laser surgery, nutrition, pain during sexual intercourse, psychosomatic disorders, psychotherapy, sexually transmitted diseases, skin disorders, stress, vulvar cancer, vulvar cysts, vulvar disorders, vulvitis, yeast infections

Vulvitis

Vulvitis simply means inflammation of the vulva—the female external genitalia. It is not a single condition but a symptom that can result from a number of different diseases, infections, injuries, allergies, and external irritants. Stress, poor hygiene, insufficient rest, and inadequate diet can increase a woman's susceptibility to vulvitis.

Except in the rare cases when it is associated with vulvar

positions that are less painful. Occasionally the clinician will recommend a psychiatric evaluation to see if the chronic pain and depression might have something to do with emotional trauma, stress, or an imbalance of neurotransmitters. Although sometimes psychotherapy may be helpful, women should ask their primary care physician to recommend a

Common causes of vulvitis

Contact dermatitis

Soaps
Laundry detergents
Vaginal sprays, deodorants, douches, and powders
Synthetic undergarments
Condoms and contraceptive foams, jellies, or creams
Bubble baths
Scented or colored toilet paper
Sanitary napkins and tampons

Diseases and disorders

Diabetes
Lichen sclerosus
Vulvar cancer

Infections

Herpes
Genital warts
Vaginitis (including yeast infections)

Infestations

Pubic lice
Scabies

Medications

Antibiotics

Lifestyle factors

Stress
Inadequate nutrition
Insufficient rest
Poor hygiene

Physical trauma

cancer, vulvitis is usually not a life-threatening condition. Even so, because it is often difficult to pinpoint a specific cause, this condition can be agonizing and frustrating to both the woman and her clinician.

Who is likely to develop vulvitis?

Vulvitis can develop in any woman who has certain allergies, sensitivities, infections, infestations, or diseases (see chart). In addition, prepubescent girls and postmenopausal women sometimes develop vulvar itching and inflammation for no obvious reason, possibly because of inadequate levels of estrogen.

What are the symptoms?

Vulvitis is characterized by redness, swelling, and often excruciating itching on the labia and other parts of the vulva. Scratching irritates the vulva even more, as does overzealous cleansing with irritating soaps. Clear, fluid-filled blisters which eventually burst and crust over are common. If vulvitis becomes chronic, there may be sore, scaly, thickened, or whitish patches. In vulvitis associated with diabetes, the vulva often looks beefy red.

How is the condition evaluated?

A clinician should be consulted about vulvitis that does not respond to simple self-help measures or is accompanied by a foul-smelling vaginal discharge. Usually diagnosing the cause of the vulvitis will involve a pelvic examination, blood tests, urine tests, and, in some cases, tests for sexually transmitted diseases. The clinician will also ask questions to see if any obvious irritants such as vaginal products or new soaps have been used. Any suspicious-looking vaginal secretions will be examined under a microscope to check for vaginal infection. A glucose test may be done if the woman has any symptoms that suggest diabetes. In addition, the clinician will also try to find out about any emotional problems that may be interfering with the woman's ability to handle stress.

Sometimes the clinician will do a biopsy of the vulva to check for precancerous or malignant cells. This is particularly likely if sores suggesting vulvar cancer are present, or if the woman is over 50 and has persistent inflammation that cannot be relieved with vaginal creams. A vulvar biopsy can usually be done in the office with local anesthesia.

How is vulvitis treated?

Sometimes vulvitis can be relieved through self-help measures. Any external irritant known to provoke vulvitis should be avoided (sometimes discovering what that might be requires a few weeks of sleuthing). Meanwhile, sitz baths with baking soda or Aveeno colloidal oatmeal can be soothing, as can warm boric acid compresses applied to the vulva. Hydrocortisone creams, which are available without prescription, can relieve itching, although they should not be used for more than a month without medical supervision (long-term use can cause tissue atrophy, which in turn can increase sensitivity and inflammation). Keeping the genital area cool, dry, and clean helps control irritation. The vulva should be washed with gentle unscented soap and water and dried thoroughly with a soft cloth or towel.

Vulvitis which does not clear up after several weeks of these treatments or which is accompanied by a foul-smelling discharge should be evaluated by a clinician. If some specific cause such as an infection can be determined, the vulvitis will usually disappear when this is treated. The clinician may prescribe a stronger hydrocortisone cream or antihistamines, either of which can provide relief to any form of vulvitis, whatever the cause. Women who are past menopause may want to consider taking estrogen replacement therapy or applying an estrogen cream.

How can vulvitis be prevented?

Not all forms of vulvitis can be prevented, particularly if they result from some underlying disease. In general, however, some vulvitis can be prevented in much the same way as vaginitis: by practicing good hygiene. This includes washing the vulva regularly with mild soap and patting it dry, not using other people's towels, and wiping from front to back (vulva to anus) after a bowel movement to avoid spreading bacteria from the rectum into the genital area.

Women with a history of vulvitis might also try switching to cotton or cotton-crotch underwear, using uncolored and unscented toilet paper, avoiding pantyhose and tight jeans, eliminating any potentially irritating vaginal products (including tampons), using a water-soluble lubricant (such as K-Y Jelly) during sexual intercourse, and avoiding sexual intercourse during a flare-up. The studies linking most of these practices to specific irritations of the vulva are sparse, but experimenting a little with clothing or hygiene products certainly cannot hurt. Getting adequate rest and nutrition and finding effective ways to deal with stress (see entry) help reduce any woman's susceptibility to vulvitis.

Related entries

Antiinflammatory drugs, biopsy, diabetes, douching, estrogen replacement therapy, genital warts, herpes, lubricants, pain during sexual intercourse, pubic lice, sexually transmitted diseases, skin disorders, stress, vaginitis, vulvar cancer, vulvar cysts, vulvar disorders, yeast infections

Weight Tables

The burning questions among weight researchers today seem to be: ▸ What range of weights for a given height is consistent with good health among adults? ▸ And do these ranges change with age? That is, is some modest weight gain during adulthood consistent with good health?

According to the 1990 *Report of the Dietary Guidelines Advisory Committee* (issued by the U.S. Department of Agriculture and the Department of Health and Human Services) and analysis done at the National Institute of Aging's Gerontology Research Center, some weight gain after age 35 is consistent with good health in both men and women. That is based on actuarial tables from life insurance companies which conclude that mortality rates overall are lowest among people who gain a few pounds per decade of adulthood. The *Guidelines* do not differentiate between the weights of men and women, which implies that women, whose bones and muscles weigh less than men's, can have a higher relative percentage of fat than men of the same height and still be considered healthy (see chart).

USDA suggested weights		
Height without shoes	**Weight without clothes**	
	19 to 34 years	**Over 35 years**
5'0"	97–128	108–138
5'1"	101–132	111–143
5'2"	104–137	115–148
5'3"	107–141	119–152
5'4"	111–146	122–157
5'5"	114–150	126–162
5'6"	118–155	130–167
5'7"	121–160	134–172
5'8"	125–164	138–178
5'9"	129–169	142–183
5'10"	132–174	146–188
5'11"	136–179	151–194
6'0"	140–184	155–199

But a few years later a study of over 115,000 nurses by Harvard University researchers threw some cold water on these recommendations. It showed that the risk of coronary artery disease is greater for women at the high end of the "normal" range as defined by the USDA *Guidelines* and lower for women who are below the low end of the "normal" range. Women of average weight had about a 50 percent higher risk of heart attack than women who weighed 15 percent less than average. And even for women within the normal range, modest weight gain after age 18 was associated with an increased risk of heart disease. Women who gained 10 pounds or less in early to middle adulthood had the lowest risk of heart attacks. The authors of this study recommend going back to the 1959 Metropolitan Life tables for "ideal weights," which make no allowances for age and recommend lower weights for women of any age (see chart page 626; subsequent Met Life weight tables are given for comparison).

One of the sticking points seems to be whether one looks at overall mortality (as the U.S. *Guidelines* do) or at heart disease, which is the greatest cause of death among women after middle age. Modest weight gain seems to be associated with a lower overall risk of dying at any given age, but also seems to raise the chances that one will die of a heart attack. Do slightly heavier people have a lower incidence of cancer and other life-threatening conditions that offsets their risk of heart disease? Perhaps, but the data are equivocal at best.

There are two things that we do know for sure: ▸ Those who gain a considerable amount of weight while passing through the adult years die at an earlier than average age. ▸ And though Americans have been getting somewhat heavier over the last few decades, their life expectancy has continued to

Comparison of 1959, 1983, and 1996 Metropolitan height and weight tables

Height without shoes	Weight without clothing		
	1959	1983	1996
4'10"	92–121	100–131	102–131
4'11"	95–124	101–134	103–134
5'0"	98–127	103–137	104–137
5'1"	101–130	105–140	106–140
5'2"	104–134	108–144	108–143
5'3"	107–138	111–148	111–147
5'4"	110–142	114–152	114–151
5'5"	114–146	117–156	117–155
5'6"	118–150	120–160	120–159
5'7"	122–154	123–164	123–163
5'8"	126–159	126–167	126–167
5'9"	130–164	129–170	129–170
5'10"	134–169	132–173	132–173

Note on 1959 table: For women 18–25 years, subtract one pound for each year under 25.

overall health more meaningfully, the number on the scale must be considered along with physical fitness, family history, lifestyle factors such as cigarette smoking and alcohol use, and current medical and psychological health.

For example, evidence is accumulating that weight may not be as important in predicting longevity as the ratio of fat to muscle. And whatever their weight, people who have large accumulations of fat around the abdomen have a risk of diabetes and cardiovascular disease far greater than that of people with large accumulations of fat around the hips or thighs. As for lifestyle, the Harvard Nurses' Study showed that cigarette smoking (which is more prevalent among lean women) is a greater risk factor for heart disease than is body weight; and while women who have more than 2 alcoholic drinks per day are at risk for many life-threatening diseases, including alcoholism, women who drink more moderately (1 to 2 drinks per day) have a lower risk of heart disease than women who do not drink at all.

From some future study or reanalysis we may learn that an active woman who does not smoke, enjoys a glass of wine with dinner, and picks up a few pounds over the years has the best chance of living a long and healthy life. But until that definitive study is published, the jury is still out on ideal weight.

Related entries

Body image, coronary artery disease, diabetes, dieting, exercise, nutrition, obesity

increase, which suggests that a few extra pounds are not a grave threat to health overall.

What factors should be considered along with weight?

The traditional weight tables were simple charts showing whether or not one weighed "too much" for one's height. Sometimes these tables were broken down by sex or differentiated by age (with some allowance for a few extra pounds in mid-life and beyond). In recent years weight tables are more likely to include measures of body fat such as the body mass index (BMI). This index indicates how much of the weight comes from muscle or bone versus fat. It is calculated by multiplying weight in pounds by 700 and then dividing the product by the square of height in inches. A woman who weighs 125 pounds and stands 5'5" (65 inches) tall, for example, would have a BMI of $(125 \times 700)/(65 \times 65)$ or about 21. A BMI higher than 25 is considered to be reason for concern. Therefore, a 5'5" woman weighing 170 pounds would have a BMI of $(170 \times 700)/(65 \times 65)$ or about 28 and would be labeled overweight by this measure. (see BMI index page 413) Ultimately, however, even weight tables derived from the BMI are based on the number that appears on a scale. And for that reason weight tables of any sort must be read with a wary eye. An individual woman should not assume she is unhealthy just because the scale registers a few pounds above or below the listed values. Weight is only one of a number of factors that help indicate a person's well-being. To evaluate

Wrinkles

Wrinkles occur because as women age, their skin tends to become drier and less elastic (see skin care). Wrinkles may be a natural part of this aging process, but that does not mean that most women are happy about them. Face lifts, dermabrasion, and chemical peels (see entries) are options available to some women for eliminating sagging skin, deep frown lines, and pitted scars. In addition, a series of collagen injections can sometimes "plump up" the surface skin, thus erasing superficial wrinkles for several months or so. Beyond these rather drastic measures, however, not much could be done about wrinkles until recently, despite millions of dollars spent in pursuit of ageless skin.

A few years ago researchers reported a drug's seemingly too-good-to-be-true ability to accomplish what phony wrinkle creams had been promising to do for years: genuinely eliminate wrinkles. This miracle drug was Retin-A (the trade name for the prescription medication tretinoin, which is a kind of vitamin A acid), which had been prescribed for years as a treatment for acne. In 1996 an emollient cream called Renova containing 0.05 percent tretinoin was approved specifically for treating wrinkles.

How does tretinoin work?

Tretinoin appears to plump up and smooth out fine lines by actually rebuilding the damaged outer layer of skin. It reverses sun damage by speeding up skin cell renewal, stimulating blood vessel growth, and restoring the skin's ability to produce collagen, a fibrous protein that gives support and elasticity to normal skin.

To prevent skin irritation, tretinoin needs to be started at low doses, which can be increased gradually. Treated areas should be covered with sunscreen.

What are the risks and complications?

Tretinoin is not a miracle cure for wrinkles. For one thing, it takes 6 weeks of regular use before wrinkles start to disappear, and once the drug is stopped, the lines tend to return. Any woman who is pregnant or breastfeeding should mention this fact to a clinician before being prescribed Retin-A or Renova.

Can any other cosmetic products smooth out wrinkles?

"Fruit acids," also known as alpha-hydroxy acids (AHAs), show some promise in smoothing out dry skin, and at 25 percent concentrations they may even thicken collagen and add elasticity to the skin. Glycolic acid, the most widely used of these acids (which are either derived from fruits or synthesized in a laboratory) is a component of numerous cosmetic products in varying concentrations. Products with concentrations of under 8 percent or so are unlikely to have much effect, however, so labels of products claiming to smooth out wrinkles should be checked carefully.

Some antiwrinkle products also include hefty concentrations of vitamin C, or ascorbic acid, on the theory that this substance might help reverse wrinkling by acting as an antioxidant, potentially reversing free radical skin damage caused by ultraviolet light (sunlight). Another theory is that vitamin C may play a role in the production of collagen. At this point, however, evidence is still too limited to determine if vitamin C has any noticeable effect on wrinkles.

Botox and other pricey approaches

Many new non-invasive fillers can be injected under the skin to temporarily plump out wrinkles and relax furrowed brows. These include Botox (*botulinum toxin*, also sold under the trade name of Myobloc), bovine collagen, various hyalouronic acid gels, and a longer-lasting filler containing tiny plastic beads suspending in bovine collagen and lidocaine called Artecoll. Other new procedures "plump and tighten" sags and bags using sound waves. These treatments can also be combined with other interventions such as chemical peels and laser resurfacing. However, most tend to be pricey, none work miracles, and, naturally, all have associated risks—particularly if provided by unskilled practitioners or used by the wrong candidate. Generally, these procedures are most effective for women 30 to 50 years of age; the better off the skin in the first place, the better the results.

How can wrinkles be prevented?

Wrinkling is a function not just of one's age but of one's hereditary makeup and habits. Some women will wrinkle at an earlier age than others no matter what they do. Other women speed up their natural rate of wrinkling by smoking cigarettes, drinking alcohol excessively, failing to maintain a nutritious diet, avoiding exercise, and allowing their weight to fluctuate drastically. A yo-yo pattern of weight gain and loss stretches the skin when weight is high and then leaves it sagging when weight is lost. Changing these behaviors while one is still young is essential for youthful-looking skin in middle age and beyond.

Ultraviolet light wrinkles, dries, and burns the skin and increases the odds of developing skin cancer, including the often deadly melanoma. Although dark skin can tolerate more sun than lighter skin, no one is immune to the deterioration in the health and appearance of the skin wrought over time by UV light. Anyone who spends time outdoors needs to wear protective clothing and use sunscreens or sunblocks every day, all year round. Women with dry skin should use a sunscreen with a sun protection factor (SPF) of 15 to 30 and reapply it before going outside.

When skin is dry, wrinkles are more apparent. Applying moisturizing creams and lotions, and hydrating the skin from the inside out by drinking plenty of fluids, can help combat dryness. Facial masks may make a woman feel pampered, but they are no more effective than moisturizers in preventing wrinkles. Antiwrinkle creams (other than Renova and possibly those containing high concentrations of alpha-hydroxy acids), collagen implants, hormone injections, and electrical stimulation are equally ineffective, although some of the newer lasers show promise for resurfacing fine wrinkles. Estrogen replacement therapy has no known effect on wrinkles or other signs of aging skin.

Dry skin needs extra protection from wind, which pulls water out of skin. In colder weather, skin should be covered as much as possible with appropriate outdoor apparel, including face or ski masks in frigid temperatures. Skin exposed to severely cold temperatures should also be coated with petroleum jelly. This is especially true for skiers and other winter athletes.

Some dermatologists think that facial exercises may be able to prevent—and perhaps even reverse—the formation of facial lines and wrinkles. For example, to prevent the chin from sagging, jut the lower teeth out into an underbite and move them up and down with the lower jaw only. To prevent lines around the eyes, close the eyes with the lower lids. From a physiological viewpoint, facial exercises *should* lessen age-related sagging, and they are definitely relaxing. Anecdotal "before" and "after" photographs are impressive, although there have been no controlled studies. Women concerned about wrinkles can do no harm by giving facial exercises a try.

Related entries

Acne, body image, cosmetic safety, cosmetic surgery, dermabrasion and chemical peels, exercise, eyelid surgery, face lifts, hair care, laser surgery, melanoma, nutrition, smoking, stress

Yeast Infections

Yeast infections are a common and often frustrating form of vaginal infection which occurs in about 1.3 million American women each year. Although effective treatments are now available without prescription—which should help cut back on the enormous number of medical dollars devoted to this condition—many women and health care providers alike are still frustrated by recurrent or chronic infections.

Yeast infections are not life-threatening, but the vaginal itching can be severe enough to make daily life a misery. In addition, if a woman has a yeast infection during childbirth, the baby can swallow yeast and develop a condition called thrush (treated with drops of nystatin).

Yeast infections are caused by one of several species of a yeastlike fungus called Candida, usually *Candida albicans.* Over the past 25 years, however, increasing numbers of women (now about 1 in 5) seem to have been developing yeast infections resulting from other species of Candida. Some investigators think that these other species might explain somewhat uncharacteristic symptoms and be slightly more resistant to standard treatments.

Who is likely to develop a yeast infection?

Although Candida are present to some extent in the vagina of most women, yeast infections can develop if the natural balance of microorganisms becomes upset so that the yeast proliferates. Women taking antibiotics to treat some other infection are at particular risk for yeast infections because the antibiotics destroy protective bacteria in the vagina which normally suppress the Candida population. Yeast infections caused by antibiotics are notoriously difficult to treat until the antibiotic is stopped. Taking steroid drugs or other immunosuppressive agents can also increase the risks of developing a yeast infection.

Pregnancy and diabetes—both of which raise the sugar content (and the pH) of the vagina—put women at risk for yeast infections. This is probably because the symptoms of yeast infections are thought to result from alcohol produced when the Candida fungus metabolizes sugar. Other commonly cited risk factors turn out to be less than certain. The jury is still out as to whether or not taking oral contraceptives predisposes a woman to yeast infections. Tight jeans, pantyhose, and other synthetic or occlusive clothing have been traditionally suspected of favoring Candida growth. It is also unclear whether or not yeast infections can be acquired from an infected sexual partner, although it makes sense to assume that they can until it is proven otherwise.

Just which women are prone to developing chronic or recurrent yeast infections is equally unclear. Traditionally, it was believed that some women have reservoirs of Candida in their intestinal tract which "reseed" the vagina after treatment. Another theory (the "vaginal relapse theory") postulated that small colonies of yeast remain in the vagina after treatment, too small to be detected in a culture but large enough to multiply later and produce new symptoms. Other investigators have speculated that women who continue to have yeast infections are being reinfected by an untreated sexual partner.

More recently, some evidence has indicated that certain women have a localized allergic reaction to Candida which predisposes them to recurrent symptoms and infections. It also appears that women infected with the AIDS virus may be more likely to have frequent or hard-to-treat yeast infections, because their immune system is chronically depressed. A woman with chronic yeast infections may want to speak with her clinician about HIV testing. Some women are mistakenly thought to have recurrent yeast infections when in fact they actually have some other form of vaginitis (such as cytolytic vaginosis) which does not respond to treatments for yeast infections.

What are the symptoms?

The classic symptoms of a yeast infection are severe vaginal itching and a thick white vaginal discharge that often looks like cottage cheese and smells sweet or bread-like. Sometimes there may be no obvious discharge and more burning than itching. The vulva and vagina are often red, swollen, and covered with the discharge, and when the infection has been present a long time, fissures or cracks may appear in the vulva. Often sexual intercourse is painful, and with chronic yeast infections this can significantly affect a woman's relationship with a sexual partner.

How is the condition evaluated?

Clinicians can easily and inexpensively diagnose yeast infections by doing a pelvic examination and then inspecting the vaginal discharge under a microscope to see if any fungi are present. This procedure is particularly important because it helps distinguish yeast infections from cytolytic vaginosis, which is often mistaken for a yeast infection. Some clinicians may also want to culture the cells from the discharge to determine the exact species of Candida that is causing the infection, especially in the case of chronic or recurrent infections. It usually takes a couple of days for a culture to be grown in a laboratory.

How are yeast infections treated?

A variety of home remedies for yeast vaginitis have been tried, particularly in the days before antifungal creams were available over the counter. These include vinegar douches, insertion of yogurt containing live acidophilus cultures, and insertion of acidophilus capsules into the vagina. These remedies in theory (and in the experience of some women) help by lowering the vaginal pH, making the environment inhospitable to yeast. There are few scientific studies of their effectiveness, but they are probably not harmful so long as their use does not unduly delay a woman's seeking medical care if symptoms persist.

Several relatively inexpensive products such as clotrimazole (Gyne-Lotrimin, Mycelex) and miconazole (Monistat) are now available without a prescription to treat mild and nonrecurrent yeast infections. Another product, Mycolog, combines an antifungal drug with cortisone to increase comfort, but this should be used for a limited time to avoid vulvar atrophy (thinning of tissues) from the steroid. The over-the-counter preparations are available in both a suppository and a cream form (inserted into the vagina with a plunger-type applicator similar to the ones used for spermicides). They should be used once a day for as many days as instructed, even if symptoms disappear after a day or two (which they usually do). The cream forms work better for women with vulvitis, since they can be spread over the vulva. Whether cream or suppository, all the over-the-counter treatments can and should be continued throughout a menstrual period, although they should not be used with tampons.

Used appropriately, the over-the-counter preparations cure about 85 percent of yeast infections, whether taken in small doses over 7 days or somewhat larger doses over 3 days. In most cases they are just as effective as the prescription medications butoconazole (Femstat) and terconazole (Terazol). If the yeast infection is particularly mild and not a side effect of taking antibiotics, a clinician may prescribe a single large dose of tioconazole (Vagistat-1), which is nearly as effective. A single dose of an oral antifungal drug, fluconazole (Diflucan), has been compared with traditional intravaginal treatments and found to be similarly effective. But because oral antifungal drugs can occasionally cause liver problems, most clinicians prefer to prescribe the oral form of treatment only for chronic or recurrent yeast infections.

If yeast infections recur after over-the-counter treatment, the clinician may prescribe terconazole (Terazol), an antifungal drug which some investigators think may be more effective in treating yeast infections not resulting from *Candida albicans*. Although it is still not clear that yeast infections are sexually transmitted, it may be worth a try for a woman with recurrent yeast infections to ask her partner to be treated as well.

A woman who has never before had a yeast infection should see a clinician first, just to make sure that her symptoms are indeed due to a yeast infection and not some other form of vaginitis or sexually transmitted disease which requires a different treatment. Women who try an over-the-counter drug and do not see improvement should also seek medical attention. Women who are pregnant should consult a clinician before trying any home remedies or over-the-counter products.

How can yeast infections be prevented?
Women with recurrent or chronic yeast infections may want to talk with their clinician about taking either ketoconazole

(Nizoral) or fluconazole on a long-term basis. Because of the side effects associated with these oral medications, however, a safer alternative may be to use clotrimazole vaginal suppositories once a week. Women who have a history of yeast infections after taking antibiotics may want to use over-the-counter antifungal remedies while taking antibiotics.

Basic hygienic practices thought to help prevent other forms of vaginitis are no guarantee against yeast infections, but they probably prevent at least some occurrences. These practices include keeping the vulva clean, dry, and cool, getting enough sleep, eating nutritious foods, and finding effective ways to handle the stress of daily living.

Related entries
Acquired immune deficiency syndrome, antibiotics, cytolytic vaginosis, diabetes, douching, pain during sexual intercourse, pregnancy, vaginitis, vulvitis

Zinc

Zinc is an essential trace mineral, which means that it is necessary in very small quantities for proper growth and functioning of the body. It plays an important role in gene expression, bone metabolism, and normal vision (particularly adaptation to darkness), and it is a component of insulin, the hormone crucial for the storage of blood sugar.

Because zinc has a number of effects on the metabolism of the sex hormones and the prostaglandins, it plays an important part in the reproductive cycle. Zinc is essential for ovulation (release of an egg from the ovary), fertilization, and, in men, for the formation of the hormone testosterone and the maturation of sperm.

Recently zinc lozenges sold over the counter have become a hot item as a possible means to relieve colds and "boost" immune system function. While some studies have indeed shown that zinc gluconate may shave a few days off the duration of the average cold, other equally solid studies suggest that they make no difference at all. Whether this lack of effect may be due to certain flavoring agents added to the lozenges remains to be determined.

Who is likely to develop a zinc deficiency?
Although no one knows the precise number of people who are deficient in zinc, mild deficiency seems to be common in many parts of the world, particularly among children, adolescents, and pregnant and breastfeeding women. Zinc deficiency in the United States is probably rare in these groups, though not unheard of.

People with poorly controlled diabetes or those who consume excessive alcohol, use diuretic drugs, or have certain liver or bowel disorders (see entry) such as celiac disease or Crohn's disease may develop a zinc deficiency. Many women who have iron deficiencies seem to have low levels of zinc as well (see anemia).

Low levels of zinc have been associated for years with anorexia nervosa (see entry), and some investigators have speculated that the altered taste and smell perception associated with zinc deficiencies may be involved in appetite loss. It is not clear whether the low levels of zinc are a cause or effect of anorexia, however.

What are the symptoms of zinc deficiency?

People without enough zinc may become susceptible to infections and skin rashes and may develop mental lethargy, a diminished sense of taste and smell, and a poor appetite.

Zinc deficiencies have been linked to an increased risk of infertility in women and, during pregnancy, to an increased risk of abnormal bleeding, miscarriage, preeclampsia, difficult labors, premature or unusually late delivery, and stillbirth, as well as to retarded growth and deformities in the baby.

What are the recommended levels of zinc?

The recommended dietary allowance (RDA) for zinc is 8 mg per day in women over 19. Pregnant women need an additional 3 mg each day, and breastfeeding women need an extra 4 mg. Women who eat a strictly vegetarian diet may require between 12 and 18 mg, depending on their age and reproductive status.

What are the best sources of zinc?

For women who are not pregnant or breastfeeding, a balanced diet that includes whole grains, fruit and vegetables, and 5 to 7 ounces of fish, poultry, or lean meat per day supplies an adequate daily intake of zinc (see chart). Prenatal vitamin and mineral supplements provide the extra amounts needed by pregnant and breastfeeding women.

People with conditions that can lead to zinc deficiencies (such as bowel disorders, anemia, and anorexia) should consult their clinician about appropriate levels of supplementation, in addition to a balanced diet. Some research has pointed to a possible role for supplementary zinc in preventing or treating inflammatory bowel disease, macular degeneration, certain skin disorders, diabetes, and premenstrual syndrome (see entries). There is some limited evidence that adding zinc to the diet of women recovering from anorexia can increase their weight gain.

Dental rinses that include zinc citrate together with chlorhexidine (Triclosan) seem to reduce gingivitis, staining, plaque, and tartar (see gum disease).

What are the risks and complications of zinc supplements?

Taking zinc as a mineral supplement can sometimes be counterproductive, particularly when supplements of zinc are mixed with other minerals. For example, some studies suggest that zinc supplements taken together with calcium car-

Good sources of zinc in the diet		
Food	Serving size	Mg of zinc
Oysters	6 medium	124.9
Lobster	3½ oz	7.9
Crab	1 cup	6.7
Pork roast	3 oz	5.1
Liver, beef	3 oz	4.6
Beef, extra-lean	3 oz	4.6
Turkey, dark meat	3 oz	3.7
Wheat germ	¼ cup	3.1
Lima beans	½ cup, cooked	2.7
Lentils	1 cup cooked	2.0
Almonds	½ cup	2.0
Split peas	1 cup cooked	2.0
Turkey, light meat	3 oz	1.8
Parmesan cheese	1 oz	1.5
Spinach	1 cup cooked	1.3
Yogurt, plain	1 cup	1.3
Tuna, in water	1 can	1.3
Brown rice	1 cup cooked	1.2

bonate or calcium citrate may reduce the body's ability to absorb both zinc and calcium. Zinc supplements can also interfere with the absorption of the antibiotic tetracycline and can severely lower blood levels of copper.

Zinc is effective in very low amounts, and consuming large doses of it (beginning at 10 to 15 times the RDA, or about 120 mg or more per day) can lead to stomach cramps, nausea, and vomiting. Over longer periods, excess zinc can damage the pancreas, lead to anemia, and reduce levels of high-density lipoprotein (HDL) cholesterol (the "good" cholesterol). Hotly debated is the role—if any—that too much zinc may play in the formation of clumps similar to the amyloid plaques found in the brains of people with Alzheimer's disease (see entry). Some animal studies have suggested that excess zinc may lead to infertility or underweight offspring (just as low levels are already known to do), but the implications for human reproduction are not known.

The best bet for most women is to get their daily zinc as part of a balanced diet. There is little need for most women to take zinc supplements at all.

Related entries

Alcohol, Alzheimer's disease, anemia, anorexia nervosa and bulimia nervosa, bowel disorders, calcium, cholesterol, diabetes, diuretics, gum disease, infertility, iron, macular degeneration, miscarriage, nutrition, preeclampsia, pregnancy, premenstrual syndrome, vitamins

For Further Information

The following listings provide a useful starting point for readers looking for referrals, support groups, or more extensive information about a given topic. Websites including information in Spanish or French have been noted with the designation "Se habla Español" or "Je parle Françoise" respectively. Although we do not list relevant books, many of the websites listed include extensive lists of recommended books and other resources.

General Resources

American College of Obstetricians and Gynecologists
409 12th Street SW
Washington, DC 20024-2188
www.acog.org

Canadian Women's Health Network
419 Graham Avenue, Suite 203
Winnipeg, Manitoba
Canada R3C 0M3
204-942-5500
www.cwhn.ca/indexeng.html
Je parle Français

Harvard Women's Health Watch
Harvard Medical School Health Publications
10 Shattuck Street
Boston, MA 02115-6011
www.health.harvard.edu

MEDLINE Plus
U.S. National Library of Medicine
8600 Rockville Pike
Bethesda, MD 20894
www.medlineplus.gov
Se habla Español

National Black Women's Health Project
600 Pennsylvania Avenue SE, Suite 310
Washington, DC 20003
202-548-4000
www.blackwomenshealth.org

National Institute on Aging
Building 31, Room 5C27
31 Center Drive, MSC 2292
Bethesda, MD 20892
301-496-1752
www.nia.nih.gov

National Latina Health Network
1680 Wisconsin Avenue NW, Second Floor
Washington, DC 20007
202-965-9633
www.nationallatinahealthnetwork.com
Se habla Español

National Women's Health Network
514 10th Street NW, Suite 400
Washington, DC 20004
202-628-7814
www.womenshealthnetwork.org

National Women's Health Resource Center
120 Albany Street, Suite 820
New Brunswick, NJ 08901
877-986-9472
www.healthywomen.org

Native American Women's Health Education Resource Center
P.O. Box 572
Lake Andes, SD 57356-0572
605-487-7072
www.nativeshop.org/nawherc.html

Planned Parenthood Federation of America
434 West 33rd Street
New York, NY 10001
800-230-PLAN
www.plannedparenthood.org
Se habla Español

Planned Parenthood Federation of Canada
1 Nicholas Street, Suite 430
Ottawa, Ontario
Canada K1N 7B7
613-241-4474
www.ppfc.ca
Je parle Français

Women's Health
52 Featherstone Street
London EC1Y 8RT
United Kingdom
020-7251-6333
www.womenshealthlondon.org.uk

Abortion

British Pregnancy Advisory Service
Austy Manor
Wootton Wawen, Solihull
West Midlands B95 6BX
United Kingdom
01564-793225
www.bpas.org

Childbirth by Choice Trust
344 Bloor Street West, Suite 502
Toronto, Ontario
Canada M5S 3A7
416-961-7812
www.cbctrust.com
Je parle Français

Marie Stopes International
153–157 Cleveland Street
London W1T 6QW
United Kingdom
020-7574-7400
www.mariestopes.org.uk

National Abortion Federation
1755 Massachusetts Avenue NW, Suite 600
Washington, DC 20036
800-772-9100
www.prochoice.org
Se habla Español

Planned Parenthood Federation of America
434 West 33rd Street
New York, NY 10001
800-230-PLAN
www.plannedparenthood.org
Se habla Español

Planned Parenthood Federation of Canada
1 Nicholas Street, Suite 430
Ottawa, Ontario
Canada K1N 7B7
613-241-4474
www.ppfc.ca
Je parle Français

AIDS

AIDSInfo
National Institutes of Health
P.O. Box 6303
Rockville, MD 20849-6303
800-HIV-0440
www.aidsinfo.nih.gov

CATIE (Canadian AIDS Treatment Information Exchange)
555 Richmond Street West, Suite 505
Toronto, Ontario
Canada M5V 3B1
800-263-1638
www.catie.ca
Je parle Français

I.C.W. (International Community of Women Living with HIV/AIDS)
2c Leroy House
436 Essex Road
London N1 3QP
United Kingdom
020-7704-0606
www.icw.org

Terrence Higgins Trust
52–54 Grays Inn Road
London WC1X 8JU
United Kingdom
0845-1221-200
www.tht.org.uk

Women Alive
1566 Burnside Avenue
Los Angeles, CA 90019
800-554-4876
www.women-alive.org

Women's Outreach Network
c/o AIDS Committee of Toronto
399 Church Street, 4th Floor
Toronto, Ontario
Canada M5B 2J6
647-340-8484
www.womenfightaids.com
Se habla Español
Je parle Français

Airbags

U.S. Department of Transportation National Highway Traffic Safety Administration
400 7th Street NW
Washington, DC 20590
888-327-4236
www.nhtsa.dot.gov/airbags

Alcohol Abuse

Al-Anon/Alateen
1600 Corporate Landing Parkway
Virginia Beach, VA 23454-5617
888-4AL-ANON
www.al-anon.org

Alcohol Concern
Waterbridge House
32–36 Loman Street
London SE1 0EE
United Kingdom
0800-917-8282
www.alcoholconcern.org.uk

Alcoholics Anonymous
Grand Central Station
P.O. Box 459
New York, NY 10163
www.alcoholics-anonymous.org
Consult phonebook for local chapter

The National Clearinghouse for Alcohol and Drug Information
11426 Rockville Pike, Suite 200
Rockville, Maryland 20852
800-729-6686
www.health.org

National Institute on Alcohol Abuse and Alcoholism (NIAAA)
6000 Executive Boulevard, Willco Building
Bethesda, MD 20892-7003
www.niaaa.nih.gov
Se habla Español

Alternative Therapies

National Center for Complementary and Alternative Medicine
National Institutes of Health
6707 Democracy Boulevard
Bethesda, MD 20892
www.nccam.nih.gov
Se habla Español

Natural Health Products Directorate
Health Canada
2936 Baseline Road, Tower A
Postal Locator: 3302A
Ottawa, Ontario
Canada K1A 0K9
613-952-2558
www.hc-sc.gc.ca/hpfb-dgpsa/nhpd-dpsn/index_e.html
Je parle Français

Alzheimer's Disease

Alzheimer's Association
919 North Michigan Avenue, Suite 1100
Chicago, IL 60611-1676
800-272-3900
www.alz.org

Alzheimer's Disease Education & Referral Center
National Institute on Aging
P.O. Box 8250
Silver Spring, MD 20907-8250
800-438-4380
www.alzheimers.org

Alzheimer Society of Canada
20 Eglinton Avenue West, Suite 1200
Toronto, Ontario
Canada M4R 1K8
800-616-8816
www.alzheimer.ca
Je parle Français

Alzheimer's Society
Gordon House
10 Greencoat Place
London SW1P 1PH
United Kingdom
020-7306-0606
www.alzheimers.org.uk

Anorexia Nervosa and Bulimia Nervosa

Anorexia Nervosa & Bulimia Association
767 Bayridge Drive
P.O. Box 20058
Kingston, Ontario
Canada K7P 1C0
613-547-3684
www.phe.queensu.ca/anab/index.html

National Association of Anorexia Nervosa and Associated Disorders
P.O. Box 7
Highland Park, IL 60035
847-831-3438
www.anad.org

National Centre for Eating Disorders
54 New Road
Esher, Surrey KT10 9NU
United Kingdom
01372-469493
www.eating-disorders.org.uk

National Eating Disorders Association
603 Stewart Street, Suite 803
Seattle, WA 98101
206-382-3587
www.nationaleatingdisorders.org

Anxiety Disorders

Anxiety Disorders Association of America
8730 Georgia Avenue, Suite 600
Silver Spring, MD 20910
240-485-1001
www.adaa.org

National Phobics Society
Zion Community Resource Centre
339 Stretford Road
Hulme, Manchester M15 4ZY
United Kingdom
0870-7700-456
www.phobics-society.org.uk

Arthritis

Arthritis Care
18 Stephenson Way
London NW1 2HD
United Kingdom
080-8800-4050
www.arthritiscare.org.uk

Arthritis Foundation
P.O. Box 7669
Atlanta, GA 30357-0669
800-283-7800
www.arthritis.org

The Arthritis Society
393 University Avenue, Suite 1700
Toronto, Ontario
Canada M5G 1E6
416-979-7228
www.arthritis.ca
Je parle Français

National Institute of Arthritis and Musculoskeletal and Skin
  Diseases
Information Clearinghouse
National Institutes of Health
1 AMS Circle
Bethesda, MD 20892-3675
877-22-NIAMS
www.niams.nih.gov

Asthma

The American Lung Association
61 Broadway, 6th Floor
New York, NY 10006
212-315-8700
www.lungusa.org

Asthma and Allergy Foundation of America
1233 20th Street NW, Suite 402
Washington, DC 20036
202-466-7643
www.aafa.org

Asthma Society of Canada
130 Bridgeland Avenue, Suite 425
Toronto, Ontario
Canada M6A 1Z4
800-787-3880
www.asthma.ca

National Asthma Campaign
Providence House
Providence Place
London N1 0NT
United Kingdom
020-7226-2260
www.asthma.org.uk

Autoimmune Disorders

The American Autoimmune Related Diseases Association
22100 Gratiot Ave.
East Detroit, MI 48021
586-776-3900
www.aarda.org

Bipolar Disorders

See Manic Depression

Birth Control

Childbirth by Choice Trust
344 Bloor Street West, Suite 502
Toronto, Ontario
Canada M5S 3A7
416-961-7812
www.cbctrust.com
Je parle Français

Marie Stopes International
153–157 Cleveland Street
London W1T 6QW
United Kingdom
020-7574-7400
www.mariestopes.org.uk

Planned Parenthood Federation of America
434 West 33rd Street
New York, NY 10001
800-230-PLAN
www.plannedparenthood.org
Se habla Español

Planned Parenthood Federation of Canada
1 Nicholas Street, Suite 430
Ottawa, Ontario
Canada K1N 7B7
613-241-4474
www.ppfc.ca
Je parle Français

Bowel Disorders

The Canadian Society of Intestinal Research
855 West 12th Avenue
Vancouver, British Columbia
Canada V5Z 1M9
866-600-4875
www.badgut.com

Crohn's & Colitis Foundation of America
386 Park Avenue South, 17th Floor
New York, NY 10016
800-932-2423
www.ccfa.org

Crohn's and Colitis Foundation of Canada
60 St. Clair Avenue East, Suite 600
Toronto, Ontario
Canada M4T 1N5
800-387-1479
www.ccfc.ca

IBS Association
1440 Whalley Avenue 145
New Haven, CT 06515
www.ibsassociation.org

National Association for Colitis and Crohn's (NACC)
4 Beaumont House
Sutton Road
St. Albans, Herts. AL1 5HH
United Kingdom
0845-130-2233
www.nacc.org.uk

Breast Cancer

American Cancer Society
1599 Clifton Road NE
Atlanta, GA 30329
800-ACS-2345
www.cancer.org

Breast Cancer Care
Kiln House
210 New Kings Road
London SW6 4NZ
United Kingdom
020-7384-2984
www.breastcancercare.org.uk

Breast Cancer Society of Canada
401 St. Clair Street
Point Edward, Ontario
Canada N7V 1P2
1-800-567-8767
www.bcsc.ca

National Alliance of Breast Cancer Organizations
9 East 37th Street, 10th Floor
New York, NY 10016
888-80-NABCO
www.nabco.org

No Hair Day
607 Franklin Street
Cambridge, MA 02139
617-876-6416
elsa.photo.net/nohairday

The Susan G. Komen Breast Cancer Foundation
P.O. Box 650309
Dallas, TX 75265-0309
800-IM-AWARE
www.breastcancerinfo.com

Breast Implants

Center for Devices and Radiological Health
U.S. Food and Drug Administration
Communications Section
1350 Piccard Avenue (HFZ-210)
Rockville, MD 20857
800-532-4440
www.fda.gov/cdrh/breastimplants/index.html

Breast Reconstruction

Bosom Buddies
40 East Schiller Street
Chicago, IL 60610-2110
877-245-1300
www.bosombuddies.org

M. D. Anderson Cancer Center
1515 Holcombe Boulevard
Houston, TX 77030
800-392-1611
www.mdanderson.org/diseases/breastcancer/breastsurgery

See also Breast Cancer

Breastfeeding

The American Academy of Pediatrics
141 Northwest Point Boulevard
Elk Grove Village, IL 60007-1098
847-434-4000

The Breastfeeding Network
P.O. Box 11126
Paisley PA2 8YB
United Kingdom
0870-900-8787
www.breastfeedingnetwork.org.uk

GotMom.com
American College of Nurse-Midwives
818 Connecticut Avenue NW, Suite 900
Washington DC 20006
202-728-9860
www.gotmom.com

International Lactation Consultant Association
1500 Sunday Drive, Suite 102
Raleigh, NC 27607
919-861-5577
www.ilca.org

Medela, Inc.
1101 Corporate Drive
McHenry, IL 60050
800-435-8316
www.medela.com

National Women's Health Information Center
U.S. Department of Health and Human Services
200 Independence Avenue SW
Washington, DC 20201
800-994-WOMAN
www.4woman.gov/breastfeeding
Se habla Español

Breathing Disorders

The American Lung Association
61 Broadway, 6th Floor
New York, NY 10006
212-315-8700
www.lungusa.org

British Lung Foundation
78 Hatton Garden
London EC1N 8LD
United Kingdom
020-7831-5831
www.lunguk.org

The Lung Association
3 Raymond Street, Suite 300
Ottawa, Ontario
Canada K1R 1A3
613-569-6411
www.lung.ca

Carpal Tunnel Syndrome

Cumulative Trauma Disorder Resource Network, Inc.
2013 Princeton Court
Los Banos, CA 93635
209-826-8443
www.ctdrn.org

Repetitive Strain Injury Association
380–384 Harrow Road
London W9 2HU
United Kingdom
0800-018-5012
www.rsi.org.uk

Cataracts

Canadian Ophthalmological Society
610-1525 Carling Avenue
Ottawa, Ontario
Canada K1Z 8R9
www.eyesite.ca
Je parle Français

Prevention of Blindness Society
1775 Church Street NW
Washington, DC 20036
202-234-1010
www.youreyes.org

Royal National Institute for the Blind
RNIB Falcon Park
Neasden Lane
London NW10 1RN
United Kingdom
0845-702-3153
www.rnib.org.uk

Cervical Cancer

Canadian Cancer Society
National Office
10 Alcorn Avenue, Suite 200
Toronto, Ontario
Canada M4V 3B1
416-961-7223
www.cancer.ca
Je parle Français

CancerBACUP
3 Bath Place
Rivington Street
London EC2A 3JR
United Kingdom
0808-800-1234
www.cancerbacup.org.uk

National Cancer Institute
NCI Public Inquiries Office
6116 Executive Boulevard, MSC8322
Bethesda, MD 20892-8322
800-4-CANCER
www.cancer.gov/cancerinformation

National Cervical Cancer Coalition (NCCC)
16501 Sherman Way, Suite 110
Van Nuys, CA 91406
800-685-5531
www.nccc-online.org

Childbirth

American Academy of Husband-Coached Childbirth
(a.k.a. The Bradley Method®)
Box 5224
Sherman Oaks, CA 91413-5224
800-4-A-BIRTH
www.bradleybirth.com

American College of Nurse-Midwives
818 Connecticut Avenue NW, Suite 900
Washington, DC 20006
202-728-9860
www.midwife.org

International Childbirth Education Association
P.O. Box 20048
Minneapolis, MN 55420
952-854-8660
www.icea.org

Lamaze International
2025 M Street, Suite 800
Washington DC 20036-3309
800-368-4404
www.lamaze.org
Se habla Español

The National Childbirth Trust
Alexandra House
Oldham Terrace
Acton, London W3 6NH
United Kingdom
0870-444-8707
www.nctpregnancyandbabycare.com

Chronic Fatigue Syndrome

The CFIDS Association of America, Inc.
P.O. Box 220398
Charlotte, NC 28222-0398
800-442-3437
www.cfids.org

Colon and Rectal Cancer

Colon Cancer Alliance
175 Ninth Avenue
New York, NY 10011
877-422-2030
www.ccalliance.org

Colon Cancer Concern
9 Rickett Street
London SW6 1RU
United Kingdom
08708-50-60-50
www.coloncancer.org.uk

Colorectal Cancer Association of Canada
180 Bloor Street West, Suite 904
Toronto, Ontario
Canada M5S 2V6
888-318-9442
www.ccac-accc.ca
Je parle Français

Congestive Heart Failure and Coronary Artery Disease

See Heart Disease

Cosmetic Surgery

American Society of Plastic Surgeons
Plastic Surgery Educational Foundation
444 East Algonquin Road
Arlington Heights, IL 60005
1-888-4-PLASTIC
www.plasticsurgery.org

Crohn's Disease and Colitis

See Bowel Disorders

Depression

Depression and Bipolar Support Alliance (DBSA)
730 North Franklin Street, Suite 501
Chicago, IL 60610-7204
800-826-3632
www.dbsalliance.org

The Mood Disorders Society of Canada
3-304 Stone Road West, Suite 763
Guelph, Ontario
Canada N1G 4W4
519-824-5565
www.mooddisorderscanada.ca
Je parle Français

National Institute of Mental Health
Information Resources and Inquiries Branch
6001 Executive Boulevard, Room 8184, MSC 9663
Bethesda, MD 20892-9663
301-443-4513
www.nimh.nih.gov

Dethylstilbestrol (DES)

DES Action USA
610 16th Street, Suite 301
Oakland, CA 94612
510-465-4011
www.desaction.org

Diabetes

American Diabetes Association
National Call Center
1701 North Beauregard Street
Alexandria, VA 22311
800-DIABETES
www.diabetes.org
Se habla Español

Canadian Diabetes Association
15 Toronto Street, Suite 800
Toronto, Ontario
Canada M5C 2E3
800-226-8464
www.diabetes.ca
Je parle Français

Diabetes UK
10 Parkway
London NW1 7AA
United Kingdom
020-7424-1000
www.diabetes.org.uk

Take Time to Care . . . About Diabetes
Office of Women's Health
Food and Drug Administration
5600 Fishers Lane
Rockville, Maryland 20857
888-463-6332
www.fda.gov/womens/taketimetocare/diabetes/default.htm

Domestic Abuse

Assaulted Women's Helpline
P.O. Box 369, Station B
Toronto, Ontario
Canada M5T 2W2
866-863-0511
www.awhl.org

National Center on Elder Abuse
1201 15th Street NW, Suite 350
Washington, DC 20005-2800
202-898-2586
www.elderabusecenter.org

National Domestic Violence Hotline
Texas Council on Family Violence
P.O. Box 161810
Austin, TX 78716
800-799-7233
TTY 800-787-3224
www.ndvh.org

National Latino Alliance for the Elimination of Domestic
    Violence
P.O. Box 672, Triborough Station
New York, NY 10035
800-342-9908
www.dvalianza.org
Se habla Español

Stop Abuse For Everyone
P.O. Box 951
Tualatin, OR 97062
www.safe4all.org

Women's Aid
P.O. Box 391
Bristol BS99 7WS
United Kingdom
08457-023-468
www.womensaid.org.uk

Endometriosis

Endometriosis Association
8585 North 76th Place
Milwaukee, WI 53223
414-355-2200
www.endometriosisassn.org
Se habla Español

The National Endometriosis Society
50 Westminster Palace Gardens
Artillery Row
London SW1P 1RL
United Kingdom
020-7222-2781
www.endo.org.uk

Epilepsy

Epilepsy Canada
1470 Peel Street, Suite 745
Montréal, Quebec
Canada H3A 1T1
1-877-SEIZURE
www.epilepsy.ca
Je parle Français

Epilepsy Foundation
4351 Garden City Drive
Landover, MD 20785-7223
800-332-1000
www.epilepsyfoundation.org
Se habla Español

The National Society for Epilepsy
Chesham Lane
Chalfont St. Peter
Bucks SL9 0RJ
United Kingdom
01494-601400
www.epilepsynse.org.uk

Fibromyalgia

Fibromyalgia Network
P.O. Box 31750
Tuscon, AZ 85751
800-853-2929
www.fmnetnews.com

Foot Care

American Podiatric Medical Association
9312 Old Georgetown Road
Bethesda, MD 20814
800-FOOTCARE
www.apma.org/foot.html
Se habla Español

Genetic Counseling

MEDLINE Plus
U.S. National Library of Medicine
8600 Rockville Pike
Bethesda, MD 20894
www.medlineplus.gov
Se habla Español

Heart Disease

British Heart Foundation
14 Fitzhardinge Street
London W1H 6DH
United Kingdom
020-7935-0185
www.bhf.org.uk/women

Heart and Stroke Foundation of Canada
222 Queen Street, Suite 1402
Ottawa, Ontario
Canada K1P 5V9
613-569-4361
www.heartandstroke.ca
Je parle Français

WomenHeart
The National Coalition for Women with Heart Disease
818 18th Street NW, Suite 730
Washington, DC 20006
202-728-7199
www.womenheart.org

Hepatitis

British Liver Trust
Ransomes Europar
Ipswich IP3 9QG
United Kingdom
01473-276326
www.britishlivertrust.org.uk

Hepatitis C Society of Canada
3050 Confederation Parkway, Unit 301B
Mississauga, Ontario
Canada L5B 3Z6
800-652-HepC
www.hepatitissociety.com
Je parle Français

Hepatitis Foundation International
504 Blick Drive
Silver Spring, MD 20904-2901
800-891-0707
www.hepfi.org

Latino Organization for Liver Awareness
888-367-LOLA
www.lola-national.org
Se habla Español

Herpes

National Herpes Resource Center
American Social Health Association
P.O. Box 13827
Research Triangle Park, NC 27709
919-361-8488
www.ashastd.org/hrc/index.html

Hyperthyroidism and Hypothyroidism

See Thyroid Disorders

Hysterectomy

The Hysterectomy Association
60 Redwood House
Charlton Down, Dorchester DT2 9UH
United Kingdom
0871-7811141
www.hysterectomy-association.org.uk

Hyster Sisters
2436 South I-35 East, Suite 376-184
Denton, TX 76205-4900
www.hystersisters.com

See also Uterine Fibroids

Incontinence

See Urinary Incontinence

Infertility

American Infertility Association
666 Fifth Avenue, Suite 278
New York, NY 10103
888-917-3777
www.americaninfertility.org

European Infertility Network
Woodlawn House
Carrickfergus, Co. Antrim.
Northern Ireland BT38 8PX
7885-138101
www.ein.org/uk.htm

Infertility Awareness Association of Canada
P.O. Box 23025
Ottawa, Ontario
Canada K2A 4E2
800-263-2929
www.iaac.ca
Je parle Français

Resolve
The National Infertility Association
1310 Broadway
Somerville, MA 02144
888-623-0744
www.resolve.org

Insomnia

National Sleep Foundation
1522 K Street NW, Suite 500
Washington, DC 20005
202-347-3471
www.sleepfoundation.org
Se habla Español

Interstitial Cystitis

Interstitial Cystitis Association
110 North Washington Street
Suite 340
Rockville, MD 20850
800-HELP-ICA
www.ichelp.com
Se habla Español
Je parle Française

Irritable Bowel Disorder

See Bowel Disorders

Kidney Disorders

American Association of Kidney Patients
3505 East Frontage Road, Suite 315
Tampa, FL 33607
800-749-2257
www.aakp.org

iKidney
c/o Hartwell Communications
1102 North Brand Boulevard #74
Glendale, CA 91202
www.iKidney.com

The Kidney Foundation of Canada
300-5165 Sherbrooke Street West
Montréal, Quebec
Canada H4A 1T6
800-361-7494
www.kidney.ca
Je parle Français

The National Kidney Foundation
6 Stanley Street
Worksop S81 7HX
United Kingdom
01909-487795
www.kidney.org.uk

Lung Cancer

The American Lung Association
61 Broadway, 6th Floor
New York, NY 10006
212-315-8700
www.lungusa.org

CancerBACUP
3 Bath Place
Rivington Street
London EC2A 3JR
United Kingdom
0808-800-1234
www.cancerbacup.org.uk

Lupus

Lupus Canada
18 Crown Steel Drive, Suite 209
Markham, Ontario
Canada L3R 9X8
800-661-1468
www.lupuscanada.org

Lupus Foundation of America, Inc.
1300 Piccard Drive, Suite 200
Rockville, MD 20850-4303
800-558-0121
www.lupus.org
Se habla Español

Lupus UK
St. James House
Eastern Road
Romford, Essex RM1 3NH
United Kingdom
01708-731251
www.lupusuk.com

Lyme Disease

American Lyme Disease Foundation, Inc.
Mill Pond Offices
293 Route 100
Somers, NY 10589
914-277-6970
www.aldf.com
Se habla Español

Macular Degeneration

The Foundation Fighting Blindness
60 St. Clair Avenue East, Suite 703
Toronto, Ontario
Canada M4T 1N5
800-461-3331
www.rpresearch.ca

Macular Degeneration Foundation
P.O. Box 531313
Henderson, NV 89053
888-633-3937
www.eyesight.org

Royal National Institute for the Blind
RNIB Falcon Park
Neasden Lane
London NW10 1RN
United Kingdom
020-7388-1266
www.rnib.org.uk

Manic Depression

Depression and Bipolar Support Alliance
730 North Franklin Street, Suite 501
Chicago, IL 60610-7204
800-826-3632
www.dbsalliance.org

Melanoma

See Skin Cancer

Menopause

A Friend Indeed
419 Graham Ave
Winnipeg, Manitoba
Canada R3C 0M3
204-989-8028
www.afriendindeed.ca

The North American Menopause Society
P.O. Box 94527
Cleveland, OH 44101
440-442-7550
www.menopause.org
Se habla Español

Midwifery

American College of Nurse-Midwives
818 Connecticut Avenue NW, Suite 900
Washington, DC 20006
202-728-9860
www.midwife.org

Miscarriage and Pregnancy Loss

The Miscarriage Association
c/o Clayton Hospital
Northgate
Wakefield, West Yorkshire WF1 3JS
United Kingdom
01924-200799
www.miscarriageassociation.org.uk

Mood Disorders

Canadian Mental Health Association
8 King Street East, Suite 810
Toronto, Ontario
Canada M5C 1B5
416-484-7750
www.cmha.ca
Je parle Français

Depression and Bipolar Support Alliance
730 North Franklin Street, Suite 501
Chicago, IL 60610-7204
800-826-3632
www.dbsalliance.org

The Mental Health Foundation
83 Victoria Street
London SW1H 0HW
United Kingdom
020-7802-0300
www.mentalhealth.org.uk

National Alliance for the Mentally Ill
2107 Wilson Boulevard, Suite 300
Arlington, VA 22201
800-950-NAMI
www.nami.org
Se habla Español

Multiple Sclerosis

Multiple Sclerosis International Federation
3rd Floor Skyline House
200 Union Street
London SE1 0LX
United Kingdom
020-7620-1911
www.msif.org
Se habla Español

Multiple Sclerosis Society of Canada
250 Bloor Street East, Suite 1000
Toronto, Ontario
Canada M4W 3P9
800-268-7582
www.mssociety.ca
Je parle Français

The National Multiple Sclerosis Society
733 Third Avenue
New York, NY 10017
800-FIGHT-MS
www.nationalmssociety.org

Nutrition

The FoodFit Company
2213 M Street NW, Suite 200
Washington, DC 20037
www.foodfit.com

Obesity

See Weight Management

Obsessive-Compulsive Disorder

Obsessive-Compulsive Foundation, Inc.
P.O. Box 70
Milford, CT 06460-0070
203-878-5669
www.ocfoundation.org

Obsessive Compulsive Information & Support Centre Inc.
204-825 Sherbrook Street
Winnipeg, Manitoba
Canada R3A 1M5
204-942-3331
www.members.shaw.ca/occmanitoba/index.htm

OCD Action
Aberdeen Centre
22–24 Highbury Grove
London N5 2EA
United Kingdom
020-7226-4000
www.ocdaction.org.uk

Occupational Health

Canadian Centre for Occupational Health and Safety
250 Main Street East
Hamilton, Ontario
Canada L8N 1H6
800-263-8466
www.ccohs.ca
Je parle Français

Institution of Occupational Safety and Health
The Grange
Highfield Drive
Wigston, Leicestershire, LE18 1NN
United Kingdom
0116-257-3100
www.iosh.co.uk

National Institute for Occupational Safety and Health
200 Independence Avenue SW
Washington, DC 20201
800-35-NIOSH
www.cdc.gov/niosh/homepage.html
Se habla Español

Osteoporosis

National Osteoporosis Society
Camerton
Bath BA2 0PJ
United Kingdom
01761-471-771
www.nos.org.uk

Osteoporosis and Related Bone Diseases
National Resource Center
1232 22nd Street NW
Washington, DC 20037-1292
800-624-BONE
www.osteo.org

Osteoporosis Society of Canada
33 Laird Drive
Toronto, Ontario
Canada M4G 3S9
800-463-6842
www.osteoporosis.ca
Je parle Français

Ovarian Cancer

National Ovarian Cancer Association
27 Park Road
Toronto, Ontario
Canada M4W 2N2
877-413-7970
www.slip.net/~mcdavis/ovarian.html

National Ovarian Cancer Coalition
500 NE Spanish River Boulevard, Suite 14
Boca Raton, FL 33431
888-OVARIAN
www.ovarian.org

Ovacome
St. Bartholomew's Hospital
West Smithfield, London EC1A 7BE
United Kingdom
020-7600-5141
www.ovacome.org.uk

Panic Disorder

See Anxiety Disorder

Polycystic Ovary Syndrome

Polycystic Ovarian Syndrome Association
P.O. Box 3403
Englewood, CO 80111
877-775-PCOS
www.pcosupport.org

Verity
The Polycystic Ovaries Self-Help Group
52-54 Featherstone Street
London EC1Y 8RT
United Kingdom
www.verity-pcos.org.uk

Postpartum Depression

Association for Post Natal Illness
145 Dawes Road
Fulham, London SW6 7EB
United Kingdom
020-7386-0868
www.apni.org

Depression After Delivery, Inc.
91 East Somerset Street
Raritan, NJ 08869
800-944-4773
www.depressionafterdelivery.com

Posttraumatic Stress Disorder

The International Society for Posttraumatic Stress Studies
60 Revere Drive, Suite 500
Northbrook, IL 60062
847-480-9028
www.istss.org

Sidran Traumatic Stress Foundation
200 E. Joppa Road, Suite 207
Baltimore, MD 21286
410-825-8888
www.sidran.org

Preconception Counseling

MEDLINE Plus
U.S. National Library of Medicine
8600 Rockville Pike
Bethesda, MD 20894
www.medlineplus.gov
Se habla Español

Premenstrual Syndrome

National Association for Premenstrual Syndrome
41 Old Road
East Peckham, Kent TN12 5AP
United Kingdom
0870-777-2177
www.pms.org.uk

Psychotherapy

Mental Health Matters
Get Mental Help Incorporated
Kenmore, WA 98028
425-402-6934
www.mental-health-matters.com

Mental Health Resource Center
National Mental Health Association
2001 North Beauregard Street, 12th Floor
Alexandria, VA 22311
800-969-NMHA
www.nmha.org

Rape

Rape, Abuse & Incest National Network
635-B Pennsylvania Avenue SE
Washington, DC 20003
800-656-HOPE
www.rainn.org

Rheumatoid Arthritis

See Arthritis

Safer Sex

Planned Parenthood Federation of America
434 West 33rd Street
New York, NY 10001
800-230-PLAN
www.plannedparenthood.org
Se habla Español

Planned Parenthood Federation of Canada
1 Nicholas Street, Suite 430
Ottawa, Ontario
Canada K1N 7B7
613-241-4474
www.ppfc.ca
Je parle Français

Playing Safely
Department of Health
Richmond House
79 Whitehall
London SW1A 2NS
0800-567-123
www.playingsafely.co.uk

Schizophrenia

Mental Health Resource Center
National Mental Health Association
2001 North Beauregard Street, 12th Floor
Alexandria, VA 22311
800-969-NMHA
www.nmha.org

National Electronic Library for Mental Health
Department of Psychiatry
University of Oxford
Oxford OX3 7JX
United Kingdom
01865-226451
www.nelh.nhs.uk

Schizophrenia Society of Canada
50 Acadia Avenue, Suite 205
Markham, Ontario
Canada L3R 0B3
888-SSC-HOPE
www.schizophrenia.ca
Je parle Français

Scleroderma

Scleroderma Foundation
12 Kent Way, Suite 101
Byfield, MA 01922
800-722-HOPE
www.scleroderma.org

The Scleroderma Society
3 Caple Road
London NW10 8AB
United Kingdom
020-8961-4912
www.sclerodermasociety.co.uk

Scleroderma Society of Canada
95 Woodfield Road SW
Calgary, Alberta
Canada T2W 5K5
www.scleroderma.ca

Sexual Abuse and Incest

Rape, Abuse & Incest National Network
635-B Pennsylvania Avenue SE
Washington, DC 20003
800-656-HOPE
www.rainn.org

Sexual Dysfunction and Sexual Response

American Association of Sex Educators, Counselors, and
  Therapists
P.O. Box 5488
Richmond, VA 23220-0488
www.aasect.org

Sexual Harassment

Equal Opportunities Commission
Arndale House
Arndale Centre
Manchester M4 3EQ
United Kingdom
08456-015901
www.eoc.org.uk

Ontario Women's Justice Network
158 Spadina Road
Toronto, Ontario
Canada M5R 2T8
416-392-3148
www.owjn.org/issues/s-harass/guide.htm

U.S. Equal Employment Opportunity Commission
1801 L Street NW
Washington, DC 20507
800-669-4000
www.eeoc.gov

Sexually Transmitted Diseases

American Social Health Association
P.O. Box 13827
Research Triangle Park, NC 27709
919-361-8488
www.ashastd.org

Planned Parenthood Federation of America
434 West 33rd Street
New York, NY 10001
800-230-PLAN
www.plannedparenthood.org/sti
Se habla Español

Planned Parenthood Federation of Canada
1 Nicholas Street, Suite 430
Ottawa, Ontario
Canada K1N 7B7
613-241-4474
www.ppfc.ca
Je parle Français

Playing Safely
Department of Health
Richmond House
79 Whitehall
London SW1A 2NS
0800-567-123
www.playingsafely.co.uk

Sjögren's Syndrome

Sjögren's Syndrome Foundation
8120 Woodmont Avenue, Suite 530
Bethesda, MD 20814
800-475-6473
www.sjogrens.com

Skin Cancer

CancerBACUP
3 Bath Place
Rivington Street
London EC2A 3JR
United Kingdom
0808-800-1234
www.cancerbacup.org.uk

The Skin Cancer Foundation
245 5th Avenue, Suite 1403
New York, NY 10016
800-SKIN-490
www.skincancer.org

Sleep Disorders

National Sleep Foundation
1522 K Street NW, Suite 500
Washington, DC 20005
202-347-3471
www.sleepfoundation.org
Se habla Español

Smoking

National Women's Health Information Center
U.S. Department of Health and Human Services
200 Independence Avenue SW
Washington, DC 20201
800-994-WOMAN
www.4woman.gov/QuitSmoking/index.cfm
Se habla Español

Quit
Ground Floor
211 Old Street
London EC1V 9NR
United Kingdom
020-7251-1551
www.quit.org.uk

QuitNet
Boston University School of Public Health
1 Appleton Street, 4th Floor
Boston, MA 02116
617-437-1500
www.quitnet.com
Se habla Español

Stroke

National Stroke Association
9707 East Easter Lane
Englewood, CO 80112
800-STROKES
www.stroke.org
Se habla Español
Je parle Français

Thyroid Disorders

The Thyroid Foundation of America
410 Stuart Street
Boston, MA 02116
800-832-8321
www.allthyroid.org

Thyroid Foundation of Canada
P.O. Box/CP 1919 Station Main
Kingston, Ontario
Canada K7L 5J7
613-544-8364
www.thyroid.ca
Je parle Français

Thyroid UK
32 Darcy Road
St. Osyth
Clacton-on-Sea, Essex CO16 8QF
United Kingdom
www.thyroiduk.org

Urinary Incontinence

The Continence Foundation
307 Hatton Square
16 Baldwins Gardens
London ECIN 7RJ
United Kingdom
0845-345-0165
www.continence-foundation.org.uk

National Association for Continence
P.O. Box 1019
Charleston, SC 29402-1019
800-BLADDER
www.nafc.org
Se habla Español

Uterine Fibroids

Fibroid Network, Sisternetwork
27 Old Gloucester Street
London WC1N 3XX
United Kingdom
08453-342461
www.fibroidnetwork.com

National Uterine Fibroids Foundation
P.O. Box 9688
Colorado Springs, CO 80932-0688
877-553-NUFF
www.nuff.org

Weight Management

Aim for a Healthy Weight
National Heart, Lung, and Blood Institute
Health Information Center
P.O. Box 30105
Bethesda, MD 20824-0105
301-592-8573
www.nhlbi.nih.gov/health/public/heart/obesity/lose_wt
    /index.htm

American Obesity Association
1250 24th Street NW, Suite 300
Washington, DC 20037
202-776-7711
www.obesity.org

Shape Up America!
c/o WebFront Solutions Corporation
15757 Crabbs Branch Way
Rockville, MD 20855
301-258-0540
www.shapeup.org

Acknowledgments

Many of the entries in *The Harvard Guide to Women's Health* were developed from information contained in *Primary Care of Women*, a textbook for physicians edited by Drs. Carlson and Eisenstat. That professional book was intended to provide an accurate, up-to-date resource for clinicians involved in the care of women. While they were developing *Primary Care of Women* (which was published in 1995 by Mosby, followed by a 2nd edition in 2002), Drs. Carlson and Eisenstat thought it would be ideal if a companion book could be created that would offer explanations and information to help women understand what their doctor was trying to convey and make women more active participants in their own health care.

Following the recommendation of Daniel D. Federman, MD, Dean for Medical Education, Harvard Medical School, the editors at Harvard University Press approached Drs. Carlson and Eisenstat with just that idea. Dr. Ziporyn, formerly an associate editor for the *Journal of the American Medical Association* and the author of many articles and books, was brought into the project to contribute her expertise as a writer, researcher, and medical historian. Thus *The Harvard Guide to Women's Health* was born.

Drs. Carlson and Eisenstat would like to express their appreciation to Isaac Schiff, MD, and Fredric D. Frigoletto Jr., MD, associate editors of *Primary Care of Women*, for their technical expertise in the creation of that book and for their continuing mentorship, professional collaboration, and support for this and many other projects. They also wish to thank their colleagues at Women's Health Associates, Massachusetts General Hospital, who have helped create a laboratory in which physicians learn from their patients the kind of information women need for good health, and from one another how to meet those needs: Joell Bianchi, MD, Claire Bloom, MD, Nancy Gagliano, MD, Pamela Hodges-Eskew RNC, Kathleen Kelly, RNC, Amsale Ketema, MD, Elizabeth Mort, MD, Mary Norato-Indeglia, RNC, Karen O'Brien, MD, Susan Oliverio, MD, Nancy Rigotti, MD, Olga Smulders-Meyer, MD, Anne Thorndike, MD, Kathleen Ulman, PhD, Barbara Woo, MD, and Marcia Zucker, MD.

Dr. Ziporyn would like to express great appreciation for the many friends and colleagues who freely shared their expertise and perspectives, including Naomi Bromberg Bar Yam, Ronald Daniel, MD, Allan Graham, MD, FACP, Robert Hayward, MD, Jeanette Jensen, DDS, Elizabeth Knoll, PhD, F. Y. Li, MD, Diane Rippa, MD, Benjamin Sachs, MD, Sean Tuttle, MD, Toni Wolf, DDS, and Marvin Ziporyn, MD. Particular gratitude goes to Alan Guttmacher, MD, and Wendy Mackinnon, MS, of the Vermont Regional Genetics Center, and to Claire Harmon, RN, BSN, MPA, without whose support, both technical and personal, this book would have been incomplete, or even uncompleted. Equally vital were the unending faith, tolerance, and generosity of Charlotte Ziporyn and of Stanley and Mary Ann Snider. Finally, Dr. Ziporyn would like to thank Eve Nichols of the Whitehead Institute for helping to bring her into this project in the first place and for offering valuable insights into the world of medical writing over the years.

The physicians who contributed chapters to *Primary Care of Women* have earned our deepest respect and gratitude. The clinical experience and state-of-the-art knowledge that each of these contributors has shared have provided the firm foundation on which this book rests. Their names and respective areas of expertise are:

Ronald J. Anderson, MD, Meredith August, DMD, MD, Johnny T. Awwad, MD, Margaret H. Baron, MD, PhD, Joshua A. Beckman, MD, Susan Bennett, MD, Bonnie L. Bermas, MD, David L. Carr-Locke, MD, FRCP, Grace Chang, MD, MPH, Tanuja Chitnis, MD, Bum-Chae Choi, MD, Barbara Ann Cockrill, MD, Karen H. Costenbader, MD, M. Cornelia Cremens, MD, Susan M. Cummings, MS, RD, Corey Stephen Cutler, MD, Michele G. Cyr, MD, David M. Dawson, MD, Sheila Ann Dugan, MD, PT, Linda R. Duska, MD, Barbara A. Dworetzky, MD, Patricia A. Fraser, MD, MPH, MS, Lawrence S. Friedman, MD, Marie Gerhard-Herman, MD, RUT, FACC, Soheyla Dana Gharib, MD, Elizabeth S. Ginsburg, MD, Julie Glowacki, PhD, Samuel Z. Goldhaber, MD, Michael F. Greene, MD, Joseph A. Grocela, MD, Janet Elizabeth Hall, MD, Linda J. Heffner, MD, PhD, Susan E. Herz, JD, MPH, Joseph A. Hill, MD, Jennifer Ho, MD, Keith B. Isaacson, MD, Linda S. Jaffe, MD, Phyllis Jen, MD, Paula A. Johnson, MD, MPH, Lee M. Kaplan, MD, PhD, Jeffrey N. Katz, MD, MS, Martha Ellen Katz, MD, Laurence Katznelson, MD, John M. Kauffman, MD, Powell H. Kazanjian, MD, Robyn S. Klein, MD, PhD, Anne Klibanski, MD, Anthony L. Komaroff, MD, FACP, Nicole B. Korbly, BA, Irene Kuter, MD, DPhil, Joseph C. Kvedar, MD, Carol Landau, PhD, Carolyn S. Langer, MD, JD, MPH, Ruth A. Lawrence, MD, Matthew H. Liang, MD, MPH, Robert C. Lowe, MD, James A. MacLean, MD, Kathryn A. Martin, MD, Kelly A. McGarry, MD, Roseanna H. Means, MD, MSC, Harold Michlewitz, MD, Felise B. Milan, MD, A. Jacqueline Mitus, MD, Anne W. Moulton, MD, Toufic I. Nakad, MD, Olivia I. Okereke, MD, Lori D. Olans, MD, MPH, L. Christine Oliver, MD, MPH, MS, Rapin Osathanondh, MD, Kristine Phillips, MD, PhD, May C.M. Pian-Smith, MD, MS, John M. Poneros, MD, Athena Poppas, MD, Janey S.A. Pratt, MD, David M. Rapoport, MD, Neeraj Rastogi, BE DNB, Nancy A. Rigotti, MD, Douglas S. Ross, MD, Raja A. Sayegh, MD, Isaac

Schiff, MD, Ellen W. Seely, MD, Julian Lawrence Seifter, MD, Margaret Seton, MD, Linda Shafer, MD, Ellen Elizabeth Sheets, MD, Jan L. Shifren, MD, Robert H. Shmerling, MD, FACP, Iris Shuey, MD, Lawrence N. Shulman, MD, Naomi M. Simon, MD, David M. Slovik, MD, Barbara L. Smith, MD, PhD, Olga Smulders-Meyer, MD, Caren G. Solomon, MD, MPH, Farzaneh A. Sorond, MD, PhD, Egilius L.H. Spierings, MD, PRD, Michael R. Stelluto, MD, Ann E. Taylor, MD, Kathleen F. Thurmond, MD, Erin E. Tracy, MD, MPH, Katharine K. Treadway, MD, Kathleen Hubbs Ulman, PhD, Adele C. Viguera, MD, May M. Wakamatsu, MD, Joyce A. Walsleben, RN, PhD, Louise Wilkins-Haug, MD, PhD, Jacqueline L. Wolf, MD, Barbara J. Woo, MD, Mylene W.M. Yao, MD

The following people provided excellent technical review of the manuscript during its revision. Bonnie Bermas, MD, Robert Blatman, M.D., Joanne Borg-Stein, M.D., Leslie Brody, Ph.D., Andrew Cole, M.D., F.R.C.P. (C.), Sue Cummings, M.S., R.N., Annekathryn Goodman, MD, Charlea Maisson, JoAnn Manson, M.D., James May, Jr., M.D., Bob Novelline, MD, Richard Penson, MD, Nelly Pitteloud, MD, Sharon Reimold, MD, Jane Sillman, MD, Sujata Somani, MD, and Stephen Sonis, D.M.D.

We would like to acknowledge the professionalism and persistence of those at Harvard University Press who have worked so hard on *The New Harvard Guide to Women's Health*. Foremost is Ann Downer-Hazell, our sponsoring editor, whose sound advice has informed every page of this new edition. Ann was ably assisted by Sara Davis, who shepherded the project through the manuscript preparation, copyediting, and production phases. Once again Amanda Heller kindly took on the job of copyediting, while Marcia Carlson agreed to prepare the index; Gwen Frankfeldt offered design expertise, and David Foss coordinated production. We are grateful to all these people for their invaluable contributions to this work. Finally, looking backward for a moment, we would like to thank Michael Fisher at HUP for his sponsorship and support during publication of the first edition, and Susan Wallace Boehmer for the editorial vision that helped make *The Harvard Guide to Women's Health* a reality.

As these Acknowledgments indicate, the contributions of over a hundred physicians and colleagues have helped make this project possible. We would like to express our utmost gratitude for the expertise and time they so generously shared. Any errors that, regrettably, may remain in the text are the responsibility of the authors.

Stephanie A. Eisenstat, MD
Karen J. Carlson, MD
Terra Ziporyn, PhD

Illustration Credits

Illustrations by Harriet Greenfield: on pages 30, 35, 39, 41, 56, 57, 62, 64, 65, 70, 71, 83, 91, 92, 93, 94, 95, 98, 112, 115, 116, 120, 121, 124, 125, 127, 142, 149, 163, 167, 169, 170, 171, 172, 173, 186, 190, 191, 195, 197, 218, 219, 225, 238, 239, 245, 255, 256, 265, 268, 269, 271, 272, 273, 294, 295, 299, 302, 307, 310, 318, 331, 332, 360, 368, 375, 380, 382, 389, 394, 399, 405, 421, 426, 428, 429, 430, 446, 454, 455, 507, 512, 513, 526, 527, 552, 557, 588, 596, 597, 601, 614

Illustrations by Susan Keller: on pages 2, 3, 13, 22, 60, 75, 76, 77, 98, 106, 109, 116, 120, 128, 134, 138, 146, 156, 161, 183, 208, 213, 216, 240, 243, 281, 287, 297, 317, 325, 327, 330, 335, 339, 362, 383, 404, 406, 414, 427, 436, 439, 450, 452, 471, 487, 499, 500, 501, 510, 514, 516, 528, 576, 591, 592, 604, 619, 620

Illustrations by Interactive Composition Corporation: on pages 1, 19, 73, 80, 97, 131, 157, 159, 226, 230, 234, 247, 249, 259, 324, 344, 345, 346, 347, 348, 349, 353, 364, 373, 418, 438, 501, 503, 511, 519, 577, 589

Illustrations reprinted by permission of Harvard University Press: on pages 159, 222, 361, 363, 559

Illustrations reprinted by permission of The American Cancer Society: on page 391

Index

Boldface type indicates a major discussion or illustration. Cross-references refer to other index entries.